D0230495

This book is to be returned on or before the last date stamped below.

LIBREX

The COMET Library
Luton & Dunstable Hospital
NHS Trust, Lewsey Road
LUTON LU4 0DZ

Tel: 01582 497201
E-mail: library@ldh.nhs.uk

Evidence-based Pediatrics and Child Health

Second edition

Updates for *Evidence-based Pediatrics and Child Health* will be regularly posted to the following website, giving the latest trial data applicable to the clinical questions addressed in the text.

www.evidbasedpediatrics.com

Evidence-based Pediatrics and Child Health

Second edition

Editor in Chief

Virginia A Moyer

Professor of Pediatrics and Epidemiology
Associate Director, Center for Clinical Research and Evidence
  Based Medicine
Department of Pediatrics
The University of Texas Houston Health Science Center
Houston, Texas, USA

Senior Associate Editor

Elizabeth J Elliott

Associate Professor, Discipline of Paediatrics
  and Child Health
University of Sydney, and
Consultant Paediatrician, The Children's Hospital
  at Westmead
Sydney, Australia

Associate Editors

Ruth Gilbert

Senior Lecturer in Clinical Epidemiology and Honorary
  Consultant Paediatrician
Centre for Evidence-Based Child Health
Centre for Paediatric Epidemiology and Statistics
Institute of Child Health
London, UK

Terry Klassen

Professor and Chair
Department of Pediatrics
University of Alberta
Edmonton, Alberta, Canada

Stuart Logan

Professor of Paediatric Epidemiology
Director, Institute of Health and Social Care Research
Peninsula Medical School
St Luke's Campus
Exeter, UK

Craig Mellis

Professor and Foundation Head of Medicine
School of Health Sciences
Bond University
Gold Coast, Queensland
Australia

David J Henderson-Smart

Director
Centre for Perinatal Health Services Research
Queen Elizabeth Research Institute
University of Sydney
Sydney, Australia

Katrina Williams

Staff Specialist
Clinical Epidemiology Unit
The Children's Hospital at Westmead
Sydney, Australia

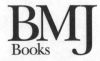

BMJ Books

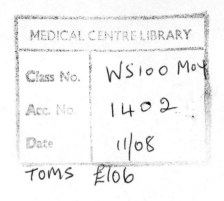

MEDICAL CENTRE LIBRARY

Class No.   WS100 Moy

Acc. No.   1402

Date   11/08

TOMS   £l06

© BMJ Books 2004
BMJ Books is an imprint of the BMJ Publishing Group

All rights reserved. No part of this publication may be reproduced, stored in a retrieval system,
or transmitted, in any form or by any means, electronic, mechanical, photocopying, recording
and/or otherwise, without the prior written permission of the publishers.

First published in 2000
By BMJ Books, BMA House, Tavistock Square,
London WC1H 9JR

First edition 2000
Second Impression 2001
Second edition 2004

www.bmjbooks.com
www.evidbasedpediatrics.com

British Library Cataloguing in Publication Data

A catalogue record for this book is available from the British Library

ISBN 0-7279-1746-3

Typeset by Siva Math Setters, Chennai, India

Printed and bound by MPG Books, Bodmin, Cornwall

Contents

Contributors

Kate Armon
The Jenny Lind Children's Department
Norfolk and Norwich University Hospital
Norwich, UK

Robert Armstrong
Department of Paediatrics
Children's Hospital and Women's Hospital
University of British Columbia
Vancouver, British Columbia
Canada

Nadia Badawi
Department of Neonatology
The Children's Hospital at Westmead
University of Sydney
Sydney, NSW
Australia

Alexandra Barratt
School of Public Health
University of Sydney
Sydney, NSW
Australia

Helen Bedford
Centre for Paediatric Epidemiology and Biostatistics
Institute of Child Health
London, UK

Carol Bower
Telethon Institute for Child Health Research
and
School of Population Health, University of Western Australia
Crawley, Western Australia
Australia

Julie C Brown
Departmant of Pediatrics
University of Washington and Children's Hospital
and Regional Medical Center
Seattle, Washington
USA

Blake Bulloch
Division of Emergency Medicine
Phoenix Children's Hospital
Phoenix, Arizona
USA

Tracey Burrell
The Langton Centre
South Eastern Area Health Service
Sydney, NSW
Australia

Phyllis Butow
Departments of Medicine and Psychological Medicine
University of Sydney
Sydney, NSW
Australia

Roberto Buzzetti
Centre for Evaluation of Effectiveness of Health Care (CeVEAS)
Modena, Italy

Patrina Caldwell
Centre for Kidney Research
The Children's Hospital at Westmead and Discipline of
    Paediatrics and Child Health
University of Sydney
Sydney, NSW
Australia

Aaron Chiu
Section of Neonatology
Department of Paediatrics and Child Health
University of Manitoba
Winnipeg, Manitoba
Canada

Jonathan Craig
School of Public Health
University of Sydney and The Children's Hospital at Westmead
Sydney, NSW
Australia

Heather M Davey
School of Public Health
Screening and Test Evaluation Program
University of Sydney
Sydney, NSW
Australia

Heather J Dean
Section of Endocrinology
Department of Pediatrics and Child Health
University of Manitoba
Winnipeg, Manitoba
Canada

Chris Del Mar
Centre for General Practice
University of Queensland
Queensland
Australia

Eugene Dinkevich
Department of Pediatrics
State University of New York – Health Science
    Center at Brooklyn
Brooklyn, New York
USA

Jon Dorling
Division of Child Health
University of Leicester
Leicester Warwick Medical School
Leicester, UK

Lex W Doyle
Department of Obstetrics and Gynaecology
The Royal Women's Hospital
Carlton, Victoria
Australia

Laurel Edmunds
The Avon Longitudinal Study of Parents and Children
Unit of Paediatrics & Perinatal Epidemiology
University of Bristol
Bristol, UK

David Elliman
Islington PCT
and
Great Ormond Street Hospital For Children
London, UK

Elizabeth J Elliott
Discipline of Paediatrics and Child Health
University of Sydney and The Children's Hospital
    at Westmead
Sydney, NSW
Australia

Jonathan HC Evans
Children and Young People's Kidney Unit
Nottingham City Hospital
Nottingham, UK

Ruth Gilbert
Centre for Evidence-based Child Health
Centre for Paediatric Epidemiology and Statistics
Institute of Child Health
London, UK

Sue Gilmour
Department of Pediatrics
University of Alberta
Edmonton, Alberta
Canada

Cathryn MA Glazener
Health Services Research Unit
University of Aberdeen Medical School
Aberdeen, UK

Roberto Grilli
Regional Health Care Agency of Emilia-Romagna
Bologna, Italy

Paul Gringras
Harper House Children's Service
London, UK

James P Guevara
Department of Pediatrics
Children's Hospital of Philadelphia
University of Pennsylvania School of Medicine
Philadelphia, Pennsylvania
USA

Louise Hartley
Child Development Centre
University Hospital of Wales
Cardiff, UK

Andrew Hayen
Centre for Epidemiology and Research
NSW Department of Health
North Sydney, NSW
Australia

David J Henderson-Smart
Centre for Perinatal Health Services Research
Queen Elizabeth Research Institute
University of Sydney
Sydney, NSW
Australia

Jordan Hupert
Division of General Pediatrics
University of Illinois at Chicago
Chicago, Illinois
USA

Kathleen Kennedy
Department of Pediatrics
University of Texas Houston Health Science Center
Houston, Texas
USA

John Keogh
Department of Obstetrics and Gynaecology
Hornsby Ku Ring Gai Hospital
Hornsby, Sydney, NSW
Australia

Robert Klaassen
Division of Hematology/Oncology
Department of Paediatrics
Children's Hospital of Eastern Ontario
University of Ottawa
Ottawa, Ontario
Canada

Terry P Klassen
Department of Pediatrics
University of Alberta
Edmonton, Alberta
Canada

Eileen J Klein
Pediatric Emergency Medicine
University of Washington and Children's Hospital and Regional
    Medical Center
Seattle, Washington
USA

Margaret L Lawson
Division of Endocrinology and Metabolism
Children's Hospital of Eastern Ontario
University of Ottawa
Ottawa, Ontario
Canada

Alessandro Liberati
Italian Cochrane Centre
University of Modena and
Centre for Evaluation of Effectiveness of Health Care (CeVEAS)
Modena, Italy

Gregory S Liptak
Children's Hospital at Strong
University of Rochester
Rochester, New York
USA

Stuart Logan
Institute of Health and Social Care Research
Peninsula Medical School
Exeter, UK

Chris Lovato
Centre for Behavioural Research and Program Evaluation
Department of Health Care and Epidemiology
University of British Columbia
Vancouver, British Columbia
Canada

Geraldine Macdonald
School for Policy Studies
University of Bristol
Bristol, UK

C Raina MacIntyre
National Centre for Immunisation Research
The Children's Hospital at Westmead and
University of Sydney
Sydney, NSW
Australia
and
Discipline of Paediatrics and Child Health
University of Sydney
Sydney, NSW
Australia

Nicola Magrini
Centre for Evaluation of Effectiveness
    of Health Care (CeVEAS)
Modena, Italy

Elise Maher
Centre for Community Child Health
Royal Children's Hospital
Parkville, Victoria
Australia

Lynnette J Mazur
Department of Pediatrics
University of Texas Houston Health Science Center
Houston, Texas
USA

Peter McIntyre
Department of Immunology and Infectious Diseases
    and National Centre for Immunisation
    Research and Surveillance
The Children's Hospital at Westmead
University of Sydney
Sydney, NSW
Australia

Maud Meates-Dennis
Department of Paediatrics
Christchurch Public Hospital
Christchurch, New Zealand

Craig Mellis
School of Health Sciences
Bond University
Gold Coast, Queensland
Australia

Silvia Minozzi
Italian Cochrane Centre
Mario Negri Institute
Milan, Italy

Anne Morris
Discipline of Paediatrics and Child Health
The Children's Hospital at Westmead
Sydney, NSW
Australia

Virginia A Moyer
Department of Pediatrics
University of Texas Houston Health Science Center
Houston, Texas
USA

Gina Neto
Division of Pediatric Emergency Medicine
Children's Hospital of Eastern Ontario
Ottawa, Ontario
Canada

Jerry Niederman
University of Illinois at Chicago
Department of Pediatrics
Chicago, Illinois
USA

Maureen E O'Donnell
Centre for Community Health and
    Health Evaluation Research
University of British Columbia
Vancouver, British Columbia
Canada

Martin Offringa
Center for Pediatric Clinical Epidemiology
Emma Children's University Hospital
Academic Medical Center
Amsterdam, The Netherlands

Arne Ohlsson
Department of Paediatrics
University of Toronto
Toronto, Ontario
Canada

David Osborn
RPA Newborn Care
Royal Prince Alfred Hospital and the University of Sydney
Sydney, NSW
Australia

Martin H Osmond
Division of Pediatric Emergency Medicine
Department of Pediatrics
Children's Hospital of Eastern Ontario
University of Ottawa
Ottawa, Ontario
Canada

Carolyn A Paris
Pediatric Emergency Medicine
University of Washington and Children's Hospital and
    Regional Medical Center
Seattle, Washington
USA

Sandi Pirozzo
School of Population Health
University of Queensland
Queensland
Australia

Martin Pusic
Centre for Community Child Health Research
University of British Columbia
Vancouver, British Columbia
Canada

Parminder Raina
Department of Clinical Epidemiology and Biostatistics
Faculty of Health Sciences
McMaster University
Hamilton, Ontario
Canada

Alison Salt
Neurodisability Service
The Wolfson Centre
Great Ormond Street Hospital for Children NHS Trust
London, UK

Connie Schardt
Medical Center Library
Duke University Medical Center
Durham, North Carolina
USA

Adam Scheinberg
Department of Rehabilitation
The Children's Hospital at Westmead
Sydney, NSW
Australia

Vibhuti Shah
Department of Paediatrics
University of Toronto
Toronto, Ontario
Canada

Jean Shoveller
Department of Health Care and Epidemiology
University of British Columbia
Vancouver, British Columbia
Canada

Holly D Smith
Department of Pediatrics
University of Texas Houston Health Science Center
Houston, Texas
USA

Martin T Stein
Department of Pediatrics
University of California San Diego
   School of Medicine
San Diego, California
USA

Kent Stobart
Department of Pediatrics
University of Alberta
Edmonton, Alberta
Canada

Gayla Swihart
Department of Health Care and Epidemiology
University of British Columbia
Vancouver, British Columbia
Canada

Shayne P Taback
Department of Pediatrics and Child Health
University of Manitoba
Winnipeg, Manitoba
Canada

Milton Tenenbein
Department of Pediatrics and Child Health
University of Manitoba
Winnipeg, Manitoba
Canada

Lyndal Trevena
School of Public Health
University of Sydney
Sydney, NSW
Australia

Kate Turcotte
Centre for Community Health and Health Evaluation Research
British Columbia Injury Research and Prevention Unit
Vancouver, British Columbia
Canada

Jon E Tyson
Department of Pediatrics
University of Texas Houston Health Science Center
Houston, Texas
USA

Sunita Vohra
Hospital for Sick Children
Toronto, Ontario
Canada

Melissa Wake
Centre for Community Child Health
Royal Children's Hospital
Parkville, Victoria
Australia
and
University of Melbourne and
   Murdoch Childrens Research Institute

Jeanette Ward
Department of Public Health
South West Sydney Area Health Service
Liverpool, NSW
Australia

Donna Waters
Faculty of Nursing, Midwifery and Health
University of Technology
Sydney, NSW
Australia

Elizabeth Waters
Centre for Community Child Health
University of Melbourne
Victoria, Australia
and
Department of Public Health
University of Oxford
Oxford, UK

Natasha M Wiebe
Department of Pediatrics
Alberta Research Centre for Child Health Evidence
University of Alberta, Alberta
Canada

Katrina Williams
Department of Clinical Epidemiology
The Children's Hospital at Westmead
Sydney, NSW
Australia

Ann Williamson
NSW Injury Risk Management Research Centre
University of New South Wales
Sydney
Australia

Sue Woolfenden
Liverpool Health Sector
Liverpool Hospital
Liverpool, NSW
Australia

Karen Zwi
School of Women's and Children's Health
University of New South Wales
Sydney Children's Hospital
Randwick, NSW
Australia

Evidence-based Pediatrics and Child Health, Second edition CD Rom

Features

Evidence-based Pediatrics and Child Health, Second edition PDF eBook

- Bookmarked and hyperlinked for instant access to all headings and topics
- Fully indexed and searchable text – just click the 'Search Text' button

PDA Edition sample chapter

- A chapter from Evidence-based Pediatrics and Child Health, adapted for use on handheld devices such as Palm and Pocket PC
- Click on the underlined text to view an image (or images) relevant to the text concerned
- Uses Mobipocket Reader technology, compatible with all PDA devices and also available for Windows
- Follow the on-screen instructions on the relevant part of the CD Rom to install Mobipocket for your device
- Full title available for purchase as a download from http://www.pda.bmjbooks.com

BMJ Books catalogue

- Instant access to BMJ Books full catalogue, including an order form

Also included – a direct link to the Evidence-based Pediatrics and Child Health update website

Instructions for use

The CD Rom should start automatically upon insertion, on all Windows systems. The menu screen will appear and you can then navigate by clicking on the headings. If the CD Rom does not start automatically upon insertion, please browse using "Windows Explorer" and double-click the file "BMJ_Books.exe".

Tips

The viewable area of the PDF ebook can be expanded to fill the full screen width, by hiding the bookmarks. To do this, click and hold on the divider in between the bookmark window and the main window, then drag it to the left as required.

By clicking once on a page in the PDF ebook window, you 'activate' the window. You can now scroll through pages using the scroll-wheel on your mouse, or by using the cursor keys on your keyboard.

Note: the Evidence-based Pediatrics and Child Health PDF eBook is for search and reference only and, aside from the free consumers sections and faces figures, cannot be printed. A printable PDF version as well as the full PDA edition can be purchased from http://www.bmjbookshop.com

Troubleshooting

If any problems are experienced with use of the CD Rom, please send an email to the following address stating the problem you have encountered:

cdsupport@bmjbooks.com

Evidence-based Pediatrics and Child Health update website

Further information and updates can be found at: http://www.evidbasedpediatrics.com

Foreword

Evidence-based medicine (EBM) is about solving clinical problems. In particular, EBM provides tools for using the original medical literature to determine the benefits and risks of alternative patient management strategies, and to weigh those benefits and risks in the context of an individual patient's experiences and values.

The term EBM first appeared in the medical literature in 1991; it has rapidly become something of a mantra. EBM is sometimes perceived as a blinkered adherence to randomized trials, or a healthcare managers' tool for controlling and constraining recalcitrant physicians. In fact, EBM involves informed and effective use of all types of evidence, but particularly evidence from the medical literature, in patient care.

EBM's evolution has included outward expansion: we now realize that optimal healthcare delivery must include evidence-based nursing, physiotherapy, occupational therapy, and podiatry – and specialization. We need evidence-based obstetrics, gynecology, internal medicine, and surgery – and indeed, urology, orthopedics, and neurosurgery. And of course, we need evidence-based pediatrics (EBP).

EBP involves use of a hierarchy of evidence, from meta-analyses of high quality randomized trials showing definitive results directly applicable to an individual patient, to relying on physiological rationale or previous experience with a small number of similar patients. The hallmark of the evidence-based practitioner is that, for particular clinical decisions, you know the strength of the evidence, and therefore the degree of uncertainty.

Unfortunately, practicing EBP is not easy. Practitioners must know how to frame a clinical quandary to facilitate use of the literature in its resolution. Evidence-based pediatricians must know how to search the literature efficiently to obtain the best available evidence bearing on their question, to evaluate the strength of the methods of the studies that they find, extract the clinical message, apply it back to the patient, and store it for retrieval when faced with similar patients in the future.

Traditionally, neither medical schools nor postgraduate programs have taught these skills. While this situation is changing, the biggest influence on how trainees will practice is their clinical role models, few of whom are currently accomplished EBP practitioners. The situation is even more challenging for those looking to acquire the requisite skills after completing their clinical training.

This text primarily addresses the needs of this last group, practising pediatricians. The text represents a landmark in a number of ways. It is among the first EBM text directed specifically at pediatricians. The book represents an effort to comprehensively address the EBM-related learning needs of this clinical community.

The book is also original in its structure. The text begins with chapters that introduce the tools for evaluating the original pediatric literature. The bulk of the text, however, provides examples of how to use the skills of the evidence-based pediatrician to address clinical problems in everyday practice. These chapters do not provide *the* answer to a clinical question. In fact, they point out that the answer today may not be the answer tomorrow, as new evidence emerges. What they do provide is an approach that clinicians can use to address questions that they currently face, and will face in the future.

The clinician may find the prospect of practising EBP daunting. Where, you may wonder, are you to find the time to identify, let alone evaluate, the studies relevant to the myriad clinical problems that you face on a daily basis? There are a number of answers to this question. One is the suggestion that there are a relatively small number of issues, perhaps one to two hundred in any individual's practice, that are important and arise frequently enough, and for which there is high quality evidence, to warrant working familiarity with the data.

Whether or not this perspective is valid – and its validity may depend on the eye of the beholder – another answer comes from the increasing bank of preprocessed EBM resources. One can consider a classification of these resources that comes with the mnemonic 4S:

- the individual *study*
- the *systematic review* of all the available studies on a given problem
- a *synopsis* of both individual studies and summaries, and
- *systems* of information.

Secondary journals such as *Evidence-Based Mental Health*, *Evidence-Based Nursing*, and *ACP Journal Club* which does the job for internal medicine – survey a large number of journals relevant to their area and choose *studies* that meet both relevance and validity screening criteria. Similarly, the *Journal of Pediatrics* summarizes selected published studies on a bimonthly basis. These journals present the results of these studies in structured abstracts or *synopses* that provide clinicians with the key information they need to judge their applicability to their own practices. Fame and fortune await the enterprising group who applies this methodology to produce evidence-based pediatrics.

If there is any chance it may be available, clinicians whose priority is efficient evidence-based practice seek a high quality systematic review rather than the primary studies addressing their clinical question. For issues of therapy, published *systematic reviews*, including those in the Cochrane Collaboration database, provide a rapidly growing repository of clinically useful *summaries*. Finally, clinicians often seek answers to questions about a whole process of care rather than a focused clinical question. Increasingly, clinicians asking these sort of questions can look to high quality evidence-based practice guidelines or clinical pathways to provide, in effect, a series of synopses that summarize available evidence. The best *systems* use computer technology to match the patient or problem characteristics with an evidence-based knowledge repository and provide patient-specific recommendations. At the same time, we must remember that recommendations can only be made for "average" patients, and the circumstances and values of the patient and family before us may differ. One way of dealing with this might be to bring the tools of decision analysis to the bedside.

Whatever the future holds for the increasing efficiency of evidence-based practice, the current text provides an introduction to a system of clinical problem-solving that is becoming a prerequisite for modern pediatric practice.

Gordon Guyatt

Preface to the 2nd edition

Elizabeth J Elliott and Virginia A Moyer

Richard Dawkins coined the term "meme" in his 1976 book *The Selfish Gene*.[1] In his foreword to *The Meme Machine*,[2] he describes a meme as "an entity that might play a role in the transmission of words, ideas, faiths, mannerisms, and fashions." A meme may represent "a set of religious beliefs, a regional accent, a new word, a mannerism, a fashion or an idea." The term, now included in the *Oxford English Dictionary*,[3] is defined as "an element of culture that may be considered to be passed by a non-genetic means." Like genes, memes can be transmitted vertically within a population, for example the passing of religious beliefs or mannerisms from parent to child, but memes also travel horizontally, like viruses in an epidemic. One example is the rapid spread of new terms such as "Y2K" over the internet. Another is the spread of a schoolyard craze – whether hula hoops, pogo sticks or yo-yos – through a generation of children the world over. A prerequisite for the transmission of a meme, whatever its nature, is the willingness of the human recipient to accept and imitate it. Committing a meme to paper (whether it be grandma's chocolate brownie recipe or the rules of a new playground game), greatly enhances the likelihood that a meme will be transmitted and the accuracy with which this is achieved.

In the context of the above definition, evidence-based medicine (EBM) could be considered a meme. It is an element of medical culture that has been passed by non-genetic means, including imitation, to clinicians around the world. The term evidence-based medicine, coined in 1991 by Sackett and colleagues at McMaster University, is defined as "the conscientious, explicit and judicious use of current best evidence in making decisions about the care of individual patients."[4] The concept of EBM fell on the fertile ground of a generation of clinicians who were overwhelmed by the exponential growth of the medical literature and needed a means of locating, making sense of, and applying relevant information to their patients. Although some clinicians appeared to shun EBM, the concept spread like an epidemic through other groups of the medical profession – both vertically, from clinician to junior doctor or student (and sometimes in the reverse direction) and horizontally, amongst peers. The principles of EBM have been committed to paper and Sackett's book, *How to Practice and Teach EBM*[5] has found its way into thousands of white coat pockets. Increasingly, clinicians have access to electronic medical databases, while specialized journals that present evidence-based summaries of the literature have flourished. In many universities EBM is now incorporated into undergraduate and graduate medical curricula and postgraduate courses on how to practise and teach EBM abound.

EBM is the subject of a series of specialty texts published by BMJ Books and including *Evidence Based Cardiology*,[6] *Evidence Based Gastroenterology and* Hepatology,[7] and *Evidence Based Pediatric Oncology*.[8] We are pleased to present the second edition of *Evidence-Based Pediatrics and Child Health*. The first edition[9] was well reviewed, well received by its readers and underwent several reprints. One reviewer[10] described the book as "a practical tutorial in the process and practice of evidence-based medicine," saying that "if any book is to persuade paediatricians to practice evidence-based paediatrics, this is it". More importantly, our colleagues assert that the book is used by clinicians to inform clinical practice and also provides a source of teaching material on "how to do EBM." The first book spawned two series on evidence-based pediatrics, in the *BMJ*[11] and the *Western Journal of Medicine*,[12] and its format has been adapted for use in a current series on evidence-based pediatrics in the *Archives of Diseases in Childhood*.[13]

Like the first edition, the second edition of *Evidence-Based Pediatrics and Child Health* is intended as a "primer" in EBM rather than a "master class". Its target audience is pediatricians, family physicians, and other healthcare workers who deal with children. It is a not a book aimed at a readership with a PhD in epidemiology and therefore avoids the use of complex statistics and obscure terminology. Neither is it a standard pediatric text. It makes no attempt to be comprehensive and neither purports to cover all conditions presenting to pediatricians, nor all possible aspects of a single disease. Rather, it aims to introduce the principles of EBM and to illustrate, with the use of "real" and exclusively pediatric cases, how to incorporate these principles into daily clinical practice. This book is purposely written in an informal, conversational tone. This is intended to convey the idea that the knowledge imparted to the reader comes from a clinical colleague who is aware that, in order to make it reasonable for a busy clinician to practise EBP, the process must be realistic, time-efficient, and have practical relevance. Although this is a multi-author book, we have tried to ensure some consistency of style and theme throughout. While the information in some chapters represents a thorough systematic review of the literature, other chapters illustrate the "quick and dirty" approach that we are all forced to use in our busy clinical practices. We thank all authors for their valuable contributions and Mary Banks, our editor, for her unfailing support.

Format and contents

The format of this book is similar to that of the first edition. Section I provides readers with the conceptual background and skills they need to practise each component step of EBM, namely identifying the need for information, asking clinical questions, and finding, evaluating, and applying the evidence. Each chapter starts with a clinical scenario, introduces the concepts involved in critical appraisal of, for example, a paper on therapy, and then demonstrates the process using publications from the literature. In keeping with the structure of the *JAMA* series "Users' Guides to the Literature"[14] we adhere to the sequence of assessing first the study's validity, then its results, and then its application to the child in question. The converse method, to start by assessing applicability to the patient and going on to assess validity only if applicability is shown, has its proponents. We are yet to be convinced that the former method is problematic. Section I also contains some chapters addressing topics that are often omitted from EBM texts. These include the assessment of quality of life, the use of scales to rank the strength of evidence, issues of clinical measurement and disagreement, and the evidence-base for various methods of continuing education. There is evidence that physician performance is enhanced for those who learn to use EBM and apply it to their clinical practice.[15,16] Also, evaluation of medical students taught EBM skills shows that this approach improves their ability to evaluate the clinical literature, and enhances life-long learning skills.[17,18]

Section II covers some routine interventions for the care and prevention of disease in children (including well child examination, immunization, and injury prevention) and Section III covers a range of common and/or important illnesses (including diabetes, asthma, and gastroenteritis) that present to pediatricians. Each is written by practising clinicians and commences with a "real world" scenario. The reader is led through the process of EBP – asking questions about the case, searching and evaluating the evidence and summarizing the answers found before applying the relevant information back to the original "case". We should stress that in resolving clinical questions the available evidence is not the only consideration. Patient and family preferences, risk aversion, cost and cultural issues, and quality of life must be considered. Different clinicians, with their own patients, in different settings, may come to conclusions that are different from those reached by the authors. We emphasize the Bayesian approach to evidence: the evidence is like a

diagnostic test in that it adds information to prior knowledge and sways clinicians a predictable and measurable distance.[19] Thus, clinicians with access to the same information may end up in a different place because their starting point was different. The important thing is to be able to make explicit the influence of the evidence (which is empiric and quantifiable) and the patients' or clinicians' prior beliefs and values (which are highly individual) on the question at hand.

The rationale behind the book's case-based format is that it is easier for readers to learn how EBP can be used in their practices if they are provided with comprehensive clinical examples. The reader should not be disappointed that the whole of pediatrics is not covered, that the information provided on each topic is not comprehensive, and that the answer to a clinical question is rarely a clear "yes" or "no". This is a book about "process." It does not try to provide all the answers, but does demonstrate how the questions posed by the chapter authors can be addressed. It also illustrates the concept that, when making any decision based on evidence, you must weigh the potential benefits against the potential harms. Thus, the book provides a framework for readers to use when managing their own patients. For easy reference and to enable repetition or expansion, summary search strategies that identify the database and search terms are "boxed". Inevitably, the search for evidence to answer a clinical question often identifies areas in which there is a lack of good evidence. This has led authors to suggest topics for future research, which appear at the end of each chapter.

All chapters that were included in the 1st edition have been updated and the 2nd edition has been expanded considerably. In Section I a new Chapter 1 provides an overview of EBM and includes discussion of some topical issues in EBM – publication bias, analysis bias, and conflict of interest. The addition of chapters on communicating evidence to patients, qualitative research, complementary and alternative medicine, and informatics is timely. Increasingly, parents come to consultations "armed" with a recent Cochrane review or other information about their child's condition downloaded from the web. We must embrace the arrival of IT and take every opportunity to help carers interpret the literature and to involve them in informed decision-making about their child's care.[20–22] Four new chapters on neonatology for the generalist have been added to Section III. The neonatal topics now covered – neonatal abstinence syndrome, pain control in the newborn, neonatal encephalopathy, outcome of prematurity and apnea – reflect societal change, the changing nature of our practices, and the rapid recent expansion in published data in neonatology.

So is EBM a passing "fad" or is it here to stay?[23] If, as Gordon Guyatt says in his Foreword to this book, "evidence-based medicine is about solving clinical problems," then clearly EBM is "a prerequisite for modern pediatric practice". More than ever, there is a legal imperative for clinicians to keep up to date so as not to risk providing suboptimal care – or ending up in the courts! In pediatrics, a delay in the use of beneficial treatments, such as antenatal steroids in preterm labor to prevent neonatal respiratory distress and avoidance of prone sleeping to minimize the risk of SIDS,[24] has previously resulted from our failure to act on the available evidence. However, we should be heartened by one recent study showing that the primary intervention was supported by evidence from at least one randomized trial or convincing non-experimental evidence in 75% of pediatric admissions.[25]

EBM is part of the e-revolution currently occurring in our health systems. The integration of evidence into our practices is made infinitely easier by access to electronic databases of the medical literature and to summarized sources of evidence. However keeping up to date is a daunting task. Over 2 million scientific papers are published each year and keeping abreast of pediatrics alone would require reading more than five journal articles every day of the year.[26] Most busy clinicians admit they have little time to read and many seek information from local "experts".[4] To add to our woes, conventional continuing medical education programs do little to improve patient care. Thus, throughout the book, the emphasis is on illustrating "shortcuts" for the busy clinician, whether to ensure good capture of the relevant literature or to evaluate its quality. For example, the reader is encouraged to use high quality "secondary" or "synthesized" evidence such as systematic reviews, when available, rather than to scour MedLine for the answer to a question of therapy. These evidence sources not only minimize the time required for searching, but provide the clinician with "predigested" information located, critically appraised, and summarized by skilled colleagues.

We hope that this book will help clinicians to more easily find and understand information relevant to patient care. EBM is not about saving money and it is not just about randomized trials. Both good clinical skills and good evidence are essential for the practice of EBM. We acknowledge that EBM does have limitations – not least of which is lack of evidence applicable to pediatrics and child health. As pediatricians, our challenge is to increase the number of clinical studies and systematic reviews addressing diseases of childhood. Similarly, it is important that we put pressure on editors of other sources of synthesized evidence, such as *ACP Journal Club*, *Evidence Based Medicine*, and *Clinical Evidence*,[27] to include more topics on pediatric and child health. As researchers, we should identify knowledge gaps and encourage the conduct of quality clinical trials of therapies for use in children.

EBM may never convince its critics, but is certainly preferable to the alternatives – including "eminence-", "vehemence-", and "confidence-" based medicine as proposed by Isaacs and Fitzgerald.[28] The future for EBP will be bright if we can both capitalize on our clinical expertise and ensure that we harvest, critically evaluate, and judiciously use the available evidence to improve patient care. We hope that this book will provide an impetus for busy clinicians to practise EBP and some practical tips to facilitate this task and ensure better outcomes for our patients.

References

1 Dawkins R. *The selfish gene, 2nd edn*. Oxford: Oxford University Press, 1976.

2 Blackmore SJ. *The meme machine*. Oxford: Oxford University Press, 1999.

3 *Oxford English Dictionary, 2nd edn*. Oxford: Oxford University Press, 1989.

4 Sackett DL, Rosenberg WM, Gray JAM, Haynes RB, Richardson WS. Evidence based medicine. What it is and what it isn't. *BMJ* 1996;**312**:71–2.

5 Sackett DL, Richardson WS, Rosenberg W, Haynes RB, eds. *Evidence based medicine. How to practice and teach EBM*. Edinburgh: Churchill Livingstone, 1998.

6 Cairns JA, Camm J, Fallen E, Gersh B, Yusuf S. *Evidence-Based Cardiology*. London: BMJ Books, 2003.

7 McDonald JWD, Burroughs AK, Feagan BG. *Evidence Based Gastroenterology and Hepatology*. London: BMJ Books, 1999.

8 Ferrers B, Philip T, Pinkerton R. *Evidence-Based Pediatric Oncology*. London: BMJ Books, 2002.

9 Moyer VA, Elliott EJ, Davis R *et al*. *Evidence Based Pediatrics and Child Health*. London: BMJ Books, 2000.

10 Phillips R. Evidence based pediatrics and child health. *Arch Dis Child* 2002;**89**:139.

11 Edmunds L, Waters E, Elliott EJ. Evidence based management of childhood obesity. *BMJ* 2001;**323**:916–19.

12 Moyer V, Elliott E. Op-Ed. How to practice evidence-based pediatrics. *West J Med* 2001;**174**:1–2.

13 Phillips B, ed. Archimedes. Towards evidence based medicine for paediatricians. *Arch Dis Child* 2003;**88**:638–42.

14 Oxman AD, Sackett DL, Guyatt GH *et al*. User's guides to the medical literature, 1: How to get started. *JAMA* 1993;**270**:2093–5.

15 Oxman AD, Thomas MA, Davis DA, Haynes RB. No magic bullets: a systematic review of 102 trials of interventions to improve professional practice. *CMAJ* 1995;**153**:1423–31.

16 Davis DA, Thomson MA, Oxman AD, Haynes RB. Changing physician performance: a systematic review of the effect of educational strategies. *JAMA* 1995;**274**:700–5.

17 Bennett KJ, Sackett DL, Haynes RB, Neufeld VR. A controlled trial of teaching critical appraisal of the clinical literature to medical students. *JAMA* 1987;**257**:2451–4.

18 Shin JH, Haynes RB, Johnston ME. Effect of problem-based, self-directed undergraduate education on life-long learning. *Can Med J* 1993;**148**:969–76.

19 Brophy JM, Joseph L. Placing trials in context using Bayesian analysis. *JAMA* 1995;**273**:871–5.

20 Dixon-Woods M, Young B, Heney D. Partnerships with children. *BMJ* 1999;**319**:778–80.

21 Jadad AR. Promoting partnerships: challenges for the internet age. *BMJ* 1999;**319**:761–3.

22 Shepperd S, Charnock D, Gann B. Helping patients access high quality health information. *BMJ* 1999;**319**:764–6.

23 Christakis DA, Davis R, Rivara FP. Pediatric evidence-based medicine: Past, present and future. *J Pediatr* 2000;**136**: 383–9.

24 Gilbert R, Logan S. Future prospects for evidence based child health. *Arch Dis Child* 1997;**75**:465–8.

25 Moyer VA, Gist AK, Elliott EJ. Is inpatient pediatric medicine evidence-based? *J Paediatr Child Hlth* 2002;**38**:347–51.

26 Davidoff F, Haynes B, Sackett D, Smith R. Evidence based medicine: a new journal to help doctors identify the information they need. *BMJ* 1995;**310**:1085–6.

27 Goodlee F, Goldmann D, Donald A *et al.* eds. *Clinical Evidence.* London: BMJ Publishing Group, published 6-monthly from 1999.

28 Isaacs, D, Fitzgerald D. Seven alternatives to evidence based medicine. *BMJ* 1999;**319**:18–25.

Glossary of terms

Algorithm An explicit description of the ordered sequence of steps to be followed in patient care under specified circumstances.

Absolute risk The probability (rate) of a specified outcome during a specified period in the control and experimental groups. Sometimes referred to as the control event rate (CER) and experimental event rate (EER) respectively. In contrast to common usage, the word "risk" may refer to adverse events (such as seizure or the need for ventilation), or desirable events (such as prevention of complications or cure).

Absolute risk difference The absolute arithmetic difference in the event rate (risk of an outcome) in the treatment (experimental) and control groups in a randomized trial. The absolute risk difference may be an: **Absolute risk reduction** (the bad outcome is less frequent in the treatment than control group); an **Absolute risk increase** (the bad outcome is more frequent in the treatment than control group); an **Absolute benefit reduction** (the good outcome is less frequent in the therapy group).

Allocation concealment A method used to ensure that the result of randomization (allocation to groups) in a trial is concealed from the individual responsible for actually allocating the patient. Concealment can be achieved by separating the randomization and recruitment process. For example randomization might be determined by a centralized agent (for example, pharmacy); by use of an on-site computer with restricted access; by use of identical, coded containers; or using sequentially numbered opaque and sealed envelopes. "Concealment" is different from "blinding".

Association A statistical relationship between two variables or events, which does not imply a causal relationship.

Baseline risk The risk (probability) that a child within a specified population will have a particular condition or disease at the present time or the risk (probability) that the child will develop a particular outcome in the future.

Best Evidence An electronic database of over 1000 abstracted articles that have been published in the journals *Evidence Based Medicine* and *ACP Journal Club*. All articles have be deemed methodologically sound and are accompanied by a commentary written by a content expert and outlining its importance and usefulness to clinical practice (www.bestevidence.org).

Bias (systematic) Any trend in the collection, analysis, interpretation, publication, or review of data that can lead to conclusions that are systematically different from the truth.

Blinding (masking): Blinding is any method used to deny investigators, patients and assessors information about allocation of patients to treatment groups. Knowledge of allocation might influence measurements, observations, or management and thereby introduce bias into a clinical trial. The terms double-blinded or triple-blinded are best avoided and it is preferable to state precisely who (assessor, investigator or patient) was blinded to group allocation.

Boolean logical operator A group of search terms (for example, "AND", "OR", and "NOT") available in MedLine (and other searchable databases), which help in refining the search strategy. For example the request "gastroenteritis AND loperamide" will give the articles common to both sets. The search "gastroenteritis OR loperamide" will give both sets of articles, while use of the term "NOT" will help exclude irrelevant articles.

Case–control study An observational study in which a group of children with an outcome of interest (for example, leukemia) and a group of children who have not experienced the same outcome are compared to see how exposure to suspected risk factors (for example, viral agents, radiation) differs between the two groups. This type of study provides a relatively quick and easy way to measure risk factors and is most useful for the study of rare diseases. However bias and confounding my influence the results and it is difficult to infer causation from this type of study.

Case report (series) Uncontrolled observational studies consisting of a report on one (or a series of) patients with an intervention and/or outcome of interest.

CINAHL (Cumulative Index of Nursing and Allied Health) An electronic database of nursing and allied health sciences literature, including health education, occupational and physiotherapy, social services at www.cinahl.com (1983–).

Clinical Evidence A publication containing summaries of evidence on questions of therapy, prepared by clinicians and epidemiologists using standardized methodology. Published by BMJ Books and updated approximately every 6 months. Predominantly relates to adult medicine but contains a section on Child Health (www.clinicalevidence.com).

Clinical practice guideline A statement designed to assist decision-making about health care for specific clinical circumstances. Although some guidelines are based on a systematic review of the literature, others are not evidence-based. In the absence of published evidence, recommendations may be based on "consensus expert opinion".

Clinically significant A finding that is clinically important. Here, "significant" means "important" (rather than statistically significant). Where the word "significant" or "significance" is used without qualification in this text, it is being used in its statistical sense.

Cochrane Library A regularly updated, electronic database containing several literature databases including the Cochrane Database of Systematic Reviews (CDSR), the Database of Abstracts of Reviews of Effects (DARE), Cochrane Central Register of Controlled Trials (CENTRAL), Cochrane Database of Methodology Reviews, and the Cochrane Methodology Register (CMR). Also contains information about the Cochrane Collaboration. It is available on CD-ROM or on the Internet with free access for all in some countries (www.cochranelibrary.com).

Cochrane Collaboration This international network (named after the epidemiologist Archie Cochrane) has a unique role in evaluating and collating health care interventions with the ultimate aim of helping people make well informed health-care decisions. The collaboration prepares, disseminates, and updates systematic reviews of the literature (for example, RCTs for interventions). This process involves searching the medical literature, classifying articles according to study type, and abstracting, analyzing and summarizing information in a standardized way.

Cochrane Central Register of Controlled Trials (CENTRAL) A database within the Cochrane Library containing all randomized controlled trials identified by the members of the Cochrane Collaboration and which may be relevant for inclusion in Cochrane Reviews. Over 370 000 trials were listed in Issue 4, 2003.

Cochrane Database of Systematic Reviews (CDSR) A database within the Cochrane Library, updated quarterly, of all systematic reviews completed by members of the Cochrane Collaboration using strict methodological criteria. It contains both completed reviews and reviews in progress (Protocols). Over 3000 reviews were listed in Issue 4, 2003.

Cochrane Methodology Register (CMR) A database of abstracts of books and articles related to methodological issues relevant to summarizing evidence about health care in systematic review.

Cochrane review *see* systematic review.

Cohort study A study that follows a group of people over time and compares outcomes in people exposed to a particular factor or intervention (for example, a vaccine or a medicine) and in people not exposed (or exposed to different levels or doses). This type of observational study is useful to determine whether a specific exposure is the *cause* of a specified outcome (often adverse). A prospective or concurrent cohort follows participants forward in time and is more reliable than a retrospective cohort study, which look back in time to ascertain whether or not participants with a particular outcome were exposed to the agent in question. Cohorts including of a single group of patients are used to evaluate prognosis. Cohort studies may also called longitudinal, prospective, incidence or follow up studies.

Co-intervention An intervention given apart from the intervention under study. When evaluating randomized controlled trials, it is important to determine whether co-interventions were applied equally to treatment and control groups.

Completer analysis Analysis of data only from children who remained at the end of the study. This contrasts to intention-to-treat analysis, which uses data from all children who were enrolled in a study regardless of whether they remained at the end of the study (see below).

Confidence interval (CI) Gives an indication of the precision of an estimate for example, of treatment effect. The 95% CI is most often reported and indicates the range of results that would be obtained 95% of the time if a study with the same size and design were repeated. This is similar to saying that the true value of an estimate (never exactly known) has a 95% chance of falling within the confidence interval.

Confounder (confounding variable) A variable (or factor) that distorts the true relationship between the study variable of interest and the outcome of interest, because it is also related to that outcome. The process of randomization should ensure equal distribution of confounders amongst study groups and hence minimize distortion of results by confounders.

Consolidated Standards of Reporting of Trials (CONSORT) Evidence based and regularly updated guidelines published by a group of editors of biomedical journals, scientists, epidemiologists and statisticians, to standardize the format for reporting of randomized controlled trials.

Controls In a randomized controlled trial with two or more interventions, controls are children in the comparison (rather than the treatment or intervention) group who are allocated to receive either a placebo, no treatment, or the current best treatment. In a case–control study the control (a member of the comparison group) is someone who does not have the outcome or disease of interest.

Cost-benefit analysis An economic assessment to determine whether the cost of an intervention is worth the benefit by measuring both cost and benefit in the same (usually monetary) units.

Cost-effectiveness analysis An economic analysis in which the effects of treatment (for example, vaccination) are converted into health terms so that the costs of treatment can be described in terms of some additional health gain (for example, prevention of rotavirus infection).

Critically appraised topic (CAT) A short summary of evidence from a one or more publications that address a specific clinical question. This allows people to share the results of critical appraisals. CATs are not systematic literature reviews (examples can be found at www.ped.med.umich.edu/ebm/cat.htm).

Cross sectional study An observational study design that involves surveying a population for an exposure, an outcome, or both at one point in time or over a specified time period. These studies are relatively easy to perform but can only establish association (not causation) and are susceptible to bias (for example, recall bias) and confounding.

Evidence-based child health A useful evidence-based health care resource at www.ich.bpmf.ac.uk/ebm/ebm.htm

Ecological study An observational study that compare summary data for example, disease prevalence between populations at a particular point in time. Bias and confounding cannot be controlled.

Effect size "Effect size" is a measure of effect used for continuous data when different scales are used to measure an outcome (for example, mood). In statistical terms, is defined as the difference in means between the intervention and control groups divided by the SD of the control (or both) group(s). For continuous outcomes (such as pain scores or height) effect size may be expressed as the standardized mean difference or weighted mean difference. However, the term "effect size" is also used generically to describe the *magnitude* of the estimate of therapeutic effect for dichotomous outcomes. In this situation the size of an effect can be expressed as a relative risk or an odds ratio.

Effectiveness A measure of the benefit from an intervention for a given health problem under *usual* practice conditions, i.e., a "real world" clinical setting. This measure takes into consideration compliance and acceptance by the patient as well as the efficacy of an intervention. It is useful for assessing the relative risks-benefits of a treatment.

Efficacy A measure of the benefit from an intervention for a given health problem under *ideal* practice conditions, i.e., in a randomized controlled trial with full patient compliance.

The size of the effect may be greater than in the real world situation.

EMBASE The electronic bibliographic database of *Excerpta Medica* – the European equivalent of MedLine – with a focus on drugs and pharmacology. Covers over 3000 journals from over 100 countries (1974–).

Event The occurrence of a dichotomous outcome that is being sought in a study (such as seizure, death, or an improvement in croup score).

Event rate The proportion of patients in each treatment group in whom an event occurs. May be expressed as control event rate (CER) or experimental event rate (EER).

Evidence-based health care The application of the principles of evidence based medicine is extended to all health-care related activities, including clinical care, purchasing, and management.

Evidence-based medicine (EBM) The conscientious, explicit and judicious use of current best evidence in making decisions about the care of individual patients (after Sackett). The practice of EBM involves integrating clinical expertise (information from history taking, examination) with the best available research evidence and including patients (with their individual preferences and values) in decision making about their health care.

Exclusion criteria Pre-specified criteria that exclude patients from enrolment in a clinical study (even if they meet inclusion criteria).

Follow up Observation of individuals or groups for health-related outcomes over a period of time. In a randomized trial loss of substantial numbers of patients to follow up may bias study results.

Forest plot A diagram representing the results of individual trials included in a meta-analysis and a summary statistic.

Funnel plot A method of plotting the sample size against the effect size of results of individual trials included in a meta-analysis, to investigate whether or not publication bias is likely to have occurred.

Grateful Med Software available through the National Library of Medicine to help non-experts search MedLine. The search can be conducted using author name, title of article, or subject.

Hazard ratio (HR) This is broadly equivalent to relative risk, but is used when the risk is not constant with respect to time. If however, the assumption is made that the risks remain in proportion between population groups in a study then, although the absolute risks (hazards) may alter as time passes, the hazard ratio between groups remains constant. The term is typically used in the context of survival over time and is then broadly equivalent to the relative risk of death. If the HR is 0·5 then the risk of dying in one group is half the risk of dying in the other group.

Heterogeneity In the context of meta-analysis, heterogeneity means dissimilarity between studies. It can be due to differences in reported effects (statistical heterogeneity), in patients, treatments or outcomes (clinical heterogeneity), or in study design (methodological heterogeneity). Heterogeneity may render pooling of data for meta-analysis unreliable or inappropriate. Statistical tests can be used to determine whether the degree of heterogeneity is greater than would be expected by chance.

Homogeneity In the context of meta-analysis, homogeneity means similarity between studies (opposite of heterogeneity).

Inception cohort A group of patients recruited as close as possible to the onset of the target disorder for example, when they developed clinical symptoms. This is the best type of cohort to examine short and long term prognosis (future outcome) of an individual with a particular disease.

Incidence The number of new cases of a condition occurring in a specified population over a specified period of time.

Intention-to-treat analysis Data from all children who were originally enrolled into a randomized controlled trial are analyzed, regardless of whether they remained until the end of the trial, withdrew from the trial, or swapped treatment groups. Intention-to-treat analysis (as opposed to completer analysis) is preferred in RCTs because it mirrors the changes to treatment and non-compliance that may occur in clinical practice. It also minimizes the risk of attrition bias that can influence results if participants are excluded from data analysis.

Kappa statistic A measure of agreement between observers that is beyond the agreement expected based on chance alone. A value of kappa > 0·8 is excellent and kappa <0·4 is poor agreement.

Likelihood ratio (LR) The LR is the ratio of likelihoods for a given test result. The LR for a test indicates the likelihood that a given test result would be expected to occur in a patient with the target disease, compared to the likelihood of that same result in a patient without that disease, i.e., a LR is the ratio of the proportions of patients with and without disease who have a given test result. LRs can help evaluate the usefulness or performance of a diagnostic test and compare it to other tests. The LR of a test with binary results can be calculated from sensitivity and specificity. LR = sensitivity/(1–specificity) for a positive test and LR = (1–sensitivity)/specificity for a negative test. The LR can be used in conjunction with the pretest probability to estimate post-test probability (the chance that a child with a particular diagnostic test result will have a particular diagnosis).

Likelihood ratio nomogram A nomogram that simplifies determination of post-test probability from pretest probability and likelihood ratio, eliminating the need for calculations. (Adapted from Fagan, *N Engl J Med* 1975;**293**:257.)

MedLine A huge database of medical articles, compiled by the United States National Library of Medicine. It indexes millions of articles from over 4000 journals published in over 70 countries and covering clinical medicine, biological sciences, health education, social and information sciences and health-related technology. MedLine is available in printed form (*Index Medicus*), on the Internet or on CD-ROM. Software to access MedLine includes PubMed and OVID (Ovid Technologies).

MeSH headings (Medical Subject Headings) The headings (terms) used by the United States National Library of Medicine to index publications in MedLine. In the MeSH system, broad subject headings branch into a series of progressively narrower headings.

Meta-analysis A statistical technique that uses quantitative methods to summarize in a single estimate the results of several studies included in a systematic review. When using this technique, studies are weighted depending on the variance of the results, the size of the study and the event rate in the study.

Morbidity rate Rate of illness but not death in a specific population.

Mortality rate Rate of death in a specific population.

N-of-1 randomized trials A trial in which the benefit and risks of a treatment are evaluated in an individual patient (a randomized trial in one individual). In such trials, the patient undergoes pairs of treatment periods organized so that one period involves the use of experimental treatment and the other involves the use of an alternate of placebo therapy. The treatments are given in a random order and the patient and the clinician are blinded to the treatment received during each period. The clinician and patient document specific outcomes during the trial. Usually the pair of treatments is given three times in order to convince the participant and clinician that a treatment is either effective, ineffective, or harmful.

Negative predictive value (NPV) The chance of not having a disease given a negative test result.

Number needed to treat (NNT) One measure of treatment effectiveness. NNT is the number of children that you would need to treat with a specific intervention for a given period of time to prevent one additional adverse outcome or achieve one additional beneficial outcome. NNT can be calculated as 1/absolute risk reduction.

Number needed to harm (NNH) One measure of harm from treatment. NNH is the number of people you would need to treat with a specific intervention for a given period of time to cause one additional adverse outcome. NNH can be calculated as 1/absolute risk increase.

Odds The odds of an outcome is the ratio of the number of people with the outcome to the number of people without the outcome.

Odds ratio (OR) OR is one measure of treatment effectiveness. It is the ratio of the odds of an outcome in the experimental or treatment group to the odds of that outcome in the control group. The closer the OR is to one, the smaller the difference in effect between the experimental intervention and the control intervention. If the OR = 1 (or the CI of the OR cross 1) then there is no difference in outcome rate in the treatment and control groups. If the OR is > (or <) 1, then the effects of the treatment are more (or less) than those of the control treatment. Note that the effects being measured may be adverse (for example, death or disability) or beneficial (for example, cure or survival). The OR is analogous to the relative risk (RR) when the events are rare; but as event rates increase, the OR becomes further and further from 1 relative to the RR.

Odds reduction The complement of odds ratio (1–OR), analogous to the relative risk reduction when events are rare.

Overview *see* **systematic review.**

Paired or matched subjects Children receiving different treatments within a study can be "matched" or "paired" to balance potential confounding variables, for example, sex and age. Study results are analyzed and presented as differences between pairs.

P value The probability that an observed difference occurred by chance, if it is assumed that there is in fact no underlying difference between the means of the observations. If this probability is < 1 in 20 (which is when the *P* value is < 0·05, i.e., under the null hypothesis), then the result is conventionally regarded as being "statistically significant".

Placebo A biologically inert treatment (looking, tasting, and given in the same way as the active treatment) that is given to the control group in a randomized, placebo-controlled trial.

Positive predictive value (PPV) The chance of having a disease given a positive test result. The value is strongly influenced by the "prevalence" of that disease in the population under study.

Post-test odds The odds of a patient having a condition once the result of the test for diagnosing that condition is available. Post-test odds = pretest odds × likelihood ratio. Post-test odds can be used to calculate the post-test probability.

Post-test probability The probability of a child having a condition once the result of the diagnostic test is available. This estimate is more useful and meaningful than the pretest probability. Post-test probability can be estimated mathematically. Post-test probability = post-test odds/(post-test odds + 1). When the likelihood ratio is known, post-test probability can be estimated by using the likelihood ratio nomogram.

Power Refers to the ability of a study reliably to detect a clinically important difference (for example, between two treatments) if one actually exists. Statistical power is a function of sample size and should be calculated before the study commences.

Pretest odds The odds of a patient having a condition before the diagnosis is confirmed. Pretest odds = prevalence/(1–prevalence). Pretest odds can be used to calculate post-test odds.

Pretest probability The estimate of the probability of a patient having a condition before the test for diagnosing that condition is performed and/or the result is available, i.e., the prevalence of that disease in the population. Clinicians often derive this estimate from their own clinical experience in their own setting, and there may be wide variation in different settings.

Prevalence The proportion of people with an outcome or a disease in a given population at a given time.

Primary evidence Evidence available from primary (original) studies, including randomized controlled trials, cohort studies, case–control studies, cross-sectional surveys, and case reports (see secondary evidence).

Protocol (Cochrane) A systematic review that is currently being undertaken by members of the Cochrane Collaboration and contains everything but the results. Protocols are listed in the Cochrane Library's Database of Systematic Reviews.

PsycLIT A database of literature, indexed like MedLine, covering the fields of psychology, psychiatry, sociology and related disciplines.

Publication bias may result for a number of reasons. Studies with positive results are more likely to be published than studies with negative results, making it appear from reviews of the published literature that certain treatments are more effective than is truly the case. Other sources of publication bias include duplicate publication, failure to publish completed trials, publication in the non-English language, and publication in journals not listed in MedLine (see Chapter 1).

Randomization A "formal chance" process (equivalent to the flip of a coin) by which children participating in a study are allocated to groups. Using this process, each child has an independent, fixed, and usually equal chance of inclusion in the intervention or comparison group. This process may be facilitated using a table of random numbers or a computer-generated sequence.

Randomized controlled trial (RCT) A trial in which participants are randomly assigned to groups. One group (the experimental or treatment group) receives the intervention being tested, and the other (the comparison or control group) receives an alternative treatment or placebo. This study design for assessment of the relative effects of an intervention is least likely to be subject to bias.

Reference standard (gold standard) diagnostic test The most widely accepted (or established) method, for diagnosing a condition. A "gold standard" provides a benchmark against which a new or proposed screening or diagnostic test can be compared. Although a gold standard usually comprises a single intervention or test, it could also be a period of follow up to observe the evolution of a child's condition, the consensus of an expert panel of clinicians, or a combination of these. In articles about diagnostic tests, the gold standard must be explicitly stated and applied independently in a blinded fashion and regardless of the results of other tests.

Relative risk (RR) (synonyms: risk ratio, or event rate ratio) The ratio of the risk of an event in the treatment group and the control group. If (RR > 1 or RR < 1, then the therapy either increases or decreases the event rate respectively. If the RR = 1 (or the CI of the RR crosses 1), then there is no significant difference between groups.

Relative risk increase (RRI) The proportional increase in risk (event rate) of an adverse outcome between children in experimental and control groups in a trial. (RRI = RR −1).

Relative risk reduction (RRR) The proportional reduction in risk of an adverse event between children in experimental and control groups in a trial. (RRR = 1−RR).

Secondary evidence (evidence syntheses, predigested evidence) Evidence from primary or original studies (see primary evidence) which has been searched out and critically appraised – often using predetermined methodology – and sometimes combined and reanalyzed. Secondary evidence may be presented in systematic reviews, meta-analyses, and literature reviews.

Sensitivity The proportion of children with a disease, who have a positive diagnostic test. Sensitivity should not to be confused with positive predictive value (see above).

Significant By convention "significant" means statistically significant at the 5% level (see statistically significant).

SnNOut When a clinical sign or diagnostic test has a high **S**ensitivity, a **N**egative result rules **Out** the diagnosis.

Specificity The proportion of children without a disease who have a negative diagnostic test. Specificity should not to be confused with negative predictive value (above).

SpPin When a sign or diagnostic test has a high **Sp**ecificity, a **P**ositive result rules **In** the diagnosis.

Standardized mean difference (SMD) A measure of effect size used when outcomes are continuous (such as height, weight, or symptom scores) rather than dichotomous. The mean differences in outcome between the groups being studied are standardized to account for differences in scoring methods (such as pain scores). The measure is a ratio, and therefore has no units.

Statistically significant The findings of a study are unlikely to be due to chance. Significance at the commonly cited 5% level ($P < 0.05$) means that the observed result would occur by chance in only 1 in 20 similar studies. Where the word "significant" or "significance" is used without qualification in the text, it is being used in this statistical sense. A finding that is statistically significant may not be clinically significant or important (see above).

Systematic review A review in which all the primary studies on a topic have been systematically identified, appraised, and summarized according to explicit and reproducible methodology. It can, but need not, involve meta-analysis as a statistical method of combining and numerically summarizing the results of the trials that meet minimum quality criteria. The *Cochrane Library* lists systematic reviews performed by the Cochrane collaboration in the Cochrane Database of Systematic reviews and in the Database of Abstracts of Reviews of Effects lists Systematic Reviews, done by others and deemed to have sound methods (see above).

Toxlit A medical database on toxicology, indexed like MedLine.

Validity The extent to which the results of a study reflect the truth (and are not affected by bias, confounding, or random error). *Internal validity* reflects the study; external validity refers to the extent to which the differences between groups reflect integrity of the study design. ***External validity*** reflects the ability to apply the results to the target (or non-study) population.

Weighted mean difference (WMD) A measure of effect size used when outcomes are continuous (such as symptom scores or height) rather than dichotomous (such as seizure or death). The mean differences in outcome between the groups being studied are weighted to account for different sample sizes and differing precision between studies. The WMD is an absolute figure, and so takes the units of the original outcome measure.

Further reading

- *Clinical Evidence*. London: BMJ Books, 2003.
- Badenoch D, Heneghan C. *Evidence-based toolkit*. London: BMJ Books, 2002.
- Cochrane Reviewer's Handbook. Glossary. Version 4.1.5, December 2003. In: *Cochrance Library* http://www.cochrane.org/resources/handbook/glossary.pdf
- Sackett D, Strauss SE, Richardson WS, Rosenberg W, Haynes B. *Evidence-based medicine. How to practice and teach EBM*. London: Churchill Livingstone 2000.

Compiled by Elizabeth J Elliott and Virginia A Moyer

Abbreviations

A&E	accident and emergency
AABR	automated auditory brainstem response
AACPDM	American Academy of Cerebral Palsy and Developmental Medicine
AAP	American Academy of Pediatrics
ABR	auditory brainstem response
ACOG	American College of Obstetrics and Gynecology
ADH	antidiuretic hormone
ADHD	attention deficit hyperactivity disorder
ADL	activities of daily living
AHRQ	US Agency for Healthcare Research and Quality
ANC	absolute neutrophil count
AOM	acute otitis media
AR	absolute risk
AR	attributable risk
ATNR	asymmetric tonic neck reflex
AVP	arginine vasopressin
BMI	body mass index
BMJ	British Medical Journal
BPD	bronchopulmonary disease
BTX–A	botulinum toxin
CAM	complementary and alternative medicine
CAT	critically appraised topic
CBC	complete blood count
CDC	US Centers for Disease Control and Prevention
CDSR	Cochrane Database of Systematic Reviews
CDSS	computer decision support system
CE	continuing education
CEBMH	Center for Evidence Based Mental Health
CENTRAL	Cochrane Central Registry of Controlled Trials
CER	control group event rate
CFU	colony forming units
CHr	reticulocyte hemoglobin content
CI	confidence interval
CINAHL	Cumulative Index of Nursing and Allied Health
CMR	Cochrane Methodology Register
CNS	central nervous system
CONSORT	consolidated standards of reporting of trials
CP	cerebral palsy
CPP	collaborative perinatal project
CPT	continuous performance tests
CRP	C– reactive protein
CSF	cerebrospinal fluid
CT	computerized tomographic (scan)
CTG	cardiotocograph
CVAS	cosmetic visual analogue scale
DALYs	disability adjusted life years
DARE	Database of Reviews of Effects
dB	decibels
DFA	direct fluorescent assay
DKA	diabetic ketoacidosis
DPNB	dorsal penile nerve block
DSM	Diagnostic and Statistical Manual
DSM–PC	Diagnostic and Statistical Manual for Primary Care
DTO	dilute tincture of opium
DTP	diphtheria–tetanus–pertussis
EBM	evidence-based medicine
EBP	evidence-based pediatrics
ECW	extracellular water
ED	emergency department
EEG	electroencephalogram
EER	experimental group event rate
EHR	electronic health record
ELBW	extremely low birth weight
EMG	electromyogram
EMLA	eutectic mixture of topical anesthetic
EP	erythrocyte protoporphyrin
EpHM	esophageal pH monitoring
EPOC	Effective Practice and Organization of Care (a Cochrane Review Group)
ER	emergency room
ESR	erythrocyte sedimentation rate
ETCO$_2$	end-tidal CO$_2$
FEV1	forced expiratory volume in 1 second
FVC	forced vital capacity
GABA	gamma-aminobutyric acid
GER	gastroesophageal reflux
GERD	gastroesophageal reflux disease
GPR	gastropharyngeal reflux
GRADE	Grades of Recommendations, Assessment, Development and Evaluation
GTT	glucose tolerance test
H2RA	H2 receptor antagonists
Hgb	hemoglobin
HIB	hemophilus influenza type B
HL	hearing loss
HMO	health maintenance organization
HR	hazard ratio
HRQOL	health-related quality of life

IAIMS	integrated advanced information management system
ICC	intraclass reliability
ICU	intensive care unit
IMP	intraesophageal impedance
IPPV	intermittent positive pressure ventilation
IQ	intelligence quotient
IT	information technology
ITB	intrathecal baclofen
i.v.	intravenous
IVF	in-vitro fertilization
LAT	lidocaine-adrenaline-tetracaine
LBW	low birth weight
LESP	lower esophageal sphincter pressure
LGG	lactobacillus GG
LP	lumbar puncture
LR	likelihood ratio
MBPS	modified behavioral pain scale
MCHC	mean corpuscular hemoglobin concentration
MCID	minimum clinically important difference
MCV	mean corpuscular volume
MDI	metered dose inhaler
MDI	mental development index
MEE	middle ear effusion
MeSH	medical subheading
MMR	measles, mumps, rubella
MMWR	Morbidity and Mortality Weekly Report
NAS	neonatal abstinence syndrome
NASS	neonatal abstinence severity score
NBW	normal birth weight
NFCS	neonatal facial coding system
NHP	national health product
NICHD	National Institutes of Child Health and Development (US)
NICU	neonatal intensive care unit
NNH	number needed to harm
NNT	number needed to treat
NPV	negative predictive value
NRT	nicotine replacement therapy
OAE	evoked otoacoustic emission
OB	occult bacteremia
OHSU	Oregon Health Sciences University
OR	odds ratio
ORS	oral rehydration solution
ORT	oral rehydration therapy
PAS	pediatric appendicitis score
PCR	polymerase chain reaction
PEER	patient's expected event rate
PEFR	peak expiratory flow rate
PKU	phenylketonuria
POE	physician order entry
PP	pulsus paradoxus

PPI	proton pump inhibitors
PPV	positive predictive value
PRSP	penicillin-resistant *Streptococcus pneumoniae*
PY	person-years
QALY	quality adjusted life years
QOL	quality of life
RCT	randomized controlled trial
RD	risk difference
RDAI	respiratory distress assessment instrument
RDW	red cell distribution width
RE	racemic epinephrine
ROC	receiver operator characteristic curve
RR	relative risk
RRI	relative risk increase
RRR	relative risk reduction
RSV	respiratory syncytial virus
SASSI	substance abuse subtle screening inventory
SBI	serious bacterial illness
SD	standard deviation
SIADH	syndrome of inappropriate anti-diuretic hormone
SIDS	sudden infant death syndrome
SMD	standard mean difference
SR	sustained release
SR	systematic review
SSEP	steady-state evoked potential
STNR	symmetric tonic neck reflex
SWC	standard wound closure
TA	tissue adhesives
TAC	tetracaine–adrenaline–cocaine
TCA	tricyclic antidepressants
TCM	traditional Chinese medicine
TIBC	total iron binding capacity
TSB	total serum bilirubin
URTI	upper respiratory tract infection
USPSTF	US Preventive Services Task Force
USTFCPS	US Task Force on Community Preventive Services
UTI	urinary tract infection
VAS	visual analogue scales
VLBW	very low birth weight
VUR	vesicoureteral reflux
WBC	white blood cell count
WES	wound evaluation score
WHO	World Health Organization
WMD	weighted mean difference
YIOS	Young Infant Observation Scale
YOS	Yale Observation Scale
ZPP	zinc protoporphyrin

This book is dedicated to our spouses and children,
and to the health of children everywhere

Section I

Finding, evaluating
and applying the evidence

1 Introduction: what is evidence?

Virginia A Moyer, Elizabeth J Elliott

Case scenario

While in town for an investment banking conference, your dearest friend from university days drops by to take you to lunch. Waiting in your office, your friend notices a book on your desk about evidence-based pediatrics and says to you, "Just what is evidence-based pediatrics?" You reply that this is a new approach in medicine that involves finding and using the best evidence available in the management of patients. Your friend is taken aback and says, "But isn't that what doctors have always done?" You contemplate how to answer.

What is EBM and haven't we always used it?

This book is one of a series of specialist books emphasizing the application of evidence to different fields of medicine. Evidence-based medicine is defined as the conscientious, explicit, and judicious use of current best evidence in making decisions about the care of individual patients. It involves integrating clinical expertise with the best available external evidence from systematic research, and incorporating this into clinical decision-making, taking into account patients' predicaments, rights, and preferences about their care.

Upon hearing this definition in a lecture, it is not uncommon for a physician in the audience to protest, "What's new about this? I have always incorporated the best evidence into my practice!" But the information we have suggests that we, as a profession, are failing to practise evidence-based medicine. There are wide variations in care that are not related to differences in populations; physician knowledge deteriorates over time; clinicians fail to seek information even when it is needed; and our usual sources of information are often outdated.

If physicians were routinely applying the best available evidence to clinical decisions, then care should be relatively similar in similar populations of patients. Empirical evidence says that this is not the case. Care varies dramatically from one locale or institution to another. Among the 14 centers of the NICHD Neonatal Research Network, the proportion of small premature infants who received indomethacin early to close the ductus arteriosus varied from 0% to 95%. The use of steroids for chronic lung disease varied from 5% to 49%.[1] Among contiguous areas in the central USA in 1995–99, the use of pneumococcal vaccine for older people varied threefold and the use of colorectal cancer screening varied fourfold.[2]

While some variation in care is undoubtedly due to uncertainty about the value of specific interventions, huge variation in the use of proven interventions is a clear demonstration that some patients do not receive evidence-based care.

Routine application of the best evidence requires firstly that physicians are aware of the best evidence. Thus, physicians must keep up with new information and changes in practice. In a study of the management of hypertension diagnosed in the workplace, some patients who were referred to their primary care practitioners for care did not receive appropriate antihypertensive treatment.[3] The most important determinant of treatment was the patient's age and the second most important determinant was the diastolic blood pressure. The fourth most important determinant was the presence of end-organ damage. The third most important determinant was not the patient's gender, insurance coverage, race, or even systolic blood pressure. It was the year the physician graduated from medical school. Clearly, we don't keep up as well as we should and this gets harder as we get older.

In addition to keeping up with what's new, incorporating best evidence into practice requires that the physician recognizes when he or she needs information. General practitioners in one study were asked how often they needed new information and where they went to get it.[4] They said that they needed information about twice a week, and obtained it from textbooks and journals. However, when the same physicians were shadowed in practice, they were found to need information up to 60 times per week. Most of the time they did not find the information they needed and when they did, they got it from colleagues. As a profession, we don't always recognize when we need information, let alone acknowledge gaps in our knowledge.

Until the latter part of the 20th century, the pace of medical discoveries was slow enough that scientists could keep up without too much effort. Much research shed light on physiologic processes, and physicians then used pathophysiologic reasoning, clinical experience, and intuition to apply the new knowledge to patient care. It was not until the last part of the century that evidence accumulated to show that using pathophysiologic reasoning to make clinical decisions could lead to disastrous results. At this time clinical research – systematic studies in human subjects – became more prominent. Now, clinical studies are accumulating so fast that no one can keep up with them even in relatively narrow subspecialties – let alone in broad fields such as pediatrics. The rapid pace of research means that textbooks are often out of date by the time they are published, and we need to rely on more current sources of information to make clinical decisions.

As a result, we are not consistently incorporating the best available evidence into our clinical decisions. Five steps typify the practice of evidence-based medicine (see Box). The first is the most critical – to recognize that we need information to address clinical problems, most commonly relating to the therapy, diagnosis, prognosis, and etiology of disease. Once an information need is recognized, a well-structured clinical question can be formulated, and that question can be used to search for information in an organized way. Since all information is not created equal, the next step is to critically appraise any information found to determine whether it is valid and applicable to the patient at hand. If so, it can be applied to the individual patient. In the case of a therapy, for example, its application must take into account the patient's baseline risk for certain outcomes and how he or she values the potential risks and benefits of the therapy. The final step is to evaluate how well we are doing with respect to current best practice and to find ways to improve our practice.

Steps in the practice of evidence-based pediatrics and child health

1. Identify information needs and structure clinical questions
2. Search for relevant information from literature
3. Evaluate the evidence found (critical appraisal) or identify lack of evidence
4. Apply the evidence to your patients
5. Evaluate your practice

The first step to embracing evidence-based medicine requires a change in attitude and awareness for most physicians. Having passed their exams, many may feel that they have "arrived" and no longer need to devote so much time and energy to learning. However, the pace of change in medicine means that rather than learn a set of basic facts in medical school, we must instead learn a framework on which to hang information. We must then learn how to keep on learning for the rest of our lives. The pace of change in information science has been just as fast (or faster) than the pace of change in other fields. The result is that, while practising evidence-based medicine really was not possible just a decade or two ago, we now have access to resources (for example, synthesized evidence) and the means to get at the resources (for example, computerized databases such as the *Cochrane Library*). The skills needed to practise evidence-based medicine are increasingly taught in medical schools. For those who graduated without these skills, courses and books (such as this one) offer an opportunity to catch up. The entire first section of this book is devoted to the steps of evidence-based medicine, from asking questions (Chapter 2) to putting it all together (Chapter 17).

What is evidence?

Simply citing the literature that supports a plan of action does not equate to practising evidence-based medicine. Practising evidence-based medicine involves being aware of the *best* evidence currently available that bears on the *specific problem* at hand. The best evidence is the evidence most likely to provide an unbiased view of the truth. Of course, we can never know the truth, but we can try to come as close as possible by performing and using well-designed and well executed studies. A hierarchy of evidence for decisions about interventions in medicine has been proposed by Guyatt *et al.*[5] with n-of-1 trials and syntheses of all relevant randomized trials on top and physiologic studies and unsystematic clinical observations at the bottom (see Box).

Hierarchy of evidence

- N-of-1 randomized controlled trial
- Systematic review of randomized trials
- Single randomized trial
- Systematic review of observational studies
- Single observational studies (cohort or case–control studies)
- Physiologic studies and physiologic reasoning
- Unsystematic clinical observations (case series, case reports, personal observations)

Adapted from *Users' Guides to the Medical Literature*, AMA Press, 2002.

N-of-1 trials entail studying the risks and benefits of a proposed therapy in the patient in whom it is to be used, in a randomized and blinded fashion. N-of-1 trials are not always possible. For example, they can only work when the intervention has temporary effects and the outcome is reversible. A classic example of the value of n-of-1 randomized, blinded trials of medication in pediatrics is for testing the effect of stimulant medications in children with ADHD.[6] N-of-1 trials may be particularly useful for studying therapy in children with rare diseases when there are insufficient children for a trial. When these trials are not possible, groups of patients must be studied. In that case, the study design least subject to bias is the randomized controlled trial. However, any one trial represents what happens with just a sample of the universe of potential subjects, and the answer might be wrong just by chance. If more than one trial has been done, the power and precision of the result can be increased if all of the available trials can be put together in a meta-analysis. Observational studies are subject to selection biases that are avoided in randomized trials, but high quality observational studies still may provide helpful evidence when RCTs are not available or are not of good quality. At the bottom of the list are methods that clearly are subject to the biases of the individual and the limitations of their knowledge (for pathophysiologic reasoning) or their experience (for unsystematic clinical observations).

Sometimes the only evidence available is of low quality. This is not an excuse to throw up one's hands in despair and declare that it is not possible to practice evidence-based medicine. One can always use *current best* evidence, even when the best is not very good. It is also important to remember that lack of evidence of effect is not equivalent to evidence of lack of effect. Recognition of the lack of evidence should be, for both physicians and patients, a strong motivator to participate in high quality research to address the deficit.

The practice of evidence-based care has been facilitated by several recent developments. Clinical epidemiologists have developed strategies to track down and assess evidence reasonably efficiently, and they have also developed ways to teach these skills to clinicians and medical students. Systematic reviews and evidence summaries are increasingly available and of high quality. Clinicians owe a great debt of gratitude to institutions and individuals who have advanced these resources. The Cochrane Collaboration in particular has been at the heart of advances in developing methods for, and producing, systematic evidence summaries.

However, the key development has been the creation of powerful information systems that can store huge amounts of information and that allow its efficient retrieval. As these systems evolve (which they seem to do every day!), they will provide evidence when and where it is needed – whether at the bedside or in the consulting room. In addition to research evidence, practitioners need a wide variety of patient-related information (history, physical exam, laboratory results) in order to make clinical decisions. If evidence from the medical literature can be provided at the same time that clinical decisions are being made, it has a fighting chance of getting used. This kind of decision support is further discussed in Chapter 15 on Informatics.

Limitations of evidence

The amount of biomedical information that is available is truly astonishing. In December 2003 the MedLine database alone contained over 14 million citations dating back about a half a century – but estimated at only about a third of the world's biomedical literature. However, much of what is available is not easily accessible, is not clinically relevant, is of poor quality, or does not pass the "so what" test when it comes to application to patient care. In contrast, the information that we need to solve a specific problem is far too often not available or hard to find. In some fields, such as pediatric oncology, the evidence is changing so rapidly that by the time questions are answered and the data are published, they are no longer relevant. Even when it is available, questions have also been raised about the quality of evidence. Some studies are never published, some studies are designed to obtain a particular result, and in a few instances, results may even be falsified.

Finding information to answer specific questions sometimes feels like looking for a needle in a haystack. The authors of one review estimate that searches by clinicians generally retrieve only a quarter to half of the relevant articles on a given topic[7] and even highly skilled librarians miss 30% or more of the relevant articles.[8] Haynes and colleagues developed and tested search strategies to improve the yield of MedLine searches on clinical topics.[9] Use of these "methodologic hedges" dramatically improves the relevance of the articles retrieved, and these terms are incorporated into PubMed in the Clinical Queries screen (see Chapter 3 on searching for more detail). These strategies can be used in other databases, but have not been specifically tested. Information that is not in MedLine may be even harder to find, and may be systematically different from the information that is more readily available.

Publication bias may arise in a number of ways. Studies published in languages other than English, or in journals that are not indexed in MedLine, may have systematically different results than their counterparts in English and in MedLine. Egger *et al.* reviewed published meta-analyses and found that non-English language trials and non-indexed trials tended to show larger treatment effects.[10] Vickers *et al.* found that studies of acupuncture from certain countries uniformly reported positive results.[11]

Substantial numbers of studies that are completed are never published. If the unpublished studies differ systematically from those that are published, then review of the literature will yield a result that is systematically different from the truth. Ten years after approval by an institutional review board, only about two-thirds of studies had been published, and results were more likely be statistically significant among the published studies.[12] Studies with significant positive results are also published more quickly than those with negative results – nearly twice as fast, according to another 10-year follow up study. Studies with indeterminate results were even less likely to be published.[13] A more worrying type of publication bias occurs when study results are intentionally suppressed. Manufacturers may attempt to suppress publication of adverse information about their products, and industry sponsors may require researchers to ask permission prior to publishing results of their studies. As a result, industry-sponsored research systematically favors the products of the sponsor.[14]

Finally, publication bias can result from *overpublication* of certain results. The results of some trials have been published as many as five times, often in such a way that it is difficult for a reader to determine that these studies are duplicate reports.[15] The resulting multiple counting of the same data (nearly always data supporting the use of a specific pharmaceutical agent) biases the literature (and any systematic literature review) in favor of the drug. The implications of these different types of publication bias for systematic reviews is tremendous. Reviews run the risk of excluding unpublished, not yet published, negative, or indeterminate results, and of being biased by duplicate publication of favorable results. Although this systematic bias has not been demonstrated for every area of medicine, this remains a vexing problem for both readers of the literature and those who perform systematic reviews.

In addition to the problem of publication bias, bias may also occur within studies. Studies may be intentionally designed to show that one treatment is superior to another. This can be done by choosing an inappropriate comparator (such as an inadequate doses of the comparator drug) or by choosing a comparator that is known to be ineffective.[15] Selection of which data to present when publishing study results may also result in bias. A recent study of discrepancies between study protocols and publications revealed that in the publications of over 80% of trials, authors either omitted planned outcomes or introduced new outcomes (the analysis of which had not been planned in the original protocol). In over 50% of the trials studied, at least one primary outcome was changed between protocol and publication.[16] This source of bias is impossible to detect at the publication stage.

A commonly cited barrier to practising evidence-based medicine is the perception that evidence simply doesn't exist for much of what we do in medicine, and especially in pediatrics. In 1978, the United States Office of Technology Assessment stated (based on no particular evidence) that "only 10–20% of all procedures currently used in medical practice have been shown to be efficacious by controlled trial."[17] In 1991, the editor of the *BMJ* repeated the claim that little of what we do in medicine is based on evidence.[18] However, this all depends on how you look at this issue. Ellis *et al.* reported in 1995 that 82% of primary treatments in a general medical ward were based on good quality evidence.[19] Using his methodology, about the same proportion of

treatments in general pediatric inpatient wards in the USA and Australia were based on good evidence.[20] For other populations, the rates are between 29% and 96%. However, these studies evaluated only the primary intervention for the primary diagnosis for consecutively admitted patients. For some settings, such as neonatal intensive care units, only a few primary diagnoses apply to the vast majority of patients, so that if evidence is available for these diagnoses, the proportion of treatments based on good evidence will be very high. Other studies have evaluated interventions in outpatient settings, or have attempted to catalog "all interventions" rather than just the primary intervention for the primary diagnosis. Among 1149 clinical actions that took place during 247 outpatient pediatric consultations, Rudolph *et al.* found that just under 50% of actions were supported by good quality evidence.[21] Although the situation is not as dismal as stated by the OTA, lack of evidence remains a problem. Certainly, no evidence is available to support many of the actions that we take in clinical care (not only interventions, but also diagnostic tests) or to answer questions about prognosis or etiology.

It takes time to develop high quality evidence, and more time to get it to publication. Studies published today report on questions that were conceived several years ago. However, many areas of pediatric practice are fairly stable – new treatments are not evolving every day, and the questions that were relevant 10 years ago remain relevant today. Frequently, outcomes are immediate (response to bronchodilators or antibiotics for example), and many conditions are common (asthma is a good example). For these illnesses, studies published today are likely to reflect current treatment options. However, for rapidly evolving fields, and for outcomes that require longer follow up, what is published today may already be out of date. Pediatric oncology provides an excellent example. Studies published today report treatments from 5–10 years ago, and better treatments are likely already to be under study. In these cases, patients should not be treated according to the results of published trials, but as *participants* in randomized trials that will become the published literature of the future.[22]

Addressing the limitations of evidence

Individual practitioners have an opportunity to address the limitations raised above. We must become "more rather than less attentive in the face of information overload".[23] Awareness of what constitutes high quality information allows us to bypass most of what is published and to use our limited reading time wisely. The first section of this book is intended to teach the necessary skills to assess the quality of evidence. The clinical chapters are intended to provide examples of how evidence-based medicine can be efficiently practised in a wide variety of ways under different circumstances. The rapid development of easily accessible sources of high quality synthesized information provides us with a magnet with which to seek the needle from the haystack.

The shortage of evidence means that we are often obliged to make decisions about patient care with less than optimal evidence. Each time we choose an option in the absence of evidence, we end up, like it or not, experimenting on our patients. Unfortunately, since we generally do not systematically collect data on the outcome of these experiments, and since these experiments are generally unplanned, we are not able to learn from them to benefit the next generation of patients. If we, as a medical community, genuinely do not know which of two options to choose, or evidence does not exist to answer our patients' pressing questions about prognosis or etiology, then we have a clear obligation to help ameliorate that situation. We should all be participating in high quality research at every opportunity and should encourage our patients to do so as well.

We can also demand accountability from the research community. A strong case can be made that all controlled trials should be registered before they begin, so that the results from unpublished trials can be sought by reviewers as they synthesize evidence. Failure to publish the results of a trial means that the patients who participated in the trial were subjected to whatever risks the trial might have entailed (as great as the risk of mortality or as small as the inconvenience of data collection) with no compensatory benefit to future patients. As consumers of research, we can demand that research be conducted and reported with the highest level of integrity.

These limitations of evidence should not be taken as reasons for nihilism. Evidence-based medicine is the application of the *current best* evidence to the care of individual patients. The alternative is to practice without the knowledge of that evidence, however flawed it may be, and thus to base practice on flawed memory, faith, and unsystematic personal experience. We owe it to our patients to do our best, recognizing the problems with the current state of the evidence, and taking responsibility for addressing these problems. We must judge the state of a body of evidence (including studies of different types) in order to quantify our degree of certainty or uncertainty in out clinical decisions. Then, we can be honest with ourselves and our patients about what we know, and genuinely practise evidence-based medicine.

Resolution of the scenario

You explain to your friend that only in the last half-century has medicine had much beyond supportive care to offer patients. Doctors in the past could depend on the knowledge they gained during their training, and could keep up by consulting with colleagues and reading the few available journals in their own specialties. You remind your friend that the explosion in biomedical knowledge has made keeping up to date a near impossible task for any one person. However, as new technology has developed to make information more and more accessible, it is again becoming possible to bring the current best evidence to bear on clinical decisions. Your friend admits to having taken advantage of technology to look up health questions on the internet and wonders about the quality of that information. Always thinking, your friend wonders out loud about investing in software to help doctors obtain and integrate evidence at the point of care.

References

1 Unpublished data. NICHD Neonatal Research Network, Generic Data Base Summary Tables, August 2003, Research Triangle Institute.

2 Dartmouth Atlas of Health Care, http://www.dartmouthatlas.org/

3 Sackett DL, Haynes RB, Gibson ES, Taylor DW, Roberts RS, Johnson AL. Hypertension control, compliance, and science. *Am Heart J* 1977;**94**:666–7.

4 Covell DG, Uman GC, Manning PR. Information needs in office practice: are they being met? *Ann Intern Med* 1985;**103**:596–9.

5 Guyatt G, Haynes B, Jaeschke R, *et al.* Introduction: The philosophy of evidence-based medicine. Chapter 1A in: Guyatt G, Rennie D, eds. User's Guide to the Medical Literature: A manual for evidence-based practice. AMA Press 2002. p7.

6 Kent MA, Camfield CS, Camfield PR. Double-blind methylphenidate trials: practical, useful, and highly endorsed by families. *Arch Pediatr Adolesc Med* 1999;**153**:1292–6.

7 Hersh WR, Hickam DH. How well to physicians use electronic information retrieval systems? A framework for investigation and systematic review. *JAMA* 1998;**280**:1347–52.

8 McKibbon KA, Walker-Dilks CJ. The quality and impact of MEDLINE searches performed by end users. *Hlth Libr Rev* 1995;**12**:191–200.

9 Haynes RB, Wilczynski N, McKibbon KA, Walker CJ, Sinclair JC. Developing optimal search strategies for detecting clinically sound studies in MEDLINE. *J Am Med Inform Assoc* 1994;**1**:447–58.

10 Egger M, Juni P, Bartlett C, Holenstein F, Sterne J. How important are comprehensive literature searches and the assessment of trial quality in systematic reviews? Empiric study. *Hlth Technol Assess* 2003;**7**.

11 Vickers A, Goyal N, Harland R, Rees R. Do certain countries produce only positive results? A systematic review of controlled trials. *Control Clin Trials* 1998;**19**:159–66.

12 Dickersin K, Min YI, Meinert C:. Factors influencing publication of research results. Follow up of applications

submitted to two institutional review boards. *JAMA* 1992; **267**:374–8.

13 Stern JM, Simes RJ. Publication bias: evidence of delayed publication in a cohort study of clinical research projects. *BMJ* 1997;**315**:640–5.

14 Lexchin J, Bero LA, Djulbegovic B, Clark O. Pharmaceutical industry sponsorship and research outcome and quality: systematic review. *BMJ* 2003;**326**:1167.

15 Rennie D. Fair conduct and fair reporting of clinical trials. *JAMA* 1999;**282**:1766–8.

16 Chan A-W, Altman D. Discrepancies between protocols and publications: evidence of outcome reporting bias in randomized trials. XI *Cochrane Colloquium Abstract* O-13, 2003.

17 Office of Technology Assessment of the Congress of the United States. *Assessing the efficacy and safety of medical technologies.* Washington, DC: US Government Printing Office, 1978.

18 Smith R. Where is the wisdom…? *BMJ* 1991;**303**:798–9.

19 Ellis J, Mulligan E, Rowe J, Sackett DL. Inpatient general medicine is evidence-based. *Lancet* 1995;**346**:407–10.

20 Moyer VA, Gist AK, Elliott EJ. Is the practice of paediatric inpatient medicine evidence-based? *J Paediatr Child Hlth* 2002;**38**:347–51.

21 Rudolf MC, Lyth N, Bundle A *et al.* A search for the evidence supporting community paediatric practice. *Arch Dis Child* 1999;**80**:257–61.

22 Cole CH. Randomized controlled clinical trials. *J Paediatr Child Hlth* 2003;**39**:161.

23 Silverman WA. The glut of information. In: Silverman WA. *Where's the evidence: Debates in modern medicine.* Oxford: Oxford University Press, 1998.

2 Asking questions

Stuart Logan, Ruth Gilbert

Case scenario	*In the middle of the night you are called to see a screaming, febrile 3-year-old child with ear pain. A number of questions arise. The medical student asks how likely is acute otitis media (middle ear infection) in this situation and what organisms are associated with this diagnosis? He also asks how you will confirm the diagnosis and whether or not you will prescribe antibiotics. You explain what outcomes might be achieved by treating the child with antibiotics (reduce pain, control fever, prevent complications, or reduce parental anxiety) and the potential harms (diarrhea, vomiting, allergic reactions, drug resistance.) Your medical student then asks why young children are susceptible to otitis media and what are the likely complications of this infection.*

The aim of evidence-based practice is to integrate clinical experience with the best available research evidence in order to make the best decisions, together with your patients. Most of the time, clinicians do this unsystematically, intuitively combining information from history, examination, and prior knowledge, and weighing up the chances of a good or bad outcome. At the heart of evidence-based practice is the belief that basing decisions on a more explicit use of the available evidence achieves better outcomes for patients.

Asking questions is the driving force for evidence-based practice. Clinicians often don't recognize the need to ask questions, particularly about procedures or interventions that are common practice. In one study, clinicians reported that they needed new clinically relevant information once or twice a week and that this was available from textbooks or journals. However, "shadowing" and direct questioning of these same clinicians in their clinical workplace identified that two questions, primarily about therapy, arose for every three patients they saw.[1]

The aim of this chapter is to help you to take the first step in evidence-based practice – identifying information needs and formulating answerable questions. This will help you decide what evidence you need to help you and your patient reach a decision about management. Framing questions will also help you to identify the type of study most likely to provide a valid answer to your question. Identifying the study type will help guide you to the best source of information.

Types of information

In clinical practice you need a range of different types of information to answer different questions. For example medical students and junior doctors frequently need *background information*, which tells about a condition or situation, but does not directly inform clinical practice. These questions are frequently in the form of "What is...?" For example, "What is otitis media?" or "What organisms are associated with otitis media?" This type of information is usually answered by recourse to a review article, textbook, or colleague. In contrast, practising clinicians most frequently ask questions related directly to patient care. These *foreground questions* include questions of therapy (the most common), diagnosis, prognosis, and harm. Foreground questions are most easily answered if they are structured and if the question type is clearly identified.

Anatomy of a foreground question

Most clinical questions can be structured in three or four parts, according to the mnemonic PICO (population, intervention, comparison, outcome).

- *Patient population.* This describes a patient or population who has similar attributes to your patient.
- *Intervention* (or *exposure*). This describes what happens or is done to that population. It might be an intervention (for example, giving antibiotics) or an exposure (for example, passive smoking).

- *Comparison.* If you want to know the effect of a treatment or exposure, you need to define a comparison group who experience a different intervention/exposure or no intervention/exposure.
- *Outcomes.* This refers to the outcomes, for example morbidity, mortality, quality of life, cost, that are likely to be most important to patients, policy-makers, service providers, or clinicians.

As a general rule, it is helpful to make sure that the parts of the question reflect a chronological sequence of events in practice.

Why structure questions?

Structuring questions helps you to find and use the best evidence to inform your clinical decisions. It forces you to think more clearly about each of the components of the question.

Patient population

It is important to define the patient population. Although the patient who prompted your question is unique, you can predict what might happen to him or her by inference from studies in populations of similar patients. When evaluating evidence, you have to decide whether the patients reported would be sufficiently similar to yours that you would be able to apply the results to your patient – or so dissimilar that the results are not applicable. The broader the population that you are prepared to consider, the more likely you are to find evidence in the literature. How you limit the populations that you are prepared to consider involves a biological or sociological judgement. This may be informed by analyses of outcomes in subgroups of patients.

Intervention/exposure

In any clinical situation there are usually many treatment options. A general literature search for treatment of otitis media will not answer your specific question and is likely to yield an unmanageable number of references. Therefore, any question about therapy should specifically define the intervention. It should also define the comparison that you are considering, whether it be an alternative therapy or no therapy. For example, if the question is about acute otitis media, the therapy options might include antibiotics, scheduled antipyretics, or both. The comparisons might include reassurance of the parents without giving any medication. For each comparison, a separate question must be formulated.

Outcomes

The process of framing questions requires that you decide which outcomes are important. This depends on the perspective and values of both the decision-maker and the patient. For example, when considering the decision about whether to treat acute otitis media, clinicians from developing countries may argue that the most important outcome is mastoiditis. This is a more common and serious complication in the children whom they see than in children from developed communities. Parents may be concerned about pain or adverse effects of antibiotics, whereas a public health physician or policy-maker may be most concerned about the costs of antibiotics and the risk of antibiotic resistance.

Question type and study design

Having structured your question, you need to identify what type of question it is: it may be about an intervention, diagnostic test accuracy, baseline risk (prevalence), prognosis, or harm. The type of question that you ask will determine the study design most likely to yield valid results. Intervention questions most often refer to therapies, but also may refer to diagnostic tests (when the issue at hand is whether or not the patient will benefit), or preventive interventions.

Structuring questions helps you decide on the most valid study design to answer your question (see Table 2.1). For example, intervention questions are best answered by randomized controlled trials (RCTs) or systematic reviews of RCTs (see Chapter 6). Questions of diagnostic accuracy are best answered by studies comparing the test to a reference standard (see Chapter 5). Questions about prognosis are best answered by cohort studies (see Chapter 4), and questions about harm or etiology may be answered by a variety of study designs (see Chapter 7). Systematic reviews of the literature are most commonly reviews of RCTs, however, systematic reviews can be performed for any of these study types (see Chapter 8).

Searching the literature

Structuring your question has made you think about the search terms needed to search the literature efficiently. As a general rule, the most useful terms to start searching define the population, the intervention or exposure, and the most valid and appropriate study design. In considering the treatment of acute otitis media for example, you could start by selecting studies relating to children, otitis media, and antibiotics and go to the *Cochrane Library* to look for a systematic review (see Chapter 3).

Table 2.1   Question type and study design

Question type	Study design likely to lead to least biased answer	Comments
Therapy/Intervention	Randomized, blinded trial	Systematic review of RCTs is ideal if of good quality
Accuracy of a diagnostic test	Independent, blind comparison to a gold standard	Usually cross-sectional or cohort design
Prognosis	Cohort study	May be prospective or historical
Harm/etiology	RCT, concurrent cohort study, case-control study	Design will be determined by nature of exposure and frequency of outcome
Baseline risk	Cohort or cross-sectional design	

Some examples of different question types are shown below.

Constructing questions

Interventions

The majority of clinical questions relate to therapeutic interventions.[2] Other types of interventions are preventive interventions and diagnostic tests, when the outcome of interest is benefit or harm to patients. Intervention questions require all four elements: population, intervention, comparison, outcome. In the otitis media example, one question of therapy might be:

Question

1. In young children with otitis media (*population*), does treatment with antibiotic and analgesics (*intervention*) rather than analgesics alone (*comparison*) result in more rapid resolution of pain (*outcome*)? **[Therapy]**

A similar question is addressed in Chapter 33.

Baseline risk

Questions of baseline risk (or prevalence) may only have two elements, namely population and outcome. In the otitis media example, one question of baseline risk might be:

Question

2. In preschool age children with fever (*population*), what is the probability of a diagnosis of otitis media (*outcome*)? **[Baseline Risk]**

A similar question is addressed in Chapter 33.

Diagnostic accuracy

Questions of diagnostic accuracy usually have three components: the patient population, the test (*exposure*) and the outcome, which is the accuracy of the diagnostic test. In the otitis media example, one question of diagnosis might be:

Question

3. In children with suspected otitis media (*population*), will a red tympanic membrane (*exposure*) help accurately diagnose otitis media (*outcome*)? **[Diagnosis]**

A similar question is addressed in Chapter 33.

With questions of baseline risk and diagnostic accuracy, the chronology rule does not always apply, because you may be asking about an "outcome" that has already occurred. In both examples above, the child already has the outcome, although it has not yet been identified.

Prognosis

Patients and parents often ask about the outcome of their condition. Questions of prognosis usually include only a population and an outcome. The description of the population includes both the patient and the exposure. In the otitis media example, one question of prognosis might be:

Question

4. In children with the first episode of otitis media (*population*), what is the likelihood of recurrent episodes (*outcome*)? **[Prognosis]**

Harm or causation

Questions of harm involve a population, an exposure, and an outcome. The comparison is generally lack of exposure and is usually unstated. In the otitis media example, one question of harm might be:

Question
5. In patients with otitis media (*population*) treated with antibiotics (*exposure*), what is the likelihood of recurrence with a resistant organism (*outcome*)? **[Harm or Causation]**

Conclusions

Careful formulation of your questions is the essential first step in the practice of evidence-based medicine. It will make the subsequent steps to clinical problem solving (searching, critical appraisal, and decision-making) more efficient. It may also illuminate the gaps in the available research evidence and help to set a relevant research agenda.

A wide range of questions arise in clinical practice, including background and foreground questions. Many clinical situations entail more than one type of question, as illustrated by the clinical scenario on otitis media. Furthermore, some questions cannot be easily answered because of lack of direct evidence. In this situation, modeling using a series of related questions may be the best available option (see Chapter 17).

Take home list

- The first step in evidence-based practice is asking a question.
- Questions may address foreground or background issues.
- Foreground questions include questions about therapy, harm or causation, diagnostic accuracy, baseline risk or prognosis.
- The type of foreground question will define the most appropriate study design.
- Most clinical questions can be structured into parts including patient population, intervention or exposure, comparison and outcome.
- Structuring a question helps you to think about specific options for intervention (and comparisons), important outcomes (to you, your patient, and society), and whether the evidence can be generalized to your patient.

References

1 Covell DC, Uman GC, Manning PR. Information needs in office practice: are they being met? *Ann Intern Med* 1985; **103**:596–9.
2 Smith R. What clinical information do doctors need? *BMJ* 1996;**313**:1062–8.

3 Finding the evidence

Virginia A Moyer, Connie Schardt

Case scenario	*A 9-year-old boy presents to your office with a 24-hour history of intermittent vomiting without diarrhea. He has also been refusing to drink much because of a sore throat. On examination, he has a markedly inflamed throat with exudates on his tonsils and enlarged cervical lymph nodes. He is actually having difficulty swallowing when you see him. You consider whether you should treat him empirically with antibiotics while you wait for his throat culture to come back, and you also wonder whether a dose of dexamethasone would help relieve his distress. Later in the day, you see a 15-month-old girl whom you know well because of her frequent bouts of otitis media. Today, she is in for a check-up, feeling fine. However, on examination you note that both of her tympanic membranes are bulging but without erythema. She has otitis media with effusion, no doubt a late effect of her most recent acute otitis media. Her mother wonders whether she should take steroids to help clear the fluid from her ears.*

The previous chapter discussed the first step of the evidence-based medicine process, that of recognizing your information needs and developing the well-structured questions that help to clarify the specific information you need. The goal of this chapter is to help with the second step in the evidence-based medicine process: that of finding information. This will provide you with the skills needed to search efficiently and effectively for the information needed. As clinicians, we are faced with a problem: in spite of knowing that we need information, and in spite of knowing that an unbelievable amount of information is out there (around 2 million new research articles are added to the world's literature every year[1]), it often seems inordinately difficult to get at the information we need, when we need it. Fortunately, this once-daunting task is becoming more feasible as new evidence-based information resources and information technology become more widely available in clinical settings. Recent curriculum changes in many medical schools emphasize a problem-based approach and self-directed learning, so that medical students are now taught how to access the evidence. This chapter will review how practising pediatricians can find current best evidence for the care of children, to solve individual patient problems when they arise, to help formulate policy, and to keep up with new evidence that has become available for application to clinical practice. In each of the clinical chapters of this book, the authors demonstrate the search strategy that they used to find valid and clinically useful information to answer the questions from clinical scenarios. The editors did not dictate the search engine or the strategies that authors were to use when searching, so you will see many different approaches, especially different approaches to searching MedLine. Most chapters start with a general search for evidence, seeking high quality systematic evidence reviews ("evidence syntheses"). Then, for each specific question, the actual search that led to the articles under discussion is shown.

We need and seek information for several reasons. We seek information to answer questions about specific patients – to decide what diagnostic test to use, what treatment to choose, and what the expected outcome might be. Another reason for seeking information is to develop comprehensive knowledge of an area, an approach most often used by researchers and specialists. Some of the time, we are simply trying to keep up with what is going on in pediatrics or in medicine in general, and most of us enjoy just browsing through journals that come in the mail. The patients whom you see and the problems encountered on a daily basis provide the best stimulus to staying current. Patients and their parents may present you with information from the media, from friends, or from their search of the internet, or they may ask questions that you want to research before answering. In fact, as information is more and more available to our patients directly, our role as physicians is expanding from simply being the source of information to being the locator and interpreter of information for our patients.[2] Depending on the type of setting in which you work, your colleagues, teachers, and students may also ask questions or provide suggestions that make you realize that your knowledge has become "time-challenged" and you need to revise or update it. A growing array of specialized information resources is available to respond to such challenges. Aided by information technology, you can have access to these at your fingertips, almost anywhere in the world.

The types of questions that are suggested by the scenario in this chapter illustrate common information needs of pediatricians. Being able to find the best evidence to answer clinical questions appropriately and efficiently is all the more important these days. With increasing demands for financial and legal accountability, evidence-based treatment may be more expensive, less expensive, or not much different from current care, but whichever it is, it must be justified.

Where to search

Where can you find the information needed to address the questions raised in clinical practice? The optimal medical information resource depends, to a large extent, on the type of question that you have asked and the time that you are reasonably able to devote to finding the answer. Are you looking for general information about a disease or condition, or is this a specific clinical question about therapy, diagnosis, prognosis, or harm? Using the structure suggested in the previous chapter, you can define the population, the exposure or intervention, and the outcome that are relevant to your question. Some sources (such as the *Cochrane Library* and *Clinical Evidence*, which are described below) are great for finding evidence about therapy and prevention and control issues, but rarely address the other areas of inquiry that you may have.

Sources of evidence

- *Clinical Evidence*
- *Cochrane Library*
- *EBM Online*
- *ACP Journal Club Online*
- *MedLine*
- Other biomedical databases
- Medical textbooks and EBM textbooks
- World wide web

Background information

To find answers to more general "background" questions (as opposed to "foreground" or focused clinical questions), textbooks, especially those published in searchable electronic versions, are often helpful. Textbooks remain an important resource for clinicians in terms of anatomy and pathophysiology, the basics of practice that usually do not change very quickly. They also provide descriptions of the classical presentations of diseases and conditions and review important practical aspects of history, physical examination, and diagnostic testing. Reviewing conditions that may present with similar findings in a good textbook can also help to broaden the differential diagnosis in more complex cases. Textbooks, however, are seldom explicit about the quality or currency of evidence used in recommendations for management, and are often very poorly referenced. Particularly for rapidly evolving aspects of management, such as laboratory diagnosis and therapeutics, printed textbooks simply cannot be trusted. There is often a passage of 4 or more years between updates of non-electronic textbooks, and many new studies will be published meanwhile. The most recent print edition of *Oski's Pediatrics*, a popular pediatric textbook, devotes several pages to otitis media, but no mention is made of the option to treat supportively rather than with antibiotics, and newer antibiotic options such as the macrolides also are not included.[3] These options have become widely known since the publication date of the book.

Fortunately, we now have access to online and CD-ROM textbooks with regular updates, such as *Scientific American Medicine* (*SAM*, http://www.samed.com/) and *UpToDate* (http://www.uptodateinc.com/). These provide reasonably current background information on many topics, in addition to answers to more specific questions. *UpToDate* is selectively updated every 4 months and is well referenced. While *UpToDate*, unlike *Clinical Evidence* and the Cochrane Database of Systematic Reviews, does not have a set of explicit methodologic quality criteria that must be met for articles to be included, it does reference many high quality studies. Unfortunately, the content of these texts primarily concerns adult patients. We await the production of a pediatric text that is similar to these two sources of information.

Although not routinely updated (in the way that *SAM* and *UpToDate* are), other textbooks are now available in searchable electronic format (*Harrison's* is available on line at http://www.harrisonson-line.com/, *Nelson's Textbook of Pediatrics* is available at the MD Consult Website, and *Oski's Pediatrics* is available in CD-ROM), which makes finding background information considerably quicker.

Another good source of current background information is general review articles, also referred to as narrative reviews, published in journals. If the journal is indexed in MedLine, such articles can be found in PubMed by limiting your search to "Review" under Publication Type. (See description of using Limits in PubMed later in this chapter.) Recent narrative reviews are often better referenced and more current than textbook chapters, but run the same risks of bias in the material selected as with a textbook chapter or any other non-systematic review.

Specific clinical questions

Busy clinicians will find that the most efficient way to answer specific clinical questions arising from individual patients is to begin with a "predigested" evidence-based resource such as *Clinical Evidence* or the Cochrane Database of Systematic Reviews, both of which are updated with methodologically sound and clinically important studies on a regular basis.

Clinical Evidence

This collection of summaries of evidence was launched in 1999. It is added to and updated every 6 months. As it is aimed at the general practitioner, the pediatric topics are those most likely to be seen in general outpatient practice. The methods used to develop the questions and the summaries are explicitly outlined in the preface to the book. The approach to developing these systematic reviews is evidence-based, similar to that outlined in Chapter 8, including comprehensive searching for published systematic reviews and primary studies, and appraisal of the quality of the evidence that is found. Recommendations for therapy are not made; rather, the evidence as the authors found it is presented, leaving the reader free to determine how it fits his or her clinical situation. In each chapter, the questions that have been addressed are shown and the interventions that were considered are listed in a hierarchy of evidence as "beneficial", "likely to be beneficial", "unknown effectiveness", "unlikely to be beneficial", and "likely to be ineffective or harmful", categories originally used by the Cochrane Collaboration. As noted previously, dividing evidence into these categories is not always straightforward, and some degree of subjectivity is likely to be present. Currently, only questions about interventions are addressed, so your questions about prevalence, diagnosis, and prognosis will not be answered by this resource. *Clinical Evidence* is published in full and concise versions every 6 months, and updated continuously on its website (http://www.clinicalevidence.com/). Access is free to developing nations, and available by subscription elsewhere. Many governmental and non-governmental agencies have made *Clinical Evidence* available free of charge to their constituents.

Evidence-Based Medicine Online and ACP Journal Club Online

If you know that the problem that you are facing has been studied recently, one alternative is to use a resource that includes only methodologically sound and clinically relevant studies, such as *Evidence-Based Medicine* (*EBM*) or *ACP Journal Club*. For both of these publications, a large number of journals (all specialties for *EBM* and internal medicine for *ACP Journal Club*) are scanned for articles describing studies that are clinically relevant and meet criteria for valid design and proper execution. Both are available online (http://www.acpjc.org/ and http://ebm.bmjjournals.com/). In addition to including only methodologically sound articles[4] and presenting the results using a structured abstract format, each article also includes a commentary written by a clinical expert that is designed to put the study findings into clinical context. Cassady and Parker pointed out the relative lack of studies involving pediatric patients in *Evidence-Based Medicine*,[5] although the editors have been working to increase the pediatric content. *ACP Journal Club* is specific to internal medicine, and thus likely to help pediatricians mainly with managing their oldest patients.

The Cochrane Library

The Cochrane Collaboration, an international organization that prepares, maintains, and disseminates high quality systematic reviews of healthcare interventions, offers a rich electronic resource for locating high quality synthesized information quickly (see Chapter 8 for a complete discussion of what constitutes a good systematic review). The *Cochrane Library* focuses almost exclusively on interventions, both therapeutic (for example, antibiotics for otitis media) and prevention and control (for example, how to reduce the incidence of teenage pregnancies). It provides little help in addressing other aspects of medical care, such as the value of a new diagnostic test or a patient's prognosis. Updated quarterly, the *Cochrane Library* is available in CD-ROM format or online (http://www.update-software.com/cochrane/), and is also available through many medical libraries with which physicians may be affiliated. The library consists of seven databases, five on evidence-based medicine and two on research methodology. All are searched every time you enter a word onto the search screen.

The centerpiece of the Library is the Cochrane Database of Systematic Reviews (CDSR), which includes the complete reports for all the systematic reviews that have been completed by members of the Cochrane Collaboration (1669 were in the 2nd issue for 2003) and the protocols, which are systematic reviews under preparation and include the background, objectives, and methods sections only (1266 were in the 2nd issue for 2003). The reviews in the CDSR are undertaken using stringent methodology and are peer reviewed prior to incorporation in the database. Each review is regularly updated as the need arises; in fact, if a review has not been property updated, it is dropped from the Library. The second section of the *Cochrane Library*, the Database of Reviews of Effects (DARE), includes bibliographic details and (when available) the abstracts of systematic reviews that have been published outside of the Collaboration (4006 were in the 2nd issue for 2003).

The third section of the Library, the Cochrane Central Register of Controlled Trials (CENTRAL), contains a growing list (the 2nd issue for 2003 had over 362 000 citations) of references to trials that Cochrane investigators have found by searching a wide range of sources, as part of completing Cochrane systematic reviews. Sources include the MedLine and EMBASE (Excerpta Medica) bibliographic databases, hand searches, and the reference lists of potentially relevant articles. While the majority of citations refer to randomized and pseudo-randomized trials, the database also includes a small number of observational studies. More clinical trials are now indexed in both CENTRAL and MedLine because of the efforts of volunteers who have hand-searched the literature for trials that were not originally indexed as trials. (MedLine adds the appropriate indexing to these trials as they are identified.) In addition, many of the trials in CENTRAL are not included in MedLine at all because they were published before 1966 or are in journals not indexed by MedLine. The two other medical databases are the Health Technology database, which contains over 3000 technology reviews, and the NHS Economic Evaluation Database, with over 11 000 economic evaluations.

The *Cochrane Library*

- Cochrane Database of Systematic Reviews (CDSR)
- Database of Reviews of Effects (DARE)
- Cochrane Central Registry of Controlled Trials (CENTRAL)
- Cochrane Database of Methodology Reviews (CDMR)
- The Cochrane Methodology Register (CMR)
- The Health Technology Assessment Database (HTA)
- The NHS Economic Evaluation Database (NHS EED)

MedLine and other bibliographic databases

MedLine is a huge bibliographic database of medical literature citations and abstracts produced by the US National Library of Medicine (NLM). Over 12 million citations, many with abstracts, are indexed from 4600 biomedical journals published in over 70 countries. In spite of its size, MedLine contains only about a third of the world's biomedical literature. This database can be used to answer both focused and background medical questions, but its size and complexity makes searching a more challenging task. Articles from the journals that are included in MedLine are read by professional MedLine indexers, who choose appropriate terms from a thesaurus of 22 000 specific terms (Medical Subject Headings or MeSH) Each article is indexed based on its content area, its publication type (review, randomized trial, etc.), on other descriptors, such as patient age (adult, child, newborn) and the language of publication. The citation elements of the article, such as author names, date of publication, and the journal name, are also indexed, so articles can also be located using these descriptors. MedLine is available free of charge to

everyone through NLM's PubMed website (http://ncbi.nlm.nih.gov/PubMed/) and for a fee from commercial vendors, such as Ovid Technologies, Inc. or Dialog.

EMBASE, the database of Excerpta Medica, although it was designed to include information covering all aspects of health care, focuses on drugs and pharmacology and has more European content than MedLine. There is some overlap between these databases, but much of their content is different. EMBASE is available for a fee from commercial vendors such as Ovid Technologies, Inc. or Dialog.

In addition to databases that are specifically medical, other databases such as PsycLIT (psychology), Toxline (toxicology), and CINAHL (nursing and allied health sciences) may be useful for specific purposes. These databases are indexed in a similar way to MedLine.

ISI Web of Science from Thomson ISI is another database to consider. It provides a different access to the medical literature through searching by cited reference to track research forward in time from a specific paper. Searching by cited reference can demonstrate the potential importance of a paper based on the number of times it has been cited and can show more recent research that is related to the cited paper. The database is multidisciplinary and can include the social sciences as well as biomedicine, biology, chemistry, and related sciences. Web of Science includes citations to some biomedical journal articles, and proceedings of symposia and conferences that are not indexed in MedLine.

Electronic databases relevant to medical care

- Cancer-CD – a combination of CANCERLIT and EMBASE cancer-related records, updated quarterly
- CINAHL – cumulative index to nursing and allied health literature from 1983 onwards
- *Cochrane Library* – provides access to systematic reviews, clinical trials, economic evaluations, and more
- Current Contents Search – provides searchable contents listings of journal issues on or before publication date, updated weekly, from 1990 on
- EMBASE – database of Excerpta Medica, focus on drugs and pharmacology, more European coverage than MedLine
- MedLine – major biomedical database for journal literature
- PsycLIT – searchable version *of Psychological Abstracts*, English language journals from 1974 onwards
- Toxline – toxicologic effects of drugs, from 1981 onwards
- TRIP Database – Turning Research into Practice; searches evidence-based resources on the internet
- Web of Science – tracks research by looking for articles that cite a specific study

Adapted from Greenhalgh T. *How to read a paper: The basics of evidence-based medicine.* London: BMJ Books, 1997.

The internet

The world wide web is an increasingly useful resource for locating current information, and one that our patients are accessing at an increasing rate. MedLine and many other databases can be accessed over the Web. A growing number of journals are available on line, including most major pediatric journals. Websites for journals provide online access to the editorials, letters, review articles, and abstracts as well as full texts of original studies, often going back 5 or more years. Most journals also provide search engines to locate articles on a particular topic. Access to full text for most journals is by subscription, although a few are available without cost. Many hospital and regional medical libraries have online subscriptions to a variety of journals, and your membership on the hospital staff or to the library may also allow you remote access to the journals. The journals' vendors may also offer to send complete copies of articles to you for a fee.

Finally, a growing number of sites on the internet contain information relevant to clinical medicine. Some pediatric textbooks are available on line, as are many clinical practice guidelines. While many of these sources contain information that is less current than some of the articles indexed by MedLine, this may well change with the rapid rate of development of the internet. Services such as MDConsult have full text versions of textbooks, many journals, drug information, and clinical guidelines. This service is available by subscription and also may be available through your local medical library. A number of websites provide links to other sites and information. The TRIP Database (http://www.tripdatabase.com/) is a good example of such a site. It has recently begun charging a subscription fee; again, your library may subscribe on your behalf. A list of websites that are explicitly concerned with evidence-based practice is shown in the Box.

World wide web resources for evidence-based medicine

- Netting the Evidence (An EBM Web Directory) http://www.sheffield.ac.uk/~scharr/ir/netting/
- Resources for Practicing EBM (PedsCCM) http://pedsccm.wustl.edu/EBJ/EB_Resources.html
- University of Rochester, Critically Appraised Topics http://www.urmc.rochester.edu/medicine/res/CATS/index.html
- University of Michigan, Evidence-Based Pediatrics http://www.med.umich.edu/pediatrics/ebm/
- University of Alberta Evidence-based Medicine Tool Kit http://www.med.ualberta.ca/ebm/ebm.htm
- Bandolier – Evidence-Based Healthcare http://www.jr2.ox.ac.uk/bandolier/
- UK Centre for Evidence-Based Medicine http://www.cebm.net/

- Centre for Evidence-Based Child Health http://www.ich.ucl.ac.uk/ich/html/academicunits/paed_epid/cebch/about.html
- Centre for Evidence-Based Mental Health http://www.psychiatry.ox.ac.uk/cebmh/
- Canadian Centres for Health Evidence http://www.cche.net/
- Finding answers to questions in Evidence-Based Medicine http://www.uib.no/isf/people/atle/ebm.htm
- Centre for Evidence-based Medicine (Toronto) http://www.cebm.utoronto.ca/

Journals and browsing to keep up to date

We have focused to this point on looking for evidence to answer specific clinical questions. If the search is successful, the evidence can be applied immediately and this can be a powerful learning experience. But what if we don't search for evidence because we don't know that we are out of date? A complementary strategy of browsing the medical literature regularly in one way or another is needed. The difficulty is that so many journals include articles relevant to pediatrics that it is impractical to review them all. Several journals have been developed specifically to present summaries of evidence, including *ACP Journal Club* (mostly internal medicine) and *Evidence-Based Medicine.* These journals are produced by the continuous scanning of a wide range of journals in a systematic way (according to explicit criteria) and publishing structured abstracts and commentaries on methodologically sound and clinically relevant studies. *ACP Journal Club* is specific to internal medicine, so does not address many topics of use to pediatricians, and *Evidence-Based Medicine* still has relatively little pediatric content as well; we await our own "evidence-based pediatrics" journal. The "Abstracts from the Literature" section in the *Journal of Pediatrics* uses a systematic approach to searching for important new evidence, but the search excludes the three largest pediatric journals (*Pediatrics*, *Archives of Pediatrics and Adolescent Medicine*, and *Journal of Pediatrics*) on the grounds that pediatricians are reading these already.

How to search

This section of the chapter will focus on the techniques that are used to search for evidence in the sources listed in the previous section. A simple and logical approach to searching consists of making several quick decisions.

- Structure your clinical question – do you need background information, or is this a focused clinical question?

- Decide whether you want a comprehensive search or a quick and dirty answer. This will help you decide the resources that will serve you best.
- Is it a question of therapy, diagnosis, prognosis, or harm? This will help you choose search terms based on study type or allow you to use built-in searching filters.
- Use your question to provide the elements of a search strategy that you can then combine using logical operators as described below.

Using Boolean logical operators

The process of searching most databases involves trying to narrow down the huge list of references by searching on the key concepts of the clinical question. You can logically combine the terms that you use to maximize the return on your investment of time. In a way that is remarkably similar to first-year algebra, you can direct the search engine to find certain sets of articles. If you want all articles that contain *either* one particular term *or* another one (say, either dexamethasone or prednisone) then you combine the two terms, using "OR" between them ("dexamethasone OR prednisone"). If instead you want only the articles that have *both* terms in them (say, all articles on meningitis and the use of steroids), then you will enter both terms, combining them with "AND" ("meningitis AND glucocorticoids"). You can also use "NOT", although this Boolean operator may cause more problems than it solves in a search. The Help pages for the *Cochrane Library*, PubMed, and most other databases have thorough discussions of how to use these operators, which you can review right at the time you need them. PubMed also has a very thorough searching tutorial on its website.

Clinical Evidence

Clinical Evidence is easily searched using common terms and Boolean operators, if needed, to combine terms. The home page has two search boxes – you will want to search the box labeled "Search current issue". Each issue builds on the previous one, so there is nothing more up to date and complete than the current issue. Using the "search these pages" box allows you to search for information *about Clinical Evidence*, rather than its contents. Your search results will be displayed with a listing of all of the topics and sections in which your term appears. Clicking on the section will bring up the full text of the topic. You can review it on screen, or print it out in pdf format. The paper version of *Clinical Evidence* has a table of contents listing the topics, and a comprehensive index. The paper copy of the Concise version comes with a CD-ROM, which contains the entire contents in a format similar to the web page.

The Cochrane Library

The *Cochrane Library* is only available online and on CD-ROM. Options for searching the *Cochrane Library* include the easy approach, which allows you to enter terms in the first search screen. You can create more complex search strategies that include Medical Subject Headings (MeSH) and Boolean logical operators. After you have entered the term or terms that represent your question, the next screen displays the results for each of the seven databases of the library, showing the number of citations. Click on the specific database that you wish to view and the next screen will list the titles of the reviews or articles that came up in your search. For the reviews in the CDSR, clicking on the title will produce the full text of the review or the protocol; for the DARE and the CENTRAL, it will produce the abstract if available, or the full citation if an abstract is not available. Clicking on "databases" or "citations" takes you back to the relevant previous lists, and you can start a new search any time just by clicking the search button.

MedLine

Clinical Evidence, the Cochrane Database of Systematic Reviews, *Evidence-based Medicine,* and *ACP Journal Club*, provide evidence that has been appraised prior to inclusion in the databases, so that you can feel reasonably confident that the information you retrieve is valid. However, when you search MedLine, you are on your own. Later chapters in this book review in detail the criteria of study design and execution that enable you to judge the quality of studies. As you search, you will want to be able to identify quickly those articles that you find in your search that are likely to yield valid answers. You can do this by applying "quick and dirty" validity checks to the titles and abstracts that you find. These are based on the criteria for critical appraisal that are covered in detail in each of the relevant chapters.

Quick and dirty validity criteria to be used while searching

- *Therapy questions.* Is this a randomized trial or a systematic review of RCTs?
- *Diagnostic tests.* Is there an independent comparison with a gold standard?
- *Prognosis questions.* Is this a cohort study with a high rate of follow up?
- *Harm questions.* Was a reasonable comparison group chosen?
- *Systematic reviews.* Was there an explicit and comprehensive search for evidence?

MedLine is readily available at the National Library of Medicine's free PubMed site (http://www.ncbi.nlm.nih.gov/PubMed). MedLine is also available through a number of commercial vendors (for example, Ovid Technologies, Inc, and Dialog), subscription services (for example, MD Consult) and web portals (for example, http://www.medscape.com/). If ready and easy access is one of MedLine's strengths,[6–8] then the skill needed to rapidly and dependably locate high quality articles that specifically address a clinical question is a weakness. A working knowledge of MedLine searching terminology and searching strategies is essential. Luckily, most hospital and university libraries offer training courses for new MedLine users, and the tutorial on the PubMed website is very useful.

The MeSH terms used by MedLine indexers to classify articles are not always intuitive or obvious to clinicians (for example, beta-blockers indexed as adrenergic beta-antagonists). Therefore, it is often helpful to search through the MeSH vocabulary before carrying out a search. The software for all search systems includes MeSH, so it is quite easy to search for appropriate terms. On the PubMed site, the MeSH database is accessible on the left side of the screen, under the heading "PubMed Services". When you enter a term that represents what you want to search, it will show you where in the MeSH tree that term resides, so that you can see all the related terms under which relevant articles may be indexed.

Depending on the topic and the scope that you are interested in covering, you may also want to take advantage of two additional features of MeSH headings. Because many articles deal predominantly with two or three topics, the indexer will indicate these topics for each citation by designating them as major subjects of the article. This can be done most simply by selecting "MeSH Major Topic" from the Fields menu under the Limits feature on the main PubMed search screen. Limiting your search to articles in which the search term has been designated as the major subject heading can be beneficial if you retrieve too many citations. However, sometimes you can miss important studies this way, because they have not been properly indexed. A trial and error approach may be needed to retrieve the best studies.

"Exploding" is another useful feature of MeSH indexing. When articles are indexed, they are classified according to the most specific MeSH heading available. Thus, if you wish to identify all articles that deal with "otitis media", including those with more specific MeSH terms such as "otitis media with effusion", then you will want to be sure that your search strategy includes exploding the term "otitis media". In the PubMed searching interface and in many other newer systems, all terms are automatically exploded, so you do not need to do this yourself. See the Box for demonstration of how exploding terms works.

MeSH tree for "otitis"

- "Otitis"
- "Otitis Externa"
- "Otitis Media"
    "Mastoiditis"
    "Otitis Media with Effusion"
    "Otitis Media, Suppurative"

If you are searching for a topic that has not been well indexed, you may want to take advantage of textword searching. Using this approach, you are simply asking MedLine to search the titles and abstracts of all of the citations for any occurrences of a certain sequence of letters, such as "effusion". This approach is particularly useful for new drugs, or for concepts such as "clinical disagreement" that have not yet been incorporated into MeSH. MeSH is updated annually, but the lag can be considerably longer for new terms. PubMed automatically searches for your terms as MeSH headings or as textwords.

If several different endings to a word may have been used, and you wish to identify them all, you can use the truncation symbol (in PubMed it is "*"; in Ovid it is "$"). For example, if you asked for RANDOM*, PubMed would search for RANDOM, RANDOMIZATION, RANDOMIZED, RANDOMISATION, RANDOMISED, and RANDOMLY. Be careful with truncation. The term "salmon:" retrieves not only words such as salmonella and salmonellosis, but the fish as well! Some systems may use symbols other than "*", such as ":" or "?".

Using the Limits menu allows you to limit the citations you retrieve in several useful ways. You can also limit the results to articles in the English language, articles that have an abstract (this gets rid of letters and editorials, but also older articles), by age of the included subjects, publication type, publication date, and other criteria.

In addition to these terms, which you will apply as you search the databases, specialized filters have been developed to make searching more efficient. Haynes and colleagues[9–10] developed a set of terms and phrases that can be added to any search in order to retrieve articles that are most likely to be methodologically sound and address the type of question you are asking. These are found at the Clinical Queries page of the PubMed website. When you click on Clinical Queries under PubMed Services, you are linked to a page on which you enter the search terms from your clinical question (an *intervention* and an *outcome*, for example) and then click on what kind of question (**therapy, diagnosis, prognosis** or **harm**) and on whether you prefer a search that is highly **sensitive** (which will net lots of studies, but many may be irrelevant) or one that is highly **specific** (which will net fewer, but more relevant studies). These filters are effective for a quick search on a clinical question, but inevitably are not

Table 3.1 Optimal search strategies for identifying studies relating to treatment, diagnosis, prognosis, or etiology using MedLine[12]

Studies	Search strategy: PubMed	Search strategy: Ovid*
Therapy		
Best single term	Clinical trial as a publication type under Limits	Clinical trial. pt.
Combination of terms with best specificity	Placebo OR (double AND blind*)	Placebo.tw. OR (double.tw. AND blind$.tw.)
Combination of terms with best sensitivity	random* OR drug therapy [SH] OR therapeutic use [SH] OR randomized controlled trial [PTYP]	Randomized controlled trial.pt. OR random$.tw. OR drug therapy.fs. OR therapeutic use.fs.
Diagnosis		
Best single term	Sensitivity	Sensitivity.tw.
Combination of terms with best specificity	(Sensitivity AND specificity) OR (predictive AND value*)	Exp "sensitivity and specificity"/ OR (predictive. tw. AND value$.tw.)
Combination of terms with best sensitivity	Diagnosis [SH] OR sensitivity OR specificity OR diagnostic use [SH]	Exp "sensitivity and specificity"/ OR diagnosis.fs. OR sensitivity. tw. OR specificity,.tw. OR diagnostic use.fs.
Prognosis		
Best single term	Cohort studies	Exp cohort studies/
Combination of terms with best specificity	Prognosis OR survival analysis	Prognosis/ OR survival analysis/
Combination of terms with best sensitivity	incidence OR mortality OR follow up studies OR prognos* OR predict* OR course*	Incidence/ OR exp mortality/ OR follow up studies/ OR prognos$.tw. OR predict$.tw. OR course$.tw. OR mortality.fs.
Harm		
Best single term	Risk	risk.tw.
Combination of terms with best specificity	Cohort OR case-control studies	Cohort.tw. OR case-control studies/
Combination of terms with best sensitivity	Cohort studies OR risk OR odds ratio* OR relative risk* OR case control*	exp cohort studies/ OR exp risk OR (oddsratio$.tw.) OR (relative risk$.tw.) OR (case control$.tw.)

*.tw. indicates textword
.pt. indicates publication type
exp indicates explode
.fs. indicates free floating subheading

perfect. If you really want to find *everything* on a topic, use Clinical Queries and also conduct a search in PubMed using the MeSH terms and limits described above.

Alternatively, you can search for a systematic review of studies. Research is ongoing to establish the best approach to identify systematic reviews and meta-analyses. Shojania and Bero[11] developed a strategy that is currently used by PubMed on its Clinical Queries page. If you click on "Systematic Review" rather than on a question type, this strategy (which you can use yourself by simply adding "AND systematic[sb]" to any search) is applied. This is intended to be a fairly comprehensive strategy, so your number of hits may be greater than you want. A more conservative strategy is to use the Limits menu, and choose "meta-analysis" under Publication Type.

MedLine can be searched in many ways, none of them perfect. What works well in one situation may not work as well in another. Combining appropriate content terms with methodology terms for reviews or for sound study designs (as in Table 3.1) will usually give you better search results. It also has to be considered, however, that such searches are bound to take some time. This is because of the general nature of this huge biomedical research database: it is so big and comprehensive that even the extensive indexing and care that is taken in preparing it are insufficient to guarantee quick and accurate retrieval for clinical uses.

Resolution of the scenario

A number of questions occur to you from your day in the office; you decide to focus on the two questions about steroid treatment:

- *In children with acute, severe pharyngitis, do steroids in addition to antibiotics versus antibiotics alone, result in more rapid resolution of symptoms without significant harm?*
- *In children with otitis media with effusion, does a course of steroids result in more rapid resolution of the "glue ear"?*

You identify these as questions of therapy, so the two sources of predigested evidence that focus on therapy may be useful: Clinical Evidence and the Cochrane Library. Checking the table of contents of Clinical Evidence, you find that the current issue does not have a chapter on pharyngitis, but it does have a chapter on otitis media with effusion.[13] This chapter lists oral steroid therapy as "likely to be ineffective or harmful" based on two systematic reviews, one addressing steroids versus placebo and the other addressing whether steroids should be added to antibiotic therapy. You feel confident that this answers your question, so you move on to the Cochrane Library to research the question about steroids for acute pharyngitis.

The term "pharyngitis" in Issue 2 of 2003 yields 25 completed reviews and four protocols in the CDSR, 13 citations in DARE and 656 citations in CENTRAL. A Cochrane review entitled "Antibiotics for sore throat"[14] appears promising. Double-clicking on this item, you find a systematic review, including information on the methodology for the review, the inclusion and exclusion criteria, the results, and a discussion. The results are presented with the findings in both textual and graphical forms, showing a modest decrease in duration of symptoms with treatment.

You move on to searching for information about steroid therapy in pharyngitis in MedLine. Using the Clinical Queries screen on PubMed, you enter the disease (pharyngitis) and the intervention (steroid) and click on "therapy". You also click on "specificity" since this will net the fewest and the most relevant studies: 22 citations are listed, two of which are randomized trials of steroids added to antibiotic therapy for acute tonsillopharyngitis,[15-16] and both show more rapid resolution of symptoms with steroid therapy. Since you see a moderate number of patients with acute pharyngitis, you would like more information about this intervention and decide to add these articles to your list of articles to pick up next time you are at the hospital library.

Your search has taken only about 30 minutes and has addressed both of your questions reasonably well.

Conclusion

In summary, while the time that we devote to updating ourselves with new developments is limited, a growing number of online resources are available so that we can use this time effectively. MedLine is more readily available than ever before and is seeding the development of specialty-specific collections. Journals that abstract only high quality,

clinically relevant articles are appearing and systematic reviews are becoming the norm. Applying these resources to clinical care on an ongoing basis after appraising the quality of information and considering how it relates to our individual patients can improve the quality of care we provide.

- New resources are rapidly emerging that make keeping up-to-date with clinically significant developments in pediatrics and child health easier than ever.
- Large bibliographic databases, such as MedLine, are becoming more accessible to practising physicians, and search strategies for locating high quality studies are now available.
- Specialty journals, such as *Evidence-Based Medicine*, that identify and abstract methodologically sound and clinically relevant studies also facilitate the ongoing process of staying current.

Take home list

- Textbooks may be a useful source of information on "background" questions but may provide biased advice and rapidly become out of date.
- Turning your clinical problem into a carefully structured question helps to guide where to search, what type of studies to look for, and what search terms to use.
- Before starting a search, decide whether you want a comprehensive search or a "quick and dirty" answer.
- A number of short-cuts to high-quality evidence such as *Evidence-Based Medicine, Clinical Evidence*, or the *Cochrane Library* are now available.

References

1 Mulrow CD. Rationale for systematic reviews. In: Chalmers I, Altman DG eds. *Systematic reviews*. London: BMJ Publishing Group, 1995.
2 Del Mar C, Jewell D. Tracking down the evidence. In: Silagy C, Haines A eds. *Evidence-based practice: primary care*. London: BMJ Publishing Group, 1998.
3 Kline M. Otitis media. In: McMillan JA, DeAngelis CD, Feigin RD, Warshaw JB, eds. *Oski's pediatrics: principles and practice, 3rd edn*. Philadelphia: Lippincott Williams and Wilkins, 1999.
4 Haynes RB. The origins and aspirations of *ACP Journal Club*. *ACP J Club* 1991;**114**:A18.
5 Cassady G, Parker L. Evidence-based medicine is not for kids. *Pediatric Academic Societies meeting, May 1–5 1998, New Orleans LA*, Abstract 1913.
6 McKibbon KA, Walker-Dilks CJ. Beyond ACP Journal Club: how to harness MedLine to solve clinical problems. *ACP J Club* 1994;**120**:A10–12

7   Haynes RB, Walker CJ, McKibbon KA, Johnston ME, Willan AR. Performance of 27 MedLine systems tested by searches with clinical questions. *J Am Med Inform Assoc* 1994;**1**: 285–95.

8   Engstrom P. MedLine free-for-all spurs questions about search value, who pays. *Medicine on the NET* 1996;**2**:1–5.

9   Haynes RB, Wilczynski N, McKibbon KA, Walker CJ, Sinclair JC. Developing optimal search strategies for detecting clinically sound studies in MedLine. *J Am Med Inform Assoc* 1994;**1**:447–58.

10 Wilczynski NL, Walker CJ, McKibbon KA, Haynes RB. Assessment of methodological search filters in MedLine. *Proc ANNU Symp Comp Appl Med Care* 1994;**17**:601–5.

11 Shojania KG, Bero LA. Taking advantage of the explosion of systematic reviews: an efficient MedLine search strategy. *Eff Clin Pract.* 2001;**4**:157–162.

12 Mckibbon, A. *PDQ Evidence-based Principles and Practices.* Ontario, Canada: BC Decker Inc., 1999.

13 Williamson I. Otitis media with effusion. *Clin Evid* 1999; **1**:94–100.

14 del Mar CB, Glasziou PP. Antibiotics for sore throat. In: Cochrane Collaboration. *Cochrane Library*, Issue 4. Oxford: Update Software, 1999.

15 Ei JL, Kasperbauer JL, Weaver AL, Boggust AJ. Efficacy of single-dose dexamethasone as adjuvant therapy for acute pharyngitis. *Laryngoscope.* 2002;**112**:87–93.

16 Marvez-Valls EG, Stuckey A, Ernst AA. A randomized clinical trial of oral versus intramuscular delivery of steroids in acute exudative pharyngitis. *Acad Emerg Med* 2002; **9**:9–14.

4 Assessing baseline risk: prevalence and prognosis

Carol Bower

Case scenario

You are working in the newborn nursery one weekend when you see a child whose face is not quite normal: the palpebral fissures are slightly upslanting and the face looks a little flat, the tone seems poor with hyperflexibility of the joints, and the child has bilateral simian creases. Although these findings are not pathognomonic for Down's syndrome, you are concerned enough to order chromosomal testing. This baby's mother is only 32 years old, and you wonder what the underlying risk of a Down's syndrome birth is among mothers this age. You also wonder whether the probability of heart disease is so high that you should get a cardiac echo, even in the absence of a heart murmur, if the baby does have Down's syndrome. You know that you will need to discuss the child's outlook for intellectual development and life span with the parents.

Pediatricians intuitively use baseline risks as they make decisions along the diagnostic, prognostic, and preventive paths of clinical practice. Knowing how common (or rare) a disease is in the population, as well as the natural history of the condition and its prognosis, is important in deciding what diagnostic tests to use, in helping parents to understand their child's condition, and in determining management.

The probability that a patient has a specific disease right now (usually called prevalence, pretest likelihood, or pretest probability) and the probability that the patient will develop a specific outcome in the future (risk or prognosis) are often misestimated by clinicians. In a survey of obstetricians and general and family physicians performing deliveries in Alabama, responding physicians significantly underestimated both survival rates and freedom from serious handicap in infants born at 23–34 weeks' gestation.[1] In this instance, counseling parents of preterm infants and the provision of appropriate perinatal care may be adversely affected by these misperceptions of baseline risk and prognosis.

This chapter aims to demonstrate how to use data to determine baseline risk, and where to find the data to assist you in diagnosis, prognosis, and preventive practice, and also in practice management and community service.

Current probability and future risk

There are two types of baseline risk: the risk or probability that a child has a disease or condition at the present time, and the risk that he or she will develop a particular outcome in the future. This division is somewhat artificial (many future events are already determined, we just don't know the answer yet!), but it is useful for understanding how to evaluate the information that you find. Current risk is often termed "prevalence" and, when used in evaluation of diagnostic tests, is understood as "pretest probability" (see Chapter 5). Future risk is what we usually term "prognosis", or the probability that a child will develop a particular outcome over a specified period of time. These types of information are usually best obtained using high quality observational studies.

Types of baseline information

In order to gather information about baseline risks, you need to have three types of information available: denominator, numerator, and exposure data. *Denominator data* describe the whole population of interest. Knowing the number of individuals in the population is useful, as is having information about the distribution of different groups within the population and about the characteristics of the region in which the population lives. *Numerator data* describe the children who have the type of problem, or outcome, of interest to you. *Exposure data* provide information about events or issues that may be linked to the outcome as a causal or risk factor, confounding factor, source of bias or effect modifier. The Box provides information about the types of data that may be relevant to these three broad areas, depending on the nature of your practice and the question that you are asking.

Examples of types of information needed to establish baseline risk

Denominator data

Population enumeration
- total number of children in your population or practice
- number of births per year in your region
- number of families
- number of hospital admissions
- number of pediatricians, hospitals, general practitioners, and other healthcare providers

Descriptive data
- by racial or ethnic groups
- by languages spoken
- by age
- by family size and structures
- by socioeconomic status
- by parental occupations

Regional information
- climatic conditions
- availability and means of transportation
- types of housing
- location and nature of parks and playgrounds
- child-care facilities
- educational institutions
- industrial and other potential environmental hazards
- availability of support services

Numerator data
- main reasons for consultation and hospitalization
- major causes of perinatal, infant, and childhood death
- features and natural history of the disease
- response to treatment
- likely outcomes

Exposure data
- rates of childhood and parental smoking, alcohol and other substance use
- pollens, and other allergens
- infectious agents

Sources of baseline information

Information on baseline risk, prognosis, and trends over time is essential to the practice of evidence-based medicine. Much of the information on denominators, numerators, and exposures will be specific to your own patient population. This type of information may need to be sought from government and other reports, which are not usually indexed in MedLine and other databases of published literature. The next Box shows the types of data sources that could be used.

Data sources
- Clinical experience
- Data from your own practice
- Vital statistics
- Special registers
- Special studies
- Government and other reports
- Published literature

As a clinician, you are aware, often subconsciously, of much of the baseline information relevant to your practice, but may be surprised at some of the data once quantified. Memory can play tricks, and there is a tendency to remember the most recent cases or cases with the most adverse outcomes more vividly than routine cases. Nevertheless, this is a valuable starting point. Data from your practice can be extremely valuable and, if your practice has a computerized system of management, such information can be readily available for analysis.

A potential problem with both of the above sources is that the number of patients may be small, particularly for rare conditions. The full spectrum of diseases, their signs, symptoms, and prognosis may not be represented, if the data are only available for a limited number of patients with a given condition, a relatively short time period, or for a single practitioner.

Vital statistics collected by your state or region should, at very least, include the number of births, deaths, census data on the population (for example, race, language, and family structure), and data on hospital admissions (or discharges). Information on a population basis for particular conditions (for example, communicable diseases), or exposures (for example, vaccination rates for the population, smoking prevalence among schoolchildren) may also be available on a regional basis. Depending on the way in which your health services are organized, data of this kind may also be readily available for your local area or nationally.

Many places have special registers of disease, for example for birth defects, cerebral palsy, mental health, and juvenile diabetes. Special studies in your region can be valuable sources of baseline data. These include outputs from pediatric surveillance units, such as the British, Canadian, New Zealand, and Australian Pediatric Surveillance Units.[2]

Searching the literature is dealt with in Chapter 3. Skill is needed in assessing the quality of the data from any source, and determining if it is relevant to your patient(s) and your practice. You will need to search for observational studies, particularly cohort studies, for data on prognosis. Data from randomized trials may be useful, but often represent highly selected populations, so that much of the information that you need will not come from randomized controlled trials.

Evaluating information on risk

Once you have located data, you need to assess their relevance and applicability to your patients and practice. A summary of issues to consider when evaluating the data is shown in critical appraisal criteria (see Box), based on guides to using articles about disease probability for differential diagnosis and for prognosis.[3,4]

In order to assess whether the study patients are representative of the underlying population, you need to consider the setting of the study, and how the patients have been recruited. If, for example, you are seeking information on the proportion of babies with Down's syndrome who have a cardiac defect, a community practice or population-based sample is likely to yield a lower proportion than a sample drawn from a tertiary hospital or a pediatric cardiology clinic, where children with Down's syndrome and cardiac anomaly are referred for evaluation and treatment. You will also need to take note of the proportion of patients eligible for inclusion in the study who actually participated, and whether those that did not participate are known or likely to be different in some systematic way from those who did participate. Also consider the inclusion and exclusion criteria for the study patients. If babies with Down's syndrome who died in the neonatal period are excluded, then the study will almost certainly be underestimating the proportion of all babies with a cardiac defect, as serious cardiac defects are an important cause of mortality in Down's syndrome.

How was the disease defined? Here you need to consider how the diagnosis was confirmed or rejected, and whether standard diagnostic criteria were used. The more objective, unbiased, consistent, and comprehensive the criteria for diagnosis, the more likely they are to be reproducible by different clinicians, in different settings, both within the one study, and between studies. Using the Down's syndrome example, echocardiography as a criterion for diagnosing congenital heart defects will provide a more exact measure than clinical examination only.

The length of follow up needs to be sufficient to allow for the occurrence and/or diagnosis of the conditions of interest. A year may be long enough to identify almost all cardiac defects in children with Down's syndrome (especially if they have had echocardiographic examination), but not sufficient to provide a good estimate of the risk of leukemia.

The completeness of follow up is also important, as outcomes might occur in patients who are lost to follow up (they may have died; or be too ill to participate), and this may bias the results.

Other factors to consider are the age and sex distribution of the study sample, the presence of other co-morbid conditions, and what treatments have been undertaken that may influence the findings.

In looking at the results, you will be interested in the different diagnoses in the case group(s), and the incidence of the outcomes of importance. Have the authors calculated confidence intervals to assist you in assessing the precision of the estimates? Remember that the size of the estimate and the confidence intervals both provide important information. A small study may not have sufficient power to produce statistically significant results, although the size of the effect, if true, would be of clinical importance, whereas a large study may provide a very precise estimate with tight confidence intervals around a clinically unimportant effect.

Finally, you need to consider how the study's findings relate to the care of your patients. You will feel more confident that the results apply to your practice if the study patients are similar to yours (if for example, the environmental, cultural and disease profile of your community is similar to those of the study). Also take note of when the study was done, as diagnostic methods and treatment regimens may have changed. This is especially relevant to studies of prognosis over a long period of time. In Western Australia, infants with Down's syndrome who were born recently have a much lower mortality (especially from congenital heart defects) when compared with infants born 1980–1985.[5]

You are now in a position to decide whether the results of this study can be used to select or avoid therapy, counsel or reassure patients, or whether you need to seek further information.

Critical appraisal criteria

Are the results valid?

- Are the study patients representative of the underlying population?
- How was the disease defined?
- Was the length of follow up adequate?
- Was follow up complete?
- Were other factors taken into account?

What are the results?

- What were the estimates of the outcomes?
- What was the precision of the estimates?

Will the results help me care for my patients?

- Were the study patients similar to mine?
- Have conditions changed since the study was done?
- How can these results be used to select or avoid therapy, counsel, or reassure patients?

Applying information on baseline risk

Making diagnoses

"Common things are common." Knowing the baseline risk of a condition in your population should raise your awareness of the condition, and thus the likelihood of making a correct and timely diagnosis. From the literature, juvenile arthritis is said to affect around 1 child per 1000.[6] However, in a population-based study in Western Australia (in which all 12-year-old children in a representative sample, regardless of symptoms, were examined by a single pediatric rheumatologist), the prevalence of juvenile arthritis was found to be four times higher (4 per 1000). Moreover, the mean time from first symptoms to definitive diagnosis was 39.9 weeks.[7,8] An appreciation of this higher baseline risk should lead to an increase in diagnostic suspicion, more timely treatment for the condition and ultimately a better outcome for children with juvenile arthritis.

It is also important to realize that the introduction of preventive measures will alter baseline risk (assuming the prevention program is effective), and thus information on trends in the prevalence of conditions over time may be relevant. Hib vaccines are known to be highly efficacious so, if vaccination rates of children against *Haemophilus influenzae* type b (Hib) infection are high, Hib will be a rare cause of meningitis.[9] Similarly, if prenatal screening with maternal serum testing and/or ultrasound examination is commonplace in your region, and pregnancies with prenatally diagnosed neural tube defects are terminated, then the baseline risk of a liveborn infant with spina bifida will be low. Also, if the use of periconceptional folate is high, then the occurrence of neural tube defects (in fetuses as well as liveborn infants) would be expected to be lower than the baseline risk before folate use was widespread.

In almost all instances, you will require more refined information than simply the overall prevalence or incidence of a condition. At the very least, prevalence or incidence by age and sex will be important in deciding if your patient is likely to have the condition. Other prior knowledge about the child may help to refine baseline risk. An example of this is demonstrated in Chapter 42, where the pediatrician wants to know the baseline risk of a urinary tract infection in an 18-month-old girl with fever. Furthermore, it is important to bear in mind the source of the data you are using to determine the baseline risk for your practice. For example, the pattern of referral to your service will have an effect on your choice of baseline risk data. If you work as a primary care pediatrician, community-based prevalence figures will be more relevant to you. However, if you work as a tertiary referral pediatrician, the prevalence of the disorder of interest is likely to be higher than in the community setting, and you will need to seek out data from studies based in tertiary referral settings.

Diagnostic and screening tests

The effect of baseline risk on the performance of a diagnostic (or screening) test is well known, and is demonstrated in Chapter 5, using auscultation for congenital heart defects as an example. This test performs much better in children with Down's syndrome, who have a high baseline risk (or pretest probability) of having congenital heart defects (about 40%), and performs much less well in a general population sample of infants, where the baseline prevalence of heart defects is <1%. It is also important to remember that for rare conditions, in the case of screening, you will probably need to seek information beyond your own practice in order to evaluate the success of the screening program. This is because, although you may be conducting an excellent program, you have too small a population ever to identify a single case.

Knowledge of baseline risk is valuable in assisting you to select appropriate screening tests for your population. Take, for example, screening for developmental dysplasia of the hip in infants. Several aspects of baseline information are required in order to assess, from the literature, whether the screening tests (the Ortolani and Barlow maneuvers) are relevant to your patient. Firstly, were the tests evaluated in a population similar to your own? Then, are the screening and subsequent diagnostic tests likely to be performed in a similar manner? Finally, you need to know the baseline risk of developmental dysplasia of the hip in your population in order to determine the post-test probability of hip dysplasia that applies to your patients. If the baseline risk (prevalence) of a condition is low in your population, it may be inappropriate to screen for it.

Treatment and prevention

Randomized controlled trials give us information on the effect of therapy, and meta-analyses such as those presented in the *Cochrane Library* give us a summary of the best evidence of effect.

Nevertheless, you will need data from non-randomized studies to assist you in determining whether the evidence is applicable to your population. To do this you will want to know whether your patients are similar to those who took part in the trial with regard to age, sex, and other relevant attributes, and the diagnostic criteria used. Then, having applied evidence-based principles to treating your patients, you will want to know if the treatment has been effective. Baseline information is important here, in order to compare the results beforehand with those obtained after the change in practice has been implemented. This is demonstrated in the practice study of otitis media referred to later in this chapter.[10]

With respect to prevention, it is important to know the baseline prevalence in your population of the condition to be prevented, as it may not be cost-effective (all other things being equal) to institute a preventive program if the condition is rare. Consider the example of maternal periconceptional folic acid supplementation, which has been shown to prevent 70% of neural tube defects in offspring.[11] You can apply this information to the baseline risk of neural tube defects in your population to ascertain the absolute reduction in risk that would result from introduction of this preventive strategy.

Between 1980 and 1995 in Western Australia, the prevalence of neural tube defects was 1·9 per 1000 births (including pregnancies terminated for fetal abnormality).[12] Thus, the absolute risk reduction in this population would be 1·33 per 1000 and, hence, the number needed to treat is 752. In other words, 752 women would need to be treated in order for one neural tube defect to be prevented. However, in the USA, the baseline prevalence of neural tube defects 1985–1994 was only 1 per 1000.[13] The absolute risk reduction in this population is thus 0·7 per 1000 births, and hence the number needed to treat to prevent one case is 1428, almost double that in Western Australia. Given the seriousness of neural tube defects and the relative simplicity of the intervention (folic acid supplements), most would still judge this a worthwhile intervention.

Prognosis

Information on prognosis usually comes from well-conducted cohort studies, in which children are followed over time to document their progress in relation to various treatments, the duration of the disease, and to identify side effects of treatment and complications of the condition. In assessing the quality of such studies, it is important to determine the population from which the cohort is drawn – for example, is it the whole population (or a random sample of it), or a hospital or clinic-based sample? – and the participation and follow up rates. The more complete the sample and the more like your population it is, the more reliable and relevant it will be for your purposes. This is demonstrated in Chapter 46, where for one of the studies on prognosis, concern was raised that not all children with cerebral palsy were followed up.[14] It was considered possible that children with cerebral palsy who were walking might be less likely to return to the clinic for follow up. Hence, basing the likelihood of walking only on children who attended clinic might result in an underestimate of the proportion of children with cerebral palsy who ultimately were able to walk.

Practice management

Baseline data are necessary to assist in ensuring that resources are available for identifying and managing conditions in your practice. If, for example, you work in a neonatal nursery serving a hospital where women on an IVF program deliver, you would need to know that the baseline risk of preterm and multiple births is increased for these women. Having accurate and current baseline data on these risks will assist you in obtaining and allocating appropriate resources to care for these high risk infants.

Baseline information will also assist you to determine if you should change management at an individual or service level. It will assist you in practice management by identifying whether a problem exists, and will allow you to assess the effect of any changes introduced. A group of general practitioners In the UK decided, on the basis of two recent reviews,[15,16] to evaluate the introduction of a "watch and wait" policy before treating otitis media with antibiotics. They needed baseline information on prescribing practices in their own setting and in a control practice before the policy was changed, so that they could determine whether the policy led to a decline in antibiotic prescriptions.[10] A fall in antibiotic prescriptions over a year was demonstrated in both practices, but the fall was much greater in the intervention practice.

Another example that demonstrates the need for collection of baseline risk information to inform management, regardless of known efficacy of a prevention strategy, relates to vaccination for rubella. In 1971, schoolgirl vaccination for rubella was introduced in Australia, to prevent congenital rubella syndrome in the offspring of these girls when they came to have children. It was assumed that the girls would have lifelong immunity following vaccination. Data from Western Australia showed a dramatic fall in children born with congenital rubella syndrome as the cohorts of vaccinated girls reached childbearing age.[17] However, over the same period, there was an increased availability of termination of pregnancy in Western Australia and there was concern that the fall in congenital rubella syndrome might be due to termination of affected pregnancies rather than primary prevention owing to vaccination. A study collecting information on terminations of pregnancy following maternal rubella infection confirmed the success of the vaccination program (rather than termination of pregnancy) in preventing congenital rubella syndrome in children born in Western Australia.[18] However, the study identified that a few children were still being born with congenital rubella syndrome.[18] Further investigation revealed that women born in Asian countries were less likely to be immune than Australian-born women and, that amongst some confirmed vaccinees, immunity waned with time. This led to two policy recommendations:

- women migrating to Australia should be vaccinated before or immediately on arrival, and
- a woman's rubella immune status should be checked in each pregnancy.[18]

Children (boys and girls) in Australia are now also vaccinated in infancy, thus increasing herd immunity and reducing the risk of exposure to wild rubella virus. Had the vaccination program not been thoroughly evaluated using information about baseline risk gathered from several sources, for more than one outcome, these changes would not have been made, children would still be born with congenital rubella syndrome, and public confidence in rubella vaccination might have fallen.

Community service

A study conducted in a defined regional center in Australia documented the role of and time spent by community-based pediatricians in the region in community activities, including advisory and management roles in child service agencies and hospitals.[19] Baseline documentation of these community service roles identified that pediatricians needed administrative, business, and management training, if they were to be able to contribute effectively to the direction of child healthcare policy in their region.

Furthermore, service advisory roles required baseline knowledge of the local risk of particular conditions, hospital admission rates, treatment, and prognosis, in order to assist in the provision of health and support facilities for children and their families in the community. A community-based project that affected health outcomes began with the collection of baseline data on injuries in public playgrounds in Cardiff, and the estimation of the number of children playing in playgrounds in order to calculate baseline injury rates per observed child.[20] In response to these data, a partnership between the local authority and pediatricians in the health service led to improvements in a number of safety features in playgrounds. A comparison of injury rates following the introduction of the improvements with the baseline rates demonstrated a significant reduction in injury, without a change in use of the playgrounds.[20]

Professional development

Information about the type of problems you most commonly see will inform you about any areas of need for further training or development of specific skills. For example, a survey of all 14 711 pediatric, non-hospital consultations over a 12-month period in a community pediatric practice in Victoria, Australia, identified that pediatricians spent most of their time dealing with children with chronic illness, chronic physical and intellectual disability, and learning and behavioral disorders.[21] If you identified that your training in any of these areas was inadequate, knowledge about the time that you are likely to spend working in the area might affect courses you attend. Further, this information can be used to help plan residency training in pediatrics and child health.

Resolution of the scenario

You realize that essentially all of your questions relate to baseline risk either in the sense of prevalence (what percentage of infants born to 32-year-old women have Down's syndrome?) or in the sense of prognosis (what is this child's prognosis for intellectual development?). You will search for this information in population-based cohort studies, and will look for studies with good follow up rates and unbiased assessment of outcome on which to base your prognostic estimates for these parents.

Future needs – how pediatricians can contribute

Appreciation of the importance and value of baseline information and data to follow trends over time should encourage you to collaborate with those who collect the information and make it available for use. This includes pediatric surveillance units, disease registries, and special surveys. The more complete these data collections, the more valuable they become. If the data you require are not available in a suitable form from these sources, it is important that you communicate with those responsible for the data, so that they know your requirements and can try to meet them.

Similarly, an appreciation of baseline risk might encourage you to set up data collections or modify existing ones based on your own practice. Although you should recognize its limitations, especially for rare diseases, such a system can address many aspects of baseline information, particularly if an easy-to-use, computerized system is established. Some examples of uses of practice data are shown in the Box.

Uses of practice data

- Describing your practice and your patients
- Evaluating treatment outcomes, trends over time, or changes in practice
- Establishing a reminder/recall system to ensure that children are screened, reviewed or vaccinated at appropriate times
- Identifying children at high risk (this might include children whose vaccinations are behind schedule, or those who have missed a screening test)
- Identifying children or families who might benefit from a new therapy or diagnostic test (this will become increasingly relevant as the genetic basis of more conditions is identified)
- Identifying patients eligible for inclusion in randomized controlled trials
- Identifying cases to notify to surveillance systems, disease registers, etc.
- Estimating the resources needed to run your practice
- Providing practice-based information to patients and their parents, for example, to encourage health-promoting activities

Baseline risk is integral to almost every aspect of pediatric practice. Information on baseline risk is not always available from the published literature, and may need to be sought from Government and other reports. Pediatricians can collect valuable baseline data from their own practice, and are encouraged to contribute to regional and national collections of data. This will help to ensure the availability of relevant, complete, accurate and up-to-date information to enhance the application of evidence-based principles to their practice.

Take home list

- Baseline risk refers to both the prevalence of a condition in a population, and to the risk of adverse outcome in children with the condition.
- Designing appropriate diagnostic and therapeutic strategies depends on reliable estimates of baseline risk.
- Estimates of baseline risk can be derived from clinical experience but evidence suggests that clinicians tend to overestimate prevalence and risk of adverse outcome.
- When using research evidence to estimate baseline risk clinicians must consider:
  - the population from which the sample is drawn and the way in which cases are defined (relative to their own population)
  - the effects of non-participation and loss to follow up on validity
  - the validity of instruments used to assess outcome.

References

1   Haywood JL, Goldenberg RL, Bronstein J, Nelson KG, Carlo WA. Comparison of perceived and actual rates of survival and freedom from handicap in premature infants. *Am J Obstet Gynecol* 1994;**171**:432–9.
2   Hall SM, Glickman M. The British Paediatric Surveillance Unit. *Arch Dis Child* 1988;**63**:344 6.
3   Richardson WS, Wilson MC, Guyatt GH, Cook DJ, Nishikawa J, for the Evidence-Based Medicine Working Group. User's Guides to the Medical Literature. XV. How to use an article about disease probability for differential diagnosis. *JAMA* 1999;**281**:1214–19.
4   Laupacis A, Wells G, Richardson WS, Tugwell P, for the Evidence-Based Medicine Working Group. User's Guides to the Medical Literature. V. How to use an article about prognosis. *JAMA* 1994;**272**:234–7.
5   Leonard S, Bower C, Petterson B, Leonard H. Survival of infants born with Down's Syndrome: 1980–1996. *Paediatr Perinatal Epidemiol* 2000;**14**:163–71.
6   Gewanter HL, Roghmann KJ, Baum J. The prevalence of juvenile arthritis. *Arthritis Rheum* 1986;**26**:599–603.
7   Manners PJ, Diepeveen DA. The prevalence of juvenile arthritis in a population of 12 year old children in urban Australia. *Pediatrics* 1996;**98**:84–90.
8   Manners PJ. Delay in diagnosing juvenile arthritis. *Med J Aust* 1999;**171**:367–9.
9   Peltola H, Kilpi T, Anttila M. Rapid disappearance of *Haemophilus influenzae* type b meningitis after routine childhood immunisation with conjugate vaccines. *Lancet* 1992;**340**:592–4.
10 Cates C. An evidence-based approach to reducing antibiotic use in children with acute otitis media: controlled before and after study. *BMJ* 1999;**318**:715–16.
11 Lumley J, Watson L, Watson M, Bower C. Periconceptional supplementation with folate and/or multivitamins to prevent neural tube defects (Cochrane Review). In: *Cochrane Library,* Issue 1. Oxford: Update Software, 1999.
12 Bower C, Ryan A, Rudy E, Cosgrove P. *Report of the Birth Defects Registry of Western Australia 1980–1998.* King Edward Memorial Hospital, Perth, No 6, 1999.
13 Centers for Disease Control and Prevention. Surveillance for anencephaly and spina bifida and the impact of prenatal diagnosis. United States, 1985–1994. *MMWR* 1996;**44** (SS-4):1–3.
14 Molnar GE, Gordon SU. Cerebral palsy: predictive value of selected clinical signs for early prognostication of motor function. *Arch Phys Med Rehabil* 1976;**57**:153–8.
15 Glaziou PP, Hayem M, Del Mar CB. Antibiotic versus placebo for acute otitis media in children. In: *Cochrane Library,* Issue 1. Oxford: Update Software, 1997.
16 Froom J, Culpepper L, Jacobs M *et al.* Antimicrobials for acute otitis media? A review from the International Primary Care Network. *BMJ* 1997;**315**:98–102.
17 Stanley FJ, Sim M, Wilson G, Worthington S. The decline in congenital rubella syndrome in Western Australia: an impact of the schoolgirl vaccination program? *Am J Pub Health* 1986;**76**:35–7.
18 Condon R, Bower C. Rubella vaccination and congenital rubella syndrome in Western Australia. *Med J Aust* 1993; **158**:379–82.
19 Hewson PH, Anderson PK, Dinning AH *et al.* The evolving role of community-based general paediatricians: the Barwon experience. *J Paediatr Child Hlth* 1999;**35**:23–7.
20 Sibert JR, Mott A, Rolfe K *et al.* Prevention of injuries in public playgrounds through partnership between health services and local authority: community intervention study. *BMJ* 1999;**318**:1595.
21 Hewson PH, Anderson PK, Dinning AH *et al.* A 12-month profile of community paediatric consultations in the Barwon region. *J Paediatr Child Hlth* 1999;**35**:16–22.

5 Assessing diagnostic and screening tests

Ruth Gilbert, Stuart Logan

The concepts

Diagnosis is the first step in clinical management. It is a powerful determinant of the investigations that you carry out on your patients, and the interventions and healthcare resources that you use. You need to make a diagnosis before you can discuss prognosis and treatment with your patient. Diagnosis may involve the interpretation of a constellation of clinical observations and tests that you undertake in order to be certain that, for example, a child has leukemia before you start chemotherapy. Alternatively, you may diagnose asthma based on a history of night-time cough and wheeze, and start treatment. Observing delay in motor milestones may raise the possibility that a child has developmental delay, but you might decide not to offer therapy until you have observed her further. Alternatively, you may diagnose a multiparous woman as being unlikely to have problems during delivery simply based on characteristics such as a previous normal delivery, vertex presentation, and no complications during pregnancy.

As these examples illustrate, diagnosis is rarely definitive. The aim of diagnosis is to give you a working hypothesis about which condition the patient is most likely to have. Clinicians often implicitly measure diagnostic uncertainty in terms such as "certain", "probably", "possibly", and "unlikely", as in the examples above. These terms are vague and their interpretation varies widely within and between clinicians. When you make diagnoses, you estimate the probability of a disease or condition.

Why estimate probabilities?

How you manage your patient varies depending on the probability of disease and how likely the patient is to benefit from treatment. You need to be pretty certain about your diagnosis of leukemia before starting chemotherapy because the consequences of treating someone who turns out not to have leukemia are serious. On the other hand, you may not be certain that a child has asthma, but consider that, on balance, the harm from unnecessarily treating someone without asthma is outweighed by the benefit of early treatment in a child who does have asthma. It is easier to determine whether you will do more good than harm if you are explicit about the probabilities of beneficial and harmful outcomes and how these are valued.

When is a test worth doing?

Tests (which include clinical observations) are the tools used to refine your estimate of your patient's probability of a particular condition. Testing is worthwhile if it changes your management or provides clinically important information about your patient's prognosis. Clinicians often intuitively decide when it is worth testing.

For example, imagine you are the director of a hospital nursery. Oxygen saturation monitors are used widely in your nursery, but not for all babies. You do not put monitors on babies who are pink and have no respiratory problems. This is because you know from experience that when the monitor shows low oxygen saturation in a well, pink appearing baby, it is most likely that the monitor is inaccurate. You always ignore the monitor in such cases and you certainly don't give oxygen. Not using monitors at all for pink, stable babies avoids lots of false alarms that annoy parents and staff.

Conversely, for babies who are blue and in acute respiratory difficulty, you do not first reach for the oxygen saturation monitor. You have calculated that, even if the monitor showed that the oxygen saturation was normal, the chance of the monitor being wrong is much higher than the chance of a blue baby having a normal oxygen saturation. You would provide oxygen anyway, and the test would not help you make this decision.

Implicitly, you have defined a middle group of babies, between those who have a very high and very low probability of hypoxia, for whom the test is useful and likely to change your action. The upper threshold is your "test:treatment"

Table 5.1   Should I test?

Implicit estimate of probability of hypoxia	Action
Blue babies – near 100% probability of hypoxia	Don't reach for monitor above this threshold. Give oxygen anyway
Test:treat threshold	
Unstable or sick babies – hypoxia quite likely	Use oxygen saturation monitor
No-test:test threshold	
Pink babies – no respiratory problems. Probability of hypoxia near 0%	Don't use monitor below this threshold. If saturation low, monitor error most likely

Table 5.2   Clinical examination in Down's syndrome-affected babies[2]

Test	Reference standard cardiac echo		
Clinical examination	Major defect	No major defect	Total
Positive	18 (a)	(b) 3	21
Negative	16 (c)	(d) 44	60
Total	34	47	81

Cardiac echo is the reference standard (sometimes referred to as the "gold standard") and clinical examination is the "test": (a) true positives; (b) false positives; (c) false negatives; and (d) true negatives.

threshold,[1] above which you will give oxygen anyway. The lower threshold is your "no-test:test" threshold, below which it is not worth testing. The test is useful only for patients at intermediate risk of disease (see Table 5.1).

Somewhere between these two thresholds is your "action threshold". This threshold is determined by the consequences of the test result, and represents the point at which the harm caused by giving oxygen to babies who are not hypoxic is equivalent to the harm of not giving oxygen to babies who are hypoxic.

What determines whether a test will change your action?

Tests are useful if they move the patient across your action threshold. Logically, you will treat patients with a probability of disease above this threshold, and not treat patients below it. In practice, your threshold may differ among patients according to their values about the harms and benefits of testing and/or treatment. For example, we do not automatically test children who have a parent with Huntington's chorea. Some families may decide that the information is beneficial while others may decide that it would cause harm to know.

You need two further pieces of information to decide whether testing is likely to move your patient across your action threshold:

- the probability of disease in your patient before you do the test (pretest probability);
- a measure of test performance (likelihood ratios or sensitivity and specificity).

Suppose you want to know how well the clinical examination (i.e., listening to the heart for murmurs) performs at separating newborns into those with a major heart defect and those without a major heart defect. Tubman *et al.*[2] recorded the result of the clinical examination in an unselected, regionally representative population of newborn babies with Down's syndrome, all of whom also underwent echocardiography (the reference standard for detection of major heart defects). The results are shown in Table 5.2.

The columns show how many babies turned out to have a major heart defect and how many did not. Major heart defects were very common (34 of 81, or 42%), as expected in babies with Down's syndrome. This is the pretest probability of major heart defect in this population. The important information for clinicians is the probability of disease *after* a particular test result (the post-test probability), which is obtained by looking along the rows. In an unselected population of babies with Down's syndrome and a positive clinical examination, 18/21 (86%) will have a major heart defect (sometimes called the positive predictive value). In the same population of babies, among those with a negative clinical examination, 16/60 (27%) will have a major heart defect (this is 1 minus the negative predictive value).

Table 5.3   Clinical examination in well term babies

Test	Reference standard cardiac echo		
Clinical examination	Major defect	No major defect	Total
Positive	18 (a)	(b) 638	656
Negative	17 (c)	(d) 9327	9344
Total	35	9965	10 000

Cardiac echo is the reference standard (sometimes referred to as the "gold standard") and clinical examination is the "test": (a) true positives; (b) false positives; (c) false negatives; and (d) true negatives.
*(see text below) the probability of a positive test among those with the disease [a/(a + c)] is the **sensitivity** of the test, and the probability of a negative test among those who do not have the disease [d/(b + d)] is the **specificity** of the test.

Clinicians want to know how a test will perform in their own patients, who may have a different pretest probability from the patients in the study. For example, you want to know the usefulness of the clinical examination in term newborns on the postnatal wards, none of whom have Down's syndrome. You find a paper reporting that the probability of cardiac malformations detected in infancy in babies born after 35 weeks gestation with no perinatal problems is 3·5 per 1000 (i.e., the pretest probability).[3] You can now redraw the table for your own population.

Given an imaginary population of 10 000, about 35 will have a major heart defect. For the moment, assume that the clinical examination performs just as well (or just as badly) in term newborns as in Down's syndrome-affected babies. This would mean that the probability of a positive test in babies with major heart defects is the same in babies with Down's syndrome as in well term babies. Similarly, the probability of a positive test in babies without major heart defects is the same in babies with Down's syndrome as in well term babies. (In fact, the test may perform differently as the type of heart defects differ. We discuss this "spectrum bias" later. The clinician's expectation of finding a defect is also likely to differ, which may affect the sensitivity of the test.)

Given this principle and the pretest probability in well term babies, you can complete Table 5.3. The probability of a positive test in the Down's syndrome-affected babies with a heart defect was 18/34 = 53% (this is the sensitivity of the test).[1] Therefore 53% (~18) of your 35 term babies will have a positive test. The probability of a positive test in those without major heart defects was 6·4% (this is the false positive rate or 1 − specificity).* (see Table 5.3 legend) Hence, 0·064 × 9965 = 638 term babies will have a positive test result. The ratio of these probabilities is called the likelihood ratio (LR) for a positive test (for example, 53%/6·4% = 8·3). Likelihood ratios reflect the performance of a test. The further a likelihood ratio is above or below 1·0, the better the test separates patients with and without the disease.

For clinicians, the important information is along the rows. When you are faced with a patient, all you know is the test result – you do not know whether the test result is correct.

Using the table, you can determine the post-test probability of disease in patients with a given test result. For example, for babies with a positive clinical examination, the post-test probability of a major heart defect is 2·7% (18/656). In other words, < 3 out of 100 newborn babies with an abnormal heart examination will actually have a major heart defect.

This example illustrates that the consequences of a positive test result can be very different depending on the pretest probability of disease. In Down's syndrome-affected babies, you would probably arrange for immediate echocardiography. In the well term population, you might instead arrange to review the baby in a few weeks. If you referred all babies with murmurs to the cardiologist immediately, cardiologists would have to see 6·6% of all newborns (656/10 000) and for every one with a major defect, 37 would be normal (100/2·7%).

In practice, clinicians use different test cut-offs to trigger a similar action (such as referral to the cardiologist) in different populations. For example, in normal term babies, you would request an immediate echo in a baby with a loud murmur, palpable thrill, who had had an episode of transient cyanosis, whereas you might postpone testing in a baby with a soft, non-radiating murmur.

Changing the cut-off for a "positive" test result

Many clinical and laboratory tests do not give clearly positive or negative results but a range of values. Clinical experience and common sense tell you that very abnormal test results are more likely to reflect true disease than those that are mildly abnormal.

For example, attainment of motor milestones can be used as a test to identify children who may have cerebral palsy. If a child is delayed in just one milestone you would probably be less anxious than if she is delayed in all milestones. Allen and Alexander[4] studied the performance of the test of delayed motor milestones in a population of 154 high risk infants born at < 32 weeks gestation. They determined the status of motor milestones when the child was 12 months old (corrected for gestation). They then did a full neurodevelopment assessment

Table 5.4   Number of delayed motor milestone, by 12 months and diagnosis of cerebral palsy at 18–24 months

Number of delayed motor milestones at 12 months	Reference standard of clinical assessment at 18–24 months		Total
	Cerebral palsy	No cerebral palsy	
Six	17	0	17
Five	4	2	6
Four	3	2	5
Three	2	9	11
Two	3	4	7
One	1	12	13
None	1	94	95
Total	31	123	154

when the child was at a corrected age of 18–24 months, and classified children into two groups: those with and those without cerebral palsy, defined as persistently abnormal tone or reflexes and functional impairment. Table 5.4 shows how increasing numbers of delayed milestones predicted the diagnosis of cerebral palsy.

You can see from the table that if you refer all children with one or more delayed milestones you would pick up virtually all (30/31) children with cerebral palsy. However, this would be at the expense of investigating 29 children who do not have cerebral palsy. If you raise the cut-off for referral to five delayed milestones, you would investigate only two children without cerebral palsy, but 10 children with cerebral palsy would be missed. This inverse relationship is common to all tests. There is always a trade-off between wrongly labeling people without the disease, and missing those with the disease.

Where you draw your cut-off for a positive test result depends on the probability of missing children and hence delaying diagnosis, the probability of wrongly labeling children without cerebral palsy, and how these consequences are valued. In this population, if you refer all babies with five or more delayed motor milestones, 21/23 (~90%) of them would turn out to have cerebral palsy (the post-test probability). However, the high risk preterm babies have a high pretest probability of cerebral palsy: 31/154 (20%).

Making the assumption that the test (delayed motor milestones) performs in the same way in babies seen in the well-baby clinic as in high risk preterm babies, you can work out the post-test probabilities that would occur in a routine clinic population. In a population of 10 000 babies seen in a well-baby clinic, there would be about 10 children with cerebral palsy (1/1000 × 10 000).[5] In the high risk preterm babies, 21/31 (67%) of the children with cerebral palsy had five or more delayed milestones as did 2/123 (1·6%) of the children without cerebral palsy. Applying these probabilities to your well-baby clinic population, you would expect to detect five or more delayed milestones in seven (10 × 67·7%)

babies with cerebral palsy and in 160 babies (9990 × 1·6%) without cerebral palsy. In other words, even using this high cut-off, only 7/167 (4%) infants referred for assessment would actually have cerebral palsy.

Using likelihood ratios

It is quicker to calculate the post-test probability of disease for a given test result according to the pretest probability of disease in different populations by using the likelihood ratio:

$$\frac{\text{The probability (likelihood) of the test result in people with the disease}}{\text{The probability (likelihood) of the test result in people without the disease}}$$

Table 5.5 shows delayed milestones and cerebral palsy with the likelihood ratios calculated for each test result.

There are two ways in which you can use the likelihood ratios to work out the post-test probability of cerebral palsy in your patient.

The easy way – with a nomogram

You can use the likelihood ratios shown in Table 5.5, together with the pretest probability, to work out the post-test probability of cerebral palsy using the nomogram in Figure 5.1.

Imagine that your patient was born at 28 weeks of gestation. He was ventilated for 4 days and had a small intraventricular hemorrhage. You estimate his pretest probability of cerebral palsy to be about 33%. On examination you find he has failed five milestones at 12 months post term. Draw a straight line joining your patient's pretest probability of cerebral palsy with the likelihood ratio for the test result you are thinking of using, to give you the post-test probability.

Table 5.5   Likelihood ratios for delayed motor milestones

Number of delayed motor milestones	Reference standard of clinical assessment	
	Calculation of likelihood ratio	Likelihood ratio
Six	(17/31)/(0/123)	Infinity
Five	(4/31)/(2/123)	7·9
Four	(3/31)/(2/123)	6·0
Three	(2/31)/(9/123)	0·9
Two	(3/31)/(4/123)	3·0
One	(1/31)/(12/123)	0·33
None	(1/31)/(94/123)	0·04

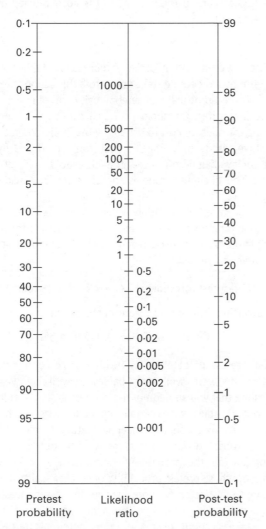

Figure 5.1   A likelihood ratio nomogram. (Adapted with permission from Fagan TJ. *N Engl J Med* 1975;**293**:257.)

By doing sums

Alternatively, you can calculate the post-test probability yourself. If you hate doing sums, skip this section.

Pre-test odds × likelihood ratio = post-test odds

First, you have to turn the pretest probability into pretest odds. This is simple if you remember that a probability of 33% (1 in 3) means that one person has the condition for every two who do not – representing an odds of 1:2 (or a half). If you want to convert an odds of 1:2 back into a probability, it would be $1/1+2 = 0.33$ or 33%. (Odds = probability/[1–probability]; probability = odds/[1+odds].)

In the example above, the child had five delayed motor milestones, for which the likelihood ratio is 7·9. The post-test probability is therefore 0·8 or 80% and you would probably want to refer this child for a full neurodevelopmental assessment. (Probability 33% = $0.33/(1–0.33) = 0.5$. Pretest odds × likelihood ratio = post-test odds = $0.5 × 7.9 = 3.95$. Post-test probability = $3.95/(1+3.95) = 0.8$ or 80%.) Contrast this with a child seen in the well-baby clinic, who was born at term with no adverse birth history. The pretest odds of cerebral palsy for this child would be about 1/1000. If we assume that the likelihood ratio would be the same in this population,

$$\text{the post-test odds} = 1/1000 × 7·9$$
$$= 0·0079 \text{ (post-test odds)}.$$

The post-test probability of cerebral palsy would be:

$$0·0079/1+0·0079 = 0·0078 \text{ or } 0·8\%$$

Hence, < 1% of babies with five delayed milestones at 12 months and no other adverse characteristics would actually have cerebral palsy. Your strategy for this child would therefore be to arrange for review in a few months time rather than immediate referral.

Using sensitivity and specificity to calculate likelihood ratios

When there are just two test results (positive and negative), you can use the "sensitivity" and "specificity" to calculate the likelihood ratio. Sensitivity refers to the column containing people with the disease: it is the probability of a positive result in people with the disease. In the cerebral palsy example, the proportion with five or more delayed milestones is 21/31 = 67%. Specificity refers to the column for people without the disease: it is the probability of a negative test result (i.e. no delayed milestones) in people without the disease (94/123 = 76%).

The likelihood ratios can then be written as:

$$\text{Likelihood ratio for a positive test} = \frac{\text{sensitivity}}{1\text{-specificity}}$$

$$\text{Likelihood ratio for a negavtive test} = \frac{1\text{-sensitivity}}{\text{specificity}}$$

In Table 5.5, we showed the likelihood ratios for each test result as this provides more information. However, you could impose a cut-off, for example above which children would be referred. If you consider all results above the cut-off as positive and below as negative, you can then calculate sensitivity and specificity or the likelihood ratios for a positive and negative test result.

Useful tips: SpPIn; SnNOut

A simple way of remembering the effect of different properties of tests is to use the mnemonic SpPIn; SnNOut.

If you use a highly **sp**ecific test, a **p**ositive result rules **in** the diagnosis, SpPIn. For example, six delayed motor milestones is 100% specific for cerebral palsy (the likelihood ratio is infinity). Hence, children with six delayed milestones can be "ruled in" as having cerebral palsy, and, given this test result, you are unlikely to treat people without the disease.

On the other hand, a highly **sen**sitive test, if **n**egative, rules the diagnosis **out**, SnNOut. A screening test for cystic fibrosis should be highly sensitive, that is, almost all children with the disease have a positive test, and there are very few false negatives. However, a large number of false positives will need to be excluded by confirmatory testing.

Calculating the no-test:test threshold and the test:treat threshold

To decide which population it is worthwhile testing, you need to calculate two thresholds for the pretest probability:

- the no-test:test threshold – below which you will not bother testing at all;
- the test:treat threshold above which you would refer anyway.

The test is worth using in patients with a pretest probability of disease between these two thresholds.

First, you need to ask yourself, how much worse would it be to miss a child with cerebral palsy than to wrongly label a child who does not have cerebral palsy? If you miss the diagnosis at 12 months, it is likely that you simply delay the diagnosis until further check-ups at 18 or 24 months. You will balance this delay against the emotional trauma of wrongly labeling a child with cerebral palsy. Suppose that you and the parents consider that the cost (or harm) of wrongly labeling a child with cerebral palsy is at least twice as bad as delaying the diagnosis in a child who does have cerebral palsy.

Your action threshold, the post-test probability of cerebral palsy at which you would refer children for investigation for suspected cerebral palsy, is equal to the costs divided by the costs + benefits:

$$2 \div (1+2) = 67\%.$$

Note that even a cut-off of five or more delayed milestones in well term babies does not take you across this action threshold as the post-test probability of cerebral palsy was only 4%.

The no-test:test threshold (in odds) can be calculated by dividing the odds for cost to benefit by the likelihood ratio (for a positive test result). Imagine that you would use five or more delayed milestones as the threshold for referring babies. The likelihood ratio is therefore 21/31 divided by 2/123 = 42. The odds of costs to benefits is 2:1. (To calculate no-test:test threshold multiply odds of costs/benefits by the likelihood ratio for a positive test. For the test:treat threshold, multiply the odds of costs/benefits by the likelihood ratio for a negative test result.)

$$\text{No-test:test threshold} = 2/1 \div 42 = 0{\cdot}048 \text{ (odds)}$$

Converting these odds into a probability, this is:

$$0{\cdot}048/1+0{\cdot}048 = 0{\cdot}045 \text{ or } 4{\cdot}5\%$$

The pretest probability (1/1000) for cerebral palsy in infants who were well term babies is well below 4·5%, suggesting that you should not use the test in this population, except for babies with certain characteristics, such as a history of hypoxic ischemic encephalopathy, which raises the pretest probability for cerebral palsy. The test is certainly appropriate for the preterm neonates born at < 32 weeks gestation, whose pretest probability of cerebral palsy is 20%.

More sophisticated methods for determining the treatment threshold include cost-effectiveness or cost-utility analyses. These take account of many more potential harms and benefits of treating and not treating and assign explicit values to each outcome.[6]

Finding a better test

Although you can increase the usefulness of tests by changing the cut-off for a positive test, sometimes you simply need a better test. You can recognize better tests by the separation of

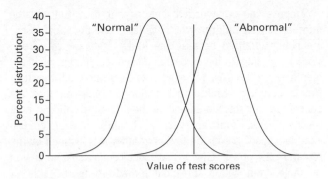

Figure 5.2 Frequency curves for test results in "normal" and "abnormal" populations

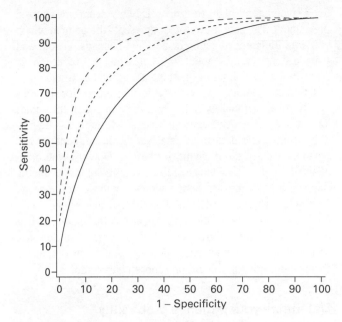

Figure 5.3 Receiver–operator curve

the distribution of the test results (or likelihood ratios) in "normal" and "abnormal" people (see Figure 5.2). A frequency distribution shows the variation in the proportion of normal people with a particular test result and of abnormal people with a particular test result.

At the test cut-off for a positive test shown by the vertical line in Figure 5.2, you will detect most of the "abnormal" group and include a proportion of the "normal" people as false positives. The less the overlap between the curves, the better the resolution of the test. If a test is perfect, the frequency distributions do not overlap at all.

Test resolution can also be summarized as a ROC curve (receiver–operator curve, Figure 5.3). ROC curves were originally developed to show the relationship of "signal" to "noise" for radio receiver operators during the early years of radio transmission. The curve shows the relationship between sensitivity (signal, on the *y* axis) and the false positive rate (noise, 1 – specificity, on the *x* axis). Each point on the curve represents a test result and the gradient of the curve at this point gives the likelihood ratio. Tests that have the best resolution have curves nearest to the top left-hand corner.

You can only improve detection of people with the disease **and** reduce erroneous labeling of people without the disease by choosing a test with better resolution (reduced overlap of test results in people with and without the disease, giving higher and lower likelihood ratios).

Summary of concepts

Use a test only if it is likely to change what you do to patients. This depends on:

● your action threshold (the probability of disease at which you would offer the intervention because it would do more good than harm);
● your patient's pretest probability of disease;
● how well the test performs (measured by likelihood ratios or sensitivity and specificity).

All tests have an inverse relationship between sensitivity and specificity.

How to use the research literature on diagnosis

The next part of this chapter is based on the concepts described so far and takes you through how to evaluate the available evidence to help you decide whether to use a test or not. We have skipped the process of deciding which tests should be considered at all, which is often informed by causal or physiologic reasoning.[7] Our focus is on how to work out whether the test will lead to a beneficial change in management so that you can use tests more effectively and efficiently.

We will describe this process in steps:

● Decide on your action threshold
● Work out your patient's probability of disease before doing the test (see Chapter 4)
● Determine the likelihood ratios for the test results from valid clinical studies
● Determine whether the post-test probability for your patient crosses your action threshold

Decide on your action threshold

The action that you are considering may be a therapeutic intervention (for example, antibiotics for a urinary tract infection) or further investigations (for example, amniocentesis for a woman at high risk of a Down's syndrome-affected pregnancy). The action threshold represents the point at which you are indifferent to acting or not, and depends on your and your patient's values about the consequences of action or inaction, before you know anything about the test result.

Pregnant women who undergo screening for Down's syndrome are familiar with the notion of an action threshold. The threshold above which a woman decides to undergo amniocentesis to determine fetal karyotype depends on her personal values about giving birth to a Down's syndrome-affected child balanced against the possibility of loss of a fetus due to amniocentesis. Some women choose to undergo amniocentesis above a risk of 1 in 100, while others would choose amniocentesis at a much lower risk (for example, 1 in 400). Sometimes service providers arbitrarily decide the action threshold rather than allowing women to decide for themselves, but still the cut-offs chosen vary widely.[8]

Determine your patient's probability of disease before testing

You can look up the pretest probability of disease based on the woman's age from published tables – approximately 1 in 130.[9] However, age is a poor test for discriminating between women with a Down's syndrome-affected fetus and those without. A much better test is to measure a combination of biochemical markers in maternal serum. (for example, the triple test). The serum test results are always combined with the woman's pretest probability based on her age, to give her post-test probability of a Down's affected pregnancy (for example, 1 in 5000). Down's syndrome screening is unusual in that the pretest probability is known fairly precisely. More often in clinical practice, clinicians need to estimate pretest probabilities based on their clinical experience of seeing similar patients and knowing what proportion ended up with the diagnosis. Unfortunately, there is evidence that clinicians often overestimate the probability of disease, fail to adequately take account of new information, base their estimates on unrepresentative patients, and bias their estimates by the patients they recall most easily.[10]

More reliable evidence can be sought from the research literature. The type of study you want could be a cohort study, cross-sectional study, randomized controlled trial, or a study evaluating a diagnostic test. Another solution is to take a range of estimates, from the published literature and estimates from you and your colleagues, and use this range as the basis for your calculations. For further discussion of this issue see Chapter 4.

Determine likelihood ratios for the test results

You seek evidence about how well a test performs from the published literature. We will work through a real-life clinical example to illustrate how you would go about this.

Suppose you are worried that in your busy unit a large number of well children who have fever and petechial rashes are being admitted because the junior staff are concerned that they might have bacterial septicemia, particularly meningococcal sepsis. You suggest to the junior staff that they should consider sending such children home but they are concerned that this would lead to them missing children with severe illness. Your approach is based on your clinical experience, so you decide to see whether it is justified by the research literature. Given that bacteremia is serious and treatable, your action threshold for admitting the child is pretty low. Roughly, you think it is 20 times worse to miss a child with bacteremia than to admit a child unnecessarily. Hence your action threshold for admission is a probability of bacteremia of about 5% ($1/20+1 = 4\cdot8$%). The probability of disease with just fever and petechiae (before testing) is about 2%.[10] Hence a negative test of "looking well" would need to give a post-test probability below 5% to send the child home.

You ask a three-part question.

Question

1. In children with fever and petechiae (*population*), who look well (*exposure*), what is the risk of bacteremia (*outcome*)?

You go to MedLine and type in terms to describe your patient group, for example, children with petechiae and the outcome, bacteremia. You try these terms before adding any search filters that will pick up papers that report evaluation of diagnostic tests. See Chapter 3 for a discussion of search filters.

sensitivity AND petechiae AND bacteremia AND child*

This search yields eight articles, one of which appears to address your question. The next thing to decide is whether you can believe the result. This involves appraising the methodology of the study to determine whether the results are likely to be valid (close to the truth).

Is the study valid?

Does the study include an independent, blind comparison with an adequate reference standard?

A reference standard ideally represents unequivocal truth and should dichotomize patients into those who definitively have the disease and those who definitively do not. For example, chromosome analysis for trisomy 21 is the reference standard for Down's syndrome. However, for most conditions, the division into those who have the disease and those who do not is an artificial cut-off in a spectrum of disease severity. For example, the reference standard for anemia in a toddler is generally quoted as Hb < 11·0 g dl^{-1}. But why not 11·5, 9·0, or 10·5? A cut-off has to be drawn somewhere to define patients who require treatment or further investigation, and those who do not. Although few reference standards are perfect, you need to judge whether the reference standard used in the article is acceptable. This will depend on what it means in terms of how closely the reference standard relates to prognosis and the potential to benefit from the intervention. The reference standard in the article by Mandl *et al.* was blood culture. This is probably the best reference standard available for bacteremia.[10]

The next step is to work out whether there was a blind comparison between the test ("looks ill or well") and the reference standard (blood culture). This means that the person interpreting the blood culture did not know whether the child looked ill or well, nor did the person making this judgement know the results of blood culture. In this instance, a blind comparison is quite likely. Unblinded comparisons are biased towards agreement. Imagine if your boss says, "Listen to this heart, I think there is a systolic murmur", you are quite likely to agree. Similarly, if she says, "This heart sounds normal", you are less likely to hear a murmur.

Tests are independent if the reference standard does not include the test or elements of the test. For example, the white cell count (test) should not be compared with a reference standard for sepsis composed of blood culture, white cell count, and clinical condition as this would produce bias in favor of agreement. In the study by Mandl *et al.*,[10] the assessment of how ill the child looked did not form part of the interpretation of the blood culture.

Did the study sample include an appropriate spectrum of patients to whom the test would be applied in practice?

You need to work out whether the test was compared in all patients, or just in those who obviously had the disease and those who obviously did not. The latter often happens. Clinicians decide to write a paper and pull out a selection of their obvious bad cases and a group of unaffected "controls". Common sense tells you that it is easy to differentiate between severe disease and no disease at all. Any reports like this should be treated with caution as they grossly overestimate the performance of the test[11] because they exclude patients at intermediate risk of disease – the group in whom you most want to use the test. This sort of study is only informative if the test shows no difference in results between abnormal and normal cases, as you then know to abandon the test.

Ideally, you need to look for a study that has evaluated the test in patients with a similar range of severity of disease as in your patients. Unfortunately, it is rarely possible to find the perfect study. A rough rule is that patients with negative results are less likely to be referred, so the proportion of false negatives is underestimated (and sensitivity is overestimated) in referral centers. There also may be an excess of patients with positive results due to other disorders that present with similar signs or co-morbidity leading to an overestimation of the proportion of false positives (thereby underestimating specificity). In primary care, where few patients have co-morbid conditions that give rise to false positive results, specificity is more likely to be overestimated. In practice, the spectrum of patients in which the test was evaluated, characterized by factors such as disease severity, co-morbidity, and age and sex of patients, usually does affect the likelihood ratio.[12–14] The likelihood ratio should therefore be thought of as an average measure of test performance.

The study by Mandl *et al.* meticulously surveyed all 24 000 patients attending an Accident and Emergency department during an 18-month period who had a temperature ≥ 38°C. They identified 411 patients with petechiae, eight of whom had bacteremia. The spectrum of patients studied is therefore likely to be similar to your own patient population.

Did the test result influence the decision to perform the reference standard?

Tests that define the reference standard may be expensive, invasive, or hazardous. That's why you want a test, so that you don't have to perform the reference standard! However, when evaluating the test, the reference standard should be performed regardless of the test result. For example, if you want to know about the performance of prenatal serum testing for babies with Down's syndrome, you want a study in which all women had amniocentesis and chromosome analysis, and the serum test had no effect on whether amniocentesis was performed or not. If women knew the results of their tests, those with a negative result might not turn up for amniocentesis and the proportion of false negatives would be underestimated.

Sometimes it is simply not feasible to perform the reference standard on all patients with a negative result. In these cases, it is possible to perform the reference standard on a random sample of patients with a negative result. For more information on the pitfalls and calculations associated with this approach see the articles by the STARD group on standards for reporting of diagnostic test studies[15] and by Begg.[16] In some studies, different reference standards are used for patients with positive and negative test results. Such studies overestimate test performance.[11]

In the study by Mandl *et al.*,[10] virtually all children (393/411) with fever and petechiae had a blood culture result available.

Given the answers to the questions so far, the study appears to be reasonably valid.

Table 5.6 Working out likelihood ratios

Test Clinical examination	Reference standard of blood culture		
	Bacteremia	No bacteremia	Total
Looks ill	6	47	53
Looks well	2	355	357
Total	8	402	410

What are the results

What is the likelihood ratio?

Now you need to calculate the likelihood ratio. In the clinical scenario, you are interested in a negative test result – a well-looking child. Likelihood ratios are not reported in this paper but you can calculate them for yourself by completing 2×2 table for "appears ill" or "does not appear ill" compared with the reference standard (bacteremia). By convention, the reference standard always goes along the top of the table and test down the side (Table 5.6).

The likelihood ratio for "looks well" is: $2/8 \div 355/402 = 0.28$
The likelihood ratio for "looking ill" is: $6/8 \div 47/102 = 6.4$

How precise is the likelihood ratio?

The authors systematically evaluated 24 000 children with fever: only eight were found to have petechiae and bacteremia, highlighting the difficulty of performing such studies. The small number of children with bacteremia means that it is important to use the upper and lower confidence interval around the likelihood ratio to guide your use of the test, rather than rely on a single estimate.[17] An approximate confidence interval for the likelihood ratio is given by the formula[15] or you can use a web-based calculator:

http://ptwww.cchs.usyd.edu.au/Pedro/CIcalculator.xls).

The 95% confidence interval likelihood ratio (0.28) for the test result "looks well" = 0.08, 0.94.

The 95% confidence interval likelihood ratio (6.4) for the test result "looks ill" = 3.9, 10.4.

Will the test help you in caring for your patients?

What is the pretest probability of bacteremia in your patient population?

As you are very concerned not to miss children with bacteremia, the pretest probability of bacteremia in your patient is critical. If your patient is similar to the patients in the study, the pretest probability would be $8/411 = 2\%$.

However, this average risk could vary depending on population characteristics such as endemicity of meningococcal disease or uptake of *Haemophilus influenzae* B vaccine. An audit of bacteremia in pyrexial children presenting to your department would help to address this question. The pretest probability will also depend on patient factors, for example, age at presentation, duration and height of fever, and previous treatment with antibiotics. See Chapter 4 on baseline risk.

What is the post-test probability of disease and does it cross your action threshold?

You can read off the post-test probability from the nomogram by joining the pretest probability of 2% and the likelihood ratio for looking well, which is 0.28. The post-test probability is about 0.6%.

The post-test probability of 0.6% is well below your action threshold of 5% for admission. A sensitivity analysis, with the use of the lower 95% confidence interval for the likelihood ratio of 0.94, produces a post-test probability of 2%, still well below your action threshold. Your options could be to do more tests (for example observe in the department for 4 hours, or perform a white cell count), or send the patient home. In practice, sending the child home involves a test of continued parental surveillance and if they don't improve, returning for reassessment.

Were the methods for performing the test described in sufficient detail to be reproducible in your practice?

Clearly your assessment of an ill child may differ from the assessment used in the study. Fortunately, the authors described what they meant by "ill" and "not ill" in some detail, so it is possible to use their criteria in your practice.

Is the test feasible, affordable, accurate, and precise in your setting?

The assessment of "ill-looking child" is likely to be reproducible and similarly precise in your practice, as many doctors in the emergency department in the study were involved in this assessment, not just one skilled researcher. If a single skilled researcher performed the test, you may find that the test would not perform as well in your own routine practice (LRs would be nearer to 1.0). For example, ultrasound examination of nuchal thickness may be highly reliable (get the same result in the same patient time and again, by the same or different observer) in the hands of a team of fetal medicine specialists, but less reliable in the hands of non-specialized ultrasonographers. If a study is based on a small number of testers, you want information on the intra-observer and interobserver variation (see Chapter 10).

Critical appraisal criteria

1 Does the study include an independent, blind comparison with an adequate reference standard?
2 Did the study sample include an appropriate spectrum of patients to whom the test would be applied in practice?
3 Did the test result influence the decision to perform the reference standard?
4 What are the results, and what is the precision of the results?
5 Will the test help you in caring for your patients?

- What is the pretest probability of disease in your patient?
- What is the post-test probability of disease and does it cross your action threshold?
- Were the methods for performing the test described in sufficient detail to be reproducible in your practice?
- Is the test feasible and affordable, accurate and precise in your setting?

Sequences of tests

If you are using tests in sequence, you can, under some circumstances, use the post-test odds of disease after the first test as the pretest odds for the second test, and use the likelihood ratio for the second test. However, this only works if the tests are completely independent. Often they are not. Tests are most likely to be independent if they measure different physiologic elements of the same condition. You can assess independence in studies in which both tests and the reference standard have been performed in a large number of patients. The likelihood ratio for the second test should be calculated twice: in patients with a "positive" result on the first test and in patients with a "negative" result on the first test. If the likelihood ratios are the same under both of these conditions, they are said to be conditionally independent of the results.[9]

The reference standard

Much of this chapter has been based on the assumption that we know what the reference standard means. However, few reference standards unequivocally define disease and no disease. More often, the reference standard is itself an arbitrary cut-off in a spectrum of disease. For example, there is no clear dividing line between children who have cerebral palsy and those who do not. All clinicians are likely to agree about a child with severe spastic quadriplegia, but where would you place children with very mild monoplegia or moderate dyspraxia?

For some tests (blood pressure, fasting blood sugar, postnatal depression) you must correlate the test result with the patient's eventual prognosis or their response to treatment, and decide at what level of severity the benefits of intervention outweigh the harms. Evidence about how test results relate to benefits of treatment can be obtained from randomized controlled trials (RCTs). If RCTs are not available, or do not relate to an appropriate patient group, cohort studies may provide useful information. Evidence relating to prognosis can be obtained from cohort studies and, sometimes, controlled trials (see Chapters 4 and 6).

Screening

Screening has been defined by the UK National Screening Committee, in 1998, as "the systematic application of a test, or inquiry, to identify individuals at sufficient risk of a specific disorder to warrant further investigation or direct preventive action, amongst persons who have not sought medical attention on account of symptoms of that disorder."[19]

Although the dividing line between clinical practice and screening is somewhat arbitrary, the key difference is an ethical one. In clinical practice patients approach professionals and ask for help. In screening programs, professionals actively encourage people to undergo a procedure on the basis that they will benefit. It is therefore important to be certain that the benefits of the program outweigh the potential harms.

A particular problem faced in screening is that it involves uncommon disorders (the prior probability of disease is low). This means that, unless there are highly specific tests, diagnostic facilities are in danger of being swamped by patients labeled positive on the screen who do not have the condition of interest. There is also evidence that some families whose children "fail" the screening test and are subsequently found not to have the condition (i.e., a false positive result) will suffer long-term problems.[18] This requires a careful approach to the way in which results of screening are given to parents and to subsequent confirmatory testing. This potential source of harm needs to be included in the overall assessment of the potential costs and benefits of any screening program.

The approach to the evaluation of tests or clinical observations outlined earlier is the same for screening tests. However, it is not appropriate to consider the performance of screening tests in isolation from other aspects of the program, such as the effectiveness of the interventions, and the availability of facilities for diagnosis and treatment. A number of criteria for evaluating potential screening programs have been suggested.[18] All seek to ensure that potential harms and benefits have been adequately weighed before a new program is embarked upon. Table 5.7 gives terms used in tests and the Box shows criteria adapted from the First Report of the National Screening Committee in the UK.

Table 5.7 Jargon buster

Feature of the test	Terms used	Alternative terms and comments
Probability of disease in the population	Pretest probability	Prevalence
Probability of disease for a given test result	Post-test probability	Positive predictive value (for a positive test result), 1 minus the negative predictive value for a negative test result
Proportion of people with the disease correctly identified by the test	Sensitivity	Detection rate, true positive rate, 1 minus false negative rate
Proportion of people without the disease correctly identified by the test	Specificity	True negative rate, 1 minus false positive rate
Test performance	Likelihood ratio	Sensitivity and specificity if results are dichotomized. Represented by ROC curves
Test agreement	Accuracy [a + d] ÷ total	Not a very useful measure

Screening criteria

Ideally all the following criteria should be met before screening for a condition is initiated.

The condition

- The condition should be an important health problem.
- The epidemiology and natural history of the condition, including development from latent to declared disease, should be adequately understood and there should be a detectable risk factor, disease marker, latent period, or early symptomatic stage.
- All the cost-effective primary prevention interventions should have been implemented as far as practicable.

The test

- There should be a simple, safe, precise and validated screening test.
- The distribution of test values in the target population should be known and a suitable cut-off level defined and agreed.
- The test should be acceptable to the population.
- There should be an agreed policy on the further diagnostic investigation of individuals with a positive test result and on the choices available to those individuals.

The treatment

- There should be an effective treatment or intervention for patients identified through early detection, with evidence of early treatment leading to better outcomes than late treatment.
- There should be agreed evidence-based policies covering which individuals should be offered treatment and the appropriate treatment to be offered.
- Clinical management of the condition and patient outcomes should be optimized by all healthcare providers prior to participation in a screening program.

The screening program

- There should be evidence from high quality RCTs that the screening program is effective in reducing mortality or morbidity.
- There should be evidence that the complete screening program (test, diagnostic procedures, treatment/intervention) is clinically, socially, and ethically acceptable to health professionals and the public.
- The benefit from the screening program should outweigh the physical and psychologic harm (caused by the test, diagnostic procedures, and treatment).
- The opportunity cost of the screening program (including testing, diagnosis, and treatment) should be economically balanced in relation to expenditure on medical care as a whole.
- There should be a plan for managing and monitoring the screening program and an agreed set of quality assurance standards.
- Adequate staffing and facilities for testing, diagnosis, treatment, and program management should be available before the screening program begins.
- All other options for managing the condition should have been considered (for example, improving treatment, providing other services).

(Adapted from the *First Report of the National Screening Committee*, Health Departments of the UK, April 1998: www.open.gov.uk/doh/nsc/nsch.htm)

Take home list

- In practice "diagnosis" does not imply certainty but always carries an implicit probability.
- Virtually all diagnostic tests, whether based on laboratory results or clinical findings, make errors.

- The probability of a test correctly predicting a condition depends on the underlying probability of the condition (pretest probability) and the test performance (measured by the likelihood ratio or sensitivity and specificity).
- The usefulness of a test depends on:
  - whether the test results result will lead to a beneficial action
  - the patient's pre-test probability of disease
  - the test characteristics.

References

1 Pauker SG, Kassirer JP. The threshold approach to clinical decision-making. *N Engl J Med* 1980;**302**:1109–17.

2 Tubman TR, Shields MD, Craig BG, Mulholland HC, Nevin NC. Congenital heart disease in Down's syndrome: two year prospective early screening study. *BMJ* 1991;**302**: 1425–7.

3 Ainsworth S, Wyllie JP, Wren C. Prevalence and clinical significance of cardiac murmurs in neonates. *Arch Dis Child Fetal Neonatal Ed* 1999;**80**: F43–F45.

4 Allen AC, Alexander GR. Using motor milestones as a multi-step process to screen preterm infants for cerebral palsy. *Develop Med Child Neurol* 1997;**39**:12–6.

5 Stanley FJ, Watson L. Trends in perinatal mortality and cerebral palsy in Western Australia, 1967 to 1985. *BMJ* 1992;**304**:1658–63.

6 Kassirer JP. Introduction – Diagnostic reading. In: Sox HC, ed. *Common diagnostic tests – use and Interpretation*. Philadelphia: American College of Physicians, 1990.

7 Reynolds TM. Down's syndrome screening in the UK (letter). *Lancet* 1996;**347**:907.

8 Hecht CA, Hook EB. The imprecision in rates of Down's syndrome by 1-year maternal age intervals: a critical analysis of rates used in biochemical screening. *Prenat Diagn* 1994; **14**:729–8.

9 Sox HC. Probability theory and the interpretation of diagnostic tests, In: Sox HC, ed. *Common diagnostic tests – use and Interpretation*. Philadelphia: American College of Physicians, 1990.

10 Mandl KD, Stack AM, Fleisher GR. Incidence of bacteremia in infants and children with fever and petechiae. *J Pediatr* 1997;**131**:398–104.

11 Lijmer JG, Mol BW, Heisterkamp S *et al.* Empirical evidence of design-related bias in studies of diagnostic tests. *JAMA* 1999;**282**:1061–6.

12 Bossuyt PM. No burial for Bayes' rule. *Epidemiology* 1997; **8**:4–5.

13 Ransohoff DF, Feinstein AR. Problems of spectrum and bias in evaluating the efficacy of diagnostic tests, *N Engl J Med* 1978;**299**:926–30.

14 Brenner H, Gefeller O. Variation of sensitivity, specificity, likelihood ratios and predictive values with disease prevalence. *Stat Med* 1997;**16**;981–91.

15 Bossuyt PM, Reitsma JB, Bruns DE *et al.* (STARD group). Towards complete and accurate reporting of studies of diagnostic accuracy: the STARD initiative. *Clin Chem Lab Med* 2003 Jan;**41**:68–73.

16 Begg CB. Biases in the assessment of diagnostic tests. *Stat Med* 1987;**6**:411–23.

17 Simel DL, Samsa GP, Matchar DB. Likelihood ratios with confidence: sample size estimation for diagnostic test studies. *J Clin Epidemiol* 1991;**44**:763–70.

18 First Report of the National Screening Committee. *Definitions and classification of population screening programmes.* London: Department of Health, 1998.

19 Marteau TM, Cook R, Kidd J *et al.* The psychological effects of false-positive results in prenatal screening for fetal abnormality: a prospective study. *Prenat Diagn* 1992;**12**:205–14.

6 Assessing therapy

Elizabeth J Elliott, Kathleen Kennedy

Case scenario
A 4-month-old infant born preterm at 31 weeks and weighing 1500 g presents to your office for a well child visit in autumn. As a newborn he had respiratory distress syndrome treated with mechanical ventilation and surfactant. His respiratory symptoms completely resolved by 1 week of age. He was discharged from the hospital at 6 weeks of age and has been well since discharge. His mother saw an article about palivizumab (respiratory syncytial virus [RSV] monoclonal antibody) in a parents' magazine and asks your advice on whether her infant should receive this preventive therapy.

Background

In clinical practice, questions of therapy/prevention arise more frequently than questions of etiology, diagnosis or prognosis.[1] Clinicians frequently ask a range of therapy questions, including the following:

- How should I treat my patient?
- Is one therapy better than another therapy (or no therapy)?
- Do the harms of therapy outweigh the benefits?
- Will the therapy be cost-effective?
- Is the therapy acceptable to the patient and family?
- Do I have the expertise and willingness to use this newly available therapy?
- Will the provider pay for this new therapy?

When any trial of a new therapy is published, the clinician must evaluate the study and decide whether or not to incorporate the therapy into his/her clinical practice.

The "best" evidence to support a therapy is the evidence that is subject to the least bias. The best study type to minimize bias in the evaluation of a therapeutic intervention is a randomized controlled trial (RCT) in human subjects. The best evidence to support a therapy comes not from a single RCT but from a systematic review that includes a meta-analysis of all RCTs that evaluate that therapy. Some clinical practice guidelines are based on a systematic review of the literature. However, in the absence of evidence, recommendations in guidelines may represent the consensus of experts. Methods have been developed to grade evidence about therapy on the basis of its validity or quality (see Chapter 9). One such method ranks a systematic review of RCTs with homogeneous results as Grade A, Level 1a, while an RCT with precise results (a narrow confidence interval) is ranked Grade A, Level 1b.[2] However, the quality of RCTs and systematic reviews varies considerably and quality cannot be assessed on the basis of study type alone.

In practice, clinical therapy decisions often have to be made in the absence of good quality information from RCTs. In pediatrics particularly there is often a lack of published evidence to guide management. Fewer RCTs are performed in children than in adults and many therapies we use have not been adequately studied or licensed for use in children. For example in the field of renal medicine, only about 7% of RCTs and 20% of systematic reviews include children (personal communication, Cochrane Renal Group). Even when reviews and trials have included children, the data validity may be insufficient to support treatment recommendations. By 2001, 113 systematic reviews including 559 RCTs were published in the *Cochrane Library* by the Neonatal Review Group.[3] In 45 (40%) of these 113 reviews, the evidence was judged to be insufficient because of small sample size, failure to assess important clinical outcomes, or lack of data for important patient subgroups. Of the primary therapeutic interventions used in pediatrics, it has been estimated that 75% of inpatient interventions (most of which were for asthma and bacterial infections)[4] and 40% of outpatient interventions[5] are based on high-level evidence.

The report of an RCT should make it clear to the reader why the study was undertaken, what methods were used, and how the data were analyzed. The way in which the results of a trial are reported can also help the reader evaluate its strengths and limitations. The Consolidated Standards for Reporting of Trials (CONSORT) statement was first published in 1996[6] by an international group of editors of biomedical journals, scientists, epidemiologists, and statisticians. It is regularly reviewed and has subsequently been revised (http://www.consort-statement.org)[7] and is now accepted by many journals. It provides authors with a standardized format for reporting the results of RCTs that includes a diagram of the flow of participants through the trial, so that their progress can be easily followed. By specifying that authors clearly describe their methods (for example, of randomization, blinding, and data analysis), the CONSORT format facilitates the assessment of trial quality.

There is evidence that the use of CONSORT improves the completeness and quality of reporting of RCTs.[8,9] The requirement for good quality reporting may also encourage researchers to design their RCTs appropriately and thus to limit the potential for bias in estimating the effectiveness of a therapy. Unfortunately, despite CONSORT, many trials are still reported inadequately.[7] The astute clinician should also be aware of the potential for conflict of interest in clinical trials. The most obvious examples are drug trials sponsored by the manufacturer of that drug. In this situation it is often difficult to know whether the investigator or the manufacturer had control over the data analysis and publication. In an attempt to address this issue, most journals now ask authors to declare any potential conflict and this statement is published with the paper.

When you are evaluating a paper about therapy, it is important to look not only at the study type and design but also the way in which the study data have been analyzed.[10] The study questions should be clearly stated, the criteria for entry and exclusion of participants should be well defined, and the primary outcome measure should be stated. Information should also be given about the sample size (and power) of the study and the methods of data analysis. Statistical tests should be appropriate for the type of data being analyzed. Flaws in study design and/or data analyses can lead to false conclusions. Chapter 2 deals with how to structure a question of therapy and Chapter 3 deals with how to find the evidence efficiently. In this chapter the relative strengths and weaknesses of study designs used to assess therapies will be discussed, as will some principles of statistical analysis of data. The RCT found in response to the case scenario above will be used to illustrate the process of critical appraisal for an article about therapy using the checklist published in the *Users' Guides to the Medical Literature*.[11,12] The critical appraisal of systematic reviews is covered in Chapter 8.

The question of whether a particular therapy should be used in an individual patient does not depend solely on whether benefits are demonstrated in published trials. Any benefits of a therapy must be weighed against the potential harms of that therapy.[13] Furthermore, the decision to use a therapy must be made in conjunction with the patient (or parent), taking into account personal preferences and how the patient values the possible outcomes.[14] All therapy options (including the option of no therapy), and the harms

and benefits of each option, should be discussed with the patient. Methods of communicating evidence to patients, including information about risk, are covered in Chapter 14. Finally, the applicability of study results to your patient will depend on a number of factors, including whether the study was conducted in a similar population to yours and the likelihood that your individual patient will benefit from the treatment. Even when good evidence is available to support a therapy, there may be considerable barriers to introducing that therapy. These include resistance from colleagues to changing their practice, lack of local expertise to deliver a therapy, or lack of approval or funding for a new drug.

Sources of information, study types, and bias

According to Sackett[15] clinicians make decisions about therapy by one of three methods. These include:

- *Induction.* Based on their own anecdotal experience or an understanding of disease mechanisms (this therapy seems to work or ought to work);
- *Deduction.* Using information from properly conducted studies; or
- *Seduction.* Relying on the word of others, for example, colleagues or drug representatives.

In the absence of properly conducted RCTs, the clinician is often forced to use information from uncontrolled or poorly controlled studies. It is important to understand the strengths and weaknesses of different study types.

The best study type is the one with the least chance of bias. Bias can be defined as any factor that will systematically influence the collection, analysis, interpretation, publication, or review of data, and lead to conclusions that are different from the truth. At least 70 types of biases have been identified[16] but there are four main sources of systematic bias that may affect the internal validity of randomized trials of healthcare interventions.[17]

- *Selection bias* occurs when there are systematic differences in the *characteristics* of comparison groups, for example disease severity.
- *Performance bias* occurs when there are systematic differences in the *treatment* received by comparison groups (apart from the therapy being evaluated).
- *Attrition bias* occurs when there are systematic difference between participants who *withdraw* from comparison groups in the trial.
- *Sampling bias* occurs when there are systematic differences between the study population and the target population, for example when trial participants are recruited from a referral center. This type of bias affects the external validity or generalizability of a trial.

Uncontrolled studies

As Chalmers said, "Studies without controls are not likely to fool anybody."[18] Uncontrolled studies, including case reports, case series, and before-after studies (that evaluate the effectiveness of a therapy by comparing the same subjects before and after its use) do not use an appropriate control group for comparison. Such studies can be done fairly quickly and cheaply and were widely used in the past. It is now recognized that these types of study are highly subject to bias. Uncontrolled studies may lead to an overestimate of therapy for a number of reasons.

● *Potential investigator bias.* Consciously or not, the investigator may determine which patients are included in the study and which therapy is given to individual patients. For example if he wants a new therapy to succeed, he may give it to less ill patients, exaggerating any benefits of therapy. Similarly, new surgical therapies may be introduced in "ideal" candidates who are likely to have better outcomes than other patients.

● *Predictable improvement over time.* Many acute diseases are self-limited, and many patients recover without therapy over time. Similarly, many chronic diseases are characterized by remissions and exacerbations and "apparent" improvement with therapy may reflect this variation. Some participants recruited because they have abnormal values for a variable under study may actually be normal individuals with chance deviations in results. Over time, their results may move back towards "normality", a statistical phenomenon known as "regression to the mean". In a before-after trial this improvement could be interpreted as a response to therapy.

● *Volunteerism.* People who volunteer for studies of new treatments may be systematically different from people who refuse consent; for example, they may be eager to please the researcher and more likely to report improvements in their symptoms.

Studies using historical controls

Some investigators use non-concurrent or historical control groups (i.e., patients who did not receive the therapy in the past) rather than concurrent controls (drawn from the same time and location as the therapy group). With this approach the benefits of therapy may be overestimated for a number of reasons:[19]

● Improvements in patient care (other than the therapy being tested) over time may lead to lower morbidity and mortality in the therapy group than in historical controls.

● Improvements in diagnostic tests may lead to earlier diagnosis and thus inclusion of healthier patients in the therapy group than in the historical control group.

● Psychological effects, such as the desire to please the investigator, may influence participant behavior in the therapy group and bias results.

● Disease virulence may decrease over time.

● Differences may exist between groups with regard to potential confounding variables, such as age, sex, or race.

Studies using concurrent non-randomized controls

The results of trials using concurrent but non-randomized controls may also be misleading. For example, there are potential differences in disease severity and medical care in controls recruited from different hospitals or even different wards in the same hospital. Within a given ward or hospital, patients whose clinicians choose to use one therapy are likely to differ from patients whose clinicians choose to use another therapy or no therapy. Equal distribution of unknown but potential confounders is very unlikely when subjects enter their groups by non-random allocation. Investigators interfering with treatment allocation may also introduce bias. Comparisons of treatment effects reported in randomized compared with non-randomized controlled trials is discussed in a systematic review by Kunz.[20] Failure of randomization resulted in large increases in estimates of treatment effects.

When differences in baseline characteristics between groups are apparent, statistical methods are often used to adjust for these differences (or confounders). However, adjustment can only be made for the factors that were recognized and adequately measured, and this information may be missing, especially for historical control groups. Thus, the clinician should be wary about the conclusions from studies using historical controls or concurrent non-randomized controls, even if such adjustments are made. For all of the above reasons, the findings of uncontrolled studies (studies with no control group) and those with non-randomized control groups may be strongly biased.

Randomized controlled trials

A randomized controlled trial is a trial in which participants are assigned to two (or more) therapy groups using a "formal chance" process and followed prospectively for the outcome of interest. In essence, each patient has the same chance as every other patient of being assigned to a particular group. RCTs incorporating a concurrent control group are the "ideal" study type to minimize bias in the evaluation of a therapy. Randomization should ensure that the distribution of potential confounders (both known and unknown) is equal between groups. However, poor quality RCTs may be subject to bias if insufficient attention is paid to the method of randomization; the concealment of allocation to groups; blinding of participants, investigators, and study assessors to therapy allocation; the methods of assessment and analysis of results; and the proportion of participants who complete the study.

The process of critical appraisal addresses each of these criteria (see below). Many published trials (and particularly older trials) do not explicitly report these important threats to validity (such as the method of randomization or whether there was allocation concealment). As discussed above, use of the CONSORT reporting method will make this information more easily accessible to the reader. When assessing RCT quality, some authors advocate the use of an overall quality score and many scoring methods have been proposed. However, correlation between these scoring systems is poor[21,22] and summary scores do not specifically identify the strengths or weaknesses of a RCT. Thus, many authors of systematic reviews for example, state the individual quality characteristics of a trial rather than give the trial an overall score.

Searching for an article on therapy

A guide to searching the literature is provided in Chapter 3. A few points should be reiterated with regard to searching for articles on therapy. As a busy clinician you should first look for summarized (synthesized) or secondary evidence (for example, systematic reviews of RCTs) before searching MedLine, Embase, and other databases for primary evidence (for example, RCTs) about a therapy. The *Cochrane Library* is the best single source of articles to guide therapy. In Issue 3 of 2003, 1754 completed reviews (and 1304 protocols) were listed in the Cochrane Database of Systematic Reviews, and 4123 reviews were included in the Database of Abstracts of Reviews of Effects. Over 378 000 clinical trials (many of them RCTs) were listed in the Cochrane Central Register of Controlled Trials (CENTRAL).

Apart from the *Cochrane Library*, there is an increasing number of sources of good quality summarized evidence on therapy. These include the BMJ publication *Clinical Evidence* (http://www.clinicalevidence.com) and related sites *Best Treatments* (http://www.besttreatments.org) and *Best Bets* (www.bestbets.org). In addition, journals such as *Evidence-Based Medicine* (http://ebm. bmjjournals.com), *ACP Journal Club* (http://www.ACPJC. org) and its electronic version *Best Evidence* (http://www.bestevidence. org) provide critical summaries of individual journal articles that are considered to be methodologically sound. Unfortunately evidence relating to child health is underrepresented in all of these sources.

Case scenario (continued)

Because you know that the Cochrane Library is a rich source of systematic reviews on neonatal therapies, you first go there and search for an article on "palivizumab" therapy for prevention of RSV infection in infants born preterm. You find one completed review that was last updated in 2001.[23] In this review, the results from one trial of palivizumab are combined with the results from three trials of polyclonal antibody. You decide to use PubMed to search for original articles evaluating the specific effects of palivizumab. Using the "Clinical Queries" function, you search for "palivizumab" and locate 17 articles. Only two of these are original reports of randomized trials, one in infants with congenital heart disease and one in preterm infants published in Pediatrics.[24] You read the latter paper to appraise its quality to see whether the therapy is useful and whether the findings are applicable to your patient. You use the criteria included in the User's Guides to the Medical Literature that explain how to determine whether the results of a study about therapy are valid[11] and whether they will help you in caring for your patient.[12]

Critical appraisal of randomized controlled trials

The assessment of an RCT involves three steps. First, you need to decide whether the trial is valid. This will depend on the type of study, the study design, and the way the data are analyzed. Then, you need to determine whether the results are important by looking at the size of the effect of the therapy. Finally you need to decide whether the trial results are applicable to your patients and whether you will use the therapy. The criteria below derive from articles published in the *Users' Guides to the Medical Literature*.[11,12] They provide a useful checklist for the critical appraisal of an RCT.

Critical appraisal criteria[11,12]

Study design

- Were patients randomized to therapy groups?
- Was therapy allocation adequately concealed?
- Were there eligible patients who were not enrolled?
- Were patients, health workers, and study personnel "blind" to therapy?
- Was sample size adequate?

Data analysis

- Were groups similar at the start of the trial?
- Were groups treated equally during the trial?

- How complete was follow up?
- Were patients analyzed in the groups to which they were randomized (intention-to-treat analysis)?
- Was unplanned interim analysis and "data dredging" avoided?

Reporting of results

- How large was the therapy effect?
- How precise was the estimate of therapy effect?
- How complete was study reporting?

Application of study findings

- Were all clinically important outcomes considered?
- Do the therapy benefits outweigh the potential harms?
- Can the results be applied to patients in my care?

Study design

Randomization

Randomization of patients to therapy groups should ensure that each child recruited to a study has an independent, fixed and equal chance of inclusion in each group. One group (the experimental, intervention, or therapy group) receives the therapy that is being tested and the other (the comparison or control group) receives either a placebo or an alternative therapy (usually the current best therapy). Randomization minimizes the risk of selection bias because the distribution of both known and unknown confounders should be similar in each group. The randomization process should be explicitly stated and must be truly random (for example, the use of a computer-generated random sequence or a random numbers table). Randomization may be simple (analogous to tossing a coin) or may involve a method, such as use of random permuted blocks, to ensure that large unintended disparities in the number of enrolled subjects do not occur between therapy groups. The size of groups need not be equal. For example, patients may be randomized to the experimental and comparison groups in the ratio of 2:1. In clinical trials individuals, sides of the body, wards, hospitals, schools, or places of work may be randomized.

- *Stratified randomization* can be used to ensure equal distribution of participants with certain known or suspected prognostic characteristics (for example, disease severity, age) to intervention and control groups. This is particularly important in trials with a small sample size, in which random allocation can result in differences between groups occurring by chance. Failure to stratify may complicate data analysis in small randomized trials.
- *Quasi-randomization* refers to non-random methods of allocating patients to a therapy group. An example is alternating allocation of patients seen in clinic to the experimental and control group. Other examples include allocation to a therapy based on the patient's medical record number or date of birth, or the day of the week that they were seen in the clinic. Quasi-randomization methods may inadvertently introduce selection bias into a trial since group assignment is predictable and may influence who is recruited for the trial. For example, use of birth dates may mean that the treatment groups differ by age. Study investigators need to be vigilant to the fact that "humans, if given the opportunity, frequently subvert the intended aims of randomization".[25]

Failure to randomize patients may influence the validity of trial results. Chalmers[26] and others[19] have shown that the effects of a therapy are overestimated in non-randomized compared with randomized trials.

Allocation concealment

If the investigator is aware of the group into which the next (or any particular) patient will be allocated, he or she may selectively recruit patients for the study. At the extreme, envelopes containing the therapy allocation (as generated centrally by the computer) may be steamed open and a patient's group assignment may be swapped with another by the treating clinician. Even if group allocation is not changed, knowledge of the therapy that a patient is to receive may influence patient management or assessment and may affect whether the patient is enrolled in the study, resulting in selection bias. Thus, the "allocation" of study participants to therapy groups must be adequately "concealed" from the individual responsible for enrolling the patient.

One way of achieving allocation concealment is to keep the randomization list in a central location removed from enrolment sites. In an individual center, the pharmacy is often used this way. Centralized randomization in a multicenter study ensures that the treating pediatrician will not be aware of the randomization sequence, and thus will not be able to predict or alter patient assignment, whether consciously or subconsciously. The importance of allocation concealment has been demonstrated.[27,28] The benefits of therapy are overestimated by about 30–40% in trials with inadequate allocation concealment, compared with trials in which there was adequate concealment.

Eligible non-enrolled subjects

According to the CONSORT guidelines, an account should be made of all eligible subjects, including those who are not enrolled in the study. The reasons for non-enrolment should be given along with clinical baseline and outcome data as feasible. This allows the reader to judge whether the study subjects were representative of subjects defined by the study's eligibility criteria.

Case scenario (continued) *In the palivizumab trial, there is no description of eligible non-enrolled patients and the progress of participants is not reported according to the CONSORT guidelines. Inclusion and exclusion criteria were clearly stated: 1502 children who were either born premature (≤ 35 weeks) or had bronchopulmonary dysplasia (BPD) requiring ongoing medical treatment were randomized in a 2:1 treatment:control ratio. Allocation concealment was ensured by use of a central telephone registration system.*

Blinding

Blinding (or masking) is a method used to deny study participants, investigators, or assessors access to any information that might influence measurement, observation, or management and thus introduce bias. Unblinded trials are usually easier to conduct than blinded trials. In RCTs the reporting of blinding is variable. Some authors report on single, double, or triple blinding. However, when this terminology is used it is often impossible to know who was actually blinded – the patient or parent, investigator, or assessor. For this reason, it is preferable to state explicitly who was blinded.[29]

Blinding is important because patients who think they are receiving an active treatment do better than patients who think they are receiving an inactive treatment or placebo. Blinding is crucial for therapy trials in which outcomes of importance are subjective and open to interpretation (for example, reporting of symptoms, mood, and adverse effects of therapy). Recording of these outcomes may be variable, depending on the assessors' inherent biases and influenced by the assessors' knowledge of the patient's therapy. Blinding is less important in therapy trials in which the primary, and perhaps only, outcome of interest is something as obvious as death. Even if the outcome is objectively measured (such as blood pressure), failure to blind the assessor to the therapy that the child received may lead to misinterpretation or misrepresentation of the measure. In a well-designed trial, participants, care givers, investigators, and assessors should all be "blinded" or unaware of the therapy that participants received.

Adequate blinding is most often achieved in drug trials, in which the experimental therapy is compared with a placebo that is identical in taste, appearance, and smell. Therapies are allocated centrally and dispensed in identical containers with coding that cannot be broken. Care must be taken to ensure that the placebo cannot be distinguished from the active drug.

Some investigators use methods to ensure that the placebo mimics the active therapy, including pretesting of compounds by blinded panels.

Investigators can bias study outcomes by changing the participant's group assignment or excluding the participant from the study. Depending on the investigator's conscious or unconscious views about the trial, the therapy and control groups may be treated and assessed differently, leading to results that may be biased in either direction. For example, unblinded investigators might look more carefully for either *adverse* or *beneficial* effects of a therapy in participants in the experimental therapy arm. Unblinded clinicians may also use other therapies more aggressively if they are aware that the subject is in the control group.

It may be impossible to blind investigators or care givers to the allocation of participants, for example in trials of a surgical procedure. This can be partly overcome by ensuring that outcome assessors and patients are blinded to the therapy. "Sham" operations are sometimes used to blind participants to their surgical versus non-surgical therapy. Although this may appear unethical to some, many clinicians feel that it is important to use whatever means are required to establish the true value of an intervention. Sometimes it is difficult to blind participants to their therapy – for example, in a comparison of intravenous versus oral rehydration. In this situation, studies blinding the investigator or assessor to the therapy that the patient received are better than completely unblinded studies.

There is evidence that lack of blinding can influence study results. For example, some participants in a trial of vitamin C versus placebo for therapy of the common cold became aware of their therapy. Vitamin C was found to be beneficial in participants who were aware that they received vitamin C but not in those who were blinded to their therapy.[30] Trials that are not adequately blinded, compared with those that are, exaggerate the effectiveness of a therapy.[28] The success of blinding can be assessed after trial completion by asking participants and investigators to guess their group assignment.

Case scenario (continued) *In the palivizumab trial, placebo administration (equal volume and identical appearance to the palivizumab) was used to blind the subjects, their parents, care givers, and investigators. The drug or placebo was given by intramuscular injection every 30 days for a total of five doses during the RSV season. While this placebo-controlled design is ideal for minimizing observer bias and differences in patient management, in this particular case, it also introduces the possibility that the rate of RSV infection was artificially increased (above what it would have been in an untreated control group) by requiring extra visits to the clinic or doctor's office.*

Sample size and power

Determination of sample size and/or study power is important for any RCT and should be performed before the study commences. The power of a study is a measure of its ability to reliably detect a clinically important difference between two therapies if a difference actually exists. Concluding "there is no difference" when a difference truly exists is termed a beta or type II error. Power (defined as 1 − beta) is a function of sample size. Researchers should aim for a sample size that will provide a power of ≥ 80% to detect a significant difference (usually $P < 0.05$) in outcome between groups. Inadequate sample size is a common problem in RCTs and may result in a true difference being missed. In one review it was reported that sample size was inadequate in 94% of 71 RCTs in which there was no statistically significant difference between interventions.[31] These RCTs were too small to detect moderate (25%) or large (50%) differences between therapy groups. Small studies with inadequate power continue to be published.[32]

The same principles apply to analysis of subgroups within trials, in which the subgroup size is too small to reliably detect a true difference between subgroups. For example, in one RCT, subgroup analysis suggested that antenatal steroids were ineffective for preventing respiratory distress syndrome in male infants.[33] This was later refuted by a meta-analysis that showed the benefits were equal in males and females when groups were of sufficient sample size.[34] Sample size also influences the precision of a result – the larger the sample size the greater the precision (as indicated by small confidence intervals). On the other hand, a very large sample size may result in a statistically significant difference in outcomes between therapy groups even when the magnitude of the difference is not clinically important. The NNT can be used to evaluate the clinical importance of the treatment effect.

Case scenario (continued)	*In the palivizumab trial, no information is given regarding sample size calculation, interim analyses, or stopping rules for the study. However, the sample size is large enough to allow for fairly precise estimates of the treatment effect. The relative risk of hospitalization with RSV infection in the palivizumab compared with the placebo group was RR − 0·45 (95% CI 0·28, 0·62).*

Data analysis

Baseline characteristics

The aim of randomization is to distribute known and unknown confounding variables equally between study groups. A confounding variable is a factor that may distort the relationship between the therapy being tested and the outcome of interest. For example, gestational age at birth, the use of day care, smoking in the house, or a family history of asthma may affect the risk of RSV infection. The "success" of randomization can be judged by looking at the similarity of the characteristics of groups after randomization at the start of the trial *(baseline characteristics)*. In most reports of RCTs, the baseline characteristics (for example, age, sex, disease severity, co-morbidity, results of laboratory and other tests) are included in Table 1 of the article. Differences between groups may be due to chance alone; however, differences may also reflect problems with the method of randomization (for example, lack of stratification or allocation concealment) and may introduce bias. If there are differences in the baseline characteristics between groups that are judged to be important, then appropriate statistical tests can be used to adjust for these differences, or potential confounders. These tests require input from a statistician and include analysis of co-variance or multiple linear regression (for continuous outcomes such as height or blood pressure) or multiple logistic regression (for binary outcomes such as dead or alive). Some statisticians suggest that such adjustments are inappropriate in randomized trials because they undermine the effect of randomization with respect to equal distribution of *unmeasured* baseline characteristics.

Case scenario (continued)	*In the palivizumab trial, the baseline characteristics shown in Table 1 are similar between the study groups and include all of the most likely confounders. Of the 15 baseline characteristics compared in this table, only "No smoker in household" is significantly different between the groups (there were more smokers in the palivizumab group). With the number of comparisons made, it is likely that this difference could have occurred by chance.*

Additional therapy during the trial

It is important to establish that groups receive similar treatment during the study, so that the only difference between groups is whether or not they receive the therapy being tested. If patients in different groups are managed differently, a statistically significant difference between the groups could be observed even if the therapy is ineffective. As outlined previously, adequate blinding will reduce the chance that the study groups are consciously or unconsciously treated differently by clinical personnel.

Case scenario (continued)	*The primary outcome reported in the palivizumab trial is the proportion of infants hospitalized with RSV. A standardized definition of hospitalization with RSV was used and included confirmation of the diagnosis with an RSV antigen test. Clinical management, including the decision to hospitalize, was left to the discretion of the clinicians caring for the patients. Blinding of the care givers, if effective, makes it unlikely that important differences in management occurred in this trial.*

Completeness of follow up

Every participant should be accounted for at the end of a trial. Withdrawal of patients from a trial or loss to follow up may invalidate trial results because patients lost to follow up may differ systematically from those who completed the trial. For example, participants may be lost from a trial because they did well and did not return for assessment. Conversely they may have done poorly and sought therapy elsewhere. Some patients lost to follow up may even have died. The CONSORT guidelines acknowledge the importance of follow up and suggest that reports of RCTs include a flow diagram that clearly shows the outcome of each participant. A follow up rate of $\geq 80\%$ is considered satisfactory.[10] Even higher follow up rates are needed in studies of rare outcomes. If loss to follow up is $> 20\%$ then the trial results may differ from the true results. In trials in which $\geq 20\%$ of participants are lost to follow up, a worst-case and best-case analysis of the data can be performed.[11] In doing this, you assume that all patients lost in the therapy arm failed therapy and that all those lost in the control arm did well and re-analyze the data to see if this changes the conclusions of the study. Similarly you could assume that all patients lost in the therapy arm did well and that all those lost in the control arm did badly.

Case scenario (continued)	*Of the 1502 infants randomized in the palivizumab trial, 16 (1%) of the patients did not complete the protocol follow up period of 150 days (seven died, four withdrew consent, and five were lost to follow up.) Longer-term follow up for assessment of reactive airway disease would have been valuable but was not undertaken.*

Intention-to-treat analysis

The way in which data from RCTs are analyzed can bias trial results. For example, inclusion only of data from participants who actually received the prescribed therapy ignores the original random allocation of participants to therapy groups (designed to ensure that patient groups are similar at baseline) and may invalidate the results. Analysis of this type determines the *efficacy* of a therapy (whether a therapy works under ideal or restricted circumstances), for example, in participants well enough or compliant enough to have *received* the therapy. In contrast, in an intention-to-treat analysis, data from all randomized participants are analyzed according to the therapy group to which they were originally allocated, even if they did not receive the therapy (for example, they dropped out of the trial, had intolerable side effects, were non-compliant with therapy, or changed to the comparison therapy). This is important because patients who are compliant have better outcomes than non-compliant patients, even if they receive a placebo.[35] Patients who withdraw from a trial are likely to differ systematically from patients who complete a trial.[10] Intention-to-treat analysis is the accepted way to analyze data in RCTs. It measures the *effectiveness* of a therapy, that is, whether the therapy works in those to whom it was *offered*. This more accurately reflects the real world situation. The disadvantage of intention-to-treat analysis is that clinically important differences may be missed if large numbers of participants change groups, drop out, or fail to comply with their assigned therapy. In this situation the results will be biased towards the null hypothesis and may fail to show a real difference between groups when a difference exists.

Case scenario (continued)

In addition to the 16 patients who did not complete the protocol follow up, 6% of the placebo group and 8% of the treatment group did not receive all the scheduled study injections. As is appropriate in an intention-to-treat analysis, the partially treated infants were included in the analysis. It appears that the infants who died or withdrew were also included in the analysis; the appropriateness of this is unclear since these infants were not evaluated fully for the primary outcome.

Interim analysis

Interim analysis of trial data should be avoided unless it is planned at the outset of the trial and "stopping rules" are clearly stated.[10] In most clinical trials, we accept a 5% chance ($P < 0.05$) that we will falsely conclude that "there is a difference" between the groups when there is truly no difference (termed an alpha or type I error). The problem with multiple interim analyses is that a statistically significant difference between therapies is very likely to be found by chance at some point *during* the trial, even if it is not found at the *completion* of the trial. The likelihood of finding a difference increases with each interim analysis if appropriate statistical adjustments in the P value are not made. Trials with a small sample size should not be analyzed or stopped until the full sample has been recruited. For example, if a trial is stopped because an interim analysis suggests an outcome is worse in the therapy group, then the results of the trial may be invalid and a larger RCT will be needed to definitively answer the question. In large trials, interim analysis may be planned to allow for detection of either adverse effects or larger than expected beneficial effects of a therapy. In this case only interim results that are highly significant should be accepted. Some trials include a provision for stopping if the interim effect size is large and the precision of the result is high.

Case scenario (continued)

Although the subject is not clearly addressed in the manuscript, there appear to have been no interim analyses. It seems unlikely that interim analyses were undertaken because enrolment occurred over a 1-month period and outcomes were not determined until 150 days after enrolment. The stopping rules were not specified in the manuscript.

Data dredging

"Data dredging" should also be avoided during analysis. The problems associated with not identifying a primary study outcome and performing multiple statistical tests on a range of secondary outcomes are discussed above. In summary, the more tests you do, the more likely you are to find at least one statistically significant result by chance.[10] If 20 comparisons are made, the probability of finding at least one P value of < 0.05 is much greater than 5%, being $1 - (1 - 0.05).^{20}$ Thus, there is a 64% chance that at least one of these comparisons will show a statistically significant difference between groups even if no true difference exists.[10] In one small trial[36] evaluating the effect of a topical emollient on transepidermal water loss in 60 preterm infants, at least 20 secondary outcomes were evaluated. Infants in whom the emollient was used had lower rates of sepsis (positive blood and CSF cultures). However, sepsis had not been identified as the primary outcome at the outset of the study. In a subsequent large RCT (n = 1191)[37] designed to evaluate the effect of the emollients on nosocomial sepsis as the *primary* outcome, the finding was not confirmed. Indeed in the second trial the rate of sepsis was higher in the therapy than the control group.

Subgroup analysis can result in a similar problem. For example, when a trial is completed investigators sometimes put participants into "new" subgroups (for example, on the basis of age or sex) to allow for comparisons between the study groups that were not originally proposed. Randomization is lost in this process and investigators make multiple statistical comparisons that were not originally planned, increasing the risk of finding statistically significant differences purely by chance. As a rule of thumb, if the primary outcome is not statistically significant between the original therapy groups, it is best to regard significant findings in secondary outcomes or subgroup analyses as hypotheses for testing in future studies rather than results.

Case scenario (continued)

Although not explicitly stated, the planned primary outcome in the palivizumab trial appears to have been the proportion of infants hospitalized for RSV infection. Multiple subgroup analyses, based on primary diagnosis (prematurity or BPD), weight, and gestational age at birth, and analyses of secondary efficacy endpoints (days of hospitalization, days of increased supplemental oxygen, rates of ICU admission, and mechanical ventilation) were evaluated. It is not clear whether these secondary hypotheses were predetermined and whether additional analyses were undertaken but not reported.

Table 6.1 A 2 × 2 table identifying children with an adverse outcome in treatment and control groups

| | | Adverse outcome | | |
		Present (case)	Absent (control)	Totals
Treatment (intervention)	Yes (treatment group)	a	b	a + b
	No (control group)	c	d	c + d
Totals		a + c	b + d	a+b+c+d

Reporting study results

Clinicians need to understand the way in which results are expressed statistically in RCTs before they can apply findings to their clinical practice. The size of the effect of a therapy and the precision of the estimate of that effect are both important. The effect of a therapy may be presented as the relative risk, risk reduction, relative risk reduction, or odds ratio of an outcome. The number needed to treat (to prevent an outcome) or to harm (to result in an adverse effect of treatment) may also be reported. The statistical significance of a difference in outcomes between groups may be expressed as a *P* value. The precision of a result is usually indicated by a confidence interval around the point estimate of the size of the effect.

When appraising a paper it is often helpful to insert the numbers of participants with an outcome into a 2 × 2 table (Table 6.1) because this facilitates calculation of the estimate of effects. The definitions of some commonly used statistical measures of effect and statistical terms are shown in Tables 6.2 and 6.3.

Effect size

"Effect size" has been used as a technical term, defined as the mean difference divided by the standard deviation.

More often, the term is less technically used to describe the size or magnitude of the therapeutic effect. The size of the effect needs to be presented clearly so that the clinician can make an informed decision about the usefulness of a therapy. Even if the difference in outcome in groups receiving an experimental and comparison therapy is statistically significant (usually defined as $P \leq 0.05$, or no greater than a 1 in 20 chance that the result is due to chance alone), you may decide that the effect is of no clinical importance. For example, a reduction of 0·3 days in average hospital stay might be statistically significant but not clinically important enough to justify a very expensive, unpleasant, or risky intervention. In contrast, a relatively modest reduction in mortality or risk of developing asthma would be a clinically significant benefit even if the therapy were expensive.

The way in which study results are presented to patients and their care givers is important (see Chapter 14). For example, some patients will understand an absolute risk and risk reduction more easily than a relative risk or relative risk reduction. For most people, perhaps with the exception of gamblers, risks are easier to understand than odds.

Case scenario (continued)

In the palivizumab trial, the absolute risk of RSV hospitalization was 48/1002 (4·8%) in the palivizumab group and 53/400 (10·6%) in the control group. The relative risk was 0·45, the relative risk reduction was 55%, and the risk difference (absolute risk reduction) was 5·8%. Using the baseline risk data from the patients enrolled in the trial, the NNT was 1/0·058 = 17.

Precision of estimates of therapy effect

The result of the study – the estimate of the therapeutic effect – is a "point estimate." The *P* value establishes a statistical significance between estimates in groups, usually considered to be significant if $P < 0.05$. The confidence interval gives the reader additional information about the precision of the estimate. Both pieces of information are required to assess the result. The 95% confidence interval (CI) is most often reported

and can be defined as the range of results that would be obtained 95% of the time if the trial were repeated many times. However, other intervals (for example, the 90% CI are sometimes reported). A CI can be calculated for any measure of the difference between groups (for example, risk difference, relative risk, odds ratio, or the difference between means or medians). As the sample size of a study increases, the estimate of effect becomes more precise, the CI narrows, and the point estimate becomes closer to the "truth." If there is no significant

Table 6.2 Some statistical measures used to express the effect of an intervention in trials with binary outcomes

Measure	Definition	Formula
Relative risk (RR)	Relative risk (RR) is the ratio of the risk (event rate) in the intervention *v* control groups. The RR is also known as the risk ratio or event rate ratio	$RR = (a/[a+b])/(c/[c+d])$
	If the therapy has no effect, the RR = 1. If the therapy decreases the event rate the RR < 1. If the CI of the RR crosses 1, then the therapy effect observed is not statistically significant	
	The RR provides clinicians with information about the relative proportion of patients in the intervention group and control group experiencing an outcome	
	The RR provides no information about the event rates or the absolute difference (magnitude) in event rates in intervention and control groups	
Relative risk reduction (RRR)	Relative risk reduction is the percentage reduction in events in the intervention group compared with the control group	$RRR = 1 - RR$ $RRR = 1 - (a/[a+b])/(c/[c+d])$
	The relative risk reduction can be misleading because it does not take into account the baseline risk of an event in groups. The RRR may be similar in two studies even if there is a large difference in absolute risk difference	
	RRR is larger than ARR, so RRR is sometimes used misleadingly, e.g., in advertising the effectiveness of a medication	
Risk difference (RD) or absolute risk reduction or increase (ARR/ARI)	The difference in risk of an outcome between the intervention and control groups (either an increase or decrease). The RD is an absolute value that is easy to calculate and to understand. The RD takes into account the baseline risk of the event in the study participants. The inverse of the RD is the number needed to treat	$RD = (c/[c+d]) - (a/[a+b])$
Number needed to treat (or harm)	The number of patients you would need to treat to see the benefit (or harm) of a therapy in one additional patient	$NNT = 1/RD$ or $1/ARR$ (or $1/ARI$)
	Risk difference between the control and intervention group (and thus NNT) depends on the baseline risks of an outcome in the patient population. If baseline risk is lower (RD smaller), NNT increases. When considering whether a therapy effect is clinically important, the NNT must be weighed against the risks and costs of the therapy	
Odds ratio (OR)	The ratio of the odds of an outcome occurring in the intervention group and the control group. If there is no difference in outcome between intervention and control groups, the OR = 1. Conventionally, for adverse outcomes eg death a favorable effect of the intervention is represented by an OR < 1 and an OR > 1 favors the control. Conversely, if the outcome is beneficial (e.g., pregnancy in infertile couples) a favorable outcome is represented by an OR > 1. The OR should be given with a 95% CI. If the CI crosses 1, then there is no statistically significant difference between groups. The OR is not easily interpreted in the clinical setting and it is often misinterpreted or mistaken for a relative risk. Only when events rates are low (the outcome is rare) can OR can be used as an estimate of the RR	$OR = (a/b)/(c/d)$

difference between groups in a trial and the CI is wide, this suggests that the study is too small to detect a clinically important effect from therapy. Conversely, if the confidence intervals are narrow and the difference between groups is not significant, the reader can be more certain that the therapy is not likely to be beneficial. The limits of the 95% CI can be thought of as the most extreme values that are plausible point estimates of the therapeutic effect.

Case scenario (continued)	*The 95% CI for the 0·45 relative risk is (0·28, 0·62). A 95% CI of (11, 36) can also be calculated for the NNT of 17.[38] These relatively narrow CIs signify good precision for these estimates and result from the large number of patients enrolled in this trial.*

Table 6.3 Commonly used statistical terms

P value	The P value quantifies the probability that an observed difference between two groups of subjects could have occurred by chance. By convention if $P < 0.05$, the difference between two groups is "statistically significant" and unlikely to have occurred by chance
Confidence interval (95% CI)	For clinical purposes, the 95% CI can be viewed as the range of results within which you can be 95% confident that the real value lies. The CI gives an indication of the precision of a result. Generally the larger the sample size, the smaller the CI

Completeness of reporting

Even well designed and well conducted trials will be less likely to be accepted if they are poorly reported since the reader will be unable to determine their validity. The CONSORT initiative[6] is an evidence-based approach to help improve RCT reporting by guiding both authors and reviewers. The CONSORT statement, consisting of a checklist and flow diagram, includes many items for which there is empirical evidence that failure to report could result in bias in the estimates of the effects of interventions. These include method of randomization, allocation concealment, blinding, and completeness of follow up. Although CONSORT is an evolving tool that will be revised as new empirical evidence becomes available, use of the statement already appears to increase the completeness of RCT reporting.[39]

Case scenario (continued)	*Many of the CONSORT criteria were followed in the reporting of this trial. Baseline characteristics of patients were included in Table 1. Outcomes were reported as event rates in therapy and control groups. A flow diagram indicating the progress of patients in the trial was not included. Some important information was omitted from the methods, including a clear statement of primary and secondary outcomes, planned secondary analyses, prospectively defined stopping rules, and information regarding eligible patients that were not enrolled and the reasons for non-enrolment. The importance of the latter will be addressed below.*

Application of study findings

Outcomes considered

A good RCT will include all clinically important (rather than proxy) outcomes. For example, when evaluating a therapy for respiratory infection, clinicians and their patients will be more interested in the rates and duration of hospital stay than the mean or maximum Fio_2 required during the hospitalization. In a well-designed trial, the outcomes of interest should be identified and explicitly stated in the planning stage and the primary outcome should be identified.

Benefits versus harms

In any RCT both the benefits and harms (including the cost) of a therapy should be evaluated. Evaluating the risks of a treatment is often problematic because the sample size in RCTs is often insufficient to detect rare adverse outcomes.[14] It may be necessary to seek information from case series, cohorts, and case–control studies in order to estimate the risk of relatively rare adverse events. As discussed above, the NNT is based on the absolute risk reduction, which depends on the subject's (or your patient's) baseline risk for developing the outcome. If your patient's baseline risk differs from the study population, your patient's baseline risk without therapy can be obtained from other cohort studies. If the relative risk reduction is assumed to stay the same for all baseline risks, the NNT can be calculated for your patient. If the risk of harm from the therapy is assumed to stay constant (these assumptions should be verified), the net benefit for a given patient can be calculated.

The number needed to treat (or harm) can be a useful way of expressing the balance between benefits and risks of a therapy. A therapy with a large NNT would only be worthwhile if the outcome prevented is important and the therapy is relatively cheap and very safe. Even if the NNT is small for a therapy, the decision to use that therapy will also require consideration of its cost and the potential for adverse effects. For example, if the NNT = 3 for 5-year survival after a liver transplant for a certain disease, this means that for every three patients transplanted, a beneficial outcome (survival) will be seen in one additional patient. However, this therapy is extremely expensive and is associated with risks of anesthesia, surgery, immunosuppression, and graft versus host disease. In this situation the clinician must, with the patient, weigh the benefits against the harms of therapy. Methods have been proposed to help clinicians decide when an effective therapy should be used.[14,40]

Application to my patients

An important consideration for the reader is whether the results of the RCT can be applied to patients outside the trial setting. Ideally, the observations made in the participants in a trial will be generalizable to other populations of interest. However, even when two groups are randomly chosen from the same population, there are likely to be differences because of random sampling variation, or chance.[10] When study subjects are not randomly selected from a population (described by the study eligibility criteria), study subjects may differ in important ways from the target population for the intervention. Thus even if an RCT is internally valid (well designed to answer the research question), its external validity, or generalizability, may be difficult to interpret. If the study patients differ considerably from those in your practice, a good approach is to ask whether there is some clear reason why, despite the differences, the findings cannot be applied to your patients.[12] The ability to use a therapy in clinical and research settings may also vary. For example, levels of compliance achieved in a trial setting may not be feasible in reality, and therapeutic success may be less impressive in the real world. Assessing the applicability of study findings is considered further in Chapter 17.

Application of evidence to the case scenario

Because there is no information given in the palivizumab trial about eligible non-enrolled patients, it is impossible to determine whether the sample of enrolled patients is representative of typical patients born at ≤ 35 weeks gestation or with BPD requiring treatment. In a large cohort study of unselected infants enrolled in a healthcare plan[41] the baseline risk (without treatment) of RSV hospitalization in infants born preterm at 23–32 weeks gestation, requiring oxygen treatment for < 28 days, and discharged outside the RSV season was 3%. (The risk might be even lower for an infant born at 31 weeks than for the group of infants born between 23–32 weeks.) If you assume that palivizumab would provide the same relative benefit (RR = 0·45) for such an infant as for infants in the trial, the ARR would be 0·03–(0·45 × 0·03) = 0·0165 (1·65%) and the NNT would be 1/0·0165 = 61. The reported frequency of adverse effects from palivizumab was very low in this trial.

However, you would also need to consider the cost and inconvenience of the therapy for 61 infants against the cost and suffering associated with one hospitalization for RSV.

You discuss the benefits and risks of palivizumab with the mother of the infant described in the case scenario. She is reluctant to subject her child to five intramuscular injections. She also says she lives a long way from the clinic, has no car and has another young child. Together you make a decision not to treat because the infant's risk of getting severe bronchiolitis is low and there would be considerable inconvenience associated with treatment.

Conclusions

Information on the beneficial and adverse effects of any new therapy should be based on good quality RCTs or systematic reviews. These study types minimize the chance that bias will influence the assessment of a therapy. Pediatricians should support the conduct of RCTs in children so that we are not forced to rely on data generated in adults. Systematic reviews of studies in children should be conducted and in reviews including both adults and children, child participants should be identified. Pediatric journals should ensure that RCTs submitted for publication are reported in the format stipulated in the CONSORT statement. This will educate readers about the qualities of a good RCT and will encourage researchers to consider the CONSORT checklist when planning a trial. Pediatricians need to be aware that the quality of RCTs is variable and that inadequate study design or inappropriate data analysis may influence trial results. They should therefore develop the skills required to critically appraise RCTs of new therapies and to decide whether trial results are applicable to their clinical setting. When reading the report of a trial, clinicians should also be aware that there is potential for publication bias, for example, trials reporting negative findings are less likely to be published (Chapter 1). Even when a new therapy is shown to be beneficial in a good quality trial, there may be considerable barriers to the use of that therapy, not least of which is resistance to change in both attitudes and clinical practices.

Take home list

- Questions of therapy arise more frequently than other foreground clinical questions.
- Randomized controlled trials or systematic reviews of RCTs provide the best (most unbiased) evidence about a therapy.
- Study validity depends on the study type and the quality of the methods and the analyses.

- Unbiased assessment of the effects of therapy requires comparison of groups with similar baseline risk of adverse outcome.
- Groups selected from different places or at different times, or selected systematically by investigators, often differ in baseline risk. This may lead to biased estimates of therapy effect.
- Random allocation leads to groups that differ on baseline risk only by chance.
- Allocation to groups should be adequately concealed from investigators or they may subvert randomization and preferentially allocate some types of participant to one therapy.
- Ideally, participants, investigators and outcome assessors should be "blind" to therapy allocation. This is particularly important for assessors when outcome measures are subjective.
- The primary outcome for an RCT should be clearly stated and should be clinically important.
- Follow up of over 80% of participants in an RCT is desirable.
- Participants should be analyzed in the groups to which they are originally allocated, regardless of whether they comply with therapy (intention-to-treat analysis). This maintains the balance of baseline risk achieved by randomization.
- The effects of treatment can be presented as a relative risk, relative risk difference, number needed to treat or odds ratio.
- The size and precision of the effect of a treatment is important. A statistically significant effect may be of no clinical significance.
- An imprecise estimate of treatment effect may fail to exclude a clinically important difference.
- The study size (and power) should be estimated at the study outset. Underpowered studies may be too small to detect an important difference between therapies.
- The applicability of trial results to other populations depends on the characteristics of that population, including their baseline risk for adverse outcomes without treatment.
- Any treatment decision should be made jointly with the patient or caregiver after weighing the risks and benefits of treatment.

Acknowledgments

Parts of this chapter are based on the chapter on therapy that appeared in the first edition of this book:

- Slinger R, Moher D. Assessing therapy. In: Moyer VA, Elliott EJ, Davis RL *et al.*(eds). *Evidence Based Pediatrics and Child Health*. London: BMJ Books, 2000.

References

1 Smith R. What clinical information do doctors need? *BMJ* 1996;**313**:1062–8.

2 Badenoch D, Heneghan C. Levels of evidence and grades of recommendations. In: *Evidence-based medicine toolkit*. London: *BMJ* Books, 2002.

3 Sinclair JC, Haughton DE, Bracken MB, Horbar JD, Soll RF. Cochrane neonatal systematic reviews: a survey of the evidence for neonatal therapies. *Clin Perinatol* 2003;**30**: 285–304.

4 Moyer VA, Gist AK, Elliott EJ. Is the practice of paediatric inpatient medicine evidence-based? *J Paediatr Child Hlth* 2002;**38**:347–51.

5 Rudolf MCJ, Lyth N, Bundle A *et al.* A search for the evidence supporting community paediatric practice. *Arch Dis Child* 1999;**80**:257–61.

6 Begg CB, Cho MK, Horton R *et al.* Improving the quality of reporting of randomized controlled trials: the CONSORT statement. *JAMA* 1996;**276**:637–9.

7 Moher D, Schulz KF, Altman DG for the CONSORT group. The CONSORT statement: revised recommendations for improving the quality of reports of parallel-group randomised trials. *Lancet* 2001;**357**:1191–4.

8 Moher D, Jones A, Lepage L for the CONSORT Group. Use of the CONSORT statement and quality of reports of randomized trials: a comparative before and after evaluation. *JAMA* 2001;**285**:1992–5.

9 Egger M, Junni P, Bartlett C, CONSORT Group. Value of flow diagrams in reports of randomized controlled trials: bibliographic study. *JAMA* 2001;**285**:1996–9.

10 Kennedy KA, Frankowski RF. Evaluating the evidence about therapies. What the clinician needs to know about statistics. *Clin Perinatol* 2003;**30**:205–15.

11 Guyatt GH, Sackett DL, Cook DJ. Users' guides to the medical literature. II. How to use an article about therapy or prevention. Are the results of the study valid? Evidence-Based Medicine Working Group. *JAMA* 1993;**270**: 2598–601.

12 Guyatt GH, Sackett DL, Cook DJ. Users' guides to the medical literature. II. How to use an article about therapy or prevention. B. What were the results and will they help me in caring for my patients? Evidence-Based Medicine Working Group. *JAMA* 1994;**271**:59–63.

13 Irwig J, Irwig L, Sweet M. *Smart health choices: how to make informed health decisions.* Sydney: Allen & Unwin. 1999.

14 Glasziou PP, Irwig LM. An evidence-based approach to individualising therapy. *BMJ* 1995;**311**:1356–9.

15 Sackett DL, Haynes RB, Tugwell P. *Clinical epidemiology: a basic science for clinical medicine.* Boston: Little, Brown and Company, 1985.

16 Sackett DL. Bias in analytic research. *J Chronic Dis* 1979; **32**:51–63.

17 Cochrane Collaboration Handbook. www.cochrane.dk/ cochrane/handbook/sources of bias in trials of healthcare

18 Chalmers TC, Schroeder B. Controls in "Journal" articles. *N Engl J Med* 1979;**301**:1293.

19 Sacks H, Chalmers TC, Smith H Jr. Randomized versus historical controls for clinical trials. *Am J Med* 1982;**72**: 233–40.

20 Kunz R, Oxman AD. The unpredictability paradox: review of empirical comparisons of randomised and non-randomised clinical trials. *BMJ* 1998;**317**:1185–90.

21 Berlin JA, Rennie D. Measuring the quality of trials: the quality of quality scales. *JAMA* 1999;**282**:1083–5.

22 Juni P, Witschi A, Bloch R, Egger M. The hazards of scoring the quality of clinical trials for meta-analysis. *JAMA* 1999;**282**:1054–60.

23 Wang EEL, Tang NK. Immunoglobulin for preventing respiratory syncytial virus infection (Cochrane Review). In: Cochrane Collaboration. *Cochrane Library*. Issue 4. Oxford: Update Sofware, 2003.

24 The Impact-RSV Study Group. Palivizumab, a humanized respiratory syncytial virus monoclonal antibody, reduces hospitalization from respiratory syncytial virus infection in high-risk infant. *Pediatrics* 1998;**102**:531–7.

25 Schulz KF. Subverting randomization in controlled trials. *JAMA* 1995;**274**:1456–8.

26 Chalmers TC, Matta RJ, Smith J Jr, Kunzler AM. Evidence favoring the use of anticoagulants in the hospital phase of acute myocardial infarction. *N Engl J Med* 1977;**297**: 1091–6.

27 Moher D, Pham B, Jones A *et al.* Does quality of reports of randomised trials affect estimates of intervention efficacy reported in meta-analyses? *Lancet* 1998;**352**:609–13.

28 Schulz KF, Chalmers I, Hayes RJ, Altman DG. Empirical evidence of bias: dimensions of methodological quality associated with estimates of therapy effects in controlled trials. *JAMA* 1995;**273**:408–12.

29 Montori V, Bhandari M, Devereaux PJ *et al.* In the dark. The reporting of blinding in randomized controlled trials. *J Clin Epidemiol* 2002;**55**: 787–90.

30 Karlowski TR, Chalmers TC, Grenkel LD, Kapikian AZ, Lewis TL, Lynch JM. Ascorbic acid for the common cold: a prophylactic and therapeutic trial. *JAMA* 1975;**231**: 1038–42.

31 Freiman JA, Chalmers TC, Smith H Jr, Keubler RR. The importance of beta, the type II error, and sample size in the design and interpretation of the randomized controlled trial: survey of 71 "negative" trials. *N Engl J Med* 1978;**299**: 690–4.

32 Moher D, Dulberg CS, Wells GA. Statistical power, sample size, and their reporting in randomized controlled trials. *JAMA* 1994;**272**:122–4.

33 Collaborative Group on Antenatal Steroid Therapy. Effect of antenatal dexamethasone administration on the prevention of respiratory distress syndrome. *Am J Obstet Gynecol* 1981;**141**:276–87.

34 Crowley P. Prophylactic corticosteroids for preterm birth. In: Cochrane Collobration. *Cochrane Library*. Issue 3. Oxford: Update Software, 2002.

35 Coronary Drug Project Research Group. Influence of adherence to treatment and response of cholesterol on mortality in the coronary drug project. *N Engl J Med* 1980;**303**:1038–41.

36 Nopper AJ, Horii KA, Sookedeo-Drost S *et al.* Topical ointment therapy benefits preterm infants. *J Pediatr* 1996; **128**:660–9.

37 Edwards WH, Connor JM, Soll RF *et al.* for Vermont Oxford Network. The effect of Aquaphor original emollient ointment on nosocomial sepsis rates and skin integrity in infants of birthweight 501–1000 grams. *Pediatr Res* 2001; **49**:388A

38 Sackett DL, Straus SE, Richardson WS, Rosenberg W, Haynes RB. *Evidence-Based Medicine: How to Practice and Teach EBM, 2nd edn*. Edinburgh: Churchill Livingstone, 2000.

39 Moher D. CONSORT: an evolving tool to help improve the quality of reports of randomized controlled trials. Consolidated Standards of Reporting Tools. *JAMA* 1998; **279**:1489–91.

40 Sinclair JC, Cook RJ, Guyatt GH *et al.* When should an effective therapy be used? Derivation of the threshold number needed to treat and the minimum event rate for treatment. *J Clin Epidemiol* 2001;**54**:253–62.

41 Joffe S, Ray GT, Escobar GJ, Black SB, Lieu TA. Cost-effectiveness of respiratory syncytial virus prophylaxis among preterm infants. *Pediatrics* 1999;**104**:419–27.

7 Assessing claims of harm or causation

Parminder Raina, Kate Turcotte

Case scenario   *New parents arrive in your office with their infant son. They have brought an article that recently appeared in* Homemaker's *magazine[1] describing a case of serious neurologic injury sustained by a little girl as a result of routine vaccination. The parents are concerned that their son is at risk for a severe reaction to the DTP vaccine. They are aware that vaccination is not mandatory in Canada, and have heard that whooping cough is no longer a disease that needs to be inoculated against. Although you generally believe that the benefits of vaccination outweigh the risks, you recall a recently published article describing current movements against vaccinations and sources of information available over the internet.[2] You decide to review the current evidence to provide the parents with the best possible advice. Knowing that there is controversy in this area, you decide to hunt down a selection of studies for comparison. Searching MedLine using the PubMed site over the internet, you find several randomized controlled trials (RCTs), cohort, and case–control studies as well as many review papers.*

Claims of harm are often made for new and even standard procedures. For example, vitamin K given at birth has been implicated in acute childhood leukemia, and more recently the measles vaccine has been accused of causing autism. Investigating such concerns requires skills for locating the evidence, evaluating the quality of the evidence, and judging the probability of a causal relationship between the exposure and the outcome. Clinicians then must decide whether the probability of benefit from the treatment outweighs the chance of sustaining harm.

This chapter will describe the process of evaluating the available literature for a question of harm, with the aim of determining whether it provides accurate and sufficient information on which to base a decision. Then with a clear picture of both the risks and the benefits of the treatment, you will be able to decide if a particular exposure should be continued or stopped.

When it appears that an exposure may cause an undesirable outcome, two aspects of the relationship between the suggested cause and the outcome must be evaluated: whether the two are really associated, and whether the association is really causal. A systematic approach to an observed association leading to the investigation of causation is presented in Figure 7.1.[3]

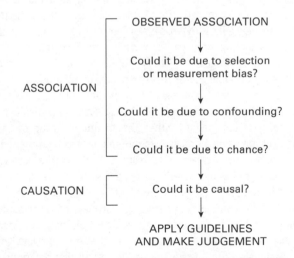

Figure 7.1 Systematic process from observed association to establishing causation

Assessing the validity of an association

A perceived association can be created or influenced by systematic problems with observation (bias), by unmeasured external variables (confounding), and by the play of chance.

Each of these threats to validity can be addressed in the design of the study as well as in its analysis. The quality of research depends upon the appropriateness of the study type and the integrity with which the research is conducted. The first section of Figure 7.1 shows the steps to determine the validity of an association prior to examining causality.

Study designs: were comparison groups clearly defined?

Study designs can minimize the threats to validity that are posed by bias, confounding, and chance. Five study designs have been used in the literature to make claims of harmful associations: randomized controlled trials (RCTs), cohort studies, case–control studies, case series, and case reports. Each study design has different strengths and weaknesses for evaluating questions of harm. A defining feature of the first three study designs is the procedure for assembling one or more comparison groups. The last two study designs are anecdotal, do not have comparison groups, and are used for hypothesis generation rather than to confirm an association. Therefore these two study types will not be addressed in this chapter.

RCTs, cohort, and case–control studies all require selection processes for enrolling participants into the study. This is an initial opportunity for ensuring the validity of the study. *Selection bias* can occur when all participants are not entered into the study based on the same inclusion and exclusion criteria. All patients meeting the inclusion criteria should be recruited; if the investigator does not recruit the patients systematically, a bias towards his or her preference may occur, perhaps selecting only patients with a high socioeconomic status. This changes the study population and limits the ability to generalize the results to a wider population.

In a *randomized controlled trial*, participants are selected prior to either the exposure or the adverse outcome. Each participant is assigned to either the treatment group or the control group using a process of random chance, to ensure that the groups are similar with respect to both the known determinants of outcome such as age and gender, as well as the determinants that have yet to be identified. This is an attempt to control for confounding variables that may influence study results, and lead to false conclusions. Selection bias is avoided because it is chance, rather than choice (conscious or unconscious) of the investigator or the patient that determines the group to which any particular patient is assigned.

The treatment group is introduced to the exposure of interest in a systematic fashion while the controls receive an alternative treatment, a placebo, or no treatment at all. RCTs are therefore prospective designs that can demonstrate a clear temporal relationship. The treatment and control groups are followed over time to identify those who develop the outcome of interest. The different frequencies of outcomes between the two groups are then compared to determine if an association is present.

Practitioners can be confident in the results if high quality RCTs consistently demonstrate an association between the exposure and the outcome. However, not all research questions lend themselves to the RCT design. An RCT may not be feasible when the outcome is rare because a large sample size is required to ensure that the outcome of interest occurs in at least a few patients. Similarly, if the latent period between exposure and outcome is long, such as exposure to radiation by mammography and breast cancer, the study period may be too long for an RCT to be carried out effectively. Furthermore, if an exposure is thought to be detrimental to health and to be without potential benefit, such as cigarette smoking, it is not ethical to assign this exposure to participants.

It is important to note that, when assessing a question of harm, not all RCTs focus on adverse events as the primary study outcome. Many RCTs studying the efficacy of a treatment do not systematically report adverse events encountered.[4] For those studies in which safety is not the primary focus, the following recommendations for reporting have been suggested[5]:

- Specify number of participants withdrawn from the study because of adverse events, per study arm and type of event.
- Use standardized scales for adverse events, or provide definitions for new scales.
- Specify the schedule for collecting safety information, tests performed, questionnaires used, and whether surveillance was active or passive.
- Specify the number of adverse events per study arm and type of event.
- Tabulate safety information per study arm and severity grade, and provide detailed description of unusual events.

Following these recommendations not only allows for the safety assessment of a given study but also allow for the meta-analysis of similar studies.

Case scenario (continued)

Two RCTs were selected for review. The first was a double-blind placebo-controlled trial involving 3450 infants in Sweden.[6] All infants were full term and healthy and were randomized to receive either a diphtheria-tetanus-pertussis (DTP) vaccine ($n_1 = 1724$) or a diphtheria-tetanus (DT) vaccine ($n_2 = 1726$).

The second double-blind RCT was conducted in Italy, again comparing two acellular vaccines ($n_1 = 4696$; $n_2 = 4672$) and one whole-cell vaccine ($n_3 = 4678$) with a placebo vaccine ($n_4 = 1555$).[7] Randomization and masking was conducted according to a specific protocol. Participants were scheduled to receive three vaccines and one booster.

Cohort studies are considered to be the best choice when it is either not possible or not ethical to randomly assign the exposure of interest. In this situation participants are enrolled into the study based on their pre-existing exposure status (exposed or not exposed). In some studies the degree of exposure is taken into account, such as the number of packs of cigarettes smoked per day or per week. At this time no one in the sample has developed the outcome of interest (i.e., everyone is disease free). Participants are then followed for a specified length of time, the appropriate follow up period being dependent on the biology of the outcome. During this period all participants are regularly monitored for signs and symptoms of the outcome.

A strength of the cohort study design is that the temporal relationship can be established between the exposure and the outcome. This is a good design for studying rare exposures because participants are selected for the study based on exposure, insuring adequate representation. Cohort studies are also appropriate for evaluating multiple disease outcomes of a single exposure. Incidence rates in the population can be measured directly, and the relative risk (RR) of the association can be calculated. Finally, serial measures can be obtained on the same participants over time. A disadvantage of the cohort study is that it can be time-consuming and costly.

Historical (retrospective) cohort studies, also known as non-concurrent cohort studies, require previously collected data to determine exposure status prior to the development of the outcome, and may also require historical data to determine outcome status. This decreases the time and cost of the study; however, it requires pre-existing data and may compromise the certainty of temporal relationship between exposure and outcome. In addition, the quality of information regarding exposure may be poor if it must be collected from old records that were not intended for this purpose.

Another disadvantage of the cohort design is that it is inefficient in the study of rare outcomes, such as rare adverse drug reactions (ADRs). When an outcome is rare a very large cohort sample is required to ensure enough cases will develop. Therefore the frequency of the outcome of interest should be considered when reviewing the results of these studies. Negative findings may be due to the limitations of this study design.[8]

Case scenario (continued)	*The first cohort study selected for consideration focused on the risk of non-neonatal seizures and encephalopathy associated with the DTP vaccine.[9] The cohort consisted of a subset of children who were enrolled in the Tennessee Medicaid program within 90 days after birth. All children had received at least one DTP vaccination by 1 year of age. Exposure was defined by time since last vaccine measured in days: 0–3, 4–7, 8–14, 15–29, and 30 +.*
	The second cohort study focused on immunization-related seizures and neurologic consequences.[10] This study used data from the National Institute of Neurological and Communicative Disorders and Stroke Collaborative Perinatal Project (NCPP) which enrolled approximately 54 000 pregnant women between 1959 and 1966. Of the children born to these women, 2766 experienced one or more seizures during the first 7 years of life. Immunization records were only complete for children who had experienced one or more seizures; therefore only these children were studied. Comparison was made between those who had recently received a vaccination and those who had not.

In *case–control studies*, participants are grouped by whether or not they have experienced the outcome of interest. Hence, they must be conducted after the outcome has taken place. Cases are identified and enrolled into the study and controls are selected from the same study population. Controls should be similar to the cases in every respect except for disease status (i.e., they are disease negative). To avoid potentially confounding effects, controls should be randomly selected and may be matched to cases based on certain characteristics such as age and gender. Confounding can also be controlled for in the analysis. The exposure status of both the cases and the controls is determined retrospectively, with the risk of uncertainty in the temporal relationship between exposure and outcome.

The case–control design is most effective when the outcome of interest is rare or takes a long time to develop. It is an efficient design in terms of cost and time, and can be used to examine the effects of multiple exposures on the outcome of interest. This study design also requires fewer participants as compared to RCT or cohort studies. However, it is not a good study design for rare exposures, as the odds ratio will systematically overestimate the true effect size,[11] and incidence rates and relative risks cannot be calculated directly.

Case scenario (continued)	*The first case–control study selected for review compared three models to investigate the temporal relationship between the pertussis vaccination and infantile spasms: association, temporal shift, and no effect.[12] Out of 269 cases identified in the National Childhood Encephalopathy Study (NCES) aged*

2–35 months, 262 met the inclusion criteria for this study. Two controls for each case were identified and matched on age, gender, and area of residence. All cases and controls were analyzed using three different exposure groupings: those exposed to the DTP vaccine alone, those exposed to the DT vaccine alone, and the those exposed to either the DTP or DT vaccines. Exposure was defined as having received a vaccine within 0–28 days prior to the adverse event or reference date (for controls.)

The second case–control study was population-based and focused on the risk of serious acute neurologic illness after immunization with a whole cell DTP vaccine.[13] Cases for this study were identified prospectively in Washington and Oregon states in the US ranging in age from 1 to 24 months. Two controls for each of the 424 confirmed cases of encephalopathy were subsequently matched on age, gender, and county of birth. Exposure was defined as having received a vaccination within 7 days prior to the adverse event, or the reference date for controls. This study used the same definition for neurologic illness as the NCES.

Each of these study designs has inherent strengths and weaknesses. The appropriateness of any study is dependent on the characteristics of both the exposure and outcome of interest. The study design that is most appropriate for the topic of investigation will provide the most reliable evidence, as long as it is of high quality. Hence a carefully conducted case–control study can provide better information than a poorly conducted RCT.

For the purpose of investigating adverse reactions to the pertussis vaccine, it is important to recognize that these are rare events. The main focus of the RCT studies was to compare the efficacy of whole cell and acellular preparations of the pertussis vaccine. Adverse reactions and safety were secondary considerations. Because the serious adverse reactions to pertussis are estimated to be very rare, it is important to consider whether or not these studies had sample sizes large enough to investigate adverse neurologic reactions.

Sample size is also a problem for cohort studies when the outcome is rare. The cohort studies presented here were population surveillance studies. Wentz *et al.*[8] estimated that if the excess risk of a serious adverse reaction is one per 140 000 vaccinations, a large multiple of 140 000 immunizations is required to study this problem. Furthermore, these studies did not have external control groups (i.e., not exposed at all), as the pertussis vaccine is in widespread use.

Thus, the best study design for investigating rare adverse reactions to the pertussis vaccine is the case–control study. Because this outcome is rare, this is the best method for ensuring an adequate number of cases, and therefore sufficient power to detect an association.

Were exposure and outcome consistently and independently measured?

When you are gathering data relevant to the exposure and outcome status of study participants, it is important to take precautions against the various different forms of *information bias*. This bias has the potential to overestimate or create an association between a vaccine and the suspected adverse outcome,[14] and can affect:

- the identification of participants' exposure or outcome status (*misclassification bias*);
- the collection of exposure and outcome data independent of each other (*measurement bias*);
- the observation of the study groups with the same amount of attention (*observer bias*);
- the collection of detailed self-reported information from the controls as well as from the exposed or case groups (*recall bias*).

In the anticipation of finding an association between a treatment and an outcome, investigators or participants may unknowingly influence the detection of an association. If an investigator is aware that a patient is in the exposed group, adverse symptoms may be more likely to be recorded. Conversely, if an investigator is aware of the absence of exposure, these same symptoms may not be given as much attention. Similarly, patients who know they are receiving an experimental treatment may be more likely to report any adverse events than the controls. The value of a placebo group is that the patients believe they may be receiving a treatment. Therefore a background measurement of the adverse events and benefits attributable to the perception of receiving a treatment can be recorded.

Preventing measurement bias can be accomplished through the use of blinding during the observation period. In RCT studies, proper blinding procedures of participants as well as investigators is highly regarded for providing unbiased observations. It is also common to blind investigators to exposure or outcome status when information is being collected for cohort or case–control studies, or when analyses are being conducted.

A disadvantage of the case–control study is that both exposure and outcome have already occurred, and it is therefore vulnerable to recall bias. Those study participants who have a personal interest in the research topic are likely to be motivated to offer detailed information and remember past events in more detail than those not concerned with the issue.

Case scenario (continued)

A recognized strength of the double-blind RCT is that all participants are subjected to the same level of scrutiny. The RCTs reviewed were both double-blind, thereby avoiding observation bias. Taranger et al. conducted telephone interviews using structured questionnaires after each of the vaccinations. Greco et al. had parents evaluate and record symptoms, with serious ADRs confirmed by physician.

The cohort study by Griffin et al. was a chart review of a subset of children who had received at least one pertussis vaccination. The medical chart abstractor for this study was not aware of the child's immunization history unless it was stated in the chart. Therefore complete blinding was not assured, and the study was vulnerable to observer bias. However detailed description was included for the identification of the neurologic events as reported on Medicaid claims, making the collection of data systematic and less subjective.

The cohort study by Hirtz et al. analyzed NCPP data, which included medical histories (including seizures) of all children at ages 4, 8, 12, 18, and 24 months and annually thereafter. Family histories were recorded at both the initial visit and the final visit when the child was 7 years old. Standardized neurologic evaluation and developmental status were performed at 4 and 12 months of age. All children were evaluated in the same standardized manner; however, immunization records were not always recorded. Therefore the rates of complications following immunization could not be determined.

The NCES study (by Goodman et al.) had an outcome of hospitalization for any one of a defined group of severe neurologic disorders. Immunization histories were provided by local sources. However, the children's development and neurologic status were not formally assessed prior to the development of their illness. Furthermore, neurologic assessment of very young children is difficult, therefore the validity of the methods used could be questionable.

Gale et al. used written immunization records to determine exposure status of participants, and blinded investigators to immunization history when confirming cases.

Was the extent of follow up appropriate?

The appropriate length of follow up is dependent on the biology of the outcome. The period between exposure and the development of signs and symptoms will dictate the appropriate follow up period for a specific topic. *Follow up bias* occurs when the follow up period is not appropriate for the outcome. If the incubation of a disease is 2 weeks, then a follow up period of 1 week will underestimate the incidence of disease. However a follow up of 4 weeks may overestimate the incidence of disease, if the outcomes observed result from some other exposure. Furthermore, patients lost to follow up can greatly affect the results of a study. It is therefore important to account for all participants at the end of a study.

Follow up is important for both RCT and cohort studies where the outcomes have yet to happen. Similarly, a defined period between exposure and outcome is important in determining exposure status in case–control studies.

Case scenario (continued)

In the case of vaccine-related adverse reactions, there is no pre-established period of time in which the reaction is expected to occur. The closer to receiving the vaccination, the stronger the evidence that an association truly exists. In the studies reviewed here, the extent of follow up varied from a few days following vaccination to several months. RCT follow up was 1 week after each vaccination in the study by Taranger et al. Greco et al. enlisted nurses to collect the parent recorded ADR information by telephone day 8 following vaccination.

For the Griffin's cohort study, follow up began after children had received the first DTP vaccination and ended with an event recorded on a medical chart, or when the child reached 36 months of age. Hirtz et al. analyzed the NCPP data that had a 7-year long-term follow up for seizures from the time of birth regardless of immunization status. They defined the post-immunization period as 14 days.

The case–control conducted by Goodman et al. using NCES data had a follow up period of up to 28 days post vaccination. Gale et al. had post-immunization follow up for 7 days.

Is there evidence of confounding?

Confounding can occur when a third variable exerts an effect on the relationship between the exposure and the outcome.[15] This third variable must:

- be a risk factor for the disease;
- be associated with the exposure;
- not be an intermediate step in the causal path between exposure and disease.

For example, lack of exercise is a risk factor for cardiovascular disease. However if a study does not control for age, the strength of the association may be artificially inflated. Younger people are more likely to be physically active because they are in better health, whereas older individuals are more limited in their activities. Furthermore, cardiovascular disease is more prevalent among the elderly than among the young. Therefore the association between lack of exercise and cardiovascular disease will be confounded by age if the study compares young vibrant active individuals with older less vibrant sedentary individuals.

Confounding can be controlled at the design stage or at the analysis stage of the study. Design level control includes randomization, matching or restriction. A major strength of the RCT study design is this ability to control confounding through randomization. Case–control studies can control for confounding by matching controls to cases based on potentially confounding variables, such as age and gender. Furthermore, inclusion and exclusion criteria are means of limiting variability among the study group, thereby limiting potentially confounding factors. Adjustment in the analysis is possible for all three study types, and includes stratification, standardization, and multivariate modeling.

It has been suggested that failure to control factors predisposing to both avoidance of vaccination and the adverse reactions under study could confound the outcome.[14] This is *confounding by indication*, and may include medical conditions and social factors.

Case scenario (continued)	*In the cohort study by Griffin et al., children whose medical charts indicated pre-existing chronic neurologic abnormality without seizures, spells that were not clearly seizures, diagnoses of failure to thrive, other non-neurologic events and miscoded records were excluded from analysis.*
	Hirtz et al. reported that only 1·4% (39) of the convulsions occurred within the defined post-vaccination period, and only 10 children had received a DTP vaccine. Three of these DTP inoculations were coupled with either polio or smallpox vaccines, which are potential confounding variables. Nine of the 10 events occurred within 2 days after receiving the inoculation; the time of occurrence for the 10th case was unknown.
	Infantile spasms were excluded from the NCES, as well as cases with a previous history of neurologic illness prior to the index date (Goodman et al.) Gale et al. did a matched-set case–control analysis to control for confounding, and reported the strength of association after adjusting for factors related to avoidance.

Is the association due to chance?

Chance is always at play when a sample of the population is being studied rather than the whole population. Sample size is a primary factor in assessing the capability of a study to estimate the truth. Large sample sizes increase the precision of the estimate and minimize the play of chance. A large confidence interval around a point estimate indicates decreased precision and increased play of chance.

The statistical power of a study is a function of the sample size. Power refers to the ability of a study to detect a relationship between an exposure and an outcome should one truly exist. Factors required to calculate power are the frequency of the outcome, the magnitude of the effect, the study design, and the sample size.[16] If an adverse drug reaction affects 1 in every 1000 people taking a medication, then a study including 1000 participants may not detect this outcome.

Case scenario (continued)	*The first RCT reported no serious reactions, while the second reported 18 serious reactions out of more than 45 000 inoculations. However these studies were primarily efficacy trials, which typically include sample sizes too small to investigate rare outcomes.[17] Sample size calculations for these studies were based on the efficacy portion of the study, not safety.*
	The two cohort studies and two case–control studies were population-based with very large sample sizes. These studies involved 38 171 children receiving over 107 000 inoculations; approximately 54 000 children; 269 cases of infantile spasms; and 424 confirmed cases of neurologic illness.
	Sample size and power issues were not addressed in the studies conducted by Griffin et al., Hirtz et al., or Goodman et al. The latter two studies analyzed data from large projects (NCPP and NCES); these issues may have been addressed in previous publications. Gale et al. calculated a power of 80%, adequate to detect a significant odds ratio of at least 2·5. Power was limited for individual diagnoses in this study.

Assessing causation

Once it has been confirmed that bias, confounding, and chance are not contributing to the observed association (i.e., that the association appears to be real), then the issue of causation can be addressed. This is the focus of the second section of Figure 7.1. A causal association implies that changes in the exposure will affect the frequency of the outcome. This cannot be established by one study alone, but by the total body of evidence available supporting Hill's Criteria of Causation.[16]

The major criteria include:

- *Temporal relationship.* Does the cause precede the effect?
- *Biologic plausibility.* Is the association consistent with our understanding of biologic mechanisms?
- *Consistency of the relationship.* Have similar results been shown in other studies?

The other considerations include:

- *Dose-response.* Does increasing the exposure lead to an increased effect?

- *Strength of the association.* What is the measured size of the risk?
- *Cessation effects.* Does the effect disappear if the exposure is removed?

It is important to note that no single criterion listed here is capable of establishing a causal association. Conversely, not all of the criteria are required for a relationship to be causal. Generally speaking, the more supporting evidence there is, the more likely the association is causal.

Does the cause precede the effect?

Temporality of an association dictates that the exposure of interest truly occurred prior to the presentation of the outcome. This is the strength of prospective studies (RCT and cohort), where the exposure is introduced to non-diseased participants at the onset of the study, and participants are then monitored for development of the outcome.

Case scenario (continued)	*The temporal relationship for the pertussis vaccination is easily determined, with the adverse reaction occurring following the inoculation. However, most studies involve infants receiving the pertussis vaccination three times before they are 1 year old, starting in the first few months. Therefore any adverse event occurring within the first year of life is likely to occur sometime after the child has been vaccinated.*

Is the association consistent with our understanding of biologic mechanisms?

Biologic plausibility of the hypothesis is supported when the etiology of events leading from the risk factor to the outcome is supported by prior knowledge. This condition is often difficult to satisfy at the time of hypothesis testing, becoming the topic of future research.

Case scenario (continued)	*Neurologic damage is a known outcome of pertussis; however, this is thought to result from the lack of oxygen and bleeding from small blood vessels consistent with severe coughing.[18,20] There has been no plausible mechanism accepted by which the pertussis vaccine could cause neurologic damage.*

Have similar results been shown in other studies?

Consistency of findings between different studies investigating the same hypothesis provides strong support for causality. It is therefore important that a particular topic be addressed more than once by independent researchers. A similar concept is that of replication, where the same study methods are used with a different sample in an attempt to produce similar results.

Case scenario (continued)	*The studies presented here all suggest the possibility of an association between the pertussis vaccine and neurologic damage; however, this outcome appears to be sufficiently rare to evade confirmation. The RCTs may not have had sufficient sample size to detect an association of such a rare outcome. One did not detect any serious reactions, while the other reported four children having a seizure out of just over 45 000 doses of the pertussis vaccine.*

The population-based cohort studies rarely achieved significance despite large numbers. Griffin et al. reported 0·9% of the study sample experienced a seizure; however, these included children with prior neurologic or developmental abnormality, prior seizure, or epilepsy. Hirtz et al. reported that of all children experiencing a convulsion, 1·4% were associated with recent vaccination, only a proportion of these being pertussis. Not all children were considered previously normal.

Goodman et al. concluded that the NCES data did not fit the model of association that they had proposed. A better fit was observed for the no-association model, with possible temporal shift of seizures in children likely to have experienced this event at some point. Gale et al. reported odds ratios as a measure of association between vaccination and serious acute neurologic illness; however, none of these attained significance.

Does increasing the exposure lead to an increased effect?

Dose-response, also known as the *biologic gradient*, refers to the concept that a small dose of the risk factor will produce a weaker reaction, whereas a larger dose will produce a stronger reaction.

Case scenario (continued)	*A dose-response relationship was mentioned in one of the studies reviewed (Taranger et al.), with minor adverse reactions being more common with subsequent inoculations. This has not been a focused topic of any of the investigations reviewed here and requires more research.*

What is the measured size of the risk?

Strengths of association can be measured by frequencies, rates, or by statistical measures such as the relative risk (RR), odds ratio (OR), or attributable risk (AR). It has been argued that strong associations are more likely to indicate a causal relationship, whereas weak associations indicate undetected bias in the study design. It is important to note that, when you are evaluating research, the quality of the study takes precedence over the reported strength of association.

The *frequency* of an event is the number of events occurring within the sample or population within a specified period of time. To compare between groups or populations, these frequencies can be expressed in *rates*, the number of events per 100 or per 1000, etc.

The quantitative strength of an association is measured using the *RR*. This measure determines the excess risk of developing the outcome of interest among the exposed group as compared to the unexposed group:

- If RR = 1, risk in exposed equals risk in unexposed, therefore no association.
- If RR > 1, risk in exposed is greater than the risk in unexposed, therefore positive association, detrimental.
- If RR < 1, risk in exposed is less than the risk in unexposed, therefore negative association, protective.

Case–control studies, however, do not contain the information required to calculate the RR directly. In this case, the *OR* is calculated to determine the odds of cases being exposed as compared to the odds of the controls being exposed. In this way the OR is used to approximate the RR for rare outcomes, and has the same interpretation as the RR.

The *AR, absolute risk difference, or absolute effect* is the rate of an outcome that the exposure is accountable for, assuming that the outcome can occur in the absence of the exposure. It is calculated by subtracting the rate of the outcome among the unexposed group from the rate of the outcome among the exposed group.[16] Interpretation is as follows:

- If AR = 0, no difference in risk between exposed and non-exposed groups.
- If AR > 0, number of cases of the outcome among the exposed group that could be prevented if the exposure was removed.

Case scenario (continued)	*The first RCT reported the frequency of adverse reactions. No major adverse reactions were observed in either group. Redness and swelling were more common among those receiving the DTP vaccine. The second RCT reported rates per 1000 doses of vaccination. Serious reactions included 12 hypotonic, hyporesponsive episodes, two cases of generalized cyanosis, and four seizures. There were no cases of anaphylaxis or encephalopathy. Seizures were reported to occur at a rate of 0·07 per 1000 doses among those receiving an*

acellular DTP vaccination and 0·22 per 1000 doses for those receiving a whole-cell DTP. There was no comparison with the control as no seizures occurred among those receiving a DT vaccine.

In the first cohort study, Griffin et al. reported the frequency of different types of seizures, acknowledging that a percentage of these individuals had potentially confounding conditions: neurologic/developmental abnormality, prior seizure, and epilepsy. These conditions, however, were not taken into consideration when the RRs were reported. Of the 38 171 charts reviewed, 0·9% (356) had a medical procedure for a seizure and two patients were hospitalized with encephalopathy. Another 359 were identified as having had a potential seizure. Rates were reported for four outcomes (febrile, afebrile, symptomatic, and potential seizures) per 1000 person-years (PY) of observation for five age groups. Four time periods (0–3, 4–7, 8–14, 15–29 days post-vaccination) were analyzed for increased risk of seizure compared to a later time period (30+ days). The greatest RRs reported were:

- *febrile seizure (0–3 days) RR 1·5 (95% CI 0·6–3·3)*
- *afebrile seizure (4–7 days) RR 2·2 (95% CI 0·5–9·9)*
- *potential seizure (15–29) RR 1·4 (95% CI 1·0–2·1).*

Hirtz et al. reported 39 children experiencing convulsions within 2 weeks following immunization. A sample of 2766 children received a DTP vaccination, nine of whom had a seizure within 2 days of receiving the vaccine. Of 40 post-immunization seizures (for all vaccine types), all but one of the seizures was febrile, 31 were brief, three were >30 minutes in duration, and six were of unknown type. Because of incomplete vaccination data, no external comparison group was used and RRs were not calculated. There were no long-term neurologic problems observed.

Goodman et al. analyzed the cases as a whole, followed by a subanalysis of the cases: previously normal (healthy) and previously abnormal (some history of specified neurologic problems). ORs were calculated for each analysis performed; however, these did not attain statistical significance. Time interval analysis showed that exposure was more likely to have occurred within a week prior to the spasm, although this too did not attain statistical significance.

Outcomes of interest reported by Gale et al. included complex febrile seizures, seizures without fever, infantile spasms, and acute encephalitis/encephalopathy. The adjusted OR was found to be 3·6 with a 95% CI of 0·8–15·2. No significant results were found for subanalyses performed.

What is the precision of the estimate of risk?

The *confidence interval* (CI) is used to assess the precision and the statistical significance of the estimate. Precision is measured by the width of the CI, which is affected by several factors including the sample size. Larger sample sizes allow for more precise estimates, indicated by narrower CIs. The CI indicates statistical significance when the value 1·0 is not contained within the range for an RR or OR, since there is a 95% certainty that the true RR or OR for the population falls within the CI range.

Case scenario (continued)

The cohort study by Griffin et al. reported one significant RR for potential seizures between 15 and 29 days post vaccination using the 30+ days group as a comparison. The 95% CI for this RR of 1·4 was 1·0–2·1. No other studies reported statistically significant results.

Does the effect disappear if the exposure is removed?

Cessation of exposure embodies the concept that removing the exposure will cause a decrease in the magnitude of the outcome, possibly disappearing altogether. This provides strong supportive evidence for a causal association; however, it is dependent on the biology of the association. For example, an individual with an allergy to aspirin will display shortness of breath or develop a rash when taking the medication. These effects will disappear if the drug is stopped, and reappear if the drug is resumed.

Case scenario (continued)

Cessation of exposure is not relevant in the study of the pertussis vaccination. Because no one predetermined length of follow up has been established, it is reasonable to assume that, once you have received an inoculation, the exposure cannot be removed.

Implications for practice

Are the results applicable to your patients?

The first issue to consider is whether the studies were appropriately conducted. This decision is based on the process of evaluating each study based on its design:

Were comparison groups clearly defined?

- Were exposure and outcome consistently and independently measured?
- Was the extent of follow up appropriate?
- Was there evidence of confounding?
- Could the association be due to chance?

If you are confident that the studies were designed and conducted in an appropriate manner you can then consider the results of the studies. Continuing to follow the process:

- Did the cause precede the effect?
- Is the association consistent with our understanding of biologic mechanisms?
- Were similar results seen among the studies?
- Did increasing the exposure lead to an increased effect?
- What was the measured size of the risk?
- What was the precision of this estimate of risk?
- Did the effect disappear when the exposure was removed?

If you are confident the study results represent the truth in the study populations, you now need to determine if these results can be extrapolated to the patients in your practice. If your patients would have met the selection criteria of the studies, then extrapolation is likely appropriate. If there were marked differences between the individuals who participated in the studies and your patients, then extrapolating these results is not appropriate.

Case scenario (continued)	*Participants in the studies reviewed here were young children of both genders. Most studies were population-based, either in the USA or the UK. Treatments varied in some studies, comparing whole cell pertussis vaccines to acellular vaccines. Some studies did not distinguish between these two types. Current practices are similar to the study treatments; therefore it is appropriate to extrapolate the results of these studies.*

Should the exposure be stopped?

To decide if the exposure should be stopped, you must believe that the treatment has the potential to cause more harm than good. To determine this, you must consider the strengths of the studies, the risk of serious adverse reactions occurring, and the consequences to the patient if the treatment were not delivered.

Case scenario (continued)	*Serious adverse events following the pertussis vaccine have been described as "so rare they defy measurement".[18] The serious reactions included hypotonic, hyporesponsive episodes, generalized cyanosis, encephalopathy, and seizures. Rates were generally small, sometime reported per number of inoculations and sometime reported per number of individuals. Significance was not attained for the ORs reported in the two case–control studies.*
	Pertussis is a contagious bacterial disease caused by Bordetella pertussis. *Infants are most susceptible to this disease, suffering the highest incidence rates and the highest hospitalization rates.[19] The case fatality rate among cases in Canada is currently 1:200. Complications of the disease can include ear infections, pneumonia, and severe neurologic sequelae. Pneumonia has been reported to occur in 15% of cases among 6-month-old infants and younger, while the rate of severe neurologic sequelae is 0·1–4%. One in 400 cases suffers permanent brain damage, and learning and behavior problems in later life have been associated with the disease.*

Conclusion

Practising physicians are periodically confronted with issues of harm as they relate to new or standard procedures. Judging the probability of a causal relationship between the exposure and the outcome requires a systematic process to weigh the harms against the benefits. The Box summarizes the criteria that are used to assess whether an exposure is associated with a harmful outcome and whether that association is likely to be causal. Using these criteria to judge published reports of potentially harmful exposures will assist you in making evidence-based judgements of the validity of such claims.

Case scenario (continued)

When they return to your office for their second visit, you explain the results of your research to the concerned parents. Pertussis is considered the most poorly controlled vaccine-preventable disease in Canada.[20] More than 4800 cases occurred in Canada during 1996, with underreporting suspected. The introduction of vaccination has allowed for the control of many infectious diseases; however, the decreased occurrence of these diseases has been perceived as decreased health risk. As the focus has shifted away from the severity of disease, more attention is being paid to the adverse reactions the vaccinations may cause. The current prevalence of pertussis is high for a preventable disease, and the severe outcomes of the disease are far more common than reactions to the vaccine.

Should the parents choose not to vaccinate their son, the risk of contracting this disease is very real and the effects of pertussis can be severe. The minor potential reactions to the vaccine are well documented, and the chance of a serious reaction is very rare. Based on this evidence, you recommend adhering to the vaccination schedule as planned.

Criteria for assessing the validity of an association, determining causality, and judging the implication for practice

Association

- Were comparison groups clearly defined?
- Were exposure and outcome consistently and independently measured?
- Was the extent of follow up appropriate?
- Is there evidence of confounding?
- Is the association due to chance?

Causation

- Does the cause precede the effect?
- Is the association consistent with our understanding of biologic mechanisms?
- Have similar results been shown in other studies?
- Does increasing the exposure lead to an increased effect?
- What is the measured size of the risk?
- What is the precision of the estimate of risk?
- Does the effect disappear if the exposure is removed?

Implication

- Are the results applicable to your patients?
- Should the exposure be stopped?

References

1 Edwards M. Your Child's Best Shot? *Homemaker's* 1999; September:113–16.

2 Sibbald B. It's wise to immunize, regardless of what the web says. *JAMC* 1999;**161**:736–8.

3 Beaglehole R, Bonita T, Kjellstrom T. *Basic Epidemiology.* World Health Organization, 1993.

4 Ioannidis JPA, Lau J. Completeness of safety reporting in randomized trials: an evaluation of 7 medical areas. *JAMA* 2001;**285**:437–43.

5 Ioannidis JPA, Lau J. Improving safety reporting from randomized trials. *Drug Safety* 2002;**25**:77–84.

6 Taranger J, Trollfors B, Knutsson N. Adverse reactions of a pertussis toxoid vaccine in a double-blind placebo-controlled trial. *Dev Biol Stand* 1997;**89**:109–12.

7 Greco D, Salmaso S, Mastrantonio P *et al.* and the Progetto Pertosse Working Group. A controlled trial of two acellular vaccines and one whole-cell vaccine against pertussis. *N Engl J Med* 1996;**334**:341–8.

8 Wentz K, Marcuse R, Edgar K. Diphtheria-tetanus-pertussis vaccine and serious neurologic illness: an updated review of the epidemiologic evidence. *Pediatrics* 1991;**87**:287–97.

9 Griffin M, Ray W, Mortimer E, Fenichel G, Schaffner W. Risk of seizures and encephalopathy after immunization with the diphtheria-tetanus-pertussis vaccine. *JAMA* 1990;**263**:1641–5.

10 Hirtz D, Nelson K, Ellenberg J. Seizures following childhood immunizations. *J Pediatr* 1983;**102**:14–18.

11 Austin PC, Mamdani M, Williams IJ. Adverse effects of observational studies when examining adverse outcomes of drugs: case-control studies with low prevalence of exposure. *Drug Safety*, 2002;**25**:677–87.

12 Goodman M, Lamm S, Bellman M. Temporal relationship modeling: DTP or DT immunizations and infantile spasms. *Vaccine* 1998;**16**:225–31.

13 Gale J, Thapa P, Wassilak S, Bobo J, Mendelman P, Foy H. Risk of serious acute neurological illness after immunization with diphtheria-tetanus-pertussis vaccine. *JAMA* 1994;**271**:37–41.

14 Fine P, Chen T. Confounding studies of adverse reactions to vaccines. *Am J Epdemiol* 1992;**136**:120–35.

15 Rothman KJ. *Modern Epidemiology.* Boston/Toronto: Little, Brown and Company, 1986.

16 Last J (ed.) *A Dictionary of Epidemiology, 3rd Edition.* New York: Oxford University Press, 1995.

17 Kraisinger M. Update on childhood immunization. *Am J Hlth-Syst Pharmacol* 1998;**55**:563–9.

18 Gangarosa E, Galazka A, Wolfe C *et al.* Impact of anti-vaccine movements on pertussis control: the untold story. *Lancet* 1998;**351**:356–61.

19 Gold R, Martell A. Childhood immunizations. In: Canadian Task Force on the Periodic Health Examination. *Canadian Guide to Clinical Preventive Health Care.* Ottawa: Health Canada, 1994.

20 Canadian Paediatric Society. *Your Child's Best Shot: A Parent's Guide to Vaccination.* Canadian Paediatric Society, 1997.

8 Assessing systematic reviews and clinical guidelines

Geraldine Macdonald

Case scenario

Recently, several parents in your practice have asked you about the use of fluoride mouthrinses for children to prevent cavities. It seems that a local dentist is encouraging parents to purchase and use these since the local water supply has little fluoride. You are not familiar with rinses, and decide to see what the medical literature has to say. You go to PubMed and enter "fluoride rinse AND caries" and, knowing that the best evidence comes from randomized trials, you limit your search to clinical trials. You get 34 hits, and quickly realize that most of them really are trials, and a scan of the abstracts reveals that some do and some do not show an effect. You know that you have neither the time nor the expertise to evaluate this whole body of literature and wonder if there is a better option.

Background

"Well read" is fast becoming an almost meaningless concept for those whose occupations require or permit them to intervene in the lives of others. There was, perhaps, a time when one person could know all there was to know about a particular discipline, or area of practice – particularly if their lives were not overly cluttered with the business of actually having to use said knowledge in day-to-day practice. Indeed, some historical figures have prided themselves on their grasp of all available knowledge, such as one Master of Balliol, who dismissed grubby, technical science, saying, "I am Master of this College; What I don't know isn't knowledge" (Henry Charles Beeching [*The Masque of Balliol*, 1878], in *The Oxford Dictionary of Quotations, 2nd edn*, Oxford: Oxford University Press, 1953;39:5).

Now that science has become respectable, however, what was previously a trickle in research has become a torrent. Nowhere is this more true than in healthcare research, where almost 2 000 000 articles are published each year.[1] Quantity, however, is not the only problem. If it were, then the task of keeping abreast would be primarily a technical challenge. The quality of published material is highly variable since the drive for productivity ("publish or perish") has not been restricted to those whose work is either "fit for the purpose" or conducted to an acceptable standard to inform clinical decision-making. Critical reviews or summaries of evidence seem the only way forward.

This chapter first considers the range of reasons why clinicians need what might be called "predigested" summaries of research in a given area, and then discusses the problems that have undermined traditional approaches to research synthesis. It then discusses the nature and features of systematic reviews and, in light of that discussion, considers the contribution of clinical guidelines.

- *Review*. A general survey of a subject or clinical issue.
- *Systematic review*. A review in which all the primary studies have been systematically identified, appraised, and summarized according to an explicit and reproducible methodology.
- *Meta-analysis*. A statistical method of combining and summarizing the results of the trials that meet minimum quality criteria in a systematic review.

Types of reviews

Narrative reviews

In the traditional review article (often called a narrative review), the authors take on the task of bringing together research reports in a given area, reading them carefully, making a judgment about their quality, and pulling out key themes or messages across all identified studies. Sometimes problems with particular studies are raised, and attention is drawn to issues that pervade research in a given area, such as unrepresentative samples or problems in measurement. On the whole, however, this rarely introduces more than a note of caution and one whose implications are not necessarily obvious to the reader. The method by which the conclusions were drawn from the evidence is seldom made clear.

Unfortunately, this approach to research synthesis is not good enough to be a basis for making clinical decisions. Narrative reviewers have generally failed to appreciate that the review process is itself prone to bias and error, and these can, and do, undermine the validity and reliability of the conclusions reached. Bias, or systematic error, can invalidate attempts to synthesize research studies in a number of ways, including failure to identify all relevant studies and failure to consider the methodologic quality of studies when drawing conclusions.

Technical competence (for example, language abilities, searching skills) and available resources can bias the process of study identification, resulting in failure to identify all relevant studies. Hard to find studies appear to be systematically different from studies that are more readily located. Publication bias has been empirically demonstrated: studies with statistically significant results are more likely to get published than studies without such results, or with "negative" findings.[2] Reasons for this can include the selective submission of papers,[3] the selective acceptance of papers,[4] database bias and citation bias (both of which can lead to a failure to locate relevant studies).[2] Thus, a strict reliance on electronic searching can result in failure to identify large numbers of relevant studies.[5] In particular, a reliance on English language sources can bias the entire review process.[2,6] The failure to identify all relevant studies can seriously threaten the validity of a review, since the studies that are not located might well push the evidence in a completely different (and often less positive) direction.

A desire to produce something that includes firm conclusions and recommendations can unduly influence decisions regarding which studies to include and which to exclude. Inclusion/exclusion criteria for studies are seldom explicitly mentioned in narrative reviews. It is therefore very difficult for a reader to know whether or not the reviewers have been successful in identifying all relevant studies: this is an example of a failure to "show one's working out". It is tempting to relax any inclusion/exclusion criteria that one might have settled on at the outset when faced with a dearth of qualifying studies unknown to the readers of the review. More subtly, where inclusion criteria are stated, it is also possible that prior knowledge of the results of studies may influence the inclusion criteria settled upon by reviewers.[2]

Cognitive and perceptual bias may distort the perceived methodologic adequacy and weight afforded to individual studies. It is not unusual for students (or clinicians) to be highly critical when it comes to scrutinizing studies that reach conclusions that they do not much care for, and methodologically forgiving when the findings favor cherished beliefs or preferences. Experts may be even less objective than non-experts and may, for example, overweight research they themselves have undertaken. As with primary research, errors made in the process of research synthesis can seriously undermine the validity of any conclusions reached. If reviews are explicit about their methods, it is at least theoretically possible for others to attempt to duplicate their work.

Systematic reviews

Although a relatively recent development, methods are now available that enable reviewers to apply scientific principles to the synthesis of research, whatever their field. Reviews produced in this way are generically referred to as systematic reviews. When augmented with statistical analyses, they are typically referred to as meta-analyses. A systematic approach to research synthesis requires two things:

● a declaration of intent, and
● transparency of methodology.

A "declaration of intent" means that reviewers take key methodologic decisions about how the review will be conducted before going to the literature. This is analogous to developing the methods for a study prior to collecting data. Clearly, given that most reviews will be conducted by those familiar with a particular field, it is likely that reviewers will be familiar with the literature. Pinning of one's methodologic colors to the mast makes it less likely that reviewers will be swayed by the reality of the available literature, and will adhere to adequate standards of evidence and synthesis. For example, on finding that randomized controlled trials are all but absent, reviewers are often tempted to revise inclusion criteria to encompass what is available, rather than what is acceptable evidence.

Transparency means making explicit to potential readers the reasoning underpinning decisions. Such explicitness is a key strategy for minimizing random error, and enabling errors (whether random or otherwise) and sources of bias to be detected. It also enables a reader to come to an informed opinion as to whether or not the review has been appropriately conducted. Transparency allows readers to draw their own conclusions about the relevance of a particular review to their working circumstances, as it spells out, for example, the kinds of participants covered by the review, the precise nature of the intervention, and so on.

One well-known source of high quality systematic reviews is the *Cochrane Library*,[7] named for Archie Cochrane, who challenged the profession of medicine in 1979 by saying, "It is surely a great criticism of our profession that we have not organized a critical summary, by specialty or subspecialty, adapted periodically, of all relevant randomized controlled trials." Reviews that are published in the *Cochrane Library* must first be approved at the "declaration of intent" stage (referred to, as in primary research, as a protocol). The Box below shows a list of the decision points in a typical Cochrane protocol.

Decision points in a protocol for a systematic review

- Objectives
- Criteria for considering studies for this review
- Types of studies
- Types of participants
- Types of intervention
- Types of outcome measures
- Search strategy for the identification of studies
- Methods of the review
- Selection of studies
- Assessment of methodologic quality
- Data management
- Data synthesis
  how to deal with incomplete data
  how to analyze binary data
  how to analyze continuous data
  whether and when to undertake a meta-analysis, and if so, what kind.

At any point in the decision-making process, different reviewers will make different choices about how to proceed. Some decisions will comprise sources of error, for example, choosing a statistical approach that is not appropriate for the task at hand. Sometimes, however, these are not matters of right or wrong but "judgment calls". For example, choices often must be made when there is no consensus on the most appropriate course of action, for example, how best to assess methodologic adequacy,[8,9] or what statistical approach to use. Protocols submitted to the Cochrane Collaboration undergo peer review at this stage, so that errors and judgments that have been made can be discussed and debated before the review is carried out. A systematic approach to research synthesis does not guarantee accuracy, nor does it completely remove subjectivity from the review process. However, well-conducted systematic reviews can minimize common sources of bias and error, generally improve the quality of research syntheses, and provide informed readers with the information needed to assess its value.

Meta-analysis

One advantage of a systematic review is the possibility of combining the results statistically to increase the number of subjects and estimate more precisely the magnitude of the effect of the intervention. This is referred to as a meta-analysis. The product of a meta-analysis can be thought of as an "average" of the results of the included studies, which has taken account of how precisely the individual results were estimated in the original studies. This will depend on the size of the original studies and the number of adverse events or spread of data, and means that those with more precise estimates (usually the bigger studies) will be given more weight in calculating the mean value. The techniques also allow the calculation of confidence intervals that will be narrower (indicating a more precise estimate) than those of included studies. In other words, by combining the data, we are able to have a better idea of the range in which the "true" size of the effect is likely to lie. The different techniques used to combine data are beyond the scope of this chapter and anyone contemplating carrying out a meta-analysis should get statistical advice.

Before carrying out a meta-analysis, it is important to be sure that the data from individual studies are sufficiently homogeneous for it to make sense to combine them. If the results of the studies are very different, it may be because the subjects, interventions, or outcomes that were measured are actually different, and combining the data from the different studies makes no sense. In conducting or reading a systematic review there are two complementary approaches to judging the heterogeneity (degree of variability) of the data – statistical and clinical. It is accepted practice to carry out statistical tests for evidence of heterogeneity, but unless the meta-analysis includes very large numbers of studies, these tests lack the power to find even important heterogeneity. In other words, there may actually be substantial heterogeneity, but this may not be demonstrated by the test, and clinical judgment is needed.

Research and clinical questions can be stated in the format of:

- a population of interest
- an intervention or exposure (and a comparison)
- an outcome (see Chapter 2).

If data are to be combined in a meta-analysis, they must come from studies in which these three elements are judged to be similar.

There should be no reason to believe that the populations in the included studies are likely to respond differently to the intervention. For example, if a systematic review of the effect of antibiotics in children with sore throats were to include some studies in which all the participants were judged to have streptococcal infections and others in which participants with positive throat cultures were excluded, one might consider it unlikely that antibiotics would have similar effects in the two groups; in this case a meta-analysis would be inappropriate. Similarly, there should be no *a priori* grounds for believing that the interventions in the included studies would have different effects. In the sore throat example above, if some studies used what are regarded as inadequate doses of antibiotics, pooling of data would not be appropriate.

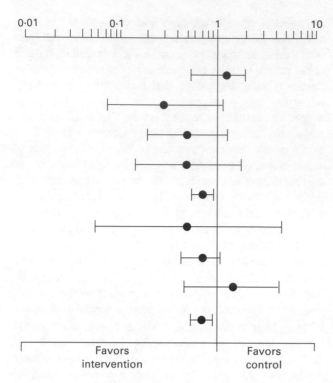

Figure 8.1 Odds ratios and 95% confidence intervals for effect of home visiting on child injury[10]

Finally, the outcome measures used in the included studies should measure the same underlying outcome. In this example one might question whether retrospective parental report of time to resolution of symptoms and direct observation by a researcher would be likely to reflect the same underlying outcome.

The results of a meta-analysis of dichotomous data (i.e., data such as the chance of cure or death) are often shown in the form of a "blobogram". Figure 8.1 shows the results of a systematic review of trials of home visiting for the prevention of injury in children in which eight studies met the inclusion criteria.[10] The odds ratio (OR) for each study is represented in the figure as a dot, with bars on either side representing the 95% confidence interval. A heavy vertical line is drawn representing an odds ratio of 1, which is the line at which there is no evidence that the intervention has either a beneficial or a harmful effect. In this case the confidence levels of all but one of the included studies cross this line, in other words they do not individually show a "statistically significant" effect. The pooled estimate is shown, again with a "blob" for the estimated effect (OR = 0·74) and lines for the 95% confidence interval (0·60–0·92). These lines do not cross the vertical line at OR = 1, so the pooled effect is statistically significant. Other types of data can also be combined statistically, although for some types (such as ordinal data) the appropriate methods remain a source of debate.

Critical appraisal of systematic reviews and meta-analyses

Given that few clinicians have the time or skills to assemble and interpret all the available evidence on important topics, it seems inevitable that we will have to rely on systematic reviews or syntheses of evidence. Unfortunately terms like "systematic review" or "evidence-based guideline" can easily be borrowed by those who either do not understand them or who do not accept the principles that underlie them. Therefore, clinicians need either to be afforded the skills to distinguish "good" from "bad" syntheses or be able to identify "quality assured" sources of research synthesis, recognizing that not every practitioner will be able critically to appraise in detail all of the scientific qualities of a systematic review. The following set of questions was developed by the Systematic Reviews Training Unit at the Institute of Child Health in London, UK, as a guide to appraising a systematic review.

Are the results valid?

- *Did the review address a sensible, clearly focused question?* Ideally, the questions framed for systematic review should be focused and limited in scope. When a problem is complex, as most clinical problems are, several questions may be needed to describe it, and a review performed for each question. It is always possible to "yoke"-related reviews and build a composite picture with individual "building blocks".

- *How likely is it that the search strategy would have missed eligible studies?* Minimally, does the search strategy attempt to cover all relevant published studies? It should demonstrate coverage of all relevant databases, and include hand-searching of relevant journals that have not already been searched – or, if appropriate, have only been searched for randomized controlled trials. Reviews should not be restricted to English unless the clinical question is unique to English-speaking countries. Have the reviewers gone to reasonable lengths to identify unpublished material?

- *Are the inclusion criteria clearly stated?* Do these cover types of study, types of participant, types of intervention, and outcome measures of interest?

- *Are the inclusion criteria relevant?* For example, in psychosocial effectiveness research, there is a fundamental problem regarding relevancy criteria. Samples are often dissimilar to those encountered in clinical practice,[11] settings are more controlled (laboratory versus "real life" settings), and outcome measures are of dubious relevance (for example, self-report rather than behavioral measures).

- *Did the method used to select studies for inclusion minimize bias?* In other words, (for a question about an intervention), was there randomization? Was the allocation of participants to groups unknown to therapists and to data gatherers or providers (i.e., double-blind)? If the study was not randomized, were all possible steps taken to ensure that the comparison groups were as similar as possible?

- *To what extent are the conclusions based on valid primary studies?* In other words, are the included studies good-quality randomized controlled trials? Where RCTs are not possible, are the studies that are incorporated (as indicated and justified in the protocol) of high quality? Assessing the methodologic quality of included studies is a contentious area.[8,9] The most significant factor in determining the quality of RCTs appears to be the extent to which allocation was adequately concealed.[12]

- *If a meta-analysis was performed, were the included studies sufficiently homogeneous to make it appropriate to pool the data?* Put simply, it is misleading to lump together apples and oranges under the generic category "fruit". Always consider both clinical and statistical heterogeneity before deciding whether or not a statistical synthesis of the data is useful or simply provides a spuriously accurate bottom line. It is important to realize that there is no infallible way of coming to this decision. Rather it is a matter of judgment, which depends partly on understanding the underlying pathophysiology of the condition and therefore subject to interpretation.

What are the results?

- *Are outcomes clinically meaningful and/or relevant to patients? Are adverse effects recorded?* While the collection of significant qualitative data is quite compatible with scientific studies, including RCTs, this is not always done.[13]

- *Do the results apply to my patients?* The results of a systematic review may not be generalizable to any particular clinical setting or group of patients (or individual patient). A good starting point is to pose the following questions: Are my patients so different from those in the review that there are likely to be important differences in treatment effect? Is the intervention in the studies in the review sufficiently similar to the treatment that I am considering? Are the outcome measures documented an adequate reflection of the outcomes of importance to my patients?

Sources of high quality systematic reviews

As indicated earlier, one source of "quality assured" systematic reviews is the *Cochrane Library*, which is produced by the Cochrane Collaboration. The Cochrane

Collaboration is an international organization that aims to prepare, maintain, and disseminate systematic reviews of healthcare interventions. One of the consequences of the exponential growth in published studies is that there is a log-jam between the acceptance of an article by a journal and its publication, so that any review article published in paper form will most likely be out of date by the time it appears. This, combined with the difficulty that many healthcare professionals face in accessing paper publications, means that the "evidence" finding its way to most practitioners may well be suspect, if not decidedly compromised by being beyond its "best-before" date. This is why the Cochrane Collaboration opted for an electronic platform for publication, with a commitment to maintain reviews regularly once published. A brief scrutiny of the *Cochrane Library* will demonstrate that this particular aspiration is not without its own set of problems, but at least readers can see when a review was last updated and what "post-review" studies are awaiting inclusion.

In the UK, the NHS Centre for Reviews and Dissemination (CRD) in York commissions systematic reviews in response to identified needs. It produces reports and "Effective Health Care Bulletins" – overviews based on systematic reviews of research on the effectiveness, cost-effectiveness, and clinical acceptability of health service interventions. In the US, evidence reports commissioned by the AHRQ use similar methods. Other strategies, more universally deployed, are the development of clinical guidelines, both nationally and locally, and the establishment of bodies such as the National Institute for Clinical Excellence (UK) to ensure the high quality of such guidelines.

This is not to say that reviews produced by the CRD, by the AHRQ, or within the Cochrane Collaboration are flawless or could not be improved upon. Indeed, the *Cochrane Library* has a "Comments and Criticisms" facility within it, in recognition of this and of the iterative nature of producing high quality evidence. It is simply that, all things being equal, these are good places to look for high quality evidence of the effectiveness of clinical interventions.

Clinical guidelines

Having access to a systematic review of high quality may be a necessary starting point for evidence-based practice, but it is unlikely to be a sufficient basis. A systematic review will not necessarily provide a clear answer to the question "What should I do with this kind of patient, with these kinds of problems, in these circumstances?" A number of other considerations, in particular how potential good and bad outcomes are valued, need to be considered. A desire for evidence-based, prescriptive guidance has led to increasing emphasis on the use of systematic reviews as a basis for the development of clinical guidelines.

Clinical guidelines (also known as "clinical practice guidelines") have been defined as "systematically developed statements to assist practitioner and patient decisions about appropriate health care for specific clinical circumstances".[14] This definition represents a move away from earlier guidance based on consensus statements of good practice, which are as susceptible to forms of bias and error as narrative reviews (albeit of somewhat different ilk). Clinical guidelines differ from systematic reviews in that they are designed specifically to influence policy and practice. Indeed, the central measure of the effectiveness of clinical guidelines must be their ability to bring about changes in the behavior of healthcare professionals, where this is at odds with the guidelines. Since it is extraordinarily rare that high quality evidence is available to support every step of management for a particular problem, guidelines necessarily go beyond the evidence.

The potential scope of influence for clinical guidelines is broad. A 1994 Health Care Bulletin on the implementation of clinical guidelines identified the following areas for which guidelines might have relevance[15]:

- to improve appropriateness of referral at the primary/secondary interface[16];
- to guide the introduction of new procedures or services;
- to promote effective health care in primary or secondary settings;
- to encourage the adoption of cost-effective interventions;
- to improve the timing and processes for the discharge of patients;
- to structure and encourage patient participation in clinical management decisions;
- to inform the development of criteria and standards for monitoring the quality of care, in particular through clinical audit.

Although different bodies may endorse different criteria in the development of clinical guidelines (perhaps reflecting, for example, differing policy concerns), there is now general agreement that the basis of high quality guidelines should be the systematic appraisal of available evidence of the effects of particular activities, whether investigations, diagnostic tests, medical treatments, or psychosocial interventions. Thus, the relationship between high quality clinical guidelines and high quality systematic reviews is a close one. For organizations such as the World Health Organization, who wish to use guidelines as part of their strategy for improving the quality of health care, it highlights the importance of ensuring that:

- their development is adequately resourced,[15,17] and
- there is strategy in place for providing the evidence that is needed to underpin guidelines, if these are to amount to more than the consensus of experts and other interested parties.

This is signally important in a field such as child health where there is a dearth of research evidence, particularly randomized controlled trials,[18] and where there is a risk that the absence of evidence will be interpreted by policy-makers as evidence of ineffectiveness.

Development of clinical guidelines

There are a number of parallels to be drawn between a systematic approach to research synthesis and a systematic approach to guideline development. Transparency and explicitness have already been discussed. What other factors influence the quality and validity of clinical guidelines for a particular area of health care? The validity of guidelines depends on their ability to result in improved outcomes for patients, when followed. This, in turn, is a function of how well appropriate evidence has been identified, scientifically synthesized and used appropriately. Many guidelines are developed on the basis of "expert opinion", but these have been shown frequently to be out of kilter with current best evidence, and are highly susceptible to bias – for example, vested interest groups (experts versus generalists, one discipline versus another). When a guideline is drawn up, a number of factors need to be considered to ensure both rigor and acceptability.[18,19]

Membership of the guideline development group

In brief, a development group needs to be composed in such a way that it can address a range of tasks. First, it needs to include all key stakeholders, including service users, a multidisciplinary perspective to avoid biased evaluation of evidence by groups with vested interests,[20] and a range of skills covering literature search and retrieval, epidemiology, biostatistics, health services research, clinical experts, writing, and editing.[19]

Identifying, assessing and synthesizing the evidence

The evidence base of guidelines is central to their validity. Relevant systematic reviews or meta-analyses are therefore needed to inform them. If not available, relevant studies should be identified and synthesized following the guidelines for systematic reviews.[1,21]

Quantifying risk and benefits

The effectiveness of a particular intervention is not the only consideration in clinical decision-making. Patients and clinicians need to take into consideration the relative effectiveness of a range of intervention options, and the risks and benefits associated with each.[22] Ease of interpretation of what are, essentially, statistical tools and measures is important for both patients and clinicians. The Royal College of Paediatrics and Child Health (RCPCH) recommends the use of measures such as the "number needed to treat",[23,24] or the likelihood of being helped[25] as more clinically useful than odds ratios, relative risks, or effect sizes. The choice of measures must, however, be determined by "fitness for purpose". Decision analyses (based on a Bayesian approach to risk) could be incorporated to develop decision-making algorithms for categories of patient with similar clinical presentation and personal utilities, i.e., preferences for one outcome over others.[26] Decision analytic methods can be used to estimate the effects of different options and decision trees used to provide a visual representation of the choices available, with their associated risks.[26,27] In more general terms, guidelines should identify exceptions (in applicability) and indicate how patient preferences are to be incorporated into decision-making[25] (see also Chapter 17).

Categorizing evidence

The evidence found may be ranked according to methodologic strength as may the resulting recommendations[28,29] (see Chapter 9).

Taking account of contextual factors

Evidence of effectiveness alone is insufficient as a basis for recommending action. This evidence requires to be considered in the light of other influences, such as the clinical or policy context in which someone is operating, the costs of alternative options,[19] and the values ascribed to the outcomes of the intervention, which may vary between different stakeholders.

Grading recommendations

Insofar as recommendations are incorporated into guidelines, the links between these and the quality of supporting evidence should be made explicit. Thus, for example, the AHRQ suggests grading recommendations as follows:[30]

- *Grade A (levels Ia, Ib)*. Requires at least one randomized controlled trial as part of the body of literature of overall good quality and consistency addressing the specific recommendation.
- *Grade B (levels IIa, IIb, III)*. Requires availability of well-conducted clinical studies, but no randomized clinical trials on the topic of recommendation.
- *Grade C (level IV)*. Requires evidence from expert committee reports or opinions and/or clinical experience of respected authorities. Indicates absence of directly applicable studies of good quality.

Recommendations in the absence of evidence

Advocates of evidence-based practice have never discounted the relevance of practice wisdom, but have urged that it be evaluated in the light of other sources of evidence, which are less susceptible to bias. Where research evidence is lacking, a component of a guideline may well have to be based on expert advice. What is important in these circumstances is that the basis of recommendations be made explicit, and the need for more secure evidence acknowledged.

Timescale for review

As with systematic reviews, clinical guidelines will have an unpredictable shelf-life, and it is important that they are regularly reviewed and, where appropriate, updated. Therefore, a quality criterion of guidelines is the identification of a timescale for review.

Because clinical guidelines are specifically designed to influence practice, some other considerations are important. Factors that are desirable in systematic reviews, but essential in clinical guidelines, include that they are written clearly, use precise definitions and unambiguous language, and are produced in a user-friendly format. Anything short of this will increase the risk that they will be misunderstood, poorly implemented, or not implemented at all. Finally, guidelines should identify the target population in accordance with scientific evidence.

Critical appraisal of clinical guidelines

Clinicians are faced with a plethora of guidelines from different sources and it may be difficult to decide which to follow. Recommendations may vary between guidelines as a result of the socioeconomic, policy, and clinical circumstances for which they are designed. However, differences may result from biased summaries or interpretation of evidence. While more recently produced guidelines are more likely to be explicitly evidence-based, few fulfill all the recommended quality criteria.[31]

A number of useful templates for the assessment of guidelines have been developed. That used by the RCPCH consists of 37 questions addressing three dimensions of guideline quality (see Box). These are designed to have yes/no answers and aim to produce not a simple summative assessment but an overview of the strengths and weaknesses of the guideline.

Dimensions and topics to be considered in the development and appraisal of clinical guidelines in pediatrics end child health

Dimension I: Rigor of development
- responsibility for guideline development
- guideline development group

- identification and interpretation of evidence
- formulation of recommendations
- peer review
- updating
- overall assessment of the development process

Dimension II: Context and content

- context
- content
- likely costs and benefits

Dimension III: Application

- guideline dissemination and implementation
- monitoring of guidelines/clinical audit
- national guidelines only (deals with issues of local relevance)

What clinical guidelines can and cannot do

Carefully developed, evidence-based guidelines can potentially bring a range of benefits to clinicians and to patients concerned with improving the quality and consistency of care.[31,32] They can provide guidance in situations when individual clinicians are unsure how to proceed; they can provide easily accessible means of updating the knowledge base of the "out-of-date" clinician, and can discourage risky practices and procedures. They may also form the basis of lay versions of guidelines, providing patients with information about the benefits and harms of a range of clinical options, enabling them to make informed decisions, as well as adding to the pressure on clinicians to make evidence-based and patient-centered decisions. Guidelines, like reviews, also alert policy-makers and patient groups to areas where there is a dearth of good-quality evidence, and can (and increasingly do) form the basis of a better use of scarce resources.[33–35] However, the quality of any particular set of guidelines will only be as useful as the evidence underpinning them and the recommendations made. As Woolf *et al.* point out, all too often the high quality scientific information necessary to make sound recommendations is unavailable.[33] When such data are not available, guidelines have as much potential to do harm as to do good. Even when available, the data require interpretation and judgment, which can provide the opportunity for bias or error to undermine the validity of some or all of the recommendations made, particularly with regard to perceptions of risks and benefits. To some extent, the incorporation of decision-analytic techniques into guidelines may go some way to addressing these problems, where evidence is available, but is unlikely to assist in its absence. At worst, if guidelines are flawed (i.e., fail to use and interpret evidence appropriately, or "act" as if the absence of evidence were unproblematic), then what is promulgated is less than optimal, and possibly harmful clinical practice.

Clinical guidelines are a growth industry. In areas where good-quality scientific evidence is absent, or where clinical pictures are complex (both of which often pertain to child health), one needs to be especially vigilant about the quality of guidelines that might be produced, hence the importance of critical appraisal. The potential of clinical guidelines to bring about harms rather than benefits (for patients, healthcare professionals and healthcare systems), and the ways in which they can be used to support professional or political interests rather than the best interests of patients led Woolf and his colleagues to the following verdict:

> The unbridled enthusiasm for guidelines, and the unrealistic expectations about what they will accomplish, frequently betrays inexperience and unfamiliarity with their limitations and potential hazards. Naive consumers of guidelines accept official recommendations on face value, especially when they carry the imprimatur of prominent professional groups or government bodies.[33]

Conclusion

The impossibility of keeping up to date in the face of the knowledge explosion means that clinicians will increasingly be forced to depend on predigested evidence. If they are to be confident that they are using the best information in caring for their patients, they must be sure that these syntheses are both valid (i.e., unbiased) summaries of the evidence, and that they are applicable to their patient population. Relying on systematic reviews or guidelines produced within the Cochrane Collaboration or other sources known to have good-quality control procedures can make this easier but there is no substitute for healthy skepticism. Centrally prepared guidelines alone are relatively ineffective at changing behavior.

Resolution of the scenario

You decide to search the Cochrane Library using the same search terms as you did for PubMed. This nets three hits, all of which are completed Cochrane reviews: one on mouthrinses, one on fluoride varnishes, and one on topical fluoride in general, all focused on children and adolescents. The last one is the most recent, having been amended only 3 months ago.[36] You note that a comprehensive search strategy was used, with appropriate inclusion and exclusion criteria, and that the quality of the studies was carefully assessed. You conclude that this is a valid systematic review and proceed to the results. The authors found 144 studies, and conclude that the benefits of topical fluoride are well-established, but potential harms have not been well-studied. Your entire search took only 15 minutes, and you feel confident that you now have up to date and comprehensive information to help you address your patients' concerns.

Take home list

- A torrent of research is published in medicine, much of it of poor quality, so that it has become impossible for clinicians to keep abreast.
- Traditional narrative summaries of research evidence are subject to bias as a result of the authors' prejudices, incomplete knowledge and frequently a lack of explicit criteria for evaluating the methodological rigor of summarized studies.
- Publication bias (the fact that the likelihood that a study will be published in a high-ranking journal, in English rather than another language or at all, is related to whether it reports "positive" results) is a constant threat to research synthesis.
- Systematic reviews are characterized by clear research questions, exhaustive attempts to identify studies, explicit criteria, including methodological criteria, for inclusion and methodological transparency.
- Guidelines can be defined as "systematically developed statements to assist practitioners and patient decisions about appropriate health care for specific clinical circumstances".
- The usefulness of guidelines depends on the rigor with which underlying evidence has been appraised, and a process of development, which takes account of a range of clinical and consumer perspectives.

Critical appraisal criteria for a systematic review

Are the results valid?

- Did the review address a sensible, clearly focused question?
- How likely is it that the search strategy would have missed eligible studies?
- Are the inclusion criteria clearly stated?
- Are the inclusion criteria relevant?
- Did the method used to select studies for inclusion minimize bias?
- To what extent are the conclusions based on valid primary studies?
- If a meta-analysis was performed, were the included studies sufficiently homogeneous to make it appropriate to pool the data?

What are the results?

- Are outcomes clinically meaningful and/or relevant to patients?
- Are adverse effects recorded?
- Do the results apply to my patients?

References

1 Mulrow C. Systematic reviews: rationale for systematic reviews. *BMJ* 1994;**309**:597–9.

2 Egger M, Davey Smith G. Meta-analysis bias in location and selection of studies. *BMJ* 1998;**316**:61–6.

3 Stern JM, Simes RJ. Publication bias: evidence of delayed publication in a cohort study of clinical research projects. *BMJ* 1997;**315**:6450–5.

4 Manuscript guidance. *Diabetologia* 1994;**25**:4A.

5 Dickersin K, Scherer R, Lefebvre C. Identifying relevant studies for systematic review. In: Chalmers I, Altmann DG eds. *Systematic reviews.* Plymouth: *BMJ* Publishing Group, 1995.

6 Egger M, Zellweger-Zähner T, Antes G *et al.* Language bias in randomised controlled trials published in English and German. *Lancet* 1997;**350**:326–9.

7 The *Cochrane Library. BMJ* Books/Update Software. Published quarterly on CD ROM.

8 Jüni P, Witschi A, Bloch R, Egger M. The hazards of scoring the quality of clinical trials for meta-analysis. *JAMA* 1999;**282**:1054–60.

9 Moher D, Pham B, Cook DJ, Moher M, Tugwell P, Klassen TP. Does quality of reports of randomised trials affect estimates of intervention efficacy reported in meta-analyses? *Lancet* 1998;**352**:609–13.

10 Roberts I, Kramer MS, Suissa S. Does home visiting prevent childhood injury? A systematic review of randomised controlled trials. *BMJ* 1996;**312**:29–33.

11 Weisz JR. Effects of interventions for child and adolescent psychological dysfunction: relevance of context, developmental factors, and individual difference. In: Luthar, SS, Burack JA, Cicchetti D, Weisz JR, eds. *Developmental psychopathology: perspectives on adjustment, risk, and disorder.* New York: Cambridge University Press, 1997.

12 Schultz KF, Chalmers I, Hayes RJ, Altman DG. Empirical evidence of bias: dimensions of methodological quality associated with estimates of treatment effects in controlled trials. *JAMA* 1995;**273**:408–12.

13 Sanders C, Egger M, Donovan J, Tallon D, Frankel S. Reporting on quality of life in randomised controlled trials: bibliographic study. *BMJ* 1998;**317**:1191–4.

14 Fields MJ, Lohr KN, eds, for Institute of Medicine. *Guidelines for clinical practice. From development to use.* Washington DC: National Academy Press, 1992.

15 Health Care Bulletin. *Implementing clinical guidelines.* York: Centre for Reviews and Dissemination, 1994.

16 Emslie CJ, Grimshaw J, Templeton A. Do clinical guidelines improve general practice management and referral of infertile couples? *BMJ* 1993;**306**:1728–31.

17 Health Care Bulletin. *Getting evidence into practice.* York: Centre for Reviews and Dissemination, 1999.

18 Royal College of Paediatrics and Child Health. *Report of the Quality of Practice Committee: Standards for development of clinical guidelines in paediatrics and child health.* London: Royal College of Paediatrics and Child Health, 1998.

19 Shekelle PG, Woolf SH, Grimshaw J. Developing guidelines. *BMJ* 1999;**318**:593–6.

20 Kahan JP, Park RE, Leape LL *et al.* Variations by speciality in physician ratings of the appropriateness and necessity of indications for procedures. *Med Care* 1996;**34**:512–23.

21 Implementing clinical practice guidelines: can guidelines be used to improve clinical practice? *Effective Health Care Bulletin, No. 8.* York: NHS Centres for Reviews and Dissemination, 1994.

22 Glasziou PP, Irwig LM. An evidence-based approach to individualising treatment. *BMJ* 1995;**311**:1356–9.

23 Sackett DL. Applying overviews and meta-analyses at the bedside. *J Clin Epidemiol* 1995;**48**:61–6.

24 Cook RJ, Sackett DL. The number needed to treat: a clinically useful measure of treatment effect. *BMJ* 1995;**310**:452–4.

25 Chalmers I. Applying overviews in meta-analysis at the bedside. *J Clin Epidemiol* 1995;**48**:67–70.

26 Lilford RJ, Pauker SG, Braunholtz A, Chard J. Decision analysis and the implementation of research findings. *BMJ* 1999;**317**:405–9.

27 Gilbert R, Logan S. Future prospects for evidence-based child health. *Arch Dis Child* 1996;**75**:465–73.

28 Colditz GA, Miller JN, Mosteller F. How study design affects outcomes in comparison of therapy. II: surgical. *Stat Med* 1989;**8**:455–66.

29 Miller JN, Colditz GA, Mosteller F. How study design affects outcomes in comparison of therapy. I: medical. *Stat Med* 1989;**8**:441–54.

30 Agency for Healthcare Research and Policy. http.//www.ahcpr.gov, 1992.

31 Effective Health Care. *Implementing clinical practice guidelines.* Bulletin No. 8. York: Centre for Reviews and Dissemination, 1994.

32 Grimshaw JM, Russell IY. Effect of clinical guidelines on medical practice: a systematic review of rigorous evaluations. *Lancet* 1993;**342**:1317–22.

33 Woolf SH, Grol R, Hutchinson A, Eccles M, Grimshaw J. Potential benefits, limitations, and harms of clinical guidelines. *BMJ* 1999;**318**:527–30.

34 Norheim OF. Healthcare rationing – are additional criteria needed for assessing evidence-based clinical practice guidelines? *BMJ* 1999;**319**:1426–9.

35 Haycox A, Bagust A, Whalley T. Clinical guidelines – the hidden costs. *BMJ* 1999;**318**:391–3.

36 Marinho VCC, Higgins JPT, Logan S, Sheiham A. Topical fluoride (toothpastes, mouthrinses, gels or varnishes) for preventing dental caries in children and adolescents (Cochrane Review). In: *The Cochrane Library*, Issue 4. Chichester, UK: John Wiley & Sons, Ltd, 2003.

9 Grading quality of evidence

Alessandro Liberati, Roberto Buzzetti, Roberto Grilli,
Nicola Magrini, Silvia Minozzi

Case scenario	The parents of a healthy, asymptomatic 5-year-old boy are very anxious about his health and ask their pediatrician about the appropriateness of undergoing a screening urine examination. You search for existing recommendations on this topic and find the book Putting Prevention into Practice: Clinician's Handbook of Preventive Services.[1] In Chapter 10, "Urinalysis", under the heading: "Recommendations of major authorities", you find the two different statements outlined below:

- American Academy of Family Physicians and US Preventive Services Task Force (USPSTF): "Routine screening of males and most females for asymptomatic bacteriuria is not recommended. The Canadian Task Force on the Periodic Health Examination and the USPSTF recommend against screening for asymptomatic bacteriuria with urinalysis in infants, children, and adolescents."
- American Academy of Pediatrics: "Urinalysis should be performed once at 5 years of age. Also, dipstick leukocyte esterase testing to screen for sexually transmitted diseases should be performed once in adolescence, preferably at 14 years of age."

You wonder what sort of evidence has been used to come to these quite different conclusions and decide to go back to the original documents to find the basis for these different recommendations. You wonder how the two Committees have looked at the evidence; whether they have used an explicit approach to classify the quality of existing studies and, if so, which elements (i.e., study design, study conduct, relevance of the outcome measures, frequency and severity of the problem to be prevented, etc.) they have considered.

Terms of reference

The evidence-based medicine (EBM) approach to searching, critically appraising and summarizing evidence has already been extensively discussed in other chapters of this book. Despite its limitations, its main and unquestionable advantage is that it makes "the rules of the game" explicit. One reason for critically appraising existing evidence on etiology, diagnosis, therapy, and prognosis is to make explicit recommendations for clinical practice (in the form of practice guidelines, diagnostic, or therapeutic clinical pathways, etc.). To decide which of these guidelines we should follow we need common criteria to assess the available evidence.

While it is generally agreed that practice guidelines should present, in an explicit way, an assessment of the quality of the evidence that supports different statements, this is still uncommon, and many guidelines are still based on an implicit process broadly defined as "consensus-based".[2] The type of evidence that is necessary varies depending on the question addressed. When effectiveness is at issue, it is agreed that randomized clinical trials (RCTs) represent the gold standard methodology. For questions of diagnosis, prognosis, or etiology, the best evidence does not come from RCTs and should rather be derived from other types of study designs.[3]

Assessment of quality of evidence aims at assessing the extent to which one can be confident that an estimate of effect is correct. Since the 1970s a growing number of organizations have employed different systems to grade the quality of evidence and the strength or recommendations; however, they have used different systems so that the same evidence can be graded in many different, and difficult to compare, ways.

Historically, the first attempt to classify levels of evidence supporting clinical recommendations was made by the Canadian Task Force on Preventive Health Care,[4] who reviewed the indications for preventive interventions and produced recommendations with an explicit grading of the supporting evidence and of the strength with which this evidence should be implemented. This approach was subsequently adopted by the US Preventive Services Task Force.[5] The original approach used by the Canadian Task Force classified RCTs as the highest level of evidence, followed by non-randomized control trials, cohort and case–control studies (representing fair evidence), comparisons between times and places with or without the intervention and, at the lowest level, "expert opinion". This approach has been widely used because it is simple to understand and easy to apply. It implicitly assumes that RCTs, no matter how small or large they are or how they are conducted, always produce better evidence than non-experimental studies, such as cohort or case–control studies. Moreover, this approach ignores the issues of precision and heterogeneity and thus is not helpful to decide what to do when results from several RCTs, or other non-experimental studies, vary among themselves.

Other schemes proposed since that of the Canadian Task Force still rely on methodologic design of primary studies as the main criterion, but have incorporated systematic reviews and meta-analyses as a hierarchically higher level of evidence above randomized control trials. While this allows for a potentially more refined way of grading of levels of evidence it still suffers from the same limitation as the attention is given to the *a priori* validity of the methodology used. More recently, schemes assessing the quality of study conduct and the consistency of results across different studies have been proposed.

The aim of this chapter is therefore:

● to review existing schemes aimed at assessing the quality of evidence supporting treatment (i.e., effectiveness) recommendations;
● to discuss the need to go beyond the assessment of the methodologic quality (whether measured *a priori* by looking at study design or *a posteriori* by looking at study conduct) to include an explicit assessment of the epidemiologic and clinical relevance of the evidence in terms of consistency, precision, and appropriateness of the outcomes measured;
● to suggest directions that research in this area should take.

It is outside the remit of this chapter to discuss and analyze ways in which *recommendations* are formulated and graded in terms of their strength as a function of the quality of evidence. As, however, there is considerable confusion between the two constructs of *grading of the evidence* and *formulation and grading of the recommendation(s)*, a brief clarification may be warranted. *Formulating recommendations and grading their strength are* more complex tasks than grading the evidence. The former, in fact, implies a trade-off between benefits and harms that can hardly be made in a fully explicit way. As recently suggested by the GRADE (Grades of Recommendations, Assessment, Development and Evaluation) Working Group,[6] *strength of recommendations* is a construct that should be based on the grading of *evidence* as starting point and then should also be based on other considerations including:

● the trade-off implied by the size of the effect of an intervention on relevant outcome(s);

● the translatability of the evidence into a specific practice setting;
● the degree of uncertainty about baseline risk in the population of interest.

For a more detailed discussion of this issue the reader should refer to a forthcoming paper by the GRADE working group.[6]

Ways to grade quality (levels) of evidence

Grading *quality of evidence* can be a useful tool for users of practice guidelines who are critically appraising the validity of what they read. This grading heavily weights the quality of the methodology used in primary studies and can be performed at the level of individual studies or of a systematic review of several individual investigations. When used for individual studies, quality assessment provides explicit criteria to separate valid from invalid studies (i.e., a dimension usually referred to as "internal or scientific validity"). When used within the context of a systematic review, grading quality of evidence can be used to assist in qualifying the recommendations to be incorporated into practice guidelines and the confidence with which they should be implemented.

In principle, *quality of evidence* can be graded according to:

● *a priori* validity of study design
● quality of study conduct
● consistency of results across studies
● clinical relevance of the study results.

Each of these approaches has benefits and risks. Assessing the validity of the recommendations as a function of the "*a priori* validity of the methodology" used in individual studies is the oldest, and still most commonly used, approach to levels of evidence classification. This was the approach originally proposed by the Canadian Preventive Task Force, followed by several other groups. The main advantages of this approach are its explicit nature and the fact that a general consensus exists regarding the hierarchy of different types of study designs in terms of their *a priori* ability to prevent bias.[4,5] On the other hand, this approach relies exclusively on issues of design (thereby ignoring issues of study conduct) and ignores the need to judge the importance of study findings in terms of their consistency and clinical and epidemiologic relevance.

It is thus fairly obvious that a much better approach would be that of assessing not only the *a priori* validity of the study methodology but also the "quality of the actual conduct" of the study. However, despite its appeal, the feasibility of this approach is seriously jeopardized by the lack of consensus regarding the appropriate indicators of study validity. This is clearly demonstrated by the lack of an agreed gold standard.

Table 9.1 Dimensions of quality explored by different schemes

Schemes	Number of levels	Study design	Quality of conduct	Consistency of results
Canadian Preventive Task Force, 1990[4]	4	✓		
US Preventive Services Task Force, 1992[5]	5	✓		
AHCPR, 1992[13]	5	✓		
Eccles *et al.*, 1995[12]	6	✓		
Adorn *et al.*, 1996[14]	7	✓	✓	
Jovell *et al.*, 1997[15]	9	✓	✓	✓
Guyatt *et al.*, 1998[16]	6	✓		✓
Oxford Centre for Evidence-based Medicine., 1998[17]	10	✓	✓	✓
National Health and Medical Research Council of Australia, 2000[18]	5 (+6)	✓	✓	✓

Not even for RCTs – which seem to be the most highly standardized type of study design – is there an agreement on whether a quality score[7] or a criteria-based system is better. Several years ago, Emerson *et al.*[8] failed to demonstrate the predictive validity of the "Chalmers" quality score" and, more recently, Juni *et al.*[9] reported substantial differences in the assessed "quality" of a paper depending on the scale used to measure it. Thus far, the only item for which there is clear empirical evidence of bias prevention is the quality of the randomization process (defined as the extent to which concealment of allocation was truly maintained).[10]

Besides the assessment of the methodologic quality of component studies, "consistency of results" across different investigations becomes an important issue. Consistency, however, does not stand alone and must be adjusted for both type of study design and quality of study conduct. Dramatically large effects may be consistently reported in studies of lower methodologic quality (i.e., from a series of observational studies), but further tests based on more rigorous designs may then indicate much smaller, if any, effect.[11] Relative to the quality of study conduct, consistency *per se* does not imply validity, as a series of individual studies can be systematically wrong, if the same biases (such as biased selection of study population or systematically inaccurate measurement) are made.

The "clinical and epidemiologic relevance" of the evidence that is available should also become an important consideration when grading quality of evidence and this issue is explicitly addressed by the new system currently under development by the international GRADE Working Group.[6]

Existing schemes to grade evidence

Table 9.1 lists nine schemes[4,5,12–18] that we have identified with respect to the dimensions that they are intended to explore. All schemes explore the dimension of the "*a priori*

study validity" but the level of details varies from the simplest approach of the Canadian Task Force (four levels) to the more complex and analytic taxonomy proposed by more recent schemes. Only four[9–12] also critically appraised the "quality of the study conduct" through predefined criteria but differed on criteria applied and on operational definitions.

"Consistency of results" is incorporated into four schemes.[8,10–12] However, heterogeneity is neither clearly nor consistently defined across schemes.

More recently, the GRADE Working Group carried out a thorough comparative assessment of six existing approaches including two – such as the Scottish Intercollegiate Guidelines Network (SIGN)[20] and the US Task Force on Community Preventive Services (USTFCPS)[20] – showing that all existing systems have important shortcomings.[21]

Some schemes (i.e., those of the Canadian and US Task Forces) separate "levels of evidence" from "strength of recommendations" (in the case illustrated in the opening scenario, for example, the evidence for the use of routine culture was Level I and the recommendation was " type E" (i.e., do not perform), while in others, the two are more closely tied).

This analysis of existing schemes suggests therefore that the "state of the art" is still far from satisfactory. Although there are three schemes available[10–12] that look at all three dimensions illustrated in Table 9.1, the main challenge for a better approach to "levels of evidence" classification seems to be how to combine the three dimensions outlined above with the "clinical and epidemiologic relevance" of the study findings.

The need to consider epidemiologic and clinical relevance

When the Canadian Task Force scale was originally proposed, RCTs were less common and requirements for drug approval were less stringent, so that evidence from RCTs was often not available. With the much wider availability of RCTs, the scales have become quite insensitive to differences in the quality of supporting evidence. As a result, it may be inappropriate to accept the presence of one or two RCTs as sufficient evidence in favor of an intervention.

Critically appraising aspects of the question addressed is also important: was the study designed to explore long-term versus short-term use of the treatment, the type of skill/experience required by the providers, and the availability of the appropriate level of care? Two issues are central here:

- the nature of the endpoint
- the appropriateness of the comparator chosen

When you are critically appraising the nature of the endpoint, whether it is hard or soft, clinical versus surrogate, and what its relationship is to the quality or quantity of life all must be considered. The other important question to be addressed is whether there are direct comparisons of different candidate interventions or only RCTs comparing each to nothing/placebo.

Strong evidence of effect does not necessarily translate into equally strong recommendations for use or, on the contrary, instances where less strong, or fair evidence, may lead to strong recommendations (for example, when there are no viable alternatives and the "do nothing" approach is not practically feasible).

For instance, when you are assessing the evidence for and against breast cancer screening on a population level, while the evidence of effectiveness is strong (the usefulness of mammography screening in women > 50 years of age is supported by several RCTs), it may still be inappropriate to recommend a screening, if the other criteria for implementation are not met. There might be insufficient well-trained radiologists to read the mammograms, pathologists to read the biopsies, or surgeons to perform appropriate surgery in a particular health district.

Similarly, if you are assessing the evidence for and against screening for visual impairment in preschool children with a view to making recommendations for a specific health district, while the evidence can be fair (as the usefulness of routine testing for amblyopia and strabismus is supported by cohort studies), it may still be worth not recommending it, if there are reasons to believe that the implementation of such screening would not do more good than harm (say, because there are not enough well-trained nurses, ophthalmologists, etc.).

Future directions and conclusions

Although more recent schemes take into account the quality of study conduct, we found no scheme that explicitly includes the clinical and epidemiologic relevance of the question addressed by the studies. Using only methodologically based quality assessment to judge the evidence supporting intervention is inadequate, especially in an area of therapy where RCTs (and thus the highest level of evidence) are commonly available. Schemes such as those discussed by Adorn *et al.*,[14] Jovell *et al.*,[15] Ball *et al.*,[17] and the NNMRC[18] are all good steps in this direction, although an effort to provide operational definitions is needed. The work currently being undertaken by the international GRADE Working Group[6,19] is addressing most of the issues discussed in this paper, and it is hoped that it may soon gain large acceptance so that documents produced by different guidelines development agencies become more explicit and their recommendations comparable.

As outlined above, the main limitation of available schemes for "grading of evidence" is their lack of proper conceptualization of all the dimensions that should be considered in deciding whether an estimate of effect is correct. Failure to recognize this carries the risk of accepting the content of irrelevant, if not misleading, guidelines.

Resolution of the scenario

Going back to the original source, you find that the US Preventive Task Force document indicates that there is evidence from both RCTs and observational studies in support of their recommendation not to perform a screening test for asymptomatic bacteriuria in infants, children, and adolescents.[5] On the contrary, the recommendation by the American Academy of Pediatrics is an unqualified "consensus statement" without any reference to the evidence supporting it.[22] Despite the limitations of existing schemes available to assess levels of evidence discussed in this chapter, we can therefore conclude that having an explicit approach aimed at grading the evidence from available studies can still be a useful screening tool, especially when you are comparing different recommendations allegedly drawn from the same type of evidence.

Take home list

- A thorough assessment of the quality of evidence that underlies recommendations or guidelines may help clinicians decide which to follow.
- Evidence should be graded not only on the basis of *a priori* validity of study design and aspects of study conduct, but also on consistency of evidence and the clinical relevance of the outcomes (end-points) assessed.
- A number of schemes are available to grade evidence but none is wholly satisfactory. Work is currently underway by an international working group to develop a new unified approach able to overcome the shortcomings of existing ones.

- The strength of recommendations should depend on the quality of evidence, judgments about the values to be ascribed to various outcomes and contextual issues such as availability of resources and impact on other services.

References

1 US Department of Health and Human Services. *Putting prevention into practice: clinician's handbook of preventive services: children and adolescents – screening. 2nd edn.* Washington DC, 1998.

2 Grilli R, Magrini N, Penna A, Mura G, Liberati A. Practice guidelines produced by specialty societies: the need for a critical appraisal. *Lancet* 2000;**355**:103–6.

3 Sackett DL, Rosenberg WMC, Gray JAM. Evidence-based medicine: what it is and what it is not. *BMJ* 1996;**312**:71–2.

4 Woolf HS, Battista R, Anderson CM *et al.* Assessing the clinical effectiveness of preventive maneuvers: analytic principles and systematic methods in reviewing clinical evidence and developing clinical practice recommendations. *J Clin Epidemiol* 1990;**43**:891–905.

5 US Preventive Services Task Force. *Guide to clinical preventive services, 2nd edn.* Baltimore: Williams & Wilkins, 1996.

6 The GRADE Working Group. Grading evidence and formulating recommendations. *BMJ* (2004, In press).

7 Moher D, Jadad A, Tugwell P. Assessing the quality of randomized control trials: current issues and future directions. *Int J Technol Assess Health Care* 1996;**12**: 195–208.

8 Emerson JD, Burdick E, Hoaglin DC, Mosteller F, Chalmers TC. An empirical study of the possible relation of treatment differences to quality scores in controlled randomized clinical trials. *Controlled Clin Trials* 1990;**11**:339–52.

9 Juni P, Witschi A, Bloch R, Egger M. The hazards of scoring the quality of clinical trial for metanalysis. *JAMA* 1999; **282**:1054–60.

10 Schultz FK, Chalmers I, Hayes RJ, Altman DG. Empirical evidence of bias: dimensions of methodological quality associated with estimates of treatment effects in controlled trials, *JAMA* 1995;**273**:408–12.

11 Sacks H, Chalmers TC, Smith R. Randomized vs historical control for clinical trials. *Am J Med* 1982;**72**:233–40.

12 Eccles M, Clapp Z, Grimshaw J *et al.* North of England evidence-based guidelines development project: methods of guidelines development. *BMJ* 1996;**312**:760–2.

13 US Department of Health and Human Services. Public Health Services, Agency for Health Care Policy and Research. *Acute pain management.* Rockville, MD: Agency for Health Care Policy and Research Publications. (AHCPR Pub 92–0038), 1992.

14 Adorn DC, Baker D, Hodges JS, Hicks N. Rating the quality of evidence for clinical practice guidelines. *J Clin Epidemiol* 1996;**49**:749–54.

15 Jovell AL, Navarro-Rubio MD. Evaluadon de la evidencia cientifica. *Med Clin (Barc)* 1997;**105**:740–3.

16 Guyatt G, Cook D, Sackett D *et al.* Grades of recommendations for antithrombotic agents *Chest* 1998; **114**(5 Suppl.): 441S–4S.

17 Ball C, Sackett D, Phillip B, Straus S, Haynes B. Levels of evidence and grades of recommendations. Centre for Evidence-based Medicine [http://cebm.jr2.ox.ac.uk/docs/levels.html].

18 National Health and Medical Research Council. How to use the evidence: assessment and application of scientific evidence. Commonwealth of Australia.2000 [http://www.health.gov.au/nhmrc/publicat/pdf/cp69.pdf].

19 The GRADE Working Group. A critical appraisal of systems for grading evidence and formulating recommendations (unpublished manuscript).

20 Harbour R, Miller J. A new system for grading recommendations in evidence-based guidelines. *BMJ* 2001; **323**:334–6.

21 Briss P, Zaza S, Pappaioannou M et al. Developing an evidence-based guide to community and preventive services–methods. The Task Force on Community Preventive Services. *Am J Prevent Med* 2000;**18**:35–43.

22 American Academy of Pediatrics. Recommendations for preventive pediatric health care. *Pediatrics* 1995;**96**: 373–4.

10 Clinical measures

Sue Gilmour, Robert Klaassen

Case scenario 1 *You are working in a pediatric emergency room as a staff pediatrician when a 2-year-old child is brought in by ambulance with a history of lethargy and large ecchymoses. There have been four recent and well-publicized deaths from meningococcal sepsis in your area and the Public Health Department has declared that the region is experiencing an epidemic of meningococcal disease. Presuming a diagnosis of meningococcal sepsis, stabilization of the patient is started and the pediatric intensive care (PICU) is notified. The parents are well aware of the recent deaths and ask you and the PICU staff about the prognosis of their child. After you leave the parents, your colleague in the PICU tells you of a new prognostic measure for meningococcal sepsis developed in Spain[1] and suggests implementing the measure in your hospital. You wonder if this measure will provide the emergency room (ER) staff with a good prognostic measure.*

Case scenario 2 *It is winter, and your general pediatric practice is seeing many preschool children (2–5 years) presenting with exacerbations of asthma. Objectively documenting these exacerbations can be difficult as the preschoolers cannot reliably cooperate with pulmonary function testing and their respiratory rates and the use of accessory muscles will vary with activity and crying. Also, the practice is arranged such that, if you do not have a clinic day, your patients will be seen by one of your colleagues. Knowing that it is difficult to obtain objective criteria for improvement in asthma symptoms in this age group and that the children may be assessed by more than one pediatrician, you wonder if there is a valid measure that can be administered by primary care providers to assess improvement in the children's asthma symptoms.*

Background

For most patients, clinical evaluation is far more powerful than laboratory evaluation in establishing diagnoses, prognoses, and therapeutic plans.[2] A clinical measure is an attempt to quantify clinical evaluation. The above clinical scenarios provide examples of the variety of issues that can arise from the use of clinical measures and their potential impact on clinical management.

In some situations, clinical information can be captured only by using a clinical measure. Evaluation of pain is a good example. When children (such as those with sickle cell disease) are treated for pain, it is hard to know how to interpret an answer of "sort of" when the physician inquires if the pain is better. Since there are no laboratory tests available for the assessment of pain, a clinical measure is needed to evaluate pain control. One of the advantages of using clinical measures over other methods is that the patient's perspective can be incorporated. If the child is cooperative, a measure

that incorporates his or her perspective is preferred. There are a number of different pain measures that have been used in this setting, including the Faces Pain Scale,[3] or a visual analogue scale (VAS) (Figures 10.1 and 10.2).

Practical, reliable, and valid clinical measures can also be used to monitor a patient's condition over time, to monitor patients as they pass through different levels of care, or as outcome measures in clinical trials assessing therapeutic options. An example of this is the Westley croup score (Table 10.1), which can be useful in the ambulatory, emergency, or inpatient setting. For croup, "hard measures" such as heart rate and respiratory rate are poorly correlated with improvement in severity.[4] The alternatives, such as oxygen desaturation or intubation, are such rare events that they are not realistic outcomes, except perhaps in very large trials. The Westley croup score is determined by adding up values from five clinical categories: stridor, retractions, air entry, cyanosis, and level of consciousness.[5] In a clinical study, a measure such as the Westley croup score is the only practical

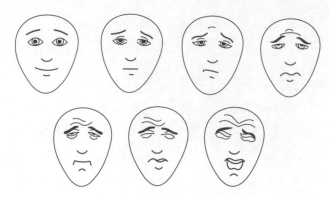

Figure 10.1 The Faces Pain Scale. In actuality each face is 6 cm high[3]

No pain		Worst pain imaginable

Figure 10.2 Visual Analogue Scale

Table 10.1 Westley Croup score[5]

Level of consciousness	
Normal (including sleep)	0
Disoriented	5
Cyanosis	
None	0
Cyanosis with agitation	4
Cyanosis at rest	5
Stridor	
None	0
When agitated	1
At rest	2
Air entry	
Normal	0
Decreased	1
Markedly decreased	2
Retractions	
None	0
Mild	2
Moderate	2
Severe	3

means of assessing a therapeutic response, and the score is a well established primary outcome in a number of croup trials.[6,7]

In this chapter, we will discuss the various categories of clinical measures, review what constitutes a good clinical measure, and explain the different methods that can be used to quantify the degree of agreement and responsiveness of a particular measure.

Table 10.2 Types of measures

Type	Examples
Binary	Presence or absence of pain
Nominal	Gender, race
Ordinal	Faces pain scale, Westley croup scale
Continuous	Pain visual analogue scale

Parameters of measures

Types of measures

Measures can be loosely classified as binary, nominal, ordinal, or continuous (Table 10.2). Asking a sickle cell patient if she did or did not have pain would provide a *binary* response, while having her point to one of the seven sequential categories of the faces scale would be using an *ordinal* measure. Nominal scales have categories (such as race or religion) that have no inherent order. *Continuous* measures have multiple categories where the intervals between each are considered equal, such as with a visual analogue scale (VAS).

Purpose

Depending on its purpose, a clinical measure can be classified as discriminative or evaluative. *Discriminative instruments* are used to distinguish between two or more groups of patients, whereas *evaluative measures* capture change over time (Table 10.3). The faces pain scale, for example, helps healthcare providers distinguish between sickle cell patients with different needs for pain control (i.e., a discriminative measure). A patient with a score of 1 or 2 may need only an oral analgesic, whereas a score of 5 or 6 may indicate the need for a morphine infusion. Some measures are suited to both purposes. The faces scale can also be used as an evaluative measure to monitor pain therapy. If the score decreases from 5 to 2, it is likely therapy such as a morphine infusion can be decreased.

Setting

The setting of a clinical measurement generally refers to the clinical environment and patient population in which the measure is intended to be used. For example, all of the pain measures mentioned so far have been used in studies involving patients with sickle cell disease,[8] but not all of the measures would be applicable to a particular patient. The faces pain scale has been used in children as young as 3 years of age, whereas visual analogue scales have been shown to be valid only in patients over 7 years of age.[3]

The setting may also affect the relevance of the individual components of a particular measure. For instance, the original

Table 10.3 What makes a good clinical measure?[28,29]

Purpose	Discriminative (distinguish groups)	Evaluative (recording change over time)
Example	Face pain scale	Croup score, faces pain scale, VAS
Reliability	Interrater reliability	Internal consistency; test-retest reliability
Validity	Content validity; discriminant validity; concordance with suitable physical examination and laboratory tests	Construct validity; convergent agreement with equivalent methods
Responsiveness	Not applicable	Statistical responsiveness; minimal clinically important difference
Interpretability	Differences between patients at a point in time can be interpreted as trivial, small, moderate or large	Differences within subjects over time can be interpreted as trivial, small, moderate or large

Table 10.4 Approaches to validity[11,29]

Approach	Description
Face validity	Do the items appear to measure what they are intended to measure?
Content validity	Is the choice of, and relative importance given to, each item of the measure appropriate for the clinical event it is supposed to measure?
Criterion validity	Does the measure produce results which are in agreement with some "gold standard" test obtained simultaneously (concurrent validity), or that will be available in the future (predictive validity)?
Construct validity	Do the results obtained confirm *a priori* hypotheses consistent with the target disorder? Are they correlated to variables and measures of the same construct to which they should be related (convergent validity)? Are they uncorrelated with dissimilar, unrelated ones (discriminant validity)?

croup score evaluated five clinical aspects of acute respiratory illness in hospitalized children.[5] For clinical trials involving outpatients with mild to moderate croup, two aspects of the score, the degree of consciousness and cyanosis, may not be applicable. As such, a modified version of the score has been suggested for outpatient settings.[9]

Reliability

The two aspects of reliability are internal consistency and reproducibility. The internal consistency of a measure relates to whether all of the components are assessing the same thing. In the case of the Westley croup score, all components should measure the severity of the croup. Thus, all the components should correlate well with each other,[10] and the score for each variable should correlate with the total score. Each component should add value to the overall measure, and should cover the spectrum of what is being measured.

The reproducibility of a measure is the extent to which it yields the same results when used repeatedly on an unchanged population. The measure should be consistent over time (test–retest and intrarater reliability) and should show agreement between different users of the same measure (interrater reliability). Reproducibility studies should be undertaken in several contrasting patient populations that are representative of the full range of possible scores in a measure. Strategies to improve reliability include observer training and/or increasing the number of items in the measure, although the latter strategy can lead to a loss of internal consistency.[11]

Validity

A valid instrument measures what it is purported to measure while minimizing systematic (non-random) error. Validity testing can be facilitated if the purpose and setting of the clinical measure are well defined. A measure may be valid for the specific purpose for which it was developed, but may not be valid for a related but different purpose. Some approaches to validity testing are summarized in Table 10.4.

The initial step in assessing validity is to consider *face validity*: does it look like the instrument measures that it intends to measure? Next look at the *content* of the measure: does it include a representative sample of items that cover the clinical concept that it is supposed to measure? *Criterion validity* is divided into concurrent and predictive validity depending on whether the measure can be correlated with a gold standard at the same time (concurrent) or in the future (predictive). Finally, if no gold standard exists, *construct validity* should be assessed by using mini-theories: does the measure correlate to another measure that measures a similar clinical event (*convergent validity*) or does not correlate with an unrelated measure (*divergent validity*)?

In addressing whether a measure is valid, it is not always feasible to apply all of the possible approaches. For discriminative instruments, both content and face validity are essential as these attributes help to distinguish groups of patients across the spectrum of a disease. When the gold standard required for criterion validity is not available, both qualitative and quantitative methods can be used to examine validity.[10] Qualitative judgments can be made about the range and content of items in the measure. Content validity addresses whether comprehensive aspects of the disease under investigation (process, outcome, or prognosis) have been covered. For example, the five clinical aspects in the croup score can be examined to see if they are reasonably comprehensive for that illness.

Quantitative evaluation of a measure involves examining patterns of relationships amongst a range of other relevant variables. To assess construct validity, a range of clinical scenarios, or constructs, are hypothesized, and the performance of a clinical measurement in these scenarios is examined. Convergent validity occurs when the measure correlates well with constructs that are related, whereas divergent validity occurs when the measure does not correlate with constructs that are unrelated. For example, the croup score has been shown to correlate with parent and physician global assessments of change.[12] It has also been shown to be highly correlated with pulsus paradoxus, a more objective measure of croup severity.[4] In terms of divergent validity, the score is poorly correlated with changes in respiratory rate and heart rate.[12] These aspects of construct and convergent validity demonstrate that the Westley croup score is representative of croup severity, and provides a good outcome for use in clinical trials.

Responsiveness

Responsiveness is the ability of a measure to detect small but important clinical changes.[14] One might assume that a measure that can discriminate among patients at a single point in time could also detect subtle changes over time. However, the requirements for a measure that can accurately divide a group up into different categories, for instance moderate versus severe croup, can differ substantially from what is needed to evaluate a change in clinical status, such as a significant clinical improvement on racemic epinephrine.[15]

Evaluative instruments must be sensitive to change and the identified change must be relevant to the patient and/or the illness.[16] The difficulty with many measures is that, although they can measure small changes between groups, the clinical relevance of the results are not intuitive.[17] To help deal with this, a minimal clinically important difference can be established. Klassen and Rowe demonstrated that a change in

the croup score of 1 point corresponds to a mild improvement in severity as judged by physicians using a global assessment scale.[12]

Interpretability

In addition to being reliable and valid, clinical measures should provide clinically applicable information. Most clinical measures use ordinal scoring or, occasionally, continuous scoring. Interpreting these scores can be difficult: is an improvement from 40 mm to 30 mm on a pain VAS really equivalent to a change from 50 mm to 40 mm?

If a measure becomes widely used, its repeated applications in different patient populations can provide some clinically-based interpretation of its scores. The faces pain scale was administered to children with acute lymphoblastic leukemia and resulted in a median raw score of 2 for children undergoing a venipuncture, 3 for an intramuscular needle insertion, and 4 for a lumbar puncture.[3] This provides clinicians with a framework for interpreting raw scores in other settings.

If an instrument is new or used in a new setting, two strategies are often used to improve its interpretability. The first is to identify the minimal clinically important difference or change. The second approach is to correlate scores of an instrument with other objective measures such as severe life events, so that some intuitive calibration of the scale can be made available.[10]

Evaluating a clinical measure

Before being introduced to wide use, a clinical measure should be evaluated for reliability, validity, and responsiveness to important clinical changes. Such evaluations should be done in the target setting. Confusion may arise because multiple approaches can be used to evaluate the same property.[14] In the following sections, we briefly discuss the indices used in the evaluation of reliability and responsiveness. We then provide some criteria for evaluating a clinical measure.

Evaluating reliability

Reliability is concerned with the consistency of measurement across time, patients, or observers. Reliability can be measured by kappa coefficient and intraclass correlation (ICC). The notion of repeatability, or internal consistency, can be measured by Cronbach's alpha.

Kappa coefficient

The kappa coefficient is used to report the reliability of instruments that have binary, nominal, or ordinal scales. The

Table 10.5 Calculation of kappa coefficient

		First rater		
		Optimal healing (exp. by chance)*	Suboptimal healing (exp. by chance)*	Total
Second rater	Optimal healing	70 (59·2)	4 (14·8)	74
	Suboptimal healing	10 (20·8)	16 (5·2)	26
	Total	80	20	100

*Values in parentheses are the expected values by chance alone if there were no difference between raters.

kappa coefficient captures the degree of agreement after accounting for the agreement that would occur by chance alone. In a study of wound healing, two raters independently evaluated 100 patients' wounds for cosmetic appearance (data shown in Table 10.5). Both raters concluded that 70 patients had optimal healing and that 16 patients had suboptimal healing, and in the remaining 14 cases the raters disagreed. The observed agreement between the two raters is (70 + 16)/100, or 86%. Of course, some of this agreement must have occurred just by chance. If the first rater generally finds that 80% of wounds have healed optimally, then, of the 74 cases rated optimal healing by the second rater, one would expect 80% of the 74, or 59·2 cases, in agreement with the first rater by chance alone. Likewise, since the first rater found 20% of the wounds suboptimal, taking 20% of the second rater's 26 suboptimal cases yields 5·2 of the cases that the two would agree on by chance alone. The total agreement expected by chance is (59·2 + 5·2)/100, which equals 64·4%. Therefore, 100% − 64·4% = 35·6% is the potential for agreement beyond what is expected by chance alone. The actual agreement beyond chance is the observed agreement minus the agreement expected by chance (86% − 64·4% = 21·6%). The kappa coefficient is the ratio of actual (21·6%) to the potential (35·6%) agreement beyond chance. In this example, kappa is 21·6%/35·6% = 0·61.

When a score has more than two categories, a weighted kappa coefficient can be used to reflect the partial agreement of categories that are close but not the same. In the croup score, chest retractions are scored as none = 0, mild = 1, moderate = 2, and severe = 3. If a study had two research assistants independently score a group of children with croup, it would be important to differentiate between a small discrepancy of just one point, and a large discrepancy such as 0 versus 3.[18]

Intraclass correlation

The ICC is used to report the reliability of instruments that are based on ordinal or continuous scales. In its simplest form, the ICC is the ratio of the true variation between subjects to the sum of all observed variation (owing to subjects, raters, and random error).[11] The ICC quantifies the signal, which is the systematic variation the instrument claims to measure, given the background noise or variation from other sources inherent to the instrument or clinical setting. As the between-subject variation is highly dependent on the population being studied, any change in the patient population will affect the ICC. Evidence of reliability in one clinical setting may not imply the same degree of reliability in a different setting with a different patient population.

Interpreting reliability

The ICC and kappa coefficients are interpreted similarly.[18] For most purposes, values greater than 0·75 may be taken to represent excellent agreement beyond chance, values below 0·40 may be taken to represent poor agreement, and values between 0·40 and 0·75 may be taken to represent fair to good agreement.[13] Both measures of reliability will be artificially low if the patients are too similar, i.e., the between-patient variation is low. This would occur, for example, if the reliability of the faces pain scale were assessed at the time of a routine sickle cell clinic visit and 90% of patients were rated as having a score of 0 (no pain). The full range of the scale would not have been used and the resulting low reliability coefficients indicate a problem in the study design rather than a problem with the scale itself.

Cronbach's alpha

Internal consistency is the concept that the individual components of a measure assess the same overall clinical construct. Cronbach's alpha can be written as a function of the number of test items and the average intercorrelation among the items. The rationale of using Cronbach's alpha as a measure of reliability is that the overall clinical measure functions as if the test were being repeatedly performed because each item is roughly measuring the same thing. This deals with some of the problems of test-retest reliability, in particular learning effects (patients remembering their previous responses leading to falsely high reliability) or patients' clinical state changing between measurements (falsely lowering reliability). Cronbach's alpha and the ICC often provide similar results, as long as the patients' clinical status remains stable between measurements.

Evaluating responsiveness

While responsiveness is increasingly accepted as a distinct and important requirement of a clinical measure, there is less agreement on the details of how to evaluate it.[10] Such evaluation essentially entails two considerations: a sensitivity to change assessment and a relevance determination. Three indices commonly used to evaluate responsiveness include a standard paired t-test, a sensitivity index of the effect size, and a sensitivity statistic in which the mean change in scores among patients receiving the intervention is judged by the variation in scores from patients who remain "stable".[14,15]

These sensitivity indices do not indicate whether the response is clinically relevant. Additional information is required for relevance determination. If the minimal clinically important change has been described, a responsiveness index can be derived by dividing this change by the standard deviation in score changes for "stable" patients.[15]

Now let us look at our original scenarios and evaluate whether or not the measures are acceptable.

Case scenario 1 (Continued)

Recalling the first scenario of prognosis in meningococcal sepsis, you review the literature and find more than 20 disease-specific measures plus general measures to evaluate illness-related mortality of meningococcal disease. You decide to evaluate the new disease specific measure from Spain, the Spanish meningococcal septic shock score (SMSSS) and compare it to a measure you have read about previously, the Glasgow meningococcal septicemia prognostic score (GMSPS).[19,20,21]

Both measures are discriminative and are used to predict outcome in meningococcal disease. The outcome for the SMSSS is death and for the GMSPS is fulminant sepsis and admission to PICU. You note that the GMSPS outcome includes but is not restricted to mortality. Both measures were developed to classify patients into homogeneous risk groups for future interventional clinical trials. Both provide ordinal scores, ranging from 0 to 10 for the SMSSS and 0 to 15 for the GMSPS (Table 10.6 and 10.7). The SMSSS was developed in a retrospective cohort study in 14 PICUs, and included a developmental cohort of 192 children consecutively admitted with presumed meningococcal sepsis and a validation sample of 158 such children.[1] The GMSPS was developed in a retrospective cohort of 123 children from which the performance characteristics were derived.[20] Subsequently, a prospective observational validation study was done including 278 children admitted to hospital or seen in the emergency room of two tertiary and four referring hospitals with confirmed or probable meningococcal disease.[21]

You consider that the SMSSS was developed retrospectively, and you note that neither inter- nor intrarater reliability were evaluated. Four of the variables are objective, but three have some subjectivity (cyanosis, Glasgow Coma Scale, and refractory hypotension). The GMSPS prospective study also does not include intra- or interrater testing and acknowledges the requirement for this testing of reproducibility.

With regard to face validity, both measures appear to be comprehensive in their selection of variables. Further review of literature reveals to you that the variables contained in the measures have been associated with disease severity and mortality.[22] From the standpoint of content validity, both measures incorporate variables that reflect the disease process and the importance given to each item corresponds to your literature review. The variables have scores that include the spectrum of disease from normal to markedly impaired. Neither measure used a simultaneous criterion standard, but both correlated well with future death. In the populations in these studies, an SMSSS score of 6 or higher had a positive predictive value (PPV) of 74%, while a GMSPS score of 11 or higher had a PPV of 56%. You note that sensitivity and specificity were calculated, which will enable you to apply the results to your own population (see Chapter 5). A receiver operator curve (ROC) curve and area under the curve (AUC) are also provided. As there is a future gold standard (death), construct validity is not a concern. The GMSPS score was compared to other severity measures (low leukocyte counts, TNF-alpha levels, low fibrinogen levels) and good correlation was found.

You consider how to interpret these measures. Neither scoring system was able to accurately predict all non-survivors. Both measures used an intuitive marker for calibration. The SMSSS stratified the patients into three risk groups for death, low risk (score ≤ 3), intermediate risk (score 4–5), and high risk (score ≤ 6). The GMSPS stratified children into high and low risk of fulminant disease requiring PICU admission (cut-off of 8).

In summary, both measures have a clear purpose, well defined setting, and have been validated. Both need to be assessed for reliability and have not been used to assess change over time. They have similar performance characteristics and discriminate well between survivors and non-survivors, although that is not the primary purpose of the GMSPS. The SMSSS does contain easily obtainable variables that are objective, but the patients and setting for this study were very ill children already admitted to the PICU and do not represent your population in the pediatric ER that includes a wider spectrum of disease. The GMSPS is designed for initial evaluation such as is done in an emergency room, and the variables are easily and quickly obtainable on initial presentation.

Case scenario 2

In the second scenario, you wondered about an evaluative measure for preschool asthma. Using PubMed and the search strategy "asthma (MAJR) AND questionnaires (MESH) AND validation studies (PT)" you search for evaluative measures of asthma in pediatric asthma. Your search finds one validated measure for preschool children that was developed for use in clinical trials (Table 10.8).[23] This measure is designed to evaluate change in asthma symptoms over time (an evaluative measure) in preschool children. The diary is completed by primary caregivers who act as proxy respondents for the children (clearly necessary in this age group). The result is expressed as an ordinal score that can range from 0 (no symptoms) up to 25 (all symptoms very severe). The diary was prospectively tested in 125 children aged 2–5 years from 13 referral clinics (mostly asthma/allergy clinics) across North America. The majority of the patients were on maintenance anti-inflammatory therapy, usually cromolyn (63% of stable and 37% of unstable patients) with only 22–30% of patients receiving inhaled corticosteroids.

Internal consistency was examined using Cronbach's alpha, which was acceptable with an alpha coefficient = 0·90.[23] Test-retest reliability was assessed by ICC. The ICC was excellent (ICC > 0·75) for the symptom and activity questions in the stable patients. The unstable patients had ICC ranging from 0·44 to 0·69 (fair to good agreement).

You judge the items to have good face validity, that is, they appear to measure relevant asthma symptoms, with questions about disease symptoms and impact. A review of the literature in both pediatric and adult evaluative measures of asthma reveals that similar types of questions have been used, assessing the asthma symptoms in the daytime, night-time, impact on activity, impact on the patient and the family.[24–26] Weighting of the questions appears similar. Therefore the content validity appears acceptable. Criterion validity is difficult to assess as there are no "gold standard" tests in this age group. Convergent validity was assessed by evaluating the relationship between the change in the measurement questions with change in the caregiver quality of life questionnaire, MD asthma severity rating, beta-agonist use, and physician and caregiver responses to a global question of change at the end of the three weeks. Change in the diary question scores were strongly correlated with beta-agonist use and only moderately correlated with other asthma measures. Discriminant validity was assessed by measuring the differences between the stable and unstable groups over all measurement questions both at the start and at 3 weeks (end of study).

Statistical responsiveness was evaluated examining the change over the 3-week period within the two groups as well as the differences between the stable and unstable groups. Statistically significant differences were demonstrated. There was no definition of minimal clinical important difference (MCID) but responsiveness was compared to days without asthma or symptom-free days, an approach that has been used in other evaluative studies.[27] Over the 3 weeks, symptom-free days varied in the "stable" group of preschoolers from 33% to 45%. The "unstable" group of children demonstrated a change from 5% to 32% of children experiencing symptom-free days. Although this is not a defined MCID, there was an attempt to place some clinical relevance to the change in measurement scores. The authors acknowledge that this is still an unacceptably low percentage of both stable and unstable children being free of asthma symptoms. No information is provided about changes that can be clinically quantified.

You consider whether this measure would be useful for your general pediatric practice. The measure was designed for clinical trials in referral clinics and most of the patients were on cromolyn for maintenance which means that the setting and some of the baseline characteristics are not similar to your patients. The questions that comprised the measure are believed to represent the symptom burden of asthma and its impact on the children and their families, as noted in several studies.[24–27] Unfortunately, the test-retest reliability in the unstable unstable patients showed only fair agreement. The authors conclude that this is because the test-retest was not performed in a stable state. The patients were on new therapy and parents were requestioned after a period of time on the new therapy so this may represent clinical improvement. Responsiveness seems reasonable and there is an attempt to compare results with the measure of symptom-free days. Perhaps further use will improve the interpretability. In sum, the measurement demonstrates adequate validity, responsiveness, and with some issues on reliability, but does use questions that are typically used in a primary pediatric setting.

Table 10.6   GMSPS (adapted from Sinclair *et al.*[19,20])

Items	Points
BP < 75 mmHg systolic, age < 4 years	3
BP < 85 mmHg systolic, age > 4 years	
Skin/rectal temperature difference > 3°C	3
Modified coma scale < 8 or deterioration	3
≥ 3 points in 1 hour	
Deterioration 1 hour before scoring	2
Absence of meningismus	2
Extending purpuric rash or widespread ecchymoses	1
Base deficit (capillary or arterial) > 8	1
Maximum score	15

Table 10.7   Spanish Meningococcal Septic Shock Score[1]

Variable	Score
Refractory hypotension	2
Base deficit > 10 mmol liter^{-1}	1
Glasgow coma scale < 8	2
Leukocyte < 4000 mm^3	1
Oliguria	1
Cyanosis	2
PTT > 150% of control	1
Maximum score	10

Table 10.8   Pediatric Asthma Caregiver Diary[30]

Overnight

How much did your child cough last night after being put to bed for the night until awaking this morning? (Check 1 response)

0 Did not cough at all	2 Coughed several times	4 Coughed almost all night
1 Coughed very little	3 Coughed frequently	5 I do not know

Daytime symptoms

How severe was your child's cough today? (Check 1 response)

0 No cough	2 Mild cough	4 Severe cough
1 Very mild cough	3 Moderate cough	5 Very severe cough

How severe was your child's wheezing today? (Check 1 response)

0 No wheezing	2 Mild wheezing	4 Severe wheezing
1 Very mild wheezing	3 Moderate wheezing	5 Very severe wheezing

How severe was your child's trouble breathing today? (Check 1 response)

0 No trouble breathing	2 Mild trouble breathing	4 Severe trouble breathing
1 Very mild trouble breathing	3 Moderate trouble breathing	5 Very severe trouble breathing

How much did your child's asthma symptoms interfere with your child's activities today? (Your child's activities could include any sort of physical activity such as running, playing, jumping, sports, bike riding, climbing, or school activities) (Check 1 response)

0 Did not interfere	2 Mildly interfered	4 Severely interfered
1 Very mildly interfered	3 Moderately interfered	5 Very severely interfered

Summary

In order to appraise the effectiveness of a therapy, it is essential to evaluate the clinical measure for which the therapy outcome is assessed (Table 10.3). The major criteria for evaluating a clinical measure are summarized below:

- *Purpose.* What is the primary purpose of the measure? Was the measure designed to be a discriminative measure and yet is being used to assess response over time?
- *Setting.* What was the original setting of the measure (i.e., when it was developed), and does it correspond to the current setting? Are there important differences in the

severity of illness, age, or method of administration between the two settings?

- *Reliability.* Is the measure internally consistent? Is the measure reproducible between raters and, if it is an evaluative measure, reproducible over time when no change occurs?
- *Validity.* Does the instrument measure what it was intended to measure? Do the items in the measure cover the important aspects of the clinical event it is trying to measure? Has the measure been compared to an available gold standard, or does it perform appropriately in a variety of clinical scenarios if no gold standard is available?
- *Responsiveness.* Does the measure detect subtle but important clinical changes? What is the minimal clinically important difference, and how does that compare with the therapeutic effect?
- *Interpretability.* What do the results mean? Has the scale been calibrated to common clinical scenarios to provide a framework to interpret the raw scores?

Resolution of the scenario 1

Despite your PICU colleague's suggestion that you adopt the SMSSS, you will discuss with the pediatric ER staff the possibility of incorporating the GMSPS measure into your assessment of patients with presumed meningococcal disease. The SMSSS remains a better prognostic measure for your PICU colleague.

Resolution of the scenario 2

In the clinic, you decide to introduce the asthma diary to your practice. Parents will complete it between office visits to help the physicians assess improvement or lack of improvement when there has been a change in asthma therapy. You hope that this will assist in providing more objective information than relying on recall when re-evaluating a preschooler with an asthma exacerbation. This new practice initiative will be reassessed in 3 months to see if it is providing useful evaluative information.

Take home list

- Textbooks may be a useful source of information on "background" questions but may provide biased advice and rapidly become out of date.
- Turning your clinical problem into a carefully structured question helps to guide where to search, what type of studies to look for, and what search terms to use.
- Before starting a search, decide whether you want a comprehensive search or a "quick and dirty" answer.
- A number of short-cuts to high-quality evidence such as *Evidence Based Medicine, Clinical Evidence*, or the *Cochrane Library* are now available.

References

1 Castellano-Ortega A, Delgado-Rodiquez M, Llora J *et al.* A new prognostic scoring system for meningococcal septic shock in children. Comparison with three other scoring systems. Intensive *Care Med,* 2002;**28**:341–51.

2 Sackett DL, Haynes RB, Tugwell P. *Clinical epidemiology. 1st edn.* Boston: Little, Brown, 1985.

3 Bieri D, Reeve RA, Champion GD, Addicoat L, Ziegler JB. The Faces Pain Scale for the self-assessment of the severity of pain experienced by children: development, initial validation, and preliminary investigation for ratio scale properties. *Pain* 1990;**41**:139–50.

4 Ausejo M, Saenz A, Pham B, Kellner JD, Johnson DW, Moher D, Klassen TP. The effectiveness of glucocorticoids in treating croup: meta-analysis. *BMJ* 1999;**319**:595–600.

5 Westley CR, Cotton EK, Brooks JG. Nebulized racemic epinephrine by IPPB for the treatment of croup. *Am J Dis Child* 1978;**132**:484–7.

6 Muhlendahl KE, Kahn D, Spohr HL, Dressler F. Steroid treatment in pseudo-croup. *Helv Paediatr Acta* 1982;**37**:431–6.

7 Kuusela A, Vesikari T, A randomized, double-blind, placebo-controlled trial of dexamethasone and racine epinephrine in the treatment of croup. *Acta Paediatr Scand* 1988;**77**:99–104.

8 Jacobson SJ, Kopecky EA, Joshi P, Babul N. Randomised trial of oral morphine for painful episodes of sickle-cell disease in children. *Lancet* 1997;**350**:1358–61.

9 Geelhoed GC, Macdonald WBG. Oral dexamethasone in the treatment of croup. *Pediatr Pulmonol* 1995;**20**:362–8.

10 Fitzpatrick R, Davey C, Buxton MJ, Jones DR. Patient-assessed outcome measures. In: Black N, Brazier J, Fitzpatrick R, Reeves B, eds. *Health services research methods.*. London: BMJ Publishing Group 1998.

11 Streiner DL, Norman GR. *Health measurement scales.* Oxford: Oxford University Press, 1989.

12 Klassen TP, Rowe PC. The croup score as an evaluative instrument in clinical trials. Abstract No. 70. *Arch Pediatr Adolesc Med* 1995;**149**:60.

13 Landis JR, Koch GG. The measurement of observer agreement for categorical data. *Biometrics* 1977;**33**:159–74.

14 Deyo RA, Diehr P, Patrick DL. Reproducibility and responsiveness of health status measures. *Controlled Clini Trials* 1991;**12**:142S–158S.

15 Guyatt G, Walter S, Norman G. Measuring change over time: assessing the usefulness of evaluative instruments. *J Chronic Dis* 1987;**40**:171–8.

16 Fisher D, Stewart AL, Bloch DA, Lorig K, Laurent D, Holman H. Capturing the patient's view of change as a clinical outcome measure. *JAMA* 1999;**282**:1157–62.

17 Todd KH, Funk KG, Bonacci R. The clinical significance of reported changes in pain severity. *Acad Emerg Med.* 1995;**2**:369–70.

18 Fleiss JL. *Statistical methods for rates and proportions. 2nd edn.* New York: John Wiley & Sons, 1981.

19 Sinclair JF, Skeoch CH, Hallworth D. Prognosis of meningococcal septicemia. *Lancet* 1987;**ii**:38.

20 Thomson APJ, Sills JA, Hart CA. Validation of the Glasgow Meningococcal Septicaemia Prognostic Score: A 10–year retrospective survey. *Crit Care Med,* 1991;**19**:26–30.

21 Riordan FA, Marzouk O, Thomson AP, Sills JA, Hart CA. Prospective validation of the Glasgow Meningococcal Septicaemia Prognostic Score. Comparison with other scoring methods. *Eur J Pediatr* 2002;**161**:531–7.

22 Baines PB, Hart CA. Severe meningococcal disease in childhood. *Br J Anesthesh* 2003;**90**:72–83.

23 Santanello NC, De Muro-Mercon C, Davies G *et al.* Validation of a pediatric asthma caregiver diary. *J Allergy Clin Immunol* 2000;**106**:861–6.

24 Powell CV, McNamara P, Solis A, Shaw NJ. A parent completed questionnaire to describe the patterns of wheezing and other respiratory symptoms in infants and preschool children. *Arch Dis Child* 2002;**87**:376–9.

25 Santanello NC, Barber BL, Reiss TF, Friedman BS, Juniper EF, Zhang J. Measurement characteristics of two asthma symptom diary scales for use in clinical trials. *Eur J Respir* 1997;**10**:646–51.

26 Asher MI, Keil U, Anderson HR *et al.* International study of asthma and allergies in childhood (ISAAC): rationale and methods. *Eur J Respir* 1995;**8**:483–91.

27 Tasche MJ, van-der-Wouden JC *et al.* Randomized placebo-controlled trial of inhaled sodium cromoglycate in 1–4-year-old children with moderate asthma. *Lancet* 1997;**350**: 1060–4.

28 McDowell I, Jenkinson C. Development standards for health measures. *J Hlth Serv Res Policy* 1996;**1**:238–46.

29 Guyatt HG. A taxonomy of health status instruments. *J Rheumatol* 1995;**22**:1188–90.

30 Santanello NC, MD, MS West Point, PA Pediatric asthma assessment: Validation of 2 symptom diaries. Table VI. PACD (completed by children 2 to 5 years old). *J Allerg Clin Immunol* 2001;**107**:S468.

11 Assessing quality of life

Elizabeth Waters, Elise Maher

Case scenario *You are working as registrar in the pediatric intensive care unit of a large tertiary referral center. One of your patients is a 10-year-old boy 1-week post bone marrow transplantation for acute myeloid leukemia. The unit head is currently conducting a research project to assess functioning and quality of life in children at discharge from the transplant unit. While reading the instruments used to assess QOL and functioning in the research project, you realize that the information obtained will also be useful to parents and carers. You wonder why these particular measures were chosen, how well they have been validated, how they will be used, and whether they are useful in clinical practice as well as in research.*

Background

Within the last few decades the concept of "good health" has moved from the "absence of disease or illness" to a more positive concept which embraces the subjective experience of well-being and quality of life (QOL). In pediatrics, as in other areas of health care, there is growing awareness that medical parameters such as mortality and morbidity are not the only important outcome variables to be considered when we evaluate child health interventions.

A QOL perspective can identify sensitive child and adolescent issues that may be affected by illness, disability, or treatment. In the past, we have assumed that the link between physiologic measurements and patient well-being is strong, i.e., if the physiologic state is shown to be improving, then overall well-being will inevitably follow. To the surprise of many, empirical research shows that the relationship is usually modest and variable,[1–3] and suggests that improvements in outcomes are more likely to occur if treatment decisions are based on both patient perspectives and clinical indicators. However, in the absence of adequate instruments, child health and overall well-being is often estimated by researchers and physicians using as a guideline their own personal reference points and experiences with similar patients. Although valuable, such assessments are not comparable for different physicians or patient groups.[4]

QOL assessment also integrates psychologic and sociologic perspectives, drawing attention to determinants of health at a range of levels. Personal factors such as attitudes, cultural background and beliefs; community factors such as family, peers, employment, and schools; and structural factors such as income distribution, educational opportunities, and employment opportunities are specifically recognized. Taking a QOL perspective and using a systematic measurement process can also provide opportunities for clinicians to promote positive health and healthy behaviors among parents, children, and adolescents.[5]

The addition of a QOL measure in clinical assessment assists in decision-making by providing information about the patient's view of what they gain or lose from treatment. Many clinicians are not familiar with the range of health-related QOL instruments available for clinical use, nor the spectrum of diseases for which they have been developed, ranging from common conditions such as otitis media to rarer conditions such as spina bifida.

Subjective QOL or well-being can be measured quantitatively and precisely. Unfortunately, the development of instruments to measure QOL in children and adolescents lags far behind that for adults, primarily due to the unique measurement challenges in children.[6–8] The language, content, and setting of instruments need to be pertinent to the activities and stages of the child's experience and development.

Definitions of quality of life for children and young people

The terms QOL, health-related QOL (HRQOL), health, and functional status are not interchangeable, nor are the instruments used to assess them. Functional status can be distinguished from the other constructs, as it tends to focus more on physical abilities or disability.[9,10] However, the terms QOL, HRQOL, and health status are more similar and are commonly confused.[11-14] In this section we will attempt to define and differentiate QOL, HRQOL, and health.

The definitions of QOL and HRQOL cited in the child health literature are often complex and difficult to operationalize.[15] For example, researchers often cite the World Health Organization's definition of QOL as "the individual's perception of their position in life, in the context of the culture and value systems in which they live and in relation to their goals, expectations, standards and concerns."[16] Other researchers develop their own definitions, such as "QOL includes, but is not limited to the social, physical and emotional functioning of the child, and when indicated, his or her family, and it must be sensitive to the changes that occur throughout development."[17] There is no commonly accepted definition of HRQOL. For example, HRQOL has been defined as "a multidimensional functional effect of an illness or a medical condition and its consequent therapy upon the child,"[18] and "a rubric, encompassing various aspects of personal experience, including physical and psychologic health, cognitive factors, social role performance, and general life satisfaction."[19]

In order to differentiate QOL and HRQOL it is useful to examine the definitions adopted in the QOL literature on adults. Although varying definitions of QOL and HRQOL have also been developed for adults, HRQOL is generally conceptualized as being a subset of QOL.[20] HRQOL refers to an individual's perception of his or her health,[21] whereas QOL refers to satisfaction with a variety of domains such as physical well-being, material well-being, productivity, emotional well-being, intimacy, safety, and community.[22]

The confusion between HRQOL and QOL appears to stem from the conceptualization of health. Health has been broadly defined by the World Health Organization as "a state of complete physical, mental, and social well-being and not merely the absence of disease or infirmity."[23] This definition, which has been influential in defining HRQOL,[24] suggests that HRQOL does not just include physical well-being but also social well-being and emotional/mental well-being. It appears that when examining perceptions of health using a broad definition of health, researchers term the construct QOL rather than HRQOL.[14] However, it is important to recognize that QOL includes not only physical well-being, social well-being, and emotional/mental well-being, but also non-health-related domains. These domains, which are dependent on age, have not been extensively researched for children, but may include parental support and home environment.[25]

HRQOL is affected in a complex way by a person's physical health, psychologic state, level of independence, social relationships, and their relationship to salient features of their environment.[26] Measures of HRQOL for children should:

- be child centered;
- employ subjective self-report where possible;
- be age-related or at least developmentally appropriate;

- have a generic core and specific modules;
- put an emphasis on health-enhancing aspects of QOL.[26]

For example, while complete cure of health problems such as epilepsy or leukemia may not always be possible, it may be possible to prevent or reduce negative emotional feelings in affected children. In children with chronic diseases in particular, psychosocial care often forms an essential part of health care. Based on assessments of HRQOL in a variety of clinical settings, psychologic care should be an essential part of routine care throughout life.[4]

Instruments used to assess QOL and HRQOL fall into three broad categories.

- *Comprehensive child health status instruments* commonly include measures of physical, psychologic, and social functioning (functional status), but may also measure well-being, illness-related stress, and social and behavioral functioning.
- *Functional status instruments* generally measure the impact of health problems on children's functioning in various roles, but do not address their subjective experience of a condition.[24]
- *Preference and utility-based instruments* measure a patient's level of satisfaction with his or her health, or preference for certain health states. The use of preference and utility-based instruments in pediatrics and child health has been vigorously debated. Firstly, it is not feasible to capture preferences from infants and very young children. Secondly, a child who has not experienced various states of health cannot possibly express a preference. Utility scores, however, can be combined with morbidity and mortality data to provide a comparative, single-weighted measure with broad applications for economic evaluation of health policy and funding.

A range of generic (Tables 11.1 and 11.2) and condition (disease)-specific (Table 11.3) measures of health status, functional health, QOL and HRQOL are available. The choice of one over another will be determined by the aims of the research study or the clinical application.[27]

Generic measures:

- permit direct comparisons between different patient populations, thereby informing policy decisions across a range of diseases;
- are generally robust, as evidenced by validation in a wide variety of situations;
- are usually subject to long and systematic development and testing, and have known measurement properties, which may not be practical for disease-specific measures.

Condition (disease)-specific measures:

- only include elements known to be relevant to the patient population under study;

Table 11.1 Generic health and quality of life instruments for children and adolescents

Measure/instrument	Concept	Study/author	Age range (years)	Respondent	Domains	No. items
Short survey for assessing health and social problems of adolescents (COOP charts)	Functional assessment/HRQOL	Wasson et al.[28]	12–21	Adolescent	Physical fitness, emotional feelings, school work, social support, family communications, health habits	6
Child Health Questionnaire (CHQ CF87/80/50)	Functional health status and wellbeing (HRQOL)	Landgraf et al.[29,30] Waters et al.[31]	10/12–18	Child/adolescent	Physical functioning, social role (emotional/behavioral, physical), general hearth, bodily pain, behavior, mental health, self-esteem, family activities and cohesion, change in health	87/80/50
Child Health Questionnaire (CHQ FF50/28)		Landgraf and Ware[29]	0–5 5–18	Parent/proxy	As above plus parent impact (time, emotional)	128 50/98
Functional Status (II)R (FSII-R/FSQ-S)	Functional status	Stein et al.[32]	0–16	Parent	Communication, mobility, mood, energy, play, sleep, eating, toileting	43 (interview)/ 14 (self-admin)
Measure of Functioning (RAHC MOF)	Functioning	Dossetor et al.[33]	10 years and over	Parent	Functional assessment by levels with categories (10 points) range: 0–100	Allocation of a category
				Clinician		Exact score
TACOOL	Functioning	Theunissen et al.[34]	8–11	Child	Pain and symptoms, functioning: social, motor, autonomy, cognitive, global emotional (negative and positive)	108
TAPQOL	Functioning/HRQOL	Fekkes et al.[35]	8–11	Parent	Pain and symptoms, functioning: social motor, autonomy, cognitive, global emotional (negative and positive)	108
			1–5	Parent		46
TAAQOL			16+	Adolescent		45
TAAQOL	Functioning/HRQOL	Vogels et al.[4]	6–15	Parent	Pain and symptoms functioning: social, motor, autonomy, cognitive, global emotional (negative and positive)	63
Quality of Wellbeing (QWB)	Functioning and wellbeing	Kaplan et al.[36]	8–15	Child/adolescent	Functioning: physical, role, cognitive; emotional wellbeing	63
			5–12	Child		18
Child Quality of Life Questionnaire (COOL)	HRQOL	Graham et al.[37]	9–15	Child/adolescent	Getting about and using hands, school, out of school activities, family, bodily symptom discomfort, worries, depression, seeing, communication, eating, sleep, appearance	15
				Mother		

Abbreviations: HRQOL, Health-related quality of life; QOL, quality of life.

Table 11.2 Generic health and quality of life instruments for children and adolescents

Measure/instrument	Concept	Study/author	Age range (years)	Respondent	Domains	No. items
Pediatric Quality of Life Questionnaire (PedsQL)	HRQOL	Varni et al.[38]	2–4	Parent	Functioning: physical, psychological, social, school and wellbeing	27
			5–7			30
			8–12			15
			13–18			15
			5–7	Child/adolescent		30
			8–12			15
			13–18			15
16D	HRQOL (16 dimensions)	Apajasalo et al.[39]	12–15	Child	Mobility, vision, hearing, breathing, sleeping, eating, elimination, speech, mental function, discomfort and symptoms, school and hobbies, friends, physical appearance, depression, distress, vitality	16
17D	HRQOL (17 dimensions)	Apajasalo et al.[40]	8–11	Child	As above excluding anxiety and including ability to concentrate, learning ability and memory	17
KINDL	HRQOL/Functioning and wellbeing	Ravens–Sieberer and Bullinger[41]	8–16	Child/adolescent	Psychological wellbeing, social relationships, physical functioning, everyday life activities	40
The Warwick Child Health and Morbidity Profile	Health status	Spencer and Coe[42]	0–5	Parent	Health status: general, acute minor illness, behavioral accident, significant illness, hospital admission, chronic illness, functional; QOL	16
Child Health and Illness Profile Adolescent Edition (CHIP-AE)	Health status	Starfield et al.[8]	11–17	Adolescent	Achievement, comfort, disorders, resilience, risks, satisfaction	153
Quality of Life Profile: Adolescent Version (QOLPAV)	QOL	Raphael et al.[5]	14–20	Adolescent	Being, belonging, becoming	54
DUCATOOL	QOL (global)	Koopman et al.[43]	School-aged	Child	Physical, emotional, social, cognitive	36
Generic Child Quality of Life measure (GCQ)	QOL	Collier et al.[44]	6–16	Child/adolescent	General affect, peer relationships, attainments, relationships with parents, general satisfaction	25

Abbreviations: HRQOL, Health-related quality of life; QOL, quality of life.

Table 11.3 Condition-specific instruments: cancer

Measure/instrument	Concept	Study/author	Age	Respondent	Domains	No. items
BASES (for children having a bone marrow transplant)	Difficult to define	Phipps et al.[45]	5–17	Parent	Somatic distress, compliance, mood disturbance, quality of interactions, activity	38
				Child		38
				Nurse		14
Perception of illness experience scale (PIE)	Functioning	Eiser et al.[46]	8–24	Parent	Functioning: physical and psychological	34
				Child		
Paediatric Oncology quality of Life Scale (POQLS)	Functioning and behavior	Goodwin et al.[47]	Pre-school/adolescence	Parent	Physical functioning, emotional distress, externalizing behavior	21
The Pediatric Cancer Quality of Life Inventory-32 (PCQL 32)	Functioning and symptoms	Varni et al.[48]	8–12	Child	Disease and related symptoms; functioning: physical, psychological, social, cognitive	32
Health Utilities Index II (HUI II)	Health preferences	Feeny et al.[49]	From birth	Child	Sensation, mobility, emotion, cognition, self-care, pain, fertility	7 items
				Parent		7
				Clinician		7
Quality of Well-being Scale	Wellbeing preferences	Bradlyn et al.[50]	0–18	Parent	Scores assigned to levels of wellbeing	3 scales; 23 symptoms
				Child		
Scale for assessing QOL of children survivors	Health status	Martinez et al.[51]	4–23	Child	Physical, psychointellectual and growth status	5
				Parent		
The Miami Pediatric Quality of Life Questionnaire	HRQOL	Armstrong et al.[52]	1–18	Parent	Competence: social and self, emotional stability	56
Play Performance Scale	Play	Lansky et al.[52–54]	6/12–16	Parent	Play: active and quiet	1

Abbreviations: HRQOL, Health-related quality of life; QOL, quality of life.

- are shorter and more appropriate to understanding the needs related to specific illnesses or problems;
- can be sensitive and specific measures of the health problems associated with a disease;
- can be especially sensitive measures of change in QOL or HRQOL.

In general, these measures are used to evaluate and compare subgroups of children. They can also be used to monitor change in the health of an individual over time. In practice, sophisticated software that efficiently scores and provides data output on the health status of individuals is not commonly available to clinicians. Thus, these instruments will be most useful for individual patients if the completion of the questionnaire is used as a discussion point between the patient and family (as appropriate) in the context of a consultation.

Whose perspective matters? Reporting by parent or child?

Although self-report questionnaires are regarded as the primary method of assessing HRQOL,[55] proxy report by a parent or another representative may be a useful alternative for young children. However, perceptions of health by two different people differ markedly, whether they be two parents, a parent and a clinician, or a parent and child.[56–58] Despite this, parent opinion is relevant and important. Parents are generally able to estimate their child's well-being, and daily monitoring of a child's well-being can alert parents to small behavioral changes or physical symptoms. However, parents may easily over or underestimate the importance that their child attributes to certain aspects of his or her well-being at a specific point in time. For example, peer-related issues may be far more important to an adolescent than parents might think they are. Moreover, parental expectations and previous experiences with the child may influence their views of the child's current health state.[4] Evidence suggests that proxy reports are more accurate for "hard" information, for example ability to dress than for subjective evaluation, for example emotional well-being.[59] Proxies report more precisely when the phenomenon in question is directly observable, requires little evaluation or opinion, is non-controversial,[59,60] or reflects usual and regular behavioral patterns.[61] Even though the opportunity for direct child reports is often limited, it is necessary to measure children's own evaluation of their health to measure QOL accurately in children.

Evaluation of instruments used to measure QOL

Reliability

A measure is judged to be reliable when it consistently produces the same results when applied to the same subjects, when there is no evidence of underlying change in the health state being assessed.[62] Reliability of an instrument is most frequently evaluated by internal consistency, internal reliability, and test–retest.[27]

- *Internal reliability* depends on the internal consistency *(homogeneity)* of the items or soles (*sets of questions within a questionnaire*). Each item is assumed to be related in linear fashion to the underlying concept being measured. Cronbach's alpha coefficient measures the average correlation among the items in the scale and the number of items in the instrument. This measure has a range of 0–1 with higher values indicating a closer correlation, which suggests that the set of questions is assessing a single domain. A low alpha coefficient (for example, < 0.5) indicates that the item does not arise from the same conceptual domain. If the coefficient is too high, it is likely to indicate that some of the items are unnecessary and the scale may be too narrow in its scope to have much validity. Coefficients > 0.7 and < 0.9 are recommended.[62–64]
- *Test–retest reliability* is assessed when the instrument is administered to the same population on two occasions and the results are compared by correlation. However, repeating a health measurement to assess its stability or reliability over time is often not as simple as repeating a measurement in the physical sciences. The main problem is that the second response to a question is likely to be affected by the previous administration of that question. Similarly, for unstable concepts such as QOL, a subjective report may change between administrations depending on what life experiences have occurred in the intervening time. However, "if the measure is to be used to predict outcomes, it must be able to predict itself accurately, and so test-retest reliability is crucial; but if it is intended to mainly measure current status, the internal structure is the most crucial characteristic."[65]
- *Agreement and association* are measures of the discrepancies between pairs of ratings such as between ratings from a mother and her child. Agreement may be assessed by examining the distribution in the score given for a particular domain between a pair of reporters. There is a general level of agreement between parent and child if the parent routinely scores higher values of health than the child. Conversely there will be lack of agreement if the parent regularly or irregularly scores in an opposite direction. Association, however, refers to the relationship between two sets of scores, for example, parent scores with child scores, and is usually tested by a correlation coefficient.

Validity

Validity is defined as the extent to which the instrument measures what it is intended to measure.

- *Content validity* consists of a subjective judgement as to whether the instrument samples all the relevant and important content or domains.[62,66] This is an important prerequisite of acceptance of a measure, although it is critiqued as "validity by assumption" because judgment of the relevance and importance of the content usually depends on the "informed opinion" of "experts".
- *Face validity* is a simplified version of content validity, and refers to the extent to which the scale appears to be a good test of the construct in question, i.e., whether the items and scales look reasonable at "face value".
- *Criterion validity* establishes whether the variable or concept can be measured with accuracy by comparison with an existing "gold standard", and whether the instrument can substitute for the "gold standard" or vice versa. Testing criterion validity involves application of the two measures simultaneously or randomly to alternate subjects, and is important when you are attempting to develop a scale that is simpler or less expensive to administer than an existing measure.[66]
- *Construct validity* requires establishing theories and testing these theories and models against the relationships of the measure. Establishing construct validity is an ongoing process because often there is no one single study that can satisfy the criteria.
- *Discriminant validity* assesses the "success" of an item to correlate more strongly with its hypothesized scale than with any other scale within a questionnaire, and provides evidence of the conceptual logic for placing an item within a particular scale relative to other scales within the instrument. A summary of the desirable psychometric attributes of health measures is provided in the Box.

Desirable psychometric attributes of health measures

Reliability

- Internal reliability
- Test–retest reliability
- Agreement and association

Validity

- Content validity
- Face validity
- Criterion validity
- Construct validity
- Discriminant validity

Instruments for measuring QOL

Potential users of QOL instruments need to know the content of the instrument, what it is aiming to measure, and its performance in various situations. For many newer instruments, this information is unpublished or performance is still being assessed. The UK Health Technology Assessment Research and Development Programme recently funded a systematic review of QOL measures in chronic diseases in childhood.[67] This review addresses the following:

- the extent to which adult measures of HRQOL are applied to evaluate healthcare interventions in children;
- the appropriateness of using adult measures in children;
- the extent to which child self-reports correspond with assessments made by parents and carers;
- the feasibility and reliability of proxy measures of various aspects of HRQOL in different disease contexts.

This review includes generic as well as condition-specific measures, and should be a useful resource for pediatricians and child health practitioners who wish to use these in practice.

Available generic,[4–6,8,28,29,32–34,36–44,54,68–71] and condition-specific measures[17,46–49,51–53,72–94] of HRQOL were drawn from the electronic published and gray (unpublished) literature. The content, relevant ages, intended respondent, domains, and length (numbers of items) of some well-validated generic instruments are summarized in Tables 11.1 and 11.2. These instruments are currently at an adequate stage of development for application in research and practice. Disease-specific instruments are available for a wide range of conditions including cancer,[17,45,47–49,51–53,95] asthma, lung, and ENT problems,[74,76,80,81,91,92,96] diabetes,[83] headache and epilepsy,[73,82,86,87,93] rheumatic disease,[77,85,94] dermatologic conditions,[78,87] short stature,[89] spinal disabilities,[75,88] and inflammatory bowel disease.[72,79,90]

Details of instruments for use in children with cancer are listed in Table 11.3. These instruments have been developed to be used and interpreted in different ways, ideally with individual patients. Their application, development, reliability, and validity data are continually being published and are not summarized here. If you are interested in using any instruments for patients with a particular condition, you should review the literature at that time for any new information on its performance.

Interpreting and reporting QOL in children

Methodologic issues to consider

Increasingly, QOL has become an important outcome measure for health care, and data are being collected in a variety of studies using a variety of instruments.[97] A systematic review has recently been conducted to examine the methods used for analyzing QOL data for use in the assessment of health care.[97] Observations from the review are noted below.

- *QOL analysis and informative dropout.* It is common for patients who are severely ill, or have the worst QOL, to drop out of studies. This is particularly problematic in longitudinal studies of QOL where survival is also an endpoint. The authors comment that dropping out may not be random, but may depend on the QOL being experienced. Incomplete follow up of patients is called "informative dropout" and it is necessary to account for this in the analysis to prevent bias.

● *Analysis of survival data adjusting for QOL*. Routine analysis of survival is commonly adjusted for patient-related variables (fixed and time-dependent covariates). If QOL data are infrequent or missing, accurate adjustment for changes in QOL is difficult. Independent modeling of QOL and survival may improve the analysis.

● *Simultaneous analysis of QOL and survival data*. If both of these endpoints are considered important, they need to be considered simultaneously. Such analysis is limited in its application to children, owing to the relative rarity of death as an outcome. However, the most powerful approach to analyzing QOL and survival data is to model the longitudinal QOL and dropout processes, which includes dropout due to death, as two simultaneous processes.[97]

Measures

Standard criteria have been developed to assist clinicians in judging the usefulness of QOL measurements in clinical studies of interventions and outcomes. The McMaster Evidence-based Medicine Working Group has developed a Users' Guide entitled *How to use articles about health-related quality of life measurements*.[1] Another, more comprehensive set of criteria has been developed to assess the value and clinical significance of QOL results presented in a clinical trial or study (see Box).[98]

Critical appraisal criteria

1   What is the value of the information?

● Does the QOL information from this study add anything to your understanding of the preferences, desires, and needs of your patients?

2   How is QOL measured?

● Are the measures used in the trial common measures, a new measure, a generic measure, a condition-specific measure, or a combination of measures such as a "battery of scales"?

3   What information is available on the validity of the measures used?

● What scales are used?
● What domains are covered?
● What are the items in the various domains?

4   How "generalizable" are the results?

● Who are the patients included in the trial and how do they relate to the general population and to your population of patients?

● Do they have similar demographic and disease severity characteristics?

5   Are the analyses appropriate?

● Were all measurements, tests and time periods reported?
● Were many of the patients at the floor or ceiling of the measures at the start of the trial?
● Is there some indication of the distribution of change (difference between baseline and follow up) in scores?
● Do only a few individuals account for all the change?
● Do some individuals show a marked change in the opposite direction from the majority?
● If means and standard deviations are reported (or medians), is there any evidence that the measure is linear?
● Do the authors indicate the number of dropouts from the study and the reasons for discontinuation?
● Is the number of patients discontinuing or reasons for discontinuation likely to have affected the results?

6   What is the clinical significance of the result?

● Has there been any effort to anchor the changes in scores reported to a more intuitive standard, such as disease severity, change over time, correlation with another measure, threshold for change, life events, or a global measure of health or health-related QOL? *Additional questions should be answered in relation to their use with children and young people*

7   Who is the respondent?

● If proxy report, what is their relationship to the child?

8   Does the instrument have face validity in its application to children, i.e., is the content child related or has the instrument been developed with the population group of children in whom it is to be used?

Interpreting and reporting QOL results in systematic reviews

HRQOL is an important endpoint in evidence-based decision-making, but it is rarely included as an outcome in pediatric studies. To raise awareness of this deficit, systematic reviewers should highlight the absence of HRQOL outcomes in trials included in their review. Prior to the conduct of systematic reviews (and trials themselves), few researchers consult the relevant population group regarding their preferred QOL outcomes. In three systematic reviews listed in the *Cochrane Library* ("Prevention and treatment of obesity in childhood",[99,100] and "Effects of smoking cessation and prevention programs children and their parents"[101]), children were consulted about appropriate outcomes during the planning of the review. Conceptual and methodologic challenges remain regarding the inclusion, analysis, and interpretation of QOL instruments in research studies and reviews.

The Cochrane Collaboration is in the process of establishing a Quality of Life Methods Working Group to provide support for systematic reviewers and others in the application and interpretation of QOL data. Although not specifically targeting those working with children, it aims to be widely consultative of individuals working in pediatrics.

QOL in children with cancer

Measures of morbidity associated with acute and chronic diseases and their treatment are likely to become increasingly important with further advances in disease management. It is now possible to collect information about children's cancer-related health status using measures such as the PCQL-32, the cancer-specific model of the Peds-QL[48] the Miami Pediatric Quality of Life Questionnaire,[52] and several other cancer-specific instruments. However, condition-specific instruments do not indicate the overall burden of disease faced by children with cancer compared to healthy children, or show the profile of ill health suffered by these children. Generic measures of child health status and HRQOL provide information on overall health and well-being that may subsequently be used to understand how characteristics of a population with disease differ from those in a normal population. Like cancer-specific measures, these generic measures of QOL extend beyond biomedical and pathologic indicators of disease progression and capture the subjective perspectives of children and their parents

In a recently published study of children receiving maintenance therapy for acute lymphoblastic leukemia (ALL)[102] the generic parent-reported Child Health Questionnaire described the poor health experienced by children across multiple domains of health and well-being in comparison to that of the normative population. The questionnaire was acceptable and feasible for use in a clinical setting, and correlated strongly and appropriately with physician-reported aspects of the children's health. Significant deficits were noted in children with leukemia across all domains of functioning, and especially in general health, physical functioning, and impact of physical health problems on social interactions. The effect of illness on mental health and well-being was less marked, indicating that, overall, parents believe their children's physical problems have the greatest impact on QOL. In this particular study, the condition-specific instrument confirmed the results of the generic instrument but did not provide any new information.

Future research needs

- Development of new HRQOL instruments which involve children in early developmental phases, provide corresponding proxy measures where required, and undergo thorough field testing in community populations.

- When such instruments are being developed, single score measures, which undervalue the complexity of HRQOL in children, should be avoided. Rather, multidimensional instruments, which allow computation of domain scores, should be adopted.

References

1. Guyatt GH, Naylor D, Juniper E, Heyland DK, Jaeschke R, Cook DJ. How to use articles about health-related quality of life measurements. *internet Communication*, 1999.
2. Wake M, Hesketh K, Cameron F. Functional health status of children with diabetes. *Diabet Med* 2000;**17**:700–7.
3. Waters EB, Wake M, Hesketh K, Ashley D, Smibert E. Health-related quality of life of children with acute lymphoblastic leukemia: parent and clinician reports. *Int J Cancer* 2003;**103(04)**:514–518.
4. Vogels T, Verrips GW, Verloove-Vanhorick SP *et al.* Measuring health-related quality of life in children: the development of the TACQOL parent form. *Qual Life Res* 1998;**7**:457–465.
5. Raphael D, Rukholm E, Brown I, Hill-Bailey P, Donato E. The Quality of Life Profile-Adolescent Version: background, description and initial validation. *J Adolesc Health* 1996;**19**:366–75.
6. Eisen M, Ware JA. Measuring components of children's health status. *Med Care* 1979;**17**:921.
7. Pless IB, Perrin JM. Issues common to a variety of illnesses. In: Hobbs N, Perrin JM, eds. *Issues in the care of children with chronic illnesses.* San Francisco: Jossey-Bass, 1985.
8. Starfield B, Riley AW, Green BF *et al.* The adolescent child health and illness profile. A population-based measure of health. *Med Care* 1995;**33**:553–66.
9. Bottos M, Feliciangeli A, Sciuto L, Gericke C, Vianello A. Functional status of adults with cerebral palsy and implications for treatment with children. *Dev Med Child Neurol* 2001;**43**:516–28.
10. Bombardier C, Tugwell P. Methodological considerations in functional assessment. *J Rheumatol* 1987;**14**:6–10.
11. Sullivan SA, Olson LM. Developing condition-specific measures of functional status and well-being for children. *Clin Perform Qual Health Care* 1995;**3**:132–9.
12. Schmidt LJ, Garratt AM, Fitzpatrick R. Child/parent-assessed population health outcome measures: a structured review. *Child Care Health Dev* 2002;**28**:227–37.
13. Schwimmer JB, Burwinkle TM, Varni JW. Health-related quality of life of severely obese children and adolescents. *JAMA* 2003;**289**:1819.
14. Stewart MG. Pediatric outcomes research: Development of an outcomes instrument for tonsil and adenoid disease. *Laryngoscope* 2000;**110**:12–15.
15. Eiser C, Morse R. A review of measures of quality of life for children with chronic illness. *Arch Dis Child* 2001;**84**:211.
16. World Health Organization. Measuring quality of life: the development of the World Health Organization Quality of Life Instrument (WHOQOL). Geneva: Division of Mental Health, World Health Organisation, 1993.

17 Bradlyn AS, Ritchey AK, Harris DV *et al.* Quality of life research in paediatric oncology: research methods and barriers. *Cancer* 1996;**78**:1333–9.

18 Ronen GM, Rosenbaum P, Law M *et al.* Health-related quality of life in childhood disorders: A modified focus group technique to involve children. *Qual Life Res* 2001;**10**:71–9.

19 Warschausky S, Kay JB, Buchman S, Halberg, A, Berger M. Health-related quality of life in children with cranifacial anomalies. *Plast Reconstr Surg* 2002;**110**:409–14.

20 Spilker B, Revicki DA. Taxonomy of quality of life. In: Spilker B, ed. *Quality of life and pharmacoeconomics.* Philadelphia: Lippincott-Raven, 1996.

21 Irrgang JJ, Anderson AF. Development and validation of health-related quality of life measures of the knee. *Clin Orthop* 2002;**1**:95–109.

22 Cummins RA, Eckersley R, Pallant J, Misajon R. Developing a national index of subjective well-being: The Australian Unity Well-being Index. *Soc Indic Res* 2003;**64**:159–180.

23 World Health Organization. Official records of the World Health Organization 1948;**2**:100.

24 Levi R, Drotar D. Critical issues and needs in health-related quality of life assessment of children and adolescents with chronic health conditions. In: Drotar D, ed. *Measuring health-related quality of life in children and adolescents: Implications for research and practice.* New Jersey: Lawrence Erlbaum, 1998.

25 Juniper EF. How important is quality of life in pediatric asthma? *Pediatr Pulmonol* 1997;**15**:17–21.

26 World Health Organization. *Measurement of quality of life in children.* Division of Mental Health. Geneva, World Health Organization, 1993.

27 Bergner M, Rothman ML. Health status measures: an overview and guide for selection. *Annu Rev Public Health* 1987;**8**:191–210.

28 Wasson JH, Kairys SW, Nelson EC, Kalishman N, Baribeau P. A short survey for assessing health and social problems of adolescents. *J Family Pract* 1994;**38**:489–94.

29 Landgraf J.M., Abetz L, Ware JA. *The CHQ user's manual. 1st edition.* Boston: The Health Institute, New England Medical Center, 1996.

30 Landgraf JM, Abetz L. Functional status and well-being of children representing three cultural groups: initial self-reports using the CHQ-CF87. *Psychol Health* 1997;**12**:839–54.

31 Waters E, Salmon L, Wake M. The Child Health Questionnaire in Australia: reliability, validity and population means. *Aust NZ J Public Health* 2000;**24**:207–10.

32 Stein RK, Jessop DJ. Functional status II(R). A measure of child health-status. *Med Care* 1990;**28**:1041–55.

33 Dossetor DR, Liddle JLM, Mellis CM. Measuring health outcomes in pediatrics: development of the RAHC measure of function. *J Paediatr Child Health* 1996;**32**:519–24.

34 Theunissen NM, Vogels T, Koopman HM, *et al.* The proxy problem: child report versus parent report in health-related quality of life research. *Qual Life Res* 1998;**7**:387–97.

35 Fekkes M, Theunissen NC, Brugman E *et al.* Development and psychometric evaluation of the TAPQOL: a health-related QOL instrument for 1–5 year old children. *Qual Life Res* 2000;**9**:961–72.

36 Kaplan RM, Debon M, Anderson BF. Effects of number of rating-scale points upon utilities in a quality of well-being scale. *Med Care* 1991;**106**:1–4.

37 Graham P, Stevenson J, Flynn D. A new measure of health-related quality of life for children: preliminary findings. *Psychol Health* 1997;655–65.

38 Varni JW, Seid M, Rode CA. The PedsQL: Measurement model for the pediatric quality of life inventory. *Med Care* 1999;**37**:126–39.

39 Apajasalo M, Sintonen H, Holmberg C *et al.* Quality of life in early adolescence: a sixteen-dimensional health-related measure (16D). *Qual Life Res* 1996;**5**:205–11.

40 Apajasalo M, Rautonen JA, Holmberg C *et al.* Quality of life in pre-adolescence: a 17-dimensional health-related measure (17D). *Qual Life Res* 1996;**5**:532–8.

41 Ravens-Sieberer U, Bullinger M. Assessing health-related quality of life in chronically ill children with the German KINDL: first psychometric and content analytical results. *Qual Life Res* 1998;**7**:399–407.

42 Spencer NJ, Coe CA. The development and validation of a measure of parent-reported child health and morbidity: the Warwick Child Health and Morbidity Profile. *Child Care Health Dev* 1996;**22**:367–79.

43 Koopman HM, Kamphuis RP, Verrips GH *et al.* The DUCATQOL: a global measure of quality of life of school-aged children (abstract). *Qual Life Res* 1997;**6**:428.

44 Collier J, MacKinlay D. Developing a generic child quality of life measure. *Health Psychol Update* 1997;**28**:12–16.

45 Phipps S, Dunavant M, Jayawardene D, Srivastiva DK. Assessment of health related quality of life in acute in-patient settings: Use of the BASES scales in children undergoing bone marrow transplantation. *Int J Cancer* 1999;**12**(Suppl.):18–24.

46 Eiser C, Havermans T, Craft A, Kernahan J. Development of a measure to assess the perceived illness experience after treatment for cancer. *Arch Dis Child* 1995;**72**:302–7.

47 Goodwin DA, Boggs SR, Graham-Pole J. Development and validation of the Pediatric Oncology Quality of Life Scale. *Psychol Assess* 1994;**6**:321–8.

48 Varni JW, Katz ER, Seid M, Quiggins DJ, Friedman-Bender A. The pediatric cancer quality of life inventory-32 (PCQL-32). I. Reliability and validity. *Cancer* 1998;**82**:1184–96.

49 Feeny D, Furlong W, Barr R, Torrance GW, Rosenbaum P, Weitzman SA. A comprehensive multiattribute system for classifying the health status of survivors of childhood cancer. *J Clin Oncol* 1992;**10**:923–8.

50 Bradlyn AS, Harris CV, Warner JE, Ritchey AK, Zaboy K. An investigation of the validity of the quality of well-being scale with pediatric oncology patients. *Health Psychol* 1993;**12**:246–50.

51 Martinez-Climent J, Sanchez VC, Menor CE, Miralles AV, Tortajada JF. Scale for assessing quality of life of children survivors of cranial posterior fossa tumors. *Med Care* 1994;**22**:67–76.

52 Armstrong FD, Toledano SR, Miloslavich K *et al.* The Miami Pediatric Quality of Life Questionnaire: Parent scale. *Int J Cancer* 1999;**12**(Suppl.):11–17.

53 Lansky SB, List MA, Lansky LL, Ritter-Sterr C, Miller DR. The measurement of performance status in childhood cancer patients. *Cancer* 1987;**60**:1651–6.

54 Lansky LL, List MA, Lansky SB, Cohen ME, Sinks LF. Toward the development of a play performance scale for children (PPSC). *Cancer* 1985;**56**(7 Suppl.):1837–40.

55 Hunt SM. Cross-cultural issues in the use of quality of life measures in randomized controlled trials. In: Staquet MJ, Hays RM, Fayers PM, eds. *Quality of life assessment in clinical trials: methods and practice.* Oxford, UK: Oxford University Press, 1999:51–68.

56 Pantell RH, Lewis D. Measuring the impact of medical care on children. *J Chronic Dis* 1987;**40**:995.

57 Hester N. Child's health self-concept scale: its development and psychometric properties. *Ans Adv Nurs Sci* 1984;**7**:45–55.

58 Kellerman J, Zeltzer L, Ellenberg L. Psychological effects of illness in adolescence: anxiety, self esteem and perception of control. *J Pediatr* 1980;**97**:126.

59 Smith S. *Measurement of quality of life, behaviour, and health outcomes in children with otitis media with effusion.* Ph.D. thesis: University of Nottingham, 1998.

60 Poggie JJ. Toward quality control in key informant data. *Human Organisation* 1972;**31**:23–30.

61 Freeman LC, Romney AK. Words, deeds and social structure: a prelimininary study of reliability of informants. *Human Organisation* 1987;**46**:330–4.

62 Streiner DL, Norman GR. *Health Measure Scales: a practical guide to their use.* New York: Oxford University Press, 1995.

63 Nunnally JC. *Psychometric Theory, 2nd edn.* New York: Basic Books, 1978.

64 Carmines E, Zeller R. *Reliability and validity assessment.* Newbury Park: Sage Publications, 1979.

65 McDowell I, Newell C. *Measuring Health. A guide to rating scales and questionnaires, 2nd edn.* New York: Oxford University Press, 1996.

66 Bowling A. *Measuring Health. A review of quality of life measurement scales. 2nd edn.* Buckingham: Oxford University Press, 1997.

67 Eiser C, Morse R. A review of measures of quality of life for children with chronic illness. *Arch Disease Child* 2001; **1084**:205–11.

68 Feeny D, Furlong W, Barr RD. Multiattribute approach to the assessment of health-related quality of life: Health utilities index. *Med Pediatr Oncol* 1998:54–9.

69 Lindstrom B, Eriksson B. Quality of life among children in the Nordic countries. *Qual Life Res* 1993;**2**:23–32.

70 Maes S, Bruil J. Assessing the quality of life in children with a chronic illness. In: Rodriguez-Marin J, ed. *Health psychology and quality of life research.* Alicante, Spain: Health Psychology Department, University of Alicante, 1995.

71 Singh G, Athreya BH, Fries JF, Goldsmith DP. Measurement of health-status in children with juvenile rheumatoid-arthritis. *Arthr Rheum* 1994;**37**:1761–9.

72 Akobeng AK, Suresh-Babu MV, Firth D, Miller V, Mir P, Thomas AG. Quality of life in children with Chrohn's Disease: a pilot study. *J Pediatr Gastroenterol Nutr* 1999;**28**.

73 Baker GA, Smith DF, Dewey M, Jacoby A, Chadwick DW. The initial development of a health-related quality of life model as an outcome measure in epilepsy. *Epilepsy Res* 1993;**16**:65–81.

74 Christie MJ, French D, Sowden A, West A. Development of child-centred disease-specific questionnaires for living with asthma. *Psychosom Med* 1993;**55**:541–8.

75 Climent JM, Reig A, Sanchez J, Roda C. Construction and validation of a specific quality of life instrument for adolescents with spine deformities. *Spine* 1995;**20**: 2006–11.

76 Creer TL, Wigal JK, Kotses H, Hatala JC, McConnaughty K, Winder JA. A life activities questionnaire for childhood asthma. *J Asthma* 1993;**30**:467–73.

77 Duffy CM, Arsenault L, Duffy KN, Paquin JD, Strawczynski HA. The Juvenile Arthritis Quality of Life Questionnaire-development of a new responsive index for juvenile rheumatoid arthritis and juvenile spondyloarthritides. *J Rheumatol* 1997;**24**:738–46.

78 Finlay AY, Lewis-jones MS, Sharp JL, Dykes PJ. Children's dermatology life quality index: cartoon version validation. *Br J Dermatol* 1998;**139**(Suppl. 51):67–8.

79 Griffiths AM, Nicholas D, Smith C *et al.* Development of a quality of life index for pediatric inflammatory bowel disease; dealing with differences related to age and IBD type. *J Pediatr Gastroenterol Nutr* 1999;**28**.

80 Gupta KY, Asmussen L, Olsen LM. The Ear Infection Survey (EIS). *Psychometric Testing of a Functional Status Measure for Young Children with Otitis Media,* 1999. Program and abstracts, 39th annual meeting of the Ambulatory Pediatric Association.

81 Henry B, Grosskopf C, Aussage P, de Fontbrune JM, Goehrs JM. Measuring quality of life in children with cystic fibrosis: The cystic fibrosis questionnaires (CFQ) (Abstract). *Pediatric Pulmonology* 1999;**S14**:331.

82 Hoare P, Russell M. The quality of life of children with chronic epilepsy and their families: Preliminary findings with a new assessment measure. *Dev Med Child Neurol* 1995;**37**:689–96.

83 Ingersoll GM, Marrero DG. A modified quality-of-life measure for youths: psychometric properties. *Diabetes Educ* 1991;**17**:114–18.

84 Juniper EF, Guyatt GH, Feeny DH, Ferrie PJ, Griffith LE, Townsend M. Measuring quality-of-life (Qol) in children with asthma. *J Allergy Clin Immunol* 1995;**95**:226.

85 Juniper EF. Assessing quality of life in adults and children with asthma and rhinitis. *ACI Internat* 1997;**9**:5–9.

86 Langeveld JH, Koot HM, Loonen MCB, Hazebroek-Kampschreur AAJM, Passchier J. A quality of life instrument for adolescents with chronic headache. *Cephalalgia* 1996;**16**:183–96.

87 Lewis-Jones MS, Finlay AY. The children's dermatology life quality index (CDLQI)-Initial validation and practical use. *Br J Dermatol* 1995;**132**:942–9.

88 Parkin PC, Kirpalani HM, Rosenbaum PL *et al.* Development of a health-related-quality of life instrument for use in children with spina bifida. *Qual Life Res* 1997; **6**:123–32.

89 Pilpel D, Leiberman E, Zadik Z, Carel CA. Effect of growth hormone treatment on quality of life of short-stature children. *Horm Res* 1995;**44**:1–5.

90 Rabbett H, Elbadri A, Thwaites R *et al.* Quality of life in children with Chrohn's disease. *J Pediatr Gastroenterol Nutr* 1996;**23**:528–33.

91 Rosenfeld RM, Goldsmith AJ, Tetlus L, Balzano A. Quality of life for children with otitis media. *Arch Otolaryngol Head Neck Surg* 1997;**123**:1049–54.

92 Usherwood TP, Scrimgeour A, Barber JH. Questionnaire to measure perceived symptoms and disability in asthma. *Arch Disease Child* 1990;**65**:779–81.

93 Wildrick D, Parker-Fisher S, Morales A. Quality of life in children with well-controlled epilepsy. *J Neurosc Nurs* 1996;**28**:192–8.

94 Wright FV, Law M, Crombie V, Goldsmith CH, Dent P. Development of a self-report functional status index for juvenile rheumatoid arthritis. *J Rheumatol* 1994;**21**: 536–44.

95 Eiser C, Havermans T, Craft A, Kernahan J. Development of a measure to assess the perceived illness experience after treatment for cancer. *Arch Dis Child* 1995;**72**:302–7.

96 Juniper E, Guyatt GH, Feeny D, Ferrie PJ, Griffith LE, Townsend M. Measuring quality of life in children with asthma. *Qual Life Res* 1996;**5**:35–46.

97 Billingham LJ, Abrams KR, Jones DR. Methods for the analysis of quality-of-life and survival data in health technology assessment. 3. *Health Technol Assess* 1999.

98 Lydick E, Yawn B. Clinical interpretation of health-related quality of life data. In: Staquet MJ, Hays RD, Fayers PM, eds. *Quality of Life Assessment in Clinical Trials*. New York: Oxford University Press, 1999.

99 Campbell K, Waters E, O'Meara S, Summerbell C. Prevention of obesity in children [Protocol]. Cochrane Collaboration. *Cochrane Library*, Issue 4. Oxford: Update Software, 1999.

100 Campbell K, Summerbell C., O'Meara S, Waters E. Treatment of obesity in childhood [Protocol]. Cochrane Collaboration. *Cochrane Library*, Issue 4. Oxford: Update Software, 1999.

101 Waters E, Campbell R, Webster P, Spencer NJ. The effects of smoking cessation and prevention programs for families and carers on child health outcomes (protocol). Cochrane Collaboration. *Cochrane Library*, Issue 3. Oxford: Update Software, 1999.

102 Waters EB, Wake M, Hesketh K, Ashley D, Smibert E. Health-related quality of life of children with acute lymphoblastic leukemia: comparisons and correlations between parent and clinician reports. *Int J Cancer* 2003; **103**:514–18.

12 Qualitative research

Donna Waters

Case scenario	*A 3-year-old is brought to the emergency department with a deep gash to the leg from a fall on old playground equipment. On taking the history, it appears that the child has received two of his scheduled diphtheria-tetanus-pertussis vaccinations in infancy but nothing since. You suggest that the child receive tetanus toxoid and immunoglobulin today because of the nature of the wound. The mother states that she would prefer her son not to have any injections and would simply like the wound seen to. Later that day you receive a call from the child's father. He is worried about his son and tells you that his wife "does not believe in vaccination". You offer to see the parents the next day at the clinic to discuss vaccination with both of them. You consider how you will respond to these parents' issues about vaccinations, and decide to go to the literature.*

Background

Many factors other than the availability of high quality evidence can impact upon the successful implementation of recommended health interventions. For single clinical questions concerning therapy or harm, quantitative evaluation of simple interventions such as improving rates of immunization might be expected to provide sufficient evidence.[1,2] In order to involve parents in decision-making regarding childhood vaccination, however, child health workers will often require a wider perspective than that offered by quantitative research '(for example, RCTs or SRs) alone. While quantitative studies may provide some insight into how health decisions are made, researchers increasingly use a blend of methods to gain a comprehensive understanding of the factors that influence health behaviors. Clinicians (and their patients) can draw on work from many disciplines for background theory or models of behavior and have available a range of qualitative and quantitative methods to investigate the whole process of clinical care, including health behavior, decision-making, education, and prevention.

Past approaches to illustrating the differences between qualitative and quantitative method have not always helped clinicians to understand their complementary or individual potential. Strauss and Corbin[3] define qualitative research as "any type of research that produces findings not arrived at by statistical procedures or other means of quantification." This definition reinforces the notion that qualitative research occupies a block of space at the opposite end of some imaginary research spectrum. Qualitative research methods are used to study real people in their natural setting and use mainly textual and observational data to describe or understand how aspects of reality impact upon their experiences. As such, qualitative research relies more on comprehensiveness than generalizability. As with all forms of systematic enquiry, the quality of qualitative research is measured by its consistency with a philosophical position and methodologic paradigm. Like quantitative research, qualitative research is not a single method but consists of several distinct methods reflecting rich and diverse origins in anthropology, psychology and sociology. Qualitative researchers do not hold a "soft" (qualitative) versus "hard" (quantitative) view of science, but would see both approaches as part of the systematic and disciplined inquiry into new knowledge.[4] While consumer input into health decisions gains momentum on all fronts, qualitative methods happily continue to provide a central methodologic platform for the participation of children and their families in the research process. The value and opportunity for qualitative research to link evidence with practice is increasingly being recognized, as a precursor to theory or question development, an adjunct to exploring or explaining process or outcome, and as a method in its own right.[5]

Critical appraisal of qualitative studies

There is much debate about whether a "checklist" approach to the appraisal of qualitative research is appropriate or even possible.[6-8] The nature of qualitative evidence is such

Table 12.1 Evaluative framework for qualitative research

Evaluative concept	Questions to ask of the study
Credibility	• Represent truth • Have meaning • Valid in context • Participants relevant to context • Researchers position is known • Framework is made explicit • Data collection methods and analysis are comprehensive and appropriate for setting • Methods used to improve 'truth' (e.g., triangulation, respondent validation, constant comparative method)
Repeatability	• Data collection and methods available for scrutiny • Comprehensive and transparent process • More than one researcher interprets data • Method of resolving differences in interpretation explained • Clear audit trail • Major concepts and themes explained and explored • Relationship to existing theory explored
Relevance	• Fits the context of your practice • Informs relationships with patients and families • Explains behaviors and decisions • Applicable to your practice

that methods openly embrace what quantitative researchers call "bias" in order to arrive at a deeper understanding of the phenomena being studied. Generalizability and reproducibility are not a requirement of qualitative methods. While an eloquent and reasoned argument for conducting systematic reviews of qualitative studies has been made,[9] others have argued that the process of synthesizing concepts and themes from qualitative enquiry is incompatible with the philosophy of the method and serves only to sanitize meaning.[8,10]

The Cochrane Qualitative Methods Group was established in 1998 to explore many of these issues[11,12] and currently offers information on a number of checklists and appraisal tools.[13,14] The *JAMA* Users Guides series[15] and the *BMJ* series[16] also offer checklists for evaluating qualitative studies. Brown[17] suggests a slightly different approach and offers an appraisal tool for evaluating the findings of single, original studies that use a non-experimental qualitative method. An overview of the type of concepts and questions given in these appraisal instruments is included in Table 12.1. In general, evaluative frameworks for qualitative research all focus on the notion of adherence to method[7,18] and use three main tenets to assess this.

Credibility

In order to determine adherence to method in qualitative research, the criteria used to judge this must be made explicit. Credibility refers to the meaning of the findings within the context of the study. In one of the checklists, this

is referred to as validity.[15] As an active part of the research process, the qualitative researcher makes his or her position known in regard to the chosen method, whether this is a theoretical or practical position, or both. For example, an ethnographic researcher might have conducted interviews in the spoken language of the teenage mothers in order to achieve greater cultural integration, or the feminist researcher might demonstrate how a study is based on the theoretical concepts and language associated with this method. The important point is that a reader can judge whether the ethnographic researcher was likely to have gained sufficient trust within that community for the observations to be regarded as credible, or that the feminist researcher was true to method. Creative or imaginative interpretation of method is acceptable, provided the researcher justifies and explains in sufficient detail for readers to judge the method and context for themselves.[4]

As in quantitative research, there are many types of sampling in qualitative method. Again, what is important is that the reader can follow the logic of how the researcher arrived at the sample, how or why categories were defined, and what the broader context of the study is (such as economic, political, or social conditions). In phenomenologic research, for example, participants are specifically chosen because they have experienced the phenomena being studied and therefore are in the best position to articulate their experience. Credibility includes what the researcher does to get closer to the "truth" in their interpretation of the findings. This extends from thematic conclusion validity,[17] which is the confidence we have that the researcher has faithfully reflected what the participant actually said or meant, to more complex techniques such as member validation,[19] and the constant comparative method.[4] In member validation, participants review their own data (such as transcripts) and provide feedback to the researcher on interpretation of meaning. The constant comparative method involves a continuous comparison of data indicators, such as text, to refine the fit to coded concepts or themes. Qualitative researchers commonly encourage readers to access more detailed information on the coding process, as publication rarely allows sufficient space for this. Direct quotes are also often cited within qualitative publications so that the researchers' interpretation of meaning is more transparent.

Repeatability

Repeatability in qualitative research is related to rigor and reliability more than to reproducibility (Table 12.1). The transcript of interviews or focus groups, coding processes, journal entries and field notes are all important tools that qualitative researchers use to maintain transparency in their work and to enable others to follow the method. This audit trail is also important for documenting personal reactions or influences on data by the researcher. The interplay of the researcher and the real world view of participants means that reproducibility of study conditions is highly unlikely. It is not even particularly desirable, as the replication aims to achieve a greater richness or depth of understanding of the social phenomena, behavior, or patient experience being studied. Variation in qualitative data is not regarded as a source of nuisance but as a means of exploring concepts and themes across an expanded range of dimensions. Qualitative researchers compare and contrast their findings with existing theory and other knowledge in order to find greater meaning through exploration of (in)consistencies, interactions, and linkages.

Other researchers also play a part in establishing rigor. Qualitative researchers will often seek verification of concepts, categorizations, and relationships through a co-investigator or independent person who analyses the same data using the same method. There are also computer programs that assist in coding and theme identification. Interpretation is confirmed or modified as a result of subsequent discussion and deliberation. In summary, data are validated for accuracy and veracity (usually by participants or other researchers), results are compared with other similar data and theories, meaning is explored (again with participants or other researchers) and eventually grouped such that themes or concepts emerge that give meaning to the findings.[17] In grounded theory for example, it is assumed that given the same theoretical perspective and similar conditions, researchers should be able to come up with the same or consistent theoretical explanations about the phenomena under investigation regardless of whether findings were conceptualized or integrated differently.[4]

Relevance

Relevance is analogous to the notion of applicability in quantitative research, and is also closely linked to clinical significance. We know that a (statistically) significant finding does not necessarily mean that the finding is clinically significant. In qualitative research, clinical significance is determined by the credibility of the findings and the new information the researcher has discovered about the meaning of these findings to our patients and their families. In qualitative research, the researcher aims to leave a clear decision trail that enables the reader to determine whether the findings are applicable and relevant. In most situations, the implementation of qualitative findings will not bring about major or immediate practice shifts. Small or incremental changes are more likely, such as influencing the way a clinician thinks about or approaches a problem in the future.[17] As such, practical or economic barriers to the implementation of qualitative research (like cost, time, and risk of harm) are usually minimal.

Issues around vaccinations

It is not uncommon for health professionals to encounter reluctance or resistance to childhood vaccination from parents or caregivers. Childhood vaccination schedules are becoming increasingly complex; they change regularly, and are inconsistent between countries. "Refusal" to vaccinate accounts for only a small percentage of the non-immunized population in the developed world, yet it is of sufficient clinical concern that when a similar scenario was posted as a "Challenging Case" on the website of the *American Journal of Developmental and Behavioral Pediatrics* in 2000, it recorded the highest number of web-based commentaries ever received at that time.[20] Parents are aware of the controversies because access to health information (and misinformation) is increasingly available through a variety of media. Childhood vaccination is just one area in which qualitative research can contribute to the understanding of parents' health decisions.

Framing answerable questions

You are not really looking forward to meeting these parents to discuss vaccination and you expect to encounter resistance to many of your suggestions. You are also unsure how to approach the literature. Framing questions of a qualitative nature can be difficult for practitioners of evidence-based health care since the language and type of question may be unfamiliar and may not sit comfortably within more established approaches. Qualitative methods generally provide a means of systematic enquiry into what have been termed "background" questions such as: *What? Why?* or *How?* Coming from a different philosophical position, qualitative research seeks to explore human experience rather than explain it. As such, qualitative questions are framed to capture the broader context of understanding and experience rather than specific concepts such as patient, intervention, comparison, and outcome. Qualitative questions are likely to include words like "perception", "meaning", "beliefs" and "experience" and sometimes appear more like the statement of a problem than a research question.[19] Basic rules still apply, however, with clear identification of the problem or question defining the type of knowledge required, informing the search strategy and determining the success of the inquiry.

You are aiming to understand *how* or *why* parents and caretakers come to make a decision not to vaccinate their child. You also want to know what parents think about communicating with a health professional on this subject. Note that the latter is not a question about health staff communicating information or educating parents – it is about the parents' experience of the communication. Your questions should be framed to uncover a broad range of research about parents' perceptions and real-world experience of making vaccination decisions. You might want to be more specific and ask, "How do teenage mothers from a particular ethnic background make decisions about vaccinating their children?" Framing a question in this way would focus a search towards a specific type of qualitative method (ethnographic studies) in which the researcher enters into the social world of teenage mothers in this culture in order to gain insight into their experiences. Thus, as in quantitative research, the formulation of the question plays an important part in finding the right information within an appropriately designed study.

Questions

1. Why do some parents/caretakers refuse or seem reluctant to accept vaccination for their children?
2. What is the most effective way to discuss immunization with parents who have made a decision not to immunize their child?
3. How can a child health clinician facilitate acceptance of childhood immunization?

General approach to finding the evidence

Conducting a keyword search of MedLine and Embase provides a starting point for finding qualitative evidence; however, success is more likely by targeting the journals of professional groups that have been consistent users of qualitative methods. The diverse nature of such groups has

meant that access to qualitative studies can be highly dependent upon discipline-specific (often non-consistent) conventions of indexing and searching. This and the relative lack of value placed on qualitative research in health care have contributed to the comparatively slow development of search strategies and filters for this method.

You consult your librarian, who suggests adding PsycInfo, CINAHL, and SocSci to your list of electronic databases and recommends that you include "qualitative" as a search term. Using "child" AND "immunization" AND "qualitative" as keywords and searching back to 1995, you retrieve 18 English language papers. The papers represent a range of qualitative studies on attitudes and perceptions of both parents and health staff towards childhood vaccination and factors influencing their decisions around immunization.

Initial inspection of your search reveals three papers dealing with service provision issues in developing countries or cultures, and a further three on vaccination registries and school-based programs. There is also a review that synthesizes 11 qualitative and 32 quantitative studies in order to identify factors influencing the uptake of vaccination in developing countries.[21] As these are not directly relevant to your questions, you move to the other papers. You note that a number refer to an earlier (1991) study into the uptake of infant immunization in two English health authorities.[22] You also retrieve this paper.

What is the evidence?

Question

1. Why do some parents/caretakers refuse or seem reluctant to accept vaccination for their children?

Interview and focus group methods were used in all eight studies of parents' decision-making about vaccination and groups containing both immunizers and non-immunizers were reported. Purposive and maximum variation sampling methods were used to ensure that fathers, other primary caretakers, and major socioeconomic and cultural groups were represented in the studies. All except two of the studies specified combinations of participant validation or independent rating/coding to verify themes identified from the audiotaped and written interview data.

You are initially surprised at the level of anxiety reported around making vaccination decisions, especially in first-time mothers;[23,24] the studies make it evident it is mainly mothers who take responsibility for these decisions. Confidence in parenting and accepting responsibility[25] were repeatedly identified as themes influencing decisions about vaccination, as were the practical lives of working parents and issues of constantly reassigning priorities in busy family lives.[23] Similarly, two of the studies had identified the theme of "building a strong immune system" as a significant maternal responsibility.[27,28] Other studies also explored this concept, as those who had chosen vaccination for their children also expressed concern about "stressing" or "overloading" the immune system by vaccination, particularly when the child was either very young or unwell.[24,27,29]

The process of considering, implementing, and maintaining vaccination decisions was explored by a number of researchers who compared and contrasted their findings with the health belief model, the transtheoretical model, and motivation theories.[23,25,27] Apart from those objecting to vaccination on religious or moral grounds, non-immunizers voiced more concerns about vaccine efficacy and side effects. In general, they perceived the risk of vaccination to be greater than the risk of a disease they had never seen, or felt was unlikely in their child.[29] This "developed world" view was explored in a study of Maori and Pacific Islander populations in New Zealand[24] in which the authors concluded that vaccination decisions are influenced by experience with childhood diseases within these cultures.

The perception of risk or threat to health appears to be partially influenced by individual knowledge and partially due to the influence of others. The view that vaccination "protected" or "prevented" disease was common. This view is not maintained, however, when a child contracts an illness for which they have been vaccinated, increasing parental concerns about vaccine effectiveness and the validity of advice from health professionals. Tarrant and Gregory[27] interviewed young indigenous mothers from remote Sioux communities in Canada. The women shared stories about children catching childhood diseases despite being vaccinated and spoke of their experience of the negative sequelae from vaccination. In contrast, relatively few parents from developed or metropolitan regions articulated the influence of media, friends, or family on their perceptions of risk.[24,25] Another study designed to capture parents' vaccination decisions following a public controversy over the safety of the combined measles, mumps, and rubella vaccine in the UK in the late 1990s highlighted the pressure parents felt from health professionals to comply with a treatment they were not convinced was safe.[28]

Exploring across a range of cultures, religions, socioeconomic groups, and primary carer combinations, the studies collectively suggest that parents may refuse vaccination for their children because concepts of severity of disease, susceptibility, and risk conflict with individual notions of parental responsibility, personal experience, knowledge, and the influence of others. Vaccination decisions are not single events, but arise at each stage of a complex vaccination schedule and with each successive child.

Question

2. What is the most effective way to discuss immunization with parents who have made a decision not to immunize their child?

The exploration of factors influencing the vaccination decisions of parents and caretakers also identified that these decisions are highly influenced by the behavior and attitudes of health professionals. A study of 58 primary healthcare practitioners in England and Wales found that some health staff perceived mothers' understanding of vaccination as emotional and irrational, while regarding their own as rational and factual.[31] Conducted by social scientists, the study also reported that health staff perceive the main "dissenters" to immunization as "educated, middle class mothers influenced by homeopathy and beliefs that immunization might undermine autoimmunity." The individual quotes, however, showed remarkably similar themes to those of parents. The studies also suggest that parents find advice from health professionals overwhelmingly lacking in balance. Parents were aware of the confusion around constantly changing vaccination schedules and recommendations, and this was also reflected in the narrative of health professionals.[1,31,32] Advice from a doctor or nurse recommending not to immunize when a child is unwell, for example, has long-term consequences on parents' and caretakers' future vaccination decisions.[22,27] From the interviews with parents, many either did not receive or did not attend to the information regarding the possibility of contracting a disease despite vaccination. Parents also found health professionals generally unwilling to acknowledge side effects, being either dismissive of them or failing to warn that they may occur. The implementation of financial incentives to meet vaccination targets in some countries,[31] opportunistic vaccination, and media rhetoric around drug companies all add to parents' feeling of distrust and their dilemma in decision-making.[28] For the British parents who were presented with media reports that the measles, mumps, and rubella vaccine was linked to Crohn's disease and autism,[28] individual commitment and parental responsibility were regarded as more important than societal benefit when the disease was perceived as a minimal threat.

These qualitative studies suggest that the most effective way to discuss vaccination with parents who have made a decision not to immunize their child might be to establish a considerate relationship. In this context, a health professional would aim to decrease levels of anxiety and distrust by including in the discussion a full and up-to-date explanation of disease susceptibility, risk, and consequence, supported by complete and factual background information.[28,33] A summary of the evidence from the qualitative literature suggests a shared decision-making approach as outlined in the Box.

An evidence-based approach to shared decision-making

Listen to the parents concerns

- Do not impose a view
- Discuss openly
- Respect individual choice
- Acknowledge their experience

Present a balanced argument

- Fully explain risk and benefit
- Include all the facts about side effects
- Explain the difference between disease control and prevention

Provide written and verbal information

- Give only written material that is factual and complete
- Allow time for it to be read
- Encourage questions
- Outline "normal" post immunization reactions

Make options available

- Clinic information
- Location
- Access times

Allow time to decide

- Acknowledge and respect parental choice
- Suggest alternative sources of information

- commencing vaccination education in the antenatal period and reinforcing in the early postnatal period;
- sending vaccination information with reminders (when these are in place) so that information is received *prior* to presentation at vaccination clinics;
- facilitating access to information and recommending only those sources of information that are known to be useful and factual and available through a variety of media – electronic (websites), written (publications), and audiovisual (videos).

Resolution of the scenario

Your review of the qualitative research evidence has increased your capacity and preparedness for a discussion with these parents. Allowing the parents to talk, you discover the mother's first experience of vaccination was a negative one: "I was not told there would be two needles and the person putting the liquid into his mouth was so rough!" It had been extremely upsetting and led the mother to investigate whether artificial vaccination "was really necessary?" Since then, pressure from various sources to immunize her son (including your offer to "catch up" on vaccination at the emergency department) had served only to strengthen her resolve to rely on "natural" immunity. Employing the principles of shared decision-making throughout your discussion, the parents leave the clinic with an affirmation of their individual right to choose but also a better understanding of childhood vaccination.

Question

3. How can a child health clinician facilitate acceptance of childhood immunization?

Collectively, the studies retrieved in response to our qualitative questions serve as a reminder to clinicians that decisions about health and illness are not always based on "faith" in medicine or hard facts from quantitative studies. The qualitative studies were conducted across a range of sociocultural perspectives arising from the experience, attitudes, and knowledge of individuals who are parents and caretakers. This broader context is important to understanding the acceptance of the principles of vaccination and decisions to immunize. Mass vaccination campaigns, for example, rely on the assumption that providing information about schedules and availability will be sufficient to improve uptake.[26] In reality, good public health and rights to informed consent within developed nations might serve as a more reliable predictor of non-compliance than compliance.[24] The qualitative literature suggests that facilitating the acceptance of childhood vaccination[28] is likely to be more successful using strategies such as:

References

1 Szilagyi P, Vann J, Bordley C *et al.* Interventions aimed at improving immunization rates. Cochrane Collaboration. *Cochrane Library*, Issue 1. Oxford: Update Software, 2003.

2 Grilli R, Ramsay C, Minozzi S. Mass media interventions: effects on health services utilisation Cochrane Collaboration. *Cochrane Library*, Issue 1. Oxford: Update Software, 2003.

3 Strauss A, Corbin J. *Basis of qualitative research: techniques and procedures for developing grounded theory, 2nd Edn.* California: Sage, 1998.

4 Philip G. Treatment interventions and findings from research: bridging the chasm in child psychiatry. *Br J Psychiatr* 2000;**176**:414–19.

5 Dixon-Woods M, Fitzpatrick R, Roberts K. Including qualitative research in systematic reviews: opportunities and problems. *J Eval Clin Pract* 2001;**7**:125–33.

6 Greenhalgh T. *How to read a paper: the basics of evidence-based medicine.* London: BMJ Books, 1997.

7 Mays N, Pope C. Assessing the quality in qualitative research. *BMJ* 2000;**320**:50–2.

8 Barbour RS. Checklists for improving rigor in qualitative research: a case of the tail wagging the dog? *BMJ* 2001; **322**:1115–17.

9 Dixon-Woods M, Fitzpatrick R. Qualitative research in systematic reviews: has established a place for itself. *BMJ* 2001;**323**:765–6.

10 Lambert H, McKevitt C. Anthropology in health research: from qualitative methods to multidisciplinary. *BMJ* 2002;**325**:210–13.

11 Popay J, Williams G, Rogers A. Rationale and standards for the systematic review of qualitative literature in health services research. *Qual Health Res* 1998;**8**:341–51.

12 Cochrane Qualitative Methods Network. Available URL: http://www.iphrp.salford.ac.uk/cochrane/homepage.htm

13 Health Care Practice Research and Development Unit, University of Salford. Available URL: http://www.iphrp.salford.ac.uk/cochrane/diss_ex.htm

14 NHS Public Health Resourse Unit. Critical Appraisal Skills Program. Available URL: http://www.phru.org.uk/~casp/resourcescasp.htm

15 *JAMA* Users Guides. Available URL: http://cche.net/usersguides/qualitative.asP

16 Greenhalgh T, Taylor R. How to read a paper. Papers that go beyond numbers (qualitative research). *BMJ* 1997;**315**:740–3.

17 Brown SJ. *Knowledge for health care practice: A guide to using research evidence.* Pennsylvania: Saunders, 1999.

18 Fossey E, Harvey C, McDermott F, Davidson L. Understanding and evaluating qualitative research. *Aus NZ J Psychiatr* 2002;**36**:717–32.

19 Jackson D, Daly J, Chang E. Approaches in qualitative research. In Schneider Z & Elliot D, eds. *Nursing Research: Methods, critical appraisal and utilisation, 2nd edn.* Sydney: Mosby.

20 Stein M. Parental refusal to immunize a 2-month-Old Infant. *Pediatrics* 2001;**107**:893–8.

21 Roberts KA, Dixon-Woods M, Fitzpatrick R, Abrams KR, Jones DR. Factors affecting the uptake of childhood immunization: a Bayesian synthesis of qualitative and quantitative evidence. *Lancet* 2002;**360**:1596–9.

22 New SJ, Senior ML. "I don't believe in needles": qualitative aspects of a study into the uptake of infant immunization in two English health authorities. *Soc Sci Med* 1991:**33**:509–18.

23 Marshall S, Swerisen H. A qualitative analysis of parental decision-making for childhood immunization. *Aus NZ J Public Health* 1999;**23**:543–5.

24 White GE, Thomson AN. "As every good mother should." Childhood immunization in New Zealand: a qualitative study. *Health Soc Care Community* 1995;**3**:73–82.

25 Sporton RK, Francis S-A. Choosing not to immunize: are parents making informed decisions? *Fam Pract* 2001;**18**:181–8.

26 McCormick LK, Bartholomew LK, Lewis MJ, Brown MW, Hanson IC. Parental perceptions of barriers to childhood immunization: results of focus groups conducted in an urban population. *Health Educ Res* 1997;**12**:355–62.

27 Bond L, Nolan T, Pattison P, Carlin J. Vaccine preventable diseases and immunizations: a qualitative study of mothers' perceptions of severity, susceptibility, benefits and barriers. *Aus NZ J Public Health* 1998;**22**:440–6.

28 Evans M, Stoddart H, Condon L, Freeman E, Grizzell M, Mullen R. Parents' perspectives on the MMR immunization: a focus group study. *Br J Gen Pract* 2001;**51**:904–10.

29 Kulig JC, Meyer CJ, Hill SA, Handley CE, Lichtenberger SM, Myck SL. Refusals and delay of immunization within Southwest Alberta: understanding alternative beliefs and religious perspectives. *Can J Public Health* 2002;**93**:109–12.

30 Tarrant M, Gregory D. Mothers' perceptions of childhood immunizations in First Nations Communities of the Sioux Lookout Zone. *Can J Public Health* 2001;**92**:42–5.

31 Alderson P, Mayall B, Barker S, Henderson J, Pratten B. Childhood immunization: Meeting targets yet respecting consent. *Eur J Public Health* 1997;**7**:95–100.

32 Pathman DE, Stevens CM, Freed GL, Jones BD, Konrad TR. Disseminating pediatric immunization recommendations: the physicians perspective. *Ambul Child Health* 1998;**4**:265–76.

33 Wilson T. Factors influencing the immunization status of children in a rural setting. *J Pediatr Health Care* 2000;**14**:117–21.

13 Complementary and alternative medicine

Sunita Vohra

Case scenario *Parents of an 8-year-old boy with juvenile rheumatoid arthritis on oral corticosteroid therapy want to "bolster" his immune system as he seems to get frequent upper respiratory tract infections. They ask you if he can take echinacea to prevent coughs and colds. Further history reveals this family is considering taking their child to a Traditional Chinese Medicine (TCM) practitioner to provide acupuncture for his chronic pain. They ask you for your opinion.*

Background

While the definition of complementary and alternative medicine (CAM) is somewhat vague and ill-defined, it is commonly accepted as a "broad domain of healing resources that encompass all health systems, modalities, and practices, and their accompanying theories and beliefs, other than those intrinsic to the politically dominant health system of a particular society or culture in a given historical period".[1] Of course, what is "complementary" in North America is mainstream or "traditional" in many parts of the world. The World Health Organization estimates most of the world's population regularly uses traditional medicine (as opposed to Western medicine).[2]

The popularity of CAM, including herbal medication use, is increasing in North America, and children are not excluded as consumers of alternative health care.[3-7] Telephone interviews of a national sample of adults revealed CAM use increased from 33.8% in 1990 to 42.1% in 1997 in the USA.[8] Between 1994 and 1999, the number of Canadians reporting CAM use in the preceding year jumped from 15% to 70%.[9,10] More recent data from the US and UK have found 20–47% of the general pediatric population have used natural health products.[11,12] This increases to 70% use in children with serious, chronic, recurrent, or incurable conditions.[13-18] Most patients use CAM in conjunction with Western medicine, not instead of it. The majority of users and parents do not inform their physicians about the use of alternative medication.[19,20] As a result, the potential for interaction exists, whether adverse or synergistic, and given its widespread use, inquiring about CAM use should become an important part of every medical history.

As natural health products are classified differently to conventional medications, they have not needed to meet current standards of scientific rigor for drug use.[3,21] However, there is evidence to suggest that many of these substances have pharmacologic and physiologic effects that warrant their formal evaluation.[3] In fact, many commonly used pharmaceuticals are derived from natural substances.[21,22]

While much of CAM may have been around for generations, the application of an evidence-based approach to CAM is new. This chapter will highlight relevant issues when CAM products and practices are being considered, in order to interpret the evidence available when you are answering clinical questions.

Issues relevant when considering natural health products (NHPs)

Generally speaking, NHPs are manufactured, sold or represented for use in the diagnosis, treatment, or prevention of a disease or disorder, restoring or correcting organic functions, or maintaining and/or promoting health.[23] National government regulatory agencies classify NHPs differently, and monitor them accordingly. In the United States, since the Dietary Supplement Health and Education Act (DSHEA) of 1994, NHPs are classified as dietary supplements and sold over the counter.[23] Herbal manufacturers are allowed to make vague "structure/function" claims (for example, "boosts the immune system") but not to treat disease. The Food and Drug Administration (FDA) may intervene only when harm has been demonstrated.[23] In contrast, in 1999 Canada created a new branch of Health Canada, now called the "Natural Health Products Directorate", that oversees NHP product quality, label claims, and standards of evidence used to support those claims.[22] Individuals may receive NHPs from a care provider, seek NHPs on the recommendation of a care provider and/or opt for "self-care" in which an individual purchases NHPs over the counter, either from a pharmacy or other commercial establishment.

According to the Natural Health Products Directorate of Health Canada,[23] NHPs encompass:

- a homeopathic preparation;
- a substance or substances used as traditional medicine, including, but not limited to, a substance used as a traditional Chinese medicine, a traditional Ayurvedic (East Indian) medicine, or a North American aboriginal medicine;
- a mineral or a trace element, a vitamin, an amino acid, an essential fatty acid, or other botanical, animal, or micro-organism derived substances.

In North America, NHP manufacturers are not yet compelled to demonstrate good manufacturing practices (i.e., such that their products are not contaminated or adulterated), quality assurance (i.e., that label claims are accurate for dosage, etc.), nor evidence of efficacy/safety prior to marketing their products. While this may change with proposed legislation, it will be some time before this change has any effect in the marketplace.

Current issues when you are considering NHPs therefore include:

- those related to species misidentification, whereby the wrong plant is collected;
- differences in growing conditions (soil, humidity, sunlight), which can affect the potency of the "active" ingredient(s);
- differences in manufacturing process, whereby different constituents are extracted depending on what part of the plant is used (roots, leaves, etc.) as well as what extraction technique is used (aqueous, alcoholic, etc.); and
- adulteration (with known pharmacologically active agents to enhance the NHP's perceived effect) or contamination (for example, with heavy metals, etc.). Combined, these factors contribute to the considerable heterogeneity in purity and potency of NHPs.

Relevant policy issues when considering CAM practitioners include: education, credentialing, licensure, regulation, scope of practice, professional accountability, and clinical governance. These issues are handled differently within and between countries (for example, Canada and USA have different provincial and state regulations respectively).[24]

Echinacea and acupuncture

For some herbal remedies, such as echinacea, there has been considerable work done to identify chemical composition.[25] There are three main species of echinacea (common name: purple coneflower) used for medicinal purposes: angustifolia, purpurea, and pallida. The constituents vary between species and are generally classified into the following groups: caffeic acid derivatives (including cichoric acid), polysaccharides, flavenoids, essential oils, polyacetylenes, alkylamides, alkaloids, and linoleic, oleic, and palmitic acids.[26,27] Preparations include liquid extracts of fresh or dried whole plant, aerial parts, root, and/or rhizome.[27] Depending on the part of the plant used, the concentration of active ingredient is likely to vary.[21] Echinacea may have its purported immune stimulant activity via increased phagocytosis, macrophage activation, and cytokine production.[27]

Traditional Chinese Medicine (TCM) is a distinct system of health care, with its own diagnostic and assessment methods, unique treatment principles, and its own language and terminology.[28] Like Western medicine, the goal of TCM is the promotion, maintenance, and restoration of health.[28] TCM is rooted in Chinese culture and considers nature and the person as a whole to be interrelated. TCM theory emphasizes the importance of *Qi*, whose action manifests as all life phenomena including physical, mental, and spiritual aspects. Disturbances in *Qi* are manifested as disease. The main modalities used in TCM are: traditional Chinese diagnosis, acupuncture/acupressure, traditional Chinese herbal remedies, traditional Chinese dietary therapy, traditional Chinese exercise therapy, and *tuina* massage.[28]

Acupuncture is a traditional Chinese medical practice in which fine needles are inserted into specific documented points believed to represent concentration of body energies. In some cases, a small electrical impulse is added to the needles (electro-acupuncture). Once the needles are inserted in some of the appropriate points, endorphins (morphine-like substances) have been shown to be released into the patient's system, thus inducing local or general analgesia.[28]

Education and licensing requirements for acupuncturists vary within and between countries. In America, in the 42 states (and the District of Columbia) that offer licensure, non-MD acupuncturists require 3 years or 1800 hours of training, including 300 hours of Chinese herbology and 500 clinical hours.[24] Of the more than 70 schools of acupuncture in the United States, 37 are accredited by and 9 are in candidacy status with the US Department of Education (DOE)-recognized Accreditation Commission for Acupuncture and Oriental Medicine.[24] Still, credentialing problems persist, in that there is state-to-state variation in scope of practice and regulation of acupuncture or Oriental Medicine.[24] In Britain, professional acupuncturists train for up to 3–4 years full time and may acquire university degrees on completion

Table 13.1 Where to find evidence about CAM

Database	Criteria	Comments	Access
National Center for Complementary and Alternative Medicine (NCCAM)	http://nccam.nih.gov/htdig/search.html	Informational website, part of US National Institutes of Health. Specific treatment information can be found at: http://nccam.nih.gov/health/bytreatment.htm	Free
AMED (Allied and Complementary Medicine Database) 1985–present	Includes peer reviewed journals & others significant to the field	Database includes English-language and European sources, journals, newspapers and books. Produced by the British Library. About 50% of the journals in AMED are indexed in MedLine	Subscription required
Natural Standard	Systematic, peer-reviewed analyses of complementary and alternative therapies: http://www.naturalstandard.com/	Evidence-based, individual studies are quality assessed with a validated scale and graded. Includes observational and experimental evidence	Subscription required

of their training.[29] All accredited acupuncture training courses include conventional anatomy, physiology, pathology, and diagnosis.[29] Professional acupuncturists have a single regulatory body, the British Acupuncture Council, while physicians who practise acupuncture may receive official qualifications from the British Medical Acupuncture Society.[30]

You wonder whether echinacea is safe and effective in children, and if it can be used in a patient with juvenile rheumatoid arthritis. Furthermore, you are uncertain if acupuncture is effective in treating chronic pain, or if children will tolerate having additional needles as part of their therapy.

Questions

1. In healthy children (*population*), does prophylactic echinacea (*intervention*) prevent upper respiratory tract infections (*outcome*)? **[Therapy]**

2a. In healthy children (*population*), does using echinacea (*intervention/exposure*) result in adverse effects (*outcome*)? **[Harm]**

2b. In children with juvenile rheumatoid arthritis (*population*), does using echinacea (*intervention/exposure*) result in adverse effects (*outcome*)? **[Harm]**

3a. In children with chronic pain (*population*), is acupuncture (*intervention*) effective in reducing pain (*outcome*)? **[Therapy]**

3b. In children with JRA/rheumatoid arthritis (*population*), is acupuncture (*intervention*) effective in reducing pain (*outcome*)? **[Therapy]**

4. In children with chronic pain (*population*), is acupuncture (*intervention*) tolerated (*outcome*)? **[Therapy]**

5. In children with chronic pain (*population*), does the use of acupuncture (*intervention*) result in adverse effects (*outcome*)? **[Harm]**

Searching for evidence

Publication bias is important to consider when searching for evidence about CAM. While this phenomenon is widely recognized in Western medical journals, whereby negative studies are less likely to be published, its bias regarding CAM research publications is the opposite. That is, CAM studies with negative results are more likely to be published in mainstream Western medical journals (for example, "MedLine"), and CAM studies with positive results are more likely to be published in smaller journals that may not be accessible on the usual search engines[30] Unfortunately, it is also true that the quality of the research published in these smaller journals may be inferior to that found in large mainstream medical journals. Table 13.1 lists three reputable databases that publish evidence about CAM that may or may not be available on MedLine.

Critical review of the evidence

Question

1. In healthy children (*population*), does prophylactic echinacea (*intervention*) prevent upper respiratory tract infections (*outcome*)? **[Therapy]**

Search strategy

- MedLine (Ovid) Echinacea AND respiratory tract infections, limit to review articles

You find several systematic reviews that examine the effectiveness of echinacea in treating and/or preventing

Table 13.2 Pediatric studies examining echinacea as URTI prophylaxis

Author (year)	Age of subjects	Inclusion criteria	Treatment	Control	Trial duration	Outcome
Freyer (1974)	8–13 years	Recurrent URTI	Combination treatment (six herbs in combination with *Echinacea angustifolia* and *E pallida* roots)	No treatment	6 weeks	Proportion with at least one infection: 69.5% treatment *v* 49% control
Helbig (1961)	1–3 years	Admitted to pediatric hospital	Same combination treatment as above	No treatment	6 weeks	Incidence of infections among non-infected children: 15/95 treatment *v* 36/100 control. Recurrences: 50/222 treatment *v* 100/227 control
Kleinschmidt (1965)	3–5 years	Referred to a health resort	Same combination treatment as above	No treatment	6 weeks	Incidence of infection: 57% treatment *v* 78% control. Duration of fever: 3·8 days treatment *v* 4·4 days control

upper respiratory tract infection (URTI). Their conclusions are slightly different, depending on which trials were included. The most recent Cochrane review on this topic included eight prevention trials and eight trials on treatment of URTI (total n = 3396).[31] The authors commented on the variation in preparations investigated and concerns with the quality of the trial reporting. Strengths of the Cochrane systematic review include a sensible clinical question and a transparent search strategy. Unfortunately, some of the primary studies included were of poor methodologic quality. Overall, the available prevention studies suggest that any prophylactic effect of echinacea preparations is likely to be relatively modest in effect size (around 15–20% relative risk reduction). Of the 16 included trials, three addressed children, aged 1–13 years (combined n = 1139)[32–34] (Table 13.2). Unfortunately all three studies reviewed the combination effects of two species of echinacea in conjunction with other NHPs, and therefore none can comment on the prophylactic effects of echinacea alone. The other systematic reviews that focused on methodologic quality found more convincing evidence of echinacea's role in URTI treatment, but not prophylaxis.

A second review of echinacea for treatment and prevention of URTI evaluated nine treatment trials and four prevention trials, after consideration of randomization, blinding, power, validity, clinical relevance of outcome measurements, inclusion and exclusion criteria, and indistinguishability of treatment and placebo.[35] The authors do not describe how the quality considerations were scored, or if they were reproducible.[37] Their decision not to do meta-analysis, based on the heterogeneity of product preparations, methods, and outcomes

measured, was appropriate. Eight of the nine treatment trials reported a benefit; the one study showing no benefit is unpublished and used insufficient doses of echinacea.[36] Data from the larger, more methodologically sound studies suggest that the number needed to treat to prevent progression to more severe symptoms among patients with first sign of a cold was five. Two of the prevention trials reported a marginal benefit, the third initially reported a benefit but later reported no benefit, and the fourth found no benefit.[36] The major methodologic weaknesses identified included: lack of objective validated measures, no clear evidence that the treatment was indistinguishable from placebo, and insufficient sample size.[36]

Pediatric data to support the use of echinacea in the treatment of URTI is limited to a retrospective study of 1280 children given parenteral *Echinacea purpurea*.[37] This study reported that treatment with echinacea can reduce the duration of infection. Further evidence of efficacy in pediatric respiratory illness was provided by Von Ulrich Freitag,[38] who found that children with pertussis showed greater improvement when given a combination of *Echinacea purpurea*, *E angustifolia*, and erythromycin than when given erythromycin alone. These two studies are limited in their application to this case scenario, in that parenteral echinacea is not available in many countries, nor do they provide evidence of efficacy for URTI prophylaxis.

Overall, the evidence seems to support that echinacea may have a role in the treatment of URTI if used early in the illness, but less so as URTI prophylaxis. At this time, there are many more adult than pediatric studies to support this conclusion.[31,35,36]

Question

2a. In healthy children (*population*), does using echinacea (*intervention/exposure*) result in adverse effects (*outcome*)? **[Harm]**

2b. In children with juvenile rheumatoid arthritis (*population*), does using echinacea (*intervention/exposure*) result in adverse effects (*outcome*)? **[Harm]**

Search strategy

- EMBASE Echinacea extract AND (adverse drug reaction OR safety), limit to child (infant to age 17 years)
- MedLine: Echinacea (to adverse effects, toxicity) OR Echinacea (limit to infant or child)

Echinacea has been purported to be an "immune stimulant" during infection for more than a hundred years.[39–41] Preclinical safety data reveal no evidence of any toxic effect in rats given many times the human therapeutic dose orally for 4 weeks.[25] The lethal dose (LD50) has been determined to be 50 ml kg^{-1} of fresh pressed juice of *E purpurea* in mice and rats.[42] Echinacea has no mutagenic activity or carcinogenicity.[25,42,43] It is felt to be safe if used for < 6–8 weeks consecutively.[21,40,44]

Known adverse effects include allergic reactions[31,44,45] and a tingling sensation on the tongue.[40] Intravenous, intramuscular, or subcutaneous injections of echinacea are frequently followed by a temperature rise of 0·5–1·0°C.[44,46] Some authors believe that this fever is an indicator of activity, secondary to macrophage release of interferon-alpha and interleukin-1.[25] The Cochrane systematic review concluded that for oral intake, the risks of serious adverse effects of echinacea seem very small.[31] More recently, 51 Australian adverse drug reports implicating echinacea were reviewed, revealing atopic individuals were overrepresented in this population.[45] The World Health Organization database (1968–1997) has 76 reports regarding echinacea extract, with acute hypersensitivity reactions (10 cases) and anaphylaxis (eight cases) as the predominant problem.[47]

A theoretical risk of hepatotoxicity was raised when Roder *et al.* identified two pyrrolizidine alkaloids (tussilagin and isotussilagin) from *E angustifolia* and *E purpurea*.[48] These alkaloids do not share this class's potential for hepatotoxicity as they do not contain the 1,2 unsaturated necine ring system that appears to be essential for the formation of the toxic intrahepatic pyrrole metabolites.[25,49] Moreover, there are no published reports of echinacea use and liver toxicity.

Owing to its putative immune modulating effects, contraindications to echinacea include tuberculosis, HIV/AIDS, multiple sclerosis, and autoimmune illnesses.[50] Children with autoimmune illness, such as juvenile rheumatoid arthritis, are typically advised not to take echinacea because its polysaccharides may increase cytokine production. One group of US investigators who are studying echinacea in children state that (in the USA) all marketed echinacea products are preserved by either alcohol or glycerin, and are therefore unlikely to contain the polysaccharides responsible for potential cytotoxicity.[51] While such precautions may be unnecessary, there is insufficient understanding of mechanism of action and insufficient regulatory control over the manufacturing process to recommend echinacea use in this population at this time.

Question

3a. In children with chronic pain (*population*), is acupuncture (*intervention*) effective in reducing pain (*outcome*)? **[Therapy]**

3b. In children with JRA/rheumatoid arthritis (*population*), is acupuncture (*intervention*) effective in reducing pain (*outcome*)? **[Therapy]**

Search strategy

- EMBASE Acupuncture AND Chronic pain, limit to child (infant to adolescent)
- Cochrane Database of Systematic Reviews: Acupuncture. mp AND Rheumatoid arthritis.mp
- Cochrane Database of Systematic Reviews: Acupuncure. mp AND pain.mp

The efficacy of acupuncture in pediatric pain has not been thoroughly evaluated. In a study reviewing perceived efficacy and acceptance in children with chronic pain, Kemper *et al.* found 70% of 47 patients (average age 16, 79% female) interviewed found the treatments helped symptoms and 67% rated the therapies as pleasant.[52] The predominant symptoms in this population were migraines, endometriosis, and reflex sympathetic dystrophy.

While the "best" evidence for effectiveness of a given intervention is provided by randomized clinical trials, it is not unusual to lack such evidence in the pediatric population. Limitations of observational studies include selection bias, whereby those who agreed to treatment may be systematically different from those who did not, and respondent bias, whereby those who agreed to be interviewed may be more likely to "acquiesce" to please the interviewer. As such, this study is best considered preliminary evidence.

There have been more studies examining the effect of acupuncture in adult chronic pain. Helms *et al.*[53] compared real acupuncture, placebo acupuncture, weekly visits with a physician, and no treatment in 43 women with primary dysmenorrhea. After 1 year, improvement was seen in 91% (10/11) in the real acupuncture group, 36% (4/11) in the placebo acupuncture group, 8% (2/11) in the no treatment group, and 10% (1/10) in the physician visit-only group. Of note was that a 41% reduction of analgesic medication use was found in the real acupuncture group and no change or increased use in the other groups.[53] A recent Cochrane review examining acupuncture for idiopathic headache included 26 trials (n = 1151) and found existing evidence supports the value of acupuncture for headache.[54]

A Cochrane review examined acupuncture and electroacupuncture for the treatment of rheumatoid arthritis (RA) in adults.[55] Two studies met inclusion criteria (n = 84). One used acupuncture and the other electroacupuncture. With acupuncture, no significant difference was found between groups for erythrocyte sedimentation rate, C reactive protein, visual analog scale for pain, visual analog scale for patient's global assessment, number of swollen joints, number of tender joints, the general health questionnaire, score on modified disease activity scale, or decrease in analgesic intake. With electroacupuncture, a significant decrease in knee pain 24 hours post treatment was reported in the experimental group when compared with the placebo group. While the reviewers' conclusions were that acupuncture has no effect on a number of subjective and objective assessments, they acknowledged their review was limited by the low number of clinical trials included and methodologic considerations, such as type of acupuncture (acupuncture versus electroacupuncture), site of intervention, and small sample size of included studies.[55]

Question

4. In children with chronic pain (*population*), is acupuncture (*intervention*) tolerated (*outcome*)? **[Therapy]**

Given the perception that most children do not "like" needles, it is reasonable to ask if children tolerate acupuncture. While randomized controlled trials are ideally suited to identify if an intervention is effective, phase I studies are more common when researchers are studying whether an intervention is feasible or acceptable.

After an observational study of pediatric pain patients found that 70% children found acupuncture "helpful" and "pleasant" (n = 47),[52] a phase I study of the feasibility and acceptability of acupuncture/hypnosis intervention for chronic pediatric pain was conducted[56]: 33 children aged 6–18 years were offered 6 weekly sessions consisting of individually tailored acupuncture treatment together with a 20 minute hypnosis session (conducted while the needles were in place). The treatment was highly acceptable (only two patients refused; > 90% completed treatment) and there were no adverse effects.[56] Both parents and children reported significant improvements in the child's pain following treatment. Children's anticipatory anxiety declined significantly across treatment sessions and the authors concluded that a combined acupuncture/hypnosis intervention was feasible for chronic pediatric pain.[56] The methodologic limitations of both of these studies include selection bias (for example, those who chose to participate are not representative of the general population) and reporting bias (without masking, participants and observers knew that they had received the intervention when assessing the outcome, and some children may have wanted to "please" by saying the treatment effect was more positive than it was). Even with these limitations, these studies provide sufficient evidence that at least some children tolerate acupuncture and that this intervention could proceed to more formal studies of efficacy in this population.

When considering why some children tolerate acupuncture, Kemper[52] comments that children and adolescents suffering from severe chronic pain that has not been relieved through mainstream treatments may be willing to undergo short-term discomfort to achieve long-term goals. Second, most persons who receive acupuncture remark on how much less painful it is than conventional needles, possibly because acupuncture needles are solid, very fine gauge needles. Third, acupuncture can use a variety of non-needle techniques, such as acupressure, to stimulate acupuncture points.

Question

5. In children with chronic pain (*population*), does the use of acupuncture (*intervention*) result in adverse effects (*outcome*)? **[Harm]**

Search strategy

● EMBASE Acupuncture AND Safety, limit to priority journals

While the "best" evidence for diagnosis or therapy may be randomized clinical trials, such trials are rarely of sufficient size to give adequate information on safety. If events are rare, they will only be detected with very large sample sizes. Thus, better evidence for safety may be obtained from large, prospective, population-based studies rather than from randomized clinical trial data alone. While case reports do not provide denominator data (i.e., how many people were harmed versus number of people exposed), they are useful to understand the range of potential safety concerns that may exist for a given therapy.

At least two large prospective studies have looked at adverse events following acupuncture.[57,58] The first collected data from 78 doctors and physiotherapists who delivered 32 000 acupuncture consultations between June 1998 and February 2000.[57] Altogether 43 "significant" events were reported, all but two of which resolved within 1 week (the other two resolved within a few weeks). According to accepted criteria, none of these events was serious (for example, no cases of hepatitis, pneumothorax, etc.). The most common events were bleeding (310 per 10 000 consultations) and needling pain (110 per 10 000 consultations).[57] A second study collected data from 574 acupuncturists who delivered 34 000 acupuncture treatments during a 4-week period[58]: 43 minor adverse events were reported, the most common of which were nausea and fainting. There were no reports of serious adverse events, defined as events requiring hospital admission, leading to permanent disability, or death.[58] Both reviews concluded that acupuncture is a relatively safe form of treatment. Of note, there was little difference regarding safety data when the acupuncture was delivered by doctors, physiotherapists, or professional acupuncturists. A review of case reports of serious or life-threatening incidents caused by acupuncture (for example, pneumothorax and lesions of the spinal cord) found that these could have been avoided if practitioners had better anatomical knowledge, applied existing anatomical knowledge better, or both.[59] In the case of CAM practices, safety may depend on the practitioner. Of course, acupuncture needles should follow national regulations governing medical devices, such as the FDA recommendation of sterile single-use needles.

Summary

Owing to differences in CAM product and practice regulation, there are unique issues that must be considered when you are evaluating CAM evidence. Herbal product quality is not assured, and it will be some time before consumers can know with confidence that label claims are accurate. CAM practices are practitioner-dependent, placing emphasis on credentialing and regulation where none may be in place. Patients are advised to inquire as to their CAM providers' education/training and experience before placing themselves in their hands. Some CAM fields have well recognized training programs and practitioners can demonstrate that they have passed nationally recognized exam standards.

While relatively less evidence may be available on CAM in children, that is not to say "no evidence" is available.[60,61] The four journals that published the largest number of pediatric NHP RCTs were so-called "mainstream" medical journals including *American Journal of Clinical Nutrition*, *Pediatrics*, *Journal of Pediatrics*, and the *Lancet*. Moreover, MedLine indexed 93·2% of these RCTs, suggesting that the RCT-level evidence is easily available to those who seek it.[60] The quality of the evidence must always be assessed, whether you are evaluating CAM or Western medicine.

Resolution of the scenario

Having read the evidence about echinacea in the role of URTI, you are not convinced echinacea is appropriate as a prophylactic agent. Moreover, as a potential immune stimulant, you advise parents that echinacea is contraindicated because of their son's juvenile rheumatoid arthritis. You also take the opportunity to educate the family about current issues regarding natural health product quality and labeling claims. You encourage them to ask questions of their TCM practitioner regarding his acupuncture training and if he holds nationally recognized credentials in this field. You tell them that preliminary evidence suggests that children with chronic pain tolerate acupuncture quite well, and that when performed by individuals with proper training, it is likely to be safe. There is insufficient evidence to recommend acupuncture in the treatment of rheumatoid arthritis. Finally, you tell the family that it was wise of them to speak to you about their child's proposed CAM use as there may be information regarding safety and efficacy that is important for them to consider before embarking on a new treatment.

Future research needs

With gaps identified in almost every aspect of pediatric CAM use, there is pressing need to collect effectiveness and safety data in children. The obstacles to CAM research that are frequently quoted include: limited clinical data, lack of standardized products, complex interventions that are highly dependent on the individual, and concerns about the applicability of traditional research methodology.[62–64] The National Center for Complementary and Alternative Medicine (NCCAM), one of the 27 institutes and centers that make up the National Institutes of Health (NIH) in the USA, supports rigorous research on CAM, trains researchers in CAM, and disseminates information to the public and professionals on which CAM modalities work, which do not, and why.[1] Criteria used by NCCAM to prioritize research opportunities include: quantity and quality of preliminary data, extent of public use, public health importance of disease being treated, feasibility, and cost.[65] Pediatric CAM research priorities have been identified as those: already widely used by children and families; already researched to some extent in animal models and adults; and having a potentially significant risk of substantial costs or side effects.[66]

Summary table

Question	Type of evidence	Result	Comment
Effect of echinacea on URTI	2 systematic reviews	Benefit for early treatment (NNT = 5), little apparent benefit for prophylaxis	Most data are from adult studies
Is echinacea harmful for healthy children or for children with JRA?	Case reports	Very few harms reported	Children with JRA advised not to take echinacea due to possible immunomodulating effects
Is acupuncture effective in reducing pain?	1 observational study (pediatric) 1 RCT 2 systematic reviews	Some supportive evidence, but not consistent in RA	Most data are from adult studies, and are not necessarily specific to JRA/RA
Do children tolerate acupuncture?	2 observational studies	Some children with chronic pain tolerate acupuncture	Bias may influence results
Is acupuncture harmful for children with chronic pain?	2 prospective observational studies Case reports	Very few serious harms were reported	Most data from adult studies

Acknowledgments

Thanks to Terry Klassen, Ellen Crumley, Sue Black, and Lauren Flintoft for their assistance in preparing this chapter.

References

1 NCCAM Clearinghouse. General information about CAM and the NCCAM. Retrieved from http://nccam.nih.gov/nccam/an/general/index.html

2 World Health Organization (WHO). *Traditional Medicine Strategy 2002–2005*. Geneva: WHO, 2002.

3 Ernst E. Herbal medicines: where is the evidence? *BMJ* 2000;**321**:395–6.

4 Eisenberg D, Kessler R, Foster C *et al.* Unconventional medicine in the United States: prevalence, costs, and patterns of use. *New Engl J Med* 1993;**328**:246–52.

5 Fernandez CV, Stutzer CA, MacWilliam L, Fryer C. Alternative and complementary therapy use in pediatric oncology patients in British Columbia: prevalence and reasons for use and nonuse. *J Clin Oncol* 1998;**16**:1279–86.

6 Spigelblatt L, Saine-Ammara G, Pless IB *et al.* The use of alternative medicine by children. *Pediatrics* 1994;**94**:811–14.

7 Northcott H, Bachynsky J. Concurrent utilization of chiropractic, prescription medicines, non-prescription medicines and alternative health care. *Soc Sci Med* 1993; **37**:431–5.

8 Eisenberg DM, Davis RB, Ettner SL *et al.* Trends in alternative medicine use in the United States, 1990–1997: results of a follow up national survey. *JAMA* 1998;**280**:1569–75.

9 Millar WJ. Use of alternative health care practitioners by Canadians. *Can J Public Health* 1997;**88**:154–8.

10 Berger E. *Berger Population Health Monitor #21*. Toronto: Hay Associates, 2000.

11 Simpson N, Pearce A, Finlay F, Lenton S. The use of complementary medicine in paediatric outpatient clinics. *Ambul Child Health* 1998;**3**:351–6.

12 Ottolini M, Hamburger E, Loprieto J *et al. Alternative medicine use among children in the Washington DC area*. San Francisco, CA: Paediatric Academic Societies, 1999.

13 Southwood TR, Malleson PN, Roberts-Thomson PJ, Mahy M. Unconventional remedies used for patients with juvenile arthritis. *Pediatrics* 1990;**85**:150–4.

14 Stern RC, Canda ER, Doershuk CF. Use of nonmedical treatment by cystic fibrosis patients. *J Adolesc Health* 1992;**13**:612–15.

15 Sawyer MG, Gannoni AF, Toogood IR, Antoniou G, Rice M. The use of alternative therapies by children with cancer. *Med J Aust* 1994;**160**:320–2.

16 Friedman T, Slayton W, Allen L *et al.* Use of alternative therapies for children with cancer. *Pediatrics* 1997;**100**:el. Available at: http://www.paediatrics.org/cgi/content/full/100/6/el

17 Grootenhuis MA, Last BF, deGraaf-Nijkerk HJ, van der Wel M. Use of alternative treatment in paediatric oncology. *Cancer Nurs* 1998;**21**:282–8.

18 Sibinga E, Ottolini M, Duggan A, Wilson M. Communication about complementary/alternative medicine use in children. *Pediatr Res* 2000;**47**:226A.

19 Sikand A, Laken M. Paediatricians' experience with and attitudes toward complementary/alternative medicine. *Arch Pediatr Adolesc Med* 1998;**152**:1059–64.

20 Canadian Pediatric Society, Drug Therapy and Hazardous Substances Committee. Toxicological risks of herbal remedies. *J Paediatr Child Hlth* 1999;**4**:536–8.

21 Gruenwald J, Brendlar T, Jaenicke C, eds. *PDR for Herbal Medicines*. Montvale, New Jersey: Medical Economics Company, 2000.

22 http://www.hc-sc.gc.ca/hpfb-dgpsa/nhpd-dpsn/index_e.html

23 http://vm.cfsan.fda.gov/~dms/supplmnt.html

24 Eisenberg DM, Cohen MH, Hrbek A, Grayzel J, Van Rompay MI, Cooper RA. Credentialing complementary and alternative medical providers. *Ann Intern Med* 2002;**137**: 965–73.

25 Bauer R, Wagner H. Echinacea species as potential immunostimulatory drugs. *Exon Med Plant Res* 1991;**5**: 253–321.

26 Mills S, Bone K. *Principles and practice of phytotherapy*. Toronto: Churchill Livingstone, 2000.

27 Boon H, Smith M. *The botanical pharmacy*. Kingston, Ontario: Quarry Press Inc., 1999.

28 Health Professions Regulatory Advisory Council (HPRAC). Traditional Chinese Medicine and Acupuncture: advice to the Minister of Health and Long-term care. April 2001. (Accessed at http://www.hprac.org/english/reports.asp)

29 Vickers A, Zollman C. ABC of complementary medicine: acupuncture. *BMJ* 1999;**319**:973–6.

30 Moher D, Pham B, Lawson M, Klassen TP. The inclusion of reports of randomized trials published in languages other than English in systematic reviews National Health Service (NHS) Research and Development Program. *Hlth Technol Assess Rep* 2003;**7(41)**:1–90.

31 Melchart D, Linde K, Fischer P, Kaesmayr J. Echinacea for preventing and treating the common cold. In: Cochrane Collaboration. *Cochrane Library*, Issue 1. Oxford: Update Software, 2002.

32 Freyer HU. Haufigkeit banaler Infekte im Kindesalter und Moglichkeiten der Prophylaxe. *Fortschr Med* 1974;**92**: 165–8.

33 Helbig G. Unspezifische Reizkorpertherapie zur Infektionsprophylaxe. *Med Klin* 1961;**56**:1512–14.

34 Kleinschmidt H. Versuche zur Herabsetzung der Infektneigung bei Kleinkindern mit Esberitox. *Ther Ggw* 1965;**104**:1258–62.

35 Barrett B, Vohmann M, Calarese N. Echinacea for upper respiratory tract infection. *J Fam Pract* 1999;**48**:628–35.

36 Lord RW. Echinacea for upper respiratory tract infections. *J Fam Pract* 1999;**48**:939–40.

37 Foster S. Echinacea: nature's immune enhancer. Rochester, Vermont: Healing Arts Press, 1991.

38 Freitag VU, Stammwitz U. Reduzierte Krankheitsdauer bei Pertussis durch unspezifisches immunstimulans. *Der Kinderarztl* 1984;**8**:1068–71.

39 Awang DVC, Kindack DG. Herbal medicine: echinacea. *Can Pharm J* 1991;**124**:512–16.

40 Castleman M. *The healing herbs*. Emmaus PA: Rodale Press, 1991.

41 Hobbs C. In: Michael Miovich, ed. *The echinacea handbook*. Institute for Natural Products Research. Oregon: Eclectic Medical Publications, 1989.

42 Schimmer O, Abel G, Behninger C *et al*. Untersuchungen zur gentoxischen potenz eines neutralen polysaccharids aus echinacea. *Z phytother* 1989;**10**:39–42.

43 Mengs U, Clare C, Poiley J. Toxicity of echinacea purpurea: acute, subacute and genotoxicity studies. *Arzneimittelforschung/Drug Res* 1991;**41**:1076–81.

44 Blumenthal M, ed. *The Complete German Commission E Monographs*. Texas: American Botanical Council, 1998.

45 Mullins RJ, Heddle R. Adverse reactions associated with echinacea: the Australian experience. *Ann Allergy Asthma Immunol* 2002;**88**:42–51.

46 Melchart D, Linde K, Worku F, Bauer R, Wagner H. *Phytomedicine* 1994;**1**:245–54.

47 Farah MH, Edwards R, Lindquist M, Leon C, Shaw D. International monitoring of adverse health effects associated with herbal medicines. *Pharmacoepidemiol Drug Saf* 2000;**9**:105–12.

48 Roder E *et al*. Pyrriolizidine in *Echinacea angustifolia* and *Echinacea purpurea*. *Dtsch Apoth Ztg* 1984;**13(2)**: 33–38

49 D'Arcy PF. Adverse reactions and interactions with herbal medicines. *Adverse Drug React Toxicol Rev* 1991;**10**: 189–208.

50 Snodgrass WR. Herbal products: risks and benefits of use in children. *Curr Ther Res* 2001;**62**:724–37.

51 Mark JD, Grant KL, Barton LL. The use of dietary supplements in pediatrics: a study of echinacea. *Clin Pediatr* 2001(May):265–9.

52 Kemper KJ, Sarah R, Silver-Highfield E, Xiarhos E, Barnes L, Berde C. On pins and needles? Pediatric pain patients' experience with acupuncture. *Pediatrics* 2000;**4**: 941–7.

53 Helms JM. *Acupuncture energetics*. Berkely, CA: Medical Acupuncture Publishers, 1995.

54 Melchart D, Linde K, Fischer P *et al*. Acupuncture for idiopathic headache. In: Cochrane Collaboration. *Cochrane Library*, Issue 2. Oxford: Update Software, 2002.

55 Casimiro L, Brosseau L, Milne S *et al*. Acupuncture and electroacupuncture for the treatment of RA. In: Cochrane Collaboration. *Cochrane Library*, Issue 1. Oxford: Update Software, 2003.

56 Zeltzer LK, Tsao JCI, Stelling C, Powers M, Levy S, Waterhouse M. A phase I study on the feasibility and acceptability of an acupuncture/hypnosis intervention for chronic pediatric pain. *J Pain Symptom Manag* 2002;**24**: 437–46.

57 White A, Hayhoe S, Hart A, Ernst E. Adverse events following acupuncture: prospective survey of 32 000 consultations with doctors and physiotherapists. *BMJ* 2001;**323**:485–6.

58 MacPherson H, Thomas K, Walters S, Fitter M. The York acupuncture safety study: prospective survey of 34 000 treatments by traditional acupuncturists. *BMJ* 2001;**323**: 486–7.

59 Peuker E, Gronemeyer D. Rare but serious complications of acupuncture: traumatic lesions. *Acupunct Med* 2002;**20**: 103–8.

60 Moher D, Sampson M, Campbell K *et al*. Assessing the quality of reports of randomized trials in paediatric complementary and alternative medicine. *BMC Paediatr* 2002;**2**:2.

61 Sampson M, Campbell K, Ajiferuke I, Moher D. Randomized controlled trials in pediatric complementary and alternative medicine: where can they be found? *BMC Pediatr* 2003;**3**:1.

62 Levin JS, Glass TA, Kushi LH, Schuck JR, Steele L, Jonas WB. Quantitative methods in research on complementary and alternative medicine: A methodological manifesto. *Med Care* 1997;**35**:1079–94.

63 Margolin A, Avants SK, Kleber HD. Investigating alternative medicine therapies in randomized controlled trials. *JAMA* 1998;**280**:1626–8.

64 Vickers A, Cassileth B, Ernst E *et al. How Should we Research Unconventional Therapies?* A Panel Report from the Conference on Complementary and Alternative Medicine Research Methodology, National Institutes of Health. *Int J Tech Asssess Hlth Care* 1997;**13**:111–21.

65 Nahin RL, Straus SE. Research into complementary and alternative medicine: problems and potential. *BMJ* 2001;**322**:161–4.

66 Kemper KJ, Cassileth B, Ferris T. Holistic pediatrics: a research agenda. *Pediatrics* 1999;**103**:902–9.

14 Communicating evidence to patients

Lyndal Trevena, Heather M Davey, Alexandra Barratt,
Phyllis Butow, Patrina Caldwell

Case scenario	*The parents of a 3-day-old baby boy approach you in the nursery of your maternity hospital and ask if you would circumcise their son before he goes home. He was born at term by normal vaginal delivery. He has had an uneventful postnatal period, is breastfeeding well, has had no jaundice and his weight is approximately 3·7 kg. Before agreeing to do the procedure you want to discuss with the parents their reasons for requesting circumcision and inform them about the risks and benefits of the procedure. You wonder how best to proceed.*

Background

The application of evidence within an individual consultation has been described as the juncture between the art and the science of medicine.[1] As a clinician you have to find and appraise the best available evidence and assimilate this with findings from the patient's clinical history and examination and knowledge about the nature of the clinical problem and its circumstances. It is also important, where possible, that you consider the preferences of parents and their child when deciding how to proceed (see Figure 14.1).[2]

The vast topic of clinical decision-making is beyond the scope of this chapter. Thus we have chosen to focus on strategies both to facilitate the effective communication of evidence to parents and children and to elicit their preferences, beliefs, and values relating to the evidence. We have approached the case scenario from the perspective of a clinician who wants to find out how to communicate evidence effectively to their patients and/or the patient's parents. We have summarized the broad principles of effective communication strategies identified in the literature. Most of this literature is not specific to the pediatric setting, but we have highlighted pediatric studies when they were identified.

At the outset, we would like to note two important issues regarding communicating evidence to parents/patients that are not discussed in detail in this chapter but deserve mention and should be borne in mind throughout this chapter. Firstly, you should ensure, where possible, that consumer information is evidence-based. An instrument called DISCERN has been developed to help readers judge the quality of written consumer health information on treatment

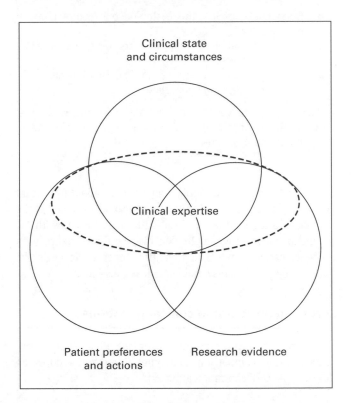

Figure 14.1 A model for evidence-based decision-making[2]

choices, and a checklist is provided in the Box.[3] In relation to the case scenario in this chapter we have used evidence on the pros and cons of circumcision provided in a clinical practice guideline that was based on a systematic review of the literature.[4]

DISCERN quality checklist for written consumer information on treatment choices

- Is the publication reliable?
- Are the aims clear?
- Does it achieve its aims?
- Is it relevant?
- Is it clear what sources of information were used to compile the publication?
- Is it clear when the information used or reported in the publication was produced?
- Is it balanced and unbiased?
- Does it provide details of additional sources of support and information?
- Does it refer to areas of uncertainty?
- How good is the quality of information on treatment choices?
- Does it describe how each treatment works?
- Does it describe the benefits of each treatment?
- Does it describe the risks of each treatment?
- Does it describe what would happen if no treatment is used?
- Does it describe how the treatment choices affect overall quality of life?
- Is it clear that there may be more than one possible treatment choice?
- Does it provide support for shared decision-making?
- Overall rating of the publication

Based on the answers to all of the above questions, rate the overall quality of the publication as a source of information about treatment choices.

Secondly, when communicating evidence about healthcare options in pediatric practice you must also take account of the ethical and legal context of local authorities.[5] Faced with the scenario above, how might you discuss the evidence with parents/patients and elicit their preferences? We begin the process by framing answerable clinical questions.

Framing answerable clinical questions

You structure three questions using the PICO (population, intervention, comparison, outcome) framework addressing three aspects of communicating evidence.

Questions

1. For parents and children making decisions about health care (*population*), are communication tools, for example decision aids, brochures/pamphlets/leaflets, videos, websites, tailored computer programs, verbal advice, structured counseling (*intervention*), more effective than no tools or other tools (*comparison*) in

increasing understanding of the evidence (*outcome*)? **[Intervention]**

2. For parents and children making decisions about health care (*population*), are available methods of representing information, for example numbers, absolute risk, relative risk, graphs, pictures/illustrations, diagrams, text words (*intervention*), more effective than no method or other methods (*comparison*) in increasing understanding of the evidence (*outcome*)? **[Intervention]**

3. For parents and children making decisions about health care (*population*), are specific tools, for example decision aids, decision analysis tools, touchscreen computers, questionnaires, question prompt sheets, rating scales (*intervention*), more effective than no tool or other tools (*comparison*) for improving parent/patient satisfaction with their decisions about management and their adherence to decisions; minimizing anxiety or decisional conflict; and increasing involvement in decision-making (*outcome*)? **[Intervention]**

Searching for evidence

Before you search for studies to answer your questions, you develop a list of possible interventions and outcomes of interest (Table 14.1). For evaluating interventions you decide to limit your search to the best available evidence, namely randomized controlled trials (RCTs) and systematic reviews of RCTs, and to exclude studies that:

- do not address the question;
- are about patient education and focus on skills and behavior outcomes (such as increasing attendance at screening) without attempting to increase understanding or knowledge;
- are concerned with counseling as a therapeutic intervention (as opposed to a method of communicating evidence); or
- are specific to communication regarding clinical trial participation.

Searching on Question 1. Effectiveness of communication tools to improve patient/parent understanding of evidence

You check the thesaurus for each intervention and outcome term and find that "cognition" is used for your outcome keywords "comprehension" and "understanding." You first search the *Cochrane Library*, combining the intervention and outcome terms as keywords and using the search strategy below. After excluding irrelevant studies you are left with nine systematic reviews and 12 RCTs.

Table 14.1   Questions about strategies for effective communication with parents/patients

Population/problem (P)	Intervention/s (I)	Comparator/s (C)	Outcome/s (O)
1. The effectiveness of communication tools to improve parent/patient understanding of 'evidence'			
Parents/patients making healthcare decisions	• Decision aids • Brochures/pamphlets/ leaflets • Videos • Websites • Tailored computer programs • Verbal advice • Structured counseling	No tool or other tools	Parent/patient • understanding • knowledge • comprehension
2. Methods for representing probabilistic information/evidence			
Parents/patients making healthcare decisions	• Numeric • Absolute risk • Relative risk • Graphical (histograms/ pie charts/line graphs, 100 faces) • Pictures/illustrations/ diagrams • Text words	No method or each other	Parent/patient • understanding • knowledge • comprehension
3. Strategies for eliciting parent/patient preferences/beliefs/values relating to 'evidence'			
Parent/patients making healthcare decisions	• Decision aids • Decision analysis tools • Touch screen computers • Questionnaires • Question prompt sheets • Rating scales	No tool or other tools	Parent/patient • satisfaction with decision • adherence to decision • anxiety • decisional conflict • involvement in decision-making

> ***Cochrane Library*: (communication) AND ((knowledge) OR (informed) OR (cognition))**
>
> • Cochrane Database of Systematic Reviews (CDSR): six systematic reviews
> • Database of Abstracts of Rerviews of Effects (DARE): three systematic reviews
> • Cochrane Controlled Trials Register (CENTRAL): 12 RCTs

Since this is a broad topic and a fairly new research area you also search MedLine, PsychInfo, and CancerLit using the Ovid interface. After excluding studies outside your criteria, you are left with 35 RCTs and nine systematic reviews to appraise.

Searching on Question 2. Methods for presenting risks and other evidence to patients/parents

You have already identified 11 RCTs that relate to this question in your earlier search. You conduct a further search of MedLine, PsychInfo, and CancerLit using keywords listed under interventions and outcomes for Question 2 in Table 14.1, along with searching personal files and finish with 14 RCTs to appraise.

Searching on Question 3. Strategies for eliciting parent/patient preferences, beliefs and values relating to the evidence

Using keywords listed under interventions and outcomes for Question 3 in Table 14.1, you search MedLine, PsychInfo, CancerLit and personal files identifying seven relevant RCTs for appraisal on Question 3.

Search summary

In total you have found 35 RCTs relevant to Question 1, 14 RCTs relevant to Question 2, and seven RCTs relevant to Question 3, as well as nine systematic reviews. As a busy clinician, you recognize that reading and critically appraising all these articles will be impossible and decide to start with the systematic reviews. For the purposes of this chapter, however, the authors have appraised and summarized all 56 RCTs and nine systematic reviews.

Critical review of the evidence

You use the quality checklist from Glasziou and Irwig[6] to appraise the 56 RCTs and the checklist from Guyatt *et al.*[7] to appraise the nine systematic reviews. Six of the systematic reviews were from the *Cochrane Library* and all nine were of reasonable quality. However, many of the RCTs did not report on the method of randomization used or follow up rates. Although blinding the outcome assessment in RCTs in this research area poses a particular challenge, this was achieved in some studies. You note that in many studies the authors chose to measure anxiety, a potentially harmful outcome of providing information, but that this was often measured over only short periods of time. Systematic reviewers also found it difficult to pool effect sizes for many of the outcomes due to heterogeneity of measures and lack of reported data. You use a grading system of A–C based on the *Cochrane Reviewers' Handbook*[8] to give each study an overall grade and exclude all studies with a C (poor quality) grading.

Question

1. For parents and children making decisions about health care (*population*), are communication tools, for example decision aids, brochures/pamphlets/leaflets, videos, websites, tailored computer programs, verbal advice, structured counseling (*intervention*), more effective than no tools or other tools (*comparison*) in increasing understanding of the evidence (*outcome*)? **[Intervention]**

After excluding poor quality studies, you are left with 24 RCTs[9–20] and nine systematic reviews[21–29] evaluating the effectiveness of various communication tools to increase patient/parent understanding of evidence. The commonly accepted definitions of these communication tools are summarized in the Box.

Definitions of communication tools discussed in this chapter

- *Tailored print information.* Printed information provided on the basis of individual data characteristics. These data may be collected by a number of methods, for example interview, computer, patient record systems, etc.
- *Decision aids.* "Interventions designed to help people make specific and deliberative choices among options (including status quo) by providing (at a minimum)

information on the options and outcomes relevant to a person's health status. They may include a decision-making support framework or exercise that allows people to synthesize the evidence with their personal values and preferences (values clarification exercise)."[28]

- *Consultation summaries.* Interventions offering video-tape, audiotape recordings, written summaries of consultation, or standardized verbal or written instructions.
- *Provider training in a patient-centered approach.* Training that promotes shared control of the clinical consultation and decisions about healthcare problems between the provider and patient. A focus in the consultation on the patient as a whole person who has individual preferences situated within social contexts.
- *Videos.* Videotape-recorded information about health-care (not providing options as would be the case with a decision aid).
- *Interactive touchscreen computer.* Computerized information (not tailored or providing options as would be the case for a decision aid).
- *Evidence-based leaflets.* Written information within a leaflet (not tailored or providing options or values clarification as would be the case for a decision aid).

The studies are grouped by intervention or type of communication tool in Table 14.2. In summary, they indicate that the provision of evidence-based information *of any type* is better than *no* information for increasing knowledge about healthcare. In general, the more tailored and interactive the method of communicating evidence, the greater the resulting level of knowledge and understanding in the parent/patient. Non-text formats such as videos, touchscreen or verbal forms of information may be better for some patients, particularly those from lower education or socioeconomic backgrounds. None of the studies found assessed whether it was more effective to give information before, during, or after the consultation. In fact, the few studies that assessed strategies within the consultation were excluded for quality reasons, indicating that it is difficult to assess the effectiveness of such strategies. Training for healthcare providers in patient-centered approaches was also an effective strategy for increasing patient understanding of evidence.

Question

2. For parents and children making decisions about health care (*population*), are available methods of representing information, for example numbers, absolute risk, relative risk, graphs, pictures/illustrations, diagrams, text words (*intervention*), more effective than no method or other methods (*comparison*) in increasing understanding of the evidence (*outcome*)? **[Intervention]**

Table 14.2 Communication tools shown to be effective in increasing parent/patient understanding of the evidence

Type of communication tool	Level of evidence	Source of evidence	Results
Tailored print information	Level I	1 review[29] of 12 RCTs	• Results not pooled but tailored print communication was better remembered, read, and perceived as relevant or credible compared with non-tailored information • Tailored information more likely to result in behavior change
Decision aids (DA)	Level I	1 review[28] of 24 RCTs	• Greater knowledge of options (WMD = 19 out of 100, 95% CI 13,25); more realistic expectations (RR = 1·48, 95% CI 1·02, 2·14); lower decisional conflict (WMD = −9·0 of 100 95% CI −15, −3); reduction in number of people who were passive in decision making (RR = 0·63, 95% CI 0·5, 0·8). Consistent trend for DAs to do no better than comparisons in affecting satisfaction with decision and decision-making process, and anxiety. Effect on decision was variable • More interactive formats such as computerized, interactive versions appear to have a greater effect size compared with audio-booklets or booklets with summary
Consultation summaries	Level I	1 review[21] of 8 RCTs and 1 additional RCT[45]*	• 83–96% of patients found summaries to be valuable. Results were not pooled but showed better recall of information, and more satisfaction with the information received. No studies found an effect on anxiety or depression. Standardized verbal instructions were better than non-standardized verbal instructions in 197 parents leaving the emergency department with a child with otitis media.[45] There was no added benefit if a written copy of the standardized instructions was supplied in addition to standardized verbal instructions
Provider training in a patient-centered approach	Level I	1 review[22] of 17 RCTs	• Improved patient satisfaction and improved consultation processes
Video	Level II	2 RCTs[9,14]	• Compared with normal practice, videos increased knowledge about options without affecting anxiety. This effect was particularly evident in low SES sub-groups
Interactive computer aids/touchscreens etc	Level II	2 RCTs[13,15]	• Compared with audio-booklet or written information, interactive computer information increases knowledge, expectations of outcomes, patient participation, and reduces decisional conflict. Patients preferred this format more than leaflets. This effect was more evident in low SES sub-groups
Evidence-based leaflets	Level II	3 RCTs[11,12,16]	• Increased knowledge compared with no leaflet. Increased reported adherence to therapy in parents of children with amplyopia

*Denotes a study in a pediatric context
SES, socioeconomic status; WMD, weighted mean difference

Five of the 14 RCTs that were appraised for this question were excluded on the basis of quality. For both written and verbal information, patients have a more accurate perception of risk if probabilistic information is presented as numbers rather than words.[30–32] In some settings, detailed written risk information (including harms) increases knowledge and satisfaction without changing anxiety.[33,34] Illustrations within narrative text compared with bullet point information can increase comprehension,[35] and cartoons in one study increased understanding, adherence, and recall in parents of children at an emergency department compared with text only information.[36] Patients can understand survival curves, when given more than one opportunity to do so.[37] Framing information in terms of either benefits or harms can affect parent/patient preferences.[38,39] There is also observational data suggesting that relative and absolute risk can also alter preferences.[40]

Questions

3. For parents and children making decisions about health care (*population*), are specific tools, for example decision aids, decision analysis tools, touchscreen computers, questionnaires, question prompt sheets, rating scales (*intervention*), more effective than no tool or other tools (*comparison*) for improving parent/patient satisfaction with their decisions about management and their adherence to decisions; minimizing anxiety or decisional conflict; and increasing involvement in decision-making (*outcome*)? **[Intervention]**

You found limited evidence on methods for eliciting parent/patient preferences and few good quality RCTs. However, with the limited evidence available, decision aids do appear to be an effective tool for eliciting preferences.[41,42] A number of trials have also shown them to be effective in improving decision-making outcomes (Table 14.2). Standard gamble and time-trade-off (where patients weigh up one health state against another) were shown in one study to be poorly predictive of preferences in men with prostate cancer.[42]

Finding evidence-based communication tools

Having established that decision aids are potentially useful tools for communicating the pros and cons of a particular treatment and for eliciting parent preferences, you want to see if such a tool is available for use with your patient's parent. A global inventory of patient decision aids is available at the Ottawa Health Decision Centre website [http://www.ohri.ca/programs/clinical_epidemiology/OPDSL/a_to_z.asp] but you find no decision aids on circumcision. There is also an extensive list of decision aids in the *Cochrane Library*[28] and, although you notice two trials have been published on circumcision decision aids,[43 44] you can't locate a copy of either tool. The Cochrane Consumer Network has an increasing list of summaries of systematic reviews for patient use, including a section on well babies and children at http://www.cochraneconsumer.com/. A new website associated with the BMJ publication *Clinical Evidence* called "Best Treatments: Clinical evidence for patients and doctors" has been established via www.bmjknowledge.com with some potentially relevant pediatric topics. Unfortunately neither of these contain entries on infant circumcision. The field of decision aids is rapidly growing and it is very likely that the availability of decision-support tools for clinicians and their patients will increase over the next few years.

You do find a Circumcision Information and Resource page at http://www.cirp.org/ which has a wide range of views, information and discussions on the topic, including a video and photographs of a circumcision. You now know that illustrations, diagrams, and other non-text formats can assist with comprehension of probabilistic information. You make a note to consider the DISCERN criteria (see the Box on page 130) when looking at this site and discussing it with your patients.

You also find the Canadian Paediatric Society Guidelines[4] on circumcision and summarize the key findings, including the potential benefits and harms of circumcision and the issues for which the evidence is absent, inconclusive or for which there is conflicting evidence of benefit or harm (Table 14.3). The summary incorporates numeric risk estimates about potential benefits and harms, where available, because you now know that patients have a more accurate perception of risk if it is presented as numbers. You include absolute as well as relative risks where possible. For instance, in relative terms, urinary tract infection is twelve times more likely in uncircumcised boys (OR 12·0). In absolute terms approximately 12 out of every 100 uncircumcised boys might get a urinary tract infection compared with 1 in 100 circumcised boys (if you take the incidence to be 1%). An example of possible components of a decision aid based on the Canadian guidelines is found in Figure 14.2.

Resolution of the scenario

In the absence of "off the shelf" communication tools on circumcision you decide you can best communicate the pros and cons of circumcision by giving the parents a written summary of the evidence you found in the medical literature. You discuss with them the key findings from the Canadian Paediatric Society and provide them with a written summary, which includes some numerical information on the absolute risks of benefits and harms (Table 14.3 or see the Box). You also provide them with the internet address for a Circumcision Information and Resource page at http://www.cirp.org/ but warn them that consumer information found on the internet about treatment choices is of variable quality. You offer to speak with them later that day after they have had a chance to read the material you have given them, which includes a copy of the DISCERN checklist.

Table 14.3   Key findings from Canadian Paediatric Society Guidelines on Circumcision[4]

Potential benefits	Potential harms	No evidence, inconclusive evidence, or conflicting evidence of benefit or harm
• Improved penile hygiene – reduced phimosis, adhesions and inflammation (usually mild) • Reduced incidence of UTI, particularly in first year of life. Overall incidence of male UTI during infancy is 1–2%. Uncircumcised males are more likely to have a UTI during infancy than circumcised male infants. OR 12·0 (95% CI 10·6–13·6) • Reduced rate of cancer of penis in circumcised men (Incidence 0·3 to 1·1 per 10^5 men per year in developed and 3–6 per 10^5 men per year in developing nations). Very few cases of penile cancer reported in men circumcised as neonates	• Procedural complications – occur in around 0·2–2% circumcisions. Bleeding is the most common (usually local and easily controlled). Infection is the second most common. Case reports of serious complications (recurrent phimosis, wound separation, urinary retention, meatal stenosis, chordee, inclusion cysts, retained Plastibell device, scalded skin syndrome, necrotizing fasciitis, sepsis, meningitis, urethral fistula, penile necrosis) exist. Better data on complication rates needed • Pain – strong evidence that neonates experience significant pain on circumcision if no anesthesia or analgesia given. EMLA, dorsal penile nerve block, or subcutaneous ring block are all effective procedures • Penile problems in childhood – usually meatal ulcers or irritation – more common in circumcised (14%) compared with uncircumcised boys (6%) $P < 0.0001$	• Penile problems reduced – no evidence of difference between circumcised and uncircumcised • Change in sexual practice/function – no evidence of any difference between circumcised or uncircumcised • Rate of HIV and sexually transmitted infections – conflicting evidence for effect of circumcision

Summary

Applying evidence effectively in practice involves synthesizing research evidence with clinical findings and patient preferences, beliefs and values. There is good evidence that a range of communication tools can increase parent/patient understanding and knowledge in healthcare decision-making. The more tailored, interactive and sophisticated these tools, the more likely it is that patients/parents will have a more accurate perception of risks, benefits, and harms of treatment options. Detailed risk information does not appear to increase anxiety but does reduce decisional conflict and increase satisfaction and participation in decision-making. Numeric risk estimates should be given where possible and written information should be supported by illustrations or diagrams to increase comprehension, adherence, and recall of information. If "state of the art" communication tools are not accessible, clinicians can be assured that simple structured verbal or written information is an effective tool.

Future research needs

The evidence about communicating with patients is growing, but a number of issues remain poorly understood. We need further research about how to communicate evidence in cross-cultural and socially disadvantaged contexts. We also have very limited knowledge about effective strategies for eliciting patient preferences and we know very little about mechanisms for combining preferences of both parents, carers or other family members, children who are patients, and their doctors in the pediatric consultation. Further research also needs to be conducted with implementation issues in mind, preferably in "real-world" clinical settings and to evaluate the impact of decision aids and tools on the quality and efficiency of pediatric healthcare.

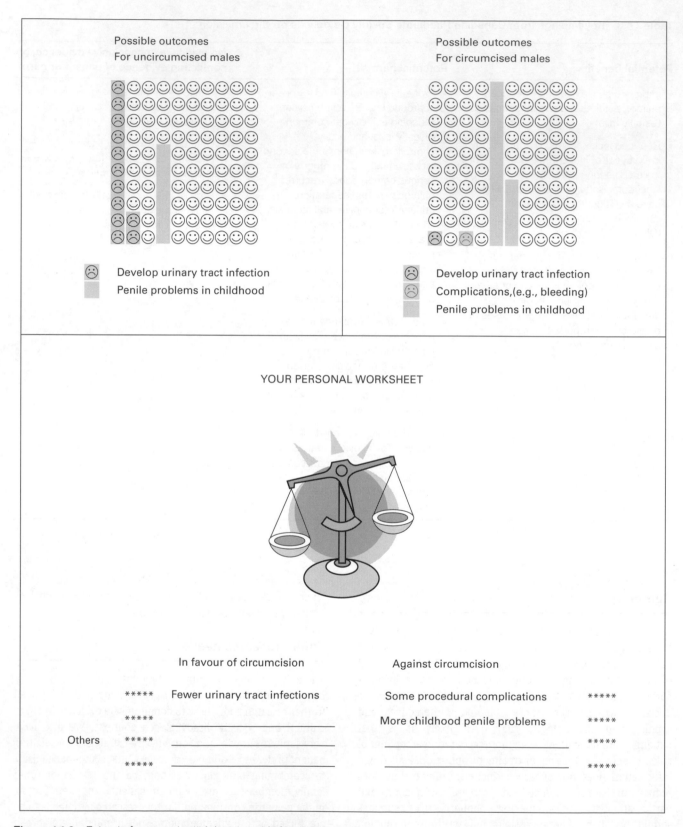

Possible outcomes
For uncircumcised males

☹ Develop urinary tract infection

Penile problems in childhood

Possible outcomes
For circumcised males

☹ Develop urinary tract infection

☹ Complications,(e.g., bleeding)

Penile problems in childhood

YOUR PERSONAL WORKSHEET

In favour of circumcision		Against circumcision	
*****	Fewer urinary tract infections	Some procedural complications	*****
*****	_____	More childhood penile problems	*****
Others *****	_____	_____	*****
*****	_____	_____	*****

Figure 14.2 Extracts from a potential decision aid about circumcision.

Take home list

- Any type of evidence-based information is better than *no* information for increasing parents/patients knowledge about health care.
- The more tailored and interactive the method of communicating evidence, the greater the resulting level of knowledge and understanding in the parent/patient.
- Non-text formats (for example, videos) of verbal information may work best for some patients.
- A wide range of communication tools is available to increase patient/parent understanding of evidence.
- For both written and verbal information, patients have a more accurate perception of risk if probabilistic information is presented as numbers.
- Detailed written risk information (including harms) may increase knowledge and satisfaction without changing anxiety.
- Illustrations (including cartoons) compared with text increase understanding of, adherence to and recall of information.
- Patients can understand survival curves when given adequate opportunity to do so.
- Framing information in terms of benefits or harms can affect parent/patient preference.
- Observational data suggest that relative and absolute risk can also frame preferences.
- Increasingly, databases of decision aids will become available.

References

1 Battista R, Hodge M, Vineis P. Medicine, Practice and Guidelines: The Uneasy Juncture of Science and Art. *J Clin Epidemiol* 1995;**48**:875–80.

2 Haynes R, Deveraux P, Guyatt G. Clinical expertise in the era of *Evidence-Based Med* and patient choice. *Evidence-Based Med* 2002;**7**:36–8.

3 Charnock D, Sheppard S, Needham G, Gann R. DISCERN: an instrument for judging the quality of written consumer health information on treatment choices. *J Epidemiol Commun Hlth* 1999;**53**:105–11.

4 Canadian Paediatric Society. Neonatal circumcision revisited. Fetus and Newborn Committee, Canadian Paediatric Society. *CMAJ* 1996(154):6.

5 General Medical Council. Seeking patients' consent: the ethical considerations, 1998.

6 Glasziou P, Irwig L, Bain C, Colditz G. *Systematic reviews in health care. A practical guide.* Cambridge: University Press, UK, 2001.

7 The *Evidence-Based Med* Working group. *Users' Guides to the Medical Literature. A manual for evidence-based clinical practice.* Chicago, IL: AMA Press, 2002.

8 Cochrane Collaboration. *Cochrane Reviewers' Handbook* 4.1.6, 2003.

9 Agre P, Kurtz R, Krauss B. A randomized trial using videotape to present consent information for colonoscopy. *Gastrointest Endosc* 1994;**40**:271–6.

10 Hopper K, Zajdel M, Hulse S *et al.* Interactive method of informing patients of the risks of intravenous contrast media. *Radiology* 1994;**192**:67–71.

11 O'Cathain A, Walters S, Nicholl J, Thomas K, Kirkham M. Use of evidence-based leaflets to promote informed choice in maternity care: randomized controlled trial in everyday practice. *BMJ* 2002;**324**:643.

12 Newsham D. A randomized controlled trial of written information: the effect on parental non-concordance with occlusion therapy. *Br J Opthalmol* 2002;**86**:787–91.

13 Rostom A, O'Connor A, Tugwell P, Wells G. A randomized trial of a computerized versus an audio-booklet decision aid for women considering post-menopausal hormone replacement therapy. *Patient Educ Counsel* 2002;**46**:67–74.

14 Hewison J, Cuckle H, Baillie C *et al.* Use of videotapes for viewing at home to inform choice in Down syndrome screening: a randomized controlled trial. *Prenat Diag* 2001;**21**:146–9.

15 Graham W, Smith P, Kamal A, Fitzmaurice A, Smith N, Hamilton N. Randomised controlled trial comparing effectiveness of touch screen system with leaflet for providing women with information on prenatal tests. *BMJ* 2000;**320**:155–60.

16 O'Neill P, Humphris G, Field E. The use of an information leaflet for patients undergoing wisdom tooth removal. *Br J Oral Maxillofac Surgery* 1996;**34**:331–4.

17 Paci E, Barneschi M, Miccimesis G, Falchi S, Metrangalo L, Novelli G. Informed consent and patient participation in the medical encounter: a list of questions for an informed choice about the type of anaesthesia. *Eur J Anaesthesiol* 1999;**16**:160–5.

18 Lewis C, Pantell R, Sharp L. Increasing patient knowledge, satisfaction, and involvement: randomized trial of a communication intervention. *Pediatrics* 1991;**88**:351–8.

19 Murray E, Davis H, Tai S, Coulter A, Gray A, Haines A. Randomised controlled trial of an interactive multimedia decision aid on hormone replacement therapy in primary care. *BMJ* 2001;**323**:1–5.

20 Lees A, Rock W. A comparison between written, verbal and videotape oral hygiene instruction for patients with fixed appliances. *J Orthodont* 2000;**27**:323–7.

21 Scott JT, Entwistle VA, Sowden AJ, Watt I. Recordings or summaries of consultations for people with cancer. In: Cochrane Collaboration. *Cochrane Library.* Issue 1. Oxford: Update Software, 2003.

22 Lewin S, Skea Z, Entwistle V, Zwarenstein M, Dick J. Interventions for providers to promote a patient-centred approach in clinical consultations. *Cochrane Database of Systematic Reviews*, 2002.

23 Edwards A, Elwyn G, Hood K. Personalised risk communication in health screening programs. *Cochrane Database of Systematic Reviews* 2002;**1**(1).

24 Walsh R A GA, Sansonfisher R W. Breaking bad news 2: What evidence is available to guide clinicians? *Behavior Med* 1998;**24**:61–72.

25 NHS Centre for Reviews and Dissemination. Informing, communicating and sharing decisions with people who have cancer. *Effect Hlth Care* 2000;**6**:8.

26 Scott JT, Entwistle VA, Sowden AJ, Watt I. Communicating with children and adolescents about their cancer. In: Cochrane Collaboration. *Cochrane Library*. Issue 1. Oxford: Update Software, 2003.

27 Toelle B, Ram F. Written individualised management plans for asthma in children and adults. In: Cochrane Collaboration. *Cochrane Library*. Issue 1. Oxford: Update Software, 2003.

28 O'Connor A, Fiset V, Rostom A *et al.* Decision aids for people facing health treatment or screening decisions. *The Cochrane Database of Systematic Reviews*, Issue 3, 2003.

29 Skinner CS, Campbell MK, Rimer BK, Curry S, Prochaska JO. How effective is tailored print communication? *Ann Behavior Med* 1999;**21**:290–8.

30 Marteau T, Saidi G, Goodburn S, Lawton J, Michie S, Bobrow M. Numbers or words? A randomized controlled trial of presenting screen negative results in pregnant women. *Prenat Diag* 2000;**20**:714–18.

31 Man-Son-Hing M, O'Connor A, Drake E, Biggs J, Hum V, Laupacis A. The effect of qualitative vs quantitative presentation of probability estimates on patient decision-making: a randomised trial. *Hlth Expect* 2002;**5**:246–55.

32 Mazur D, Merz J. Patients' interpretations of verbal expressions of probability: Implications for securing informed consent to medical interventions. *Behaviour Sci Law* 1994;**12**:417–26.

33 Garrud P, Wood M, Stainsby L. Impact of risk information in a patient education leaflet. *Pat Educ Counsel* 2001;**43**:301–4.

34 Kreuter M, Bull F, Clark E, Oswald D. Understanding how people process health information: A comparison of tailored and nontailored weight-loss materials. *Hlth Psychol* 1999;**18**:487–94.

35 Michielutte R, Bahnson J, Dignan M, Em S. The use of illustrations and narrative text style to improve readabilty of health education brochure. *J Cancer Educ* 1992;**7**:251–60.

36 Delp C, Jones J. Communicating information to patients: The use of cartoon illustrations to improve comprehension of instructions. *Acad Emerg Med* 1996;**3**:264–70.

37 Armstrong K, Fitzgerald G, Schw J. Using survival curve comparisons to inform patient decision-making. *J Gen Intern Med* 2001;**16**:482–5.

38 Gurm H, Litaker D. Framing procedural risks to patients: is 99% safe the same as a risk of 1 in 100? *Acad Med* 2000;**75**:840–2.

39 O'Connor A. Effects of framing and level of probability on patients' preferences for cancer chemotherapy. *J Clin Epidemiol* 1989;**42**:119–26.

40 Malenka D, Baron J, Johansen S, Wahrenberger J, Ross J. The framing effect of relative and absolute risk. *J Gen Intern Med* 1993;**8**:543–8.

41 Kennedy A, Sculpher M, Coulter A *et al.* Effects of decision aids for menorrhagia on treatment choices, health outcomes and costs. *JAMA* 2002;**288**:2701–8.

42 Souchek J, Stacks J, Brody B *et al.* A trial for comparing methods for eliciting treatment preferences from men with advanced prostate cancer: results from the initial visit. *Med Care* 2000;**38**:1040–50.

43 Maisels J, Hayes B, Conrad S, Chez R. Circumcision: the effect of information on parental decision-making. *Pediatrics* 1983;**71**:453–4.

44 Herrera A, Cochran B, Herrera A, Wallace B. Parental information and circumcision in highly motivated couples with higher education. *Pediatrics* 1983;**71**:233–4.

45 Isaacman D, Purvis K, Gyuro J, Anderson Y, Smith D. Standardized instructions: do they improve communication of discharge information from the emergency department? *Pediatrics* 1992;**89**:1204–8.

15 Health informatics

Martin Pusic

Case scenario   *You are the sole clinician on a 12–member committee charged with selecting a new hospital information system for your Children's Hospital. Information systems' specialists and hospital administrators dominate the committee. To date, the discussions have centered on "business cases" and "operational efficiencies." You wonder if this new system can have an impact on measurable patient health outcomes.*

Background

As a sector, health care has been slow to adopt information technology.[1] The reasons for this delayed embrace of information technologies is unclear though it may be due to the more complex nature of the final product. In this chapter, we will explore the impact of health informatics on the use of research evidence in health care. Haynes has defined "health informatics" as "being concerned with improving the retrieval, synthesis, organization, dissemination and application of...information for health care."[2] Notice that this definition encompasses both *information* (for example, a patient's blood pressure) and *research evidence* or *knowledge* (drug X lowers blood pressure). Many health informatics theories, methods, and techniques are concerned with the interplay between information and knowledge.[3] In this chapter, we will explore the impact of health informatics on the application of research evidence to health care, and focus on the assessment of information systems used to improve health outcomes. We will only briefly touch on the important contributions of health informatics to the dissemination of research evidence through digital libraries, and the use of educational technology in continuing medical education, as these are addressed in other chapters.

Computer support of healthcare processes began with large mainframe computers that housed administrative databases. Gradually, more and more healthcare enterprises have changed their processes to take advantage of advances in information systems. Of particular interest to practitioners of evidence-based medicine is the evolution of integrated advanced information management systems (IAIMS). In 1982 the US National Library of Medicine (NLM) established a funding program whose objective was to "to help organizations build institution-wide computer networks that link and relate library systems with individual and institutional databases and information files for patient care, research, education, and administration."[5] Over the succeeding 20 years, the NLM granted over $50 million to 42 large academic healthcare institutions to plan and get into operation effective information infrastructures. The supported projects varied a great deal as individual institutions grappled with local realities and ever-changing technological capabilities and standards. Gradually a generalizable model of a state-of-the-art healthcare information system has emerged.[6]

Figure 15.1 shows one version of an IAIMS system. Key components include:

- modular *subsystems* for radiology, laboratory, oncology, etc.;
- *order entry* – standardized process for entering orders; allows computer decision support and critiquing;
- *result review* – standardized interface for reviewing results from the subsystems as well as context-appropriate knowledge resources;
- *health library browser and MedLine database*;
- *drug database*;
- *clinical data repository* – containing physical copy of all patient information including a copy of relevant ancillary subsystem information;
- *event monitor* with clinical decision rules – each time data are requested or stored, an event is triggered which results in the application of relevant logic rules.

A component that is missing from this diagram is an electronic messaging interface for communication between a clinician and another peer or with a patient.

Elson *et al.* propose that most clinical activity can be viewed through an "industrial production" model in which

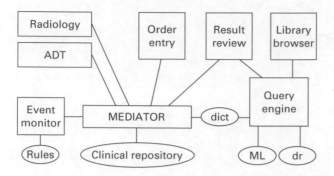

Figure 15.1 Component model of an integrated advanced information management system for health care enterprises. Each component is described in the text. Key features from an evidence-based practice standpoint include the direct incorporation of library and MedLine (ML) access into the hospital information system. Also important are the "rules" and "order entry", each of which allow research evidence to influence the delivery of health care (reproduced with permission of Elsevier)
ADT = Admission Discharge Transfer database
dict = Standardized dictionary
dr = drug database

the fundamental process is the clinical decision.[7] Substrates for this process include information that is dependent on the clinician (elicited signs and symptoms; clinical knowledge, skills and attitudes; knowledge of the patient) and on external sources (medical record, medical literature and compendia, consultations). Elson argues that successful clinical decisions are best made within well-considered *systems* where the finite limits of human cognition are taken into account.

The model in Figure 15.2 is useful in categorizing the way in which information systems can improve clinical decision-making.

In the succeeding sections, we will list some examples of these techniques with measures of their individual effects on healthcare processes and patient outcomes. We will then review the synthesized evidence for the use of these interventions (Table 15.1).

Perception

Proper diagnosis and management requires that a clinician has at hand the information and knowledge required for a sound clinical decision. However, this depends on the clinician first perceiving which information is required for the decision at hand.[7] *Unmet* information needs can result in suboptimal and potentially even unsafe decisions.[8] *Unrecognized unmet* information needs are especially problematic, since the level of uncertainty cannot be factored into the decision.

Charles Friedman showed 72 clinicians a series of clinical vignettes of difficult internal medicine patients.[9] Using a statistical model, he demonstrated that it could take up to 28 reviews by different clinicians before all *plausible*

diagnostic possibilities had been raised. Clearly the process of generating a comprehensive differential diagnosis can be beyond the abilities of a single physician, a fact recognized by our system of multiple consultations and second opinions for difficult cases. However, computer information systems can help.

The "QMR" system used an ingenious algorithm modeled on the clinical reasoning of a single University of Pittsburgh internist.[10] The program takes historical and physical findings and generates a differential diagnosis. It does this by using a large database of "evoking strengths", "importance" and "frequencies" of findings seen in diseases within its domain. A pathognomonic finding has a high evoking strength, while a finding that is commonly seen in a given disease also increases the weighting given to that disease in the differential diagnosis. An important finding that is absent will downgrade a specific disease within the differential diagnosis. Friedman *et al.* prospectively studied this system by having medical students, residents, and attending physicians consider 36 written case vignettes based on actual patients with difficult internal medicine diagnostic problems.[11] The correct diagnosis appeared on 39·5% of subjects' hypothesis lists before consultation with QMR and 45·4% after consultation. The improvement was greater for students than for attending physicians but were statistically significant for each group. However, the labor-intensive, often biased, process of entering findings limits its utility in actual clinical practice.

ISABEL is a knowledge support tool for the generation of pediatric differential diagnosis developed by the Isabel Medical Charity (http://www.isabel.org.uk/). Using a proprietary algorithm that searches pediatric textbooks, the

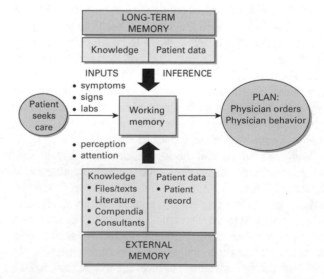

Figure 15.2 Industrial production model of medical decision making (modified from Elson *et al.*, 1997 reproduced with permission of Elsevier)[7]

Table 15.1 Component of clinical decisions and use of interventions

Component of clinical decision	Informatics technique
Perception	Diagnostic support programs Sensory aids
Attention	Clinical decision support systems • reminders • clinical alerts
Clinical knowledge	Embedded knowledge • physician order entry • disease management systems • medical calculators
Knowledge of the patient	Patient access to electronic health record Electronic messaging
Medical record	Electronic guideline implementation Structured data entry Natural language processing Data mining
Medical literature	Information retrieval Computer aided instruction

program determines 15 diagnoses that should be considered in the differential diagnosis for a given symptom or sign. Ramnarayan compared the results of an ISABEL consultation to the final diagnosis determined by the clinicians caring for 100 admitted acutely ill children.[12] The final diagnosis appeared within the 15-item differential generated by ISABEL 95% of the time in this evaluation, which was conducted by one of the architects of ISABEL. More extensive independent evaluation is lacking at this time.

There are a number of other information applications that improve a clinician's ability to perceive physical phenomena. The CT scan is the classic example since the technology that made this breakthrough possible is not a new type of imaging transducer but rather the capacity to process the tremendous amounts of information generated by multiple datasets from axial images. Information systems that help the clinician perceive all relevant inputs to a given decision are likely to be beneficial.

Attention

It is not enough that all of the information and knowledge required to make a decision be present if this happens too late to help the patient. Information systems can quickly bring information that requires a decision to the clinician's attention. This has been one of the most successful areas for the application of information systems.

An excellent example is in the area of "clinical alerts" – situations outside the norm that might require action. Consider the specific case of a low potassium level for a patient on digoxin. This situation leaves the patient at heightened risk of dysrhythmia. At the Brigham and Woman's hospital in Boston, as well as at many others, when the abnormal potassium result is entered into the laboratory information system, a specially encoded message is sent to a separate computer program entitled the "event monitor".[13] This program is a compendium of rules of the form "IF << abnormal situation >> THEN << do something >>. In the case of our example, all rules that have to do with potassium levels would be run through. The specific rule "IF K < 3·2 and patient on digoxin THEN page resident" would fire. The covering resident receives an alphanumeric page with an appropriate message prompting a clinical action. Note that this system requires a comprehensive patient database that knows which patient is on digoxin and which resident is covering that patient. A prospective cross-sectional evaluation of this system showed it being used 2300 times per month by 780 different clinicians.[14] The top 100 users (mainly housestaff) made 75% of the requests for notification of specific laboratory results.

Bates *et al.* systematically reviewed the use of information technology to *detect adverse events*.[15] They identified nine studies in which an informatics intervention was compared with a gold standard (usually manual chart review). They found that informatics techniques could be effectively applied for the detection of nosocomial infections and adverse drug events. The informatics technique had reasonable sensitivity but high false positive rates resulted in poor specificity in some of the trials. They concluded that computerized detection of adverse events would be widely practicable in the near future as more, higher quality data is available in a digital form. In a before-after comparison, the same group showed that, when used in combination with physician order entry, clinician alerts reduced medication errors by 55% (decrease from 10·7 per 1000 patient-days to 4·9; $P = .01$) with a concomitant decrease in potential adverse drug events.[16]

Timely *immunization* of children is another area in which clinicians have the requisite knowledge but may not be able to attend to the details of ensuring that all eligible patients receive their vaccinations. Within a larger systematic review of computer reminders in preventive care, Shea *et al.* showed that computer-printed reminders generated from patient data (i.e., without active human input) can effectively increase patient compliance with vaccination schedules.[17] In nine predominantly adult patient randomized controlled studies, the odds ratio (OR) for vaccination was 3·09 (95% CI 2·39–4·00) when computer reminders are compared with no reminders at all. Manual reminders (for example, telephone calls or postcards) were less effective (2·46; 95% CI 1·86–3·25). Of note, there appeared to be no additional benefit to combining manual with computer reminders.

Clinician knowledge

The ideal clinician would be all-knowing. However, the cognitive abilities of even the most capable clinician are finite. Our medical education systems have recognized this fact in gearing their curricula towards teaching the students "*how* to know" rather than "*what* to know". Information systems allow shifting of the knowledge repository function from the clinician's brain to external locations that are still easily accessible.

This externalization of knowledge seems to work best when the knowledge is embedded in the system of care.[18] A simple example is the use of *computerized advice on drug dosages*. Clinicians are frequently in the position of initiating and monitoring potentially toxic drug therapy for acutely ill patients. They have the knowledge of how to prescribe the medications but frequently cannot attend to the calculation and monitoring details involved. Computer programs can use sophisticated models to calculate optimal amount and timing of drug doses.

A Cochrane review[19] looked at the results of 15 trials involving 1229 patients in which computerized advice was compared with "standard" care (in which the clinician alone monitored drug therapy.) They showed that clinician's behaviors were positively influenced and that patient outcomes improved significantly with the computerized intervention. Specific outcomes noted were:

- faster time to achieve therapeutic control (standardized mean difference −0·44, 95% CI −0·70 to −0·17);
- decreased risk of toxic drug levels (risk difference −0·12, 95% CI −0·24 to −0·01);
- decreased risk of adverse reactions (risk difference −0·06, 95% CI −0·12 to 0·00);
- decreased length of hospital stay (standardized mean difference −0·32, 95% CI −0·60 to −0·04).

The main drugs assessed were theophylline, anticoagulants, and aminoglycosides. While this review demonstrates the potential benefits of this approach, it should be generalized with caution. There is no age breakdown – in fact many of the studies excluded children. In addition, the studies considered medications with narrow therapeutic windows, which are less commonly prescribed to children in modern practice. Measured benefits may be fewer with safer medications.

An opportune moment to bring external clinical knowledge into the decision-making process is when a physician communicates clinical orders. Evidence-based guideline information and clinical logic can be built into electronic prescription software. Information systems of this type are referred to as *physician order entry* (POE) *systems*.[20] POE systems can:

- integrate information about the patient's current status including medications;
- present clinical alerts;
- present current research evidence and guideline information;
- provide dosage calculations;
- block dangerous or otherwise suboptimal orders;
- provide a simple method for updating default drug choice or dosing regimes.

POE systems have been shown to improve a number of process and clinical outcomes including reduction in serious medication errors,[15] reduction in length of stay and hospital charges,[21] and reductions in pharmacy, radiology, and laboratory turn-around times.[22]

Christakis *et al.*[23] randomized clinicians to either receive evidence-based prompts or not when computer-prescribing antibiotics for otitis media in an outpatient clinic. The main outcome variable was proportion of patients treated for the traditional 10 days versus a more evidence-based 5–9 day course. They found that the intervention group was more likely to comply with the evidence-based suggestion: 44% (95% CI 36, 52) versus 10% (0, 20).

Tierney *et al.* carried out one of the most important studies.[21] The Regenstrief Medical Record System connects a large number of hospitals and clinics in Indiana. This system was one of the first to enable POE. In 1993, the investigators carried out a cluster-randomized study comparing the patients cared for by resident teams on three POE enabled wards with those at three comparable control sites. The main outcome measure was total inpatient charges per hospital admission. The menus of the POE system were specifically designed to encourage cost-effective ordering (for example, patient costs for each alternative were prominently displayed; for some complaints, only the most cost-effective tests were presented as options). The system also had a decision support feature that warned the clinician of allergies and potential drug interactions. In examining 5219 eligible admissions, they found that total hospital charges were 12·7% ($887) less in the intervention group. The savings seemed to be driven by a 0·89 day reduction in the length of stay though this difference was not statistically significant. The analysis did not take into account the cost of the computer system. When using the POE system, the house staff required 5·5 extra minutes per patient to write orders.

More recently, Mekhjian *et al.* did a series of before-after studies during the roll-out of POE at selected Ohio State University Health Systems (OSUHS) hospitals.[22] Unlike the custom-developed Regenstrief System, the OSUHS system was based on a commercial system. It was, however, "extensively" modified using vendor-supplied tools to meet specific local needs. The system provided an interface for all test and medication ordering as well as for consult requests and requisitions. Of note, the system included more than 450 evidence-based order sets. Neither length of stay nor total cost per admission changed by a clinically significant amount. Several process outcomes improved including number of transcription errors, medication turn-around times, radiology procedure completion times, and laboratory result reporting times.

Clinician knowledge of the patient

As clinicians are freed from the role of fact repository, they can focus on perhaps their most important function – communicating with the patient. While computers lack advanced communication skills, they can nonetheless help clinicians know their patients better.

Kuperman *et al.* performed an interesting study at the Brigham and Women's in an outpatient primary care clinic.[24] They had the patients check the accuracy of their own data in the Electronic Health Record. The data items dealt with their health maintenance profile (Pap smear, cholesterol screening, etc.), medications, and allergies. The patients were given paper forms to correct their own data in the EHR. Using the forms from 80 patients of one practitioner (collected non-consecutively), they showed that over a third of the patients had new information to contribute to their own charts. At a pediatric emergency department, Porter *et al.* had 100 parents independently supply five past medical history data points.[25] Compared with a pediatrician interview, subjects correctly entered the data at least 94% of the time. Language issues were the main barriers to even better performance.

Information technology can enable electronic communication between clinicians and their patients. Web-messaging applications are just beginning to make their way into mainstream clinical care. The early results, mainly demonstration projects with user satisfaction surveys, are promising.[26,27]

Medical record

Digitization of the patient record is thought to have significant benefits for clinicians and their patients. Computerized records can be more accessible than paper ones.[13] Multiple users can access the record simultaneously from diverse geographic locations. Data quality can be improved using "validity checks" that make it impossible, for example, to enter a birth date that would make a patient 200 years old. Well-encoded computer data is easily reusable in other contexts and serves as a key substrate for computer decision support systems (CDSS) and POE.

Demonstrating the benefit of electronic health records *per se* to patient relevant outcomes has been difficult. Most trials and systematic reviews have centered on evaluating clinical decision support systems and/or physician order entry with the electronic record being an enabler for these functions. Relatively few studies have tried to tease out the independent effect of replacing paper records.[28]

It may however take more clinician time to collect data with an electronic patient record. Sullivan and Mitchell conducted a systematic review of prospective trials in which a computer had been introduced for use by a nurse or physician in a primary care setting.[29] They noted that consultation length could increase by as much as 100% in some cases, though the average increase is probably closer to 1–3 minutes. The issue is an important one as systems have been abandoned because of this.[30]

The electronic entry of data in a consistent, legible, structured format is an important benefit in and of itself. In four studies of computerized guideline implementations in which the level of documentation was assessed, it was felt to have improved in all four.[31] Having data in a machine-readable format enables two new technologies that are in their infancy: data mining and natural language processing. In *data mining*, large quantities of data are automatically run through computer algorithms looking for statistically significant associations.[32] In *natural language processing*, the computer interprets natural language (for example, the impression section of a radiology report) and converts it to a standardized encoded form.[33] These techniques hold promise for biosurveillance of nosocomial infections, adverse drug events, and injury prevention.[15]

Considerable evaluation is required before we can be certain that EHRs justify their considerable cost. Issues such as patient confidentiality and privacy, the impact of computers on the human interaction between clinicians and their patients, organization-level success factors are only now being evaluated rigorously.[34,35]

Medical literature

The research evidence-base for a given decision is expanding exponentially. Application of this research base to the point of-care is an ongoing challenge. A number of studies have looked at the information needs of physicians during clinical care. Physicians have an unmet information need for two-thirds of the patients they see, half of which could be met by searching MedLine.[36] Osheroff *et al.* at the University of Pittsburgh had an anthropologist observe 17 hours of clinical activity that involved the care of 90 patients.[8] Over this time period, students, residents, and attending physicians generated 77 questions that could be answered by a knowledge resource such as MedLine or a textbook. Hersh *et al.* did a systematic review to assess the effectiveness of information retrieval systems for physicians.[36] He found that, in the six long-term evaluation trials identified, physician use varied from 0·3 to 9·0 MedLine searches per month. Note that this review predates much of the recent emphasis on evidence-based practice. Identified barriers to performing more searches include: the physical distance to a resource (an issue that the IAIMS initiative addresses by installing MedLine right in the clinical information system) and the retrieval inefficiency of the resource.[7] With a minimum of training, physicians can make literature searches that often match the sensitivity and precision of those performed by medical librarians.[36] Very few studies have measured the impact of information retrieval systems in terms of patient outcomes. Most evaluations purporting to measure patient outcomes have instead reported physician impressions: for example, "the information supplied helped me form a better treatment plan." In Hersh's review, three studies assessed this surrogate outcome and found that the information led to a perceived positive impact on patient care 40–86% of the time.[36]

Clinical librarians are trained librarians who participate in clinical ward or outpatient rounds. The idea is to "provide quality-filtered case-specific information directly to health professionals to support clinical decision-making".[37] In a systematic review, Winning and Beverley found 33 descriptive and 16 evaluative studies.[37] The majority of the programs were in hospital settings in the USA. While attitudes towards the intervention were largely positive, little high quality evidence was found documenting an impact on patient outcomes. In addition, no studies have documented the cost-effectiveness of such a program.

Other important areas of informatics research in the area of information retrieval include identifying optimal indexing schemes, retrieval algorithms and user interfaces to ensure proper query formulation.

Do clinical computer systems improve clinical decision-making?

Challenges in evaluating information systems

Synthesizing the evidence to determine whether these systems are effective in improving health care is complicated by several challenges. Let us consider the difficulties of creating an evaluation design for a given information intervention.

Cramer *et al.* performed a systematic review of randomized controlled trials of computer-based delivery of health evidence.[38] In their review they assessed over 500 articles and ultimately included 57 randomized controlled trials and 10 systematic reviews. They excluded trials of administrative systems (for example, reminders to keep an appointment) and calculators. In assessing the quality of included studies, they noted that it is generally not possible to "blind" subjects or assessors to the group assignment.

Blinding is a large component of any assessment of quality: for example, the Jadad score assesses RCT quality on a scale from 0 to 5 but, if blinding is not possible, the maximum score is 3. Indeed, the Cramer review found that the median quality score for the included studies was 2.

Another problem is *allocation concealment*. Ideally, potential subjects and study personnel should not know, ahead of entering the study, to which group they will be assigned. Subconscious bias to enrol favorable subjects to the intervention group could influence the outcome of the study. Cramer found that allocation concealment could not be assessed in 51 of the 57 studies. These problems with blinding and allocation concealment may result in a bias favoring the intervention.

Working in the opposite direction is *contamination*. Physicians randomized to receive health evidence by computer will often speak to "control" physicians about the evidence thus spreading the intervention to the control group. Cramer found evidence of this in 35 of the studies. Contamination can be decreased by using a *cluster randomized* design in which the unit of randomization is a natural cluster of subjects (for example, a clinic or all the patients of a single practitioner), but there is a tradeoff because these designs are less efficient than non-cluster designs.[39] Thus the investigator must decide at which level to randomize: by institution as a whole, by clinic, by practitioner, or by patient. Cramer found that, in 19 of the 57 studies, investigators violated the rule "analyze what you randomize", an error that biases the results in favor of the intervention.

Finally, it can be difficult to *generalize* the findings from an informatics study.[40] It can be difficult to isolate exactly which part of the system was responsible for the observed effect. Transporting a system to another institution can be impossible – many of the best CDSSs are based on homegrown health information systems that have taken decades to mature and are inextricably linked to their particular setting. Even when hardware and software are transportable, the necessary supporting culture may not be. Ash *et al.* have listed a number of factors necessary for successful implementation of a POE with organizational factors dominating the list.[34] Finally, these systems are very costly with most implementations being in large healthcare institutions where the cost can be justified.

Systematic reviews of health informatics interventions

Keeping in mind these difficulties, what is the evidence for the use of health informatics interventions? There are relatively few Cochrane reviews in this area. Table 15.2 shows the number of protocols and completed reviews available at this time. Cramer *et al.* performed a systematic review of computer systems designed for the delivery of health research evidence.[38] Their review excluded administrative reminder systems, drug dosage calculators, and medical record systems. Only randomized trials or systematic reviews of RCTs were considered. They identified 57 RCTs and 10 systematic reviews up to the end of 2001. As mentioned above, the assessed quality of the studies was low due to lack of blinding and poor reporting of methods of allocation

Table 15.2 Systematic reviews dealing with informatics from the Cochrane Database Effective Practice and Organization of Care Group

Title	Authors	Status	Comment
Printed educational materials	Freemantle N, Harvey EL, Wolf F, Grimshaw JM, Grilli R, Bero LA	Review completed 1997; updated 2002	"The effects of printed educational materials compared with no active intervention appear small and of uncertain clinical significance"
On-screen computer reminders	Gordon RB, Grimshaw JM, Eccles M, Rowe RE, Wyatt JC	Protocol	
Computer-generated paper reminders	Gorman PN, Redfern C, Liaw T, Carson S, Wyatt, JC, Rowe RE, Grimshaw JM	Protocol	
Interventions to implement prevention in primary care	Hulscher MEJL, Wensing M, van der Weijden T, Grol R	Review: most recent substantive update 1996	"There is currently no solid basis for assuming that a particular intervention or package of interventions will work. Effective interventions to increase preventive activities in primary care exist, but there is considerable variation in the level of change achieved, with effect sizes usually small or moderate"
Interventions aimed at improving immunization rates	Szilagyi P, Vann J, Bordley C, Chelminski A, Kraus R, Margolis P, Rodewald L	Review: August 2002	"Reminders were effective for childhood vaccinations (OR = 2·02, 95% CI = 1·49, 2·72), childhood influenza vaccinations (OR = 4·19, 95% CI = 2·07, 8·49). Patient reminder/recall systems in primary care settings are effective in improving immunization rates"
Computerized advice on drug dosage to improve prescribing practice	Walton RT, Harvey E, Dovey S, Freemantle N	Review completed 2001	"This systematic review provides evidence to support the use of computer assistance in determining drug dosage. Further clinical trials are necessary to determine whether the benefits seen in specialist applications can be realized in general use"

concealment used. They found evidence of publication bias: the number of studies favoring control groups was significantly lower than expected.

The authors grouped the studies by whether the outcome measures were based on *process of care* or a *patient health outcome* (i.e., outcomes of direct importance to a patient's well-being). For process outcomes, they were able to assess 29 trials. They found that the targets of the computer intervention, patients or providers, adhered to the best evidence recommendation 57% of the time with a computer-based intervention compared with 52% in the control group (FE OR 1·28; 95% CI 1·24, 1·32) (see Figure 15.3). For patient outcomes, there was no improvement with computer systems (FE OR 0·86; 95% CI 0·66, 1·12). However, there were comparatively few studies[12] with small patient numbers so this result is far from definitive (see Figure 15.4).

Cramer also reviewed 10 systematic reviews. Unfortunately, the majority were flawed, having scores of 4 or less out of 7 on the Oxman/Guyatt scale of methodologic quality. The main flaws were incomplete searches of the literature, imprecise inclusion criteria, and potentially biased study selection. The majority of the reviews did not attempt meta-analysis, citing the difficulties in combining disparate outcomes.

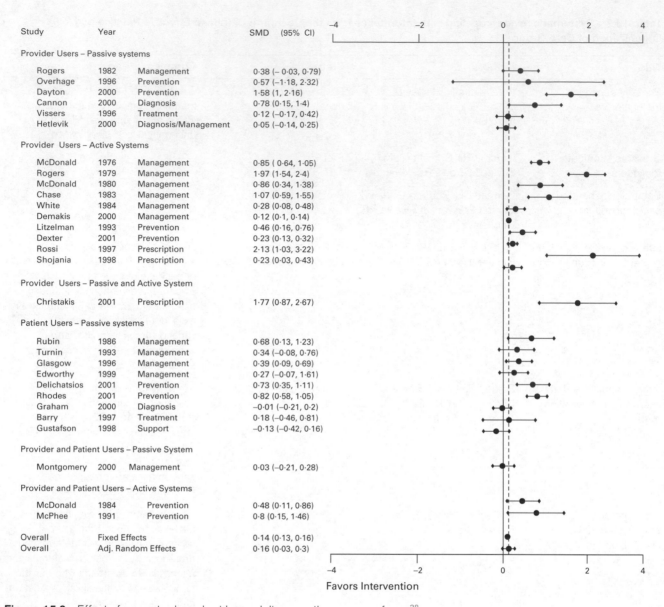

Study	Year		SMD (95% CI)
Provider Users – Passive systems			
Rogers	1982	Management	0·38 (− 0·03, 0·79)
Overhage	1996	Prevention	0·57 (−1·18, 2·32)
Dayton	2000	Prevention	1·58 (1, 2·16)
Cannon	2000	Diagnosis	0·78 (0·15, 1·4)
Vissers	1996	Treatment	0·12 (−0·17, 0·42)
Hetlevik	2000	Diagnosis/Management	0·05 (−0·14, 0·25)
Provider Users – Active Systems			
McDonald	1976	Management	0·85 (0·64, 1·05)
Rogers	1979	Management	1·97 (1·54, 2·4)
McDonald	1980	Management	0·86 (0·34, 1·38)
Chase	1983	Management	1·07 (0·59, 1·55)
White	1984	Management	0·28 (0·08, 0·48)
Demakis	2000	Management	0·12 (0·1, 0·14)
Litzelman	1993	Prevention	0·46 (0·16, 0·76)
Dexter	2001	Prevention	0·23 (0·13, 0·32)
Rossi	1997	Prescription	2·13 (1·03, 3·22)
Shojania	1998	Prescription	0·23 (0·03, 0·43)
Provider Users – Passive and Active System			
Christakis	2001	Prescription	1·77 (0·87, 2·67)
Patient Users – Passive systems			
Rubin	1986	Management	0·68 (0·13, 1·23)
Turnin	1993	Management	0·34 (−0·08, 0·76)
Glasgow	1996	Management	0·39 (0·09, 0·69)
Edworthy	1999	Management	0·27 (−0·07, 1·61)
Delichatsios	2001	Prevention	0·73 (0·35, 1·11)
Rhodes	2001	Prevention	0·82 (0·58, 1·05)
Graham	2000	Diagnosis	−0·01 (−0·21, 0·2)
Barry	1997	Treatment	0·18 (−0·46, 0·81)
Gustafson	1998	Support	−0·13 (−0·42, 0·16)
Provider and Patient Users – Passive System			
Montgomery	2000	Management	0·03 (−0·21, 0·28)
Provider and Patient Users – Active Systems			
McDonald	1984	Prevention	0·48 (0·11, 0·86)
McPhee	1991	Prevention	0·8 (0·15, 1·46)
Overall	Fixed Effects		0·14 (0·13, 0·16)
Overall	Adj. Random Effects		0·16 (0·03, 0·3)

Favors Intervention

Figure 15.3 Effect of computer-based evidence delivery on the process of care[38]

The one methodologically sound systematic review, by Hunt *et al.* (Oxman/Guyatt score 7/7), evaluated studies in which a CDSS was used in a clinical setting by a healthcare practitioner and was evaluated in a prospective, controlled trial.[41] For physician performance, they found that 43/65 studies showed benefit. The main applications tested were drug-dosing and preventive-care systems. Only one out of five diagnostic systems proved effective. When the outcome is measured at the patient instead of the physician, six of 14 studies were found to be beneficial. The authors note that the studies that did not find a difference tended to be underpowered.

Summary

Health informatics interventions can help clinicians practice in an evidence-based fashion. Elson proposed a model that takes into account the capabilities of modern information systems and the finite capacity of even the finest physician to process information and knowledge. Computer programs such as Isabel and QMR that generate differential diagnoses from a list of clinical signs and symptoms can help clinicians *recognize* the diagnostic possibilities of a given patient. These programs can be as accurate as practising clinicians. Computer reminders and alerts that focus a clinician's

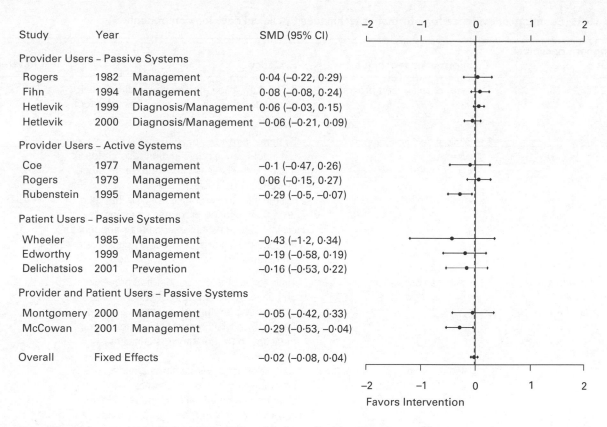

Figure 15.4 Effect of computer-based evidence delivery on the patient health outcomes[38]

attention have been very successful, especially in the domain of detection and management of potential adverse drug events. Information systems allow us to store *clinical knowledge* off-line to be accessed at the point of care when needed. One of the most effective techniques for bringing research and guideline evidence to the clinician is through physician order entry systems that interact with the physician at the time of decision-making. Information systems can help clinicians know their patients better. Patients' interaction with health research evidence and their own medical records can only improve the level of information quality for shared decision-making. The electronic patient record can enable efficient communication with patients and other providers, although issues of privacy and confidentiality still need to be worked through. The *medical record*, when electronic, enables a number of novel population-level interventions such as biosurveillance. Finally new indexing and retrieval information technologies will facilitate the flow of *medical library* information throughout modern health information systems. The studies supporting these statements are summarized in Table 15.3.

Evaluations of these technologies are much more difficult to carry out than, for example, drug trials. Blinding, allocation concealment, and contamination between study groups are all problems to be confronted. Generalizability beyond the study location can be difficult since information technologies may behave differently in different clinical environments. Results depend a great deal on social and cultural factors that can be difficult to assess using quantitative methods. Indeed, social science has a great deal to contribute in determining the optimal forms of information systems in health care. Nonetheless, good evaluations have shown that present day technologies can improve both clinician performance and patient outcomes.

Resolution of the scenario

You return to your committee meeting armed with the evidence that computer information systems probably do improve patient health outcomes to a measurable degree. Well thought out physician order entry systems and computer decision support systems are especially likely to be helpful. Small-scale projects enabling patient-provider messaging might prove interesting. You are quite sanguine about the limitations of the evidence and the difficulty in generalizing it to your home institution. You urge the committee to proceed cautiously, taking into account social and cultural factors as well as cost issues.

Table 15.3 Summary of evidence for informatics techniques by clinical decision component

Component of clinical decision	Informatics technique	Evidence	References
Perception	Diagnostic support programs	RCTs show mild improvement in differential diagnosis when clinician aided by computer program; trainees benefit most	11,12
Attention	Clinical decision support systems: • reminders	Systematic reviews of RCTs show that computer reminders can improve immunization rates in adults; not necessarily as effective for other preventive health care	17
	• clinical alerts	Systematic reviews of RCTs show that drug dosage monitoring programs can improve clinical outcomes; time-series trials suggest that computerized alerts can decrease adverse drug event rates	14,15,19
Clinical knowledge	Physician order entry	Time series studies suggest that process outcomes such as length of stay, hospital charges and lab turnaround times improve; the few RCTs in which patient outcomes were measured have not shown significant improvement	21,22,38
	Disease management systems	Can be effective with asthma and diabetes programs showing particular promise	38
	Medical calculators	Sophisticated medical calculators have been shown to improve process of care outcomes based on randomized controlled trials	19
Knowledge of the patient	Patient access to electronic record	Small prospective cohort studies suggest that having patient input may improve data quality	24
	Electronic messaging	Encouraging early descriptive studies show that it is feasible and may be well-received by patients	26,27
Medical record	Electronic guideline implementation	Systematic reviews of RCT show a mild effect of computerized recommendations on process of care variables, but too few studies to be certain of impact on patient outcomes	29,31,38
	Structured data entry	Prospective cohort studies show good data quality when compared with gold standards but no head-to-head comparisons with paper charts	28,31
	Natural language processing Data mining	Experimental studies show promise	32,33
Medical literature	Information retrieval	Barriers exist to the full integration of bibliographic databases into clinical workflow; need more studies of the impact of ready access to knowledge resources on patient outcomes	36

References

1 Landro L. Wired patients. *Wall Street J* 1 July, 2003. New York, Dow Jones & Co.
2 Haynes RB, Hayward RS, Lomas J. Bridges between health care research evidence and clinical practice. *J Am Med Inform Assoc* 1995;**2**:342–50.
3 Shortliffe EH, Blois MS. The computer meets medicine and biology: emergency of a discipline. In Shortliffe EH, Perreault LE, eds. *Medical Informatics: computer applications in healthcare and biomedicine.* New York: Springer-Verlag, 2001.
4 Coiera E, Tombs V. Communication behaviors in a hospital setting: an observational study. *BMJ* 1998;**316**:673–6.

5 Florance V, Masys D. *Next-generation IAIMS: binding knowledge to action*. N01–LM-9-3523. Washington, DC: Association of American Medical Colleges, 2002.

6 Hripcsak G. IAIMS architecture. *J Am Med Inform Assoc* 1997;**4**:S20–S30.

7 Elson RB, Faughnan JG, Connelly DP. An industrial process view of information delivery to support clinical decision-making: implications for systems design and process measures. *J Am Med Inform Assoc* 1997;**4**:266–78.

8 Osheroff JA, Forsythe DE, Buchanan BG, Bankowitz RA, Blumenfeld BH, Miller RA. Physicians' information needs: analysis of questions posed during clinical teaching. *Ann Intern Med* 1991;**114**:576–81.

9 Friedman CP, Gatti GG, Murphy GC *et al*. Exploring the boundaries of plausibility: empirical study of a key problem in the design of computer-based clinical simulations. *Proc AMIA Symp* 2002;275–9.

10 Miller RA, Pople HE, Jr, Myers JD. Internist-1, an experimental computer-based diagnostic consultant for general internal medicine. *N Engl J Med* 1982;**307**:468–76.

11 Friedman CP, Elstein AS, Wolf FM *et al*. Enhancement of clinicians' diagnostic reasoning by computer-based consultation: a multisite study of 2 systems. *JAMA* 1999;**282**:1851–6.

12 Ramnarayan P, Kapoor RR, Coren M *et al*. Measuring the impact of diagnostic decision support on the quality of clinical decision-making: development of a reliable and valid composite score. *J Am Med Inform Assoc* 2003;**10**:563–72.

13 Tang PC, MacDonald CJ. Computer-based patient-record systems. In: Shortliffe EH, Perreault LE, eds. *Medical Informatics: computer applications in health care and biomedicine*. New York: Springer-Verlag, 2001.

14 Poon EG, Kuperman GJ, Fiskio J, Bates DW. Real-time notification of laboratory data requested by users through alphanumeric pagers. *J Am Med Inform Assoc* 2002;**9**:217–22.

15 Bates DW, Evans RS, Murff H, Stetson PD, Pizziferri L, Hripcsak G. Detecting adverse events using information technology. *J Am Med Inform Assoc* 2003;**10**:115–28.

16 Bates DW, Leape LL, Cullen DJ *et al*. Effect of computerized physician order entry and a team intervention on prevention of serious medication errors. *JAMA* 1998;**280**:1311–16.

17 Shea S, DuMouchel W, Bahamonde L. A meta-analysis of 16 randomized controlled trials to evaluate computer-based clinical reminder systems for preventive care in the ambulatory setting. *J Am Med Inform Assoc* 1996;**3**:399–409.

18 Lomas J. Diffusion, dissemination, and implementation: who should do what? *Ann NY Acad Sci* 1993;**703**:226–35.

19 Walton RT, Harvey E, Dovey S, Freemantle N. Computerised advice on drug dosage to improve prescribing practice. *Cochrane Database Syst Rev*. CD002894, 2001.

20 Leapfrog Group for Patient Safety. Computerized Physician Order Entry. http://www.leapfroggroup.org/index.html. 2003.

21 Tierney WM, Miller ME, Overhage JM, McDonald CJ. Physician inpatient order writing on microcomputer workstations. Effects on resource utilization. *JAMA* 1993;**269**:379–83.

22 Mekhjian HS, Kumar RR, Kuehn L *et al*. Immediate benefits realized following implementation of physician order entry at an academic medical center. *J Am Med Inform Assoc* 2002;**9**:529–39.

23 Christakis DA, Zimmerman FJ, Wright JA, Garrison MM, Rivara FP, Davis RL. A randomized controlled trial of point-of-care evidence to improve the antibiotic prescribing practices for otitis media in children. *Pediatrics* 2001;**107**:E15.

24 Kuperman GJ, Sussman A, Schneider LI, Fiskio JM, Bates DW. Towards improving the accuracy of the clinical database: allowing outpatients to review their computerized data. *Proc AMIA Symp* 1998;220–4.

25 Porter SC, Silvia MT, Fleisher GR, Kohane IS, Homer CJ, Mandl KD. Parents as direct contributors to the medical record: validation of their electronic input. *Ann Emerg Med* 2000;**35**:346-52.

26 Mandl KD, Feit S, Pena BM, Kohane IS. Growth and determinants of access in patient e-mail and internet use. *Arch Pediatr Adolesc Med* 2000;**154**:508–11.

27 Liederman EM, Morefield CS. Web messaging: a new tool for patient-physician communication. *J Am Med Inform Assoc* 2003;**10**:260–70.

28 Thiru K, Hassey A, Sullivan F. Systematic review of scope and quality of electronic patient record data in primary care. *BMJ* 2003;**326**:1070.

29 Mitchell E, Sullivan F. A descriptive feast but an evaluative famine: systematic review of published articles on primary care computing during 1980–97. *BMJ* 2001;**322**:279–82.

30 Margolis CZ, Warshawsky SS, Goldman L, Dagan O, Wirtschafter D, Pliskin JS. Computerized algorithms and pediatricians' management of common problems in a community clinic. *Acad Med* 1992;**67**:282–4.

31 Shiffman RN, Liaw Y, Brandt CA, Corb GJ. Computer-based guideline implementation systems: a systematic review of functionality and effectiveness. *J Am Med Inform Assoc* 1999;**6**:104–14.

32 Brossette SE, Sprague AP, Hardin JM, Waites KB, Jones WT, Moser SA. Association rules and data mining in hospital infection control and public health surveillance. *J Am Med Inform Assoc* 1998;**5**:373–81.

33 Friedman C, Alderson PO, Austin JH, Cimino JJ, Johnson SB. A general natural-language text processor for clinical radiology. *J Am Med Inform Assoc* 1994;**1**:161–74.

34 Ash JS, Stavri PZ, Kuperman GJ. A consensus statement on considerations for a successful CPOE implementation. *J Am Med Inform Assoc* 2003;**10**:229–34.

35 Van Der Meijden MJ, Tange HJ, Troost J, Hasman A. Determinants of success of inpatient clinical information systems: a literature review. *J Am Med Inform Assoc* 2003;**10**:235–43.

36 Hersh WR, Hickam DH. How well do physicians use electronic information retrieval systems? A framework for investigation and systematic review. *JAMA* 1998;**280**:1347–52.

37 Winning MA, Beverley CA. Clinical librarianship: a systematic review of the literature. *Hlth Info Libr J* 2003;**20**(Suppl.1):10–21.

38 Cramer K, Hartling L, Wiebe N *et al. Computer-Based Delivery of Health Evidence: A Systematic Review of Randomized Controlled Clinical Trials and Systematic Reviews of the Effectiveness on the Process of Care and Patient Outcomes.* Final Report to the Alberta Heritage Foundation for Medical Research. 2003. http://www.ahfmr.ab.ca/grants/docs/state_of_science_reviews/Klassen_Review.pdf

39 Chuang JH, Hripcsak G, Heitjan DF. Design and analysis of controlled trials in naturally clustered environments:

implications for medical informatics. *J Am Med Inform Assoc* 2002;**9**:230–8.

40 Randolph AG, Haynes RB, Wyatt JC, Cook DJ, Guyatt GH. Users' Guides to the Medical Literature: XVIII. How to use an article evaluating the clinical impact of a computer-based clinical decision support system. *JAMA* 1999;**282**:67–74.

41 Hunt DL, Haynes RB, Hanna SE, Smith K. Effects of computer-based clinical decision support systems on physician performance and patient outcomes: a systematic review. *JAMA* 1998;**280**:1339–46.

16 Continuing education

Susan Woolfenden, Jeanette Ward

Case scenario   *You are head of the pediatrics department in a non-teaching hospital in an urban region with a catchment population of approximately 400 000. One of your busiest salaried general pediatricians submits an application to you for conference leave. Not only is the conference in Paris in the spring but it is heavily subsidized by private sector interests and dominated by clinical topics most suitable for sub-specialists rather than general pediatricians. Back-to-back keynote scientific addresses are scheduled early in the day without opportunity for discussion or questions, yet there are generous periods of free time for tourist activities. Registrants will receive one-third of their required points for continuing education for that year by attending. The scientific planning committee comprises eminent international experts in their respective sub-specialties but no generalists. You are sympathetic but cynical enough to imagine that location, price, generous points, and clinical curiosities rather than defensible educational need may underpin the pediatrician's request. You realize that you are at a loss as to how to challenge it further or convey a different expectation for the future.*

Background

For decades, commentators external to medicine have expressed concern about the organization of continuing education (CE) for those who, having secured postgraduate clinical qualifications such as College Fellowship or Board certification, then are launched into independent practice with few skills in lifelong learning and only limited access to CE programs based on sound educational principles. To medical educators, reliance on passive conveyancing of new knowledge is scarcely adequate to maintain professional standards:

> The traditional conceptual framework justifying continuing medical education is that it exposes physicians to new medical information, increases physician knowledge, changes physician behavior and favorably alters patient outcomes. It has further been assumed that completion of the first step guarantees the last three.[1]

Learning is the charter of education. Changes in the learner may be:

- cognitive (knowledge acquisition);
- skills-based (such as better skills in physical examination, problem-solving, interviewing or test-ordering), or
- attitudinal (an acquired internal state that influences the choice of personal action).

When integrated, these changes in knowledge, skills, and attitudes combine as improved "competence" (what can be done) and "performance" (what actually is done). Clinical performance itself is a purposeful action, seeking to improve patient healthcare outcomes. Therefore, the ultimate goal of learning for any pediatrician is better outcomes for patients as a result of time taken out from practice to learn.

Continuing education has been defined as

> processes aimed at improving healthcare outcomes through learning, either by individual efforts or as part of activities, products and services developed by CE providers. Learning may result in the maintenance or enhancement of professional competence and performance or in healthcare organizational effectiveness and efficiency. Thus, in today's healthcare milieu, many people consider continuing education of health professionals to be a vehicle for changing not only an individual professional's behavior but also the functioning of the health care system.[2]

Elsewhere in this book, Macdonald (Chapter 8) considers the importance of evidence syntheses such as systematic reviews and guidelines, while Williams and Mellis (Chapter 17) describe clinical decision-making and how evidence can be applied in practice. This chapter is designed to complement these other chapters by considering CE more broadly, particularly the evidence-base for CE design and the best choices pediatricians can make about CE to enhance their commitment to evidence-based practice.

This chapter examines "formal" as well as "informal" learning, although the distinctions are becoming increasingly (and appropriately) blurred. Generally, the chapter focuses on "intentional" rather than "coincidental" learning, the latter an important but serendipitous byproduct of professional experience but never, by definition, driven by planning or premeditation. As a final introductory caveat, this chapter resists the temptation to construct problems of professional effectiveness as exclusively "educational" either in origin or solution. While more "system-based" innovations are being promoted in health services management, this chapter emphasizes the responsibility of pediatricians as individuals to plan continuing episodes of learning in ways that ensure relevance to their professional practice and maximize positive outcomes.

Formal learning: insights from a growing empirical literature

"Formal" learning commonly refers to that which results from organized educational activities that are held under institutional auspices, involve "teachers" brought together by a CE provider, and typically require intention, attention, registration, and time away from practice by the pediatrician.

Over 20 years ago, Stein's seminal review article promoted a wider recognition of the need to apply educational theory to formal CE.[3] All eight studies he selected for his review had changed physician behavior in a desired direction. One also had demonstrated improved patient outcomes. He identified four elements common to these educational interventions, namely:

- *Needs assessment.* All studies examined unmet need in knowledge, performance, or outcomes. The target physician audience was specified as part of the needs assessment. Stein concluded that involvement of learners in program planning enhanced educational effectiveness.
- *Clear goals and objectives.* In all eight studies, educational objectives were clear to learners and teachers (such as presenters, instructors, small-group tutors, designers of educational resources) through explicit statements or implicit messages about the clinical problem being addressed.
- *Relevant learning methods with an emphasis on active participation.* Instruction focused on competence and performance, not simply knowledge acquisition. Active learner participation was characteristic of each study, almost always achieved through small group learning.
- *Systematic effort to evaluate.* No study assumed learner benefit. All applied a protocol to determine change in learner performance and, since each study had established a baseline of performance, it was possible to deliver an objective and sound evaluation.

Stein's four educational elements are robust and have been used ever since as pragmatic operating principles by forward-thinking CE providers and occasionally by astute clinical colleges such as the Royal Australian College of General Practitioners in their accreditation of CE (http://www.racgp.org.au/qa-cpd/). Like the EBM revolution elsewhere in clinical medicine, there now is a substantive body of empirical literature, which, when synthesized, builds upon Stein's initial insights about the characteristics of effective CE. This evidence is summarized next.

A compelling body of knowledge about effective CE

Although reviews of the effectiveness of continuing education had been published in the 1970s,[4,5] two publications from McMaster University in 1984 set a new benchmark in how we elucidate and synthesize an evidence base for CE.[6,7] Hence, the strengthening interface between clinical epidemiology with its exacting methodological standards and the increasing sophistication of CE research provides near-definitive evidence of continuing education effectiveness.[8-10] By focusing exclusively on those studies deploying randomized controlled designs; objectively assessing physician performance and/or patient outcome, and reporting these educational endpoints for at least 75% of physician participants, each successive version of these systematic reviews has synthesized evidence from a rigorous and increasing pool of admissible research. Recently published guidelines will assist researchers committed to contributing to this knowledge base to meet requisite methodologic standards for generalizability and publication.[11,12]

The body of evidence about continuing education is impressive. Readers will find the Cochrane Effective Practice and Organization of Care (EPOC) Review group a very useful resource. EPOC undertakes systematic reviews of educational, behavioral, financial, organizational, and regulatory interventions designed to improve clinical care and the systems in which health professionals provide such care. The Box lists systematic reviews that have been completed by the EPOC Review Group and protocols for others that are under way (http://www.epoc.uottawa.ca).

Examples of relevant EPOC reviews (The *Cochrane Library* 2003, Issue 2)

(http://www.epoc.uottawa.ca)

Completed reviews

- Continuing education meetings and workshops: effects on professional practice and healthcare outcomes
- Audit and feedback versus alternative strategies: effects on professional practice and healthcare outcomes

- Audit and feedback: effects on professional practice and healthcare outcomes
- Educational outreach visits: effects on professional practice and healthcare outcomes
- Local opinion leaders: effects on professional practice and healthcare outcomes
- Teaching critical appraisal skills in healthcare settings

Protocols

- Manual paper reminders: effects on professional practice and healthcare outcomes
- Computer-generated paper reminders: effects on professional practice and healthcare outcomes
- Interventions to improve the use of diagnostic tests
- Interventions to improve antibiotic prescribing practices in ambulatory care
- Interventions to improve antibiotic prescribing practices for hospital inpatients
- On-screen computer reminders: effects on professional practice and healthcare outcomes
- Tailored interventions to overcome identified barriers to change

It now is generally accepted that not all CE is equally effective in achieving education outcomes. Specifically, CE can be divided into three categories:

CE interventions with little or no effect

- didactic education
- distribution of unsolicited printed material

CE interventions of variable effectiveness

- audit and feedback, if personalized and especially if done in "real time"
- work-based interventions by respected peers or opinion leaders
- problem-based learning

Consistently effective continuing education interventions

- reminder systems
- peer coaches providing one-on-one educational programs about prescribing (also known as "academic detailing")
- multifaceted interventions combining a number of previously listed interventions, particularly if interactive and reinforced at the point of care.

Thus, little evidence supports popular but ill-founded beliefs that traditional approaches to CE (such as conferences) will lead to significant improvements in physician performance.[13] A recent systematic review of 32 studies showed that interactive workshops achieve significant changes to professional practice rather than didactic sessions which, on their own, are unlikely to lead to sustainable learning or behavioral change.[14]

In view of the compelling evidence-base, it is unsurprising that commentators despair at the persisting investment in passive continuing education strategies, repeatedly inviting more educationally sound programs and a more rigorous research agenda.[15]

However, it also is reasonable to challenge the generalizability of these studies across medical disciplines (for example, from general practice to pediatrics); across content (for example, from cancer screening to management of acute ischemia) or across healthcare settings (for example, from health maintenance organizations to fee-for-service systems). For example, problem-based learning is used widely in the teaching of medical students; however, a recent systematic review of six controlled trials on problem based learning for CE found only limited evidence that it increased participants' knowledge and performance or patients' health outcomes.[16] In addition, only a minority of these published studies has been conducted outside the UK or North America.[17]

Applying an evidence-based approach to formal CE

At this point, readers may want to pause and reflect upon their most recent formal CE education activity. Was it consistent with the evidence-based outlined above? Did it meet educational need? Was active learning encouraged? What feedback was provided? How was the intervention evaluated? Practical guidance follows to help readers apply an evidence-based approach to the formal CE in which they engage.

Needs assessment

The term "needs assessment" refers to any systematic approach to collecting and analyzing information about the educational needs of individuals or organizations.[18] While a shared "hunch" by CE providers may be a common starting point for CE planning, a more considered approach will select from a larger repertoire of methods such as:

Global needs assessment

- national or regional health problems
- role of the target learner group in a changing healthcare environment

METHODS: national/regional mortality/morbidity data; health goals and targets; priorities; population and health trends; literature review

Discipline-oriented needs assessment

- current outcomes compared with ideal
- current practice
- current competence
- component knowledge, skills, attitudes

METHODS: market research; random representative surveys; objective or unobtrusive assessment of current practice; expressed need (popular courses); learner representatives or advisors; expert opinion; consumer/ patient surveys; task analysis; critical incident monitoring; medicolegal case studies; focus groups

Individual-oriented needs assessment

- individual practitioner behavior
- individual practitioner competence
- individual knowledge, skills, attitudes

METHODS: learner-centered self-diagnostic tools; self-assessment; self-audit; as above at individual level with sufficient sample size to minimize instability of estimates.

The most useful needs assessment will apply more than one method, especially complementary quantitative and qualitative methods, and bear in mind its utility as a baseline for evaluation. One caution however:

> There's a general tendency today to equate needs assessment with surveys in general and with questionnaires in particular. Most experts in the field believe, however, that needs assessment achieves the most meaningful results if data are collected from multiple sources by using multiple techniques."[18]

This is especially pertinent given consistent evidence of the inability of physicians to self-assess educational needs.[19,20]

CE providers should translate need into specific educational objectives and choose instructional methods that should match the need and promote learning. While CE researchers are inclined to undertake purposive needs assessment, it appears uncommon to establish need in a deliberate and detailed manner in "routine" CE planning. Needs assessment is not only useful for ensuring meaningfulness and relevance of the program; it confirms need for the program objectively and can "prime" the target audience to the topic, generating new expectations about educational need. Needs assessment is a prerequisite for any quantitative comparison for program evaluation.

Program planning and instructional design

Choosing educational interventions

Interactive learning is crucial to effective CE. Small group learning in "break-out" sessions and ample time for questions and discussion are important complements to didactic teaching. Subsequent systematic reviews conducted with exquisite methodologic precision confirm Stein's original insights. Learners cannot sit around passively at seminars absorbing content and expect their professional practice to change. Even if it is occasionally effective for some learners, it most certainly is inefficient. Effective CE is resource-intensive,

time-demanding, and equally exhausting for speakers and learners. Some argue that "off-the-shelf" didactic lectures ought to be abandoned in CE. Suggestions for achieving interaction during conventional CE programs follow.

Interactive options for CE

- Ample question time after didactic presentations
- Problem-based discussion groups or case studies in "break-out" rooms
- Case review (in pairs in large lecture theaters)
- Skills sessions and skills stations
- Discussion of case studies in pairs
- Computer-assisted audience participation (for example, keypad sessions)
- Mini-residencies or mini-sabbaticals
- Peer coaches providing one on one educational programs

Those planning CE might also consider opportunities to augment formal education with clinic-based support structures such as reminders or clinical protocols or algorithms upon return to the workplace. Audit and feedback also can be considered as a promising approach to needs assessment as well as reinforcement of learning, especially when individualized and benchmarked against group norms. Readers are encouraged to read the relevant EPOC reviews as described previously in this chapter.

CE providers also may need to adopt a more sophisticated understanding of "opinion leaders". While didactic lectures delivered by an eminent medical authority may be standard CE fare, there are new ways of identifying and engaging those who are "educationally influential" in specific CE interventions. "Opinion leaders" are hypothesized to facilitate behavior change by raising awareness and swiftly advocating innovation within defined professional networks.[21,22] Indeed, seminal work by Hiss and his colleagues[21] has shaped a number of subsequent descriptive and interventional studies.[23–26] As none has yet been conducted with networks of pediatricians, attributes of "opinion leaders" may be usefully considered in the design of innovative CE for this group. As 88% of respondents to a survey of Australian surgeons recently agreed "there are colleagues who influence me in such a way that I think of changing my practice (and sometimes I do)",[27] this suggests considerable salience for this professional community of the theoretical construct of "opinion leaders". As described elsewhere in this chapter, rigorous evaluation of their deployment in CE especially should determine what they do when facilitating change in the workplace and how they do it.

Assuring evidence-based content

Pediatricians ought to expect that educational content will reflect the extant basis of clinical evidence. No systematic study has been conducted of CE content and its relationship to available evidence. As in clinical practice, it is likely that speakers present varied views about optimal health care, not always presenting an impartial and valid synthesis of the clinical evidence. There are three immediate implications of this situation.

● CE should be linked to an explicit evidence-base. Curricula for continuing education programs ought to be linked to evidence-based guidelines; systematic reviews and other evidence-based resources. If evidence is insufficient for a particular clinical intervention being promoted by the speaker, mechanisms for independent review may be needed. A checklist has been developed to inform continuing education content.

Checklist for evidence-based continuing education content

● Is there sufficient evidence to incorporate use in routine practice?
● Is there sufficient evidence to abandon use in routine practice?
● Is there insufficient evidence either to incorporate or abandon?

● Perhaps more controversially, there is little community benefit to be achieved by designing CE that modifies clinical behavior if the evidence underpinning the clinical intervention is weak. In general, maximal patient benefit will be achieved when clinicians offer treatments for which evidence from systematic reviews or randomized controlled trials exists because there is a compelling extant case for their effectiveness in changing patient outcomes. When evidence is weaker (narrative summaries for example), less confidence can be placed *a priori* in subsequent outcomes when such treatments are adopted in practice.

● Furthermore, there may be genuine equipoise about whether or not specific educational or organizational strategies are effective in imparting relevant evidence and promoting significant improvements in learning and/or clinical practice. Perhaps the evidence base is flimsy or the context in which care occurs is challenging. The discipline of "implementation research" is undertaken to answer these sorts of questions. If there is any major concern about the validity of the evidence for CE effectiveness when applied to a particular context, then consideration must be afforded the desirability of a collaboration with "implementation researchers" to design a study that will itself contribute to the body of knowledge about CE. Measuring the effects of single episodes of CE add little to the knowledge base of continuing education. Experimental designs, including cluster randomized trials (CRTs) and randomized control trials (RCTs) should be considered.[28] The design of such studies needs to consider factors such as estimation of sample size and intracluster correlation coefficients for both effectiveness and efficiency outcomes.[29]

Resources for effective continuing education

Readers may be concerned about implementing evidence-based rather than conventional (and relatively cheap) CE programs. While evidence-based interventions might increase CE costs, "…it is also important to determine the cost of failing to offer such education and of the current level of expenditure on continuing professional education using techniques of unproven effectiveness".[30]

The increased global attention to clinical governance, better quality in health care and implementation of evidence-based guidelines provides a natural alliance of common interests. For these reasons, it is highly likely that CE providers will work much more closely with guidelines developers, purchasers, and those interested in implementing evidence in practice.[31–34] Efficiencies in resource allocation can be created through collaborations at the local level between these various vested interests.[35]

Evaluation

The simplest definition of evaluation is "an undertaking to determine the worth of something".[36] Learners and CE providers have a responsibility to evaluate to what extent the CE activity has enhanced competence, performance or patient outcomes. Every individual pediatrician can develop a critical capacity to compare their intended learning objectives in registering for a CE activity and the achieved outcomes. Providing feedback to the CE provider would influence future planning.

Selection of evaluation design should incorporate the anticipated objectives and available resources. An accepted hierarchy of educational outcomes, for continuing education evaluation is listed from least to most clinically relevant, is as follows:

● attendance
● satisfaction ("happiness") indices
● cognitive gain
● skills acquisition
● attitudinal shifts
● competence (what can be done under ideal circumstances)
● performance (what is done at the workplace)
● patient outcomes.

Examples from pediatrics

Literature searches can readily retrieve useful and relevant examples of CE for pediatricians. For example, an elegant needs assessment reported by Garrett et al.[37] describes a program in which all pediatricians and pediatric registrars (residents) in New Zealand (n = 236) first were surveyed about self-reported use of asthma action plans. Findings will inform CE and workplace interventions to promote adherence as well as clinical research in response to variations identified in responses.[37] Another needs assessment conducted in the USA found that 1165 pediatricians' intention to adopt guidelines about hepatitis B vaccine was independently predicted by gender, beliefs, and information sources.[38] When a CE response is being planned to implement such guidelines, these findings could be used to target programs more precisely.

Two studies show the impact of innovative CE interventions modeled on quality improvement approaches to increase childhood immunization rates. A physician-led quality improvement initiative directed by an immunization task force achieved significant increases in preschool immunization rates in 10 private pediatric practices, demonstrating the effect of an organizational commitment to CE through feedback.[39] Schlenker et al.[40] observed an increase in childhood immunizations rates from 43% to 86%, temporally associated with systematic implementation of feedback. Evans et al.[41] reported a controlled trial involving 22 public health clinics to evaluate the impact of staff training in continuing, preventive care for asthma. Guidelines were included at intervention sites. In both the first and second follow up years, there were significant improvements in access, continuity, and quality of care. This intervention had demonstrable educational impact and should be considered a guiding evidence-based strategic direction by those in similar circumstances.[41]

Clark et al.[42] designed and implemented an innovative program for pediatricians to enhance asthma outcomes. From 1276 pediatricians initially advised of the study, 74 agreed to randomization. After baseline measures, those pediatricians allocated to the intervention group participated in an interactive seminar offered three times over a 4-month period (maximum 12 participants per seminar) as a 2 to 2·5 hour face-to-face program of lectures, video, case studies, and active discussion. Self-reported measures of clinical behavior showed significant changes. Parents recalled changes in educational aspects of their consultations and therapeutic decisions and, among low income patients seen by intervention pediatricians, significantly fewer ED visits were made in the follow up period. Even this relatively brief CE intervention achieved desirable changes in health service utilization and greater patient compliance unlikely to be attributable to any other intervention. Although tempered by selection bias, this study provides strong evidence for the effectiveness of a multifaceted CE program to achieve better pediatric practice and patient outcomes.[42]

In a state-wide study conducted in North Carolina,[43] 147 pediatricians performing child abuse evaluations were randomized to receive readings and tailored written feedback based on up to five chart reviews per clinician (n = 72) and/or to a control group that received only readings (n = 75). The main outcome measures were quality of documentation and physician knowledge (by self-administered survey). However, the attrition of clinicians from behavioral outcome measurements in the study was high. Other confounders swamped the impact of the tailored intervention. Needs assessment for this intervention was reported in detail elsewhere.[44]

Gielen et al. reported a randomized controlled trial involving 31 pediatric residents in a hospital to evaluate the effect of a multifaceted CE intervention on injury prevention counseling for parents: 18 residents received the intervention, which included seminars, an information pack, and interactive workshops; 13 were in the control group. Both groups attended a didactic session on injury prevention counseling; 117 parents were subsequently seen by the residents who had the intervention and 73 were seen by the control group. Parents who had been seen by residents who had had the intervention reported that they received significantly more injury prevention counseling and were more satisfied with the help they received than those seen by the control group. There was not, however, a demonstrated change in the parents' knowledge, beliefs and home safety behaviors. The researchers argued that this may have been because the low income families may face many barriers such as cost that mitigated uptake of safety practices.[45]

Although not implemented with pediatricians, a recent randomized controlled trial that evaluated a multifaceted education program in adolescent health care for Australian general practitioners is worthy of special mention.[46] In this rigorous study, 108 self-selected GPs were grouped into eight geographical clusters by practice location to minimize contamination and maximize efficiency of the delivery of the intervention. Clusters of similar size were randomized to the intervention or control. The intervention offered a 6-week curriculum that included evidence-based primary and secondary educational strategies such as role play with feedback, modeling practice with opinion leaders, and the use of checklists. GPs then took part in a standardized scenario of a depressed 15-year-old girl exhibiting health risk behavior (played by a trained drama student). Clinical skills and self-perceived competency and knowledge were assessed using validated assessment tools and questionnaires. The doctors completing the intervention showed substantial gains in knowledge, clinical skills, and self perceived competency when compared with controls. These CE gains were sustained at 12 months.[46]

These examples give an insight into the scope and science of formal CE for pediatricians. This next section examines the emerging interest in "informal" learning.

Informal learning: an evolving concept

By contrast to "formal learning", so-called "informal learning" is characterized by its initiation by the learner, often in the absence of continuing education provider units or academic institutions. Examples of informal learning conventionally include self-study, reading, and discussion with colleagues. That these efforts could be as planned and deliberate as formal activities is belied somewhat by the term "informal".

Learner preferences and informal learning habits

Physicians typically choose reading as their first response to a patient problem encountered in practice.[47] Other influential sources of information with which to solve problems include consultants, although previous training also predominates. Specialists appear to be influenced especially by medical journals and scientific conferences, while GPs are more influenced by medical newspapers and postgraduate meetings.[48] Physicians at risk of professional isolation are those in solo practice and older graduates.[49]

In CE, learning style and other more stable personality characteristics appear to combine with context-specific motivation to learn. Traditional undergraduate curricula and the teaching methods typically employed in medical education may place an enduring impediment upon self-directed learning. While learning style and instructional preferences have been the focus of research, interventional studies suggest they play less of a role in predicting educational outcomes than would first appear.[50,51]

In an educational experiment involving 13 matched pairs of North American medical schools providing continuing education to primary care physicians about cardiovascular risk factor management, learners were randomized to receive additional information about the characteristics of change and learning.[52] Self-assessed intention-to-change predicted learning outcomes among these physicians, irrespective of additional information to address barriers to behavioral change. Planned change remains an important if poorly understood phenomenon in both "formal" and "informal" continuing education.[52] These empirical insights – and other reflections upon experiences in facilitating "informal" CE – challenge the crude linearity of the needs assessment–objectives–instruction–evaluation model promoted for "formal" CE.

Workplace learning is even less well understood.[53] Yet the distinctions may be blurring, given the increasing interest in work-based professional development, particularly when it augments organizational goals and purposes. Concepts and practical tools recently developed to support informal workplace learning are described briefly below.

Contract learning was introduced briefly in workplace continuing education in California.[54] Parboosingh and his colleagues[55,56] have developed a robust process for learners to identify their individual learning needs, plan programs, and monitor impact. The concept of learning profiles has generated considerable interest across other medical disciplines. Practice-based small group CE, another approach applicable to disciplines beyond family practice, is being developed in Canada.[57] Another innovation, peer visits, has its origins in general practice[58] but has made in-roads into other disciplines.[59] To enact a philosophical commitment to evidence-based practice, evidence carts have been introduced on wards to promote "informal" CE, which benefits from immediate access to evidence.[60] Less ambitious perhaps, "educational prescriptions" have been advocated by others as a useful support for work-placed learning.[61]

Building better bridges between formal and informal learning

Effective CE should be neither haphazard nor determined by conference locations. Effective CE should be planned according to objective evidence of need, responsive to individualized differences in learning and current performance, reinforced, and subjected to evaluation at some level. The potential of a combined approach exploiting the sound evidence in support of needs-based and reinforced "formal" CE with frequent learning opportunities and feedback in the workplace is promising. Individual physicians will benefit from micro-skills development in critical appraisal and self-direction while their employers create and nurture "learning organizations".[62,63] Information "overload" can be reduced while learners receive both sensitive and specific data about their performance and outcomes, in order to plan "informal" educational pursuits or seek "informal" CE programs which match their need.

Self-directed learning skills

- Formulating clear learning objectives
- Reading to solve problems
- Highly selective browsing
- Establishing and maintaining a personal information system
- Carrying out self-assessments
- Executing personal behavior modification

adapted, Sackett *et al.* (2nd ed)[61]

CE providers are on the verge of achieving a model of continuing education first envisaged over a decade ago:

> First, we should encourage and facilitate physician efforts to structure their individual learning. Second, physicians do a lot of self-directed learning, but often don't view their

problem-solving as formal learning. They don't organize it, they don't dignify it, so the trick is to get them to put it into some kind of planned activity. Third, a learning plan can offer a structure under which physicians can view their natural learning as effective and measurable. Fourth, it would be a good idea to develop a self-directed "supermarket" where CME educators would offer all kinds of goodies such as journal clubs, self-assessment plans, learning contracts, telephone referral systems, faculty consults, computer programs etc., in a kind of setting that would encourage individual physicians to come and shop and get what they need. The key to the success of self-directed learning is deliberate efforts to change behavior, attitudes, and skills, rather than random, haphazard learning. If we can take self-directed physicians learning from something which just happens, and has a low rating because it doesn't get Category 1 credit, to a deliberate project by designing, planning and involving the individual in that plan, then we will have something powerful. The idea was also proposed of using role models, finding physicians who are good at self-directed learning, who do learn in a planned, effective ways, and using them to teach other physicians those skills.[64]

As demonstrated throughout this book, judicious and critical reading of evidence that matters will reduce demand on pediatricians' limited time and accelerate evidence-based practice. Similarly, highly selective pursuit of CE that itself has been designed using evidence generated through "implementation research" will characterize the practice of pediatrics in the 21st century.

Summary

If readers have concluded that pediatricians may be paying registration fees and giving up scarce time to participate in CE unlikely to make a significant difference to patient care, they are not alone. What now needs to happen in CE depends on pediatricians themselves and their heads of department like the one described in the case scenario at the beginning of this chapter.

Continuing education is the link between new advances in health care and the individual patient–doctor consultation. Better CE is needed to improve physician performance and achieve better patient healthcare outcomes. Pediatricians ought to demand quality CE that is responsive to their needs, transparently evidence-based, both in its instructional design as well as its content, and examined for impact and quality control.

Lifelong learners are not perpetual conference registrants. Through undergraduate and postgraduate training, future generations of pediatricians will be better equipped to diagnose their own learning needs and plan CE that maximizes return in terms of better health for their patients. In turn, hospitals, learned colleges, and other CE providers ought to develop systems that audit care in a non-threatening manner and provide feedback to actively learning practitioners. If we abandon those CE programs that are ineffective, a ready source of funds to support these multifaceted interventions would be available. Better links between CE researchers and learners will ensure innovative approaches are subjected to experimental evaluation, minimizing the potential for wasting money on ineffective programs. Increased academic rigor will ensure that the steady progress made since the 1980s in our collective understanding about effective continuing education will continue to grow. Indeed:

> As practitioners become increasingly involved in research, the lines between research and practice may be expected to blur. Testing theory during routine program evaluation provides valuable data to use in making day-to-day program planning and design decisions, but it also adds to the common pool of knowledge to be shared by researchers and practitioners across disciplines. Such active participation in research tends to render pointless the intellectually created schisms between research and practice and "science" for "knowledge" versus "science for practical improvement."[65]

Resolution of the scenario

You stand for election as chairperson of your society's continuing education committee and lead the development of a policy to promote more effective learning activities for pediatricians. This policy exerts considerable influence on the design of CE and receives international recognition. Your staff members are among the first to notice better health outcomes for their patients as a result of more responsive CE planning.

Acknowledgments

In addition to incorporating the science of effective continuing education from the published literature, this chapter also reflects discussions with Dr David Pencheon, Professor Jeremy Grimshaw, Professor Dave Davis and Dr Jane Young. None of these is responsible for any errant views expressed in this chapter, however. We also thank Anne Taylor-Vaisey at the University of Toronto RDRB/CME database for support in literature retrieval. We acknowledge and recommend to readers the related website (http://www.cme.utoronto.ca) as well as EPOC reviews available through the *Cochrane Library*.

References

1 Berg A. Does continuing medical education improve the quality of medical care? A look at the evidence. *J Fam Pract* 1979;**8**:1171–4.
2 Suter E, Green J, Grosswald S *et al*. Introduction: defining quality for continuing education. In: Green J, Grosswald S, Suter E, Walthall D, eds. *Continuing education for the health professions*. San Fransisco: Jossey-Bass, 198.

3   Stein L. The effectiveness of continuing medical education: eight research reports. *J Med Educ* 1981;**56**:103–10.

4   Bertram D, Brooks-Bertram P. The evaluation of continuing medical education: a literature review. *Health Educ Monographs* 1977;**5**:330–62.

5   Lloyd J, Abrahamson S. The effectiveness of continuing medical education: a review of the evidence. *Eval Hlth Prof* 1979;**2**:251–80.

6   Davis D, Haynes R, Chambers L, Neufeld V, McKibbon A, Tugwell P. The impact of CME: a methodological review of the continuing medical education literature. *Eval Hlth Prof* 1984;**7**:251–83.

7   Haynes R, Davis D, McKibbon A, Tugwell P. A critical appraisal of the efficacy of continuing medical education. *JAMA* 1984;**251**:61–4.

8   Davis D, Thomson MS, Oxman A, Haynes R. Evidence for the effectiveness of CME: a review of 50 randomized controlled trials. *JAMA* 1992;**268**:1111–17.

9   Davis D, Thomson M, Oxman A, Haynes R. Changing physician performance: a systematic review of the effect of continuing medical education strategies. *JAMA* 1995;**274**:700–5.

10 Oxman A, Thomson M, Davis D, Haynes R. No magic bullets: a systematic review of 102 trials of interventions to improve professional practice. *Can Med Assoc J* 1995;**153**:1423–31.

11 Education Group for Guidelines on Evaluation. Guidelines for evaluating papers on educational interventions. *BMJ* 1999;**318**:1265–7.

12 Hutchinson L. Evaluating and researching the effectiveness of educational interventions. *BMJ* 1999;**318**:1267–9.

13 Davis D, O'Brien M, Freemantle N *et al*. Impact of formal continuing medical education: do conferences, workshops, rounds, and other traditional continuing education activities change physician behavior or health care outcomes? *JAMA* 1999;**282**:867–74.

14 Thomson O'Brien MA, Freemantle N, Oxman AD, Wolf F, Davis DA, Herrin J. Continuing education meetings and workshops: effect on professional practice and health care outcomes. Cochrane Collaboration. In: The *Cochrane Library* Issue 3. Oxford: Update Software, 2002.

15 Moore D, Green J, Jay S, Leist J, Maitland F. Creating a new paradigm for CME: seizing opportunities within the health care revolution. *J Cont Educ Hlth Prof* 1994;**14**:4–31.

16 PBA Smits, JHAM Verbeek, CD de Buisonje. Problem based learning in continuing medical education: a review of controlled evaluation. *BMJ* 2002;**324**:153–156

17 Davis D. Global health, global learning. *BMJ* 1998;**316**:385–9.

18 Moore D, Cordes D. Needs assessment. In: Rosof A, Felch W, eds. *Continuing medical education: a primer*. Westport: Praeger, 1992.

19 Sibley J, Sackett D, Neufeld V *et al*. A randomised trial of continuing medical education. *New Engl J Med* 1982;**306**:511–15.

20 Tracey J, Arroll B, Richmond D, Barham P. The validity of general practitioners" self-assessment of knowledge: cross sectional study. *BMJ* 1997;**315**:1426–8.

21 Hiss R, McDonald R, Davis W. Identification of medical influentials in small community hospitals. *Proc Conference Res Mod Edu* 1978;**17**:283–5.

22 Rogers EM. *Diffusion of innovations, 4th edn*. New York: Free Press, 1995.

23 Locock L, Dopson S, Chambers D, Gabbay J. Understanding the role of opinion leaders in improving clinical effectiveness. *Soc Sci Med* 2001;**53**:745–7.

24 Soumerai SB, McLaughlin T, Gurwitz JH *et al*. Effect of local medical opinion leaders on the quality of care for acute myocardial infarction: a randomised controlled trial. *JAMA* 1998;**279**:1358–63.

25 Guadagnoli E, Soumerai SB, Gurwitz JH *et al*. Improving discussions of surgical treatment options for patients with breast cancer: local medical opinion leaders versus audit and performance feedback. *Breast Cancer Res Treat* 2000;**61**:171–5.

26 Flottorp S, Oxman A, Bjorndal A. The limits of leadership: opinion leaders in general practice. *J Hlth Serv Res Policy* 1998;**3**:197–202.

27 Young JM, Hollands M, Ward JE, Holman CDJ. Promoting evidence-based surgery: is there a role for opinion leaders? *Arch Surg* 2003 (in press).

28 Shadish W, Cook T, Campbell D. *Experimental and quasi experimental designs for generalised causal inference*. Boston: Houghton Mifflin, 2002.

29 Campbell MK, Mollison J, Grimshaw JM. Cluster trials in implementation research: estimation of intracluster correlation coefficients and sample size. *Stat Med* 2001;**20**:391–9.

30 Muir Gray JA. *Evidence-based healthcare: how to make health policy and management decisions*. London: Churchill Livingstone, 1997.

31 Moore D. Moving CME closer to the clinical encounter: the promise of quality management and CME. *J Cont Educ Hlth Prof* 1995;**15**:135–45.

32 Dodek P, Ottoson J. Implementation link between clinical practice guidelines and continuing medical education. *J Cont Educ Hlth Prof* 1996;**16**:82–93.

33 Haines A, Donald A. *Getting research findings into practice*. London: BMJ, 1998.

34 Donen N. No to mandatory continuing medical education, yes to mandatory practice auditing and professional educational development. *Can Med Assoc J* 1998;**158**:1044–6.

35 Grimshaw J, Ward J, Eccles M. Getting research into practice. In: Pencheon D *et al*. eds. *Oxford textbook of public health*. Oxford: OUP (in press).

36 Green J. Evaluation. In: Rosof A, Fetch W, eds. *Continuing medical education: a primer*. Wesport: Praeger, 1992.

37 Garrett J, Williams S, Wong C, Holdaway D. Application of asthma action plans to childhood asthma: a national survey. *NZ Med J* 1997;**110**:308–10.

38 Pathman D, Konrad T, Freed G, Freeman V, Koch G. The awareness-to-adherence model of the steps to clinical guideline compliance. *Med Care* 1996;**34**:873–99.

39 Sinn J, Morrow A, Finch A. Improving Immunization rates in private pediatric practices through physician leadership. *Arch Pediatr Adolesc Med* 1999;**153**:597–603.

40   Schenkler T, Sukhan S, Swenseon C. Improving vaccination coverage through accelerated measurement and feedback. *JAMA* 1998;**280**:355.

41   Evans D, Mellins R, Lobach K *et al.* Improving care for minority children with asthma: professional education in public health clinics. *Pediatrics* 1997;**99**:157–64.

42   Clark N, Gong M, Schork A *et al.* Imapct of education for physicians on patient outcomes. *Pediatrics* 1998;**101**:831–6.

43   Socolar R, Raines B, ChenMok M, Runyan D, Green C, Paterno S. Intervention to improve physicians documentation and knowledge of child sexual abuse: a randomised controlled trial. *Pediatrics* 1998;**101**:817–24.

44   Socolar R. Physician knowledge of child abuse. *Child Abuse Negl* 1996;**20**:783–90.

45   Gielan AC, Wilson ME, McDonald EM *et al.* Randomized trial of enhanced anticipatory guidance for injury prevention. *Arch Paediatr Adolesc Med* 2001;**155**:42–9.

46   Sanci LA, Coffey CM, Veit FC *et al.* Evaluation of the effectiveness of an educational intervention for general practitioners in adolescent health care: randomised controlled trial. *BMJ* 2000;**320**:224–30.

47   McClaran J, Snell L, Franco E. Type of clinical problem is a determinant of physicians self-selected learning methods in their practice settings. *J Cont Educ Hlth Prof* 1998;**18**:107–18.

48   Allery L, Owen P, Robling M. Why general practitioners and consultants change their clinical practice: a critical incident study. *BMJ* 1997;**314**:870–4.

49   Barham P, Benseman J. Participation in continuing medical education of general practitioners in New Zealand. *J Med Educ* 1984;**59**:649–54.

50   Curry L, Putnam W. Continuing medical education in Maritime Canada: the methods physicians use, would prefer and find most effective. *Can Med Assoc J* 1981;**124**:63–6.

51   Lacoursiere Y, Snell L, McClaran J, Duanto–Franco E. Workshop versus lecture In CME: does physician learning method preference make a difference? *J Contin Educ Hlth Prof* 1997;**17**:141–7.

52   Masmanian P, Daffron S, Johnson R, Davis D, Kantrowitz M. Information about barriers to planned change: a randomised controlled trial involving continuing medical education lectures and commitment to change. *Acad Med* 1998;**73**: 882–6.

53   Brlgley S, Young Y, Littlejohns P, McEwaen J. Continuing education for medical professionals: a reflective model. *Postgrad Med J* 1997;**73**:23–6.

54   University of Southern California. Self-directed learning for physicians at the University of Southern California. In: Knowles M *et al. Andragogy in action: applying modern principles of adult learning.* San Francisco: Jossey-Bass, 1984.

55   Parboosingh J. Learning portfolios: potential to assist health professionals with self-directed learning. *J Cont Educ Hlth Prof* 1996;**16**:75–81.

56   Campbell C, Parboosingh J, Gondocz S *et al.* Study of physicians use of a software program to create a portfolio of their self-directed learning. *Acad Med* 1996;**71**:S49–S51.

57   Premi J, Shannon S, Hartwick K *et al.* Practice-based small group CME. *Acad Med* 1994;**69**:800–2.

58   Ward J, Barnes R, Bell S. Interpractice visits by general practitioners: implications of a pilot project for quality assurance in general practice. *Med J Aust* 1990;**152**:349–52.

59   Toghill P. Continuing medical education: where next? *BMJ* 1998;**316**:721–2.

60   Sackett D, Straus S. Finding and applying evidence during clinical rounds: the evidence cart. *JAMA* 1998;**280**:1336–8.

61   Sackett D, Haynes RB, Guyatt G, Tugwell P. How to get the most from and give the most to continuing medical education, In: *Clinical epidemiology: a basic science for clinical medicine, 2nd edn.* Boston: Little, Brown, 1991.

62   Fox R, Bennett M. Learning and change: implications for continuing medical education. *BMJ* 1998;**316**:466–8.

63   Weight T, Phipps K, Jackson N. Clinical governance and education and training. In: Lugon M, Secker-Walker J, eds. *Clinical governance: making it happen.* London: RSM Press, 1999.

64   Fink D. Outstanding examples of innovative methods. *Mobius* 1983;**3**:70–7.

65   Masmanian P, Williams R, Desch C, Johnson R. Theory and research for the development of continuing education in the health professions. *J Cont Educ Hlth Prof* 1990;**10**:349–65.

17 Using evidence to inform decisions

Katrina Williams, Andrew Hayen, C Raina Macintyre, Craig Mellis

Background

Like medical practitioners from all disciplines, child health experts are now consulting, researching, developing policies, and managing services in the era of evidence-based practice (EBP). In the last decade, systems for appraising qualitative and quantitative evidence have become widely used, and ways of handling information have been developed to facilitate access to evidence. The ongoing challenge is to incorporate this evidence into decision-making processes to improve the health and well-being of children and their families.

Medical decision-making is not straightforward. Nearly all decisions, whether related to clinical practice, public health policy, service planning, or research, are made in conditions of uncertainty. In addition, complex questions such as those about risk/benefit ratios, questions about implementation of evidence at an individual and population level, as well as questions about the cost-effectiveness of health interventions arise. Furthermore, decisions need to incorporate individual and social values and preferences.

This chapter summarizes some of the key points from previous chapters to illustrate the types of information that are needed for decision-making. It also illustrates how evidence can be used to inform clinical practice and public health policy. We discuss the strengths and potential barriers to these approaches, being mindful of the many tensions in healthcare provision and the diverse environments within which clinicians and families function.

Summary of steps from previous chapters

Asking questions

Although the process of making decisions is complex it can be, at least in part, broken down into the critical decision. These points can then be further deconstructed to frame answerable questions, a key to decision-making. This process sometimes gives the impression that EBP is oversimplified and not related to "real" clinical and public health situations. However, it is the ability to deconstruct the most complex problems into as many bite-sized and digestible pieces and to prioritize issues appropriately that are the core skills of good clinicians, public health physicians, managers, and evidence-based researchers alike.

Different health professionals working in different settings are likely to generate different questions. The questions that pediatricians need to answer to provide good patient care can be categorized according to the type of information that is required to answer them, a process that is described in Chapter 2. In the clinical chapters that follow (Section III), questions are categorized by type: questions of baseline risk and prognosis, questions of therapy, questions about diagnostic tests, and questions about causation and harm. What the clinician then needs is evidence that both answers the question and is translatable to their individual patient.

The questions that child public health experts will ask include questions about screening, health promotion, and prevention of disease. In Section II the different types of questions asked have been categorized and include questions about the performance of screening tests and programs and the effectiveness of prevention approaches. What the public health expert then needs is evidence that both answers the question and is translatable to the target population.

Clinicians and public health experts often find that the answers obtained from this process are complex and may even raise further questions that need to be answered. While this can be frustrating, awareness of this lack of information provides important impetus for future research.

Finding evidence

How to find evidence has been dealt with in Chapter 3 on searching for the evidence. As shown in several of the chapters (for example, Chapters 20 and 46), searching for evidence using electronic databases is fallible. It is not always possible to find relevant information, even when you are certain it is there. This may be because the evidence is presented as part of other studies for which more general search terms apply, or it may be that there is no standardized search term available for concepts such as "early intervention". Electronic searches are neither 100% sensitive nor 100% specific. The same trade-off between sensitivity and specificity exists in selecting search terms as exists in setting cut-offs for screening and diagnostic tests. In spite of these problems, it is important to be as comprehensive as possible. Explicitly stated, reproducible methods of searching are crucial to allow meaningful discussion about implications of findings. In all cases it is most efficient to search first for high quality, predigested, or synthesized evidence.

Appraising the evidence: validity

Once sought and found, evidence must be appraised in order to determine its validity and applicability to the clinical situation or population. Much of Section I of this book addresses issues of validity (closeness to the "truth") of the published evidence: specifically, is the stated result free of bias and confounding? Appraisal methods vary with the type of evidence being assessed. These methods are outlined in the chapters addressing different types of evidence, and practical examples are shown in the chapters that follow. Critical appraisal is crucial for all forms of evidence, including synthesized evidence.

In medical research the ideal of perfect study methodology is rarely (if ever) met. The nature of research dictates that many studies will have both methodologic strengths and weaknesses. Decisions about the usefulness of a study need to be made from a balanced consideration of these strengths and weaknesses with special attention to weaknesses that would make study findings invalid.

The right evidence for the right questions

Chapter 4 describes the ways in which data can be gathered to develop baseline risk and prognosis. Pretest probabilities (also called baseline risk) are necessary to apply test results to your patients or population. Since pretest probability is such an important determinant of post-test probability, it is crucial to use probabilities that are appropriate to your own practice. This may require local study or practice review.

Prognosis is the estimated risk (probability) of outcomes of interest. Prognosis provides children and families with information about potential outcomes, allows development of adequate and appropriate services, and allows application of treatment outcomes to the individual or specific populations (see below). Prognosis requires good quality prospectively gathered information from cohort studies or trials with suitable length of follow up and outcome measures.

For diagnostic decision-making the most useful information for the clinician and the child and the family comes from a combination of the pretest probability and the likelihood ratio (LR) of clinical findings and test results, to yield a "post-test" probability. LRs and their use are discussed in Chapter 5.

For deciding about therapeutic interventions or prevention strategies, information about treatment or prevention effects

can be summarized in a variety of ways, each useful for different types of decision-making, as described in chapter 6.

Application of evidence

Having determined that evidence is likely to be valid, the next task is to see how applicable it is and consider ways in which it can be used to inform decision-making. In each clinical chapter, some of the issues of applicability are addressed as they pertain to the clinical problems being faced. Guidelines for assessing applicability have been developed[1] and key aspects of the assessment are listed in the Box.

Criteria for applicability of data from studies to individual patients

Biologic
- Are there pathophysiologic differences in the illness under study that may lead to a diminished treatment response?
- Are there patient differences that may diminish the treatment response?

Social and economic
- Are there important differences in patient/parent compliance that may diminish the treatment response?
- Are there important differences in provider compliance that may diminish the treatment response?

Epidemiologic
- Do my patients have co-morbid conditions that significantly alter the potential benefits and risk of the treatment?
- Are there important differences in untreated patients' risk of adverse outcomes that might alter the efficiency of treatment?

Many factors other than the probabilities of disease and health outcomes affect decision-making, including the interpretation of risk. Individuals interpret risks differently and ascribe different values to risk. Importantly, the physician's perception of risk and the patient or parent's perception of risk may differ widely.[2] In Chapter 14, communicating evidence to patients is discussed. The way in which risk is communicated, as well as the risk itself, is likely to influence decision-making.

Individuals also have different attitudes towards health services. Practical considerations such as access to services, availability of services and/or financial constraints of the service or the family will also influence decisions.

As well as assessing applicability in a general or qualitative way,[3] available clinical, health service, and research information can be incorporated into decision modeling to tailor information to individual patients and populations, as we discuss below.

The decision-making process

Information can be put together to inform clinical decision-making in two different ways. The first way is to synthesize *similar* types of information, as is done in a systematic review. This process is discussed in detail in Chapter 8. The second requires that many *different* types of information be combined.

One common problem is reconciling the average with the individual. Patients and their parents are most concerned about what happens to themselves and their families. We therefore have to try to convey the meaning of numbers gathered from populations in a way that can be interpreted for each individual. The term "decision analysis" has been coined to describe the formal process of using available evidence to quantitatively answer clinical questions and is one way of trying to achieve the "individualization" of evidence.

Models for combining different types of information are emerging, some of which will be discussed below. The types of decision-making models presented in this book are largely based on probabilities derived from published evidence. Another possible way to synthesize disparate sources of information is through the use of Bayesian methods.[4]

It is sometimes helpful to draw a diagram of the whole process of making a clinical decision, from presenting problem to treatment plan. You can then identify the decision points, see where you will need to estimate baseline risk and determine probabilities of various outcomes, consider the relevant values (at the least, yours and your patient's), and plan how to combine these sensibly. These concepts are familiar to clinicians, but the majority of decisions made by clinicians are made intuitively rather than by thinking through the process in a quantitative manner.

Diagnostic decision-making

Combining the pretest probability of disease with the test characteristics (i.e., how well the test distinguishes the diseased from the non-diseased – see Chapter 5) will tell you how likely the disease is. Before deciding to test or treat, it is important to consider whether the test result will affect your future decisions. For example, a patient's pretest probability might be so small that, even after a positive test result, the post-test probability would be too low to justify consideration of treatment. At the other extreme, a patient's pretest probability might be so great that even a negative test result will result in a post-test probability of disease that is so large that you will ignore the result and decide to treat. In either case, you should decide not to test, because testing will not affect your next decision.

Before applying an LR to a child to determine the post-test probability of disease, it is important to note that LRs can vary for different populations, because diagnostic tests can perform differently in different populations. An example of this is given in Chapter 20 on assessing development. In addition, as described in Chapter 5 and Chapter 42 on urinary tract infections, it is not appropriate to use LRs for several tests in series if the tests are not independent of each other.

A post-test probability provides an estimate of diagnostic certainty. Knowledge of the prognosis of the diagnosis, practical issues, the child's or parents' values, and your own values will all affect the action you take on the basis of that probability. For example, in a clinical situation in which the family of a child you were assessing for "fever without focus" do not have a telephone or car, you are likely to set a lower threshold probability for investigation and treatment for bacterial infection (following history-taking and examination) and thus are more likely to perform further investigations, compared with a family with a child with identical presentation who can readily access services if the clinical situation changes. That is, you are correctly altering your "test threshold" depending upon factors unrelated to the child's clinical picture. The probability at which you make a decision about investigation will also be affected by the nature of the investigation, including invasiveness, potential harm, and cost. In addition, the probability (or threshold) at which you make a decision about treatment will be affected by the available evidence about treatment efficacy and the consequences of not treating.

Decision-making for interventions

The same principles apply to incorporation of evidence from effectiveness studies into clinical decision-making as those that have been discussed for diagnostic tests, i.e., a result that shows that a treatment is effective indicates that the treatment will improve the desired outcome for a greater proportion of children than the proportion of children who will improve if not given therapy (control) or other treatment. Since we know the treatment will not be effective for all children, children and parents being offered known effective treatments are simply being offered an increased post-treatment probability of improvement compared to their baseline risk of improvement, and not a sure-fire cure.

Outcomes from intervention studies can be presented as relative risk, relative risk reduction, absolute risk reduction, and number needed to treat (NNT) (see Chapter 6). Different people (clinicians and patients/parents) prefer different presentations of these outcomes. However the outcome is presented, it can be used to generate an individualized risk of the outcome with treatment, but first you need to have an estimate of the child's baseline risk without treatment (also known as patient's expected event rate [PEER] or "absolute risk in the absence of treatment" or "control event rate"). If a trial reports risks for subgroups, then this information can be used to estimate a child's risk from that of the most similar subgroup. For example, in children with acute otitis media, those with either a temperature $> 37 \cdot 5°C$ or vomiting are more likely to be distressed or to have disturbed sleep for 3 days after seeing a doctor than children without either of these symptoms.[5] In this study children with fever or vomiting were also shown to be more likely to benefit from immediate use of antibiotics than those without either symptom.[5] From this information you would consider prescribing antibiotics immediately for children with fever or vomiting, but not for those without these symptoms. If subgroup risk is not available, an alternative is to estimate risk from similar patients from a population cohort study.

The relative risk reduction (RRR) can be used to modify the patient's baseline risk to obtain the patient's risk of the outcome after treatment, by multiplying the PEER by the RRR. Alternatively, an individualized absolute risk reduction (ARR) (also known as risk difference) is the difference between the patient's risk with treatment and the patient's risk without treatment, and its inverse is the individualized NNT. The individualized NNT can also be generated using the formula $NNT = 1/(PEER \times RRR)$.[3]

If a patient-specific baseline risk is not available from controlled trials or cohort studies, then clinical knowledge can be used to adjust the risk for the typical control patient in the study to a patient specific risk. This is done by assigning a number (f_t) that estimates a patient's risk relative to the typical patient in the control group of the study.[3] If your patient is at more risk than those in the control groups in the trials then f_t will be > 1, and conversely it will be < 1 if your patient is at less risk. Clinical experience can be used to estimate the value of f_t. An individualized NNT can be calculated by dividing the NNT by f_t.[3]

In a similar way, the patient's risk from an adverse outcome from a treatment can be assessed to calculate an individualized patient specific number needed to harm (NNH). The individualized NNT and NNH can be used to calculate patient's likelihood of being helped versus being harmed by considering the ratio[3]:

1/(individualized NNT): 1/(individualized NNH)

NNT and NNH are not "fixed quantities" and depend on an individual patient's risk of adverse outcomes, which could, for example, be affected by age or the severity of illness or your diagnostic certainty. Recent research suggests that these relative treatment effects are usually relatively uniform for patients whose baseline risks are different[7,8] but this is not always the case. Risk difference can be expected to vary symmetrically, increasing as baseline risk increases and decreasing as baseline risk decreases, in situations where relative risk measures are constant for different baseline risk.[6] As a result NNT and NNH will also vary with increase or decrease in baseline risk. However, unlike NNT and NNH, which depend on reductions in absolute risk, RR and RRR tend to be reasonably constant across levels of risk. It has been suggested that treatment effects are more likely to be uniform for patients with different baseline risk for "secondary" interventions, which are designed to slow a disease's progress, but this may be less likely for "tertiary" interventions.[8]

In situations in which you are uncertain about how to calculate some of the individualized ratios that were discussed above, a sensitivity analysis could be performed. This is done by substituting a range of clinically plausible values into the equations above.

Decisions about therapy will also be influenced by the parents' previous experience of the risk of the treatment, potential benefits, and potential harms. For example, a family who have experienced an adverse event from treatment with another child will perceive the potential risks of the treatment quite differently from a family who have not had this experience.

Different models to allow risks and benefits of treatments and patient values to be incorporated into decision-making have been suggested. Sinclair proposes a model that incorporates a threshold NNT for making decisions about treatment. This threshold is constant for different baseline risk, so decisions about treatment will vary for individuals with different baseline risk in line with variation in NNT.[6] Sinclair has further developed this model so that the risks and benefits of treatments and the values ascribed to these can be used to calculate an adjusted threshold NNT for treatment.[6] With such a model, complex interactions and values can be incorporated into treatment decision-making. Glasziou and Irwig[9] propose a model for weighing up benefit and harm that involves consideration of the reduction in relative risk of the adverse outcome, the risk of adverse outcomes, and also the relative valuation of the outcomes. They suggest using quality of life after harm that is caused by treatment, and compare this to the predicted benefit from treatment. McAlister *et al.*[3] suggest that patients use a scale that ranges from 0 (death) to 1 (normal health), to put values on both the possible harm that may arise from treatment as well as the possible harm that may arise if they are not treated. They recommend that this procedure should be repeated on more than one occasion to check the stability of the patient's values.[3] In child health, these values would often need to be elicited from the child's parent or carer. Once elicited, these values can be combined to obtain a measure of the patient's preference for treatment versus no treatment, called the "severity factor".

As all clinicians know, having made the decision to treat or not treat is only the beginning of the decision-making process. In decision analysis terms, the child's progress will feed back into your ongoing decision-making by changing the probabilities of diagnostic certainty and benefits or harms of treatment that you initially generated.

In many areas of pediatric practice, children with multiple problems (co-morbidities) are common. When we are dealing with children and families with multiple problems, both the pediatrician and family may have to prioritize problems and consider interactions between problems before applicability of therapy can be decided. Models to guide this sort of decision-making will require much more complex combinations of all the relevant issues already discussed.

Public health decision-making

To bring together decision-making for public health interventions cost effectiveness analysis is used. This allows a value to be placed on a program for the community. Public perception about the risks and benefits of public health programs such as vaccination is also an important determinant in making decisions about their implementation.

Once public health programs are established, the pediatrician is not usually faced with dilemmas of choice. However, parents may still feel that they need to tailor the "population" decision to their child. The impact on vaccination uptake in the UK after claims that the MMR vaccine caused autism, despite the strong beliefs of public health and medical authorities of the safety of the vaccine, indicates that parents' perceived risk of side effects will influence their decision-making.[10,11]

Problems with applicability

Biologic applicability

In children, the major applicability problem is the absence of evidence. Many studies either do not include children or do not provide outcomes for different age groups. In particular, the relative lack of good research data on numerous interventions in children is a barrier to decision-making about appropriate therapies. This is partly the result of the ethics of research in young children. In many instances where clinical trial data are available for adults, only observational epidemiologic data (such as case–control studies) are available for children. This means that pediatricians need to generalize high level evidence from adults without certainty of the appropriateness of the results to their patients, or rely on lesser evidence from observational studies.

In the very young we also lack good information on the true value of the history and physical examination since this is obtained from a third party (usually the mother), and the examination is often limited (due to lack of cooperation). The result is that in pediatrics there is not only a relative paucity of information relating to prior probabilities, but also limited information on the post-test probability (following history and examination) and prior to laboratory investigations.

Social and economic applicability

Parental values, access to services, and/or financial constraints of the service or the family will play a role in the applicability of study findings to a child and his or her family. In addition, the physician's perception of risk and the patient or parent's perception of risk may differ widely.[3] Bogardus *et al.* have postulated five dimensions of risk to help clinicians understand the issues and challenges for discussing risk with patient/parents. These are the:

- identity (are the risks known?)
- permanence (are the risks temporary or permanent?)
- timing (immediate or delayed?)
- probability (likelihood for the individual), and
- value (perceived importance for the individual) of the risk.

Not only does the clinician need to decide which risks to discuss but also how best to discuss them. This means clinicians need to have a good understanding of the different types of risk (absolute versus relative) and be comfortable with qualitative and quantitative expression of these risks (for example, "rare" or "infrequent" and "< 5%").

In order to improve the communication of risk, Bogardus *et al.* recommend a combination of formats to communicate these complex concepts to patients and parents with wide variations in abilities, needs, and preferences. These formats include using both qualitative and quantitative expression of risk, the use of non-medical risk equivalents (like framing the risk of problems from a test in terms of the risk of injury on the sports field), and graphic presentation of risk. See Chapter 14 for further discussion about communicating evidence to patients.

Accurate communication of the concept of risks and benefits is essential to ensure the patients/parents have available to them the information necessary to make informed decisions regarding interventions and tests. The development of measures and models that allow translation of population data to the individual, as described above, will also make this process easier.

Epidemiologic applicability

Parents, clinicians, and society are more concerned about the potential harm of all tests and interventions in children. Acute side effects are often viewed as a relatively intolerable additional burden of suffering rather than a necessary risk of the therapeutic intervention. Long-term side effects are of more concern in children than in an older population because of the potential increased risk to developing organ systems. Thus, the pediatrician generally needs to spend more time discussing the available evidence relating to harm from both interventions and diagnostic tests, and dealing with uncertainty when this information is not available.

Summary

Evidence-based pediatrics can be used in many different ways including planning health services; determining training needs; planning preventive initiatives; and in everyday clinical consultations. The use of evidence in clinical and other decision-making is not a straightforward process. However, pediatricians are in the unique position of being able to interpret and translate evidence into clinical practice in a way that takes into account an individual's values and needs. Use of evidence in this way is our best chance of improving the use of services and the well-being of children.

As the field of evidence-based medicine has matured, better tools and methods have been developed that reflect the complexity of these processes. Many of these methods now safeguard against the inappropriate use of evidence that many clinicians feared when EBM was first presented. Clinical decision support tools such as computerized prescribing programs and web-based decision support systems are more widely used in clinical practice, but pitfalls of EBM in the clinical setting still exist and need to be discussed so that they can be addressed. The methods described above are time-consuming, and might be easier to implement with computerized decision aids. Researchers need to be pressured into providing information in a format that is useful to clinicians, public health physicians and policy-makers.

Translating evidence into best clinical or public health practice requires the bringing together of research methods (qualitative and quantitative), statistical approaches (Bayesian and frequentist), and knowledge from many different disciplines and paradigms. It also requires communication and synergy between many sectors involved in the care of children and their families, which often operate in isolation but are crucially interdependent. These include the individual patient and physician, the society in which they exist, the clinical scenario, the public health system, the hospital and acute care system, government and health policy-makers, and researchers. Efforts to improve dialogue and information transfer between these many sectors would advance the use of evidence in practice at all levels.

The rest of the book provides examples of how to apply these principles. Some examples are brief and illustrate how to find and use best evidence quickly. Others offer a more comprehensive approach. The approach you choose will depend both on the nature of the problem you are managing, the purpose for which you are seeking evidence, the ease with which you can access information, the availability of evidence and the time you have available.

Take home list

- Pediatric care will be compromised if existing evidence is ignored, and new evidence is not generated.

- Clinicians should first seek good quality summary studies (such as meta analyses/systematic reviews and evidence based guidelines) and clinically useful summary statistics (such as number needed to treat).
- Establishing a study's validity and applicability is crucial before clinical implementation of the study's findings.
- Decisions about the usefulness of a study require balanced consideration of the study's strengths and weaknesses.
- Prioritizing critical parts of the decision making process will help you frame answerable questions.
- Methods are improving for combining similar and different types of evidence.
- For balanced decision making, benefits must always be weighed against potential harm of any intervention, including the "no treatment" option.

References

1 Dans AL, Dans LF, Guyatt GH, Richardson S. Users' guides to the medical literature: XIV. How to decide on the applicability of clinical trial results to your patient. Evidence-Based Medicine Working Group. *JAMA* 1998;**279**:545–9.

2 Bogardus ST, Jr., Holmboe E, Jekel JF. Perils, pitfalls, and possibilities in talking about medical risk. *JAMA* 1999;**281**:1037–41.

3 McAlister FA, Straus SE, Guyatt GH, Haynes RB. Users' guides to the medical literature: XX. Integrating research evidence with the care of the individual patient. Evidence-Based Medicine Working Group. *JAMA* 2000;**283**: 2829–36.

4 Bland JM, Altman DG. Bayesians and frequentists. *BMJ* 1998;**317**(7166):1151–60.

5 Little P, Gould C, Moore M, Warner G, Dunleavey J, Williamson I. Predictors of poor outcome and benefits from antibiotics in children with acute otitis media: pragmatic randomised trial. *BMJ* 2002;**325**:22.

6 Sinclair JC. Weighing risks and benefits in treating the individual patient. *Clinics Perinatol* 2003;**30**:251–68.

7 Furukawa TA, Guyatt GH, Griffith LE. Can we individualize the "number needed to treat"? An empirical study of summary effect measures in meta-analyses. *Int J Epidemiol* 2002;**31**:72–6.

8 McAlister FA. Commentary: relative treatment effects are consistent across the spectrum of underlying risks usually. *Int J Epidemiol* 2002;**31**:76 7.

9 Glasziou PP, Irwig LM. An evidence-based approach to individualising treatment. *BMJ* 1995;**311**(7016):1356–9.

10 Ramsay ME, Yarwood J, Lewis D, Campbell H, White JM. Parental confidence in measles, mumps and rubella vaccine: evidence from vaccine coverage and attitudinal surveys. *Br J Gen Pract* 2002;**52**:912–16.

11 Streefland PH. Public doubts about vaccination safety and resistance against vaccination. *Hlth Policy* 2001;**55**:159–72.

Section II

Evidence for routine practices: screening/prevention

18 The well child

Eugene Dinkevich, Jerry Niederman, Jordan Hupert

Case scenario

Your general pediatric practice has just purchased a computerized record system that allows you to input reminders for preventive measures that you and your colleagues should include in each health supervision visit. After discussing the American Academy of Pediatrics' (AAP) Health Supervision Guidelines, you realize that members of your group emphasize different maneuvers for any specific visit. Moreover, some of your partners eliminate the 9-month and the 21-month health supervision visits, because they feel that they are not helpful, while others recommend monthly visits for infants. You decide that you must determine how many health supervision visits are necessary and which preventive measures performed during health supervision are effective in improving health outcomes. Among the differences in opinion that come up during your discussions are how best to screen for tuberculosis (skin test for all versus only for high risk children), whether and how to screen for elevated lead levels, how to manage hip "clicks" (differentiated from "clunks"), and whether to screen adolescents for scoliosis.

Background

Well-child care is an important component of preventive services available to children. In the USA, the practice of both preventive care (well-child care), and therapeutic care (treatment of intercurrent and chronic illness) is the domain of a general pediatrician. In Canada and Great Britain, as well as in many other European countries, pediatricians are predominantly trained to practice as hospital-based specialists providing therapeutic care, while general practitioners and public health nurses are responsible for preventive care, including well-child care.[1] In the European model, compared to the US model, the target of preventive care shifts from the individual to the community.[2] Community preventive needs may then be addressed by public health nurses who make home visits (United Kingdom),[3] provide preventive services in day-care centers and schools (Norway, France, The Netherlands), and by free public health centers (Japan, France, Sweden).[4–7] Canada, like the USA, relies on private physicians to provide preventive services, although these services are also available through community health centers staffed by nurses.[8]

Although the reasons for mandating the same physician to provide preventive and therapeutic care in the US are largely related to the politics and social pressures at the turn of the 20th century, the result is that general pediatricians spend as much as 40% of their time providing well-child care.[9,10]

The American Academy of Pediatrics published its first Health Supervision Guidelines in 1967. These guidelines were revised in 1974, 1977, 1982, 1985, 1988, and in 1993.[11] These guidelines were a product of activist pediatricians and have not received the critical scrutiny such widely practiced guidelines deserve.[12,13] This criticism, as well as the need to address "new morbidities" including behavioral, emotional, developmental, and psychosocial problems lead to the development of the *Bright Futures, Guidelines for Health Supervision of Infants, Children and Adolescents problems*.[14,15] The *Bright Futures* were published in 1994 by the US Maternal and Child Health Bureau in collaboration with over 20 organizations concerned with preventive health services for children. While the original *Bright Futures* guidelines have been revised twice since 1994 and expanded to include guides for mental health, oral health, and nutrition, they are still mainly based on consensus and expert opinion rather than the evidence of their effectiveness.[16]

Objectives, structure and content of well-child care

The major objective of well-child care is maintenance of health and prevention of disease. This is traditionally accomplished through repeated medical evaluations of healthy children. The basic unit of well-child care is the health supervision visit, which serves to identify and address disease states and related conditions that may lead to disease. Any health supervision visit can be divided into three major components: screening, health promotion and disease prevention, and patient management and follow up.[17] The content of each health supervision visit is age specific.

In a well-child care visit, screening takes place on four levels:

Levels of screening at well-child care visits

- History-gathering, including medical, psychosocial, and developmental history
- Physical examination, including the general examination, and vision and hearing tests
- Observation of parent–child interaction
- Age-specific laboratory testing

The effectiveness of screening by history-taking and the well-child physical examination have been questioned.[18] Recommendations for the frequency and content of the screening physical examination vary from country to country, from full examination at every visit in the USA to only brief examinations after an initial full examination in the UK.[19,20] While both the AAP guidelines and the *Bright Futures* guidelines provide a list of consensus-based, recommended topics for psychosocial screening, time pressures often limit this review.[21,22] Doctors and nurses tend to emphasize medicophysical concerns, while parents are more frequently concerned with psychosocial issues.[23,24] Parental demographic characteristics, socioeconomic status, and longitudinal care affect the likelihood of disclosure of psychosocial information.[25] Recommendations for routine laboratory screening likewise vary significantly.

Health promotion and disease prevention is traditionally accomplished through age-specific counseling referred to as "anticipatory guidance". While the Health Supervision Guidelines recommend which age-specific topics should be discussed with parents, the actual practice of anticipatory guidance varies widely among different settings and physicians.[26,27] A number of studies have attempted to measure the effectiveness of anticipatory guidance, with most studies focusing on a specific preventive intervention, such as counseling about injury prevention or literacy promotion.

The final component of well-child care is management and follow up of the issues that arise during screening. This component will not be considered further in this chapter.

Framing relevant and answerable questions

The case scenarios suggest a number of questions concerning the practice of well-child care and its effectiveness. You frame each one in the format of a focused clinical question in order to better plan your search for evidence.

Questions

1. In healthy children (*population*), does lowering the number of health supervision visits (*intervention*), compared with the standard recommended schedule (*comparison*), result in worse health outcomes (*outcome*)? **[Therapy]**
2. Among normal full-term babies (*population*), does group well-child care (*intervention*) offer advantages over individual well-child care (*comparison*) with respect to mother–child interaction, development, and health services use (*outcomes*)? **[Therapy]**
3. In children presenting for a routine exam (*population*), what is the diagnostic accuracy of a tuberculosis questionnaire (*intervention*), compared with performing a PPD (Mantoux) test (*comparison*), in diagnosing TB infection (*outcome*)? **[Diagnosis]**
4. In infants and young children presenting for a routine exam (*population*), what is the diagnostic accuracy of a community-specific lead poisoning risk-assessment questionnaire (*intervention*), compared with a blood lead level (*comparison*), in diagnosing lead poisoning (*outcome*)? **[Diagnosis]**
5. In babies (*population*), what is the diagnostic accuracy of a hip "click" detected by the Ortolani and Barlow techniques (*intervention*), compared with orthopedic intervention or long-term follow up (*comparison*), in diagnosing developmental dysplasia of the hip (*outcome*)? **[Diagnosis]**
6. In healthy children (*population*), what is the diagnostic accuracy of the Adams forward-bend test (*intervention*), compared with *x* ray (*comparison*), in diagnosing idiopathic scoliosis (*outcome*)? **[Diagnosis]**

Critical review of the evidence

Question

1. In healthy children (*population*), does lowering the number of health supervision visits (*intervention*), compared with the standard recommended schedule (*comparison*), result in worse health outcomes (*outcome*)? **[Therapy]**

Searching for the evidence

- *Cochrane Library:* well-child care OR well baby care OR child health supervision
- MedLine: "Child Health Services"[MeSH] AND well-baby AND child health supervision. Limit to: All child 0–18 yrs, clinical trials, English, Human. Use: related articles feature of PubMed

You begin your search with sources of "predigested" evidence that are already critically appraised. No relevant citations are identified in the *Cochrane Library*. Your search of MedLine yields two documents, the second of which is pertinent to your question.[28] Using the related features option of PubMed yields over 100 papers (since no limits can be applied with this feature), but the third paper in the list is pertinent to your question.[29]

The first study you appraise, performed at the University of Rochester from 1971 to 1973, was a randomized, controlled trial of healthy term newborns during their first year of life.[28] The investigators compared the standard schedule of six health supervision visits (with either a pediatrician or a nurse practitioner) to three visits. The three-visit schedule also included two visits to a nurse for immunization, but no physician or pediatric nurse practitioner contact. The outcome variables included measurement of maternal knowledge of child rearing, maternal satisfaction with the care, compliance with recommendations, and abnormalities detected or missed. An independent physical examination was performed at 15 months by a non-study physician to detect any previously undetected abnormalities. This study took place in both public clinic and private practice settings.

Two hundred ninety-seven babies were enrolled, 146 from the clinic setting and 151 from private practice; 246 (83%) completed the study. The reasons for withdrawal from the study were similar in the standard schedule and three-visit groups. Maternal competence with child rearing was higher in the private practice setting than in the clinic setting, but was unrelated to the number of visits. Mothers in both study groups appeared highly satisfied with their child's care with mean scores of 5·9–6·5 on a 7-point scale. Interestingly, parents who received care in the private practice setting were more satisfied with the reduced visit schedule: 6·5 versus 5·9 ($P < 0.004$), while parents who brought their children to the clinic were more satisfied with the standard schedule: 6·5 versus 6·0 ($P < 0.025$). While maternal compliance with physician recommendations was higher in the private practice setting versus the clinic setting (74·6 versus 26·7%, $P < 0.001$), it was unrelated to the number of visits. Two hundred and twenty-six (92%) children received a complete physical examination by an independent physician at the conclusion of the study: 27 (12%) were found to have previously undetected physical abnormalities; 55% of these were on the six-visit schedule. All abnormalities were minor and only four required treatment.

In summary, this study compared the standard six-visit schedule with a reduced three-visit schedule in private practice and clinic practice settings. There was no significant difference between the two groups on any of the health measures evaluated by this study. Although these outcomes were proxy measures of quality of care and longer term outcomes are unknown, the author concluded that the two schedules were equally effective in achieving objectives of well-child care in the first year of life.

The second study is a Canadian trial that randomized healthy newborns to receive either 10 or five visits in the first two years of life.[29] This more recent trial focused on psychosocial and developmental outcomes, reflecting the shift in the objectives of well-child care over the last several decades. Subjects were randomized to either the standard or the reduced visit groups. Outcomes included the Mental Development Index (MDI) of the Bayley scales of infant development, the Home Observation for Measurement of the Environment (HOME), the Hulka Infancy Questionnaire (HIQ) to assess maternal anxiety, and a standardized questionnaire measured parental satisfaction with health care.[30–33] This study also employed an independent physician to carry out a complete physical assessment of the children at the end of the study. The study was large enough to detect clinically important differences in the rate of undetected physical abnormalities between the groups. Five hundred and seventy babies were enrolled and 466 (82%) completed the study. Dropouts were equivalent between groups. The five-visit group had a mean of 6·19 well-baby visits compared with 7·89 visits for the 10-visit group. No significant differences were found in the MDI, HOME, HIQ, or parental satisfaction scores, or in the number of major or minor abnormalities found between the two groups.

The results of the two studies were remarkably similar in that there were no clinically important differences found between the reduced schedule and the standard schedule groups. The authors concluded that the number of scheduled well-child visits may be safely decreased from 10 to five without loss of efficacy for the outcomes measured. As your practice setting is similar to that of the study, you feel that these results are applicable. In addition, because the authors used standardized assessments of development and home environment, you have confidence in the validity of the outcomes they chose to measure.

Question

2. Among normal full-term babies (*population*), does group well-child care (*intervention*) offer advantages over individual well-child care (*comparison*) with respect to mother–child interaction, development, and health services use (*outcomes*)? **[Therapy]**

Searching for the evidence

- PubMed
- Mother-child Relations "[MeSH] AND "Child Health Services" [MeSH] AND "Peer Group" [MeSH]. Limit to: All child 0–18 yrs, clinical trials, English, Human. Use: related articles feature of PubMed

The strategy for the search of group well-child care reveals one citation. Using the related articles' feature of PubMed you identify five citations that are pertinent to this question[35–39] but you note that the three articles by Taylor *et al.* describe different aspects of the same randomized trial. Two studies randomized patients to either individual (IWCC) or group (GWCC) well-child care. You decide to restrict your analysis of the evidence to these randomized trials.

First described by Lucy Osborn and F Ross Wooley, group well-child care is designed to provide anticipatory guidance and counseling to a group of several families simultaneously.[34] This approach allows sufficient time to counsel parents on more issues and to provide social support, which may improve mother–child interaction and decrease social isolation.[40,41]

Rice *et al.* randomized patients in groups of four to assure similar ages for each well-child care group, while Taylor *et al.* randomized individual subjects. Study completion rate was 88% for the study by Rice *et al.* and 67% for the study by Taylor *et al.* Both studies employed an intention-to-treat analysis, but owing to the nature of the study, neither the subjects nor the controls were blind to the intervention received. Moreover, for the Taylor *et al.* study, the same nurse practitioners provided care for both the IWCC and the GWCC groups. This may have introduced bias if the nurse practitioners treated the two groups differently. No report of co-interventions was given for either study, and both the GWCC and the IWCC were similar in most respects at the beginning of the study. Study outcomes were measured by observers blinded to the study arm.

There were no significant differences between the IWCC and GWCC for utilization measures, mother–child interaction, child development, or maternal outcomes. These two studies suggest that group well-child care is as effective as individual well-child care in low risk middle class and high risk low socioeconomic status families.

Question

3. In children presenting for a routine exam (*population*), what is the diagnostic accuracy of a tuberculosis questionnaire (*intervention*), compared with performing a PPD (Mantoux) test (*comparison*), in diagnosing TB infection (*outcome*)? **[Diagnosis]**

Searching for the evidence (tuberculosis)

- MedLine (PubMed Clinical Queries): Dx and specificity: tuberculin AND questionnaire AND child

The first of the diagnostic test questions concerns screening for tuberculosis and specifically the value of a risk assessment questionnaire to preclude performing a Mantoux test on children with sufficiently low risk of TB exposure. You have read the AAP's[42] and the CDC's recommendations.[43] Both recommendations suggest using a risk questionnaire, but you would like to see some primary evidence that this would work in a practice setting.

Your search using PubMed Clinical Queries results in five articles, three of which describe using questionnaires in children coming for routine well child care. One study was done in a small study population and there were only four children with reactive Mantoux tests.[44] Another well done study provides useful information regarding the utility of a questionnaire, but uses a risk assessment questionnaire that is more extensive than the questionnaire recommended by the AAP.[45]

The paper you choose to review provides adequate data to assess the questionnaire's performance as a screening test. This study by Ozuah *et al.*[46] was done in New York City among a population with a reported high prevalence of tuberculosis. The parents were asked to respond to three questions:

1 Has your child had any contact with a case of TB?
2 Was any household member including your child born in or has any household member, including your child, traveled to areas where TB is common (for example, Africa, Asia, Latin America, and the Caribbean)?
3 Does your child have regular (for example, daily) contact with adults at high risk for TB (i.e., those who are HIV infected, homeless, incarcerated, and/or illicit drug users)?

The questionnaire was considered positive if any one of the three questions was answered affirmatively.

The study met validity criteria. There was an independent and blind comparison of the questionnaire with the reference standard – Mantoux skin test (Table 18.1). The skin test was performed in all children, regardless of the questionnaire result, and, although the prevalence was expected to be higher than that of your practice, the children were clinically without symptoms and coming for routine examinations, as would the children in your practice.

The results of the risk questionnaire screening, given in the table, demonstrate a positive LR = 6·3 [95% CI 5·3, 7·5] and a

Table 18.1 Mantoux skin test

Positive response to any NYCDOH questions	Mantoux skin test	
	+	−
Yes	23	390
No	4	2503
Total	27	2893

Table 18.2 Lead poisoning risk assessment questionnaire

CDCs questionnaire				CDCs questionnaire with local modifications			
Sensitivity	Specificity	Positive LR	Negative LR	Sensitivity	Specificity	Positive LR	Negative LR
0·32	0·80	1·57 (0·77, 3·19)*	0·86 (0·63, 1·17)*	0·90	0·32	1·31 (1·09, 1·56)*	0·33 (0·09, 1·25)*

*95% confidence interval

negative LR = 0·17 [95% CI 0·07, 0·42]. In your population with an estimated prevalence of 0·5% asymptomatic TB infection, and with an average patient panel of 3000 children, the questionnaire would significantly reduce the number of children needing a Mantoux skin test. If the questionnaire's performance is similar in your population you would need to skin test 431 children (rather than 3000), and would find 13 of the expected 15 children with positive Mantoux reactions. Two children with positive skin tests would be missed using this approach. You decide that this might be efficient and plan to speak with your colleagues regarding implementation of the questionnaire in your practice.

Question

4. In infants and young children presenting for a routine exam (*population*), what is the diagnostic accuracy of a community-specific lead poisoning risk-assessment questionnaire (*intervention*), compared with a blood lead level (*comparison*), in diagnosing lead poisoning (*outcome*)? **[Diagnosis]**

Searching for the evidence (lead poisoning)

- MedLine (PubMed Clinical Queries): Dx and specificity: lead poisoning AND questionnaire AND children

Having, again, reviewed guidelines published by the AAP[47] and a potential questionnaire suggested by the CDC,[48] you do a similar search using PubMed Clinical Queries to find justification to adopt a screening questionnaire designed to exclude blood lead testing of those children at sufficiently low risk for lead exposure. Although you are not going to find all the literature related to this question by using Clinical Queries, you will filter "in" well designed, high validity articles. Your search yields 16 English language articles. Reading through the abstracts of the articles reveals inconsistent answers – some studies suggest the questionnaire is a useful first step to reduce the number of children needing blood tests and other

studies suggest no value in screening with a questionnaire. However, several studies modified the Centers for Disease Control questionnaire to reflect the epidemiology of lead exposure in local communities, and all of these studies reported improving the sensitivity of the questionnaire with these modifications.

Only a single study provided complete information to fully assess the questionnaire's performance in children with high ($\geq$ 10 micrograms dl^{-1}) and low (< 10 micrograms dl^{-1}) blood lead levels. This study by Snyder *et al.*[49] looked at the CDC's risk items that focused on older homes in poor repair, industrial source, and home hobby exposures. Also, they added questions that selected risk factors particular to their community such as history of oral exposure to paint or dirt, using home medicinal remedies that are contaminated with lead powder, and a history of migrating from or living in Mexico or Central America. The risk factors were identified retrospectively in their patient population, and validated prospectively in a separate patient cohort. The results comparing the CDC questionnaire and the focused community risk questionnaire are shown in the Table 18.2 for lead levels $\geq$ 10 micrograms dl^{-1}. The prevalence of elevated blood lead levels in their population was 7·7%.

Although at first glance the improved sensitivity with the community-focused questionnaire suggests better case finding, it is at only a modest savings owing to reduced specificity. The positive LRs are similar for both questionnaires, so regardless of prevalence, the two versions perform equally and yield similar post-test probabilities. This is a good study and suggests that you should perform blood lead testing based only on the community prevalence and that risk-assessment questionnaires will not improve case finding as the prevalence of elevated blood lead levels decreases.

Question

5. In babies (*population*), what is the diagnostic accuracy of a hip "click" detected by the Ortolani and Barlow techniques (*intervention*), compared with orthopedic intervention or long-term follow up (*comparison*), in diagnosing developmental dysplasia of the hip (*outcome*)? **[Diagnosis]**

Searching for the evidence (hip click)

MedLine

- PubMed → Clinical Queries → Diagnosis → Specificity → hip AND click*
- PubMed → Clinical Queries → Diagnosis → Sensitivity → hip AND click*
- PubMed → hip AND click*
- Review of references in articles found in above searches and review of references in the AAP[50] and Canadian Guidelines[51]

Your initial search uses the "specificity" filter of PubMed Clinical Queries and retrieves two articles, neither of which address your question. You then choose the "sensitivity" filter (which relaxes the methodologic filtering criteria a bit) and your search recover 38 articles, 10 of which appears potentially relevant to your question. Finally, you search PubMed without the Clinical Queries filters and retrieve 58 articles, 11 of which appear relevant. You decide to do the last, more general search without methodologic filters, as you are concerned that some of the older articles may not have included in their abstracts terms that the filtering system looks for. Perusal of the references of those articles and the AAP and Canadian guidelines yields other, potentially relevant, articles, with the literature going back many decades. You decide to critically appraise two of the methodologically most sound and applicable articles on each side of the argument.

During your reading, you note that a positive Ortolani sign is referred to as a "click" in the early literature.[52] Later a positive Ortolani or Barlow sign is referred to as a dislocation or some other term denoting actual hip movement. The term "click" became synonymous with "soft-tissue clicks."[53] This was the type of "click" you were interested in learning about. You find approximately an equal number of articles supporting and rejecting the view that a "hip click" is a finding consistent with DDH in some babies.

You note in your review of the literature that there are essentially two types of studies – those in which the study population included all babies born during a specified period and those that included only babies with positive findings. In neither type of study was correlation of the hip examination among examiners mentioned. There was no mention of blinding among those who performed the exam and those who evaluated the gold standard. The gold standard in most studies was the need for orthopedic intervention. However, criteria for intervention varied among studies.

One of the most extensive studies was conducted by Boeree and Clarke.[54] The study describes a DDH screening protocol in Southampton, England. All infants born at the Princess Anne Maternity Hospital from June, 1988 to December, 1992 (26 952 infants) were examined at birth for

Table 18.3 Diagnostic accuracy of hip click detection

Test*	Orthopedic intervention	
	+	−
Hip click	15	938
No hip click	26	25 853
Total	41	26 791

*Those with frank hip instability on exam were not included

DDH by a pediatrician using the Ortolani and Barlow techniques. Those with dislocatable or dislocated hips were double diapered and received an ultrasound at 10–16 days of age. Those with a hip click, or in one of the "high risk" groups (breech, family history, foot deformity) received an ultrasound at 4–6 weeks. All babies with a dislocatable/dislocated hip, a hip click, or in the high risk category were referred to the Hip Screening Clinic where they received both an ultrasound examination and an examination by an orthopedic surgeon. Ultrasound criteria for diagnosing a dysplastic hip were not mentioned. The clinic attendance rate was 95·8% of the 1894 infants referred. Infants without any sign or not in the high risk category at birth were followed by general practitioners. Any baby missed during the neonatal screening or who developed signs later were also referred to the Hip Screening Clinic. Clinically significant DDH was defined in babies who eventually required a Pavlik Harness or surgery for correction. The authors did not document follow up exams for those babies not referred to the Hip Screening Clinic. They mentioned that "to their knowledge" no child born in the Southampton district during the period of the study was treated elsewhere for late-presenting DDH. This approach to dealing with test-negative patients is not uncommon among the DDH studies. The implication is that the population of the study catchment area is stable and that the investigators would be in a position to hear of any previously undetected cases.[55]

There were 120 infants (0·4%) with hip instability and 953 infants (3·5%) with a hip click referred to the Hip Screening Clinic: 34 patients identified with a hip click (4%) were lost to follow up. The results are recorded in Table 18.3. The 120 infants with hip instability on neonatal exam are not included. Most of those with DDH in the "no hip click" group were in the high risk group.

The results of the study demonstrated that detection of a click in an infant with otherwise normal hips had a positive LR of 10 (95% CI 7, 16). Given the overall prevalence of 0·0015, the post-test probability for DDH given detection of a hip click was 0·015 (95% CI 0·01, 0·02). When the test was negative, the LR was 0·66 (0·52, 0·83) and the post-test probability was 0·001 (95% CI 0·0008, 0·0012). Given these results, a positive test is considerably more useful clinically than a negative test, as the negative LR is not very different from 1. The logical conclusion from this study, even with all methodologic concerns mentioned above, is that detection of a hip click is clinically important.

Jones and Powell (orthopedic surgeon and radiologist, respectively) conducted a prospective study from January to December 1987 of infants born from a "relatively stable population" in Wales.[56] Senior house officers examined all infants and referred for orthopedic exam by Jones (and imaging with ultrasound and/or *x* ray) those with dislocatable/dislocated hips, "clicking" hips, or anyone in the "high risk" group mentioned above in the Boeree and Clarke study. From a birth cohort of 3879 infants, 406 were referred. The babies were examined by Jones within 7 days of detection by the house officer, but it is not clear when the babies who required intervention actually received it, though the implication is that the intervention was at the time of the orthopedic exam. There were 159 babies referred with a hip click in one or both hips, six of whom had a Graf type III or IV type hip on ultrasound (0·038 of the babies with hip click and 0·0016 of the sample overall) and were treated with an Aberdeen splint. The positive LR for a hip click, not including the babies with dislocatable/dislocated hip = 6·5 (3·2, 13); the negative LR = 0·77 (0·60, 0·98). Given a DDH prevalence (not including those with frankly dislocatable/dislocated hips) of 0·006, the corresponding post-test probabilities were 0·04 (0·02, 0·07) and 0·004 (0·0036, 0·006), for a positive and negative hip click test, respectively. It is interesting to note that the disease prevalence among babies the total non-dislocatable/dislocated hip population is four times that of the Boeree and Clarke study. The LRs, however, are remarkably similar. There are a few possible explanations for the disease prevalence variation including: natural statistical variation, more lenient criteria for bracing (lowering the threshold for disease definition), and the populations are somewhat different. As in the previous study, babies with a normal exam and not in the "high risk" group were assumed not to have DDH. Long-term follow up was not part of this study.

On the other side, there are a number of studies that present results demonstrating hip clicks as a normal variant. In a recent study by Bond *et al.* 50 infants with hip clicks persisting after 3 months of age were investigated by orthopedic exam and ultrasound.[53] All infants had normal exams (negative Ortolani and Barlow signs) and ultrasounds. There was no mention of long-term follow up. Using the rule of 3/N for a study that finds no events, the 95% confidence interval is (0, 0·06), among those with a hip click.

An older, though frequently referenced study by Sommer,[57] was conducted in Odense, Denmark using a birth cohort of 5060 infants born between May 1965 and May 1967. A total of 17 babies had a positive Ortolani sign and 99 had a "dry click," a term which appears be the same as "hip click" used in the studies discussed above, where the hip is stable on examination. None of the 99, all but two of whom had

an *x* ray at a year of age and followed until they were walking, had DDH. The 95% CI is 0, 0·02. There was no discussion of false negatives (i.e., babies who had a normal examination but may have been in a "high risk" category [see above]).

The clinical practice guideline from the AAP mentions that hip clicks (termed "benign hip clicks" or "adventitial click") "in the newborn period do not lead to later dysplasia."[50] If the click is detected at 2 weeks follow up, one may consider ultrasonography or orthopedic referral at 3–4 weeks of age. The Canadian Task Force guidelines refer to the hip click as a "less widely accepted risk factor."[51] There is no further discussion of the hip click. At least two of the three articles referenced after the statement are from studies that purportedly demonstrate DDH in some babies with only hip click as a finding.[58,59]

It is clear to you that the controversy has not been resolved, but there is a reasonable concern that a persistent hip click may be associated with DDH. While you may not be able to convince those who regard the hip click as a normal variant, you plan on obtaining ultrasounds at 4–6 weeks in any baby with a persistent hip click at the 2-week visit.

Question

6. In healthy children (*population*), what is the diagnostic accuracy of the Adams forward-bend test (*intervention*), compared with *x* ray (*comparison*), in diagnosing idiopathic scoliosis (*outcome*)? **[Diagnosis]**

Searching for the evidence (forward bend)

MedLine

- PubMed → Clinical Queries → Diagnosis → Specificity → scoliosis AND (forward bend OR adams)
- PubMed → Clinical Queries → Diagnosis → Sensitivity → scoliosis AND (forward bend OR adams)

Your search using "specificity" retrieves six articles, three of which appear to be relevant. When you broaden your search with "sensitivity" you retrieve 13 articles, with only those three addressing your question.

You notice from your review that the three studies defined clinically significant scoliosis at three different Cobb angles: 10°, 20°, and 40°. The variation depended on whether or not the investigators believed back bracing was clinically efficacious or depended on the target population, primary care versus referral care (see below). As the clinical implications of missing scoliosis most likely increase with the severity of the curvature, you would order an *x* ray and/or refer to orthopedics a child with a positive forward bend test

Table 18.4 Adams forward-bend test[60]

Adams	Scoliosis (≥ 10°)	
	+	−
+	27	175
−	5	2493
Total	32	2668

Table 18.5 Adams forward-bend test[61]

Adams	Scoliosis (≥ 20°)		LR* (95% CI**)
	+	−	
+	49	21	2·3 (1·6, 3·2)
−	4	31	0·1 (0·05, 0·3)
Total	53	52	

*LR, likelihood ratio; **CI, confidence interval

whose post-test probability is at least 10%, 2%, and 0·5%, for a 10°, 20°, and 40° angle, respectively.

The first article by Karachalios *et al.*[60] was set on the Grecian island of Samos, was school-based, and scoliosis was defined as an angle ≥ 10°. All 2700 students, 8–16 years old, were screened with the forward bend test and all had x rays performed. It is not mentioned if there was an independent and blind comparison of examination and x ray results. The forward bend examination was not described. Each student was examined by two orthopedic surgeons. If there was clinical disagreement, a third orthopedic surgeon was consulted. Interexaminer agreement was not reported. The results are given in Table 18.4.

The LR for a positive test was 13 (95% CI 10, 16), and for a negative test was 0·17 (95% 0·07, 0·37). Using the study prevalence of scoliosis (0·011), the post-test probabilities for a positive and negative test were 0·14 (95% CI 0·11, 0·16) and 0·003 (95% CI 0·001, 0·007), respectively.

You have some concern that the forward bend test may not give the same results (i.e., would have a different set of likelihood ratios) in your hands compared to those of an orthopedic surgeon. However, you perform the test frequently and feel that if there are differences, they are likely to be small. Assuming the prevalence of scoliosis in your population is similar to the study population, both the post-test probability and the lower limit of the 95% CI for the post-test probability exceed your clinical threshold for ordering an x ray and/or referral to orthopedics. The results of this study suggest that the Adams forward-bend test is a relatively powerful test when positive.

The study by Cote *et al.*[61] defined a clinically significant scoliosis angle ≥ 20°. Two investigators examined 105 (87 girls) consecutively referred patients with a mean age of 15·5 years (SD = 4·8). All but two (with congenital scoliosis) had adolescent idiopathic scoliosis and 26 had already undergone some treatment for the condition. Full-spine posteroanterior and lateral x ray (gold standard) was performed on all patients and evaluated by a third independent investigator. The Adams forward-bend test was fairly well described in the methods section, so you feel confident you could reproduce it. All patients were independently assessed by both examiners and had a spine x ray. Reproducibility of the Adams test in multiple settings was not measured in the study, but

interexaminer reliability was measured. The interexaminer coefficient (k) was 0·61 (95% CI, 0·44–0·78) for the detection of a thoracic hump using the Adams test. This represents moderate agreement between examiners. The study results are shown in the Table 18.5.

The results suggest that a negative Adams test modifies the pretest probability significantly more than a positive test. The likelihood ratio (LR) for a negative test was 0·1. A correspondingly strong LR for a positive test would be 10. As the LR was only about 2, little diagnostic information is gained from a positive test. You are concerned that the usual severity of scoliosis in your practice is quite different from that encountered in the referral clinic of this study. LRs can be affected by the severity spectrum such that a study investigating a large proportion of severely affected children may generate a lower specificity and a higher sensitivity than when the test is administered in a general population. For that reason, it is not possible to estimate the post-test probability for your population even if you get a reasonable estimate of prevalence of patients with a scoliotic curve ≥ 20°.

The study by Goldberg *et al.* was designed to directly address the conclusion of the US Preventive Services Task Force that no recommendation could be made either for or against scoliosis screening (in particular, using the Adams forward-bend test).[62] The study setting was the primary and post-primary school systems in Dublin, Ireland. Only girls (10–14 years old) were included in this study, as these authors had previously concluded that the incidence of clinically significant scoliosis in boys was too low to justify screening.[63]

Examinations were done at school. If positive, the girl was referred to the hospital-based scoliosis clinic. At the hospital clinic, the girls were re-examined and then tested with a scoliometer, a device that measures the degree of truncal rotation. A posteroanterior spine x ray with Cobb angle measurement was obtained in premenarchal girls with a thoracic hump of 8° (by scoliometer) or a loin hump of 10°, and in post-menarchal girls with a thoracic hump of 10° or a loin hump of 15°. Clinically significant scoliosis was defined as a curve ≥ 40° at diagnosis or subsequently, a substantially higher angle than in the previous two studies appraised above. In their experience, Goldberg *et al.* found no benefit to bracing at lower angles, and therefore regarded surgery as the only effective corrective measure.[63] Of 8686 girls initially enrolled,

5179 (59%) were followed up for re-examination 1–4 years later. Only this cohort was used to calculate the diagnostic characteristics of the screening test. The investigators defined their "test" as the entire filtering process down to and including the scoliometer measurement. Only those with scoliometer angles that met the criteria mentioned above had x rays. "Test-negative" patients were followed up with re-examination over the next 1–4 years to detect false negatives. For *your* purposes, the "test" is the initial screening Adams forward-bend test. The gold standard, therefore, is all the rest of the filtering process up to and including the scoliometer and x ray (in those who were scoliometer positive). The investigators attempted to detect false negatives through long-term follow up so that sensitivity and specificity could be estimated from these data. Although you have some concerns about loss to follow up, you decide that the methods used are likely to be valid, so you go on to examine the results.

Similar to results in the Cote *et al.* study, a negative Adams test in the Goldberg *et al.* study appeared to be more clinically useful than a positive test. This was so, even though the LR for a positive Adams test was relatively high at 8·5. The key to understanding this lies in considering both the prevalence of the study cohort and the severity of disease as defined by the investigators. In this study, clinically significant scoliosis was defined as a curve $\geq 40°$. The prevalence of disease in the Dublin school population who attended long-term follow up was 0·1%. If the Adams test were positive, the LR of 8·5 would increase the probability of clinically significant scoliosis to 0·9%. While both the post-test probability and the lower end of its 95% CI cross your clinical threshold for x ray and/or referral, you are somewhat taken aback that for every patient with a curve $\geq 40°$ more than 100 will have an x ray and/or be referred needlessly (Table 18.6). However, that is the cost of screening for a disease (scoliosis as defined as a curve $\geq 40°$) with an extremely low prevalence.

In the case of a negative test, it appears that the pretest probability is irrelevant, since no patients with a negative test had scoliosis. In fact, the matter is more complex owing to the lack of precision in the LR for a negative test, due to the small number of girls with a curve $\geq 40°$. The 95% CI for the negative-test LR ranged from 0 to 0·89. Using the Dublin prevalence of 0·1%, the upper end of the 95% CI for the corresponding post-test probability is 0·09%, not clinically different from the pretest probability.

You are also concerned that the authors excluded from the diagnostic test calculations any girl who did not return for a follow up exam. The number of test-positive patients listed in the table assumes that all girls who tested positive returned. If that was not the case, assuming that those who initially tested positive were at least as likely to return for follow up as those who initially tested negative, the LRs for positive and negative tests are 14·2 and 0, respectively. These "worst-case scenario" results are not *clinically* different from those listed in the table, and therefore do not affect your assessment of the usefulness

Table 18.6 Adams forward-bend test[62]

Adams	Scoliosis ($\geq 40°$)		LR* (95% CI**)
	+	–	
+	6	612	8·5 (5·6, 9·7)
–	0	4561	0 (0, 0·89)
Total	6	5173	

*LR, likelihood ratio; **CI, confidence interval

of this test. Given that any amount of abnormality on the Adams test would be interpreted as positive and given the rather significant level of curvature that defined clinically significant scoliosis ($\geq 40°$), it is reasonable to assume that you would not miss any cases. As demonstrated above, when a disease with very low prevalence is screened for, even a moderate change in the number of false positives has little clinical effect on the LRs, unless the specificity is very high. Thus, you could conclude that the Adams test would perform similarly in your clinical setting.

You are amazed at the variety of approaches taken in defining clinically relevant scoliosis. It is clear that the school-based studies are most applicable to your practice. Given the current practice in your medical community of bracing children with curvature angles significantly less than 40°, the first study by Karachalios *et al.* appears to be the most applicable currently to your practice. However, you would like to learn more about the efficacy of bracing. Further research may define more clearly the benefit of bracing and you will try to review the literature from time to time.

Resolution of the scenario

At your next staff meeting, you report that you found no evidence to support the current AAP recommendation for 20 visits by the 21st birthday. The two studies that addressed this issue concluded that a reduced visit schedule had no detrimental effect on child health. You therefore recommend that a reduced visit, well-child care schedule be encouraged, but that the practice allow individual physicians to schedule visits as they deem appropriate. Finally, you report evidence that showed group well-child care to be as effective as individual well-child care with respect to psychosocial issues. You and your partners agree to consider, at the next staff meeting, providing parenting advice and behavior counseling in groups. The meeting is about to be adjourned – early, for once – when one of your colleagues asks what you found out through your review of the evidence for routine well-child screening. For the four tests you evaluated, the studies you reviewed were at least minimally methodologically valid. You don't plan to incorporate the lead questionnaire into your electronic reminder system, but will plan to use the TB questionnaire. Controversies around the hip-click and forward bend tests serve to remind you to recheck the literature routinely in these areas.

Future research needs

Thirty years ago, Yankauer issued a challenge to pediatricians to provide well-child care with clear, clinically meaningful outcomes.[64] Future research is needed to validate the content of the well-child visit as well as the currently published recommendations from the AAP, the US Preventive Services Task Force, the Canadian Task Force on Periodic Health Examination, and other authoritative organizations.

Summary table

Question	Type of evidence	Results	Comments
Lowering the number of health supervision visits	Randomized controlled trials[28,29]	No difference found between standard and reduced visit schedule	Reduced visit schedule found to be as effective as standard schedule
Group versus individual well-child care	Randomized controlled trials[35–39]	No difference found between groups on use, maternal child interaction, child development, or maternal outcomes	In Taylor's study, large drop-out rates in the GWCC group may have interfered with study's ability to show differences since primiparous women had higher scheduling rates
Risk assessment for tuberculosis	Prospective cohort assessed with a questionnaire with PPD as gold standard[46]	Positive LR = 6·3 (5·3, 7·5) negative LR = 0·17 (0·07, 0·42)	With prevalence < 1%, NPV high enough to substitute the questionnaire for universal PPD placement
Risk assessment for lead poisoning	Prospective cohort assessed with a questionnaire with blood lead level as gold standard[49]	CDC questionnaire: positive LR 1·57 (0·77, 3·19) Negative LR 0·86 (0·63, 1·17) CDC questionnaire with local modifications: positive LR 1·31 (1·09,1·56) Negative LR 0·33 (0·09, 1·25)	Neither questionnaire demonstrates a statistically significant negative LR (the 95% CIs cross 1) and is therefore unable to differentiate between children with and without lead poisoning
Diagnostic accuracy of hip "click" on newborn exam in detecting developmental dysplasia of the hip	1. Population-based prospective cohort[54] 2. Population-based prospective cohort[56] 3. Babies with persistent hip clicks for three months[53] 4. Population-based prospective cohort[57]	1. Positive LR = 10 (7,16); negative LR = 0·66 (0·52, 0·83) 2. Positive LR = 6·5 (3·2, 13); negative LR = 0·77 (0·60, 0·98) 3. Test positive data only. No DDH out of 50 patients (PPV). 95% CI (0, 0·06) 4. PPV = 0/99 [0, 0·03]	1. Even though the diagnostic test characteristics of hip click detection are good (especially for a positive test), given the very low prevalence, the PPV is quite low. However, the clinical intervention (a hip ultrasound) is mild 2. LRs remarkably similar, lending support to the test accuracy 3. Examined by orthopedic surgeon and by ultrasound 4. Followed until patients were walking. Confirmed with x ray
Diagnostic accuracy of the Adam's forward-bend test in detecting idiopathic scoliosis	1. Prospective school-based cohort[60] 2. Prospective referral cohort[61] 3. Prospective school-based cohort[62]	1. Positive LR = 13[10,16] negative LR = 0·17 [0·07, 0·37] 2. Positive LR = 2·6 [1·3, 3·2] negative LR = 0·1 [0·05, 0·3] 3. Positive LR = 8·5 [5·6, 9·7] negative LR = 0·1 [0, 0·89]	1. Scoliosis defined at > 10°. Given population base and scoliosis definition, perhaps most applicable to a general pediatric practice 2. Scoliosis defined at ≥ 20°. Probable problem with spectrum bias 3. Scoliosis defined at ≥ 40°. Not the current clinically applicable definition of scoliosis. Clinical utility of this definition depends on effect of bracing

References

1 Child Health in 1990: The US compared to Canada, England and Wales, France, The Netherlands and Norway. Proceedings of a conference, Washington, DC, March 18 and 19, 1990. *Pediatrics* 1990;**86**(Suppl.):1025–7.

2 Miller CA. Summation and commentary. Recommendations of the Workshop on Children with Special Needs. *Pediatrics* 1990;**86**(Suppl.):1124–7.

3 Goodwin, S. Child health services in England and Wales. *Pediatrics* 1990;**86**(Suppl.):1032–6.

4 Lie SO. Children in the Norwegian health care system. *Pediatrics* 1990;**86**(Suppl.):1048–52.

5 Manciaux M, Jestin C, Fritz M, Bertrand D. Child health care policy and delivery in France. *Pediatrics* 1990;**86** (Suppl.):1037–43.

6 Verbrugge HP. Youth health care in the Netherlands: a bird's eye view. *Pediatrics* 1990;**86**(Suppl.):1044–7.

7 Chaulk CP. Preventive health care in six countries: models for reform. *Hlth Care Financ Rev* 1994;**15**:7–19.

8 Pless IB. Child health in Canada. *Pediatrics* 1990; **86**(Suppl.):1027–32.

9 Baker JP. Women and the invention of well-child care. *Pediatrics* 1994;**94**:527–31.

10 Hoekelman RA. Well-child care revisited. *Am J Dis Child* 1983;**137**:1057–60.

11 Committee on Psychosocial Aspects of Child and Family Health. American Academy of Pediatrics. *Guidelines for health supervision III.* Elk Grove Village, Illinois: American Academy of Pediatrics, 1997.

12 Pless IB. Screening tests in the office practice: implications from the Canadian Periodic Health Examination Task Force Report. In: Charney E, ed. *Well-child care. Report of the seventeenth Ross roundtable on critical approaches to common pediatric problems.* Columbus, OH: Ross Laboratories, 1986.

13 Pless IB. Screening tests in the office practice: implications from the Canadian Periodic Health Examination Task Force Report. In: Charney E, ed. *Well-child care. Report of the seventeenth Ross roundtable on critical approaches to common pediatric problems.* Columbus, OH: Ross Laboratories, 1986.

14 Haggerty RJ. Child Health 2000: new morbidities in the changing environment of the children's needs in the 21st century. *Pediatrics* 1995;**96**:804–12.

15 Green M, ed. *Bright Futures: Guidelines for Health Supervision of Infants, Children and Adolescents.* Arlington: VA:National Center for Education in Maternal and Child Health, 2000.

16 Dinkevich E, Ozuah PO. Well-child care: effectiveness of current recommendations. *Clin Pediatr (Phila).* 2002;**41**: 211–17.

17 Osborn LM. Effective well-child care. *Curr Probl Pediatr* 1994;**24**:306–26.

18 Hoekelman RA. An appraisal of the effectiveness of child health supervision. *Curr Opin Pediatr* 1989;**1**:146–55.

19 The Canadian Task Force on the Periodic Health Examination. *The Canadian guide to clinical preventive health care.* Ottawa: Canadian Government Publishing, 1994.

20 Well-child care. In: *Healthy children: investing in the future.* Publication OTA-H-345. Washington, DC: Office of Technology Assessment, US Congress, 1988.

21 Kittredge D, Olson R. Well-child counseling by pediatric residents: topics raised, time spent and parent satisfaction. *Am J Dis Child* 1998;**142**:396.

22 Wissow LS, Roter DL, Wilson MEH. Pediatrician interview style and mothers' disclosure of psychosocial issues. *Pediatrics* 1994;**93**:289–95.

23 Korsh BM, Negrete VF, Mercer AS, Freemon B. How comprehensive are well-child visits? *Am J Dis Child* 1971; **122**:483.

24 Hinkson GB, Altemeier WA, O'Connor S. Concerns of mothers seeking care in private pediatric offices: opportunities for expanding services. *Pediatrics* 1983;**72**: 619–24.

25 Wissow L, Larson S, Roter D, Wang M, Hwang W, Luo X, Johnson R. Longitudinal care improves disclosure of psychosocial information. *Arch Pediatr Adolesc Med.* 2003; **157**:419-24.

26 Norkin Goldstein EN, Dworkin PH, Bernstein B. Time devoted to anticipatory guidance during child health supervision visits: how are we doing? *Ambulatory Child Hlth* 1999;**5**:112–20.

27 Reisinger KS, Bires JA. Anticipatory guidance in pediatric practice. *Pediatrics* 1980;**66**:889–92.

28 Hoekelman RA. What constitutes adequate well-baby care? *Pediatrics* 1975;**55**:313–26.

29 Gilbert JR, Feldman W, Siegel LS, Mills DA, Dunnett C, Stoddart G. How many well-baby visits are necessary in the first 2 years of life? *Can Med Assoc J* 1984;**130**: 857–61.

30 Satter JM. *Assessment of children's intelligence and special abilities, 2nd edn.* Boston, MA: Allyn and Bacon, 1981.

31 van Doornininck WJ, Caldwell BM, Wright C, Frankernburg WK. The relationship between twelve-month home stimulation and school achievement. *Child Devel* 1981;**52**: 1080–3.

32 Liptak GS, Hulka BS, Cassel JC. Effectiveness of physician-mother interactions during infancy. *Pediatrics.* 1977;**60**: 186–192.

33 Zhzanski SJ, Hulka BS, Cassel JC. Scale for measurement of "satisfaction" with medical care: modifications in content, format and scoring. *Med Care* 1974;**12**:611–20.

34 Osborn LM, Wooley FR. The use of groups in well-child care. *Pediatrics* 1981;**67**:701–6.

35 Rice RL, Slater CJ. An analysis of group versus individual child health supervision. *Clin Pediatr* 1997;**36**:685–9.

36 Dodds M, Nicholson L, Muse B, Osborn LM. Group health supervision visits more effective than individual visits in delivering health care information. *Pediatrics* 1993;**91**: 668–70.

37 Taylor JA, Davis RL, Kemper KJ. A randomized controlled trial of group versus individual well child care for high-risk children: maternal-child interaction and developmental outcomes. *Pediatrics* 1997;**99**:e9.

38 Taylor JA, Davis RL, Kemper KJ. Health care utilization and health status in high-risk children randomized to receive group or individual well child care. *Pediatrics* 1997;**100**:e1.

39 Taylor JA, Kemper KJ. Group well-child care for high-risk families: maternal outcomes. *Arch Pediatr Adolesc Med* 1998;**152**:579–84.

40 Crockenberg SB. Infant irritability, mother responsiveness and social support influences on the security of infant–mother attachment. *Child Devel* 1981;**52**:857–65.

41 Telleen S, Herzog A, Kilban TL. Impact of a family support program on mother's social support and parenting stress. *Am J Orthopsychiat* 1989;**59**:410–18.

42 American Academy of Pediatrics, Committee on Infectious Diseases update on tuberculosis skin testing of children. *Pediatrics* 1996;**97**:282–4.

43 Centers for Disease Control and Prevention. Targeted tuberculin testing and treatment of latent tuberculosis infection. *MMWR Morb Mortal Wkly Rep.* 2000;**49**(RR-6):1–51.

44 Christy C, Pulcino ML, Lanphear BP and McConnochie KM. Screening for tuberculosis infection in urban children. *Arch Pediatr Adolesc Med* 1996;**150**:722–6.

45 Froehlich H, Ackerson LM, Morozumi, PA *et al.* Targeted testing of children for tuberculosis: validation of a risk assessment questionnaire. *Pediatrics* 20001;**107**:e54.

46 Ozuah PO, Ozuah TP, Stein REK *et al.* Evaluation of a risk assessment questionnaire used to target tuberculin skin testing in children. *JAMA* 2001;**285**:451–3.

47 American Academy of Pediatrics, Committee on Environmental Health. Screening for elevated blood lead levels. *Pediatrics* 1998;**101**:1072–8.

48 Centers for Disease Control and Prevention. *Screening Young Children for Lead Poisoning. Guidance for State and Local Public Health Officials.* Atlanta, GA, CDC, 1997.

49 Snyder DC, Mohle-Boetani JC, Palla B, Fenstersheib M. Development of a population-specific risk assessment to predict elevated blood lead levels in Santa Clara County, California. *Pediatrics* 1995;**96**:643–8.

50 American Academy of Pediatrics, Committee on Quality Improvement, Subcommittee on Developmental Dysplasia of the Hip. Clinical practice guideline: early detection of developmental dysplasia of the hip. *Pediatrics* 2000;**105**: 896–905.

51 Patel H. Canadian Task Force on Preventive health care, 2001 update: screening and management of developmental dysplasia of the hip in newborns. *CMAJ* 2001;**164**: 1669–77.

52 Motta F, Calori A, Savoldi E, *et al.* Ultrasonography in the early diagnosis of congenital dysplasia of the hip. *Ital J Orthop Traumatol* 1986;**12**:117–24.

53 Bond CD, Hennrikus WL, Della Maggiore E. Prospective evaluation of newborn soft tissue hip clicks with ultrasound. *J Pediatr Orthop.* 1977;**17**:199–201.

54 Boeree NR, Clarke NMP. Ultrasound imaging and secondary screening for congenital dislocation of the hip. *J Bone Joint Surg [Br]* 1994;**76-B**:525–33.

55 Dunn PM, Evans RE, Thearle MJ, *et al.* Congenital dislocation of the hip: early and late diagnosis and management compared. *Arch Dis Child* 1985;**60**:407–14.

56 Jones DA, Powell N. Ultrasound and neonatal hip screening: a prospective study of "high risk" babies. *J Bone Joint Surg [Br]* 1990;**72**:457–8.

57 Sommer J. Atypical hip click in the newborn. *Acta Orthop Scandinav* 1971;**42**:353–6.

58 Garvey M, Donoghue VB, Gorman WA, *et al.* Radiographic screening at four months of infants at risk for congenital hip dislocation. *J Bone Joint Surg (Br)* 1992;**74**:643–4.

59 Jones DA. Importance of the clicking hip in screening for congenital dislocation of the hip. *Lancet* 1989;**1**: 599–601.

60 Karachalios T, Sofianos J, Roidis N *et al.* Ten-year follow up evaluation of a school screening program for scoliosis. Is the forward-bend test an accurate diagnostic criterion for the screening of scoliosis? *Spine* 1999;**24**:2318–24.

61 Cote P, Kreitz BG, Cassidy DJ *et al.* A study of the diagnostic accuracy and reliability of the scoliometer and Adams forward-bend test. *Spine* 1998;**23**:796–803.

62 Goldberg CJ, Dowling FE, Fogarty EE, *et al.* School scoliosis screening and the United States Preventive Services Task Force. An examination of long-term results. *Spine* 1995;**20**: 1368–74.

63 Goldberg C, Fogarty EE, Blake NS, *et al.* School scoliosis screening: a review of 21,000 children. *Ir Med J* 1987; **80**: 325–6.

64 Yankauer A. Child health supervision – is it worth it? *Pediatrics* 1973;**52**:272–9.

19 Universal newborn hearing screening

Melissa Wake

Case scenario

A 21-month-old girl presents because her mother is concerned that she isn't yet saying any single words, unlike most other children in her playgroup. On further enquiry, mother reports that, although the child does not seem to understand or say any words, she uses gestures to indicate her needs, enjoys pretend play with her doll, is affectionate with her parents and older sister, and enjoys games such as "peek-a-boo". On your examination, she can stack a four-block tower and scribbles with a pencil. Visual reinforcement audiometry confirms a sloping hearing loss in both ears, with moderate loss in the low frequencies deteriorating to severe loss in the high frequency range. The child's parent-held record indicates that she passed her universal newborn hearing screen in both ears. Universal newborn hearing screening was introduced throughout your region nearly 3 years ago. You wonder if this was a congenital hearing loss that was missed by the program (i.e., a false negative), or whether it may have developed since. You also decide to have a look at just how effective newborn hearing screening programs really are – something you've not thought to question previously.

Background

Congenital hearing loss can wreak devastating effects on an otherwise healthy, normal child. The US Agency for Health Care Research and Quality (AHRQ) recently noted that:

> the average deaf student graduates from high school with language and academic achievement levels below those of the average fourth-grade student with normal hearing. Average reading scores for hard-of-hearing students graduating from high school are at the fifth-grade level. The lag in reading performance has remained virtually unchanged since it was first carefully measured in the early 1960s.[1]

Hearing-impaired children are also reported to exhibit more behavioral problems than hearing controls.[2–4] Like most chronic conditions, impacts go well beyond the child; for example, parents of hearing-impaired children report higher levels of stress than parents of hearing children,[5,6] and there is some evidence that severity of a child's hearing loss is negatively related to parental marital satisfaction.[7]

An invisible handicap, congenital hearing loss is traditionally detected late – often only after a child has become a "late talker", in many cases well after the age of 2 years – by which time the complex building blocks of language should already have been largely in place. The overall prevalence is about 1 in 1000 babies. Affecting about 1 in 3000 healthy newborns, the incidence is much higher in special populations such as graduates of the neonatal intensive care unit and children with Down's syndrome, craniofacial malformations, and/or other specific risk factors for hearing loss. Because the risk factors may be more readily detected than the hearing loss itself, these children are often diagnosed earlier than healthy babies without risk factors – who, paradoxically, may have the most to gain from early diagnosis.

With the advent of simple-to-use portable equipment, it is now possible to objectively screen the hearing of a newborn over the space of a few minutes and with only brief training. Universal newborn hearing screening programs have therefore been implemented throughout many parts of the world, including the USA and England. However, the technology is sophisticated and cannot be piggy-backed onto an existing test (in the way that, for example, hypothyroidism screening was able to use the same blood spot as the traditional Guthrie test), and universal newborn hearing screening programs are therefore expensive. Do they work, and are they worthwhile?

Permanent childhood hearing impairment may be described across many dimensions – by its severity, by the anatomical site of abnormality, by presence or absence of risk factors, by the timing of onset, and/or by etiology. The target of universal newborn hearing screening programs is congenital permanent hearing loss, which is usually considered to include deafness that develops at or very soon after birth (for example, related to prematurity, birth asphyxia, or severe jaundice). Both congenital and acquired losses may be progressive, i.e., may worsen over time. Permanent hearing losses may be due to outer or middle ear abnormality (conductive losses), cochlear abnormality (the most common site of abnormality detected through newborn screening programs) or neural problems (exceedingly rare in healthy babies, but accounting for up to 10% of permanent losses in NICU graduates).

Hearing impairment is often described as the pure tone average hearing threshold in the better ear across a number of frequencies (usually 0·5, 1, 2, and 4 kHz) and is expressed as dB HL (decibels hearing loss) on a logarithmic scale. Based on the distribution of the normal curve, <15 dB HL is considered "normal" and therefore the optimal level of hearing for normal language development.[8] A loss of 35–40 dB HL or more in the better ear is usually considered to be educationally significant. However, since neither the lower limit above which detriment to speech and language occurs nor the point at which early intervention does more good than harm is known, cut-off points vary and are somewhat arbitrary. A typical hearing loss classification subdivides hearing losses into mild (for example, 25–39 dB HL), moderate (for example, 40–69 dB HL), severe (for example, 70–94 dB HL) and profound (for example, ≥ 95 dB HL).[9]

Two technologies are widely available to screen newborns for hearing loss at the bedside. Evoked otoacoustic emission (OAE) screening assesses the tiny responses that arise from the cochlear outer hair cells as they transduce sound to the inner ear, and requires a small probe to be placed briefly in each ear canal in turn. Automated auditory brainstem response (AABR) screening assesses the evoked potentials generated by the auditory nerve and the auditory pathway within the brainstem in response to brief sounds. It requires temporary placement of small skin electrodes, and either an ear muff or a probe in the baby's ear. OAE screening tends to be somewhat cheaper and quicker, while AABR can detect deafness due to auditory neuropathy (in which the outer ear functions normally, giving rise to normal OAE responses) and has a lower refer rate (i.e., lower false positive rate).

Framing answerable clinical questions

You are now concerned that your state's universal newborn hearing screening program may be falsely reassuring parents, and wonder how many children with congenital hearing losses are not detected by universal newborn hearing screening programs. You are also aware that parents in your practice have been worried when their child failed the newborn hearing screen, even though they subsequently passed a diagnostic hearing test. You want to know how many children are falsely referred, and how many of these parents

worry and/or have anxiety about this. Most of all, you want to know that it's all worthwhile – do newborn hearing screening programs actually make a difference to the long-term outcomes of otherwise-healthy children?

As always, you need to reframe these thoughts into answerable questions. Each question should include the patient/population; the intervention, event, or exposure (and comparison, if relevant); and the outcome of interest. The questions raised by these scenarios are related specifically to diagnosis, risk, and therapy. You formulate the following questions.

Questions

1. Do babies with congenital hearing loss (*population*) who undergo universal newborn hearing screening programs (*intervention*) have better language and quality of life (*outcomes*) than babies born in areas without such programs? **[Intervention]**

2. What is the sensitivity of universal newborn hearing screening programs (*outcome*) in detecting congenital hearing losses in healthy newborns (*population*)? **[Diagnosis]**

3. In parents (*population*) of babies with false positive screens in newborn hearing screening programs (*exposure*), what is the likelihood of anxiety, worry, and other negative emotions (*outcome*) compared to parents whose babies pass the screen (*comparator*)? **[Harm]** What proportion of parents is likely to experience unnecessary concern due to false positive screens?

Searching for evidence

Neither the BMJ publication *Clinical Evidence* nor the *ACP Journal Club* offer relevant titles. In the *Cochrane Library* (Issue 3, 2003), you enter the search term "hearing screening" and net one protocol on universal neonatal hearing screening versus selective screening[10] – but unfortunately this offers insufficient information to address your questions, and the 10 trials identified by the Cochrane Central Register of Controlled Trials are not relevant. However, the Database of Abstracts of Reviews of Effects (DARE) in the *Cochrane Library* yields four reviews, of which two seem particularly relevant.[11,12] In 1997, Davis *et al.* completed a critical review of the role of neonatal hearing screening in the detection of congenital hearing impairment for the UK Health Technology Assessment series. More recently, the US Agency for Healthcare Research and Quality (AHRQ, the health services research arm of the US Department of Health and Human Services) commissioned a systematic review of newborn hearing screening for the US Preventive Services Task Force. This was published by *JAMA* in abbreviated form in 2001[12] and in full at http://www.ahrq.gov/clinic/serfiles.htm.[13]

Because there has been an explosion of international literature on newborn hearing screening since 1997, the Davis critical review may already be out of date. You therefore take the 2001 AHRQ systematic review as your starting point for looking at the evidence to answer each of your questions, backed up by Medline searches for Australian literature that may shed additional light on your own local situation. In addition, a Google search of Australian web pages entering the term "child screening" directs you to a 2002 Australian National Health & Medical Research Council (NHMRC) document titled *Child Health Surveillance and Screening: A Critical Review of the Evidence* (http://www.nhmrc.gov.au/publications/synopses/ch42syn.htm), which contains a chapter on sensorineural hearing loss.

Critical review of the evidence

You begin by considering the criteria for appraising a systematic review, which are discussed in Chapter 8 on assessing systematic reviews and clinical guidelines. Systematic reviews require a declaration of intent and a transparency of methodology, and (like practice guidelines) depend on their currency and the quality of evidence available. The AHRQ systematic review posed four questions:

1 Can universal newborn hearing screening accurately diagnose moderate-to-profound sensorineural hearing impairment?
2 Does identification and treatment prior to the age of 6 months improve language and communication?
3 What are the potential adverse effects of screening and of early treatment?
4 What are the overall benefits versus harms?

Although not a Cochrane review, it appears to meet major Cochrane decision points and to have been well conducted with regard to prespecifying questions and inclusion/exclusion criteria, searching widely using appropriate search terms and individual contacts with experts, data extraction using prespecified criteria developed and recently updated by the US Preventive Services Task Force, assessment of methodological quality, and transparency of methodology.

Question

1. Do babies with congenital hearing loss (*population*) who undergo universal newborn hearing screening programs (*intervention*) have better language and quality of life (*outcomes*) than babies born in areas without such programs? **[Intervention]**

Very early detection of hearing loss should change several aspects of life for children with hearing impairment. Infants can be fitted with hearing aids, so that they effectively experience a lesser degree of hearing loss from very soon after birth. Second, early intervention should be qualitatively different, in that it can be geared towards promoting normal language in a developmentally-appropriate child (a *prevention model*), rather than towards ameliorating the language deficits that are otherwise virtually always present at presentation (a *treatment model*). Third, these infants may be early candidates for procedures such as cochlear implantation to permanently bypass the site of hearing loss. All these activities are geared primarily towards allowing the child the chance to achieve normal language and communication skills, which may be seen as the primary adverse outcome for hearing loss from which associated problems flow.

Before you address the question of whether newborn hearing screening leads to better outcomes, you want to know just how bad things are for school-aged children not exposed to newborn hearing screening programs. For otherwise healthy children, is hearing loss really still such a disability in this era of sophisticated hearing aids, cochlear implantation, and early intervention techniques? You are aware that outcomes are often very poor, but also that much of the current literature is based on biased samples, so that children with profound losses and those attending special educational settings are overrepresented in widely quoted figures such as those published annually by the American Gallaudet Research Institute.[14] Australian children generally have excellent access to hearing aids and to early intervention services – perhaps they do better? A population-based study of 7–8-year-old children with congenital aided hearing loss living in the state of Victoria indicates not: language scores are about 1·5 standard deviations lower than that of children in normative populations, even in the absence of intellectual disability (Table 19.1).[15]

Unfortunately, it is immediately clear that no randomized controlled trials examining long-term outcomes have been conducted. The AHRQ systematic review sought evidence that language outcomes of infants with hearing impairment are better when a newborn screening program is in place. The one controlled trial of universal newborn hearing screening reported higher rates of detection of children under 6 months of age,[9] but has not yet reported on language outcomes for these children at later ages. Only one study to date has compared language performance of hearing-impaired children born in hospitals with universal hearing screening programs with hearing-impaired children born in hospitals without such programs, and this study included just 25 children in each group.[16] The differences between the two groups were striking: 56% of the screened group, compared to 24% of the unscreened group, had language scores in the normal range at 2–4 years, and mean standard language scores were 18–21 points higher (mean expressive language score 82·9 *v* 62·1;

Table 19.1 Outcomes for a population sample of 7–8-year-old children with aided congenital hearing loss and without intellectual disability, compared to standardized measures for same-age normative populations[15]

	Congenital hearing loss			Population			
	N	Mean	SD	N	Mean	SD	P
Language							
CELF Total	83	76·5	21·3	2450	100	15	<0·0001
CELF Receptive	85	80·7	22·3	2450	100	15	<0·0001
CELF Expressive	83	73·8	21·5	2450	100	15	<0·0001
PPVT	85	77·8	17·9	2725	100	15	<0·0001
Adaptive skills							
Vineland	85	93·3	18·0	3000	100	15	<0·001
Health-related quality of life							
CHQ Physical Summary	81	53·5	9·7	865	52·4	7·2	0·2
CHQ Psychosocial Summary	81	49·2	9·6	865	53·1	8·2	<0·001
School functioning							
Academic skills	83	2·4	0·74	96	1·4	0·50	<0·0001
Temporal sequential processing abilities	83	2·1	0·59	96	1·4	0·46	<0·0001
Linguistic skills	83	2·5	0·69	96	1·4	0·51	<0·0001
Coordination skills	83	2·2	0·53	96	1·5	0·41	<0·0001
Attitude towards work	83	2·1	0·74	96	1·5	0·42	<0·0001
Creative skills	83	2·2	0·49	96	1·7	0·41	<0·0001

Abbreviations: CELF, Clinical Examination of Language Fundamentals-3; Vineland, Vineland Adaptive Behavior Scales; CHQ, Child Health Questionnaire; School Functioning, School Functioning, Questionnaire

mean receptive language score 81·5 *v* 66·8; mean total language score 82·2 *v* 64·4, all *P* < 0·001). However, the study was deemed to be of poor quality, based on potential uncontrolled baseline differences between the groups, lack of blinding, and lack of information about exclusion criteria or loss to follow up.[12]

Therefore, you need to reconsider the approach to your main question. Your fall-back position is to find good, unbiased, population-based prospective studies to address your new question, "Is early detection of moderate or greater congenital hearing loss associated with better language outcomes than late detection?" These also seem to be in short supply. The AHRQ systematic review cited a further eight poor to fair papers reporting retrospective findings from three early intervention programs comparing early- and late-identified children with impaired hearing from within their respective programs. Each of the three programs concluded that earlier diagnosis was associated with improved language outcomes during the preschool years. One of the six papers from the Colorado Newborn Hearing Screening Project[17] has been particularly influential in convincing policy makers and funding bodies internationally to subsequently fund universal newborn hearing screening programs. In this paper, Yoshinaga-Itano reported significantly higher receptive, expressive and total language scores for children identified ≤ 6 months versus > 6 months of age (mean total language quotients 79·0 *v* 63·8

(all children), 91·3 *v* 70·2 (children with IQ ≥ 80), and 59·6 *v* 51·7 (children with IQ < 80), all *P* < 0·001; mean language quotients in normative population 100, SD 15).

The systematic review criticized all eight papers for using convenience samples, not stating clear inclusion criteria, non-blinded outcome assessment, and lack of intention-to-treat analyses (i.e., increasing the chance of bias by only including results for children who had remained with the program to outcome). As a result, the task force "rated the strength of evidence linking early treatment with improved language function 'inconclusive' and the quality of evidence as 'fair/poor'".[12] While you accept that this is not a satisfactory state of affairs, you feel reassured by the uniformity of the findings of benefit and the lack of evidence of harm.

The AHRQ systematic review did not examine health-related quality of life (HRQOL) outcomes for children with hearing loss. A brief Medline search using the terms "quality of life" OR "health status", AND "neonatal screening", "hearing disorders", "deafness" OR "hearing loss, sensorineural", limited to infants and children, identifies no papers addressing this issue. This seems a major omission. The ultimate, though often unstated, aim of screening programs is to improve health status and long-term quality of life. In the absence of randomized controlled trials of newborn hearing screening, outcome studies of HRQOL in older children would provide a baseline against which improvements following the introduction of newborn hearing screening programs could later be judged. Longitudinal modeling might then shed light on the proportions of outcome variance in HRQOL that might, or might not, reasonably be expected to be modified by very early detection.

Question

2. What is the sensitivity of universal newborn hearing screening programs (*outcome*) in detecting congenital hearing losses in healthy newborns (*population*)? **[Diagnosis]**

Sensitivity values are usually derived from knowledge of how a screening test performs against a gold standard. Essentially, it requires knowledge of the true positive rate and of *either* the false negative rate *or* the prevalence of the condition in the population setting. If true positive and false negative rates cannot be accurately determined (for example, because there is no gold standard diagnostic test suitable for use at a population level), then sensitivity can be estimated from detection rates of the screening program compared to the underlying prevalence – if this is known.

For congenital hearing loss, you immediately see that no population studies have tested newborn hearing screening programs against an adequate concurrent gold standard. You realize that this is not really surprising – there *is* no true gold standard for newborn hearing, since the gold standard is a subjective response to pure-tone audiometry (i.e., a person indicating he/she can hear a sound of a particular frequency and loudness), which is totally unreliable in newborns. With this in mind, three types of study might provide convergent evidence:

- concurrent validation of the newborn screen against objective physiological tests such as diagnostic auditory brainstem response (ABR) and/or steady-state evoked potential (SSEP) testing;
- delayed validation of the newborn screen against behavioral testing when the child is old enough (usually about 8 months of age); and
- comparison of program detection rates against estimated prevalence derived from retrospective population-based ascertainment of hearing losses believed to be congenital.

Concurrent ABR or SSEP gold standard testing is not feasible at a population level, since the target condition (congenital hearing loss > 40 dB HL in the better ear) is rare with an estimated prevalence in healthy newborns of just one in every 2–3000. Therefore, if you assumed 90% sensitivity, about 20–30 000 babies would need concurrent diagnostic ABR or SSEP (which takes about an hour with a sleeping or sedated baby) to find a single baby with the target condition who was missed by the screening program. Studies using concurrent electrophysiologic tests as a quasi-gold standard have addressed yield and false positive rates reasonably well, but have been far too small to adequately tackle sensitivity.[18–21]

One well-conducted prospective study has attempted to estimate program sensitivity of a newborn screening program against subjective hearing levels in older infants. The Multicenter Consortium on Identification of Neonatal Hearing Impairment[22] measured the sensitivity and specificity of OAE and AABR in the neonatal period against visual reinforcement audiometry at ages 8–12 months (the youngest age at which behavioral audiometry becomes possible). Even though NICU babies were heavily oversampled, the yield for non-NICU babies could still be estimated at 1 in 2348 low-risk infants (0·42/1000). Overall, the protocol (OAE followed by AABR) missed 11% of ears with moderate to profound permanent hearing loss in the better ear at 8–12 months. However, this study is now a decade old and you are aware that screening technologies have moved rapidly in that time. Further, this study might have overestimated prevalence since there is no way to know whether hearing losses present at 8–12 months were truly present in the newborn period.

You decide to verify this estimate by looking at the best available studies of detection rates from screening programs against the best available epidemiologic studies ascertaining underlying prevalence. The AHRQ systematic review identified two good-quality studies addressing detection rates, the Wessex Universal Neonatal Hearing Screening Trial[9] and the New York State Universal Newborn Hearing Screening Demonstration Project.[23] To identify one case, 2794 and 2041 low-risk newborns were screened in the respective studies (0·35/1000 and 0·49/1000 respectively). The overall yields, including both low- and high-risk infants, were 1·08/1000 and 0·70/1000 respectively. The Wessex study remains the only controlled quasi-randomized trial of universal newborn hearing screening versus "standard practice" in an area with a high-risk detection system already in place, and was able to convincingly demonstrate much earlier detection and intervention in the universally screened group compared to the "standard practice" group.

You next try to estimate underlying prevalence of congenital hearing loss > 40 dB HL in the better ear. You exclude several studies which based their estimates on the findings of universal newborn hearing screening programs,[12,24,25] since this would artificially ensure 100% sensitivity. You examine three well-conducted retrospective epidemiologic studies that comprehensively tried to ascertain prevalence of congenital hearing losses at a population level – the Trent Ascertainment Study[26] from England, a study of children born in the Austrian Tyrol 1980–1994,[27] and the Victorian Infant Hearing Screening Program[28] from Australia, which may have relevance for your own local situation. The

Trent and Victorian studies both estimated the prevalence of permanent hearing losses > 40 dB HL that were probably congenital to be about 1·1/1000, with the Austrian estimate (using the oldest data) marginally higher at 1·27/1000 newborns.

Finally, therefore, you are ready to construct a 2 × 2 table to estimate sensitivity (it will also let you estimate specificity, positive predictive value, negative predictive value, etc.). You take your base prevalence to be 1·1/1000, the yield to be 0·89/1000 (the midpoint of the Wessex and New York State projects), and the referral rate to be 1·6/1000 (from the Wessex study, since the New York State project lost many children before the second-stage screen). This leads to Table 19.2.

From this table, you derive a program sensitivity of 89/110 = 81%, specificity of 98 379/99 890 = 98%, false positive rate of 94%, and positive likelihood ratio of 0·81/0·015 = 54.

Because of the pace of technological development and expertise, you also look for more up-to-date information on large programs. Knowing that a national population-based English Newborn Hearing Screening Program is in the implementation phase, you find posted a recent presentation given by the Director of the English program, Professor Adrian Davis, reporting on 40 504 babies (97% coverage of all births) screened in 12 sites (http://www.nhsp.info/presentations/panLondon210703/AD Talk.pdf). Slide 72 of this talk reports that the yield of bilateral cases (> 40 dB HL) is 40/40 504 (1/1000) and of unilateral cases is 25/40 504 (0·6/1000). You submit an email query to the program via the homepage of this same website, and the email reply gives an updated figure of 71 bilateral cases for the first 74 740 babies (0·95/1000) screened by the program. With such large numbers and again assuming a baseline prevalence of 1·1/1000, you accept that program sensitivity of new programs should probably now run at close to 90%.

However, your own Australian state program recently reported a detection rate of just 0·68/1000 babies

Table 19.2 2 × 2 table to estimate sensitivity and specificity of a universal newborn hearing screening program using a two-stage OAE/AABR protocol for well babies and AABR/AABR protocol for NICU babies

	Congenital hearing loss > 40 dB HL		
	Yes	No	Totals
Failed screening protocol	89	1511	1600
Passed screening protocol	21	98 379	98 400
Totals	110	99 890	100 000

screened.[29] This seems rather low, given that you are now confident that the prevalence of congenital moderate or worse hearing loss in Australia is the same as elsewhere – about 1·1/1000.[20] However, with only 12 708 babies screened so far, the 95% confidence interval is wide (0·31–1·28/1000) and includes the expected detection rate of 0·9–1·0/1000. You conclude that the program needs to run for another year or two before the true detection rate can be more precisely estimated.

Question

3. In parents (*population*) of babies with false positive screens in newborn hearing screening programs (*exposure*), what is the likelihood of anxiety, worry, and other negative emotions (*outcome*) compared with parents whose babies pass the screen (*comparator*)? **[Harm]** What proportion of parents is likely to experience unnecessary concern due to false positive screens?

Screening for childhood conditions can lead to lasting distress and misperceptions about the child's health, even when diagnostic testing reveals no abnormality. A classic example is the long-term impact of innocent cardiac murmurs, with many parents continuing to perceive and treat their child as vulnerable and different, long after a structurally normal heart has been demonstrated to them.[30,31] False positive screens for Down's syndrome devastate many mothers in the early stages of pregnancy, until the diagnosis can be definitively excluded by chorionic villus sampling or amniocentesis some weeks later.

Not surprisingly, the only controlled trial addressing this question for newborn hearing screening identified by the AHRQ systematic review was the Wessex study.[9] Parents in the screened and unscreened groups were reported to experience similar overall general anxiety levels, but published details are scant.

You reframe your question to ask whether parents of babies with false positive screens (*population*) in newborn hearing screening programs (*exposure*) report more anxiety, worry, and/or other negative emotions (*outcome*) than parents whose babies who pass the screen (*comparator*). Several papers address this question. The Wessex study noted that the program did not lead to increased maternal state, or trait anxiety, or more negative attitudes toward the baby 2–10 months after a failed screen, compared with mothers whose babies passed the screen.[32] However, it did not report on *ongoing* parent concern about hearing, language, or development, or more specific residual anxieties than can be measured with the State-Trait Anxiety Inventory. Three other reasonable quality studies did note more self-reported distress and worry in parents whose babies failed than those whose babies passed immediately after the screen, but this was generally not severe and usually subsided once diagnostic audiology confirmed normal hearing.[33–35] Significant or lasting anxiety was reported by 3·5–14% of parents whose babies had false positive screens. This sounds like a lot of parents, until you extrapolate from the AHRQ's estimate of 254 false positive results per 10 000 babies to estimate that 0·09–0·35% of all parents (i.e., 3·5–14% of 2·54%) will experience significant or lasting anxiety due to false positive screens. This equates to 1–3 parents suffering unnecessary anxiety for every baby correctly diagnosed. Given that such anxiety is usually mild and time-limited, you feel that this is probably acceptable – but make a note to yourself to look out for studies examining longer term impacts on parent concern about child hearing, language and well-being.

Resolution of the scenario

With approximately 10% of congenital hearing losses missed by universal newborn hearing screening programs, it is possible that this child had a moderate or greater hearing loss at birth that was genuinely missed by your local program. Perhaps more likely, she may have been born with a mild hearing loss (25–40 dB HL, which would not be detected by the program) that has since worsened somewhat. Alternately, she may have a true acquired loss (estimated prevalence 0·15/1000),[28] though she has no obvious precipitant (such as meningitis, head injury, high dose aminoglycoside). Multidisciplinary assessment may help determine which of these scenarios is most likely.

She is referred for a full assessment and diagnostic workup, including cranial imaging, genetic evaluation including testing for mutations in the Connexin 26 and Pendrin genes, ophthalmologic examination, ENT assessment, and detailed audiologic assessment of the child, her sister, and both parents. She is also referred for immediate entry to an early intervention program and for fitting of digital hearing aids. Her parents accept counseling as to possible causes and prognosis of her hearing loss, but at this stage decline advice about risks of recurrence in future children on the basis that their family is complete and they have enough to adjust to right now. Over this period you see the child and her parents several times and your impression of an intelligent child living with articulate, caring, and involved parents strengthens. Knowing that family involvement is one of the strongest predictors of outcome so far identified,[36] you feel reasonably optimistic about this child's long-term language development.

Overall, while disappointed about the quality of the evidence relating to newborn hearing screening programs, you are convinced that the evidence points to greatly increased early detection rates and most likely to improved outcomes, with an acceptably low false negative rate and limited parent distress due to false positive screens.

Future research needs

- Many states and countries are implementing large-scale newborn hearing screening programs in the period 2000–2005. Given that a randomized controlled trial seems unlikely ever to be conducted, either of two possible research designs would help determine the long-term impacts of universal newborn hearing screening:
  - *within region* – comparing outcomes for population cohorts of children with congenital hearing losses born before and after implementation of the program;
  - *between region* – comparing outcomes for parallel population cohorts of children with congenital hearing losses born in regions with and without a program.

- Outcome studies should follow population cohorts of children into the school years, and broaden their focus to include quality of life.

- Longer term studies should examine potential harms of newborn hearing screening programs, including:
  - parental anxieties and concerns relating to true and false positives;
  - implications (such as tympanostomy tubes) of early detection of middle ear effusion that would otherwise have gone unnoticed;
  - impact and management of mild (25–40 dB HL) congenital hearing losses detected as a result of programs where the target condition is moderate or greater losses.

- Research (preferably randomized controlled trials) would be useful into optimal management strategies for congenital hearing losses detected in the first 6 months of life.

Summary table

Question	Type of evidence	Results	Comments
Do newborn hearing screening programs result in better outcomes?	Systematic review	No evidence for or against improved language or quality of life outcomes with earlier detection	1 good quality RCT showing earlier detection; 8 poor-to-fair quality observational studies, no RCTs of outcomes
What is the sensitivity of screening programs in detecting infants with congenital hearing loss?	3 prospective observational studies	Sensitivity probably around 90%, specificity around 98%	Rapid evolution of screening technologies and low prevalence make stable estimates difficult
What is the likelihood of emotional distress in parents of infants with false positive screening tests?	4 observational studies	About 1–3 parents experience unnecessary significant or lasting anxiety for every child correctly diagnosed	No studies of longer term outcomes

References

1 Helfand M, Thompson D, Davis R, McPhillips H, Homer C, Lieu T. *Newborn Hearing Screening. Systematic Evidence Review Number 5* (Contract 290-97-0018 to the Oregon Health & Science University Evidence-based Practice Center, Portland, Oregon). AHRQ Publication No. 02-S001. Rockville, MD: Agency for Healthcare Research and Quality; 2001.

2 Davis A, Hind S. The impact of hearing impairment: a global health problem. *Int J Pediatr Otorhinolaryngol* 1999; **49**(Suppl.1):S51–S54.

3 van Eldik TT. Behavior problems with deaf Dutch boys. *Am Ann Deaf* 1994;**139**:394–9.

4 Vostanis P, Hayes M, Feu MD, Warren J. Detection of behavioural and emotional problems in deaf children and adolescents: comparison of two rating scales. *Child Care Health Devel* 1997;**23**:233–6.

5 Meadow-Orlans KP. Stress, support, and deafness: Perceptions of infants' mothers and fathers. *J Early Intervention* 1994;**18**:91–102.

6 Meadow-Orlans KP. Sources of stress for mothers and fathers of deaf and hard of hearing infants. *Am Ann Deaf* 1995;**140**:352–7.

7 Henggeler SW, Watson SM, Whelan JP, Malone CM. The adaptation of hearing parents of hearing-impaired youths. *Am Ann Deaf* 1990;**135**:211–16.

8 Northern JL. Hearing and Hearing Loss in Children. In *Hearing in Children, 4th edn.* Baltimore: Williams and Wilkins, 1991.

9 Wessex Universal Neonatal Hearing Screening Trial Group. Controlled trial of universal neonatal screening for early identification of permanent childhood hearing impairment. *Lancet* 1998;**352**:1957–64.

10 Puig T, Municio A, Universal neonatal hearing screening versus selective screening as part of the management of childhood deafness (Protocol for a Cochrane Review). In: *Cochrane Library*, Issue 3. Oxford: Update Software, 2003.

11 Davis A, Bamford J, Wilson I, Ramkalawan T, Forshaw M, Wright S. A critical review of the role of neonatal hearing screening in the detection of congenital hearing impairment. *Health Technol Assess* 1997;**1**:1–177.

12 Thompson DC, McPhillips H, Davis RL, Lieu TL, Homer CJ, Helfand M. Universal newborn hearing screening: summary of evidence. *JAMA* 2001;**286**:2000–10.

13 Newborn Hearing Screening: Systematic Evidence Review. Pub. No. AHRQ02–S001. http://www.ahrq.gov/clinic/uspstfix.htm.

14 Gallaudet Research Institute. Regional and National Summary Report of Data from the 2000–2001 *Annual Survey of Deaf and Hard of Hearing Children & Youth.* Washington, DC: GI, Gallaudet University, 2002.

15 Wake M, Hughes EK, Poulakis Z, Collins C, Rickards FW. Outcomes of mild-profound congenital hearing impairment at 7–8 years: a population study. *Ear Hear* 2004;**25**:1–8.

16 Yoshinaga-Itano C, Coulter D, Thomson V. The Colorado Newborn Hearing Screening Project: effects on speech and language development of children with hearing loss. *J Perinatol* 2000;**20**(Suppl.8):S132–S137.

17 Yoshinaga-Itano C, Sedey AL, Coulter DK, Mehl AL. Language of early- and later-identified children with hearing loss. *Pediatrics* 1998;**102**:1161–71.

18 Smyth V, McPherson B, Kei J *et al.* Otoacoustic emission criteria for neonatal hearing screening. *Int J Pediatr Otorhinolaryngol* 1999;**48**:9–15.

19 McNellis EL, Klein AJ. Pass/fail rates for repeated click-evoked otoacoustic emission and auditory brain stem response screenings in newborns. *Otolaryngol-Head Neck Surg* 1997;**116**:431–7.

20 Jacobson JT, Jacobson CA. The effects of noise in transient EOAE newborn hearing screening. *Int J Pediatr Otorhinolaryngol* 1994;**29**:235–48.

21 Schauseil-Zipf U, von Wedel H. [Hearing screening using acoustically evoked brain stem potentials in newborn infants and infants]. *Klinische Padiatrie* 1988;**200**:324–9.

22 Norton SJ, Gorga MP, Widen JE, Folsom RC, Sininger Y, Cone-Wesson B, Vohr BR, Fletcher KA. Identification of neonatal hearing impairment: a multicenter investigation. *Ear Hear* 2000;**21**:348–56.

23 Prieve BA, Stevens F. The New York State Universal Newborn Hearing Screening Demonstration Project: introduction and overview. *Ear Hear* 2000;**21**:85–91.

24 Aidan D, Avan P, Bonfils P. Auditory screening in neonates by means of transient evoked otoacoustic emissions: a report of 2,842 recordings. *Ann Otol Rhinol Laryngol* 1999; **108**(Suppl.6):525–31.

25 Watkin PM, Baldwin M. Confirmation of deafness in infancy. *Arch Dis Child* 1999;**81**:280–9.

26 Fortnum H, Davis A. Epidemiology of permanent childhood hearing impairment in Trent region, 1985–1993. *Br J Audiol* 1997;**31**:409–46.

27 Nekahm D, Weichbold V, Welzl Muller K. Epidemiology of permanent childhood hearing impairment in the Tyrol, 1980–1994. *Scand Audiol* 2001;**30**:197–202.

28 Russ SA, Poulakis Z, Barker M, Wake M, Rickards F, Saunders K, Oberklaid F. Congenital hearing loss in Victoria, Australia: A prospective epidemiologic study. *Int J Audiol* 2003;**42**:385–90

29 Bailey HD, Bower C, Krishnaswamy J, Coates HL. Newborn hearing screening in Western Australia. *Med J Austr* 2002; **177**:180–5.

30 Bergman AB, Stramm SJ. The morbidity of cardiac non-disease in school children. *N Engl J Med* 1967;**267**: 1008–13.

31 Young PC. The morbidity of cardiac nondisease revisited. Is there lingering concern associated with an innocent heart murmur? *Am J Dis Child* 1993;**147**:975–7.

32 Kennedy C. Controlled trial of universal neonatal screening for early identification of permanent childhood hearing impairment: `coverage, positive predictive value, effect on mothers and incremental yield. *Acta Paediatr* 1999; (Suppl.432):73–5.

33 Clemens CJ, Davis SA, Bailey AR. The "false positive" in universal newborn hearing screening. *Pediatrics* 2000;**106**: 7–11.

34 Watkin PM, Baldwin M, Dixon R, Beckman A. Maternal anxiety and attitudes to universal neonatal hearing screening. *Br J Audiol* 1998;**32**:27–37.

35 Barringer DH, Mauk GW. Survey of parents perceptions regarding hospital-based newborn hearing screening. *Audiol Today* 1997;**9**:18–19.

36 Moeller MP. Early intervention and language development in children who are deaf and hard of hearing. *Pediatrics* 2000;106(3). http://www/pediatrics.otg/cgi/content/full/ 106/3/43

20 Assessment of developmental delay

Louise Hartley, Alison Salt, Paul Gringras, Jon Dorling

Case scenario *A 7-year-old boy is referred to the child development center with concerns about developmental delay. On assessment, he is found to have moderate mental retardation (IQ 50). His parents are considering having another child.*

Background

Developmental delay is a common problem in pediatrics with an estimated population prevalence as high as 10%.[1-4] Developmental delay refers to a heterogeneous group of conditions that affect social, motor, communication, and cognitive skills, in isolation or in combination, and result from the consequences of genetic, chromosomal, infective and a variety of other processes.

There is no consensus on the choice of medical investigations for developmental delay. Clinicians have been shown to differ widely in the way they investigate children who present with developmental delay. A recent paper described the range of investigations requested by pediatricians in the London area when presented with the same common clinical scenario of a 3-year-old boy presenting with moderate developmental delay. The number of tests ordered by each pediatrician ranged from none to 15. Overall, 26 different medical investigations were selected. The four most common tests chosen were chromosome analysis, fragile X testing, amino acids, and thyroid functions. The cost of investigations chosen ranged from £0–1181 with a median cost of £386. Factors influencing the variations in clinical practice included a lack of consensus in the medical literature, and personal experience causing a biased, non-evidence-based approach to investigations.[5]

Over the last 10 years fragile X syndrome has been recognized as the second most common cause of mental retardation after Down's syndrome. The clinical features were first described as a triad of post-pubertal symptoms: moderate mental retardation with an IQ range 35–50, and elongated facies, with large everted ears and macro-orchidism.[6] This triad of symptoms has been said to be seen in 60% of fragile X males, and the variation in their severity is wide even within families. In males, early symptoms are speech and language delay, hyperactivity with short attention span, poor eye contact, a reluctance to be touched, and confused speech. Female heterozygotes for fragile X syndrome are either normal carriers or show a broad clinical spectrum with one-third being intellectually impaired.

Sutherland reported a reproducible cytogenetic test for the condition in 1977,[7] but since 1991 molecular diagnosis has been possible and is becoming the preferred method of testing.[8]

In this chapter, we provide a model for clinicians for thinking through the issues involved in assessment of developmental delay and a way of incorporating evidence into your thinking. As the topic is very large, we have chosen one common example to illustrate the process. The prevalence of a particular disorder in different patient groups or populations will influence the outcome of any diagnostic investigations (see Chapter 5). Thus, our results may not be generalizable to every situation, but our methods will be.

Framing answerable clinical questions

Perhaps one of the most common questions asked in a child development clinic is about diagnosis in a child with global developmental delay or mental retardation. The following questions come to mind.

- What is the benefit of making an early diagnosis: would it alter management and what "bad outcomes" would be prevented?
- Is there likely to be an identifiable underlying genetic cause of relevance to future pregnancies/siblings?
- What is the likelihood of fragile X?
- Do children with fragile X present in this way?
- How will family history (for example, of mental retardation or psychiatric illness) or dysmorphic features on examination alter the yield from diagnostic investigations?

● Should all children presenting with global developmental delay be tested for fragile X?

Your questions can be refined to structured, specific questions.

Questions

1. In a school-aged boy *(population)* with moderate mental retardation *(exposure)*, what is the risk of a problem, such as hypothyroidism or an inborn error of metabolism, that will improve with specific intervention *(outcome)*? **[Baseline Risk]**
2. In a 7-year-old boy *(population)* with mental retardation who does not have a diagnosis remediable to specific interventions *(exposure)*, what is the risk of fragile X *(outcome)*? **[Baseline Risk]**
3. In a boy with mental retardation *(population)*, and "no dysmorphic features" *(negative test result)*, what is the risk of fragile X *(outcome)*? **[Baseline Risk]**
4. In a boy with mental retardation *(population)*, with dysmorphic features *(positive test result)*, what is the risk of fragile X *(outcome)*? **[Baseline Risk]**
5. In a boy with mental retardation *(population)*, does knowing the diagnosis of fragile X *(exposure)* improve his parents' ability to plan and cope *(outcome)*? **[Intervention/Therapy]**

Searching for evidence

You start with a search for systematic reviews and other critically appraised and predigested evidence. You reach for the most concise source you know of, the British publication *Clinical Evidence*,[9] but there is no chapter on child development.

Searching for evidence syntheses

● *Clinical Evidence*: not covered
● *Cochrane Library*: "development AND child"
● MedLine (Ovid) "child development" limited to guideline: "Fragile X" limited to guideline

Next you examine the *Cochrane Library* for information on developmental assessment in children. Entering the search terms "development AND child" nets 375 completed reviews and 149 protocols. On review of these, however, you find that none specifically addresses investigation of developmental problems in children. The Database of Abstracts of Reviews of Effects (DARE) in the *Cochrane Library* has no reviews on the topic of developmental disorders in children.

Next, you go to MedLine, still seeking a high-quality evidence synthesis. You use the limit setting facility, choosing "meta-analysis" from the "publication type" options and apply this limit to the MeSH headings "fragile X" and "child

development". No publications are found. You change your limit to "review", finding eight publications but no relevant guidelines. Because no relevant synthesized evidence exists to help answer your questions you develop specific search strategies.

Critical appraisal of the evidence

Question

1. In a school-aged boy *(population)* with moderate mental retardation *(exposure)*, what is the risk of a problem, such as hypothyroidism or an inborn error of metabolism, that will improve with specific intervention *(outcome)*? **[Baseline Risk]**

Search

● MedLine (PubMed Clinical Queries): development AND child [prognosis and specificity] then development AND child [diagnosis and specificity]

To answer your first question, you start your search looking for a prospective, population-based cohort design or cross-sectional study that will provide the relevant prevalence for treatable conditions likely to present as non-progressive mental retardation at the age of 7 years. Hypothyroidism and some inborn errors of metabolism are the most common of the few remediable conditions that you believe may present at this age. Your careful search of MedLine using PubMed reveals no studies that specifically address your question. This is not surprising as these conditions have a very low prevalence and very large studies would be required. You change your search to look at diagnosis and specificity but again find no studies specifically addressing the question. You decide to look at textbooks as a possible alternative source of this type of information.

Typically the proportion of children with severe mental retardation found to have an organic cause is reported as 55–57%.[10–12] The major identifiable causes of severe mental retardation as reported in major textbooks are shown in the box below.

Major identifiable causes of severe mental retardation

● Chromosomal abnormalities overall: 30%
● Down's syndrome: ≈ 20%
● Fragile X syndrome: 1–6%
● All other identifiable anomalies: 4–5%
● Endocrine and metabolic causes: 3–5%
● Identifiable multiple congenital anomalies: 4–5%

- Injury (including teratogens, pre-, peri-, and postnatal injuries): 15–20%
- CNS malformations (such as neural tube defects, hydrancephaly, microcephaly, and hydrocephalus): 10–15%

In your child, with moderate mental retardation at age 7, congenital hypothyroidism and phenylketonuria (PKU) should have been excluded at birth. The results of these screening tests could be reviewed before proceeding with further investigation. A hand search of books in the library tells you that congenital hypothyroidism is by far the most common cause of hypothyroidism in children, occurring in 1:4500 live births. Your hand search of updates in current pediatric practice reveals a review of large US screening programs[13] that suggests with careful follow up 1:35 000 children screened may be missed (either through procedural errors or because of the nature of their disease and screening procedure used – for example, in hypothyroidism associated with low TSH). However, all of these children had presented symptomatically by 3–4 months.

The most common cause of acquired hypothyroidism that may present in childhood is autoimmune thyroiditis. This condition has a reported prevalence of 0·3–1·5 cases per 1000 population (all ages). Presentation of this condition is usually insidious over 3 or 4 years and is associated with other symptoms, especially growth failure. However, after the age of 3 years, hypothyroidism does not lead to mental retardation. Therefore, although you are unable to find any primary research evidence, your review of current knowledge in recent textbooks suggests that treatable hypothyroidism presenting at this age is extremely unlikely.

Are there any treatable inborn errors of metabolism that are likely to present with mental retardation at this age? Again neonatal screening programs for PKU and galactosemia will pick up the most common remediable conditions. Maple syrup urine disease and homocystinuria are likely to present earlier and with characteristic associated features. Mucopolysaccharidoses with less prominent physical features (for example, Morquio's syndrome) may present with relatively asymptomatic mental retardation but treatment options (for example, bone marrow transplantation) are still limited.

Therefore it would appear that there is little evidence to support investigation for hypothyroidism or for inborn errors of metabolism in children with asymptomatic mental retardation. There is, therefore, little evidence that investigation for remediable conditions at this age will be very fruitful.

Question

2. In a 7-year-old boy *(population)* with mental retardation who does not have a diagnosis remediable to specific interventions *(exposure)*, what is the risk of fragile X *(outcome)*? **[Baseline Risk]**

Table 20.1 Results of MedLine and EMBASE search

Terms	MedLine	EMBASE
1. Preval*	17 3743	14 0473
2. Fragile x.tw.	2316	2117
3. exp "Fragile-X-Syndrome"	2382	2341
4. 2 or 3	2763	2609
5. 1 and 4	145	149

Search

- MedLine 1966 to present and EMBASE (Ovid): fragile X (text or MeSH heading) AND prevalence

The results of this search are given in Table 20.1.

In considering the clinical outcome of fragile X, you need to know the prevalence of fragile X in a population of children with moderate learning difficulty. In this case, the initial starting points are choosing both the best estimate for fragile X prevalence in the general population, and then the best estimate for fragile X amongst children with learning disabilities.

From the papers found in your search, 24 are relevant to the question and describe population-based studies of the prevalence of fragile X. It quickly becomes clear that changes in technology have resulted in profound changes to prevalence estimates in this condition. The first estimates of the prevalence of fragile X syndrome, based on cytogenetic testing, were 1/1000–1/2600 for males. The later cloning of the fragile X mental retardation gene (FMR1) in 1991 enabled an accurate molecular diagnosis. Since cytogenetic testing lacks sensitivity and specificity with both false positive and false negative cases, prevalence studies before 1991 that used cytogenetic analysis should be excluded.

From the 12 studies remaining you select the three studies that best meet the following criteria:

- Was case definition clear?
- Was case ascertainment complete?
- Were details of non-responders/non-tested clear?
- Was the population studied representative of that from which your case came?
- Did prevalence estimates include confidence intervals and take into account the possibility of different disease rates in the non-responders?

From these you decide to start with the Murray *et al.* study[14] as being most suitable to answer your question because it was limited to boys, used a population rather than an institutional sample, and only tested people aged 18 or younger. Your concerns about the suitability of this publication relate to issues of case definition and incomplete uptake of testing. The principal problem with the case definition is that the degree of mental retardation in this population, and the distribution of IQs, is not known. The low prevalence of fragile X suggests that this is a relatively low risk population, or higher IQ, sample than other studies. With regard to incomplete testing, only 70% of children with special educational needs were tested and no information is available about non-responders. However, the prevalence estimate of fragile X from this study would only be affected if children with fragile X were less or more likely to participate. Calculations that vary the assumed relative prevalence in the non-participating group (half or double that of the participating group) give a prevalence range between 1/3990 and 1/6171 respectively. These estimates overlap with estimates from other studies identified by your search (1/6045 in de Vries *et al.*[15] and 1/5000 in Turner *et al.*[16]) Using the same method, the range of prevalence in Murray's learning disabled boys sample lies between 1/162 and 1/250 respectively (0·6–0·4%).

You then read the study by Crawford *et al.*[18] One advantage of this study is that it looks at a population of 7–10 year olds, i.e., similar in age to your child. This is a population of African-American males and the prevalence is higher than in the Caucasian studies at 1 in 2545, although the confidence intervals overlap with other studies (1/5208–1/1289). However the study is flawed by the low participation rate of 43%. Because of your concerns about these papers, you read the study by de Vries as well.[15] The advantage of this study is that the learning disabled population was stratified into mild and moderate/severe learning difficulty. Unfortunately, the calculations in this paper excluded those who already had a diagnosis of fragile X. These cases need to be included to develop accurate prevalence figures. In addition, the figures calculated will vary depending on which denominator is used. Assuming a similar prevalence of fragile X among the 30% of non-responders and adding known fragile X and new diagnoses to the numerator produces an estimate of prevalence of fragile X for mild mental retardation of 1/50 (95% CI 1/32–1/125) and 1/40 for moderate/severe mental retardation (95% CI 1/30–1/62). In your 7-year-old child presenting with moderate intellectual impairment you could estimate the prior probability of his having fragile X as somewhere between 1/40 and 1/250, and you would therefore need to test between 40 and 250 children to find one child with fragile X.

Questions

3. In a boy with mental retardation *(population)*, and "no dysmorphic features" *(negative test result)*, what is the risk of fragile X *(outcome)*? **[Baseline Risk]**

4. In a boy with mental retardation *(population)*, with dysmorphic features *(positive test result)*, what is the risk of fragile X *(outcome)*? **[Baseline Risk]**

Search

● MedLine (PubMed Clinical Queries): fragile X, diagnosis and specificity

To answer these questions, you access the internet in the library and decide to search MedLine at the PubMed site on the Clinical Queries screen, which uses methodological search filters to enable rapid retrieval of sound clinical studies (see Chapter 3).

Using "specificity" in order to confine your search to the most relevant and sound studies about diagnostic tests, you enter "Fragile X" into the search "box" and identify 60 papers. You quickly discard 53: 43 address technical issues of molecular and cytogenetic tests and the other 10 look at premature ovarian failure in FRAXA premutation, female brain volumes in quantitative neuroimaging in fragile X patients, the prevalence of fragile X in specific groups, and the healthcare economics and philosophy of predictive testing for fragile X.

You select the papers that evaluate the precision with which physical or behavioral (phenotypic) features can predict fragile X. Three of these papers used cytogenetic tests as their reference diagnostic test and, as already discussed, you know this to be unreliable. Four of these papers used molecular tests as the reference and clinical criteria to select which children among a population of mentally retarded children would have the highest probability of testing positive for fragile X.[15,17,19] The study by Teisl *et al.*[19] looked only at behavioral features, so you also exclude that one.

The paper by Giangreco *et al.*[17] sets out to refine previously defined checklists of physical and behavioral characteristics associated with fragile X, to provide simplified criteria for fragile X syndrome testing in children. They develop a six-item checklist with a scoring system as shown in Table 20.2.

In this study, a score of 5 or more, of a possible total score of 12, was found to identify all children with fragile X. To appraise this article critically, you consider the identification of these features as a "diagnostic test" for fragile X, with molecular testing as the gold standard, and use the guidelines from Chapter 5.

In this study all patients underwent the reference test, which is the molecular PCR technique to quantify the triplet repeat expansion in the FMR1 gene. The major weakness of this study is that it was done retrospectively, and there is no mention in the methods section of whether the people applying the "diagnostic test" were blinded to the fragile X molecular status of the patients. If the clinical testers were

Table 20.2   Six-item checklist and scoring system[17]

Characteristics checklist	Score		
	0	1	2
Mental retardation	IQ > 85	IQ > 70–85	IQ < 70
Family history	None	Maternal female with psychiatric disorder	Maternal history of X-linked mental retardation
Elongated face	Not present	Somewhat	Present
Large or prominent ears	Not present	Somewhat	Present
Attention deficit hyperactivity disorder	Not present	Hyperactivity	Present
Autistic-like behavior + tactile defensiveness, perseverative speech, hand flapping, poor eye contact	Not present	One behavior	More than one behavior

not blinded, the potential for biased assessment is high. Also, although the patients were both primary and secondary referrals to the service in the study, it is not clear if the provision of the genetic testing at the time of the study was unique to this service. If this were the case, then the service may have attracted a differentially selected sample, and the results may not be generalizable. In addition, all the children were referred specifically for fragile X testing and therefore (as the clinical features of fragile X are well known to clinicians) the children referred would already have had a high prevalence of fragile X. This may have affected test performance. The scoring system is clear but some of the physical features such as long face and large/prominent ears are subjective, and no absolute measurements are given so that the test could be applied objectively. Some of the behavioral characteristics may also be open to interpretation. The data necessary for the calculation of likelihood ratios (LRs) are presented in the paper as shown in Table 20.3.

In this study a negative result (those with a score < 5) will effectively *rule out* a diagnosis of fragile X because it is a high sensitivity test. An alternative way of looking at the information gathered is to consider the likelihood ratios (LR) generated for both positive and negative scoring system results. The negative LR of 0 leads us to the same conclusion as drawn above, i.e., if a child has a low score on the clinical assessment, he does not have fragile X.

- Pretest probability (prevalence) = (a+c)/(a+b+c+d) = 12/335 = 3·5%
- Post-test probability (from nomogram) = 8%

The calculated positive LR in this study is 2·5 (95% CI 2·2–2·9). In general, LRs of 2–5 only generate small changes in probability. Indeed this diagnostic test shifts the pretest probability of 3·5% to a post-test probability of having fragile X of 8·2%, i.e., with a score of ≥ 5, the chance of having fragile X will only increase by about 5%.

Table 20.3   Calculation of likelihood ratios

Score	Fragile X +	Fragile X −	Totals
Test score +	12	129	141
Test score −	0	194	194
Totals	12	323	335

- Sensitivity = a/(a+c) = 12/12 = 100%
- Specificity = d/(b+d) = 194/323 = 60%
- Likelihood ratio for a positive test result (LR+) = sens/(1 − spec) = 100/40 = 2·5
- Likelihood ratio for a negative test result (LR−) = (1 − sens)/spec = 0/60 = 0

The de Vries paper[15] used a similar scoring system. De Vries *et al.* used the phenotypic criteria as described by Laing *et al.*[20] and included family history of intellectual handicap, personality, prominent ears, elongated face, and body habitus. Scores were divided into three groups:

- low risk, when dysmorphic features suggested another diagnosis;
- medium risk, in the absence of dysmorphic features; and
- high risk, in the presence of typical fragile X syndrome characteristics.

This sample contained many adults in whom the phenotype is more characteristic than in children; nevertheless, the outcome of clinically looking at the cases and scoring them was similarly impressive. None of the low or medium scoring males had fragile X, with all the fragile X cases scoring in the high range (Table 20.4). This was a prospectively collected sample with examiners blind to the fragile X result.

With a high score as the cut-off, a standard 2 × 2 table has been constructed (Table 20.5).

Table 20.4 Phenotype scores in males

Phenotype score	Males
Low	0/223
Moderate	0/555
High	9/92
Total	9/870

Table 20.5 Standard 2 × 2 table

Score	Fragile X +	Fragile X −	Totals
Test score +	9	83	92
Test score −	0	778	778
	9	861	870

From the table, sensitivity, specificity, and positive and negative likelihood ratios can be calculated:

- Sensitivity = a/(a+c) = 9/9 = 100%
- Specificity = d/(b+d) = 778/861 = 90%
- LR for a positive test result (LR+) = sens/(− spec) = 100/10 = 10
- LR for a negative test result (LR−) = (1 − sens)/spec = 0/90 = 0

The LR in the de Vries study was high, (10; 95% CI 8·5–12·7), confirming our suspicion that the patients in his population showed more distinct features (analogous to having more severe disease and being older). Given that the confidence intervals for these positive LRs do not overlap it is unlikely that the variation is due to chance. This indicates how test performance, including LRs, can vary when a test is applied to different populations.

Tuncbilek's[21] study confirms the findings of both Giangreco and de Vries. Although this is a referred population, it is a prospective study in which the clinicians were blinded to the molecular diagnosis at the time of evaluation, which used the checklist devised by Hagerman *et al.*[22] The patients were again divided into three groups based on the checklist score and all the fragile X positive patients were in the high risk group. The advantage of this study is that the population studied was children only.

Although none of these studies is ideal, they all show that children who do not have the fragile X chromosomal abnormality can be correctly identified clinically, and that having clinically identified features increases the likelihood of a positive genetic test.

With an understanding of the possible prior probability of fragile X in your population, you can calculate whether identifying characteristic phenotypes ("the diagnostic test") will help in weighing the likely chance of missing children with the diagnosis against testing many children unnecessarily.

If your population were similar to that described by Murray,[14] a prevalence of 0·4% (the lowest possible estimate of prevalence), and the "diagnostic test" performed in the same way as described by Giangreco,[17] with an LR of 2·5, the post-test probability of having fragile X would have increased from 0·5% to 1·0%. However, the high sensitivity of the test suggests that, instead of testing 250 children before finding one child with fragile X, you could exclude 150 children (60%) from testing with minimal risk of missing a case.

De Vries *et al.*[15] suggest that, in a population of children with moderate or severe mental retardation, a higher prevalence may be expected (the highest estimate being of 3·3%). The prevalence in a population of moderately retarded children, in whom other diagnoses are not apparent, can be estimated from de Vries by excluding those with known diagnosis from the denominator, giving an estimate of the prevalence of 4%. The post-test probability therefore increases to 10%. In this case you would need to assess 24 children to find one with fragile X, nine children would be tested unnecessarily, and 14 could be excluded from testing.

Question

5. In a boy with mental retardation (*population*), does knowing the diagnosis of fragile X (*exposure*) improve his parents' ability to plan and cope (*outcome*)? **[Intervention Therapy]**

To answer this intervention question, you need evidence from either randomized controlled trials (RCTs) or cohort studies. You start by searching fragile X and parent mental health, limiting your search to controlled trials and cohort studies. Although you find some potentially relevant studies about these issues, you do not find anything directly related to the diagnosis of fragile X. Revising your search to "fragile X AND family" you find an article about family experience of the diagnosis of fragile X.[23] This is a retrospective questionnaire survey of parents of children with fragile X. The study has deficiencies in using a self-selected group of parents and the response rate is low (274 of 460 returned surveys fulfilled the criteria for the study). However, the number of respondents was high and the survey enabled the parents to describe the positive and negative outcomes for them of the diagnosis of fragile X. These are itemized in Table 20.6 which presents the most common values associated with making a diagnosis of fragile X in children with developmental delay.

Table 20.6 Parental perception of the benefits and challenges of a diagnosis of fragile X

Positive/benefits	Negative/challenges
Understanding the child and his/her behaviors and learning what to do for him/her	Having to reframe one's life, expectations for the child, and hopes for the future, not knowing how best to raise a child with fragile X syndrome
Finding out the cause of the child's problems, relieving guilt	Experiencing negative emotions (grief, loss, worry, guilt)
Informed reproductive decisions for self and the extended family	Effects on reproduction
Finding support networks and the services available	Difficulties gaining access to services and information, finding professionals who know about fragile X syndrome
Raising awareness/educating others	Explaining to others, dealing with others' responses/stigma
Hope for a cure	No cure/treatment
Personal growth	Stress on family members: dealing with the impact the diagnosis had on family members
	Dealing with insurance issues

Resolution of the scenario

In your 7-year-old child presenting with moderate intellectual impairment, you are now able to estimate the prior probability of his having fragile X as somewhere between 1/40 and 1/250; you would therefore need to test between 40 and 250 children to find one child with fragile X.

From the information you found to answer questions 3 and 4 you know that using a clinical scoring system may be helpful. According to the Giangreco study,[17] if this child had a score of < 5 for the features described, you could feel confident to rule out fragile X and not proceed to molecular testing.

As there is no well-established treatment option here, the benefit to the patient directly of making a diagnosis is marginal. The benefit of using this "clinical diagnostic test" is that children will not be subjected to an unnecessary blood test, and parents will be spared the anxiety of awaiting the results. There would also be benefits in reducing the cost of investigation. Currently a molecular test for fragile X costs approximately £100. In the lower prevalence example, not testing 150 children would save £15 000.

Although you are unable to find any evidence to support this specifically in relation to fragile X, you know from clinical experience that the resolution of diagnostic uncertainty can provide much relief and put a halt to further investigations as to the cause of the developmental delay (which may benefit patients in that they will not be subjected to more tests). It is clear that for the parents and relatives, the identification of female carriers may allow informed choice as to whether or not to proceed with at-risk pregnancies. The decisions that are made depend on the population from which the child comes and the values that the tester and the parents put on having a diagnosis versus the disadvantages of unnecessary testing.

Future research needs

- Evidence is needed to clarify the adverse effects of availability of this type of genetic information, so that parents and relatives can make informed choices about testing.
- Large prospective studies are needed of the prevalence of different causes of mental retardation in children.
- Blinded, prospective evaluations of the clinical signs of fragile X are needed to give more precise information on which to base decisions about the usefulness of investigation.

Summary table

Question	Type of evidence	Result	Comment
In a 7-year-old boy with moderate mental retardation			
What is the risk of a remediable condition?	Review of textbooks; no evidence from studies	Children with remediable mental retardation rarely present at this age	
What is the risk of fragile X?	2 prospective cohort studies	1/40 to 1/250 children with mild/moderate mental retardation	Differing populations with respect to degree of mental retardation and IQ distribution
What is the risk of fragile X, with and without dysmorphic features?	1 prospective/1 retrospective study	LR+ = 10 LR− = 0 LR+ = 2·5 LR− = 0	Prospective study, more high risk, and retrospective study open to bias
Does knowing the diagnosis help parents to plan and cope?	Retrospective study	Description of benefits and challenges of a diagnosis	Self-selected responders, low response rate (60%)

References

1 Drillen CM, Pickering RM, Drummond MB. Predictive value of screening for difficult areas of development. *Dev Med Child Neurol* 1988;**30**:294–305.

2 Smith D, Simmons ER. Rational diagnostic evaluation of the child with mental deficiency. *Am J Dis Child* 1975; **129**:1285.

3 Simeonsson RJ, Sharp MC. Developmental delays. In: Hoekelman RA, Friedman SB Nelson NM, Seidel HM, eds. *Primary paediatric care, 2nd edn.* St. Louis: Mosby-Year Book, 1992.

4 Batshaw ML. Mental retardation. *Pediat Clinics N Am* 1993;**40**:507–21.

5 Gringras P. Choice of medical investigations for developmental delay: a questionnaire survey. *Child Care Health Devel* 1998;**24**:267–76.

6 Fryns JP. X-Linked mental retardation and the fragile X syndrome: a clinical approach. In: Davies KE, ed. *The fragile X syndrome.* Oxford: Oxford University Press, 1989.

7 Sutherland GR. Fragile sites on human chromosomes: demonstration of their dependence on the type of tissue culture medium. *Science* 1977;**197**:265.

8 Fu YH, Kuhl DPA, Pizzuti A *et al.* Variation of the CGG repeat at the fragile X site results in genetic instability: resolution of the Sherman paradox. *Cell* 1990;**67**:1047–58.

9 *Clinical Evidence.* BMJ Publishing Group and American College of Physicians-American Society of Internal Medicine, updated every 6 months from 1999.

10 Broman S, Nichols PL, Shaughnessy P. Kennedy W. *Retardation in young children: a developmental study of cognitive deficit.* Hillsdale, NJ: Lawrence Erlbaum.

11 Gustavson KH, Holmgren G, Jonsell R, Son Blomquist HK. Severe mental retardation in children in a northern Swedish county. *J Mental Defic Res* 1977;**21**:161–81.

12 Einfield SL. Clinical assessment of 4500 developmental delayed individuals. *J Mental Defic Res* 1984;**28**: 129–42.

13 Fisher DA. Effectiveness of newborn screening programs for congenital hypothyroidism: prevalence of missed cases. *Pediatr Clin N Amer* 1987;**34**:881–90.

14 Murray A, Youings S, Dennis *et al.* Population screening at FRAXA and FRAXE loci: molecular analyses of boys with learning difficulties and their mothers. *Hum Mol Genet* 1996;**5**:727–35.

15 De Vries BBA, van den Ouweland AMW, Mohkamsing S *et al.* Screening and diagnosis for the fragile X syndrome among the mentally retarded: an epidemiological and psychological survey. *J Hum Genet* 1997;**61**:660–7.

16 Turner G, Robinson H, Webb T, Wake S. Prevalence of fragile X syndrome. *Am J Med Genet* 1996;**64**:196–7.

17 Giangreco CA, Steele MW, Aston CE, Cummins JH, Wenger SL. A simplified six-item checklist for screening for fragile X syndrome in the paediatric population. *J Pediatr* 1996;**129**:611–14.

18 Crawford DC, Meadows KL, Newman JL *et al.* Prevalence of the fragile X syndrome in African-Americans. *Am J Med Genet* 2002;**110**:226–33.

19 Teisl JT, Reiss AL, Mazzocco MM. Maximising the sensitivity of a screening questionnaire for determining Fragile X at-risk status. *Am J Med Genet* 1999;**83**:281–5.

20 Laing S, Partington M, Robinson H, Turner G. Clinical screening score for the fragile X (Martin-Bell) syndrome. *Am J Med Genet* 1991;**38**:256–9.

21 Tuncbilek E, Alikasifoglu M, Boduroglu K, Aktas D, Anar B. Frequency of Fragile X syndrome among Turkish patients with mental retardation of unknown aetiology. *Am J Med Genet* 1999;**84**:202–3.

22 Hagerman RJ, Amiri K, Cronister A. Fragile X checklist. *Am J Med Genet* 1991;**38**:283–7.

23 Bailey DB Jr, Skinner D, Sparkman KL. Discovering fragile X syndrome: family experiences and perceptions. *Pediatrics* 2003;**111**:407–16.

21 Immunizations

Helen Bedford, David Elliman

Case scenario	*An 8-week-old baby boy is brought by his mother for his first set of immunizations – diphtheria, tetanus, pertussis (whole cell vaccine is used in your jurisdiction), Hib, conjugate meningococcal C, and oral polio vaccines. His mother has heard that the whooping cough vaccine can sometimes cause convulsions. She also tells you that her older, 4-year-old son had a febrile convulsion when he was 14 months old. She is concerned that this may put her baby at greater risk of a convulsion after his immunization, in particular the pertussis component. She also wants to know whether her 4-year-old son should receive the booster vaccines which are now due – diphtheria, tetanus, acellular pertussis, and oral polio.*

Background

Most countries have well established immunization programs, comprising anything between six and 10 individual vaccines given on several occasions throughout childhood. The majority of countries have national or state recommendations issued by government or expert bodies. The use of some vaccines is based on high-quality evidence acquired in an era when research conformed to the current standards of evidence-based medicine. However, some vaccines were introduced at a time when the principles of evidence-based practice had not been formulated. Recommendations on the use of such vaccines may have been based on limited research and the timing of doses developed through custom and practice. As time has progressed, immunization regimens have been modified in the light of experience of their use in millions of children and good post-marketing surveillance and research. This is particularly important when considering relatively rare adverse events or the use of vaccines in particular sub-groups of the child population.

This former circumstance has been highlighted by the introduction and withdrawal of a simian-derived rotavirus vaccine. Research prior to its introduction reported it to be effective with no serious adverse reactions. Close monitoring after its introduction showed that the vaccine appeared to be associated with an increased risk of intussusception. Use of the vaccine was suspended while this was investigated and the vaccine was subsequently withdrawn.

An area that is particularly difficult to address is that of contraindications. In most studies of childhood vaccines, children with any significant illness, and sometimes with a family history of particular illnesses, tend to be excluded. Often it is not until the vaccine has been introduced on a large scale in the general population that its use in groups considered at high risk of adverse reactions is considered. Major examples of this are the use of vaccines in premature infants and those who are immunosuppressed. There is an increasing body of research in these groups. On the other hand, the further immunization of children who have had an adverse reaction has received little systematic attention. Even less research has gone into whether a family history of a condition might make a child more likely to suffer an adverse reaction. Over time experience builds up and perhaps research is conducted, so more definitive advice can be given. This is reflected in changing recommendations.

Advice on contraindications may vary from country to country or from time to time. Adverse events such as seizures have been reported following pertussis vaccination and so children at risk of seizures have often been excluded from receiving the vaccine. However, with time and the experience that these reactions do not appear to cause long-term harm, a less conservative approach has been adopted. Table 21.1 shows how advice about pertussis immunization in the presence of a personal or family history of convulsions has changed over time in the UK.

Febrile convulsions are a relatively common occurrence in early childhood. Harker reported that by the time they reached 5 years, 3% of children had experienced at least one such convulsion.[1] The incidence peaked between 9 and 21 months and was very low before 6 months. It is important to bear this in mind when you are considering the association with immunizations, as they may not be given at the same

Table 21.1   Change over time on advice about pertussis immunization in the presence of a personal or family history of convulsions in the UK

Year	Advice
1972	"Very rarely encephalopathy may occur after the administration of whooping cough vaccine; babies with a history of fits or with evidence of other abnormality of the central nervous system should therefore not receive this vaccine."
1982	"Vaccination should not be carried out in children who have: (a) a history of any severe local or general reaction (including a neurological reaction) to a preceding dose; (b) a history of cerebral irritation or damage in the neonatal period, or who have suffered from fits or convulsions. There are certain groups of children in whom whooping cough vaccination is not absolutely contraindicated but who require special consideration as to its advisability. These groups are: (a) children whose parents or siblings have a history of idiopathic epilepsy; (b) children with developmental delay thought to be due to a neurological defect; (c) children with neurological disease. For these groups the risk of vaccination may be higher than in normal children but the effects of whooping cough may be more severe, so that the benefits of vaccination would also be greater. The balance of risk and benefit should be assessed with special care in each individual case."
1992	"Children with problem histories When there is a personal or family history of febrile convulsions, there is an increased risk of these occurring after pertussis immunisation. In such children, immunisation is recommended but advice on the prevention of fever should be given at the time of immunisation. In a recent British study, children with a family history of epilepsy were immunised with pertussis vaccine without any significant adverse events. These children's developmental progress has been normal. In children with a close family history (first-degree relatives) of idiopathic epilepsy, there may be a risk of developing a similar condition, irrespective of vaccine. Immunization is recommended for these children."

ages in all countries, and therefore the background rate of febrile convulsions at the time of immunization may vary enormously. Another factor requiring consideration is that the type of whooping cough vaccine in use varies. Before 1990, whole cell pertussis vaccine was the norm, whereas by 2000, many industrialized countries had changed over to acellular vaccines.

The risk of having a convulsion following a pertussis-containing vaccine, whatever the cause, is known as the absolute risk. In order to address this mother's concerns, you will need to know the "attributable risk", i.e., the risk of a convulsion occurring due to the vaccine. This is the absolute risk minus the background risk, i.e., the risk without the vaccine.

Framing answerable clinical questions

The child's mother accepts that the whole cell pertussis vaccine is effective and rarely causes side effects. However, she wonders whether her children are at increased risk of adverse reactions following the vaccine because her elder son has a personal history of having had a febrile convulsion or possibly at increased risk of complications of the disease itself. To tackle this problem, it is easiest to consider it in bite-sized chunks. You rephrase these questions in a structured format as follows:

> ### Questions
>
> 1. In infants (*population*), does pertussis disease (*exposure*) cause convulsions (*outcome*)? **[Harm]**
> 2. In infants (*population*), is pertussis vaccine, whole cell and acellular (*intervention*), causally associated with convulsions (*outcome*)? **[Harm]**
> 3. In infants with a family history of febrile convulsions (*population*), is the risk of convulsions increased (*outcome*) after pertussis vaccine (*exposure*)? **[Harm]**
> 4. In children with a history of febrile convulsions (*population*), is pertussis vaccine (*intervention*) causally associated with an increased risk of convulsions (*outcome*)? **[Harm]**

Searching for evidence

Taking these specific clinical questions, you decide to search PubMed and the Cochrane Database of Systematic Reviews (CDSR) together with available national guidelines from a number of countries. You choose the MeSH terms listed in the box that pertain to your clinical questions.

MeSH subject headings

1.	Whooping cough OR pertussis	18 518
2.	Seizures OR convulsions OR fits OR infantile spasms	59 107
3.	1 AND 2	233
4.	Whooping cough vaccine OR pertussis vaccine	4607
5.	2 AND 4	169
6.	Family history OR personal history	36 634
7.	5 AND 6	12

Critical review of the evidence

You are able to review the immunization practice guidelines from four countries. Traditionally these guidelines have not been presented in an explicit evidence-based format.

- **USA guidance.** The report of the Committee on Infectious Diseases of the American Academy of Pediatrics[2] states that children with a personal history of seizures have an increased risk of seizures after receipt of DTP. There is no evidence that these vaccine-associated seizures induce permanent brain damage, cause epilepsy, aggravate neurologic disorders, or affect the prognosis for children with underlying disorders. However, it is recommended that pertussis immunization of children with recent seizures should be deferred until a progressive neurological disorder is excluded. Infants with well-controlled seizures may be immunized with acellular pertussis vaccine. Antipyretics should be considered at the time of the vaccine and every 4 hours for the ensuing 24 hours. In children with a family history of seizures, pertussis vaccine is not contraindicated. Although the risk of seizures after immunization with DTP in children with a family history of seizures is increased, these seizures are usually febrile in origin and generally have a benign outcome. Because a substantial number of children have a family history of seizures, DTaP is recommended for them otherwise there would be a large proportion of the population unprotected. In the USA, only acellular pertussis vaccine is available.
- **UK guidance.** Advice from the Joint Committee on Vaccination and Immunisation as stated in Immunisation against Infectious Disease 1996[3] is that, even where there is a personal or family history of febrile convulsions or epilepsy, pertussis vaccine should be given. In the presence of a still evolving neurological problem or poorly controlled epilepsy, immunization should be postponed until the condition is stable. In the UK, whole cell vaccine is usually used for the primary course and acellular vaccine for boosters.
- **Canadian guidance.** The Population and Public Health Branch, Centre for Infectious Disease Prevention and Control[4] recommends that neither afebrile nor febrile seizures are a contraindication to pertussis-containing vaccines. As evidence suggests there is little difference in the incidence of adverse events following receipt of DTaP and DT vaccines, and an evolving neurological condition is not considered a contraindication to acellular pertussis vaccine. In Canada only acellular pertussis vaccine is available.
- **Australian guidance.** The National Health and Medical Research Council[5] recommends that pertussis vaccine should be given to children with "stable neurological disease (including controlled epilepsy), or a family history of idiopathic epilepsy or other familial neurological disorders." They recommend deferring the vaccine in the presence of active or progressive neurological disease, not so much because the vaccine may cause harm, but because neurological deterioration may be incorrectly attributed to the vaccine. In Australia only acellular pertussis vaccine is available.

As the search of CDSR added nothing extra, you examine the articles you found in PubMed with regard to each individual question.

Question

1. In infants (*population*), does pertussis disease (*exposure*) cause convulsions (*outcome*)? **[Harm]**

Convulsions have long been recognized as a complication of pertussis disease.[6] Similar rates have been reported from population-based studies in different industrialized countries, with higher rates among younger patients. In one US population-based study of all 5865 cases of pertussis reported in 1984 and 1985, detailed clinical information was available for 80% cases. The overall rate of seizures was 1·7%. For infants less than 6 months of age, it was 2·6%, and for 6–11 month olds 3%.[7] In the 1977/78 UK pertussis epidemic, 2295 cases of clinical pertussis were reported in West Glamorgan. The rate of seizures was 0·6% (n = 14). In four of these cases there was a prior history of seizures.[8] Higher rates of seizures were reported from one study in which the effects of age and vaccination status were analysed. Similar high rates were reported for unvaccinated children aged under 18 months and 18 months and older (12·5% and 11·1% respectively), while the rate among vaccinated children was 1%.[9] Although this was a population-based study, the numbers of children included were relatively few, particularly in the older unvaccinated group (n = 36). In an analysis of over 8000 cases of pertussis notified over a 6-month period in 1974/75 in the UK, the reported rate of seizures was 0·4%

overall and 4% among those hospitalized.[10] A larger proportion of children under 1 year of age was hospitalized (42%) compared with children over the age of one year (4%).

These studies and accounts are based on official notifications of whooping cough disease. As this is only part of the total burden of disease and probably the most severe end of the spectrum, the complication rate is probably overestimated. However, in the absence of what would need to be a large expensive prospective cohort study, this is the best available evidence.

Question

2. In infants (*population*), is pertussis vaccine, whole cell and acellular (*intervention*), causally associated with convulsions (*outcome*)? **[Harm]**

Almost since its first introduction there have been reports of neurological events following pertussis immunization. Madsen[11] reported two infants who died convulsing within hours of receiving an early preparation of the vaccine and there have been many reports since then. However, for many decades these were case reports or case series and shed little light on the incidence of such events following the vaccine (absolute risk), let alone the risk that was actually due to the vaccine (attributable risk). The search identified 169 potentially relevant references. However, only three were population-based or controlled studies that allowed calculation of the incidence of convulsions due to pertussis vaccination.

In 1981, Cody et al.[12] described a study in which 784 doses of DT vaccine and 15 752 doses of DTP (whole cell) vaccine were given. All children were followed up for reactions within 48 hours. Nine children had one or more convulsions following DTP vaccine giving an absolute risk of 1 in 1750. This figure is quoted in many subsequent publications. Follow up of eight of these children revealed no significant adverse outcomes.[13]

Using a passive reporting system over a 7-year period, Pollock and Morris[14] reported 15 convulsions (14 febrile) within 2 days of the administration of DTP vaccine and one convulsion (febrile) following DT. This difference occurred in spite of roughly equal numbers of courses of DT and DTP vaccine being given. Hospital admissions in the same geographics area over 1 year of this period were analyzed. There was no significant difference in admissions due to convulsions following DTP and DT vaccines, thus supporting the authors' hypothesis that the difference seen over the 7-year period was likely to be due to reporting bias.

Of children enrolled in the National Institute of Neurological and Communicative Disorders and Stroke Collaborative Perinatal Project[15] (NCPP) between 1959 and 1966, 2766 had one or more seizures prior to age 7 years. Ten children had a convulsion within 6 days of DTP vaccine, one of whom had had smallpox vaccine at the same time.

One of the largest studies of the causes of severe acute neurological problems was the National Childhood Encephalopathy Study. Writing in 1988[16] Miller et al. concluded that the relative risk of convulsions after DTP whole cell vaccine was 3·3 (95% CI 1·4–8·2). However, this study only looked at complex convulsions. Similarly a study by Walker et al.[17] excluded children with febrile convulsions.

Shields et al.[18] reported that changing the age of pertussis immunization from 5, 6, 7, and 15 months to 5 weeks, 9 weeks, and 10 months in Denmark was associated with no change in pattern or rates of epilepsy or infantile spasms. However, there was an increase in reports of febrile convulsions. They calculated that in 5·9% of all children having a febrile convulsion between 28 days and 24 months of age, the febrile convulsion was due to pertussis immunization.

A number of more recent studies have examined groups of children such as those receiving Medicaid, attending Health Maintenance Organizations (HMO) or other well defined populations. Griffin et al.[19] reported that the relative risk of febrile seizures within 3 days of DTP immunization was 1·5 (95% CI 0·6–3·3) in comparison with a control period. The wide confidence interval reflects the size of the study. Using the same methodology among a larger population, Chen et al.[20] reported an increased risk of seizures on the same day as receiving DTP (RR 2·1; 95% CI 1·1–4·0). They assumed they were mostly febrile. Further analysis of the same population revealed an increased risk of febrile seizures on the day of immunization (RR 5·70; 95% CI 1·98–16·42).[21] The long-term outcome for these children was no different from that of children with febrile seizures not associated with immunization. There was no increased risk of afebrile seizures. Gale et al.[22] conducted a case–control study looking at serious neurological disorders within 7 days of DTP immunization. They found no statistically significant increase in incidence (OR 1·1; 95% CI 0·6–2·0), but excluded simple febrile seizures. Using linked databases and children as their own controls, Farrington et al.[23] examined the risk of being admitted to hospital with a febrile convulsion within 3 days of receiving DTP immunization. They found there was an increased risk, but this only reached statistical significance in children receiving the third dose (RI 3·0; 95% CI 1·6–5·5). The absolute risk in these children was 1 in 8500 doses and the attributable risk 1 in 12 500. When children were divided into those aged above or below 28 weeks, it was only the older age group whose increased risk achieved statistical significance (RI 2·7; 95% CI 0·8–8·6 in those 28 weeks or younger and RI 3·0; 95% CI 1·6–5·5 in those older than 28 weeks). This age distinction is very important to note as, in the UK, children should receive DTP immunizations at 2, 3, and 4 months and ought to have completed their course by 28 weeks, if not well before. In many other countries, including the USA and Canada, on the other hand, the immunizations are recommended at 2, 4, and 6 months, so many, if not most, children will be receiving their third dose when older than 28 weeks. Using similar methodology applied to a Canadian population, Roberts et al.[24] reported an increased risk of hospital admission with non-epileptic convulsions within 7 days of DTP immunization (P 0·0019). The authors do point out that they do not know why some children were not immunized, but it may be because they are deemed to be at higher risk of suffering a febrile convulsion after vaccination. If this were so, the reported increased risk would be lower than that for the whole of the population.

From the above we can conclude that there is conclusive evidence of an increase in febrile seizures in the first day or so following receipt of DTP containing the whole cell vaccine. Is this also true following DTaP (acellular pertussis) vaccines?

Using the Vaccine Adverse Events Reporting System (VAERS), and considering children aged 15 months to 7 years old, Rosenthal et al.[25] found that the occurrence of both fever and convulsions was commoner within 72 hours of receiving DTP than DTaP vaccine (7·5 and 1·7 per 10 000 v 1·9 and 0·5 per 10 000). Olin et al.[26] compared the rate of seizures following DTP vaccines containing either whole cell or acellular pertussis vaccines. Most children were vaccinated at 3, 5, and 12 months. There were fewer convulsions following all the DTaP vaccines used in the trial than following the vaccines containing whole cell pertussis (RR after 2 component vaccine was 0·46 [95% CI 0·18–1·20]; RR after 3 component vaccine was 0·15 [95% CI 0·03–0·68]; RR after 5 component vaccine was 0·31 [95% CI 0·40–0·94]). Using data from one HMO, Jackson et al.[27] found an incidence of febrile convulsions within 2 days of DTaP to be 1 per 19 496 immunizations in children < 2 years old. Immunizations were normally administered at 2, 4, 6, and 15 months, and 5 years. The greatest risk followed the doses given at 15 months, which is what one might expect in view of the known distribution of incidence of febrile convulsions by age.

Can this comparative data on the incidence of convulsions following acellular vaccines be extrapolated to what might happen when the vaccines are given at 2, 3, and 4 months? A trial in the UK showed that to be a false assumption. While the acellular vaccine had fewer side effects than the conventional vaccine in older children, there was little difference when it was given at the UK standard ages of 2, 3, and 4 months.[28] The study was too small to examine the effects on the risk of convulsions, but there was a higher incidence of high fever in the children receiving the whole cell vaccine.

In considering the quality of these studies, you recognize that convulsions occur in infants whether or not they have been immunized. Most studies performed have not had a control group or a reliable estimate of age-dependent background rates of convulsions. Those studies with control data allow the risk of convulsions attributable to the whole cell vaccine to be calculated. There are no studies large enough to estimate the absolute risk of febrile convulsions after acellular vaccines; however, there are data that compare acellular and whole cell vaccines. No studies with sufficient power were performed at the ages pertussis immunization is given in the UK.

Question

3. In infants with a family history of febrile convulsions (*population*), is the risk of convulsions increased (*outcome*) after pertussis vaccine (*exposure*)? **[Harm]**

Many children attending special immunization clinics are referred because there is a family or personal history of febrile or afebrile convulsions.[29–33] In the past, some national recommendations, for example, those of the UK, have included a personal history of convulsions and a family history of epilepsy as absolute contraindications to pertussis vaccination.[34] However, over time these absolute contraindications have changed to "special considerations" and now the vaccine is positively recommended in children with such histories.[35]

The search only revealed 12 articles that addressed the issue of a personal or family history. All of these were either case series or uncontrolled observational studies.

The Monitoring System for Adverse Events Following Immunization (MSAEFI) in the USA is a passive reporting system that preceded the current Vaccine Adverse Events Reporting System (VAERS). In the period 1979–82, there were 219 reports of febrile convulsions and 44 reports of non-febrile convulsions in patients following DTP vaccine containing whole cell pertussis vaccine. In those answering questions about personal and family histories of convulsions, such histories were more common in these patients[36]: 13·9% of cases with a febrile convulsion (2·1% of those with a non-neurological event) had a personal history of convulsions and 27·3% a family history (6·0% of those with a non-neurological event). Of cases with a non-febrile convulsion, 17·6% had a personal history of convulsions compared with 2·1% of those with a non-neurological event and 14·8% a family history (6·0% of those with a non-neurological event). This implies that a personal or family history of convulsions is commoner than would be expected in those suffering a convulsion after DTP; however, the limitations of the reporting system mean that this conclusion should be treated with caution.

Livengood *et al.*[37] used data from the same system and looked at a personal history of convulsions over the period 1979–86 and a first-degree family history of convulsions in 1985–86. They came to similar conclusions, with similar caveats. Blumberg *et al.*[38] described 60 children reported to them after a severe adverse event within 48 hours of DTP vaccine. Of the total group of 60 children, six had a personal history of convulsions and 15 a family history. Of the children who had a convulsion following DTP vaccination, six had a personal history of convulsions and 13 a family history. The authors concluded that these may be risk factors for convulsions following the vaccine.

Between 1959 and 1966, 54 000 pregnant women were enrolled in the National Institute of Neurological and Communicative Disorders and Stroke Collaborative Perinatal Project (NCPP).[15] Children were followed up at regular intervals: 39 children had a convulsion within 2 weeks of vaccination (nine had a convulsion after receiving DTP vaccine, all within 2 days). In nine of the 39 children (23%) there was a family history of seizures, whereas a family history was present in 14% of the total group of children with febrile seizures and in 7% of the remaining group of NCPP children. Data from the National Childhood Encephalopathy Study[39] showed that children who were reported to have had an acute neurological illness were more likely to have a family or personal history of convulsions than controls. However, in none of those with a personal history and in only one with a family history of convulsions was the onset within 7 days of DTP. It is not possible from the data presented to assess whether this was due to the fact that children with such histories were not given the vaccine, as was the advice at the time, or whether they were given the vaccine, but were not at increased risk of this outcome.

Most prospective data comes from the experience of specialist immunization clinics[29–32] but in only two of these was it possible to identify the outcome of those children with a family history of seizures who had gone on to receive pertussis containing vaccines after being seen in the clinic. In one series, 57 children with a positive family history were given DTP vaccine.[31] One child had a reaction described as a "collapse". The same child had a febrile convulsion following a subsequent DT vaccination. DT vaccine was given to nine children with positive family histories. One had a febrile convulsion and another, an apneic attack. In the second series, 77 children with positive family histories were given DTP and none had a significant reaction.[32]

As there are no controlled trials looking at the rate of convulsions following whooping cough vaccine in children with a family history of convulsions, you must rely on tenuous indirect evidence that such a history is commoner in children suffering convulsions after the vaccine. However, the overall quality of the evidence is poor.

Question

4. In children with a history of febrile convulsions (*population*), is pertussis vaccine (*intervention*) causally associated with an increased risk of convulsions (*outcome*)? **[Harm]**

There are no formal trials of giving pertussis vaccine to children with a personal history of convulsions. As pertussis vaccine is associated with a small risk of convulsions, it is not unreasonable to think that there might be a higher risk of convulsions following pertussis vaccination than in children with no such history. Indeed, some of the evidence[36–38] cited in response to question 2 indicates that this is likely. The only prospective studies are uncontrolled, but they are still useful in guiding clinical practice. In an early publication Livingston stated that 96 children with febrile convulsions were given pertussis inoculations and 10 had a recurrence.[40] All 96 have been observed for at least 10 years and none has developed epilepsy. He also reported that although pertussis immunization temporarily increased the frequency of seizures in a few cases out of a group of 284 children, their long-term outcome was no different from those not given the immunization. Unfortunately, little detail is given, so it is not possible to know whether differences in outcome may have been missed.

Experience from special immunization clinics suggests that if there is an increased risk it is low. Ramsay *et al.*[31] and Ko *et al.*[32] each describe nine children with a personal history of convulsions none of whom had convulsions nor a significant adverse event after receiving pertussis vaccine.

Gold *et al.*[33] described their experience of 42 children who had a convulsion following a vaccine, 38 of them after DTPw vaccine. Thirty five received further immunizations, one with DTPw and 28 with vaccines including acellular pertussis. None had a convulsion. The conclusions from this study have to be guarded as this group represents an unknown proportion of those who had adverse events following immunization.

You realize that there is little evidence to address this question. What is available is uncontrolled and the numbers are small. All that can be said is that the risk of convulsions following pertussis vaccination is low, even when there is a personal history of seizures.

Summary

Your review of the literature suggests a causal association between whole cell pertussis vaccine and febrile convulsions. Following acellular pertussis vaccine, febrile convulsions occur less commonly but it is not clear whether this differs significantly from the background rate. None of the studies comparing DTaP and DT have had sufficient power to detect a small increased risk of convulsions. It is important to remember that the risk of febrile convulsions with or without vaccine is age dependent. In this scenario, the two children are outside the major risk period. Studies examining whether a personal or family history of convulsions increases the risk of convulsions due to pertussis vaccine have major limitations. However, knowing that there is a genetic component to the susceptibility to febrile convulsions and that pertussis vaccine is a potent cause of fever, there is a biological plausibility to the possibility that such histories increase the risk. All the evidence suggests that there are no long-term adverse consequences, unlike after the disease.

While the whole cell vaccine may be more efficacious, it also carries a higher risk of convulsions. Therefore in those countries where whole cell pertussis vaccine is the norm, it may be worth considering substituting acellular vaccine. Whatever the decision, it would be appropriate to give advice about the management of a fever in these children. Many clinicians would advise giving a 48-hour course of antipyretic following the immunization. While there is no direct evidence that this reduces the risk of convulsions, there is strong evidence it reduces the incidence of fever in younger children and so may be of benefit in this case.[41]

Resolution of the scenario

On the basis of your review of the literature you advise the mother that it is appropriate for her children to receive pertussis vaccines at the appropriate times. For the older boy you would advise that he receives the acellular pertussis vaccine along with the other routine immunizations. For the younger child the decision is slightly more difficult.

Future research needs

As more and more countries move towards the routine use of acellular pertussis vaccine, which is associated with a lower risk of febrile convulsions in the main risk period, it is unlikely that further research studies alone will shed more light on this issue. More important will be large scale well-designed post-marketing surveillance based on record linkage.

Summary table

Question	Type of evidence	Results	Comments
In infants (*population*), does pertussis disease (*exposure*) cause convulsions (*outcome*)?	Observational studies and routine surveillance	Pertussis disease causes convulsions, but the rate is not accurately known	Because these studies and accounts are based on official notifications of disease, the complication rate is probably overestimated. However, these data are still valuable
In infants (*population*), is pertussis vaccine, whole cell and acellular (*intervention*), causally associated with convulsions (*outcome*)?	Scope of evidence ranges from case series to self-controlled case series	Pertussis vaccine is associated with convulsions. The rate is age-dependent	The evidence for the incidence of convulsions following whole cell pertussis vaccine is robust whereas that for acellular vaccines is much weaker
In infants with a family history of febrile convulsions (*population*), is the risk of convulsions (*outcome*) after pertussis vaccine (*exposure*) increased?	Majority were case series, with one case control and one prospective cohort study	Where there is a family history of febrile convulsions, convulsions after pertussis vaccine are more common	The standard of evidence is poor but highly suggestive of a link. This is in keeping with what might be expected from first principles in view of the fact that the vaccine is known to cause a temperature and febrile convulsions have a strong genetic component
In children with a history of febrile convulsions (*population*), is pertussis vaccine (*intervention*) causally associated with an increased risk of convulsions (*outcome*)?	Case series	Convulsions are more common after pertussis vaccine if there is a personal history of convulsions	There is little evidence and that available is limited to uncontrolled studies with small numbers. However, the evidence does show that the risk of convulsions following pertussis vaccine is low even with a personal history of convulsions

References

1 Harker P. Primary immunisation and febrile convulsions in Oxford 1972–5. *BMJ* 1977;**2**:491–3.

2 American Academy of Pediatrics. Pertussis. In: Pickering LK, ed. *Red Book: Report of the Committee on Infectious Diseases. 25th edn*. Elk Grove Village, IL: American Academy of Pediatrics, 2000.

3 Department of Health. *Immunisation against Infectious disease*. London: HMSO, 1996.

4 Population and Public Health Branch, Centre for Infectious Disease Prevention and control. *Canadian Immunization Guide. 6th edn*. Canadian Medical Association, 2002. http://www.hc-sc.gc.ca/pphb-dgspsp/publicat/cig-gci/pdf/cdn_immuniz_guide-2002-6.pdf

5 National Health and Medical Research Council. *The Australian Immunization Handbook. 7th edn*. NHMRC, 2001.

6 West C. *Lectures on the Diseases of Infancy and Childhood, 3rd edn*. London: Longman, Brown, Green and Longmans,1854.

7 Centers for Disease Control. Pertussis. *MMWR* 1987;**36**: 168–171

8 Effect of a low pertussis vaccination uptake on a large community. Report from the Swansea Research Unit of The Royal College of General Practitioners. *BMJ* 1981;**282**: 23–6.

9 Vesselinova-Jenkins CK, Newcombe RG, Gray OP *et al*. The effects of immunisation upon the natural history of pertussis. A family study in the Cardiff area. *J Epidemiol Comm Hlth* 1978;**32**:194–9.

10 Miller CL, Fletcher WB. Severity of notified whooping cough.*BMJ* 1976;**1**:117–19.

11 Madsen T. Vaccination against whooping cough. *JAMA* 1933;**101**:187–8.

12 Cody CL, Baraff LJ, Cherry JD, Marcy SM, Manclark CR. Nature and rates of adverse reactions associated with DTP and DT immunizations in infants and children. *Pediatrics* 1981;**68**:650–60.

13 Baraff LJ, Shields WD, Beckwith L, *et al*. Infants and children with convulsions and hypotonic-hyporesponsive episodes following diphtheria-tetanus-pertussis immunization: follow up evaluation. *Pediatrics* 1988;**81**:789–94.

14 Pollock TM, Morris J. A 7-year survey of disorders attributed to vaccination in North West Thames region. *Lancet* 1983;**1**:753–7.

15 Hirtz DG, Nelson KB, Ellenburg JH. Seizures following childhood immunizations. *J Pediatr* 1983;**102**:14–18.

16 Miller D, Wadsworth J, Ross E. Severe neurological illness: further analyses of the British National Childhood Encephalopathy Study. *Tokai J Exp Clin Med* 1988; **13**(Suppl.):145–55.

17 Walker AM, Jick H, Perera DR, Knauss TA, Thompson RS. Neurologic events following diphtheria-tetanus-pertussis immunization. *Pediatrics* 1988;**81**:345–9.

18 Shields WD, Nielsen C, Buch D, Jacobsen V, Christenson P, Zachau-Christiansen B, Cherry JD. Relationship of pertussis immunization to the onset of neurologic disorders: a retrospective epidemiologic study. *J Pediatr* 1988;**113**:801–5.

19 Griffin MR, Ray WA, Mortimer EA, Fenichel GM, Schaffner W. Risk of seizures and encephalopathy after immunization with the diphtheria-tetanus-pertussis vaccine. *JAMA* 1990; **263**:1641–5.

20 Chen RT, Glasser JW, Rhodes PH *et al*. Vaccine Safety Datalink project: a new tool for improving vaccine safety monitoring in the United States. The Vaccine Safety Datalink Team. *Pediatrics* 1997;**99**:765–73.

21 Barlow WE, Davis RL, Glasser JW *et al*. Centers for Disease Control and Prevention Vaccine Safety Datalink Working Group. The risk of seizures after receipt of whole-cell pertussis or measles, mumps, and rubella vaccine. *N Engl J Med* 2001;**345**:656–61.

22 Gale JL, Thapa PB, Wassilak SG, Bobo JK, Mendelman PM, Foy HM. Risk of serious acute neurological illness after immunization with diphtheria-tetanus-pertussis vaccine. A population-based case-control study. *JAMA* 1994;**271**:37–41.

23 Farrington P, Pugh S, Colville A *et al*. A new method for active surveillance of adverse events from diphtheria/tetanus/pertussis and measles/mumps/rubella vaccines. *Lancet* 1995;**345**:567–9.

24 Roberts JD, Roos LL, Poffenroth LA, Hassard TH, Bebchuk JD, Carter AO, Law B. Surveillance of vaccine-related adverse events in the first year of life: a Manitoba cohort study. *J Clin Epidemiol* 1996;**49**:51–8.

25 Rosenthal S, Chen R, Hadler S. The safety of acellular pertussis vaccine vs whole-cell pertussis vaccine. A postmarketing assessment. *Arch Pediatr Adolesc Med* 1996;**150**:457–60.

26 Olin P, Rasmussen F, Gustafsson L, Hallander HO, Heijbel H. Randomised controlled trial of two-component, three-component, and five-component acellular pertussis vaccines compared with whole-cell pertussis vaccine. Ad Hoc Group for the Study of Pertussis Vaccines. *Lancet* 1997;**350**: 1569–77.

27 Jackson LA, Carste BA, Malais D, Froeschle J. Retrospective population-based assessment of medically attended injection site reactions, seizures, allergic responses and febrile episodes after acellular pertussis vaccine combined with diphtheria and tetanus toxoids. *Pediatr Infect Dis J* 2002;**21**: 781–6.

28 Miller E, Ashworth LA, Redhead K, Thornton C, Waight PA, Coleman T. Effect of schedule on reactogenicity and antibody persistence of acellular and whole-cell pertussis vaccines: value of laboratory tests as predictors of clinical performance. *Vaccine* 1997;**15**:51–60.

29 Hall R, Williams ALJ. Special advisory service for immunisation. *Arch Dis Child* 1988;**63**:1498–500.

30 Newport MJ, Conway SP. Experience of a specialist service for advice on childhood immunisation. *J Infect* 1993;**26**: 295–300.

31 Ramsay M, Begg N, Holland B, Dalphinis J. Pertussis immunisation in children with a family or personal history of convulsions: a review of children referred for specialist advice. *Hlth Trends* 1994;**26**:23–4.

32 Ko MLB, Rao M, Teare L, Bridgman GCB, Kurian A. Outcome of referrals to a district immunisation advisory service. *CDR* 1995;**5**:R146–R149.

33 Gold M, Goodwin H, Botham S, Burgess M, Nash M, Kempe A. Re-vaccination of 421 children with a past history of an adverse reaction in a special immunisation service. *Arch Dis Child* 2000;**83**:128–31.

34 CNO(77)3. Department of Health and Social Services. *Immunisation against Infectious Disease*. London: HMSO, 1977.

35 Department of Health. *Immunisation against Infectious disease*. London: HMSO, 1992.

36 Stetler HC, Orenstein WA, Bart KJ, Brink EW, Brennan J-P, Hinman AR. History of convulsions and use of pertussis vaccine. *J Pediatr* 1984;**107**:175–9.

37 Livengood JR, Mullen JR, White JW, Brink EW, Orenstein WA. Family history of convulsions and use of pertussis vaccines. *J Pediatr* 1989;**115**:527–31.

38 Blumberg DA, Lewis K, Mink CM, Christenson PD, Chatfield P, Cherry JD. Severe reactions associated with diphtheria-tetanus-pertussis vaccine: detailed study of children with seizures, hypotonic-hyporesponsive episodes, high fevers, and persistent crying. *Pediatrics* 1993;**91**:1158–65.

39 Miller D, Wadsworth J, Diamond J, Ross E. Pertussis vaccine and whooping cough as risk factors in acute neurological illness and death in young children. *Dev Biol Stand* 1985;**61**:389–94.

40 Anonymous. Should the child with convulsive disorders be immunised against pertussis? *J Pediatr* 1953;**43**:746–50.

41 Ipp MM, Gold R, Greenberg S, *et al.* Acetaminophen prophylaxis of adverse reactions following vaccination of infants with diphtheria-pertussis-tetanus toxoids-polio vaccine. *Pediatr Infect Dis J* 1987;**6**:721–5.

22 Injury prevention in the clinical setting

Karen Zwi, Ann Williamson

Case scenario

You are called to the emergency department (ED) for the third time in a week to see a child who has sustained a serious injury. The first call was to assess a 4-year-old child who was in a house fire and had severe burns; the second was an 18-month old child who sustained a fractured radius-ulna from falling down the stairs in his home. On this occasion, the paramedics have brought in a 9-year-old boy involved in a motor vehicle collision. His left pupil is fixed and dilated and he is deeply comatose. A CT scan reveals an epidural hematoma and he is rushed to the operating room. His parents inform you that he was not wearing a seat restraint at the time of the crash. You wonder whether these incidents could have been prevented and what you as a practising pediatrician can do to help. You have heard a talk on injury prevention, and are aware that the most effective prevention programs are collaborative efforts between engineers, legislators, and other agencies. But what is the role of clinicians and health professionals in preventing injuries in children? You decide to conduct a literature review to identify injury prevention programs that are effective in the clinical setting, such as the emergency department or the consulting room.

Background

Unintentional injuries are the leading cause of death for children and youth (1–19 years), accounting for more than 13 000 deaths each year in the USA. Here we address the effectiveness of injury prevention strategies focused at the level of the individual and delivered in clinical settings, both primary care (for example, physician offices, clinics) and acute care (for example, emergency departments, hospitals).

Framing answerable clinical questions

You frame your questions in terms of the population (children), the interventions, and the outcomes of interest. Framing questions in this way helps to focus your thinking and guide your search for evidence (see Chapter 3).

Questions

1. Are injury prevention interventions based in the clinical setting (*interventions*) effective in improving safe behaviors (*outcome*) in children (*population*)? **[Therapy]**

2. Are injury prevention interventions based in the clinical setting (*interventions*) effective in decreasing the frequency and/or severity of childhood injuries (*outcome, population*)? **[Therapy]**

3. Are injury prevention interventions based in the clinical setting (*interventions*) effective for specific childhood injuries only (*outcome*)? **[Therapy]**

Searching for evidence

You go to the Cochrane Database of Systematic Reviews and specifically search on "child injuries". You find the protocol for a systematic review of this topic, but no completed review.[1] You next try an EMBASE search, using the terms "child injuries" and "clinical settings" and discover a published review covering exactly the topic you are interested in.[2]

You examine the systematic review of the literature, which has explicit inclusion criteria and search strategy. It includes only randomized controlled trials (RCTs) of interventions in clinical settings. The authors have assessed the quality of the articles and each article has been independently reviewed by two authors. You therefore decide that this systematic review is likely to be a valid summary of the data. This chapter summarizes and updates the systematic review and provides an example of the application of systematic reviews to preventive care issues.

Studies were included in the systematic review if:

- the intervention was designed to prevent unintentional injuries to children or adolescents under 20 years of age;
- the intervention was delivered in a "clinical setting," such as a physician's office, a clinic, an emergency department, or a hospital;
- participants were assigned randomly to the intervention and control groups; and
- the study collected empirical data on injuries or safety practices (for example, seatbelt use).

Databases searched included the Cochrane Controlled Trials Register, MedLine, EMBASE, CINAHL, and dissertation abstracts. There were no language restrictions. Also searched were the bibliographies of published reviews,[3–8] a website (http://depts.washington.edu/hiprc/childinjury/) that has reviewed, summarized, and tabulated the effectiveness of numerous injury prevention interventions, and presentation abstracts from four World Conferences on Injury Prevention and Control.[9–12] Last, authors of relevant trials were contacted, as were members of national and international injury prevention organizations. You decide to try the same search to see if there are new trials since the systematic review was published, but restricting your search to the years between 1998 and 2003.

In the systematic review, data on study design, participants, and interventions were independently extracted by two researchers. Three important elements of study design were considered:

- *Allocation concealment.* How well is the group to which the next recruited subject will be allocated concealed from the person enrolling subjects?
- *Blinded outcomes assessment.* Are study outcomes assessed without knowledge of group assignment?
- *Loss to follow up.* Is the withdrawal or exclusion of subjects after randomization adequately described?

Poorly conducted trials tend to overestimate the treatment benefits as compared with well conducted trials.[13,14] This occurs because design flaws, on average, lead to overestimates of the benefits of an intervention. The adequacy of allocation concealment is particularly important; it has been shown that intervention effects may be exaggerated by as much as 30–40% when allocation is not adequately concealed.[13,14] Chapter 6 discusses evaluation of randomized trials in more detail.

The authors explored whether variations in study results were related to the study population, intervention characteristics, or study design. Using Review Manager 3·1, meta-analyses were performed to combine odds ratios across studies, using fixed effects models. A significance level of 10% was used to test for heterogeneity. For cluster randomized trials, subject numbers were reduced to an "effective sample size" to take into account the cluster randomization,[15] using an estimate of the intraclass correlation coefficient (0·017) from a published trial involving randomized clinical practices.

In total, 10 330 unduplicated citations were identified, of which 103 were potentially eligible. The full texts of 101 studies were reviewed; two were available only in abstract. Twenty-one trials[16–36] (reported in 20 papers and two abstracts) met all inclusion criteria, however, one trial was excluded as it was still in progress. Of the remaining studies, 79 were excluded after full text review, and two trials were excluded based on information provided by investigators. Responses were received from the investigators of 18 (86%) of 21 eligible trials, from which one additional trial was identified. Your search reveals only one new trial[37], and the full publication for a trial referred to in the original review as in progress.[23]

Of the 21 randomized controlled trials that met the inclusion criteria,[16–36] the majority assessed the effect of an intervention on safety behavior, rather than on injury occurrence. Outcomes assessed included: motor vehicle restraint use; bicycle helmet use; safe tap water temperature; smoke alarm ownership; and a variety of safety practices designed to protect young children from injuries in the home (categorized as "child-proofing" the home). The most recent study[37] evaluated an intervention involving adolescents designed to promote seat belt and bicycle helmet use, and to prevent driving after drinking, traveling in cars with an impaired driver, binge drinking, and carrying a weapon.

Motor vehicle restraint use

Motor vehicle occupant injuries are one of the leading contributors to injury mortality and morbidity among children and teenagers. Observational evidence indicates that when used, infant car seats, toddler safety seats, and seat belts for older children and adolescents reduce the risk of serious injury or death by about 70%, 47%, and 45%, respectively.[3]

Ten trials have evaluated clinic-based interventions designed to promote car restraint use (see Table 22.1).[16–25] All the interventions provided information and encouragement to parents, although the extent of the educational component varied substantially. Two trials involved limited education, instead focusing on non-educational interventions. One of these trials evaluated lending car seats (at no charge) to mothers of newborns.[24] The other evaluated a year-long reinforcement program that involved parking lot monitors, verbal reminders from staff, and other incentives for use.[25]

Overall, the studies showed that families who received the experimental intervention were more likely to use a safety

Table 22.1   Promoting child-related safe behavior in clinical settings[55]

Prerequisites for behavior change	Examples	Possible interventions in clinical settings
Knowledge of the relative safety of a particular behavior or situation (knowledge of the behavior/situation)	Does the parent know about the evidence that bicycle helmets can prevent serious head injury?	General information on the safety benefits of the behavior
Belief that the change should be made (attitudes about the behavior)	Does the parent believe that bicycle helmets promote safety? (behavioral belief) Does that parent believe that preventing head injury is important (outcome evaluation)	Specific information on the benefits of the safe behavior that relates to the parent/family's individual circumstances and focuses on the information most likely to persuade them to adopt the behavioral belief
Belief that others expect the behavior to occur (subjective norms)	Does the parent believe that people they know expect their child to wear a bicycle helmet? (normative belief) Does the parent think that other people's opinions about their child's helmet wearing are important? (motivation to comply with norms)	Information presented on the attitudes of others about the behavior, e.g., public opinion, medical opinion etc. (this is likely to have most impact where there are rules or regulations that encourage or enforce wearing)
Belief that the behavior is possible in my case (perceived behavioral control)	Does the parent think that it will be possible to get the child to wear the helmet? Can the parent afford to buy a helmet?	Information on methods of overcoming potential problems, e.g., how to adjust the helmet, tips on how to persuade the child to wear it. This could include hands-on demonstrations, provision of appropriate and inexpensive helmets

restraint for their children than were families receiving the control intervention, but only immediately following the intervention. The differences between intervention and control groups diminished at longer follow up. Compared with no intervention, short-term car restraint use (< 6 months after intervention) was 28% more likely after education alone, although this result was not statistically significant. Statistically significant effects were seen in the trial that evaluated free car seat loans;[24] however, this was not sustained over even a comparatively short follow up period of 4–6 weeks. At this time, fewer intervention group parents were using car seats, and around one-third were not using them correctly. More sustained statistically significant results were seen from a trial involving a year-long reinforcement program.[25] At 6 months, the intervention group used car seats in 38% compared with 11% in the control group; at 12 months 35% compared with 30% used car seats. In this study, parents observed using appropriate child car seats were rewarded, and those who were not were provided with education.

Interventions delivered in the clinical setting promoted child car seat use in the short term. The reduction of effect over time occurred partly because control subjects increased their restraint use to the same level as intervention subjects, and partly due to a decline in use in the intervention group.

Over time, the control group may have received sufficient counseling, whether through usual well-child care, community programs, or other sources, to motivate them to use car restraints. Because the clinical intervention accelerated restraint use, however, children in the intervention group were protected earlier, and thus longer, than those in the control group.

These studies also demonstrate the beneficial effects of resource provision (i.e., free car seats) and of reinforcement on promoting and maintaining behavior change, as documented elsewhere.[38] One study compared loaning car seats with a no-loan group,[23] and only one study provided more than a single information session.[24] It is not surprising then, that there was comparatively little benefit shown in studies of promotion of child restraint use. None of the studies assessed motor vehicle crash-related injuries. While a large body of observational and laboratory research has linked car restraint use with a substantially reduced risk of injury,[3,39] these studies were not designed to detect changes in comparatively low frequency events like crash-related injuries.

Most of the RCTs evaluating promotion of child car seat use occurred in the USA before the introduction of legislation making child restraints in motor vehicles compulsory. Two of the trials[23,24] used similar methods of information provision in conjunction with a car seat loan scheme before and after the introduction of legislation. Neither study showed significant effects of the intervention. However, in the later study[23] both intervention and control groups had much higher usage of the seats, both immediately and in the longer term compared with the earlier study and compared with most of the other studies conducted before the compulsory legislation. This suggests that it was the legislation rather than the interventions that were most responsible for the increase is car seat usage.

Given that current restraint use is 60–85% across the United States,[40] and is even higher in other developed countries, the results of these trials may not be relevant to the current situation in countries with compulsory child restraint legislation. In these countries, parents who do not use car restraints for their children, despite the legislation, are likely to be harder to influence than were the subjects of these trials. There is a need for additional studies to explore the reasons for non-compliance, particularly since evidence from Australia indicates that around 45% of under 6-year-olds killed in motor vehicles were not appropriately restrained, despite three decades of compulsory child restraint legislation.[41] It is likely that the optimal solutions to correct and consistent car restraint use, however, will come from engineering and regulatory changes that make child restraints built-in safety features that are as easy to use as car safety belts.[42,43]

Bicycle helmet use

Bicycle crashes are a major cause of injury and death among school-aged children and adolescents, with most hospitalizations and deaths attributable to head injuries.[44] Observational studies estimate that bicycle helmets reduce the risk of head injuries after crashes by at least two-thirds.[39]

Two trials evaluated the effect of counseling school-aged children and their parents about bicycle helmet use in clinical settings.[26,27] These brief interventions included information, persuasion, and a list of stores that sold helmets. In one trial, the intervention was delivered by the emergency physician who treated the child for a bicycling injury,[26] and in the other trial by the child's pediatrician during well-child care.[27] The trials, individually and combined, showed almost no effect on subsequent helmet purchases 2–3 weeks after counseling. In the studies, the likelihood of purchasing a helmet after intervention was only increased by 10%, and this difference was not statistically significant.

A third trial compared two ways to subsidize helmet ownership in low-income families: free bicycle helmets versus a $5 copayment for a helmet.[28] Consistent bicycle helmet use was not statistically significantly different among children whose families were required to make a copayment compared with children given a free helmet. It is possible, however, that requiring a copayment may have led to fewer families

accepting a helmet, as clinics requesting copayment distributed fewer helmets than did those providing free helmets (218 v 288). The authors did not report how many families refused helmets or how the different distribution methods affected the number of helmets distributed.

In summary, individual counseling does not appear to increase bicycle helmet ownership or use. Counseling in the clinical setting may have failed because only isolated, one-time counseling sessions were offered, which neither actively reinforced the wearing message nor addressed key issues such as negative peer attitudes toward helmet use.[45] In contrast to office-based interventions alone, community-based educational interventions that have included clinical counseling as one component of a broader effort have shown positive effects on childhood bicycle helmet ownership and use, and particularly strong effects if the children were riding with other children or adults who were wearing helmets.[46]

Safe tap water temperature

The leading cause of burn hospitalization among children under 5 years in developed countries is scalds.[47] Hot tap water scald burns can be prevented by setting household water heaters at or below 120–130° F (48·9–54·4° C).[48] The incidence of such burns has declined, possibly because of legislation mandating maximum preset temperature settings of 120° F for new hot water heaters. Families with older heaters, heaters with malfunctioning thermostats, and in circumstances where the thermostat has been reset to an unsafe temperature remain at risk.

Six trials evaluated the effect of interventions delivered in the clinical setting on lowering, testing and/or maintaining a safe hot water temperature.[18,21,22,29–31] Five trials tested educational interventions.[18,21,22,29,30] Three trials included the provision of a free thermometer to test hot water temperature,[22,29,31] and one directly compared the effects of providing or not providing a thermometer, in addition to advice and information.[31]

Families were more likely to test and lower the temperature setting of their household water heaters when provided with information and education on hot water safety and burn prevention. All five trials of education reported positive effects, with a greater than two-fold likelihood of lowering the tap water temperature (or of testing) and of having a safe hot water temperature. There was statistically significant variation among the trials, however, largely because of one trial,[30] which showed much greater differences between intervention and control groups. Unlike the other trials, this trial had weaknesses in all measured aspects of study design, and such flaws may have exaggerated the estimate of benefit.[13,14] Provision of a thermometer in addition to advice on safe tap water temperature increased the likelihood that the water temperature would be tested.[31]

Smoke alarm ownership

Residential fires are the second leading cause of injury deaths among young children. Owning a smoke detector has been estimated to reduce the risk of death in a residential fire by more than two-thirds.[49]

Seven trials evaluated the effect of counseling interventions in the clinical setting on smoke alarm ownership.[18,21,22,30,32–34] Six trials counseled prospective parents or families of young children in preventive care settings,[18,21,22,30,32,33] and one trial counseled the families of children hospitalized for burns.[34]

Five trials reported increased smoke alarm ownership after clinical counseling,[18,22,30,32,33] while two reported no significant effects.[21,34] When results were combined, smoke alarm ownership was 1·6 times more likely in counseled families, compared with families that received usual care. (This estimate may be biased upwards, however, because of the inability to include outcome data from one trial that found no significant effects.)

One trial that found no significant effect on smoke alarm ownership (and also reported outcome data) evaluated the impact of a teaching booklet added to routine hospital discharge teaching for children with burn injuries.[34] This hospital-based trial, however, was methodologically strong compared with the other trials. Inadequate allocation concealment and unblinded outcomes assessment in the other trials may have exaggerated the effects of the interventions.

Trials that included subsidies such as discount coupons[30] or discounted smoke alarms,[32,33] as well as counseling, had positive effects. Smoke alarm ownership was 2·1 times more likely in families who received both counseling and discounted alarms, compared with control families who received neither. Low-income families, who are least likely to own smoke alarms,[50] may require assistance to overcome cost barriers. Trials of community programs involving home visits to distribute free smoke alarms have reported large increases in smoke alarm ownership[51] and decreases in fire-related injuries.[52]

Strategies to child-proof the home

Among children under 5 years, falls, poisonings, cuts, burns, smoke inhalation, drowning, suffocation, and choking cause at least two-thirds of all unintentional injuries. Many of these injuries occur in the home, where young children spend most of their time. Household risk factors for injuries to young children include unprotected stairs, windows, and fireplaces, and inadequately stored household cleaning agents, medications, matches, and sharp objects.

Six trials evaluated the effect of counseling families to child-proof their homes, all of which targeted families with children under 5 years.[18,32,33,35,36] All trials involved a short term intervention including information and advice,[18,32,33,35,36,53] and three of these also evaluated the effect of offering free or discounted safety devices.[32,33,35] In one of the interventions, the information provided was specific for the age of the child[18] and in another the initial information was reinforced by follow up telephone counseling.[35] The outcome measures in these trials ranged from tests of safety knowledge[18] self-reported safety practices and use of safety equipment,[32,33,35,36] and observations of safety practices and equipment use through home visits.[18,53] One study assessed changes in the number of injuries following the intervention.[33]

Overall, there appeared to be only modest positive effects of the interventions on safety practices. In one trial, parents who had been provided three individualized safety information sessions at three monthly intervals showed significantly increased recognition of standard hazards for small children and had slightly reduced number of household hazards one month after the last information session.[18] Two trials showed significantly higher self-reported use of safety equipment and safety practices in the group who were provided safety information[32,36] and in two trials observed safety practices and equipment use were significantly better in the intervention group.[18,53] None of the studies that looked at injuries showed significant differences between information and no-information groups.[18,33]

In summary, the evidence suggests that clinical counseling has modest but positive effects on most home safety practices designed to child-proof the home. The trials that produced the largest changes tended to reinforce the safety information[18,53] or provide access to relevant safety equipment.[32,36] It is possible that comparatively small effects were found as the scope and intensity of the interventions may not have been adequate to motivate parents to reduce household hazards, or that study families were overwhelmed by the number and variety of safety practices recommended. High cost, difficulty in obtaining recommended safety devices,[54] the need for technical skills and tools to install devices, and residence in rental accommodation should be recognized as important barriers to implementing advice about home safety, particularly for low-income households.[4]

Trials in this review also do not establish that clinical interventions aimed at making homes safer for children will reduce injuries. Such interventions may fail to reduce injuries if they do not change safety practices, or if changes in these practices do not affect injuries. This review provides some support for the first explanation. There is also a lack of observational studies demonstrating that general home safety measures are associated with a reduction in childhood injuries. For example, although the widespread use of child-resistant containers for medications and household chemicals has reduced childhood poisonings,[48] any added effect of locking away such containers has not been evaluated.

Strategies to reduce risky behavior in adolescents

One recent trial focused on interventions to reduce risky behavior in 12–20 year-olds undergoing treatment for injury in the ED.[37] Using behavior change counseling, this trial targeted a range of risky behaviors including seat-belt use, bicycle helmet use, driving after drinking, traveling in cars with an impaired driver, binge drinking and carrying a weapon. The study participants were followed up at 3 and 6 months. Results included reduction in injury-related risk behavior, specifically in seat belt and bicycle helmet use, but no difference in re-injury rate. The effect lasted for the full 6 months of the follow up period. The study authors argued that the emotional distress and recent occurrence of the injury increased the susceptibility to address behavior change. In addition, adolescents were encouraged select a risky behavior applicable to their own experience. This study demonstrates that clinical settings can be extremely good opportunities to target subjects who are receptive to safety messages.

Summary and implications for practice and research

There are a number of factors to consider in understanding why some injury interventions are more likely than others to be successful in clinical settings. The ultimate aim of these interventions is to reduce injury occurrence. This is usually through encouraging safe behavior in parents of young children, or in the child or adolescent for older groups.

Behavior change is difficult to achieve under any circumstances, especially when it is voluntary. The intention to behave safely usually requires the person to

- understand what safe behavior is;
- believe that unsafe behavior should be changed;
- believe that change is achievable; and
- believe that others, such as peers, support change.

The Box describes the major prerequisites for behavior change and relates them to the types of child safety interventions possible in clinical settings. These prerequisites are based on the Theory of Planned Action, which describes how attitudes, subjective norms and behavioral intentions combine to predict behavior.[55] This theory has been used in a range of settings to guide methods of promoting behavior change and is relevant to the types of interventions that are possible in clinical settings. As evident from this review, most interventions involve information, counseling, demonstrations, and access to safety equipment.

Behavior change is more likely if

- a greater number of the prerequisites are met as none is sufficient to bring about behavior change individually;
- specific information relevant to the person's situation and salient to their beliefs about the possibility of achieving behavior change is provided, rather than general, knowledge-based information, which may increase awareness about the safety problem, but is unlikely to induce behavior change;
- the person's previous experience of injury is relevant to the intervention as this may enhance the person's appreciation of the need for safe behavior – this is particularly relevant to clinical settings where a recent injury is the reason for attendance and may consequently present a prime opportunity to encourage behavior change;
- the safety equipment is made readily available, free or at low cost;
- the safe behavior messages are repeated and reinforced opportunistically, which may be possible at follow up visits in clinical settings.

Effects on safety practices

For most types of safety practice evaluated, counseling and other interventions in the clinical setting resulted in a greater likelihood of safe practice. For example, car restraint use, smoke alarm ownership, and maintenance of a safe hot tap water temperature were more likely to be adopted following interventions delivered in the clinical setting. Interventions delivered in the clinical setting, however, were not clearly effective in increasing bicycle helmet use or increasing the use of practices designed to protect young children in the home.

Conclusions regarding the effect of counseling and other interventions delivered in the clinical setting on childhood injuries rely on linking evidence between trials of the effectiveness of counseling on safety practices and observational studies of the association of safety practices with reductions in injury. Previous reviews of observational studies report beneficial effects of these and other safety practices on childhood injury occurrence.[3,4,39,48] Thus, there is indirect evidence that individually focused interventions in the clinical setting are effective injury prevention strategies.

Effect on childhood injuries

Only two randomized trials reviewed collected data on the effect of counseling in the clinical setting on childhood injuries.[18,33] These studies reported little or no effect on minor injuries, and the reduction in hospitalizations, though clinically important, was not statistically significant. Because hospitalizations are costly, however, clinical interventions that produce only modest effects on hospitalization rates would nevertheless be worthwhile if the interventions could be implemented cost effectively. Trials to determine the effects of counseling on injury frequency or severity, and that also consider costs in relation to effect and benefit, are needed.

Factors that may influence the effectiveness of interventions

Evidence from health education research describes three types of factors that can be modified by health education: predisposing, enabling, and reinforcing factors.[38] Trials that had the greatest effect on safety practices used a combination of these strategies – for example, by combining education with reinforcement or with the provision of free or subsidized safety devices. As future clinical interventions to improve child safety are developed, practitioners should be aware that counseling alone should raise awareness of the problem and knowledge of how to solve it, but is unlikely to alter behavior in the long term.

The clinical interventions that appeared most effective – those involving advice, demonstrations, subsidized safety equipment, and reinforcement through repeated messages and visits, incentives, and rewards – are time-consuming. Yet, the time available to the average clinician for injury prevention is limited. The busy clinician should consider focusing injury prevention counseling on practices where a beneficial effect is most likely to result. It would be reasonable to emphasize correct and consistent car restraint use, installation and maintenance of smoke alarms, and testing and maintenance of a safe tap water temperature.

Careful consideration of the target population is also important. For example, there is limited evidence to support injury prevention counseling for bicycle helmet ownership. These were the only trials, however, that specifically targeted school-age children and their parents.[26,27] The lack of impact may reflect differences in the responsiveness of families of school-aged children to safety counseling, compared with pregnant women or parents of newborns.

Study populations differed according to the baseline level of safe practice. For most safety practices, greater effects were noted in trials in which baseline use was low. These trials were usually implemented prior to legislative interventions mandating safe practice. It is reasonable to assume that when only a small proportion of the population has adopted a safety practice, many more people can be influenced to adopt the practice simply by providing information, advice, and persuasion. When 90% of the population has already adopted a practice, however, it is likely that the remaining families are prevented from doing so less by lack of awareness and more by other substantial barriers such as cost, access, language, or culture. In these instances, low-cost availability of safety devices, and education sensitive to the local culture and available in the local language, may be critical.

The clinical setting may not be suitable for implementing the entire range of information, modeling, resources, and reinforcement required to change safety practices. Clinical interventions may be more effective if delivered in the context of broader community, legislative, engineering, and regulatory changes. In many communities, physicians and other health professionals have provided leadership for effective injury prevention programs and legislation.[3,4] Clinicians may consider playing an advocacy role as a means of preventing injuries, while continuing to support behavior change with clinical interventions.

Conclusions

Given that most young children are seen regularly for well-child care, immunizations, and minor illnesses, the clinical setting offers numerous opportunities for interventions to promote childhood safety practices. Pregnant women, through participation in regular prenatal visits and classes, also form a ready target population for strategies designed to protect their infants. Emergency departments and hospitals are potential settings for injury prevention strategies in those for whom an emergency visit may provide the only opportunity to receive preventive services, such as adolescents or families with limited access to care.

Physicians caring for children have long recognized the importance of injury prevention counseling.[56,57] Offering guidance to prevent injuries to infants, children and adolescents has been recommended by professional societies,[58–60] government agencies,[61] and national task forces.[3,4,62] This review has assisted in clarifying the evidence with regard to effective interventions in certain injury types, and has highlighted large gaps in the evidence. Clinical injury prevention interventions have important resource implications, including time and effort devoted to the intervention and the costs of pamphlets, equipment, and other materials. Estimates of the likely benefits of clinical interventions on safety practices and injury occurrence contribute to cost-effectiveness analyses and to policy decisions about implementation and funding.

Resolution of the scenario

The systematic review and subsequent studies found that individual-level interventions delivered in the clinical setting may be successful in increasing certain safety practices, including motor vehicle restraint use, smoke alarm ownership, and safe tap water temperature. You are encouraged that injury prevention counseling during clinical interactions with parents and families may be relevant and effective. Furthermore, you are interested to find out more about the local community initiatives addressing childhood injury prevention through collaborative multi-agency programs, which are likely to be most effective in reducing the number of children with injuries seen in the ED.

Future research needs

The systematic review identified numerous randomized controlled trials that have evaluated the effectiveness of individual-level interventions in the clinical setting in improving safety practices. Gaps in the evidence, however, remain. For example, despite their importance as causes of injury, no trials evaluating clinical interventions designed to prevent motorcycle, pedestrian, drowning, or firearm injuries were identified, and only one designed to prevent alcohol-related injuries was identified. Further, there is a need for trials that evaluate the effects of clinical interventions on injury occurrence. Research is also required on strategies to optimize the effectiveness of counseling in different target populations, for example, parents of injured children and families of school-aged children. Finally, research is needed on how best to implement clinical interventions in the context of broader community, legislative, engineering, and regulatory efforts.

Acknowledgments

This chapter is based on the chapter on injury prevention that appeared in the first edition of this book:

Macarthur C, DiGuiseppi C, Roberts I, Rivara F. Injury Prevention and Control. In: Moyer VA, Elliott EJ, Davis RL *et al.*, eds. *Evidence Based Pediatrics and Child Health*. London: BMJ Books, 2000.

Summary table

Intervention	Type of evidence	Result	Comment
Motor vehicle restraint use	10 trials: 8 involved education and encouragement to parents through use of pamphlets, nurse/physician encouragement, videos, car seat demonstrations; 2 involved non-educational interventions through loaning of car-seats to newborns, parking lot monitors and incentives for use	Motor vehicle restraint use more likely in the short term (within 6 months of intervention) but diminished over time. Non-educational outcomes most effective (over 5-fold more likely)	Legislation making car restraints for children mandatory has made a much larger impact on restraint use than may be possible in an intervention in a clinical setting
Bicycle helmet use	3 trials: 2 involved either ED physician or pediatrician counseling school-aged children and parents, plus list of helmet stores; 1 trial compared free with subsidized helmet provision	Bicycle helmet purchase no different 2–3 weeks after intervention; helmet use no different if helmet free as compared with subsidized	It is likely that bicycle helmet use messages need repeated reinforcement to be successful, especially in the light of the age of children who need to wear them
Safe hot water temperature	6 trials: 5 tested counseling about ensuring safe hot water temperature; 3 included provision of a free thermometer	Counseling produced more than 2-fold likelihood of having safe hot water temperature; greater effect if thermometer provided free	Legislation is likely to have a large impact here, although provision of a way of helping parents comply with the legislation (e.g., a thermometer) can be shown to be most effective
Smoke alarm ownership	7 trials: 6 tested counseling of prospective parents and parents of young children in preventive care settings; 1 provided education material for families with children hospitalized with burns	Counseled families were 1·6 times more likely to own a smoke alarm (may be exaggerated effect due to methodological issues), with the greatest effect when smoke alarm subsidized; no significant effect in families with children with burns	Providing information on smoke alarms and subsidizing them is clearly effective, although we also need to ensure that the alarms supplied are installed and maintained
Strategies to child-proof the home	6 trials: all provided counseling and information about child-proofing; 4 provided more intensive interventions such as telephone reinforcement or home safety checks; 3 included subsidized safety devices; 1 involved a brief poisoning prevention talk and handout in the ED	Interventions had modest effects on home safety knowledge and practices. There were no significant effects on safe storage of cleaning agents, medications and matches, and no significant differences in injury occurrence or health care attendance. Best results if safety information reinforced and access to safety equipment provided	It should not be overlooked that increasing the knowledge of parents about safety practices is an important first step towards changing safety behavior and practices

References

1 DiGuiseppi C, Roberts I. Interventions in the clinical setting for preventing unintentional injuries among children and teenagers aged 0–19 years (Protocol for a Cochrane Review). In: *Cochrane Library*, Issue 4. Chichester, UK: John Wiley & Sons, Ltd, 2003.

2 DiGuiseppi C, Roberts I. Individual-level injury prevention strategies in the clinical setting. In *The Future of Children: Unintentional Injuries in Childhood*. Los Altos, California: The David and Lucille Packard Foundation, 2000;**10**(1).

3 US Preventive Services Task Force. Counseling to prevent motor vehicle injuries. In DiGuiseppi C, Atkins D, Woolf S, Kamerow D, eds. *Guide to clinical preventive services, 2nd edn.* Washington, DC: US: Government Printing Office, 1996.

4 US Preventive Services Task Force. Counseling to prevent household and recreational injuries. In DiGuiseppi C, Atkins D, Woolf S, Kamerow D, eds. *Guide to clinical preventive services, 2nd edn.* Washington, DC: US: Government Printing Office, 1996.

5 Bass JL, Christoffel KK, Widome M *et al.* Childhood injury prevention counseling in primary care settings: a critical review of the literature. *Pediatrics* 1993;**92**:544–50.

6 Ciliska D, Hayward S, Thomas H *et al.* A systematic overview of the effectiveness of home visiting as a delivery strategy for public health nursing interventions. *Can J Public Hlth* 1996;**87**:193–8.

7 Munro J, Coleman P, Nicholl J *et al.* Can we prevent accidental injury to adolescents? A systematic review of the evidence. *Injury Prevent* 1995;**1**:249–55.

8 Towner E, Simpson G, Jarvis S, Dowswell T. *Health promotion in childhood and young adolescence for the prevention of unintentional injuries.* London: Health Education Authority, 1996.

9 *First World Conference on Accident and Injury Prevention.* Final program. Stockholm, Sweden, September 17–20, 1989.

10 *The Second World Conference on Injury Control.* Abstracts: Workshops, oral presentations, poster sessions. Atlanta, Georgia, May 20–23, 1993.

11 *Third International Conference on Injury Prevention and Control.* Presentation abstracts. Melbourne, Australia, February 18–22, 1996.

12 *Fourth World Conference on Injury Prevention and Control.* Book of abstracts, Vol. I and II. Amsterdam, Netherlands, May 17–20, 1998.

13 Schulz KF, Chalmers I, Hayes RJ, Altman DG. Empirical evidence of bias: dimensions of methodological quality associated with estimates of treatment effects in controlled trials. *JAMA* 1995;**273**:408–12.

14 Moher D, Pham B, Jones A *et al.* Does quality of reports of randomised trials affect estimates of intervention efficacy reported in meta-analyses? *Lancet* 1998;**352**:609–13.

15 Hauck WW, Gilliss CL, Donner A, Gortner, S. Randomization by cluster. *Nurs Res* 1991;**40**:356–8.

16 Miller J.R, Pless IP. Child automobile restraints: evaluation of health education. *Pediatrics* 1977;**59**:907–11.

17 Scherz, R.G. Restraint systems for the prevention of injury to children in automobile accidents. *Am J Publ Hlth* 1976;**66**:451–6.

18 Kelly B, Sein C, McCarthy P.L. Safety education in a pediatric primary care setting. *Pediatrics* 1987;**79**:818–24.

19 Greenberg LW, Coleman AB. A prenatal and postpartum safety education program: influence on parental use of infant car restraints. *Develop Behavior Pediatr* 1982;**3**:32–4.

20 Moffit PB. *Effects of a child auto restraint education and loan program on restraint use* (dissertation). Salt Lake City, UT: University of Utah, 1981.

21 Williams GE. *An analysis of prenatal education classes: an early start to injury prevention* (dissertation). Kansas City, UT: University of Kansas, 1988.

22 Barone VJ. *An analysis of well-child parenting classes: the extent of parent compliance with health-care recommendations to decrease potential injury of their toddlers* (dissertation). Kansas City, KS: University of Kansas, 1988.

23 Christophersen ER, Sosland-Edelman D, LeClaire S. Evaluation of two comprehensive infant car seat loaner programs with 1-year follow up. *Pediatrics* 1985;**76**: 36–42.

24 Christophersen ER, Sullivan MA. Increasing the protection of newborn infants in cars. *Pediatrics* 1982;**70**:21–5.

25 Liberato CP, Eriacho B, Schmiesing J, Krump M. SafeSmart safety seat intervention project: a successful program for the medically-indigent. *Pat Educ Counsel* 1989;**13**: 161–70.

26 Cushman R, Down J, MacMillan N, Waclawik H. Helmet promotion in the emergency room following a bicycle injury: a randomized trial. *Pediatrics* 1991;**88**:43–7.

27 Cushman R, James W, Waclawik H. Physicians promoting bicycle helmets for children: a randomized trial. *Am J Publ Hlth* 1991;**81**:1044–6.

28 Kim AN, Rivara FP, Koepsell TD. Does sharing the cost of a bicycle helmet help promote helmet use? *Inj Prevent* 1997;**3**:38–42.

29 Shapiro MM, Katcher ML. Injury-prevention education during postpartum hospitalization. *Am J Dis Child* 1987; **141**:382.

30 Thomas KA, Hassanein RS, Christophersen ER. Evaluation of group well-child care for improving burn prevention practices in the home. *Pediatrics* 1984;**74**:879–82.

31 Katcher ML, Landry GL, Shapiro MM. Liquid-crystal thermometer use in pediatric office counseling about tap water burn prevention. *Pediatrics* 1989;**83**:766–71.

32 Clamp M, Kendrick D. A randomised controlled trial of general practitioner safety advice for families with children under 5 years. *BMJ* 1998;**16**:1576–79.

33 Kendrick D, Marsh P, Fielding K, Miller P. The Nottingham Safe at Home project: a controlled intervention study of childhood injury prevention in primary care. *BMJ* 1999; **318**:980–3.

34 Jenkins HML, Blank V, Miller K *et al.* A randomized single-blind evaluation of a discharge teaching book for pediatric patients with burns. *J Burn Care Rehabil* 1996;**17**:49–61.

35 Dershewitz RA, Williamson JW. Prevention of childhood household injuries: a controlled clinical trial. *Am J Publ Hlth* 1977;**67**:1148–53.

36 Woolf A, Lewander W, Filippone G, Lovejoy F. Prevention of childhood poisoning: efficacy of an educational program carried out in an emergency clinic. *Pediatrics* 1987;**80**: 359–63.

37 Johnston BD, Rivara FP, Droesch RM, Dunn C, Copass MK. Behavior change counseling in the Emergency Department to reduce injury risk: a randomized controlled trial. *Pediatrics* 2002;**110**:267–74.

38 Green LW, Kreuter MW. *Health promotion planning: an educational and environmental approach, 2nd ed.* Mountain View, CA: Mayfield Publishing Co, 1991.

39 Rivara FP, Grossman DC, Cummings P. Injury prevention: first of two parts. *N Engl J Med* 1998;**337**:543–8.

40 National Highway Traffic Safety Administration, Department of Transportation. Children – Traffic Safety Facts, 1996 [http://www.nhtsa.dot.gov/people/ncsa/].

41 Williamson A, Irvine P, Sadural S. Analysis of motor vehicle-related fatalities involving children under the age of six years 1995–2000. Report for Motor Accidents Authority, July, 2002 [http://www.maa.nsw.gov.au, 2002].

42 Roberts I, DiGuiseppi C. Children in cars. *BMJ* 1997; **314**:392.

43 Department of Transportation, National Highway Traffic Safety Administration. Federal Motor Vehicle Safety Standards. *Child Restraint Systems; Child Restraint Anchorage Systems* [http://www.nhtsa.dot.gov/cars/rules/rulings/UCRA-OMB-J08/FinalRule.html].

44 Sacks JJ, Holmgreen P, Smith SM *et al.* Bicycle-associated head injuries and deaths in the United States from 1984 through 1988. How many are preventable? *JAMA* 1991; **266**:3016–18.

45 DiGuiseppi C, Rivara F, Koepsell T. Attitudes toward bicycle helmet ownership and use by school-age children. *Am J Dis Child* 1990;**144**:83–6.

46 DiGuiseppi C, Rivara F, Koepsell T, Polissar L. Bicycle helmet use by children: evaluation of a community-wide campaign. *JAMA* 1989;**262**:2256–61.

47 Erdmann TC, Feldman KW, Rivara FP, Heimback DM, Wall HA. Tap water burn prevention: the effect of legislation. *Pediatrics* 1991;**88**:572–7.

48 Rivara FP, Grossman DC, Cummings P. Injury prevention: second of two parts. *New Engl J Med* 1998;**337**: 613–8.

49 Runyan CW, Bangdiwala SI, Linzer MA *et al.* Risk factors for fatal residential fires. *N Engl J Med* 1992;**327**: 859–63.

50 Roberts I. Smoke alarm use: prevalence and household predictors. *Inj Prevent* 1996;**2**:263–5.

51 Schwarz DF, Grisso JA, Miles C, Holmes, JH, Sutton RL. An injury prevention program in an urban African-American community. *Am J Publ Hlth* 1993;**83**:675–80.

52 Mallonee S, Istre GR, Rosenberg M, Reddish-Douglas M, Jordan F, Silverstein P, Tunnell W. Surveillance and prevention of residential-fire injuries. *N Engl J Med* 1996;**335**:27–31.

53 Gielen AC, McDonald EM, Wilson MEH, Hwang W, Serwint JR, Andrew JS, Wang M. Effect of improved access to safety counseling, products and home visits on parents' safety practices. Results of a randomized trial. *Arch Paediatr Adolesc Med* 2002;**156**:33–40.

54 Paul CL, Redman S, Evans D. The cost and availability of devices for preventing childhood injuries. *J Paediatr Child Hlth* 1992;**28**:22–6.

55 Quine L, Rutter DR, Arnold L. Persuading school-age cyclists to use safety helmets: Effectiveness of an intervention based on the Theory of Planned Behavior. *Br J Hlth Psychol* 2001;**6**:327–345.

56 Wheatley GM. Child accident reduction: a challenge to the pediatrician. *Pediatrics* 1948;**2**:367–8.

57 Shaffer TE. Accident prevention. *Pediatr Clin N Am* 1954; **1**:421–32.

58 Committee on Injury and Poison Prevention, American Academy of Pediatrics. Office-based counseling for injury prevention. *Pediatrics* 1994;**94**:566–7.

59 American Medical Association. *Guidelines for adolescent preventive services (GAPS): recommendations and rationale.* Chicago, IL: AMA, 1994.

60 American College of Obstetricians and Gynecologists. Automobile passenger restraints for children and pregnant women. Technical Bulletin no. 151. Washington, DC: ACOG, 1991.

61 US Department of Health and Human Services. Healthy people 2000: national health promotion and disease prevention objectives. Washington, DC: US Public Health Service, 1991. (DHHS Publication no. (PHS;91 50212.)

62 Green M ed. *Bright futures: guidelines for health supervision of infants, children, adolescents.* Arlington, VA: National Center for Education in Maternal and Child Health, 1994.

23 Childhood obesity

Laurel Edmunds, Elizabeth Waters

Case scenario

A very overweight 10-year-old girl turns up in your outpatient clinic with her parents. She is the younger of two girls, her mother is a little overweight and manages her weight relatively well. Her father is of normal weight. However, her mother's two sisters, brother, and grandmother are obese and there is a family history of type 2 diabetes and heart disease. Her parents report the child's behavior is deteriorating and that she is becoming isolated from her peers. Her mother has tried to implement dieting strategies following advice from a primary care provider (health visitor), but these have not halted her increasing weight gain. Her parents are concerned that she will "end up like mum's family"; the girl says that she is unhappy about her size because she gets teased and has trouble making friends. Her mother asks whether her health is at risk and how she can be helped.

Background

In 1998, the World Health Organization (WHO) designated obesity as a global epidemic.[1] The International Obesity Task Force (IOTF) is currently compiling a report for WHO on childhood obesity and Ebbeling *et al.*[2] have recently published a comprehensive background paper. For adults, effective treatment is limited, and population prevention strategies targeting physical activity, nutrition, and educational strategies have been promoted as the most effective methods of reducing the societal and health burden of obesity. Treatments for individual children are thought to be more effective, although the studies are few and samples often small and homogeneous. Lifestyle behaviors that contribute to and sustain obesity in adults are less established in children and may be more amenable to change. Weight management and improvements in physical activity, reductions in sedentary behaviors and improvements in dietary intake, and addressing social and mental health concerns are the short- and long-term objectives. Population prevention strategies delivered at the community, school, preschool, and at the environmental levels are required for achievements to be sustained.

Evaluating weight status in children is problematic as there remain no standardized and agreed definitions for obesity in children. Body status is frequently described using the Body Mass Index (BMI), (weight [kg]/height [m]^2). Use of BMI percentiles has been suggested because of their ease and accuracy of measurement. International BMI charts have been developed with cut-offs equivalent to those for adults, that is, a BMI > 25 indicates overweight and a BMI > 30 indicates obesity.[3] Adoption of these cut-offs has been suggested as a more consistent way of monitoring weight change and making comparisons in populations.[4] Although BMI is not a perfect measure in children (because weight is used as a numerator and children accumulate fat-free mass as they grow), it does correlate moderately to strongly with estimates of fatness.[5] Additional information about adiposity status can be gained from measures such as skinfold thickness; measurement of body composition[6] and the efficacy of waist circumference is being explored. We have described children as overweight when BMI is greater than the 85th percentile, or more than the overweight IOTF cut-off where available, as these are internationally comparable.[7] While "obesity" is a commonly used term, the term "overweight" is less stigmatizing and goes some way to mitigate against often harmful labeling. However, because the term obesity is in common usage and is a better search term (thesaurus term) it has been used in connection with research throughout this chapter for consistency. Within UK studies, the 85th percentile refers to charts drawn up in 1990 and so there are and will be increasing numbers of children beyond 15% (and beyond 5% for the 95th percentile). The situation is similar with the National Health and Nutrition Examination Surveys (NHANES), where cut-offs were established in 1977, when the National Centre for Health Statistics (NCHS) charts were revised.

Framing answerable clinical questions

From the scenario, several thoughts occur to you.

- How typical is it to be obese at 10 years of age?

- What are the current and long-term effects of being overweight at this age?
- Is this child likely to stay overweight?
- What strategies do you have available to manage her weight?
- What role do schools have with respect to either prevention or treatment interventions?

From these thoughts you develop the following questions.

Questions

1. In 6–12-year-old children (*population*), what is the prevalence (*event*) of obesity (*outcome*)? **[Baseline Risk]**

2. In children who are overweight (BMI > 85th percentile) (*population/exposure*), what is the risk of current and future psychosocial problems (*outcome*)? **[Baseline Risk and Prognosis]**

3. In children who are overweight (BMI > 85th percentile) (*population/exposure*), what is the risk of future health problems (*outcome*)? **[Prognosis]**

4. In children who are overweight (BMI > 85th percentile) (*population/exposure*), what is the risk of obesity in adulthood (*outcome*)? **[Prognosis]**

5. In obese pre-adolescent children (*population*), are family-based methods (*intervention*) effective for weight reduction (*outcome*)? **[Therapy/Intervention]**

6. In children (*population*), are school-based programs (*intervention*) effective for prevention and treatment of obesity without risk of harm (*outcome*)? **[Therapy/ Intervention]**

Searching for evidence

For each individual question, evidence can be sought from documents that synthesize the evidence and provide broader summaries, such as systematic reviews and evidence-based practice guidelines. Both provide an efficient source of evidence that can be critically appraised (see Chapter 8). If evidence summaries do not address your questions, evidence can be sought from primary studies.

Searching for evidence syntheses

- *Clinical Evidence*
- *Cochrane Library*: "child" AND "obesity" AND ("treatment" OR "prevention")

Clinical Evidence has a limited child health section and, unfortunately, childhood obesity is not included. You search the *Cochrane Library* using the terms "child AND obesity"

with "prevention" and "treatment". You find three published systematic reviews in the Cochrane Database of Systematic Reviews (CDSR), "Interventions for preventing eating disorders in children and adolescents",[8] "Interventions for preventing obesity in children",[9] and "Interventions for treating obesity in children".[10] There is one additional review of randomized controlled trials (RCTs), which specifically included studies of childhood obesity prevention or treatment in the Database of Abstracts of Reviews of Effects.[11] You search the Cochrane Controlled Trials Register to identify any potential research trials that may have been excluded from the previous reviews, and find two more recent trials.[12,13] The Health Technology Assessment category of the *Cochrane Library* provides you with the most recent systematic review of the intervention literature: "The prevention and treatment of childhood obesity".[14] You also find a review of behavior modification,[15] and a review[16] and meta-analysis of physical activity[17] for the treatment of childhood obesity, by searching other databases (see below).

You also search relevant pediatric professional journals and organizations for clinical guidelines. The internet site for *Pediatrics* provides recommendations for the evaluation and treatment of overweight children that were compiled at a meeting of experts in 1998 (http://www.pediatrics.org).[5] The UK-based Royal College of Paediatrics and Child Health and the UK National Obesity Forum also carry an advisory document "An approach to weight management for children and adolescents (aged 2–18 years) in primary care" (http://www.rcpch.ac.uk/publications),[18] and there are SIGN guidelines "Obesity in children and young people". The Scottish Guideline Agency has published "Management of obesity in children and young people" (http://www.show. scot.nhs.uk/sign/guidelines/published/index.html). The UK-based Health Development Agency has also published a systematic review of "Weight management: an analysis of reviews of diet, physical activity and behavioural approaches". In 2003 a draft of the Australian National Health and Medical Research Council "Guidelines for treatment of childhood overweight and obesity" was completed and is now available at http://www.health.gov.au/nhmrc.

To answer questions 1–4 you move away from reviews of the intervention literature to primary studies and systematic reviews, where available, of childhood predictors and longitudinal outcomes. You search the electronic databases MedLine, CINAHL, EMBASE, and PsycINFO using the terms shown in the search strategy (see below), and limiting the search to English publications from 1966 to March 2003. The articles obtained from your search of electronic databases provide you with national surveys, longitudinal growth studies, and other studies investigating obesity in childhood including a systematic review of childhood predictors of adult obesity.[19] You also find two interesting references[20,21] that seem relevant to your questions about treatment, which did not appear in your search of the Cochrane database and you hear of a recently published book chapter[22] through a personal communication.

Search strategy for electronic databases

Number of references found

- WINSPIRS on Silverplatter: "child" AND "obesity" and "treatment" OR "prevention" AND "intervention" and limited to "review" (publication type or do   Treatment 15
  Prevention 18
- Searches: Q1: in addition to child* and obesity add "prevalence" OR "survey"   188
- Q2: add "social"   597
- Q3 and 4: add "risk"   145
- Papers selected on the relevance of their titles and then abstracts

Critical review of the evidence

Question

1. In 6–12-year-old children (*population*), what is the prevalence (*event*) of obesity (*outcome*)? **[Baseline Risk]**

Baseline risk is best measured in large surveys that are not likely to have missed significant sectors of the population. Large, good quality national surveys provide valid evidence for within-country comparisons over time. However, measures are not necessarily consistent between countries, which makes between-country comparisons problematic, hence the development of IOTF cut-offs. Evidence from the NHANES[23] in the USA, the National Study of Health and Growth (NSHG)[24] in the UK and three Australian surveys[25] all suggest there have been increases in the prevalence of obesity and overweight in both young children and adolescents in these developed countries. Additionally, the distribution of overweight appears to have skewed to the right over time, suggesting that children who are already overweight are getting fatter. In the USA, the proportion of children aged 6–11 years who were overweight (BMI > 95th percentile) increased from 3·9% to 16·0% for boys and from 4·3% to 14·5% for girls between the 1963/65 and 1999/00 surveys.[23] A large community-based US study also clearly illustrated the trend toward increasing weight gain in children, with an observed increase of 2 kg from the 1970s to 1980s and 5 kg from the 1980s to the 1990s measured during childhood.[26] In the UK, the National Study of Health and Growth studied anthropometric data of primary school-aged children over a 20-year period. Using the IOTF cut-offs, changes between 1974 and 1984 were minimal; however, increases between 1984 and 1994 were marked: prevalence of overweight in English boys changed from 5·4% to 9·0% (obesity 1·7%) and in English girls from 9·3% to 13·5% (obesity 2·6%). Scottish children had higher prevalence of both overweight and obesity than the English children.[24]

A more recent estimate of overweight in a nationally representative survey of UK 5-year-olds has shown that 18·7% are > 85th percentile and 7·2% are > 95th centile.[27] In the Australian surveys in 1969, 1985, and 1997 with 7–15 year-olds, the prevalence of overweight and obesity were relatively constant in the first period, but have doubled over the latter time periods.[25] In summary, you conclude that there have been marked increases in the prevalence and extent of obesity in developed countries over the last 30 years, which have increased more steeply according to more recent data collection points. Similar trends are now being observed in developing societies.[28]

Question

2. In children who are overweight (BMI > 85th percentile or IOTF overweight cut-off) (*population/exposure*), what is the risk of current and future psychosocial problems (*outcome*)? **[Baseline Risk and Prognosis]**

Prognosis is best evaluated using large cohort studies. You find evidence from case–control studies,[29–32] a review,[33] and from nationally representative longitudinal cohort studies[34,35] and conclude that children who are overweight may also suffer psychological problems as the stigma of overweight and obesity continues to worsen.[36] Children as young as 6 years may be labeled negatively,[29] suffer rejection and become socially isolated, or acquire a distorted body image.[30] Obese adolescents and young adults fare less well in terms of school-age education and have lower marriage rates over time.[32,35] Severely obese children and adolescents have impaired quality of life, similar to those diagnosed with cancer.[37] The social outcomes for obese adults can also be poor: the obese, particularly women, are less likely to be selected at interview[31] are more likely to have left full-time education earlier, are less likely to receive financial support from their family while at college, and earn less.[33] You are pleased that the methods used by the case–control studies will have reduced potential bias by using hypothetical shapes, standardized videos, and appropriate statistical analyses. You conclude that the overweight child has a significantly increased risk of psychosocial and psychological problems than the child of normal weight; however, inadequate evidence is available to allow quantification of this risk. More recently, the issues associated with social outcomes have strengthened the call for childhood obesity to be considered a societal problem[38] and not just the responsibility of individuals.

The reviews include evidence from established longitudinal studies suggesting that being obese increases the risk of cardiovascular disease in adulthood, diabetes in childhood and adulthood, and premature mortality. Childhood obesity has been examined in relation to childhood hyperinsulinemia, hypertension, and dyslipidemia. Odds ratios observed for very overweight children (BMI > 95th centile) were: 2·4 for elevated diastolic blood pressure, 3·0 for elevated LDL cholesterol, 3·4 for elevated HDL cholesterol, 4·5 for elevated systolic blood pressure, 7·1 for elevated triglycerides, and 12·6 for decreased fasting insulin. Two or more risk factors were present in 58% of the very overweight children.[39]

Questions

3. In children who are overweight (BMI > 85th percentile) (*population/exposure*), what is the risk of future health problems (*outcome*)? **[Prognosis]**

Persistent overweight and obesity in childhood and adolescence is a major health concern as children are predisposed to adult consequences such as hypertension, dyslipidemia, impaired glucose homeostasis, steatohepatitis, and sleep apnea with some concerns specific to childhood, for example orthopedic disorders and accelerated skeletal and pubertal development.[40] Increasing numbers of children are also now presenting with type 2 diabetes.[41] Obesity in childhood also increases the risk of the metabolic syndrome (a cluster of diseases including obesity, hypertension, dyslipidemia, and glucose intolerance) in adulthood. Obesity established in childhood may be more harmful than adult-onset obesity, as the risk of metabolic syndrome is lower with later onset obesity.[42] Higher levels of energy intake in childhood are also associated with a significantly increased risk of non-smoking-related cancers in later life.[43] Similarly, long-term follow up of overweight adolescents (13–18 years) suggests that they have an increased risk of coronary heart disease, atherosclerosis (relative risk [RR] for men, 2·3), and diabetes; an increased risk for colorectal cancer and gout in men, and an increased risk of arthritis in women. After 55 years of follow up, overweight in adolescence was found to be predictive of many adverse health consequences including those already mentioned and independent of adult weight.[32,44] You conclude that the overweight child is at significantly increased risk of current and future disease and this provides an additional reason for offering treatment.

Question

4. In children who are overweight (BMI > 85th percentile) (*population/exposure*), what is the risk of obesity in adulthood (*outcome*)? **[Prognosis]**

The risk of adult obesity is twice as great for overweight compared with non-overweight children.[45] The likelihood of tracking (constancy of an individual's expected weight relative to population percentiles) increases with later age at onset and increasing severity of obesity.[46] The odds ratio for adult obesity associated with obesity in adolescence is 17·5 (95% Cl, 7·7–39·5) for obesity at 15–17 years of age.[45] Persistence is greatest for those most overweight and for males, and even moderate overweight is associated with excess mortality and morbidity in adulthood.[47] A review of the persistence of obesity in children indicated that 26–41% of obese preschoolers and 42–63% of obese school-age children became obese adults.[48] Children who are very overweight are increasingly likely to stay overweight as measured by either BMI or skinfold thickness.[6,48–53] Evidence from a systematic review of risk factors for obesity[19] and two birth cohort studies (the UK 1958 Cohort Study[54] and 854 subjects followed from a health maintenance organization in Washington State[55]) showed that those with overweight or obese parents have a higher risk of obesity (79% of 10–14-year-olds with at least one obese parent were obese), regardless of whether the family associations of obesity had genetic or environmental determinants. However, analyses of the UK, 1947 Thousand Family cohort suggested that frame size, rather than fatness, was tracking (measured by bioelectrical impedance).[56] Current weight status is therefore a useful indicator of a child's predisposition to adult obesity. These findings are important as they also demonstrate that obesity in adulthood is not an inevitable outcome for obese children.

Identifying children at risk of persistent obesity is an inexact science. Current body status, having an obese parent, and the period of adiposity rebound based on BMI changes may be predictive.[57] BMI increases after birth, decreases around the age of 2 years, and increases again between the ages of 3–8 years. This second increase is termed the period of adiposity rebound (AR), and may be predictive of adult obesity.[57] Longitudinal studies from England,[58] France,[57] Ohio,[59] Czechoslovakia,[60] Sweden,[61] and Switzerland[49] suggest that children who rebound around the age of 5 years are fatter in adolescence and adulthood compared with those who rebound around the age of 8 years. These studies also show that by the age of 8, the oldest age for adiposity rebound, most children have found the percentile line that they will follow until growth ceases.[57] Rebound may have the potential to help identify a child who is on a trajectory for future obesity before the clinical criteria for obesity are met. Although there are concerns about the applicability of using adiposity rebound,[62] you conclude that measures of weight and height taken between the ages of 3 and 8 years may be valuable for calculating BMI and BMI percentiles in early childhood, and determining whether there was early rebound.

Question

5. In obese pre-adolescent children (*population*), are family-based methods (*intervention*) effective for weight reduction (*outcome*)? **[Therapy]**

The best evidence of effectiveness for interventions is obtained from controlled trials, as they are more likely to minimize the effect of systematic bias than are other study designs. Based on your examination of the background literature for childhood obesity, you conclude that early intervention is likely to produce better outcomes for individual children and population groups of children, and therefore look for systematic reviews of trials that include children aged 5–12 years. You find seven reviews. The Cochrane review of treatment interventions[10] included 18 RCTs and the Effective Health Care systematic review of obesity prevention and treatment[14] included 34 RCTs in children and adolescents. Two systematic reviews of the psychological aspects include 42[15] and 11[11] studies. A second review of pediatric treatment interventions[16] was not designed as a systematic review, and there are also two meta-analyses, one for treatment components[63] and a second for physical activity effectiveness.[17] There is considerable overlap in the studies included in these reviews. The 31 RCTs from the five reviews of obesity treatment, which include children < 12 years and are family-based, are summarized in Table 23.1. You surmise from them that treating childhood obesity is complex. To answer your question on the effectiveness of family-based treatments, both the content and the duration of the intervention need to be considered. You use their relative success to rank the RCTs in Table 23.1.

Many of the published intervention studies have small sample sizes, restricted follow up and provide inadequate descriptions of randomization methods.[10,14,16,63,64] Psychological and sociodemographic factors tend to be ignored. Comments on the methodology of the trials are summarized by the reviewers. Although follow up in these trials ranges from 0–10 years, in general follow up was only about 1 year. Each trial confirms the importance of diet, activity, and behavior change as components of obesity treatments. In the summary of evidence, one review[16] also considered the positive effects of treatment on metabolic parameters and on psychological well-being. Several different dietary approaches have been successful at reducing calorie intake and improving eating behavior, including restricting dietary intake by 30%, providing nutrition information, calorie counting, the Traffic Light Diet, a protein-sparing modified fast, and increasing fiber (Table 23.1). However, comparisons between different dietary methods have not been conducted. Although most of the effect on energy balance is achieved by reducing intake, the addition of activity improves sustained weight management.[16] Again different supervised and unsupervised activity regimes have been included (exercise information, daily exercise instructions, aerobic exercise, lifestyle exercise, increasing activity, and decreasing sedentary behavior).[10,14,16,17] The addition of behavior modification to dietary behaviors appeared to improve weight management at the family/individual level,[15] and more successful results were observed with initially heavier children.[65] The prevalence of eating disorders post-treatment is unknown. This would require significant follow up time and very few investigators were able to do this. One study[66] reported that after 10 years, 4% of 158 individuals treated for obesity as children had received treatment for an eating disorder.

You conclude that emphasis should be placed on behavioral treatments that are individualized, and that the circumstances in which the intervention is delivered and by whom[67] may be as important as its content. Some children will be more at risk for adverse adult outcomes than others. Behavior change to improve weight management is a long-term objective. Currently, obesity treatments for children do not differ in content from adolescent and adult treatments, although they appear to be more effective.[14,64]

In summary, you find that family-based treatment interventions have equivocal results and the limited evidence currently available provides indications of what may be effective rather than certainties.[10] Results are typically reported as group means, and so individual outcomes are not available. Some interventions appear to be working, but there is no clear consistency in effectiveness, even for similar interventions. The modest observed effects on weight or fat loss suggest that overweight may be resistant to treatment. This may relate in part to the complexity of the interventions required to show an effect, and in part to the fact that the intervention does not alter the context of the environment that generated the obese child. Interventions are more likely to show success when the included sample is compliant, and the background circumstances are less contaminated by underlying environmental determinants. For example, the more successful studies[10,14–16] commonly sample families from backgrounds that tend to be white, middle class, and who are better motivated to attend obesity reduction pediatric clinics. However, involving parents, employing behavioral strategies, providing dietary education, targeting a

Table 23.1 Interventions of family-based treatment of obesity in children <12 years

Study (all RCTs) (author, year, country, ref)	Age in years (n)	Content and/or strategy for intervention & comparison groups	Length of intervention: duration (follow up)	Effect on outcomes
Epstein *et al*, 1985, USA[10,14,17,63]	8–12 (41)	1. Diet + aerobic exercise 2. Diet + lifestyle 3. Diet + muscular exercise	12 months (10 years)	1. −10·9% overweight 2. −17·9% overweight 3. +12·2% overweight
Epstein *et al*, 1981, USA[15,16,63]	6–12 (76)	1. Parent & child 2. Child 3. Non-specific	8 months (10 years)	1. −15·3% overweight 2. +4·5% overweight 3. +14·3% overweight
Johnson *et al*, 1997, USA[14]	8–17 (28)	1. 7-week nutrition then 7-week exercise 2. 7-week exercise then 7-week nutrition 3. Control	14 weeks (5 years)	1. and 2. both significantly lower than 3.
Flodmark *et al*, 1993, Sweden[10,14–16]	10–11 (44)	1. Family therapy 2. No family therapy 3. Control	14–18 months (2 years)	1. 5% BMI >30 2. No significant differences from control at 26 months 3. 29% BMI >30
Epstein *et al*, 2000, USA[10,14]	8–12 (52)	1. Problem-solving taught to parents 2. Problem-solving taught to child 3. Standard family treatment	6 months (2 years)	2. and 3. had greater decrease in BMI score
Epstein *et al*, 2000, USA[10,14]	8–12 (76)	1a. ↑ in activity; high dose 1b. ↑ in activity; low dose 2a. ↓ in sedentariness; high dose 2b. ↓ in sedentariness; low dose	6 months (2 years)	All significant decrease in % overweight from baseline
Epstein *et al*, 1994, USA[10,14–16]	8–12 (40)	1. Mastery 2. No mastery	12 months (2 years)	1. better than 2. at end of Rx, no significant differences at follow up
Nova *et al*, 2001, Italy[14]	3–12 (185)	1. General advice on diet and activity 2. 1400 calories + guidelines for physical activity	? (1 year)	Significant reductions in % overweight in 2.
Epstein *et al*, 1984, USA[14–16,63]	8–12 (53)	1. Parent training 2. No parent training 3. Control	2 months (1 year)	1. = 2.; 1. & 2. better than 3.

(Continued)

Table 23.1 (*Continued*)

Study (all RCTs) (author, year, country, ref)	Age in years (n)	Content and/or strategy for intervention & comparison groups	Length of intervention: duration (follow up)	Effect on outcomes
Braet et al., 1997, Belgium[14]	7–16 (93)	1. Individual therapy 2. Group therapy	7 90 min sessions + 7 family follow up sessions (1 year)	1. and 2. both significant reduction in % overweight
Goldfield et al., 2001, USA[14]	8–12 (24)	1. Individual + group treatment 2. Group treatment	6 months (1 year)	1. and 2. both significant decrease in % overweight, no difference between 1. and 2., but 2. more cost-effective
Warschburger et al., 2001, Germany[10,14]	9–19 (197)	1. Diet, exercise + cognitive behavioral training 2. Diet, exercise + muscle relaxation training	6 weeks (1 year)	1. and 2. both significant decrease in % overweight, no difference between 1. and 2.
Kirschenbaum et al., 1984, USA1[4,15]	9–13 (30)	1. Parents and children together 2. Children only 3. Control	? (1 year)	1. and 2. both significant lower weight than 3; 1. and 2. not significantly different from each other at 1 year
Epstein et al., 1995, USA[10,14–17]	8–12 (61)	1. Reinforced for ↑ in activity 2. Reinforced for ↓ in sedentariness 3. Reinforced for both	4 months (1 year)	2. better than 1. and 3.
Israel et al., 1985, USA[10,14–16]	8–12 (33)	1. Parent training 2. No parent training 3. Control	2 months (1 year)	1. and 2. better than 3.
Stolley et al., 1997, USA[14]	7–12 (65)	1. Culturally specific program diet and importance of activity 2. General health program and stress reduction	12 weeks (1 year)	Significant difference if daily calories from fat in 1.
Epstein et al., 2001, USA[14]	8–12 (26)	1. Diet + increased fruit and vegetables 2. Standard diet	6 months (1 year)	No significant differences in children, parents in 1. significant decrease in overweight

(*Continued*)

Table 23.1 *(Continued)*

Study (all RCTs) (author, year, country, ref)	Age in years (n)	Content and/or strategy for intervention & comparison groups	Length of intervention: duration (follow up)	Effect on outcomes
Senediak and Spence, 1985, Australia[10,14–16,63]	6–13 (24)	1. Rapid schedule behavior modification 2. Gradual schedule behavior modification 3. Attention control 4. Control	1–4 months (7 months)	1. and 2. better than 3. and 4.
Graves *et al*, 1988, USA[10,14,15]	6–12 (?)	1. Problem-solving 2. Behavioral group 3. Instruction group	8 weeks (6 months)	1. and 2. significantly better than 3. for weight, % overweight and BMI; 1. better than 2.
Owens *et al*, 1999, USA[17]	7–11 (74)	1. Exercise 2. Control	4 months (none)	1. significantly lower increase in visceral fat than 2.
Golan *et al*, 1998, Israel[10,14]	6–11 (60)	1. Parents as change agents 2. Children as change agents	12 months (none)	1. significantly better than 2. on BMI centile and dietary behaviors
Hills and Parker, 1988. Australia[16,17,63]	Prepuberty (20)	1. Exercise 2. No exercise	4 months (none)	1. significant reductions in weight and skinfolds
Epstein *et al*, 1985 USA[10,14,16,63]	5–8 (19)	1. Behavior modification 2. Education	12 months (none)	1. better than 2.
Epstein *et al*, 1985, USA[10,14,16,17,63]	8–12 (23)	1. Diet + exercise 2. Diet	12 months (none)	1. better than 2. for body weight
Wheeler and Hess, 1976[16,63]	2–10 (28)	1. Behavior modification 2. Control	7 months (none)	1. better than 2.
Aragona *et al*, 1975, USA[15,16,63]	5–11 (13)	1. Response cost + reinforcement 2. Response cost 3. Control	3 months (11 months)	1. and 2. showed better results after Rx, but no significant differences at 11 months
Israel *et al*, 1994, USA[8,10,14,15]	8–13 (34)	1. Enhanced child self-regulation 2. No enhanced child self-regulation	6 months (3 years)	No significant differences
Duffy and Spence, 1993, Australia[10,14–16]	7–13 (27)	1. Cognitive therapy 2. Progressive relaxation	2 months (8 months)	No significant differences

(Continued)

Table 23.1 *(Continued)*

Study (all RCTs) (author, year, country, ref)	Age in years (n)	Content and/or strategy for intervention & comparison groups	Length of intervention: duration (follow up)	Effect on outcomes
Figueroa-Colon et al., 1993, USA[9,63]	7–17 (19)	1. Protein-sparing modified fast 2. Hypocaloric balanced diet	15 months (none)	No significant differences
Gropper and Acosta, 1987, USA[9]	6–12 (8)	1. Fiber supplement 2. Placebo	2 months (none)	No significant differences
Bacon and Lowrey, 1967, USA[9]	5–17 (20)	1. Drug therapy (fenfluramine) 2. Placebo	2 months (none)	No significant differences

Studies are ranked in order of content and length of intervention in descending order of effectiveness of intervention.
NB. All but the last study included some form of nutrition/diet and physical activity regimen.

reduction of sedentary behaviors and increasing physical activity appear to be beneficial strategies.

It appears that parents probably have an important role in supporting their children up to 8 years of age, even if their own obesity is intractable.[10,64] For example, food choices in preschoolers are influenced by television advertising[13] and weight management in obese children can be improved by making television viewing contingent on physical activity.[12] There are conflicting results from interventions that treat parents and children together, but some evidence exists for the effectiveness of family therapy in preventing overweight children from progressing to severe obesity.[65]

Assessing the family's readiness to address the problem is recommended, but there are no screening or assessment tools currently available for children in the context of their families (one for adolescents is currently under development in the US).[5] An appropriate way forward may be to assess comprehensively family dietary and activity behaviors. Changes in lifestyle behaviors should be undertaken in small steps so that the family can accommodate and appreciate changes as appropriate.[5] Supplementary activities may include family therapy, counseling, support, and strategies to improve parental and child psychological well-being.[5,20] The provision of additional clinical services may include access to dieticians, particularly those with training in physical activity management, family therapists, and psychologists who specialize in nutrition, physical activity, and health.

Question

6. In children (*population*), are school-based programs (*intervention*) effective for prevention and treatment of obesity without risk of harm (*outcome*)? **[Therapy]**

You identify four reviews of school-based programs for the prevention of obesity in children, including the Effective Health Care review,[14] a review of school-based studies for the prevention of cardiovascular disease,[20] and two reviews of school-based treatments for obesity.[21,22] You base your conclusions on the effectiveness of school-based strategies on the evidence contained in 15 prevention and five treatment studies.

Prevention programs in schools are targeted at whole school populations and have the potential to change the school environment. Two randomized controlled trials that targeted decreasing television viewing, or aerobic exercise had significant effects on BMI and skinfold thickness. The first (Grades 4 and 5) was well designed, theory based, ran for 8 months, and reduced BMI by 0·45, skinfold thickness by 1·47 mm and waist circumference by 2·30 cm. The second (preschool children) was self-selecting and ran for 7 months. Triceps skinfolds decreased for both groups, but in the exercise group they decreased from 12·2% at baseline to 8·8%

($P = 0.058$), whereas that of the control group was not significant ($11.7-9.7\%$, $P = 0.179$), and a greater effect was observed for girls. A quasi-experimental field trial (Grades 4 and 5), with six intervention schools and eight matched control schools, used The Eat Well and Keep Moving Program.[68] This program is integrated into the curriculum, provides materials for families and the food services, and includes a wellness program for all school staff. Although it is not an RCT, you conclude that this is the most comprehensive school-based intervention to date. A smaller study (one intervention and one control school; Grades 3–5), using physiological outcomes, appeared less effective. Although low numbers (44 subjects in intervention school in analyses) may have resulted in lack of statistical power, the intervention was of low intensity. However, most school-based obesity prevention studies addressed risk factors for cardiovascular disease rather than obesity or overweight.

In your previous search of EMBASE, you located a recent review of interventions to prevent cardiovascular disease that only included studies with a comparison group,[20] randomized allocation, and children up to 12 years. Direct comparison between studies was not possible owing to the limited amount of information published in the review. However, the authors attempted to derive quantitative effects to give a weighted effect ratio (Table 23.2). Weighted effect ratios were derived by adding the significant effects (defined as a comparison with a $P < 0.05$ in favor of the intervention group) in each intervention and dividing this by the total number of comparisons made between the groups in each intervention, i.e., all significant effects/all possible effects. Unweighted effect ratios were calculated from cell averages by study outcome (for example, diet, BMI). The weighted and unweighted effect ratios were then averaged and ranked to provide a relative comparison by outcome of intervention effects. Effects across all studies (n = 16; age range 8–15 years) were more consistent for smoking (80%) and cognitive outcomes (65%) than for behavioral and physiologic outcomes (fitness 36%; diet 34%; lipids 31%; physical activity 30%; blood pressure 18%, and adiposity 16%). This means that, for example, more significant effects were found for smoking than for adiposity. You know that the effect ratio has limitations, as it does not incorporate intensity, sample characteristics or size, method, and quality. You decide to include information from an additional review,[22] as meta-analysis is not possible.

The studies you find on MedLine include three reviews of school-based controlled trials[16,21,22] and one meta-analysis of treatment components.[63] Unfortunately, the inclusion criteria for studies within each of these are not easily comparable, and there is a lack of data to allow detailed comparison across the studies. The studies provide definitions of overweight and obesity, but the process by which children were selected is generally not included. Sallis *et al.*[22] reviewed the five available treatment studies for children under the age of 12 years (Table 23.2).

Again, comments on the trials are summarized in the reviews and you conclude the following: in all five treatment studies, the intervention had significant effects, with a reduction of 10% in the extent of overweight in the intervention group. However, few studies instigated changes in the school environment. The characteristics of individuals leading the intervention were an important factor in their success, as has been noted elsewhere in physical activity health promotion research.[67] Follow up studies were not carried out, and so little is known about maintenance of weight reduction over time. In general, you observe that the efficacy of treatment interventions is improved when a mix of components known to impact on weight reduction (i.e., increased physical activity, diet or nutrition change/education, attention to cognitive or behavioral psychological aspects, and parental involvement) are included and are conducted with younger children and their families.

Schools provide daily contact with children during term and have the potential for early identification and treatment of obesity. Schools also provide opportunities for social interaction with peers and staff, as well as a safe environment, and the potential to provide healthy school lunches and facilities for physical activities with trained staff. They can also create strong linkages with the local community, local government, and industry. One important harm associated with treatment interventions that may have limited their implementation in schools, as proposed by Sallis *et al.*, is the potential stigmatization of overweight children. Unfortunately, this adverse outcome is rarely measured systematically[22]; however, children have voiced fears of being teased or embarrassed if peers knew of their participation in a weight-loss program at school.[69] You therefore conclude from the available evidence that it is unrealistic to expect positive health outcomes from school interventions in isolation from the wider community. However, it is likely that the strongest opportunities for long-term change will occur with prevention strategies that address societal and whole school approaches, particularly those where the effects of stigmatization can be minimized.

Schools are less desirable as a treatment location; but, school-based prevention interventions, anchored within the normal curriculum or health-promoting school framework, which aim to reduce CVD risk factors, show promise. Commonly, these interventions involve a more multifaceted whole-child approach including diet, physical activity, and other educational and psychological issues, rather than focusing on single components. Corresponding efforts, emphasizing activity and building self-esteem, may minimize inadvertent increase of eating disorders.

Table 23.2 Interventions of school-based prevention and treatment of obesity in children aged 5–12 years

Study (author, year, country, ref)	N	Study type	Intervention content						Length of intervention	Effect on outcomes
			Physical activity	Nutrition	Psychology	Parents	Theory/ model			
Gortmaker et al. 1999, USA[14]	2103	A	+	+		+	+	3 years	T v C: Significant decreases in fat intake P = 0·04, increases in fruit and veg intake P = 0·01 and fiber P = 0·05, same decrease in TV viewing P = 0·05
Donnelly et al., 1996, USA[14]	236	B	+	+			+	2 years	T v C: No differences in body weight or body fat, cholesterol, insulin, or glucose; HDL cholesterol significantly greater
Robinson, 1999, USA[14]	390	B	+				+	8 months	T v C: −1·47 mm triceps skinfold, −2·3 cm waist circumference
Mo-Suwan et al., 1998, Thailand[14]	292	B	+					30 weeks	T and C: decrease in BMI and triceps skinfold; BMI increase slowed; BMI increase in girls
Muller et al., 2001, Germany[14]	297	B	+	+		+		1 year	T v C: BMI not significant; triceps T < C; P < 0·01
Sahota et al., 2001, UK[14]	613	B	+	+				1 year	Effect not significant
Luepker et al., 1996, USA[20]	5106	C	+	+				3 years	ER: 30/49 (61%)
Resnicow et al., 1992, USA[20,22]	3066	C		+	+			3 years	ER: 9/22 (41%) significant for BMI, cholesterol, BP, dietary behavior
Harrell et al., 1996, USA[14,20]	1274	C	+		+			8 weeks	ER: 6/16 (38%)
Walter et al., 1998, USA[20]	1105	C	+	+	+			5 years	ER: 5/15 (33%)
Bush et al., 1989, USA[20,22]	1041	C	+	+	+			4 years	ER: 19/73 (26%) no effect on BMI or skinfolds
Sallis et al., 1993, USA[14,20]	550	C	+	+				2 years	ER: 6/36 (17%)
Vandongen et al., 1995, USA[20]	1147	C	+	+				9 months	ER: 13/140 (11%)

(Continued)

Table 23.2 (*Continued*)

Study (author, year, country, ref)	N	Study type	Intervention content					Length of intervention	Effect on outcomes
			Physical activity	Nutrition	Psychology	Parents	Theory/ model		
Dwyer et al., 1983, USA[20,22]	500	C		+	+			1 year	ER: 13/140 (11%)
Walter et al., 1988, USA[20,22]	2283	C	+	+	+			5 years	ER: 1/13 (8%) not significant on BMI
Brownell and Kaye, 1982, USA[21,22]	77	D	+	+	+	+		10 weeks	T: −15% overweight; C: +3% overweight
Foster et al., 1985, USA[21,22]	89	D	+	+	+	+		12 weeks	T: −5% overweight; C: +0.3% overweight
Ruppenthal and Gibbs, 1979, USA[21,22]	42	D	+	+	+			5 months	T: −11.4% overweight; C: not significant
Seltzer and Mayer, 1970, USA[21,22]	350	D		+	+			5–6 months	T: −11% overweight; C: −2% overweight
Epstein et al., 1978, USA[22]	6	D		+	+			3 months	T: −5.6% overweight; C: subject is own C

NB. Studies are ranked by effect ratio or intervention components then length of intervention.
Study type: A – Quasi-experimental obesity reduction; B – RCT obesity prevention; C – CVD prevention; D – Obesity treatment.
Outcomes: ER – effect ratio: number of positive effects for each component/total comparisons for all components between groups within a study[52]; T – treatment; C – control.

Resolution of the scenario

You note that your patient is already overweight (BMI > 85th centile), and her preschool weight check indicated early adiposity rebound (the BMI was between the 75th and 97th centiles). You explain to the girl and her parents that her current weight, in conjunction with her weight at 5 years and a genetic predisposition to obesity, suggests that a gradual trend towards adult obesity is likely. You explain that there is evidence that weight management in children has both short- and long-term positive effects, but in order to achieve long-term weight management, changes in lifestyle behaviors are necessary. You stress that improved family dietary habits and involving the family in the child's management are important, but that increasing physical activity, particularly lifestyle activities, and decreasing sedentary behavior (including watching television) are crucial for long-term weight maintenance. You comprehensively assess the family's dietary and activity behaviors, and together plan a program to encourage gradual behavioral changes. You also suggest family therapy and support to help maintain self-confidence and self-esteem, and provide strategies for increasing physical activity. You initially arrange monthly follow up meetings to help establish/support new behaviors, with longer intervals between meetings if progress is satisfactory.

Future research needs

Although this chapter summarizes the best evidence currently available, the validity and generalizability of many studies remain questionable, particularly for obesity treatment. Available RCTs may be non-generalizable owing to sampling problems – the best research in the field has been conducted in populations who are most likely to respond to interventions, tending to be white, more middle class, better motivated, better educated families. Unfortunately, these studies have rarely been repeated in other communities; however, some of these issues are likely to be addressed in the future. Furthermore, the failure to report vital and important psychological and social factors in studies, and the wide range of interventions tested, makes comparison of studies difficult. Intuitively, nutrition/diet and physical activity components are included in most programs and, more recently, behavior modification has been used and appears to be beneficial. The impact of programs on adverse outcomes is rarely considered, and studies evaluating long-term outcomes beyond one year are virtually non-existent.

The questions that remain largely unanswered by the available evidence are:

- What is the role of social health and mental health interventions in collaboration with the necessary focus on dietary change, food choices, physical activity, and sedentary behaviors in the prevention and management of childhood overweight and obesity? Similarly, what is the role of psychosocial factors such as self-esteem or family dysfunction in the development and management of obesity?
- What are the optimal parenting techniques and/or parenting involvement in treatment and management approaches to child and adolescent overweight and obesity?
- What is the role of very low energy diets, pharmacotherapy and bariatric surgery in childhood and adolescent obesity?
- What is the minimum intervention required for effective weight management program for children and adolescents in primary care?
- What are the family characteristics which promote success in treatment of childhood overweight and obesity?
- What sociocultural influences need to be considered in the planning and implementation of interventions, and what interventions are most effective for culturally different populations?
- What is the influence and role of sectors such as the built and open environment, housing, transport, media and advertising, processed food industries, health, or pharmaceutical industry, in promoting healthy lifestyles and behaviors?

The population, governments, non-governmental organizations, industry and research agencies now need to urgently recognize that:

- Childhood obesity has reached epidemic proportions and, as such, requires commensurate resources in prevention and treatment in order to achieve change for individual families and the population.
- Treatment of childhood obesity is a relatively new science necessitating careful review of the evidence base in terms of what appears to be effective as well as carefully designed and evaluated innovative programs of research.
- Research funding should be weighted towards prevention rather than treatment interventions, given that obesity in adulthood is often intractable, and the evidence of effectiveness of treatment in reducing or stabilizing weight in children is limited.
- Innovative non-RCT interventions with a rigorous external evaluation may also provide useful evidence.
- Qualitative research performed within intervention studies will provide evidence about the views of participants (families and providers) to interventions and may highlight why interventions are more successful or less successful.
- School-based programs for the prevention and treatment of obesity in children should consider: children's developmental stages; the use family-inclusive programs of integrated within the school curriculum; school policy; environmental context, and broader community activities. They also need to consider the needs of school staff and resources in terms of their capacity to support and deliver programs, as well as conjoint outcomes.

- The cost-effectiveness of treatment programs for children and their families needs to be incorporated into programs of research or non-research action. Cost measures need to include family and community opportunity costs over the short and long term.
- Appropriate short- and long-term outcomes need to be defined for children, rather than using conventional or adult-oriented outcomes. Weight loss (or failure to gain) may not be an appropriate measure of therapeutic interventions for growing children, and behaviors such as habitual physical activity, healthy eating, and improved psychosocial outcomes are likely to be more meaningful in children until their growth and development stabilize.
- Interventions are likely to be more relevant, successful, and less harmful if they are pretested with groups similar to those intended to receive the intervention.

Critical appraisal should indicate whether studies were conducted as was intended, i.e., that all participants received the study intervention as intended. If variation is observed, researchers should consider the implication of this on the estimate of effectiveness of the intervention.

Summary table

Question	Type of evidence	Result	Comment
What is the prevalence of obesity?	National surveys for children < 12 years	All evidence shows an increase in the prevalence of overweight and obesity	Increasing societal trends in industrialized countries and now developing countries
Are overweight children at greater risk of psychosocial consequences?	Cross-sectional studies	Overweight/obesity has detrimental effects on psychological well-being	Children and young adults show many negative effects due to their overweight; the psychological effects are immediate and persist
Are overweight children at greater risk of current and future disease?	Longitudinal and cross-sectional studies	Childhood obesity results in current indicators, such as detrimental lipid profiles and type 2 diabetes and higher risk status for future obesity, metabolic syndrome, CVD, and NIDDM	Children and young adults show many negative medical consequences of overweight impacting on health outcomes in adulthood
Is being overweight as a child likely to persist?	Growth studies, longitudinal community studies	Children with a BMI > 85th centile, an obese parent, and an AR around 5 years are more likely to be persistently overweight	These indicators are useful for identification purposes
Are family-based methods for reduction in childhood obesity in pre-adolescent children effective?	Family-based RCTs	Effective components: improving diet and dietary behaviors; increasing lifestyle physical activity and decreasing sedentary behaviors; family involvement	Treatment effects are limited but more successful with children compared with their parents; far more research is required to establish effective strategies
What are the benefits and harms of school-based prevention and obesity treatment programs?	School-based obesity prevention RCTs and CVD prevention interventions	Obesity prevention studies show a positive effect, CVD prevention studies show mixed effects. Treatment studies showed some positive effects	Targeting decreasing sedentary pastimes and improving the diet at school in generic studies for prevention appear promising; schools are not suitable locations for treatment because of stigmatizing of those treated

References

1 WHO. *Obesity: preventing and managing the global epidemic.* Geneva: WHO, 1998.

2 Ebbeling CB, Pawlak DB, Ludwig DS. Childhood obesity: public-health crisis, common sense cure. *Lancet* 2002;**360**: 473–82.

3 Cole TJ, Bellizzi MC, Flegal KM, Dietz WH. Establishing a standard definition for child overweight and obesity worldwide: international survey. *BMJ* 2000;**320**:1240–3.

4 Jebb SA, Prentice AM. Single definition of overweight and obesity should be used. *BMJ* 2001;**323**:999.

5 Barlow SE, Dietz WH. Obesity evaluation and treatment: expert committee recommendations. *Pediatrics* 1998;**102**:E29.

6 Lohman TG. *Advances in body composition assessment.* Champaign, IL: Human Kinetics, 1992.

7 Wang Y, Wang JQ. A comparison of international references for the assessment of child and adolescent overweight and obesity in different populations. *Eur J Clin Nutr* 2002;**56**: 973–82.

8 Pratt BM, Woolfenden SR. Interventions for preventing eating disorders in children and adolescents. In: Cochrane Collaboration. *Cochrane Library*, Issue 1. Oxford: Update Software, 2003.

9 Campbell K, Waters E, O'Meara S, Kelly S, Summerbell C. Interventions for preventing obesity in children (Cochrane Review). In: *Cochrane Library*, Issue 4, 2003. Chichester, UK: John Wiley + Sons Ltd.

10 Summerbell C, Waters E, Edmunds LD *et al.* Interventions for treating obesity in children. In: Cochrane Collaboration. *Cochrane Library*, Issue 3. Oxford: Update Software, 2003.

11 Hardeman W, Griffin S, Johnston M, Kinmonth AM, Wareham NJ. Interventions to prevent weight gain: a systematic review. *Int J Obes* 2000;**24**:131–43.

12 Faith MS, Berman N, Heo M *et al.* Effects of contingent television on physical activity and television viewing in obese children. *Pediatrics* 2001;**107**:1043–8.

13 Borzekowski DL, Robinson TN. The 30-second effect: an experiment revealing the impact of television commercials on food preferences of preschoolers. *JADA* 2001;**101**:42–6.

14 Effective Health Care: *The prevention and treatment of childhood obesity.* NHS Centre for Reviews and Dissemination, University of York, York Publishing Services, 2002.

15 Jelalian E, Saelens BE. Empirically supported treatments in pediatric psychology: Pediatric obesity. *J Ped Psych* 1999;**24**:223–48.

16 Epstein LH, Myers MD, Raynor HA, Saelens BE. Treatment of pediatric obesity. *Pediatrics* 1998;**101**:554–70.

17 Epstein LH, Goldfield GS. Physical activity in the treatment of childhood overweight and obesity: current evidence and research issues. *Med Sci Sports Exerc* 1999;**31**(Suppl.): S553–9.

18 Gibson P, Edmunds L, Haslam DW, Poskitt E. An approach to weight management in children and adolescents (2–18 years) in primary care. *J Fam Hlth Care*, 2002;**12**:108–9.

19 Parsons TJ, Power C, Logan S, Summerbell CD. Childhood predictors of adult obesity. *Int J Obes* 1999;**23**:(Suppl.8).

20 Resnicow K, Robinson TN. School-based cardiovascular disease prevention studies: Review and synthesis. *Ann Epidemiol* 1997;**7** (Suppl.):S14–S31.

21 Story M. School-based approaches for preventing and treating obesity. *Int J Obes* 1999;**23**:S43–S51.

22 Sallis JF, Chen AH, Castro CM. School-based interventions for childhood obesity. In: Cheung LWY, Richmond JB, eds. *Child health, nutrition and physical activity.* Champaign, IL: Human Kinetics, 1995.

23 Ogden CL, Flegal KM, Carroll MD, Johnson CL. Prevalence and trends in overweight among US children and adolescents, 1999–2000. *JAMA* 2002;**288**:1728–32.

24 Chinn S, Rona RJ. Prevalence and trends in overweight and obesity in three cross sectional studies of British children, 1974–94 *BMJ* 2001;**322**:24–6.

25 Booth ML, Chey T, Wake M *et al.* Change in the prevalence of overweight and obesity among young Australians, 1969–1997. *Am J Clin Nutr* 2003;**77**:29–36.

26 Berenson GS, Srinavisian SR, Bao W. Precursors of cardiovascular risk in young adults from a biracial (black-white) population: The Bogalusa Heart Study. *Ann NY Acad Sci* 1997;**817**:189–98.

27 Reilly JJ, Dorosty AR, Emmett PM. Prevalence of overweight and obesity in British children: cohort study. *BMJ* 1999; **319**:1039.

28 Popkin BM, Doak CM. The obesity epidemic is a worldwide phenomenon. *Nutr Rev* 1998;**56**:106–14.

29 Staffieri JR. A study of social stereotype of body image in children. *J Pers Soc Psychol* 1967;**7**:101–4.

30 Stunkard AJ, Burt V. Obesity and the body image: II, age at onset of disturbances in the body image. *Am J Psych* 1967;**123**:144–7.

31 Pingitore R, Dugoni BL, Tindale RS, Spring BSO. Bias against overweight job applicants in a simulated employment interview. *J Appl Psychol* 1994;**79**:909–17.

32 Sargent JD, Blanchflower DG. Obesity and stature in adolescence and earnings in young adulthood. Analysis of a British birth cohort. *Arch Pediatr Adolesc Med* 1994;**148**: 681–7.

33 Dietz WH. Childhood weight affects adult morbidity and mortality. *J Nutr* 1998;**128**:411S–414S.

34 Freedman DS, Dietz WH, Srinavisian SR, Berenson GS. The relation of overweight to cardiovascular risk factors among children and adolescents: the Bogalusa Heart Study. *Pediatrics* 1999;**103**:1175–82.

35 Gortmaker SL, Must A, Perrin JM, Sobol AM, Dietz WH. Social and economic consequences of overweight in adolescence and young adulthood. *N Engl J Med* 1993; **329**:1008–12.

36 Latner JD, Stunkard AJ. Getting worse: the stigmatisation of obese children. *Obes Res* 2003;**11**:452–56.

37 Schwimmer JB, Burwinkle TM, Varni JW. Health-related quality of life of severely obese children and adolescents. *JAMA* 2003;**289**:1813–19.

38 Schwartz MB, Puhl R. Childhood obesity: a societal problem to solve. *Obes Rev* 2003;**4**:57–71.

39 Freedman DS, Dietz WH, Srinavisian SR, Berenson GS. The relation of overweight to cardiovascular risk factors among

children and adolescents: the Bogalusa Heart Study. *Pediatrics* 1999;**103**:1175–82.

40 Yanovski JA, Yanovski SZ. Treatment of pediatric and adolescent obesity. *JAMA* 2003;**289**:1851–53.

41 Arslanian S. Type 2 diabetes in children: Clinical aspects and risk factors. *Horm Res* 2002;**57**(Suppl.1):19–28.

42 Vanhala M, Vanhala P, Kumpusalo E, Takala J. Relation between obesity from childhood to adulthood and the metabolic syndrome: population based study. *BMJ* 1998; **317**:319.

43 Frankel S, Gunnel DJ, Peters TJ, Maynard M, Davey Smith G. Childhood energy intake and adult mortality from cancer: The Boyd Orr cohort study. *BMJ* 1998;**316**:499–504.

44 Must A, Jaques PF, Dellal GE, Bajema CJ, Dietz WH. Long-term morbidity and mortality of overweight adolescents. A follow up of the Harvard Growth Study of 1922 to 1935. *N Engl J Med* 1992;**337**:1350–5.

45 Whitaker RC, Wright JA, Pepe S, Seldel KD, Dietz WH. Predicting obesity in young adulthood from childhood and parental obesity. *N Engl J Med* 1997;**337**:869–73.

46 Guo SS, Wu W, Chumlea WC, Roche AF. Predicting overweight and obesity in adulthood from body mass index values in childhood and adolescence. *Am J Clin Nutr* 2002; **76**:653–8.

47 Must A. Morbidity and mortality associated with elevated body weight in children and adolescents. *Am J Clin Nutr* 1996;**63**:445S–447S.

48 Serdula MK, Ivery D, Coates RJ, Freedman DS, Williamson DF, Byers T. Do obese children become obese adults? A review of the literature. *Prev Med* 1993;**22**:167–77.

49 Gasser T, Zeigler P, Seifert B, Molinari L, Largo R H, Prader A. Prediction of adult skinfolds and body mass from infancy to adolescence. *Ann Human Biol* 1995;**22**:217–33.

50 Clarke WR, Lauer RM. Does childhood obesity track into adulthood? *Crit Rev Food Sci Nutr* 1993;**33**:423–30.

51 Casey VA, Dwyer JY, Coleman KA, Valadian I. Body mass index from childhood to middle age: a 50-y follow up. *Am J Clin Nutr* 1992;**56**:14–18.

52 Mossberg HO. 40 year follow up of overweight children. *Lancet* 1989;**67**:401–3.

53 Rolland-Cachera M-F. Onset of obesity from the weight/stature^2 curve in children: the need for a clear definition. *Int J Obes* 1993;**17**:245–6.

54 Lake JK, Power C, Cole TJ. Child to adult body mass index in 1958 British Birth Cohort: associations with parental obesity. *Arch Dis Child* 1997;**77**:376–81.

55 Whitaker RC, Pepe S, Wright A, Seidel KD, Dietz WH. Early adiposity rebound and the risk of adult obesity. *Pediatrics* 1998;**101**:E5.

56 Wright CM, Parker L, Lamont D, Craft AW. Implications of childhood obesity for adult health: findings from thousand families cohort study. *BMJ* 2001;**323**:1280–4.

57 Rolland-Cachera M-F, Cole TJ, Sempe M, Tichet J, Rossignol C, Charraud A. Body mass index variations: centiles from birth to 87 years. *Euro J Clin Nutr* 1991;**45**:13–21.

58 Duran-Tauleria E, Rons RJ, Chinn S. Factors associated with weight for height skinfold thickness in British children. *J Epidem Commun Hlth* 1995;**49**:466–73.

59 Siervogel RM, Roche AF, Guo SM, Mukherjee D, Chumlea WC. Patterns of change in weight/stature^2 from 2 to 18 years. *Int J Obes* 1991;**15**:479–85.

60 Prakopec M, Bellisle F. Adiposity in Czech children followed from 1 month of age to adulthood: Analysis of individual BMI patterns. *Ann Human Biol* 1993;**20**:517–25.

61 He Q, Karlberg J. Probability of adult overweight and risk change during the BMI rebound period. *Obes Res* 2002; **10**:135–40.

62 Dietz WH. "Adiposity Rebound": reality of epiphenomenon. *Lancet* 2000;**356**:2027–8.

63 Haddock CK, Shadish WR, Klesges RC, Stein RJ. Treatments for childhood and adolescent obesity. *Ann Behav Med* 1994;**16**:235–44.

64 Gill TP. Key issues in the prevention of obesity. *Br Med Bull* 1997;**53**:359–88.

65 Flodmark CE, Ohlsson T, Ryden 0, Sveger T. Prevention of progression to severe obesity in a group of obese schoolchildren treated with family therapy. *Pediatrics* 1993; **91**:880–4.

66 Epstein LH, Valoski A, Wing RR, McCurley J. Ten-year outcomes of behavioral family-based treatment for childhood obesity. *Hlth Psych* 1994;**13**:373–63.

67 Biddle SJH, Fox KR, Edmunds L. *Physical activity promotion in primary health care in England.* London: Health Education Authority, 1994.

68 Donnelly JE, Jacobsen DJ, Whatley J *et al.* Nutrition and physical activity program to attenuate obesity and promote physical and metabolic fitness in elementary school children. *Obes Res* 1996;**4**:229–43.

69 French SA, Story M, Perry CL. Self-esteem and obesity in children and adolescents: A literature review. *Obes Res* 1995; **3**:479–90.

24 Youth smoking cessation: school-based approaches

Chris Lovato, Gayla Swihart, Jean Shoveller

Case scenario

The local school superintendent has contacted you for advice regarding a school-based youth smoking cessation program. You are aware that youth smoking rates are increasing in your community. A number of programs are offered for adult smokers through the local Cancer Society, but the school has questions about whether these interventions are appropriate for youth. Before making recommendations to the school, a number of questions come to mind. What approaches have been demonstrated to be successful in helping youth quit smoking? What kind of results can be expected from school-based approaches? What new approaches hold promise?

Background

Smoking is the major leading preventable cause of premature death. The World Health Organization estimates that among industrialized countries, where smoking has been common, smoking is estimated to cause over 90% of lung cancer in men and about 70% of lung cancer among women. Worldwide, tobacco causes approximately 8.8% of deaths (4.9 million) and 4.1% of Disability Adjusted Life Years (DALYs) (59.1 million). The escalation of the tobacco epidemic is illustrated by comparing these estimates for 2000 with those for 1990: there are at least a million more deaths attributable to tobacco, with the increase being most marked in developing countries.[1] Between 50 and 75% of teenagers living in countries belonging to the Organization for Economic Cooperation and Development try smoking. Half of these adolescents will become addicted to nicotine and one in two smokers will die from the effects of tobacco.[2]

Nicotine addiction can be overcome. Many smokers have great difficulty quitting, however, because the addiction is so powerful. Smokers who are successful in quitting usually need to make several quit attempts, and former smokers are at risk of relapsing. Seventy-three percent of adult daily smokers in the United States began smoking between the ages of 13 and 17 years.[3] Thus, the adolescent years represent a critical time during which to intervene both with programs to prevent uptake of smoking, and with cessation programs to interrupt nicotine addiction as early as possible.

Framing answerable clinical questions

The primary question arising from the scenario relates to the efficacy of school-based (not clinic-based) cessation programs. The question can be formulated to identify the population in question, the intervention to be evaluated and the desired outcomes (see Chapter 2).

Question

1. Among adolescent smokers (*population*), do school-based cessation programs (*intervention*) result in cessation of cigarette smoking (*outcome*)? **[Therapy]**

Searching for evidence

You start by searching for synthesized evidence in systematic reviews and evidence-based guidelines. Because this is such an important question, you decide to also conduct a search for primary literature so that you can provide the superintendent with the most directly relevant and evidence-based answer as possible. You initially try a narrower search strategy, but find that this topic is not well indexed and you lose too many potentially relevant hits. Because you will be providing expert advice for the community, you choose to make the search as comprehensive as possible. You go first to the *Cochrane Library* and *Clinical Evidence* for reviews related to smoking, and then you use a broad search strategy for MedLine, PubMed, EMBASE, Cumulative Index to Nursing & Allied Health (CINAHL), and Web of Science. To reduce the number of articles to those specific to the question of interest, you scan the article titles (and if necessary review the abstract) to identify those that describe school-based smoking cessation interventions for adolescents.

You focus on identifying studies that have a control or comparison group; this eliminates a substantial number of studies that used a single-group design. In addition, you find that there is substantial overlap in the databases, and so hits are often repeats from other databases. For example, a search using EMBASE generates 10 relevant hits, four of which are repeats from other databases. Finally, you retrieve the relevant articles, most of which can be read or downloaded and printed directly from the internet database.

Search strategy

Smoking cessation OR Tobacco control [MeSH terms] AND Adolescents [MeSH]; smoking, prevention, AND/OR schools [text words], limited to English, human, 1993–present.

In some databases, the search can be further limited to peer-reviewed journal articles (PsychInfo) or type of publication (journal articles, chapters). In some cases (for example, CINAHL, EMBASE), the search can be limited by age range; therefore Adolescents is not required as MeSH term or keyword.

- *Cochrane Library*: nine reviews, two protocols
- *Clinical Evidence*: One chapter
- MedLine (PubMed): 17 hits
- EMBASE: six new hits
- CINAHL: two new hits
- Web of Science: no new hits
- PsychInfo: three new hits
- CDC.gov: no new hits

Critical review of the evidence

Among the nine adolescent tobacco control reviews listed in the *Cochrane Library*, you find one review on school-based programs for preventing smoking, and others on community interventions for preventing smoking in young people, mass media interventions for preventing smoking in young people, and interventions for preventing tobacco sales to minors. You also find protocols (unfinished reviews) on the impact of advertising on adolescent smoking behaviors and on tobacco cessation interventions for young people. Two other potentially relevant reviews are identified – "Self-help interventions for smoking cessation" and "Antidepressants for smoking cessation" but you note that they do not address issues related to adolescent populations. The chapter in *Clinical Evidence* discusses physician advice, nicotine

replacement, and cessation targeted for high-risk individuals, but none of the studies they review addresses adolescent populations. However, you do identify a literature review on school-based cessation that was published in a previous edition of *Evidence-based pediatrics and child health*.[4]

Among the 17 relevant hits found on MedLine (Pubmed), three are descriptions of programs, eight provide background information, one does not include adolescents in the sample, and five are cessation intervention outcome studies (true hits). One of the two new hits on CINAHL is a commentary on an outcome study found in the MedLine search, and is not a true hit. Of the six hits on EMBASE, two provide background information and three are true hits. Of the three apparently relevant hits found on PsychInfo, one provides background information and two intervention outcome studies (true hits). In total, 11 cessation intervention outcome studies and 16 relevant background studies are identified in this search, as well as several general reviews of youth tobacco cessation.

Study design and outcome measures

In all, you have found 11 intervention studies published between 1993 and 2003 that report on the evaluation of a school-based smoking cessation program for adolescents.[5–17] In addition to these articles, you have a look at several review articles and book chapters that describe approaches to school-based cessation programs in order to gain background information in the area of smoking cessation. Two studies that used a single-group design are retrieved from your broad search because they focus on nicotine replacement therapy for adolescents, a new and emerging area in which there is limited research.[11,15]

Many intervention studies do not explicitly describe a theoretical basis for the interventions tested; however, the terms used to describe the approaches and the variables measured suggest that Social Learning Theory, the Health Belief Model, the Transtheoretical Model of Change, and cognitive behavioral approaches have been applied. Glanz, Marcus-Lewis and Rimer[18] provide an excellent review of these and other health behavior theories in a book entitled *Health behavior and health education: theory, research and practice*.

Five studies used a randomized approach in assigning units (students, classes, or schools) to different experimental groups.[5,6,13,16,17] Six studies used quasi-experimental designs.[7–10,12,14] Two studies you specifically chose to include focus on nicotine patch therapy.[11,15] As is typical of school-health research, classrooms or groups within schools were most frequently used as the unit of randomization. Those studies that randomly assigned individuals, classrooms, or schools to experimental groups and based the statistical analysis on the unit of randomization have the strongest design[5,6,13,16,17] for assessing this intervention question, since confounding variables are controlled through randomization.

All 13 studies report short-term (0–6 months) cessation or reductions in smoking as the outcome, and five of the 12 studies report long-term (≥ 6 months) cessation.[6,11,13,15,17] You are most interested in studies that report long-term cessation rates of 6 months or more, [6,11,13,15,17] knowing that those reporting short-term cessation rates are not as reliable because of the high likelihood of smoking relapse. The studies reporting a reduction in the number of cigarettes are relevant, but cessation is the primary outcome of interest.

All the studies rely upon self-reported outcome data. Nine of the studies also reported verification of smoking cessation using physiological measures,[5,7,8,10–12,15–17] and one study used a bogus-pipeline procedure.[13] The bogus pipeline is a set of data collection procedures that are meant to motivate study participants to truthfully answer questions about their smoking behavior. Participants are led to believe that their answers will be verified by a biochemical or physiological test. You much prefer the studies that validate self-report data with physiological data or at least use the bogus pipelines because of the potential inaccuracies in self-reported data.

In addition to these study design issues, you focus on two key issues in reviewing the evidence related to intervening with adolescent smokers: recruitment of participants and the content of the intervention. One of the most difficult issues related to adolescent cessation programs is the challenge of recruiting young smokers to participate in an intervention.[19,20] A study investigating this issue reported that student smokers in Australia (n = 863) felt that recruitment to cessation programs would be enhanced by increasing the availability of programs in the school setting; making programs available at low or no cost, and enrolling a large number of highly supportive friends in the program.[19] The primary factor inhibiting recruitment to a school smoking-cessation program was fear that friends, teachers, and especially parents would find out that the student smoked.

Most studies you review do not provide detailed information related to recruitment methods in schools. Several studies noted recruitment to be a challenging issue. Other research regarding recruitment approaches in schools suggests that active recruitment, which includes person-to-person contact, may be more effective than traditional methods, such as posters and other media-type announcements.[20]

The challenge of recruiting adolescents for cessation programs has implications for both research and practice. For those professionals implementing programs, it suggests the need for special attention to recruitment efforts. For the purpose of interpreting research, it indicates that unless study participants are randomly selected from a pool of smokers and there is a reasonable recruitment rate (60% or better), the results have low generalizability since there is a high self-selection bias.

The interventions vary substantially, but three basic types emerge: group-based, nicotine replacement therapy, and (more recently) computer-based interventions. Few articles reviewed included a description of the theoretical basis for intervention development. The lack of clearly documented interventions in many published studies creates a difficulty for both researchers and practitioners, since interpretation of results and replication of the intervention are difficult, if not impossible, to achieve. Based on the wide use of peer-led models, it appears that the Social Learning Theory provided the basis for many interventions. Other theories that appear to drive the development of some interventions include the Health Belief Model, Transtheoretical Model of Change, and cognitive behavioral approaches. A brief description of interventions according to the type of intervention follows.

In adult populations, cessation rates for community-based programs typically range between 5 and 10%. Although the research evidence in younger populations is very limited, the cessation rates reported range considerably, but are reported as high as 34% at 12-months post-testing.[17] At 6 months post-testing, most cessation rates drop to between 5 and 17%.[11,13] It is important to keep in mind that the "shelf-life" of smoking-cessation programs is shorter for adolescents than for adults, since the language and styles reflected in intervention materials change more rapidly for younger generations. Program planners should be prepared to consider updated, new, and innovative programs on an ongoing basis.

When you are selecting interventions, it is important to consider cultural factors that influence health-related behaviors, including smoking.[21] Awareness and sensitivity to cultural diversity should be reflected in planning and implementing a school-based cessation program. Huff and Kline provide helpful suggestions for practitioners working with ethnic/cultural communities (see Box).[21] Most of the publications reviewed provide no specific information that would help to evaluate the cultural relevance of program interventions. The population served cannot be described with any degree of certainty. In most of the studies reviewed, the authors did not note the participation of community members in the development of the intervention methods or implementation.

Cultural issues in smoking cessation

- Be aware of the many ways of perceiving, understanding, and approaching health and disease processes across cultural and ethnic groups, and that cultural differences can and do present major barriers to effective healthcare intervention.
- Be aware of the possible barriers that might be encountered if the program is targeted to a community primarily composed of first-, second-, or even third-generation people. Acculturation processes affect these groups in different ways.
- Seek to become more culturally competent and sensitive. The process is ongoing, and you always should be striving to increase and improve your abilities to work in a variety of cross-cultural settings.

Interventions and their impact

Group interventions

The majority of programs have more than six sessions with most sessions lasting between 40 and 50 minutes. Most programs included 10 sessions generally implemented over an 8- to 10-week period, while the longest program was 20 sessions. Of the studies reviewed, three reported 12-month follow up observations[6,15,17] and three studies reported only immediate follow up[7,9,12] In the remaining studies, the timing of follow up observations ranged between 20 weeks and 6 months.

- Project EX is an eight-session cessation program that addresses topics such as reasons for using and quitting smoking, the harmful substances in tobacco, managing withdrawal, maintenance strategies, and avoiding relapse. The program is implemented over a 6-week period and also involves activities such as games and "talk shows". Project EX was evaluated in a three-group experimental design: clinic-only, clinic plus a school-as-community component, and standard care control group. The evaluation included 335 smokers, which the authors indicate make it the largest controlled field trial conducted to date (2001).[16] Eighteen schools were assigned to each condition using a block design that involved factor scores derived from school demographics, arranging schools along a single factor score continuum and then randomly assigning adjacently scored schools to one of the three groups. At 3-month follow up (5 months after the program quit date) 17% of the smokers participating in the two groups who received the program had quit smoking for at least the past 30 days as compared to 8% in the control group. Self-reports were biochemically validated.

- Project Towards No Drug Abuse (TND) is a high school drug abuse prevention curriculum that contains 12 40-minute interactive sessions and addresses smoking, marijuana, hard drug, and violence-related behavior such as carrying weapons. Topics addressed include active listening, myths and denials, chemical dependency, self-control, positive and negative thought and behavior loops, and decision-making and commitment. Sussman *et al*[17] report the results of three experimental trials of TND. A total of 2468 high school students from 42 schools were surveyed. The first trial tested the impact of the TND classroom in alternative high schools. The curriculum was delivered alone or in combination with a set of antidrug activities outside the classroom. No reduction effects, relative to controls, were found on the prevalence of cigarette smoking. The second trial examined whether or not TND would generalize to the regular high school context. No evidence for a reduction was found in the prevalence of smoking in the second

study. The third trial tested the relative effectiveness of a health educator-led and a self-instruction version of TND, as compared to the standard anti-drug program. At 12-month follow up, prevalence reduction in smoking was 27% for the health educators-led group. In a review article by Sussman[22] it is reported that, in this third study at 12-month follow up, 34% of students in the health educator group had quit smoking compared to 21% in both self-instruction and control conditions.

- Not on Tobacco (NOT) is a teen smoking cessation program developed by the American Lung Association. The core program is 10 50-minute sessions with four booster sessions at the end of the program. A 2-year efficacy evaluation and a study that focuses on level of addiction and cessation outcomes involved 627 and 365 high school students, respectively.[8,10] The first study was conducted in 40 Florida schools using a matched design in which each NOT school was matched to a brief intervention school (n = 627).[8] NOT schools were selected and then a brief intervention school was matched based on community and school demographics. The brief intervention consisted of a 5–10 minute session with scripted quit smoking advice and self-help brochures. NOT participants reduced cigarette consumption by at least 50% from baseline. Overall, the immediate quit rate for NOT was 21·7% and 12·6% at 5·2 months post-program (validated with carbon monoxide testing). Interestingly, further analysis suggested that NOT was more effective for females than for males. Although males showed significant quit attempts in both experimental groups, NOT females were more likely to actually quit smoking. In the follow up study examining nicotine dependence and its impact on quit rates, researchers compared NOT with the same brief intervention.[10] The brief intervention was effective only with low-dependent smokers, while NOT was effective with smokers who had a range of nicotine dependence, including high-dependent smokers.

- A high school-based program consisting of eight sessions over a 6-week period was implemented during the school day and tested in a study that included a total of 74 participants.[5] The sessions addressed team-building skills, problem solving, and practising solutions with a quit date set on the sixth session. The last two sessions focused on relapse and withdrawal. In an evaluation of this program Adelman randomized students into intervention and wait-list control groups. The control group received informational pamphlets on how to quit smoking. Saliva cotinine was used to validate self-reports. Immediately following the program the classroom group was significantly more likely to be smoke-free (59% *v* 17%) and to have reduced mean number of cigarettes per day (7·0 *v* 1·0). Four weeks later these differences persisted: smoke-free (52% *v* 20%)

and reduction in mean number of cigarettes per day (6·6 *v* 1·6). At 10 weeks 41% of the classroom group were smoke-free; at 20 weeks this dropped to 31%. Once participants in the pamphlet group underwent the classroom intervention, their cessation rates were similar to the initial group: 31% at the end of the curriculum and 27% at 10-week follow up.

- "Tobacco, no thanks!" (TNT) had six sessions and used a combination of materials from other current smoking-cessation programs. An evaluation of the TNT compared peer-led groups with adult-led groups with a total of 93 Grade 11 and 12 students in seven US high schools. Students were divided into three groups of 6–12 participants; groups led by college-age instructors, by regular classroom teachers, and a control group that had no intervention at all but one school. Prince[14] reported that immediately following completion of a six-session class, 17% of intervention participatns reported quitting smoking. At the 1-month follow up, 18% of all participants reported they had quit smoking.

- The Tobacco Education Group (TEG) and Tobacco Awareness Program (TAP) are part of a two-step program based on the Stages of Change Model. TEG was designed for adolescents not yet thinking about quitting (i.e., precontemplative or contemplative stages) and TAP is intended for adolescents who want to quit smoking (i.e., preparation, action, and maintenance stages). The programs consist of 8 1-hour sessions. The program for teens thinking about quitting sought to motivate them to quit. The curriculum included reasons for smoking and consequences of tobacco use. The quit smoking curriculum addresses topics such as consequences of smoking, triggers for smoking, pitfalls to expect during and after quitting, and methods for quitting. Weight management is also addressed in this program. An evaluation study was conducted using data from 351 students in six schools who participated in the program over a 2-year period.[7] Over one-half (57%) of the students who participated in TEG had been caught smoking cigarettes and were required to attend the program to avoid suspension. With the exception of a few students who were assigned to TAP by administrators, students who participated in TAP did so on a voluntary basis. In this study students were recruited into the control group. Both intervention groups decreased tobacco use as compared to the control group. At immediate post-test, 12% of the TEG, 15% of the TAP, and 0% of the control group had quit smoking. Self-reported use was biochemically validated. The mean reduction of cigarettes for non-quitters at post-test was 18% for TEG and 24% for TAP.

- A school-based multiple risk factor reduction curriculum for Grade 10 students included 20 sessions that focused on physical activity, nutrition, stress, personal problem solving, and cigarette smoking. Each student was asked to carry out a self-change project. Tenth graders from four high schools (n = 1447) in two districts participated in an evaluation study conducted by Killen and colleagues.[12] Within each district, schools were matched for size and distribution of ethnic groups. One school was assigned at random to receive the intervention and one school served as a control. Measurements were collected at baseline and at 2 months after completion of the intervention. There was no significant difference between groups in the proportion of regular smokers who reported cessation at 2-month follow up. Carbon monoxide was used to validate self-reports. However, the authors report that only 5·6% of baseline experimental smokers in the control group had quit smoking at follow up as compared to 10·3% in the intervention group.

- A peer-led smoking prevention program that involved 6 hours of classroom time was evaluated by Hamm.[9] The program focused on 1320 Grade 7 students in four US schools, and was designed to provide social skills to resist pressures to smoke. In a study by Hamm of a group receiving a peer-led smoking prevention program, 4% quit smoking compared to 2% in a control group.[9] A comparison between quitters, youth with no change in their smoking status, and new users indicated that the program had a significant effect on smoking behavior. Although measurement may have occurred immediately following the program, the exact timing of measurement was not specified.

Nicotine replacement therapy

In the area of adult smoking cessation, one of the most significant treatment developments has been the use of nicotine replacement therapy (NRT); however, there are few studies addressing the effectiveness of NRT among adolescent populations.

- Smith provides the first published report on the use of NRT patches in adolescent smokers who were trying to quit.[15] In a single-group study design, the patch was distributed weekly to 22 students at five public high schools in the US. The intervention also included weekly group counseling strategies that took place at the school. Only one of 22 (5%) participants remained smoke-free (carbon monoxide confirmed). During the eighth and final week of patch therapy, three of 22 (14%) participants had reported not smoking (carbon monoxide confirmed). Among those who had not quit smoking, significant decreases in reported daily consumption of cigarettes were observed at 3 months (from 22 to 5 cigarettes) and 6 months (from 22 to 9 cigarettes); however, significance levels are not reported. Also, the mean number of cigarettes smoked per day was higher at the 6-month follow up, as compared to the 3-month follow up. The one participant who returned the 12-month survey had remained abstinent.

- A second single-group study of NRT tested 6 weeks of patch therapy with follow up visits at 12 weeks and 6 months.[11] Hurt and colleagues tested this approach among adolescents who smoked at least 10 cigarettes per day. Adolescents aged 13–17 years (n = 101) were instructed on the use of the patch and were given self-help materials from the package insert used in the over-the-counter product. In addition, 10–15 minute individual counseling was provided. A non-randomized, single-group study was conducted in which daily diaries were collected and carbon monoxide testing performed during weekly visits that occurred during the 6 weeks of patch therapy. Additional follow ups were made at 12 and 26 weeks. Smoking abstinence was 11% at 6 weeks and 5% at 6 months. The authors conclude that the nicotine patch program was not effective for smoking cessation.[11]

Computer-based interventions

Computer-based interventions are a relatively new area and there are a limited number of studies testing this approach with youth cessation.

- Pallonen reports on a comparison of two different computer-based smoking-cessation interventions in 88 students randomized to one of two intervention groups.[13] One intervention was based on the Transtheoretical Model of Change and was designed to be an interactive and individualized cessation expert system, while the other was a computerized version of a program developed previously by the American Lung Association ("Tobacco Free Teens"). Six months after a computer-based intervention the researchers observed a 6% cessation rate. There were no significant differences between the individualized group format and a non intervention group. Immediate cessation rates ranged from 14 to 20% at several different observation points during program implementation.
- An experts system based on the Transtheoretical Model of Change was tested on Grade 9 students. The program was designed to prevent teens from becoming smokers and help those who smoked to quit.[6] Participants received three class lessons delivered to all students in the classroom and three sessions with an interactive computer program. An evaluation involved 4227 students in 26 schools. Schools were randomly assigned to intervention and control groups. No differences in quit rates were seen among students at 12-month and 24-month follow ups.[6]

Summary

Based on the limited evidence you have found, strategies can be identified that provide direction for implementing school-based cessation interventions. It is important to note, however, that smoking-cessation programs in general tend to have low success rates. Based on a comprehensive review of 66 adolescent tobacco use cessation trials, Sussman[22] reports the mean quit-rate at a 3–12-month average follow up among interventions was 12% compared to approximately 7% across control groups.

Recruitment is clearly one of the most challenging facets of school-based cessation programs. Intervention packages for schools need to provide guidance and specific procedures, describing how to best recruit young people in this setting. Research suggests that recruitment is enhanced by active and direct, person-to-person methods that are complemented by more traditional approaches, such as bulletins and newspaper announcements. Ensuring that programs are available at low or no cost and include students' supportive friends also will facilitate recruitment.

Group intervention approaches that include structured sessions appear to hold more promise than approaches that rely solely on self-help. This recommendation is consistent with the Cochrane review on self-help intervention for smoking cessation, which concludes that self-help materials may provide a small increase in quitting compared to no intervention.[23]

There does not appear to be a clear advantage to peer versus adult leadership; however, more research is needed in this area before any final conclusions are made. Though based on evidence of the importance of peer support among adolescents, it is recommended that smoking-cessation interventions incorporate some form of peer involvement.

Although there have been no published reports of controlled studies on "quit and win" strategies for adolescents, numerous jurisdictions have provided monetary incentives to encourage adolescents to quit smoking.[24] Smoking-cessation contests appear to have high immediate success rates. However, they are costly and result in relatively low long-term cessation rates.[22]

Participatory approaches that involve youth in the development and implementation of programs will help to ensure the cultural relevance of interventions within a variety of communities. Most published studies on school-based interventions have been conducted in the USA; thus, results should be generalized with caution at an international level.

There is a lack of research evidence examining cost-effectiveness of school-based cessation programs in comparison with clinical or other community-based settings. Schools are likely to compare well with other sites for youth cessation interventions, because of the availability of low-cost or no-cost space, better access to students and their peers (as supporters or program leaders), and minimal transportation costs.

Two new approaches that may hold promise for the future include NRT and computer-based interventions. A Cochrane review concludes that all the commercially available forms of NRT increase quit rates approximately 1·5–2-fold.[25] For some adolescents, NRT may be a useful component of a smoking-cessation intervention; however, there is currently a lack of evidence regarding effectiveness in this population. More research is needed in this area and should take into consideration the unique aspects of youth addiction.

Computer-based interventions represent a relatively new innovation in community approaches in health promotion. There is very little research evidence regarding their effectiveness in either adult or adolescent populations. Pallonen demonstrated impressive recruitment rates (80%) using this mode of delivery in a school-based study; however, cessation rates at 6-month follow up were only 6%, and the Aveyard study found no cessation benefit for an interactive computer program.[6,13]

Resolution of the scenario

You meet with the school superintendent to discuss how to proceed with a school-based smoking-cessation program. You explain the limitations of the evidence currently available in the literature and discuss the list of recommendations you have developed, based on the available evidence (see Summary of Evidence). You suggest a behavioral intervention that is appropriate to the cultural background of students. It is critical that the program includes a follow up component that supports maintenance of cessation rates. At minimum, a maintenance program of 6 months after the intervention is essential.

You recommend that the cessation program be offered at school as part of a comprehensive tobacco-control program that includes prevention and a non-smoking policy. The cessation program should be offered at no cost and should be targeted to youth who smoke on either a daily or an occasional basis. Recruitment of students should be by person-to-person contact and confidentiality must be assured to encourage enrolment. The program should not be offered during class time where there is a mix of smokers and non-smokers and confidentiality cannot be maintained. The cessation program should be group-based, have a peer-support component and be led by individuals with special training in this area. For program evaluation, students should ideally be randomized to interventions and a control group should be included. Outcome measures should be clearly defined and should include reduction in the number of cigarettes smoked and cessation of smoking in the short term (3 and 6 months) and long term (12 months).

Future research needs

In comparison to the literature on adult smoking cessation, the number of studies that address the effectiveness of youth smoking-cessation interventions is limited. The majority of tobacco cessation programs for adolescents have not been rigorously evaluated.[22,26,27,28,29] In particular, there are very few published studies examining school-based cessation programs, and many of those available have methodological limitations. Those studies that have been conducted vary widely in scientific quality and effectiveness in smoking-cessation rates.[27] Many interventions that have been evaluated provide limited evidence due to weak study designs (for example, non-randomized designs, no control group), and a detailed description of the intervention and implementation are not typically available in the literature.

Research is needed on intervention approaches that have:

- a sound theoretical basis;
- recruitment procedures that ensure a representative and non-biased sample;
- full descriptions of the intervention and implementation, including recruitment;
- randomized control group designs;
- standardized outcome measures; and
- long-term follow up of at least 12 months.

Specific research questions that should be addressed include:

- What are the most effective methods for recruiting teens into smoking cessation programs?
- Is nicotine replacement therapy effective in aiding cessation among teens? Is this approach more effective for certain types of smokers?
- What approaches are effective for teens who are "occasional" or "social" smokers?
- Are computer-based approaches to cessation an effective mechanism for teens?

Summary table

Strategies	Rating*	Impact/Evidence
Structure and content		
Group-based interventions that include structured sessions rather than self-help approaches are preferable with youth in school-based settings	B	A Cochrane Systematic Review of self-help materials (adult literature) concludes that they may provide a small increase in quitting compared to no intervention[23]; Sussman *et al.* found that 34% of adolescents in a health educator group quit smoking, compared to 21% of those who used self-help, and 21% who were in a control group[17]
A maintenance phase (e.g., at least 6 months post-quit date) is essential for a successful smoking cessation program	B	Evidence for this recommendation is based on cessation programs in general and is an accepted standard of practice. Based on results of 22 studies with immediate post-program and an average 8-month follow up Sussman reports an average relapse rate of 36% among adolescents[22]
School-based Quit & Win smoking cessation contests should only be used as adjuncts to group-based interventions with structured sessions	B	Diguisto suggests that cessation contests may be a useful recruitment tool, but cautions that there is no evidence to indicate that they contribute to long-term cessation rates[24]
School-based smoking-cessation interventions should incorporate a peer support component	B	Gillespie *et al.*, reported that recruitment to smoking-cessation programs would be enhanced by participants having a large number of highly supportive friends also enrolled in the program[19]
Implementation		
Smoking-cessation programs for schools should be implemented with guidance and detailed procedures on how to best recruit youth using active and direct, person-to-person methods, complemented by traditional media	B	One of the most critical issues related to adolescent cessation programs is recruitment. Research regarding recruitment approaches in schools suggests active recruitment that includes person-to-person contact may be more effective than traditional methods, such as posters and other media-type announcements[20]
Cessation programs can be led by peers or professionals who are specifically trained in this area, preferably health professionals	B	Prince demonstrated that groups led by same-age peers trained in smoking-cessation techniques produced the same results as a program delivered by trained adult professionals[14]
School-based programs should maintain individual smokers' privacy and confidentiality because many youth do not want their parents/guardians to know that they smoke	B	The primary factor inhibiting recruitment to a school smoking-cessation program was fear that friends, teachers, and especially parents, would find out that the student smoked[19]
New approaches		
Computerized interventions have been demonstrated as feasible for high school students; however, there is currently a lack of evidence regarding effectiveness	B	Pallonen *et al.*, tested two computerized self-help adolescent smoking-cessation programs.[13] Cessation rate was 6% at 6-month follow up. High recruitment and participation rates suggest the approach is highly feasible in this population. A second study by Aveyard found that a computer-based approach was not effective[6]
Nicotine replacement therapy does not appear as promising for adolescents as it is for adults	B	The findings from two single-group studies both found the patch was not effective with adolescents.[11,15] There do not appear to be any dangerous side effects for adolescents. Adolescents may respond differently to the nicotine patch and they may smoke for different reasons than adults
General		
Schools should provide youth with access to cessation programs as part of a comprehensive tobacco control program	C	
Schools should be used as settings for delivering youth smoking-cessation interventions owing to the availability of low-cost or no-cost space, better access to students and their peers, and minimal transportation costs	C	

*The evidence supporting the strategies is rated as follows:
A: Consistent, positive findings from trials (experimental or quasi-experimental with random assignment) with adolescents in school settings
B: Some evidence with adolescents in school settings
C: Based on best professional opinion or expert panel consensus with evidence sometimes drawn from other populations or settings and from well-developed theories

References

1   World Health Organization. *The world health report 2002 – reducing risks, promoting healthy life.* Geneva: WHO, 2002.

2   World Health Organization. *The world health report 1999 – combating the tobacco epidemic.* Geneva: WHO, 1999.

3   Institute of Medicine, Committee on Preventing Addiction in Children and Youth. *Growing up tobacco free: preventing nicotine addiction in children and youth.* Washington, DC: National Academy Press, 1994.

4   Lovato C, Shoveller J. Youth smoking cessation: school-based approaches. Moyer VA, ed. In: *Evidence based pediatrics and child health.* London: BMJ Books, 2000.

5   Adelman WP, Duggan AK, Hauptman P, Joffe A. Effectiveness of a high school smoking cessation program. *Pediatrics* 2001;**107**:50.

6   Aveyard P, Sherratt E, Almond J, Lawrence T Lancashire R, Griffin C, Cheng KK. The change-in-stage and updated smoking status results from a cluster-randomized trial of smoking prevention and cessation using the transtheoretical model among British adolescents. *Prevent Med* 2001;**33**: 313–24.

7   Coleman-Wallace D, Lee JW, Montgomery S, Blix G, Wang DT. Evaluation of developmentally appropriate programs for adolescent tobacco cessation. *J School Hlth* 1999;**69**: 314–19.

8   Dino G, Horn K, Goldcamp J, Fernandes A, Kalsekar I, Massey C. A 2-year efficacy study of Not On Tobacco in Florida: an overview of program successes in changing teen smoking behavior. *Prevent Med* 2001;**33**:600–5.

9   Hamm NH. Outcomes of the Minnesota Smoking Prevention Program. *Psycholog Rep* 1994;**75**:880–2.

10 Horn K, Fernandes A, Dino G, Massey CJ, Kalsekar I. Adolescent nicotine dependence and smoking cessation outcomes. *Addict Behav* 2003;**28**:769–76.

11 Hurt RD, Croghan GA, Beede, SD, Wolter TD, Croghan IT, Patten CA. Nicotine patch therapy in 101 adolescent smokers. *Arch Pediatr Adolesc Med* 2000;**154**:31–7.

12 Killen JD, Telch MJ, Robinson TN, Maccoby N, Taylor CB, Farquhar JW. Cardiovascular disease risk reduction for tenth graders. *JAMA* 1998;**260**:1728–33.

13 Pallonen UE, Velicer WF, Prochaska JO *et al.* Computer-based smoking cessation interventions in adolescents: description, feasibility, and six-month follow up findings. *Substance Use Misuse* 1998;**33**:935–5.

14 Prince F. The relative effectiveness of a peer-led and adultled smoking intervention program. *Adolescence* 1995;**30**:187–94.

15 Smith TA, House RF Jr, Croghan IT *et al.* Nicotine patch therapy in adolescent smokers. *Pediatrics* 1996;**98**:659–67.

16 Sussman S, Dent CW, Lichtman KL. Project EX: outcomes of a teen smoking cessation program. *Addict Behav* 2001;**26**: 425–38.

17 Sussman S, Dent CW, Stacy AW. Project Towards No Drug Abuse: A review of the findings and future directions. *Am J Hlth Behav* 2002;**26**:354–365.

18 Glanz K, Marcus-Lewis F, Rimer BK, eds. *Health behavior and health education: theory, research and practice.* San Francisco: Jossey-Bass, 1990.

19 Gillespie A, Stanton W, Lowe JB, Hunter B. Feasibility of school-based smoking cessation programs. *J School Hlth* 1995;**65**:432–7.

20 Peltier B, Telch MJ, Coates TJ. Smoking cessation with adolescents: a comparison of recruitment strategies. *Addict Behav* 1982;**7**:71–3.

21 Huff R, Kline M. Tips for the practitioner. Huff R, Kline M, eds. In: *Promoting health in multicultural populations; a handbook for practitioners.* Thousand Oaks: Sage Publications, 1999.

22 Sussman S. Effects of sixty-six adolescent tobacco use cessation trails and seventeen prospective studies of self-initiated quitting. *Tobacco Induced Dis* 2002;**1**:35–81.

23 Lancaster T, Stead LF. Self-help interventions for smoking cessation. In: Cochrane Collaboration. *Cochrane Library*, Issue 3. Oxford: Update Software, 1999.

24 Diguisto, E. Pros and cons of cessation interventions for adolescent smokers at school. In: Richmond RL, ed. *Interventions for smokers: An international perspective.* Baltimore: Williams and Wilkins, 1993.

25 Silagy C, Mant D, Fowler G, Lancaster T. Nicotine replacement therapy for smoking cessation. In: Cochrane Collaboration. *Cochrane Library*, Issue 3. Oxford: Update Software, 1999.

26 Burton D. Tobacco cessation programs for adolescents. Richmond R, ed. In: *Interventions for smokers: an international perspective.* Baltimore, MD: Williams and Wilkins, 1993.

27 Lamkin L, Davis B, Kamen A. Rationale for tobacco cessation interventions for youth. *Prevent Med* 1998;**27**:A3–A8.

28 Mermelstein R. Teen smoking cessation. *Tobacco Control*, 2003;**12**(Suppl.1):i25-i34.

29 Backinger CL, Leischow SJ. Advancing the science of adolescent tobacco use cessation. *Am J Hlth Behav* 2001;**25**: 183–90.

25 Sudden infant death syndrome

Milton Tenenbein

Case scenario

Expectant parents have been referred to you because they are concerned about the sudden infant death syndrome (SIDS). They are expecting their first child in 5 months and their best friends have just lost their baby to SIDS. They read in a pamphlet obtained at their prenatal class that the risk for SIDS can be decreased by having their baby sleep in the supine position, refraining from smoking cigarettes, and by taking care not to overbundle their baby. While they intend to "do anything to protect their baby", they have concerns because, as a student, the mother had been taught that the supine position risks choking, both parents smoke, and the grandmother-to-be has told them that there is a risk for infection if newborns are not kept warm. The parents-to-be are requesting your opinion.

Background

SIDS is "the sudden death of an infant under one year of age that remains unexplained after a thorough case investigation, including performance of a complete autopsy, examination of the death scene and review of clinical history."[1] It is the most common cause of death between 1 and 12 months of age in the developed world but its etiology is unknown. The peak age for SIDS is 12 weeks with 80–90% occurring during the first 6 months of life.[2,3] Many non-modifiable risk factors have been associated with SIDS including young maternal age, low birth weight, shorter gestation, no prenatal care, single marital status, higher parity, low socioeconomic status, and admission to a neonatal intensive care unit.[2–5] However, recent research has demonstrated that modifiable infant care practices are associated with the risk of SIDS. These are the crux of our current case scenario.

Framing answerable clinical questions

The parents are asking three questions which can be framed in the following manner:

Questions

1. Do infants (*population*) who are put to sleep on their backs (*intervention*) have a decreased risk for SIDS (*outcome*)? **[Therapy]**

2. Do infants (*population*) who are exposed to cigarette smoke (*intervention*) have an increased risk for SIDS (*outcome*)? **[Etiology/Harm]**

3. Do infants (*population*) who are bundled in layers of sleep wear and bed coverings (*intervention*) have an increased risk for SIDS (*outcome*)? **[Etiology/Harm]**

Searching for evidence

Search strategy

- American Academy of Pediatrics website
- *Cochrane Library:* sudden infant death
- MedLine (Grateful Med)

  1. sudden infant death AND prevention and control, limited to ENGLISH language, human subjects and randomized controlled trials
  2. sudden infant death AND etiology, limited to ENGLISH language, human subjects and randomized controlled trials
  3. sudden infant death AND prevention and control, limited to ENGLISH language, human subjects and case–control trials

You are aware that these interventions are supported by pediatric medical societies such as the American Academy of Pediatrics and by the public health establishment. However, you have never assessed the evidence. Your first thought is to refer to your textbook of pediatrics, which is the current edition, but it is unhelpful because the data in question are too recent. You decide to peruse the American Academy of Pediatrics website where you discover their SIDS statement.[6] It is an impressive review with 120 citations in its reference list. However, it is not a systematic review, but several citations from the reference list are promising.

You then decide to search the Cochrane database. The Cochrane Database of Systematic Reviews, the Database of Abstracts of Reviews of Effects and the Cochrane Central Register of Controlled Trials have five, two and 12 hits respectively, but none is relevant to your questions. Your MedLine searches result in few hits using "randomized trial" as a search term, but more when you substitute "prevention and control" and "case–control studies". Many of these are promising. Before leaving the Grateful Med site you supplement your search by adding practice guidelines and reviews mainly for their reference lists.

Critical review of the evidence

Not finding any randomized controlled trials does not surprise you because of the nature of the problem. The questions that you are trying to answer involve simple interventions to prevent a rare outcome (death due to SIDS) in a normal and healthy population. A randomized controlled trial would be at least challenging if not totally unfeasible and likely unethical.

In this situation, a case–control study is the most feasible design[19] but a cohort study design could also be considered. The five studies on sleeping position,[7–11] the four on cigarette smoking,[15–18] and the four on thermal environment[7,9,19,20] are all case–control studies. The criteria for judging a case–control study are found in Chapter 7 on assessing harm, as well as in the *JAMA Users' Guides to the Medical Literature IV*.[21]

The primary guides that assess the validity of the results are the comparability of the case and control groups, comparability of data collection for these two groups, and whether follow up was sufficiently long and complete. The secondary guides include whether the temporal relationship is correct and whether there is a dose-response relationship.

Are the case and control infants similar?

In all 11 studies,[7–11,15–20] cases and controls were similar in age, as this was the primary criterion for matching. Cases and controls were also similar for geographic location as this was a further matching criterion but differed in terms of gender and race. However, there was no matching for known risk factors such as maternal age, prenatal care, single marital status, parity, and socioeconomic status. This avoids the problem of overmatching.

Were the outcome and exposure data collected in the same way for both the SIDS and control infants?

Since the outcome is death, there is no risk for an inappropriate assignment to the control group. The exposure data were collected in the same way in each study, in one instance by questionnaire,[15] and in the other eight by structured home interview. Home interview decreases the likelihood of misinterpretation of the questions. Interval between death and data collection varied from several days[7] to many weeks.[8,9,15] As the interval becomes longer, concern regarding recall bias increases. In all studies, data from the case and control infants were collected at the same time. However, some degree of recall bias is inevitable as parents who have just lost a child are likely to recall events leading up to the death differently from parents who have a healthy child.

Was the follow up sufficiently long and complete?

This is to ensure that subjects initially designated as controls are not ultimately cases. In all studies, the investigators were promptly notified of all infant deaths; therefore they would be aware of any control that had become a case. Furthermore, as the definition of SIDS includes 1 year of age as a cut-off point, the likelihood of missing the change from control to case is remote.

Other criteria

The criterion of a temporal relationship between exposure and outcome is not a concern because all exposures precede the outcome when the latter is death. A dose-response relationship was shown for sleeping position[10] and for cigarette smoking.[15–18] Dose-response was not specifically examined in the studies on thermal environment.

A major concern regarding a case–control design is the issue of confounding variables.[19] For SIDS, these would include non-modifiable risk factors such as young maternal age, low birth weight, shorter gestation, no prenatal care, single marital status, higher parity, low socioeconomic status, and admission to a neonatal intensive care unit.[2–5] The two methods of addressing the issue of confounding variables is to demonstrate comparability between the case and control groups or to use statistical techniques to adjust for differences. For SIDS, there is no comparability between case and control groups for these risk factors; therefore employing statistical techniques to control for these differences is the only option. On review of these 11 case–control studies,[7–11,15–20] you find that the major confounding variables mentioned above were adjusted for in the analysis in most instances.

Table 25.1   Relationship between prone sleeping position (cases) and SIDS

Citation	Year	Location	Cases	Controls	OR	95% CI
7	1990	England	67	144	8·8	7·0/11·0
8	1992	New Zealand	485	1800	3·7	2·91/4·70
9	1992	Tasmania	40	79	4·58	1·48/14·11
10	1996	England	195	780	9·58	4·86/18·87
11	1996	Scotland	201	276	6·96	1·51/31·97

Table 25.2   Fall in SIDS rates observed with decrease of prone sleeping position

Citation	Year	Location	% Prone sleeping		SIDS rate		PNDR	
			PRI	PSI	PRI	PSI	PRI	PSI
12	1992	England	58	28	3·5/1000	1·7/1000	–	–
13	1993	Netherlands	60	10	1·04/1000	0·44/1000	4·08/1000	2·74/1000
14	1994	New Zealand	43	5	4·0/1000	2·3/1000	6·2/1000	3·6/1000

Abbreviations: PNDR, postnatal death rate; PRI, pre-intervention; PSI, post-intervention

Your review of these studies using specific criteria[21] finds that these criteria for validity are reasonably met. Therefore it is now appropriate to examine the results.

Sleeping position

You review the five case–control studies that examine the relationship between sleeping position and SIDS.[7–11] In all, the prone sleeping position was a significant risk factor (Table 25.1). The consistency of these findings in studies from disparate geographic locations (New Zealand, Tasmania, Scotland, and two different parts of England) adds strength to the association of the prone sleeping position as a risk for SIDS. Further strengthening this relationship was that in one study, a type of a "dose-response relationship" was found. The side sleeping position was found to have a slight but increased risk (OR 2·01; 95% CI 1·38, 2·93) that was not as severe as the prone position (OR 9·58; 95% CI 4·86, 18·87).[10]

You discover another type of evidence in the review articles located in your MedLine search. These studies[12–14] document a decrease of SIDS in populations where the supine sleeping position is encouraged as a public health intervention (Table 25.2). As before, these studies originate from different countries, adding further strength to this observation. In two of these studies, the effect upon the postneonatal death rate is also documented.[12,14] Significant decreases were found in both populations. This is relevant for the mother's concern that the supine position might increase the rate of aspiration. In one of these studies the infant death rate from aspiration actually fell from 7·9/1000 to 2·5/1000 during the same

time period. However, data derived from observational studies do not provide evidence as strong as that from randomized trials and parents should be counseled accordingly.

Cigarette smoking

You found four case–control studies[15–18] that examine the relationship between exposure to cigarette smoke and SIDS (Table 25.3). Prenatal, postnatal, and combined pre- and postnatal exposures were studied. A significantly increased risk for SIDS was found for all three of these exposures. An observed dose-response relationship strengthens this association. The risk for SIDS increases with the number of cigarettes smoked, the number of smokers in the infant's environment, and whether the infant is exposed both prenatally and postnatally. The studied cohorts originated from the USA, California, England, and New Zealand. This further strengthens both the validity and the generalizability of this association.

Thermal environment

Two of the case–control studies examine the relationship between thermal environment and SIDS.[7,9] One from England[7] studied 67 cases and 144 controls while the other from Tasmania[9] involved 41 cases and 79 controls. Both considered the amount of infant clothing and bedding in terms of thermal resistance and the average room temperature. Both groups found a significantly increased relative risk of SIDS in infants with higher thermal insulation.

Table 25.3 Relationship between prenatal, postnatal and combined prenatal and postnatal exposure to cigarette smoke and SIDS

Citation	Year	Location	Cases	Controls	PRE		POE		CE	
					OR	95% CI	OR	95% CI	OR	95% CI
15[a]	1992	USA	234	2884	–	–	2·22	1·29/3·78	4·07	3·03/5·48
15[b]	1992	USA	201	3254	–	–	2·40	1·49/3·83	2·94	2·12/4·07
16	1993	NZ	485	1800	4·09	3·28/5·11	2·41	1·92/3·02	–	–
17	1995	California	200	200	–	–	3·50	1·81/6·75	–	–
18	1996	England	195	780	2·1	1·24/3·54	2·50	1·48/4·22	2·93	1·56/5·48

[a]white infant
[b]black infant
Abbreviations: NZ, New Zealand; PRE, prenatal exposure; POE, postnatal exposure; CE, combined exposure

This finding was independent of sleeping position in the Tasmanian study.[9] In one study there was a significantly increased likelihood that the heating had been on all night.[7] The other investigators actually measured the room temperature but found no difference between cases and controls. However, two subsequent case control studies addressed the issue of whether overheating, as a risk factor for SIDS, was independent of sleep position.[19,20] One from Tasmania (also by Ponsonby *et al.*) studied 58 cases and 120 controls,[19] while the other from New Zealand had 393 cases and 1592 controls.[20] Both found that overheating was a risk factor for infants only in the prone position and make the point that this position interferes with normal heat loss by reducing the surface of the face exposed for heat loss. These data do not support overheating in the absence of the prone sleeping position as a risk factor for SIDS.

Resolution of the scenario

You are now better equipped to answer these parents' three questions. You advise them that there is strong evidence to support the prone sleeping position as a risk factor for SIDS. You further advise them that there is suggestive and reasonable evidence that this sleeping position does not increase the risk for fatal aspirations. You have strong evidence that exposure to cigarette smoke both prenatally and postnatally increases the risk for SIDS, that there is an additive effect for prenatal and postnatal exposure, and that the risk increases with the number of cigarettes smoked. You have found that the evidence for overheating as a risk factor for SIDS applies to babies in the prone sleeping position. Nevertheless, overheating should be avoided and you advise the parents that the infant should be lightly clothed for sleep and the bedroom temperature should be kept comfortable for a lightly clothed adult.

Future research needs

The discovery that sleeping position is a key risk factor for SIDS was an enormous breakthrough. Implementation of this simple intervention saves lives. However, prone sleeping position is not the cause of SIDS and thus research is needed. First and foremost, the etiology of SIDS needs to be elucidated. Also, SIDS is well known as being more frequent among certain ethnic groups, typically the aboriginal groups in several western countries. We need to find out why this is so.

Summary table

Question	Type of evidence	Result	Comment
Does supine sleeping decrease the risk of SIDS?	5 case–control studies, 3 studies of changes in SIDS rate after change to supine sleeping	Moderate to marked increased risk with prone position, slight increase with side position; fall in rates after change in routine sleep position	Studies in various geographic locations, no compensatory rise in other causes of death
Does exposure to cigarette smoke increase the risk of SIDS?	4 case–control studies	Increased risk with increasing exposure compared to no exposure	Studies in varied geographic locations
Does thermal stress increase the risk of SIDS?	4 case–control studies	Increased risk with increased thermal insulation for babies in the prone position	Appears to be a risk factor only for the prone position

References

1 Willinger M, James LS, Catz C. Defining the sudden infant death syndrome (SIDS): deliberations of an expert panel convened by the National Institute of Child Health and Human Development. *Pediatr Pathol* 1991;**11**:677–64.

2 Little RE, Peterson DR. Sudden Infant death syndrome epidemiology: a review and an update. *Epidemiol Rev* 1990;**12**:241–6.

3 Goldberg J, Hornung R, Yamashita T, Wehrmacher W. Age of death and risk factors in sudden infant death syndrome. *Austral Paediatr J* 1986;**22**(Suppl.1):21–8.

4 Kraus JF, Greenland S, Bulterys M. Risk factors for sudden infant death syndrome in the US Collaborative Perinatal Project. *Int J Epidemiol* 1989;**18**:113–20.

5 Hoffman HJ, Damus K, Hillman L, Krongrad E. Risk factors for SIDS. Results of the National Institute of Child Health and Human Development SIDS Cooperative Epidemiological Study. *NY Acad Sci* 1988;**533**:13–30.

6 Kattwinkel J, Brooks J, Keenan ME, Malloy M Changing concepts of sudden infant death syndrome: implications for infant sleeping environment and sleep position. *Pediatrics* 2000;**105**:650–6.

7 Fleming PJ, Gilbert R, Azaz Y *et al.* Interaction between bedding and sleeping position in the sudden infant death syndrome: a population based case-control study. *BMJ* 1990;**301**:85–9.

8 Mitchell EA, Taylor BJ, Ford RPK *et al.* Four modifiable and other major risk factors for cot death: The New Zealand study. *J Paediatr Child Hlth* 1992;**28**(Suppl.1):S3–S8.

9 Ponsonby AL, Dwyer T, Gibbons LE, Cochrane JA, Jones ME, McCall MJ. Thermal environment and sudden infant death syndrome: case–control study. *BMJ* 1992;**304**:277–82.

10 Fleming PJ, Blair PS, Bacon C *et al.* Environment of infants during sleep and risk of the sudden infant death syndrome: results of 1993–5 case–control study for confidential inquiry into still births and deaths in infancy. *BMJ* 1996;**313**:191–5.

11 Brooke H, Gibson A, Tappin D, Brown H. Case–control study of sudden infant death syndrome in Scotland. *BMJ* 1997;**314**: 1516–20.

12 Wigfield RE, Fleming PJ, Berry PJ, Rudd PT, Golding J. Can the fall in Avon's sudden infant death rate be explained by changes in sleeping position? *BMJ* 1992;**304**:282–3.

13 de Jonge GA, Burgmeijer RJF, Engelberts AC, Hoogenboezem J, Kostense PJ, Sprij AJ. Sleeping position for infants and cot death in the Netherlands 1985–91. *Arch Dis Child* 1993;**69**: 660–3.

14 Mitchell EA, Brent JM, Everard C. Reduction in mortality from sudden infant death syndrome in New Zealand: 1986–92. *Arch Dis Child* 1994;**70**:291–4.

15 Schoendorf KC, Kiely JL. Relationship of sudden infant death syndrome to maternal smoking during and after pregnancy. *Pediatrics* 1992;**90**:905–8.

16 Mitchell EA, Ford RPK, Stewart AW *et al.* Smoking and the sudden infant death syndrome. *Pediatrics* 1993;**91**:893–6.

17 Klonoff-Cohen HS, Edelstein SL, Lefkowitz ES *et al.* The effect of passive smoking and tobacco exposure through breast milk on sudden infant death syndrome. *JAMA* 1995; **273**:795–8.

18 Blair PS, Fleming PJ, Bensley D *et al.* Smoking and the sudden infant death syndrome: results from 1993–1995 case–control study for confidential inquiry into stillbirths and deaths in infancy. *BMJ* 1996;**313**:195–8.

19 Ponsonby A-L, Dwyer T, Gibbons LA, Cochrane JA, Wang F-G. Factors potentiating the risk of sudden infant death syndrome associated with the prone position. *N Engl J Med* 1993;**329**:377–82.

20 Williams SM, Taylor BJ, Mitchell EA. Sudden infant death syndrome: insulation from bedding and clothing and its effect modifiers. *Int J Epidemiol* 1996;**25**:366–75.

21 Levine M, Walter S, Lee H, Haines T, Holbrook A, Mover V. Users' guides to the medical literature IV. How to use an article about harm. *JAMA* 1994;**271**:1615–19.

Section III

Common pediatric conditions

26 Fever in the young infant

Gina Neto

Case scenario

A 6-week-old boy presents to the emergency department with a history of fever for one day. His mother states that he felt hot to touch but she did not measure the temperature. He has been feeding well and there has been no change in his behavior pattern. He has had a clear nasal discharge and occasional cough for several days. His 3-year-old sister has a "cold". He was born at term after a healthy pregnancy and had an unremarkable neonatal course. He has been well until this illness. He has not received any immunizations. On examination, he has a rectal temperature of 39°C, heart rate 120, blood pressure 90/50, respiratory rate 36. He is alert and active, with good color, and appears well hydrated. He has a clear nasal discharge, but the remainder of the examination is unremarkable.

Background

The febrile infant is a common problem and accounts for a large number of ambulatory care visits. Young infants often present with non-specific symptoms and it is difficult to distinguish between young infants with a viral syndrome and those with early bacterial illness. It is also important to recognize that serious infections in young infants may present without fever.

Most febrile illnesses in infancy are secondary to viral infections and are self-limited.[1–5] Although serious bacterial illness (SBI) is relatively uncommon, if it is not promptly diagnosed and treated, serious morbidity and mortality may result. In the first month of life, the predominant bacterial organisms involved are those acquired from the birth canal; most commonly group B streptococcus and *Escherichia coli*, and less often *Staphylococcus aureus*, *Listeria monocytogenes* and other Gram-negative enteric bacteria. These organisms remain the common bacterial pathogens for the infant 4–12 weeks of age. Other organisms such as *Streptococcus pneumoniae* and *Neisseria meningitidis* may be also seen in these older infants. *Haemophilus influenzae* type b infection is now uncommon due to widespread immunization but may still occasionally be seen in the very young, unimmunized population. *Escherichia coli* is the most frequent pathogen in urinary tract infections (UTI). *Salmonella* spp., *Campylobacter* spp., and *Shigella* spp. are the common causes of bacterial enteritis.

The rate of SBI in young infants with fever is about 8% overall and is higher in the 0–4 week age range (13%) than in 4–8 week infants (8%). Rates of SBI are highest in the very youngest infants, < 2 weeks old (25%). The overall rates of bacteremia and meningitis are 2% and 0·8% respectively, with the highest rates again seen in the youngest infants.[5–11]

Owing to difficulty in making a clinical diagnosis of bacterial infections in the infant, it has been recommended that febrile infants < 3 months of age undergo a complete work-up for sepsis (including lumbar puncture), be admitted to hospital, and receive parenteral antibiotics for at least 48 hours pending culture results.[12] Although this conservative approach minimizes the risk of infectious complications, it leads to unnecessary hospitalization and treatment for many infants. An important question is how to determine which infants are at low risk of serious bacterial illness and can be managed safely as outpatients.

Definitions

- *Fever.* Usually defined as a rectal temperature > 38°C. For infants < 3 months old this value is approximately two standard deviations above the mean.[13] Most studies that focus on the febrile infant have used this definition.
- *Young infant.* The infant < 90 days of age. Some studies include only infants < 8 weeks of age.
- *Neonate.* The infant < 4 weeks of age.
- *Serious bacterial infection* (SBI). Meningitis, bacteremia, UTI, pneumonia, bone and joint infections, skin and soft tissue infections, and bacterial enteritis.

Framing answerable clinical questions

Your questions should be structured in a manner that will help to focus your search. From the issues that arise in the scenario, you frame the following questions.

Questions

1. In the assessment of young infants (*population*), can axillary and tympanic temperature measurements (*exposure*) accurately identify infants with fever (*outcome*)? **[Diagnosis]**
2. In young infants with fever (*population*), does the level of fever (*exposure*) identify infants with SBI (*outcome*)? **[Diagnosis]**
3. In young infants with fever (*population*), is the response to the administration of antipyretics (*exposure*) useful in identifying infants with bacterial versus viral infections (*outcome*)? **[Diagnosis]**
4. In young infants with fever (*population*), can clinical assessment (*exposure*) identify infants with SBI (*outcome*)? **[Diagnosis]**
5. In young infants with fever (*population*), can laboratory investigations (*exposure*) help identify infants at risk for SBI (*outcome*)? **[Diagnosis]**
6. In the evaluation of the young febrile infant (*population*), is a chest *x* ray (*exposure*) helpful to identify infants with SBI (*outcome*)? **[Diagnosis]**
7. Can febrile infants 28–90 days old at low risk for SBI (*population*) be managed as outpatients (*intervention*) with no increase in morbidity (*outcome*)? **[Therapy]**
8. Can febrile infants 28–90 days old at low risk for SBI (*population*) be managed without antibiotics (*intervention*) with no increase in morbidity (*outcome*)? **[Therapy]**
9. What is the accuracy of the low risk criteria (*exposure*) for predicting SBI (*outcome*) in febrile infants < 28 days old (*population*)? **[Diagnosis]**

Searching for evidence

Because many of these questions are interrelated, you decide to combine your searches for the answers to these questions. You begin by looking for sources of evidence that are already appraised. You search the *Cochrane Library* (2003, Issue 2) for systematic reviews on the topic. In the Database of Abstracts of Reviews of Effects (DARE) you find "A systematic review of the literature to determine optimal methods of temperature measurement in neonates, infants and children". The Cochrane Controlled Trials Register gives you five references that are relevant for your therapy questions.

You search MedLine for papers on diagnosing fever, diagnosing and managing infection, and find several hundred records that you quickly scan through for relevant studies. You also find an American Academy of Pediatrics Practice Guideline on the management of infants and children with fever without source. You know that high-quality guidelines may answer your questions, or at least can provide you with many references.

Search criteria

- *Cochrane Library* (Issue 2, 2003): fever AND infant
- *Best Evidence*: no chapter
- MedLine (OVID):

  - For diagnostic test questions about fever: exp *fever/di (Diagnosis) AND exp infant
  - For diagnostic test questions about SBIs: exp *bacterial infections/di (Diagnosis) AND exp infant AND exp fever
  - For therapy questions: exp antibiotics AND exp *fever AND exp infant Practice Guidelines AND exp infant

Critical review of the evidence

Question

1. In the assessment of young infants (*population*), can axillary and tympanic temperature measurements (*exposure*) identify infants with fever (*outcome*)? **[Diagnosis]**

Studies to determine which method of temperature measurement is most accurate should provide a blind comparison of various types of measurement to a gold standard (the "true" body temperature). Looking through the references you found from your searches and the guideline, you note that most studies use the rectal temperature as the gold standard for practical clinical use.

Parents frequently prefer axillary temperatures. You find a systematic review by Craig *et al.*[14] that compared the temperature measured at the axilla with the rectal temperature. Forty studies were reviewed and 20 were included in the meta-analysis. Of these, nine studies were in neonates. The pooled mean temperature difference (rectal minus axillary) for neonates was 0·17°C (95% CI, −0·15°C to 0·50°C). It is important to note that these studies were conducted in healthy newborn infants and the results may not be applicable to febrile infants.

No studies compared axillary to rectal temperatures in infants < 3 months old exclusively; however, you identify five prospective studies that included infants. The sensitivity of the axillary temperature for detecting fever (rectal temperature of > 38°C) ranged from 28% to 73% (i.e., 28–73% of the infants with fever would have been detected by the axillary temperature), and the specificity from 94% to 100% (i.e., 94–100% of afebrile patients were correctly identified by the axillary temperature). The likelihood ratios for a positive test (fever by axillary measurement) ranged from 12 to infinity, which implies that, if a patient has fever measured by axillary temperature, it is likely to be real. However, the poor likelihood ratio for a negative test (0·29–0·68) implies that absence of axillary fever is no guarantee of an afebrile infant.

Next, you look at the reliability of tympanic temperature measurement. You find 14 studies that addressed this issue, used an independent comparison of the two measurements, and included infants < 3 months old. The tympanic temperature detected fever in 24–97% of febrile children. One study that only included infants < 3 months old found a sensitivity for the tympanic measurement of 60%[15] (with rectal temperature elevation as the gold standard). Overall, these studies had widely varying results, so you are concerned that tympanic temperature measurement is not accurate or reliable.

One of the recent systematic reviews[16] compared ear temperatures with rectal temperatures in children, with 31 comparisons included in the meta-analysis. Of these, 15 comparisons included infants < 3 months. Overall, the pooled mean temperature difference was 0·29°C (95%CI, −0·74°C to 1·32°C). Although the difference in mean temperature is small, the wide confidence interval implies that tympanic temperature does not reliably agree with the rectal temperature.

Often parents will attempt to assess fever by touching their child's forehead or cheeks, so you evaluate the four studies that compared tactile assessment by the parent with rectal temperature. The sensitivity was variable and not very high (tactile assessment of fever did not detect 18–54% of febrile children), but the specificity ranged from 77–98%. This indicates that like axillary temperature, tactile assessment may be useful to rule in a fever when it is present, but does not reliably rule out fever.

You conclude that when parents say that their baby has a fever as measured by axillary, tympanic, or tactile means, you should be concerned about the baby. Parental report that the baby has not been febrile, however, is not reassuring.

Question

2. In young infants with fever (*population*), does the level of fever (*exposure*) identify infants with SBI (*outcome*)? **[Diagnosis]**

You seek studies that evaluate the likelihood of SBI for a range of temperatures in which children were evaluated regardless of the height of the fever. Studies that include a "clinically septic" category of infants (negative cultures but clinically suggestive symptoms and signs) may be biased in favor of the usefulness of the height of fever (and other signs) as diagnostic tests.

You review four studies that looked at predictors of bacteremia in the febrile infant and included temperature as a variable. These studies evaluated febrile infants < 8 weeks who were admitted for possible sepsis. None of these found a relationship between height of temperature and the presence of SBI.[17–20]

You find two studies that specifically address the relationship between temperature and the presence of SBI. These are limited in that they are retrospective studies. The rates of SBI (positive culture) are compared at different levels of fever. The rate of SBI rises with height of fever in both infants < 4-weeks old and < 4–8-weeks old.[21, 22] However, the sensitivity of hyperpyrexia (fever > 40°C) to detect SBI is only 21%, and the specificity is 97%. The likelihood ratio is 7. Hence, although you will have a higher level of suspicion with higher fever, this is not a reliable diagnostic test for SBI.

Question

3. In young infants with fever (*population*), is the response to the administration of antipyretics (*exposure*) useful in identifying infants with bacterial versus viral infections (*outcome*)? **[Diagnosis]**

You find four prospective studies that relate the response to fever to the etiology of the fever, in a manner that does not allow the response to antipyretics to influence the final diagnosis. In these studies, antipyretics decreased body temperature just as well among infants with a viral illness as among those with bacteremia or meningitis, and the degree of defervescence was similar in each situation.[6,23–25] You decide that the response to antipyretics will not help you distinguish bacterial from non-bacterial causes of fever in young infants.

Question

4. In young infants with fever (*population*), can clinical assessment (*exposure*) identify infants with SBI (*outcome*)? **[Diagnosis]**

The initial clinical assessment of the infant involves deciding if the child appears "toxic" or "septic". The clinical features that define toxicity include irritability, lethargy, and decreased social interaction. There also may be signs of compromised circulation with poor perfusion and cyanosis, and/or respiratory distress. However, young infants may have serious illness in the absence of signs of toxicity. In this age group, meningitis can present with non-specific symptoms and without signs of meningeal irritation.

You find four studies in hospitalized infants < 8 weeks being evaluated for sepsis that assess the value of "toxic appearance" in identifying serious bacterial illness.[17–19,26] The sensitivity of toxic signs in predicting SBI ranged from 11% to 100%. This wide range of sensitivity may represent the variability of clinical experience and the difficulty in evaluating the young infant.

You are concerned that the assessment of the infant by history and physical examination is very subjective so you look for studies that attempt to make the assessment more

Table 26.1 The Yale Observation Scale[27]

Observation variable	Normal (1 point)	Moderate impairment (3 points)	Severe impairment (5 points)
Quality of cry	Strong, normal tone *or* content, not crying	Whimpering, sobbing	Weak, moaning, high pitched
Reaction to parents	Cries briefly, stops *or* content, not crying	Cries off and on	Continual cry *or* hardly responds
State variation	If awake, stays awake If asleep, arouses easily	Eyes close briefly, awakes with prolonged stimulation	Falls to sleep, cannot be aroused
Color	Pink	Pale extremities, acrocyanosis	Pale, cyanotic, mottled, ashen
Hydration	Skin, eyes normal; mucus membranes moist	Skin, eyes normal; mouth slightly dry	Skin doughy, tented; dry mucus membranes; sunken eyes
Response to social overtures	Smiles, becomes alert	Brief smile, alerts briefly	No smile, anxious, dull, expressionless; can't be alerted

objective through the development of observation scales. The Yale Observation Scale (YOS) (Table 26.1) was developed by McCarthy *et al.*[27] to predict serious illness in the febrile child age < 24 months. In this scale, the child is assigned a score for each of six observable characteristics. Scores vary from a minimum of six to a maximum of 30, and 10 is the cut-off for "serious illness".

Is the YOS useful in predicting bacterial infection in the young infant? Four studies have evaluated the use of this scale in febrile infants. In these studies, serious illness was defined as the presence of a positive laboratory test (cultures, chest *x* ray.) The infant's clinical appearance did not influence whether bacterial cultures were obtained. If clinical signs had influenced whether tests were obtained, bacteremic babies who did not look very sick would have been missed, overestimating the sensitivity of the test. In a study of 503 infants, 5·4% of well-appearing febrile infants aged 28–90 days of age had SBI.[28] Using the YOS, Baker *et al.* showed that 67% of infants with SBI appeared well, with a YOS score < 10.[29] In a second study, Baker *et al.*[4] showed similar results with 66% of infants with SBI having a YOS score < 10. As the study periods overlap, some patients may have been included in both studies. These studies suggest that changes in behavior related to sepsis may be subtle and difficult to discriminate with a standardized scoring scale.

Because young infants have a limited range of behavior owing to their relative neurologic immaturity, the Young Infant Observation Scale (YIOS) was developed for use in infants < 8 weeks of age. Bonadio studied this scale in 242 infants < 8 weeks of age who presented with fever. Infants with SBI had a higher mean score (nine of a maximum of 15) compared to those who did not (five of 15), and a YIOS score 7 detected 76% of infants with serious illness.[30]

The evidence from these large prospective studies shows that observation scales are not adequately sensitive to identify young infants with serious illness.

Question

5. In young infants with fever (*population*), can laboratory investigations (*test*) help identify infants at risk for SBI (*outcome*)? **[Diagnosis]**

You find several studies evaluating the value of a variety of laboratory parameters in identifying infants with SBI. Investigations most commonly used included complete blood count, urinalysis, and stool analysis. What is the diagnostic value of these tests in predicting SBI? As with other diagnostic tests, you seek studies that make an independent and blind comparison of the laboratory parameters to the outcome of SBI.

The complete blood count (CBC) and specifically the white blood cell count (WBC), the absolute number of band forms (absolute band count), and the ratio of band forms to polymorphonuclear neutrophils are often used to help predict SBI. Your search yields seven studies that evaluate the CBC, and in which the CBC was not used as part of the criteria either for the diagnosis or for obtaining a blood culture (the gold standard for diagnosis). You find four prospective[18,19,31,32] and three retrospective studies.[3,26,33] None found a significant relationship between either the WBC or the absolute band count and the presence of SBI. In one study,[32] the absolute neutrophil count (ANC) was significantly higher in young infants with bacterial infections than infants with viral infections ($10·3 \ v \ 3·3 \times 10^9 \ P < 0·01$).

The overall sensitivity of a WBC > 15 000 for SBI was low at 31–52%, and specificity of the elevated WBC was 77–96%. Of the different parameters, the absolute band count had the highest sensitivity (86–88%). The WBC alone is not a good predictor for SBI.

The most frequent SBI diagnosed in young infants is UTI, The overall incidence of UTI in the febrile infant < 3 months old ranges from 3·2–7·5%.[5,33–35] Of all febrile infants with SBI, approximately 25% will have UTI.[4,36,37] The diagnosis of UTI is discussed in Chapter 42.

Bacterial enteritis is seen in 0·8–3% of febrile infants.[2,4,20,26,33] Approximately 10% of SBI is due to bacterial enteritis. Both historical features and microscopic evaluation of the stool have been used to predict bacterial enteritis in children with diarrhea. You find three prospective studies from the 1980s on this topic.[38–40] These studies included children < 4 years old. A study[38] of historical features revealed a high sensitivity for a history of abrupt onset of frequent diarrhea with no vomiting. The sensitivity of this characteristic was 86% but this feature had low specificity of 60% (likelihood ratio of 2). Therefore, while a positive test might commonly be false, a negative test gives you information that may lower your suspicion for bacterial enteritis. On the other hand, a WBC > 5/hpf on microscopic examination of the stool, a test that had high specificity (86–90%) in all three studies, substantially increases your suspicion of bacterial enteritis. Lack of white blood cells in the stool, however, does not rule out bacterial enteritis (sensitivity 40–73%).

Question

6. In the evaluation of the young febrile infant (*population*), is a chest x ray (*exposure*) helpful to identify infants with SBI (*outcome*)? **[Diagnosis]**

A chest x ray is often recommended for the evaluation of febrile infants even in the absence of respiratory symptoms. Pneumonia is found in infants with fever 1·6–6·3% of the time.[1,2,4,5,34] Viral chest infections are often not distinguishable from bacterial infections by radiographic findings.[41] Despite this, most studies consider the following radiographic findings to be indicative of pneumonia: hyperinflation plus peribronchial thickening, pulmonary infiltrates, lobar consolidation/atelectasis, and pleural effusion.

You find five studies that have examined the value of the chest radiograph in the febrile young infant with and without respiratory symptoms. Three were prospective studies, one was a retrospective study, and one had both a retrospective and a prospective component. A chest x ray was obtained in all patients evaluated in these studies. Different combinations of the following respiratory symptoms were included in the various studies: tachypnea, rales, rhonchi, grunting, cough, nasal flaring, wheezing, and rhinorrhea. In four of the studies,[42–45] the sensitivity of respiratory symptoms for radiographically defined pneumonia was above 90%. You conclude that in the absence of respiratory symptoms, the likelihood of pneumonia is low and a chest radiograph is not required in these infants.

Question

7. Can febrile infants 28–90 days old at low risk for SBI (*population*) be managed as outpatients (*intervention*) with no increase in morbidity (outcome)? **[Therapy]**

Although the traditional approach of working up and hospitalizing all febrile young infants[12] minimizes the risk of infectious complications, it leads to the unnecessary hospitalization of many infants.

Your search results in 16 studies looking at this issue. Initial studies retrospectively attempted to identify clinical predictors of infection in the febrile young infant. Subsequently, criteria were combined and applied to this population in order to identify a subgroup of infants who are at low risk for SBI. These criteria have been applied prospectively in several well-designed clinical trials.

As previously discussed, individual laboratory tests and clinical criteria are not sufficiently sensitive to detect all SBI in young infants. However, the same criteria have high negative predictive values, in part due to the relative rarity of SBI in most populations. It may be possible to combine clinical and laboratory criteria and identify a group of infants who are at low risk for SBI and can therefore potentially be managed as outpatients.

The first study to use this approach was by Dagan *et al.*[31] This study looked at infants < 2 months of age who were hospitalized with fever of unknown source. Specific clinical and laboratory criteria were used to define a low risk group. These criteria are known as the Rochester criteria and have been applied in various studies (see Box).[46]

Rochester Low Risk Criteria

Previously healthy febrile infants < 60 days of age are considered to be at low risk for serious bacterial infection if the following criteria are met:

- Infant appears well, non-toxic
- Infant has been previously well

  ○ born at term (> 37 weeks)
  ○ no antenatal or perinatal antimicrobial therapy
  ○ no treatment for unexplained hyperbilirubinemia
  ○ not hospitalized longer than the mother at birth
  ○ no previous hospitalizations

○ no recent antibiotic use
○ no chronic or underlying diseases

● Infant has no evidence of bacterial infection

○ no skin, soft tissue, bone, joint, or ear infection

● The following laboratory parameters are met:

○ WBC count 5000–15 000/mm^3
○ absolute band count < 1500
○ urinalysis WBC count < 10/hpf
○ stool WBC count < 5/hpf (if infant has diarrhea)

A review by Klassen and Rowe of diagnostic tests for febrile infants < 3 months of age found 10 studies that looked at the diagnostic evaluation of the febrile infant.[47] Of these, two were prospective studies that used the Rochester criteria.[31,46] When the data from the two studies were combined, the negative likelihood ratio was calculated as 0·03. A patient with SBI was 33 times less likely to meet the Rochester criteria than a patient without SBI. This results in a decrease in the estimated rate of SBI from 7% to 0·2% among those who meet the criteria.

In 1992, Baraff *et al.* published a systematic review of bacterial infections in young infants.[48] They searched English language publications from 1972 to 1991. Only original studies that reported the prevalence of SBI in febrile infants defined as low or high risk based upon clinical appearance and laboratory tests were included, a total of 14 studies. If the Rochester criteria were used, 464 of the 1068 infants would be considered low risk. In this group, there were only four infants with SBI: three with bacteremia and one with bacterial enteritis. The risk of SBI in the low risk group was 1·4%, the risk of bacteremia 1·1%, and meningitis 0·5%.

Baskin *et al.*[28] evaluated 503 low risk febrile infants between 28 and 90 days of age. All infants received a full sepsis evaluation including lumbar puncture and were treated with intramuscular ceftriaxone. The criteria used to define a low risk patient were different from previous criteria. A higher WBC was used (WBC < 20 000) and cerebrospinal fluid analysis (CSF WBC < 10), and chest radiographs were included. There were a total of 27 infants with SBI (5·4%). At follow up all patients were clinically improved. The higher rate of SBI in this study may be related to the higher WBC in their low risk criteria.

Bonadio *et al.* evaluated 534 febrile infants using the Milwaukee protocol.[7] The criteria were: normal physical examination, normal laboratory data (CSF WBC < 10; CBC WBC < 15 000, normal urinalysis, and normal chest radiograph); reliable caretaker with telephone and transportation. All low risk infants received intramuscular ceftriaxone (50 mg kg^{-1}) and had 24-hour follow up. The one patient with SBI in the low risk group (bacteremia) did well.

The low risk criteria used in these studies have high sensitivities ranging from 86% to 100%, with lower specificities. The likelihood ratio from the meta-analysis by Baraff is 2. Given that a febrile infant 28–90 days old has an average baseline risk for SBI of ~10%, if this infant meets low risk criteria the risk of SBI is decreased to 2% (post-test probability). The probability of bacteremia in this infant also changes from a baseline risk of 4% to 0·8% in the low risk infant. Many physicians may feel comfortable managing children as outpatients when the risk is this low.

A recent retrospective study by Bachur *et al.*[49] reviewed 5279 febrile infants < 90 days of age and derived a decision tree to predict SBI. Using the clinical variables sequentially (positive urinalysis, WBC > 20, temperature > 39·6 and age < 13 days) they identified infants at low risk for SBI with sensitivity (82%) and negative predictive value (98·3%) similar to the Rochester low risk criteria.

Question

8. Can febrile infants 28–90 days old at low risk for SBI (*population*) be managed without antibiotics (*intervention*) with no increase in morbidity (*outcome*)? **[Therapy]**

The best evidence addressing this issue comes from a series of prospective observational studies. There are no randomized clinical trials that address this issue.

In a retrospective review, Wasserman[50] questioned the need for hospitalization in febrile infants < 3 months of age. Of 443 infants evaluated for fever, five infants who were not initially treated with antibiotics had SBI, and all had good outcomes. In 1994, Jaskiewicz *et al.* conducted a prospective cohort study to appraise the Rochester criteria.[8] Of 437 low risk infants, five had SBI (three UTI, two bacteremia). In this study, over one-third of the infants in the low risk group did not receive antimicrobial therapy and all did well. Of the five infants with SBI, four did not receive any antibiotics initially and had no adverse outcomes.

Baker *et al.*[4] published a controlled study of outpatient management of febrile infants aged 29 through 56 days of age without antibiotics. Infants were defined as low risk according to the following criteria: normal physical examination, infant observation score < 10; WBC < 15 000, urinalysis WBC < 10; CSF WBC < 8; normal chest *x* ray. The low risk infants were randomly assigned to either inpatient or outpatient groups. Neither group received antibiotics. There was one SBI (0·4%–bacteremia) in the low risk group of infants. This child was in the inpatient observation group and did well. A recent study by Baker continues to support the outpatient management of the febrile infant without antibiotics.[5] The low risk criteria were as in the previous study. There were 101 of 422 infants who met low risk criteria, and 94 of these did not receive antibiotics. There were no patients with SBI and no adverse outcomes in the low risk group.

Question

9. What is the accuracy of the low risk criteria (*exposure*) for predicting SBI (*outcome*) in febrile infants < 28 days old (*population*)? **[Diagnosis]**

In your review of the literature you note that infants < 28 days old are considered a different population from infants 28–90 days old. Traditionally this group has been treated differently based on immunologic and neurologic immaturity.[51] It is more difficult to evaluate the young infant for toxic signs,[30] and the baseline risk of SBI is higher in this age group. Crain and Gershel reported on 46 febrile infants < 2 weeks of age and noted a rate of SBI of 32% with bacteremia/meningitis in 8·7%.[52] In a retrospective study by Bonadio, the rate of SBI was 12% in the 0–4 week group compared to 6% in the 4–8 week group.[53] Wasserman also noted higher rates of SBI, bacteremia and meningitis in the < 2-week-old infant.[50]

Febrile infants < 30 days have been excluded from several studies using low risk criteria. Practice guidelines published in 1993 recommended that all infants < 28 days of age have a sepsis evaluation including lumbar puncture and be hospitalized for parenteral antibiotics.[54] Subsequently, several studies have shown that although the overall risk of SBI is higher, the Rochester criteria may be able to identify low risk febrile infants < 1 month old.

In the study by Jaskiewicz *et al.*,[8] of the 931 infants evaluated there were 436 infants who were < 30 days old. In this subgroup, two of 227 low risk infants had SBI. The sensitivity of the Rochester low risk criteria was 94%, and specificity was 56%. This gives a likelihood ratio (LR) for the low risk criteria of 0·1.

In 1994, Chiu *et al.* conducted a prospective study in febrile neonates in which all infants received a complete assessment for sepsis, including lumbar puncture.[9] Infants were considered to be low risk for SBI if they met the low risk criteria (no evidence of bacterial infection, WBC 5000–15 000, normal urinalysis, normal ESR/CRP). The LR for these low risk criteria was 0·5. Chiu *et al*[11] reported on another 250 febrile infants < 28 days of age, and the LR for the low risk criteria was 0·04.

Baker *et al*[55] retrospectively applied the Philadelphia low risk criteria (WBC < 15, band to neutrophil ratio < 0·2, UA < 10 WBCs/hpf, CSF < 8 WBCs/hpf, normal chest *x* ray) to 254 infants 3–28 days of age. The sensitivity for the low risk criteria was 84% with a negative predictive value in their population of 95·4%. The likelihood ratio for the low risk criteria was 0·33. A similar retrospective study by Kadish *et al.* applied both the Philadelphia criteria and the Boston criteria (WBC < 20, UA < 10 WBCs/hpf, CSF < 10 WBCs/hpf) to a group of infants < 28 days of age.[56] The

sensitivities for the low risk criteria were 87% and 82% respectively, and the likelihood ratio for the low risk criteria was thus 0·2.

Infants < 28 days of age have a higher baseline risk of SBI (32%) and bacteremia (9%) than infants 1–3 months of age. The likelihood ratio for the low risk criteria in this age range appears to be about 0·2. Applying the low risk criteria lowers the probability of SBI and bacteremia in the low risk infants to 6% and 2% respectively. Hence, the evidence suggests that the criteria used to select infants at low risk for bacterial infection can also be applied to the infant < 28 days of age but that there is a higher risk of SBI in the younger, low risk infants.

Resolution of the scenario

This baby has been healthy until now, with no previous hospitalizations and had an uneventful neonatal course, but now is febrile without other significant findings on physical examination. Your review of the evidence suggests that you will not be able to say with certainty that this baby has SBI, but that negative tests help you modify your estimate of the likelihood of SBI. You start by considering your threshold for treating this baby, based on the risks of missing an SBI balanced against the risks, discomforts, and costs of treating an infant who may have SBI. If you and his parents decide that he should be treated if his chance of having an SBI is greater than 1 in 50, then your test/treat threshold is 2% (see Chapter 5).

The pretest probability that an unselected 6-week-old with fever has an SBI is around 10%. This child's clinical appearance gives him a score of 6 on the Yale Observation Scale; applying the LR for a negative test of between 0·15 and 0·67, you modify your estimate of SBI from 10% (pretest) to between about 2% and 7% (post-test). This is not sufficient to change your plan to test and treat. You obtain a CBC and urinalysis, but decide not to get stool studies or a chest x ray since he has no diarrhea and no respiratory symptoms. The high sensitivities of symptoms for bacterial enteritis and pneumonia suggest that disease is not present if the symptoms are not present. Many authors recommend obtaining blood and urine cultures at the same time, so as not to miss any infants at all with SBI.[54]

If he has a normal WBC and band count, and a negative UA, he meets the Rochester low risk criteria. You apply the LRs from the studies of the Rochester Criteria to his pretest likelihood of 10% (you cannot use the likelihood generated by the YOS because clinical appearance is part of the Rochester Criteria, so these are not independent). The LRs for a "low risk" on the Rochester Criteria range from 0·2 to 0, so your estimate of post-test probability of SBI ranges from a worst case of 2% to a best case of 0%. Given your treatment threshold of 2%, you decide that you feel comfortable sending this patient home, after you assure yourself that his parents understand the situation and are willing to follow up closely.

Future research needs

Studies are needed to address the following questions:

- Does the use of empiric antibiotics prevent infectious complications in low risk infants who are subsequently found to have SBI? Do the benefits outweigh the risks?
- What is the morbidity in infants who have been initially managed as outpatients and who are subsequently found to have SBI?

- Will the development of bacterial antigen detection diagnostic tests help in the management of these infants?
- Further research is needed in determining whether the low risk criteria can be safely applied in the very young infant.

Summary table

Question	Type of evidence	Result	Comment
Accuracy of axillary, tympanic, and tactile temperature assessment	Cross-sectional studies Comparison with rectal temperature (24 studies) Systematic Reviews (3 studies)	None is accurate. If elevated temperature is found by any of these means, the patient probably has fever	Rectal temperature remains the gold standard for clinical use
Can height of fever predict SBI?	Comparison with culture results (2 studies)	Higher rate of SBI when higher temperature	Not useful for diagnosis
Can response to antipyretics predict SBI?	Comparison with culture results (4 studies)	No difference in response between viral and bacterial infections	Not useful for diagnosis
Can clinical assessment predict SBI?	Comparison of YOS with culture results (5 studies)	LRs YOS > 10: 2·3–5·4, < 10: 0·2–0·6	Useful for excluding SBI, but not for predicting SBI
Can laboratory tests predict SBI?	Comparison of tests to culture results (6 studies)	LRs WBC > 15 000: 2–11, < 15 000: 0·6–0·9	Elevated WBC alone cannot predict SBI
Can clinical symptoms predict absence of pneumonia (hence, need for CXR)?	Blind comparison of respiratory symptoms to CXR results (5 studies)	Sensitivity of respiratory symptoms for pneumonia high (> 90% in 4 of 5 studies)	CXR not needed in the absence of respiratory symptoms
Can low risk infants be managed as outpatients?	No RCTs Observational cohort studies	LRs low risk criteria: 0–0·2	Low risk infants have probability of SBI (2%), bacteremia (0·8%)
Can low risk infants be managed without antibiotics?	No RCTs Observational cohort studies	No adverse outcomes described	Need large RCT to determine benefit/harm of antibiotics
Can infants < 28 days be managed the same way as older infants?	No RCTs Observational cohort studies	LRs low risk criteria: 0–0·5	Baseline risk higher in neonates Low risk infants have probability of SBI (6%), bacteremia (2%)

References

1 Rosenberg N, Vranesich, P, Cohen, S. Incidence of serious infection in infants under two months with fever. *Ped Emerg Care* 1985;**1**:54–6.

2 Krober MS, Bass JW, Powell JM, Smith FR, Dexter S, Seto Y. Bacterial and viral pathogens causing fever in infants less than 3 months old. *Am J Dis Child* 1985;**139**:889–92.

3 Berkowitz CD, Uchiyama N, Tully SB *et al.* Fever in infants less than two months of age: spectrum of disease and predictors of outcome. *Ped Emerg Care* 1985;**1**:128–35.

4 Baker M, Bell L, Avner J. Outpatient management without antibiotics of fever in selected infants. *N Engl J Med* 1993;**329**:1437–41.

5 Baker DM, Bell LM, Avner JR. The efficacy of routine outpatient management without antibiotics of fever in selected infants. *Pediatrics* 1999;**103**:627–31.

6 Bonadio W, Bellomo T, Brady W, Smith D. Correlating changes in body temperature with infectious outcome in febrile children who receive acetaminophen. *Clin Ped* 1993;**32**:343–6.

7 Bonadio WA, Hagen E, Rucka J, Shallow K, Stommel P, Smith D. Efficacy of a protocol to distinguish risk of serious bacterial infection in the outpatient evaluation of febrile young infants. *Clin Ped* 1993;**32**:401–4.

8 Jaskiewicz JA, McCarthy CA, Richardson AC *et al.* Febrile infants at low risk for serious bacterial infection. An appraisal of the Rochester criteria and implications for management. *Pediatrics* 1994;**94**:390–6.

9 Chiu CH, Lin TY, Bullard MJ. Application of criteria identifying febrile outpatient neonates at low risk for bacterial infections. *Ped Inf Dis J* 1994;**13**:946–9.

10 Broner CW, Polk SA, Sherman JM. Febrile infants less than eight weeks old: predictors of infection. *Clin Ped* 1990;**29**:438–43.

11 Chiu CH, Lin TY, Bullard MJ. Identification of febrile neonates unlikely to have bacterial infections. *Ped Inf Dis J* 1997;**16**:59–63.

12 Long SS. Approach to the febrile patient with no obvious focus of infection. *Ped Rev* 1984;**5**:305–15.

13 Herzog LW, Coyne LJ. What is fever? Normal temperatures in infants less than three months old. *Clin Ped* 1993;**32**:142–6.

14 Craig JV, Lancaster GA, Williamson PR, Smith RL. Temperature measured at the axilla compared with rectum in children and young people: systematic review. *BMJ* 2000;**320**:1174–78.

15 Selfridge J, Shea SS. The accuracy of the tympanic thermometer in detecting fever in infants aged 3 months and younger in the emergency department setting. *J Emerg Nursing* 1993;**19**:127–30.

16 Craig JV, Lancaster GA, Taylor S, Williamson PR, Smith RL. Infrared ear thermometry compared with rectal thermometry in children: a systematic review. *Lancet* 2002;**360**:603–9.

17 Roberts KB, Borzy MS. Fever in the first eight weeks of life. *Johns Hopkins Med J* 1977;**141**:9–13.

18 Caspe WB, Chamudes O, Louie B. The evaluation and treatment of the febrile infant. *Ped Inf Dis J* 1983;**2**:131–5.

19 King JC, Berman ED, Wright PF. Evaluation of fever in infants less than 8 weeks old. *South Med J* 1987;**80**:948–52.

20 Crain E, Shelov SP. Febrile infants: predictors of bacteremia. *J Ped* 1982;**101**:686–9.

21 Bonadio W. Incidence of serious bacterial infections in afebrile neonates with a history of fever. *Ped Inf Dis J* 1987;**6**:911–15.

22 Bonadio W, McElroy K, Smith D. Relationship of fever magnitude to rate of serious bacterial infections in infants aged 4 to 8 weeks. *Clin Ped* 1991;**30**:478–80.

23 Yamamoto L, Widger H, Flinger D. Relationship of bacteremia to antipyretic therapy in febrile children. *Ped Emerg Care* 1987;**3**:223–7.

24 Weisse M, Miller G, Brien J. Fever response to acetaminophen in viral vs bacterial infections. *Ped Inf Dis J* 1987;**6**:1091–5.

25 Torrey S, Heinritig F, Fleisher G. Temperature response to antipyretic therapy in children. Relationship to occult bacteremia. *Am J Emerg Med* 1985;**3**:190–6.

26 Bonadio WA, Smith DS, Sabnis S. The clinical characteristics and infectious outcomes of febrile infants aged 8 to 12 weeks. *Clin Ped* 1994;**33**:95–9.

27 McCarthy PL, Sharpe MR, Spiesel SZ *et al.* Observation scales to identify serious illness in young children. *Pediatrics* 1982;**70**:802–9.

28 Baskin M, O'Rourke E, Fleisher G. Outpatient treatment of febrile infants 28–90 days of age with Intramuscular ceftriaxone. *J Ped* 1992;**120**:22–7.

29 Baker M, Avner J, Bell L. Failure of infant observation scales in detecting serious illness in febrile 4–8 week old infants. *Pediatrics* 1990;**85**:1040–3.

30 Bonadio WA, Hennes H, Smith D *et al.* Reliability of observation variables in distinguishing infectious outcome of febrile young infants. *Ped Inf Dis J* 1990;**12**:111–14.

31 Dagan R, Powell KR, Hall CB, Menugus MA. Identification of infants unlikely to have serious bacterial infection although hospitalized for suspected sepsis. *J Ped* 1985;**107**:855–60.

32 Kupperman N, Walton E A. Immature neutrophils in the blood smears of young febrile children. *Arch Pediatr Adolesc Med* 1999;**153**:261–266.

33 Bonadio WA, Smith DS, Carmody J. Correlating CBC profile and infectious outcome: a study of febrile infants evaluated for sepsis. *Clin Ped* 1992;**31**:578–82.

34 Crain EF, Gershel JC. Urinary tract infections in febrile infants younger than 8 weeks of age. *Pediatrics* 1990;**86**:363–7.

35 Hoberman A, Chao H, Keller DM, Hickey R, Davis HW, Ellis D. Prevalence of urinary tract infection in febrile infants. *J Ped* 1993;**123**:17–23.

36 Bauchner H, Philipp B, Dashefsky B. Prevalence of bacteriuria in febrile children. *Ped Inf Dis J* 1987;**6**:239–42.

37 DeAngelis C, Joffe A, Willis E. Hospitalization vs outpatient treatment of young febrile infants. *Am J Dis Child* 1983;**137**:1150–2.

38 DeWitt TG, Humphrey KF, McCarthy P. Clinical predictors of acute bacterial diarrhea in young children. *Pediatrics* 1985;**76**:551–6.

39 Fontana M, Zuin G, Paccagnini S *et al.* Simple clinical score and laboratory based method to predict bacterial etiology of acute diarrhea in childhood. *Ped Int Dis J* 1987;**6**:1088–91.

40 Paccagnini S, Zuin G, Galli L, Quaranta S, Principi N. Occult blood and faecal leukocyte tests in acute infectious diarrhoea in children. *Lancet* 1987;**1**:442.

41 McCarthy PL, Spiesel SZ, Stashwick CA, Ablow RC, Masters SJ, Dolan TF. Radiographic findings and etiologic diagnosis in ambulatory childhood pneumonias. *Clin Ped* 1981;**20**:686–91.

42 Losek JD, Kishaba G, Berens RJ, Bonadio WA, Wells RG. Indications for chest roentgenogram in the febrile young infant. *Ped Emerg Care* 1989;**5**:149–52.

43 Crain EF, Bulas D, Bijur PE, Goldman HS. Is a chest radiograph necessary in the evaluation of every febrile infant less than 8 weeks of age? *Pediatrics* 1991;**88**:821–4.

44 Bramson RT, Meyere TL, Silbijer ML, Blickman JG, Halpern E. The futility of the chest radiograph in the febrile infant without respiratory symptoms. *Pediatrics* 1993;**92**:524–6.

45 Singhi S, Dhawan A, Kataria S, Walia BNS. Clinical signs of pneumonia in infants under 2 months. *Arch Dis Child* 1994;**70**:413–17.

46 Dagan R, Sofer S, Philip M, Shachak E. Ambulatory care of febrile infants younger than two months of age classified as being at low risk for having serious bacterial infections. *J Ped* 1988;**112**:355–60.

47 Klassen T, Rowe P. Selecting diagnostic tests to identify febrile infants less than 3 months of age as being at low risk for serious bacterial infection: a scientific overview. *J Ped* 1992;**121**:671–6.

48 Baraff LJ, Oslund SA, Schriger DL, Stephen ML. Probability of bacterial infection in febrile infants less than three months of age: a meta-analysis. *Ped Inf Dis J* 1992;**11**:257–64.

49 Bachur RG, Harper MB. Predictive model for serious bacterial infections among infants younger than 3 months of age. *Pediatrics* 2001;**108**:311–16.

50 Wasserman GM, White CB. Evaluation of the necessity for hospitalization of the febrile infant less than three months of age. *Ped Inf Dis J* 1990;**9**:163–9.

51 Wilson CB. Immunologic basis for increased susceptibility of the neonate to infection. *J Ped* 1986;**108**:1–9.

52 Crain EF, Gershel JC. Which febrile infants younger than two weeks of age are likely to have sepsis? A pilot study. *Ped Inf Dis J* 1988;**7**:561–4.

53 Bonadio WA, Webster H, Wolfe A, Gorecki D. Correlating infectious outcome with clinical parameters of 1130 consecutive febrile infants aged zero to eight weeks. *Ped Emerg Care* 1993;**9**:84–6.

54 Baraff LJ, Bass JW, FJeisher GR *et al.* Practice guideline for the management of infants and children 0–36 months of age with fever without source. *Pediatrics* 1993;**82**:1–11.

55 Baker MD, Bell LM. Unpredictability of serious bacterial illness in febrile infants from birth to 1 month of age. *Arch Ped Adolesc Med* 1999;**153**:508–11.

56 Kadish HA, Loveridge B, Tobey J, Bolte RG, Corneli HM. Applying outpatient protocols in febrile infants 1–28 days of age: can the threshold be lowered? *Clin Ped* 2000;**39**:81–8.

27 Fever without focus in the older infant

Blake Bulloch

Case scenario

A 5-month-old male is brought to you with a fever of 40·9°C. This child has been previously well with normal behavior other than being slightly irritable. He has had no rhinorrhea, cough, or difficulty breathing. His appetite has been good with no vomiting or diarrhea and his mother claims she has changed a wet diaper four times today. She has not noticed any rashes and he does not seem to have any discomfort. There is no history of previous medical problems other than a "cold" a few weeks earlier. He has had his first two immunizations including that against Haemophilus influenzae type b (Hib). On examination he is alert, active, and happy, sitting contentedly on his mother's lap. He is well hydrated with normal color, no rashes, and is not toxic in appearance. Blood pressure is 90/68; heart rate 108; respiratory rate 22. The physical examination is entirely benign, including normal neurologic, respiratory, circulatory, abdominal, and musculoskeletal examination. You wonder whether he might have "occult" bacteremia, recalling the controversy that this subject generates in discussions among your colleagues. His mother wants to know if he needs an antibiotic because of the fever.

Background

Occult bacteremia is a term used to describe febrile children with bacteremia who otherwise appear well clinically. Traditionally, young children have been divided into two age groups, those < 3 months of age and those between 3 months and 3 years of age. Children < 3 months of age are most at risk for bacterial infections acquired through the birth canal (Group B streptococci, *Escherichia coli*, *Staphylococcus aureus*, and *Listeria monocytogenes*). Studies focusing on the incidence of bacteremia in this age group have defined a rectal temperature of ≥ 38°C to be indicative of a fever.

Children between the ages of 3 months and 3 years are susceptible to occult bacteremia but the causative organisms change (*Streptococcus pneumococcus*, *Salmonella* spp. and *Neisseria meningitides*). In this age group, studies have used a temperature cut-off of ≥ 39·0°C. In children between the ages of 3 months and 3 years the incidence of occult bacteremia has been reported to range from 3% to 12%. Patients with occult bacteremia are at risk of developing focal infections, such as pneumonia, septic arthritis, osteomyelitis, urinary tract infection, septicemia, and meningitis. While clinical practice guidelines were published in 1993 to help physicians manage children at risk for occult bacteremia, much remains unknown surrounding their ideal management.[1]

The management of febrile children is a common problem encountered by physicians. In children between the ages of 3 months and 3 years there are approximately 0·80 visits for fever ≥ 38°C per child-year. About one quarter of these are for fevers ≥ 39°C.[2]

Framing answerable clinical questions

Several questions come to mind with regard to managing this patient. Is this child's fever due to a viral illness or could he be bacteremic? Do clinical examination findings or laboratory tests help you determine this? You also wonder about the possibility of a urinary tract infection, pneumonia, or meningitis with this degree of fever. Finally, should this child be treated with antibiotics until the results of any tests are known? The first step is to reframe these questions into a structured format. Each question should contain the following elements: the patient/population; the intervention, event, or exposure (and comparison, if relevant); and the outcome of interest. The questions are formulated as follows.

Questions

1. In a young child between 3 and 36 months of age (*population*) with a fever and no apparent focus of infection (*exposure*), what is the probability that the child is bacteremic (*outcome*)? **[Baseline Risk]**

---

2. If a young child with a fever and no apparent focus of infection (*population*) is bacteremic (*exposure*), what is the probability of developing a focus of infection (*outcome*)? **[Prognosis]**

3. In young febrile children with a fever and no focus (*population*), will empiric antibiotic treatment, either oral or parenteral compared with no treatment (*intervention*), decrease morbidity or mortality (*outcome*)? **[Therapy]**

4. In a young child between 3 and 36 months of age with a fever and no apparent focus of infection (*population*), what is the accuracy of the clinical examination (*test*) for detecting bacteremia (*outcome*)? **[Diagnosis]**

5. In the child with fever and no focus of infection (*population*), can the height of the fever (*event*) predict the presence of bacteremia (*outcome*)? **[Diagnosis]**

6. In a young child between 3 and 36 months of age with a fever and no apparent focus of infection (*population*), what is the accuracy of the white blood cell count or absolute neutrophil count (*test*) for detecting bacteremia (*outcome*)? **[Diagnosis]**

7. In febrile young children (*population*), what is the accuracy of a blood culture (*test*) for detecting bacteremia (*outcome*)? **[Diagnosis]**

8. In a young child between 3 and 36 months of age (*population*), what is the accuracy of clinical signs (*test*) for detecting pneumonia (*outcome*)? **[Diagnosis]**

9. In a young child between 3 and 36 months of age (*population*), what is the accuracy of urinalysis (*test*) for detecting UTI? **[Diagnosis]**

10. In a young child between 3 and 36 months of age (*population*), what is the effect of the heptavalent pneumococcal conjugate vaccine (*intervention*), on the risk of occult pneumococcal bacteremia (*outcome*)? **[Therapy]**

Searching for evidence

● MedLine (PubMed): occult bacteremia AND LA-English AND practice guideline

Clinical practice guidelines represent an attempt to summarize a large body of knowledge into a concise, easy-to-use synopsis of relevant information. Therefore, you decide to start your search by looking for a practice guideline that comments on the management of young children at risk for occult bacteremia. You find one article entitled, "Practice guidelines for the management of infants and children 0 to 36 months of age with fever without source".[1] Like all sources of evidence, practice guidelines (as well as other sources of predigested evidence) can be assessed to determine whether they have been performed in a valid manner. In this case, it appears that the authors conducted a comprehensive

search, but there are no explicit inclusion and exclusion criteria and no description of how many reviewers examined each article and how disagreements between reviewers, if any, were resolved. Without the specifics of the search, we as readers can't duplicate it or determine if important articles are likely to have been missed. No attempt to assess the quality of different studies used in systematic reviews is reported in this guideline. Also, the final algorithm for management of these children only involves the use of antibiotics; there is no option that involves withholding antibiotics. Therefore, all important options are not clearly specified and outlined in the guideline. Given these concerns about the validity of this guideline, you decide that their recommendations may not be entirely evidence-based and that opinions of the panel may have influenced the final guidelines. However, they do identify several interesting articles that you may want to look at more closely in answering some of your questions. You go on to perform specific searches for each of your questions.

Critical review of the evidence

Question

1. In a young child between 3 and 36 months of age (*population*) with a fever and no apparent focus of infection (*exposure*), what is the probability that the child is bacteremic (*outcome*)? **[Baseline Risk]**

● MedLine (PubMed, clinical queries): "occult bacteremia" AND "epidemiologic studies"

This search identifies 48 articles, five of which are directly relevant to your question. Four of the studies are randomized trials of management of children with fever and no focus. These studies were performed prior to the introduction of the immunization for Hib. The prevalence of occult bacteremia in children with fever and no focus ranged from 2·3% to 11·6%.[3-6] This wide range brings up the question of whether risk has changed since the introduction of vaccine against Hib. A study by Lee and Harper directly addresses this issue.[7] This is the first large prospective study to determine the prevalence of bacteremia since the introduction of the immunization for Hib. The study took place in the emergency department (ED) of an urban, tertiary care, children's hospital. The authors studied 9465 well-appearing children 3–36 months of age with a documented ED temperature of ≥ 39·0°C, and followed them prospectively until the results of the blood cultures (an objective and unbiased outcome measure) were known. They found that 149 of 9465 (1·57%) febrile children had positive cultures. Of these *Streptococcus pneumoniae* accounted for 137 (92%), *Salmonella* spp. (5%), *Neisseria meningitidis* (1%), and others (2%).[7]

Schuchat *et al.* described the epidemiological features of bacterial meningitis in the United States five years after Hib conjugate vaccines were introduced for routine immunization of infants.[8] The median age of persons with bacterial meningitis increased from 15 months in 1986 to 25 years old in 1995, largely as a result of a 94% decrease in the number of cases of *H influenzae* meningitis.

Question

2. If a young child with a fever and no apparent focus of infection (*population*) is bacteremic (*exposure*) what is the likelihood of developing a focus of infection (*outcome*)? **[Prognosis]**

Our previous search identified a meta-analysis that involved four randomized controlled trials. These trials followed children between 3 months and 3 years of age with a temperature ≥ 39·0°C and no focus of infection.[3–6] Their outcome measure was the development of a serious bacterial infection which were defined as pneumonia, persistent bacteremia, urinary tract infection, cellulitis, enteritis, septic arthritis, osteomyelitis, meningitis, and septicemia. These studies were done in the era prior to the widespread use of *Haemophilus influenzae* type b immunization and, although some of the children had been treated, serious bacterial infections occurred relatively infrequently. Only 244 (3·1%) of a total of 7899 patients at risk for occult bacteremia in the randomized trials were bacteremic, 17 (0·2%) developed a serious bacterial infection including 7 (0·1%) who developed meningitis.[3–6]

As seen above, some children remain bacteremic even if they do not develop a focus of infection. Harper *et al.* studied 559 children with unsuspected bacteremia.[9] From this group, 90 had initially been sent home without antibiotics. At follow up 12 of the 90 (13%) had a newly diagnosed focus of infection and 19 (21%) remained bacteremic. In the randomized controlled trial by Jaffe, eight children were initially sent home on placebo; they were subsequently identified as bacteremic and samples were recultured. One was persistently bacteremic and the remainder had spontaneously resolved (87·5%).[4] Therefore, it appears that between 70% and 87·5% of episodes of occult bacteremia will resolve spontaneously.

Question

3. In young febrile children with a fever and no focus (*population*) will empiric antibiotic treatment, either oral or parenteral (*intervention*), decrease morbidity or mortality (*outcome*)? **[Therapy]**

- *Cochrane Library*, 2002 issue 4: bacteremia

When faced with a child at risk for occult bacteremia, you are actually faced with two general choices; do no testing (and either treat all children at risk or not based on clinical judgment) or perform tests on these children and guide your treatment decisions based on the test results. The harm is treatment of children without bacteremia; the benefit is avoiding deterioration due to delayed diagnosis. For all tests used, the aim is to reduce the number treated unnecessarily because they do not have bacteremia, to minimize the delay waiting for the test result, and most importantly, minimize the number of children with bacteremia who are missed by the test (false negatives) and who will only be picked up when symptoms worsen.

The ideal treatment of children at risk for occult bacteremia is controversial.[9,10–15] A good place to start your search is the *Cochrane Library* where you find three reviews in the Database of Abstracts of Reviews of Effects DARE).[16–18] All three of these articles are systematic reviews that were performed in a valid manner with a focused clinical question with clear criteria for inclusion. The validity of the studies was appraised only in the first systematic review.

The first review addressed the issue of efficacy of empiric antibiotic treatment in children at risk for occult bacteremia.[16] In order for an article to be included in this analysis the following prespecified criteria had to be met:

- The population had to be children between the ages of 3 months and 3 years with a fever of ≥ 39°C and no focus of infection on initial assessment, and a blood culture had to be obtained.
- The study had to be a randomized controlled trial.
- The outcome measured had to be a serious bacterial infection. These included meningitis, pneumonia, periorbital cellulitis, septic arthritis, osteomyelitis, or persistent bacteremia.
- The intervention studied had to be either (a) an antibiotic versus no antibiotic, or (b) an oral antibiotic versus a parenteral antibiotic.

Based on the above criteria, four articles were identified that contained all the specified criteria.[3–6] The Jadad scale was used to assess the validity of the randomized, controlled trials. This scale measures randomization, double blinding and withdrawals and dropouts.

Children were excluded if they had a focus of infection, a known or suspected sensitivity to the antibiotics being used, had received antibiotics or diphtheria-pertussis-tetanus immunization in the preceding 48 hours, had the stigmata of a specific viral infection, were immunodeficient, or looked septic. The goal of this meta-analysis was to determine the effectiveness of antibiotics in reducing the probability of serious bacterial infection in, firstly, all patients at risk for occult bacteremia, and secondly those patients identified as bacteremic. Two of the studies compared antibiotics to no antibiotics or placebo and the other two compared intramuscular ceftriaxone to an oral antibiotic.

There were a total of 7899 children of whom 244 were found to be bacteremic (3·1%). The use of antibiotics compared to placebo revealed no significant effect (odds ratio [OR] = 0·60; 95% CI 0·10–3·49) of preventing serious bacterial infections in all children at risk. Likewise, the use of intramuscular versus oral antibiotic revealed no significant difference (OR = 0·38; 95% CI 0·12–1·17) in preventing serious bacterial infections.

However, when outcomes were compared only for those patients identified as bacteremic post hoc, the treatment effect improved dramatically. The use of antibiotics compared to placebo had an OR of 0·34 (0·05–2·34) while the use of intramuscular versus oral antibiotics had an OR of 0·25 (0·07–0·89). Therefore, if it were possible to identify bacteremic children on presentation then treating them with an intramuscular antibiotic would prove useful. You would only need to treat 17 children with ceftriaxone versus oral antibiotic to prevent one case of serious bacterial infection.[16]

The second systematic review addressed whether oral antibiotics prevent meningitis and serious bacterial infections in children with *Streptococcus pneumoniae* occult bacteremia.[17] Since Hib has largely disappeared as a result of immunization, this meta-analysis focused only on children with *S pneumoniae* occult bacteremia. Both retrospective and prospective reports were included if they contained information on children with *S pneumoniae* bacteremia treated as outpatients, and if they contained information on the occurrence of serious bacterial illness (SBI) on follow up.

They found an OR of 0·51 (95% CI; 0·12–2·09), indicating that oral antibiotics did not prevent *S pneumoniae* meningitis. The very wide confidence interval is likely due to the rarity of the outcome.

Rothrock *et al.* in another systematic review also reviewed whether parenteral antibiotics are more effective than oral antibiotics in preventing serious bacterial infections and meningitis.[18] Based on an OR for orally treated children of 1·48 (95% CI; 0·5–4·3), they concluded that the ratios of serious bacterial infections and meningitis did not differ between children who were treated with oral and parenteral antibiotics.

As can be seen from the results of the first systematic review, if children could be identified at presentation as bacteremic or not, the number of children we would need to treat to prevent one bad outcome would be reduced. If we approach the problem in this way, then all the following diagnostic questions will help us determine the risk of any particular child being bacteremic and whether we will choose to empirically treat.

Question

4. In a young child between 3 and 36 months of age with a fever and no apparent focus of infection (*population*), what is the accuracy of the clinical examination (*test*) for predicting bacteremia (*outcome*)? **[Diagnosis]**

● MedLine (PubMed; clinical queries): occult bacteremia AND observation scale

In this case we wanted to eliminate any studies that used subjective measures of the child's appearance and focus on objective measures. This search identified an article entitled "Efficacy of an observation scale in detecting bacteremia in febrile children three to thirty-six months of age treated as outpatients."[19] This study prospectively followed 6611 febrile children between the ages of 3 and 36 months with no focus of infection, who had an initial observational score calculated. All the children had blood cultures obtained on the initial visit and the results of the cultures were independently compared to the results of the Yale Observation Scale (YOS). This validated scale (described in Chapter 26) was developed to determine if a febrile child's appearance could predict the presence or absence of serious illness.[20] Of the 6611 children, 192 were bacteremic (2·9%). Although the YOS score was significantly higher in children with bacteremia than in those without bacteremia ($P < 0·0001$), 70% of the patients with bacteremia had the minimum score of 6. At various cut-off points for the YOS, the sensitivity ranged from 0·5% to 28·6%, with the best likelihood ratios for positive tests being 2·1 (for a score of > 8). These results were confirmed by Kuppermann *et al.* who analyzed 109 patients with occult pneumococcal bacteremia.[21] They found the median YOS to be 6 for all patients with and without pneumococcal bacteremia, with 69% of all patients with bacteremia having the lowest possible score of 6.

However, what we want to do is rule out bacteremia since our default strategy is to treat all the children at risk for bacteremia. If the test is sensitive then a low YOS score would rule out the disease in question (in this case bacteremia). Since 70% of all children with bacteremia have a score of 6, the YOS is not very sensitive and does not help us rule out bacteremia.

On the other hand, the specificity ranged from 82·5% for a YOS of > 8 to 98·8% for a score > 12. If a test is highly specific it will help us rule in the disease. In this case a YOS > 12 has a specificity of 98·8%. If your strategy were to watch and wait, a higher score on the YOS could be useful in redirecting your approach since the test is highly specific. Unfortunately, a score of 12 or greater occurs in only 3·7% (76 of 2027) of children at risk for bacteremia.[19]

Question

5. In the child with fever and no focus of infection (*population*), can the height of the fever (exposure) predict the presence of bacteremia (*outcome*)? **[Diagnosis]**

● MedLine (PubMed; clinical queries): occult bacteremia AND temperature

This search retrieves 14 articles and reveals that many studies have shown some correlation between the height of a fever and the presence of bacteremia. You have come across additional relevant articles on this subject in your previous searches.

In the era before *H influenzae* immunization, Jaffe prospectively looked at the rectal temperature as an indicator of bacteremia.[22] A total of 955 children between the ages of 3 and 36 months with a temperature $\geq 39 \cdot 0°C$ were enrolled, had rectal temperatures performed, and blood cultures obtained. There were 27 positive blood cultures. The authors constructed a receiver operator characteristic curve (ROC) of rectal temperature as a predictor of bacteremia and found the curve to be relatively flat, plotting near the 45° line (i.e., likelihood ratio [LR] of 1·0 for any temperature). This means that there was no temperature cut-off point at which the desired combination of a high sensitivity and a low false-positive rate occurred (see Chapter 5).

However, with the decreased prevalence of Hib bacteremia, you decide to examine the study by Lee and Harper who studied the prevalence of *S pneumoniae* bacteremia by temperature.[7] They grouped the children into five different temperature ranges and found that there was an increased prevalence of bacteremia at higher temperatures. When compared with the 39·0–39·4°C temperature group, the 40·0–40·4°C, 40·5–40·9°C, and the 41·0–42·0°C temperature groups showed significantly higher risks for bacteremia with ORs of 1·90 (95% CI: 1·13–3·21), 2·6 (95% CI: 1·5–4·5), and 3·7 (95% CI: 1·9–7·3).

Kuppermann analyzed a sample of 4384 children at risk for occult pneumococcal bacteremia participating in a prospective, randomized trial of antibiotic use. He found that the risk of bacteremia increased from 1·2% at a temperature < 39·5°C to a risk of 4·4% at a temperature $\geq 40 \cdot 5°C$.[21]

Hence, as a child's temperature increases so does the likelihood of pneumococcal bacteremia. However, as illustrated above, it only increases the chance of being bacteremic from a baseline of approximately 1·5% to 5%. There is no data correlating the height of fever with the possibility of being bacteremic from other organisms.

Question

6. In a young child between 3 and 36 months of age with a fever and no apparent focus of infection (*population*),

can the white blood cell count or absolute neutrophil count (*test*) identify the presence of bacteremia (*outcome*)? **[Diagnosis]**

● MedLine (PubMed; clinical queries): occult bacteremia AND Blood cell count

This strategy retrieves a total of 27 articles. Lee and Harper examined only cases of bacteremia due to *S pneumoniae* in a cohort of 9465 children between the ages of 3 months and 3 years who had a fever $\geq 39 \cdot 0°C$ and no focus of infection (our population of interest).[7] The gold standard for the diagnosis of pneumococcal bacteremia was a positive blood culture, and the WBC count was independently compared to this. The sensitivity of a WBC count $\geq 15\,000/mm^3$ was 86%. That is, 86% of bacteremic children had a WBC count $\geq 15\,000/mm^3$. The specificity of the WBC count was 77% so that approximately 77% of non-bacteremic children had a WBC $< 15\,000\,mm^{-3}$. These results can be converted to likelihood ratios.

The Evidence-Based Medicine Working Group published a rough guide to the interpretation of likelihood ratios as follows[23]:

● An LR of > 10 or < 0·1 generates a large and often conclusive change in pretest to post-test probability.
● LRs of 5–10 and 0·1–0·2 generate moderate shifts in pretest to post-test probability.
● LRs of 2–5 and 0·2–0·5 generate small changes in probability.
● LRs of 1–2 and 0·5–1 alter probability to a small degree.

Using the data from the Lee and Harper study we calculate the likelihood ratio for a WBC count $\geq 15\,000\,mm^{-3}$ to be 3·74 (sensitivity/(1 – specificity) or 0·86/0·23). This generates a small change in the post-test probability of bacteremia. The likelihood ratio for a negative test is 0·18 ((1 – sensitivity)/specificity or 0·14/0·77). This will likely generate a moderate change in the post-test probability of bacteremia.

The prevalence or pretest probability of bacteremia is 137/9465 or 1·45%. Using the LR nomogram (see Chapter 5), you can determine the post-test probability of bacteremia. The LRs at various cut-offs for the WBC can be calculated, and then applied to different pretest likelihoods for bacteremia. How useful the WBC count is will depend on your treatment threshold, i.e., whether the WBC result will change your clinical action. Table 27.1 illustrates the post-test likelihoods for pretest likelihoods of 3% and 5%.

The absolute neutrophil count (ANC) can be examined in the same way. Kuppermann *et al.* in a prospective study determined that an ANC cut-off of $\geq 10\,000$ cells mm^{-3} had a sensitivity of 76% (95% CI 66%, 84%) for detecting pneumococcal bacteremia and a specificity of 78% (95%

Table 27.1 Post-test probabilities for pre-test probabilities

WBC count	Likelihood ratio for this cut-off of WBC count	Post-test probability if pretest probability is 3% (%)	Post-test probability if pretest probability is 5% (%)
≥ 5000/mm³	1·06	3·2	5·3
≥ 10 000/mm³	1·75	5·1	8·4
≥ 15 000/mm³	3·74	10·4	16·4
≥ 20 000/mm³	6·00	15·7	24·0

CI 76%, 79%).[20] Therefore the likelihood ratio for an ANC ≥ 10 000/mm³ is 3·45 (sensitivity/(1 – specificity) or 0·76/0·22). This generates a small change in the post-test probability of bacteremia. The likelihood ratio for a negative test is 0·31 (1 – sensitivity/specificity or 0·24/0·78) which will also generate a small change in the post-test probability of bacteremia.

No study was identified that reported the WBC counts for cases of bacteremia other than those caused by *S pneumoniae* in the post Hib era.

Question

7. In febrile young children (*population*), what is the accuracy of blood culture (*test*) for identifying the presence of bacteremia (*outcome*)? [Diagnosis]

- MedLine (PubMed; clinical queries): "blood culture" AND bacteremia AND probability

You notice that all of these studies use the blood culture result as the gold standard for the diagnosis of bacteremia, and wonder if you can determine just how "gold" this standard is. Because the blood culture is considered the "gold-standard" for the diagnosis of bacteremia, there is no other standard with which to compare the blood culture and calculate its sensitivity and specificity. Aronson reviewed the literature on the performance of a single blood culture compared with a positive result on any of a series of repeated cultures. He wanted to find the optimal number of cultures to obtain.[24] With this approach, the sensitivity of a single blood culture was 80% with a specificity between 95% and 99% depending on the clinical scenario. The false-negative rate (1 – sensitivity) was 20%, but it could be decreased to 0·8%, if three cultures were obtained.

Many of the organisms that traditionally cause occult bacteremia, including *S pneumoniae, H influenzae*, and *N meningitidis*, are fastidious organisms, which makes them more difficult to culture. Additionally, these organisms are often present in the blood in low concentrations of < 10–15 organisms ml⁻¹, making small volume sampling less likely to be successful and causing underestimation of the number of bacteremic children.[25] The volume of blood collected in

children for culture is often small, in the magnitude of 0·5–1·5 ml. In contrast, adults often have between 7·5 and 10 ml drawn per culture.

Assuming that a single blood culture has a sensitivity of 80% and a specificity of 99%, then the LRs for a negative test would be 0·20. Hence, if a blood culture is obtained on a child with a 3% pretest probability of being bacteremic and the result is negative, there is still a 0·5% chance the child is bacteremic. In reality, this is likely to be lower than the truth as comparison with the same reference standard (i.e., BC *v* BC) will overestimate test accuracy. Therefore, the negative likelihood ratio in this calculation will be further away from 1·0 than is truly the case.

Question

8. In a young child between 3 and 36 months of age (*population*), what is the accuracy of clinical signs (*test*) for detecting pneumonia (*outcome*)? [Diagnosis]

- MedLine (PubMed; clinical queries): clinical predictor AND pneumonia AND child

Leventhal studied clinical predictors of pneumonia in a prospective study that took a cohort of children who were going to have a chest radiograph obtained as part of their diagnostic evaluation for either fever or respiratory symptoms.[26] A questionnaire, which determined the presence or absence of historical events and clinical findings, was completed prior to the results of the chest radiograph being known. Pneumonia was defined as a positive infiltrate on the radiograph determined by a radiologist blinded to the clinical information. This study prospectively examined the usefulness of 29 single signs or symptoms of pneumonia in children. Tachypnea was the only physical examination sign that significantly predicted pneumonia with a sensitivity of 81% and a specificity of 60% (LR = 2). However, no single finding or group of findings was 100% sensitive in predicting pneumonia.

In this same study, 41 children had a fever but no pulmonary findings, defined as respiratory distress, tachypnea, and rales or decreased breath sounds. Of these

41 children with no findings, none had pneumonia on chest radiograph.

Question

9. In a young child between 3 and 36 months of age (*population*), what is the accuracy of urinalysis (*test*) for detecting urinary tract infection (*outcome*)? **[Diagnosis]**

This question is addressed in Chapter 42 complete with a search strategy and results. The evidence presented in that chapter reveals a prevalence of urinary tract infection (UTI) in febrile children without a focus of infection to be 3% in males < 1 year of age and 2% in males > 1 year. In females < 1 the prevalence was 7% and, if > 1 year, 8%.

Children can be screened for the presence of a UTI by urinalysis and Chapter 42 shows the sensitivity, specificity, and LRs for the different components of the urinalysis. Suffice it to say here that a patient with a completely normal urinalysis has a very low probability of a UTI. In determining if a child has a UTI you can use either a positive leukocyte esterase or positive nitrite test which will improve the sensitivity of the urinalysis to 99·8% (95% CI 99–100%) at the expense of a lower specificity of 70% (95% CI 60–92%). That is to say that there will be more false-positive results.[27]

Question

10. In a child between 3 and 36 months of age (*population*) what is the effect of the heptavalent pneumococcal conjugate vaccine (*intervention*), on the risk of occult pneumococcal bacteremia (*outcome*)? **[Therapy]**

- MedLine (PubMed; clinical queries): Heptavalent pneumococcal conjugate vaccine AND Effectiveness

This search retrieves six articles of which one is entitled "Efficacy, safety, and immunogenicity of heptavalent pneumococcal conjugate vaccine in children".[28] In this study children were randomized 1:1 to receive heptavalent pneumococcal conjugate vaccine or meningococcus type C conjugate vaccine at ages 2 months, 4 months, 6 months, and a booster at 12–15 months. The primary endpoint was the efficacy of the vaccine against invasive pneumococcal disease, defined as a positive culture from a normally sterile body fluid in a child presenting with an acute illness compatible with pneumococcal disease. A total of 37 868 children were enrolled. The participants were masked and the physicians performing the clinical evaluations were unaware of which vaccination the child had received.

At the end of the study there were 52 cases of invasive disease in the pneumococcal group. Of these, 49 were in controls and three were in the heptavalent pneumococcal conjugate vaccine group (analyzed by intention to treat). This translated into an efficacy of 93·9% (95% CI 79·6%, 98·5%; *P* < 0·001). They also performed an analysis that compared the risk of invasive disease regardless of pneumococcal serotype (including those not covered by the vaccine) and found an 89·1% (95% CI 73·7%, 95·8%; *P* < 0·001) reduction in total pneumococcal disease burden in children who had one or more doses of the heptavalent pneumococcal conjugate vaccine. This translates into an absolute risk reduction of 0·0024 or a number needed to treat (NNT) of 417 (1/ARR). In other words, you would need to treat 417 children with the pneumococcal vaccine to prevent one case of invasive streptococcal disease.

These results are interesting as the strains of pneumococcus covered by the vaccine are the same organisms associated with antibiotic resistance. With the widespread use of the heptavalent pneumococcal conjugate vaccine the incidence of occult bacteremia is likely to decrease to a level much less than the current 1–2% seen in the post *H influenzae* era. Whether in practice this will be true awaits a trial similar to that performed by Lee and Harper as discussed above.

Resolution of the scenario

Your patient is 5 months of age with a fever and no apparent focus of infection, and Hib immunization is widely used in your community. Therefore, the probability that he is bacteremic is about 1·5%. His temperature of 40·9°C increases his risk of bacteremia to approximately 5%. Based on his clinical description he would get a YOS score of 6, which is not useful in detecting occult bacteremia. If he is bacteremic with S pneumoniae there is a 70–87·5% chance of spontaneous resolution, and meningitis is extremely rare as a complication in these children (0·1%).[3–6] If any diagnosis other than meningitis is delayed for a short time it is unlikely to result in serious morbidity. You elect to get a white blood cell count because if the WBC is ≥ 15 000 mm[−3] then there is a 16% chance that he is bacteremic. However, if the WBC is < 15 000 mm[−3], his probability of bacteremia falls to 1%, so this test will aid you in making a decision if your threshold for treatment is in the range of 10–15%. He has no signs of respiratory distress and no abnormal findings on chest auscultation, so you do not order a chest x ray. Because he is a male < 1 year of age, his risk of a UTI is approximately 3%, similar to his risk of bacteremia, and you decide to obtain urine testing. Antibiotics do not appear to be useful in preventing serious bacterial infections, so you decide not to treat at this stage but you will follow this child closely until the resolution of his illness.

Future research needs

With the current practice of widespread empiric antibiotic use there has been an increase in the prevalence of organisms resistant to current antimicrobials.[29,30] A more selective approach to antibiotic use would be desirable for patients at risk. As discussed under the section on treatment, if children could be identified as bacteremic on their initial visit then the use of intramuscular ceftriaxone would be beneficial in decreasing the incidence of serious bacterial infections. Some

work has been done using the polymerase chain reaction (PCR) attempting to identify bacteremic patients within 6 hours.[31,32] This process involves the detection of bacterial DNA in the child's serum. However, it is not currently available in a reliable, automated, cost-effective form.

Summary table

Question	Type of evidence	Result	Comment
Baseline risk of bacteremia	Cohort studies or randomized controlled trial	1–2% risk	Reduced since introduction of immunization to *H influenzae* type b
Probability of developing focal infection if bacteremic	Large cohort studies	Meningitis: 3%. SBI: 7%	70–87.5% of all cases of bacteremia will resolve spontaneously
Effectiveness of treatment with antibiotics	Systematic review	The use of antibiotics versus no antibiotics has an OR of 0.60 (95% CI 0.10–3.49) and ceftriaxone versus oral antibiotic has an OR of 0.38 (95% CI 0.12–1.17) in preventing SBIs in all children at risk for occult bacteremia	No evidence that antibiotics are effective in preventing SBI and meningitis in children at risk for occult bacteremia
Usefulness of clinical exam in identifying bacteremic children	Cohort study of comparison of YOS with blood culture	YOS > 8, LR = 2.1	Not a very useful test as most children will have a score of 6
Usefulness of height of fever in identifying bacteremic children	Large cohort studies	Risk of pneumococcal bacteremia increase from 1.5% at a temperature of 39.0°C to 5% at a temperature of $\geq$ 40.5°C	There is some association with height of fever and bacteremia
Usefulness of WBC count in detecting bacteremia	Large cohort study	LR of WBC count $\geq$ 15 000/mm^3 is 3.74	If pretest probability of bacteremia is 3% then a WBC count of $\geq$ 15 000/mm^3 gives a post-test probability of 10% and if < 15 000/mm^3 only 0.5%
Reliability of blood culture as gold standard for bacteremia	Cohort study with repeated measures in same patient	Sensitivity and specificity of a single blood culture v. repeated blood cultures are 80% and 99%, respectively, which gives an LR for a negative culture of 0.20	The finding of a negative blood culture does not completely rule out bacteremia
Accuracy of clinical exam in detecting pneumonia	Cohort or cross-sectional study	Tachypnea best predictor of pneumonia; LR = 2 No single or group of clinical findings is 100% sensitive in predicting pneumonia.	If a child has no findings referred to the respiratory system unlikely to have pneumonia
Accuracy of urinalysis in detecting a UTI	Large cohort or cross-sectional studies	Sensitivity = 99.8% (see Chapter 42)	A normal urinalysis results in a very low probability of UTI
Efficacy of heptavalent pneumococcal conjugate vaccine	RCT	79–98% reduction in cases of invasive pneumococcal disease	With widespread use may completely change assessment and management of febrile children at risk for occult bacteremia

References

1 Baraff LJ, Bass JW, Fleisher GR *et al.* Practice guidelines for the management of infants and children 0 to 36 months of age with fever without source. *Pediatrics* 1993;**92**:1–12.

2 Finkelstein JA, Christiansen CL, Platt R. Fever in pediatric primary care: occurrence, management, and outcomes. *Pediatrics* 2000;**105**:260–6.

3 Carroll WG, Farrell MK, Singer JI *et al.* Treatment of occult bacteremia: a prospective randomized clinical trial. *Pediatrics* 1983;**72**:608–12.

4 Jaffe DM, Tanz RR, David AT *et al.* Antibiotic administration to treat possible occult bacteremia in febrile children. *N Engl J Med* 1987;**317**:1175–80.

5 Fleisher GR, Rosenberg N, Vinci R *et al.* Intramuscular versus oral antibiotic therapy for the prevention of meningitis and other bacterial sequelae in young, febrile children at risk for occult bacteremia. *J Pediatr* 1994;**124**:504–12.

6 Bass JW, Steele RW, Wittler RR *et al.* Antimicrobial treatment of occult bacteremia: a multicenter cooperative study. *Pediatr Infect Dis J* 1993;**12**:466–73.

7 Lee GM, Harper MB. Risk of bacteremia for febrile young children in the post-*Haemophilus influenzae* type b era. *Arch Pediatr Adolesc Med* 1998;**152**:624–8.

8 Schuchat A, Robinson K, Wenger JD *et al.* Bacterial meningitis in the United States in 1995. *N Engl J Med* 1997;**337**:970–6.

9 Harper MB, Bachur R, Fleisher GR. Effect of antibiotic therapy on the outcome of outpatients with unsuspected bacteremia. *Pediatr Infect Dis J* 1995;**14**:760–7.

10 Lieu TA, Schwartz JS, Jaffe DM, Fleisher GR. Statistics for diagnosis and treatment of children at risk for occult bacteremia: clinical effectiveness and cost-effectiveness. *J Pediatr* 1996;**118**:21–9.

11 Downs SM, McNutt RA, Margolis PA. Management of infants at risk for occult bacteremia: a decision analysis. *J Pediatr* 1991;**118**:11–20.

12 Ros SP, Herman BE, Beissel TJ. Occult bacteremia: is there a standard of care? *Pediatr Emerg Care* 1994;**10**:264–7.

13 Baraff LJ. Management of infants and children 3 to 36 months of age with lever without source. *Pediatr Ann* 1993;**8**: 497–504.

14 Long SS. Antibiotic therapy in febrile children: "Best laid schemes". *J Pediatr* 1994;**124**:585–8.

15 Yamamoto LG, Worthley RG, Melish ME, Seto DSY. A revised decision analysis of strategies in the management of febrile children at risk for occult bacteremia. *Am J Emerg Med* 1998;**16**:193–207.

16 Bulloch B, Craig WR, Klassen TP. The use of antibiotics to prevent serious sequelae in children at risk for occult bacteremia: a meta-analysis. *Acad Emerg Med* 1997;**4**:679–83.

17 Rothrock SG, Harper MB, Green SM *et al.* Do oral antibiotics prevent meningitis and serious bacterial infections In children with *Streptococcus pneumoniae* occult bacteremia? A meta-analysis. *Pediatrics* 1997;**99**:438–44.

18 Rothrock SG, Green SM, Harper MB *et al.* Parenteral vs oral antibiotics in the prevention of serious bacterial infections in children with *Streptococcus pneumoniae* occult bacteremia. A meta-analysis. *Acad Emerg Med* 1998;**5**:599–606.

19 Teach SJ, Fleisher GR and the Occult Bacteremia Study Group. Efficacy of an observation scale in detecting bacteremia in febrile children three to thirty-six months of age, treated as outpatients. *J Pediatr* 1995;**126**:877–1.

20 McCarthy PL, Sharpe MR, Spiesel SZ *et al.* Observation scales to identify serious illness in febrile children. *Pediatrics* 1982;**70**:802–9.

21 Kuppermann N, Fleisher GR, Jaffe DM. Predictors of occult pneumococcal bacteremia in young febrile infants. *Ann Emerg Med* 1998;**31**:679–87.

22 Jaffe DM, Fleisher GR. Temperature and total white blood cell count as indicators of bacteremia. *Pediatrics* 1991;**87**:670–4.

23 Jaeschke R, Guyatt GH, Sackett DL for the Evidence-Based Medicine Working Group. Users guides to the medical literature. III. How to use an article about a diagnostic test. B. What are the results and will they help me in caring for my patients? *JAMA* 1994;**271**:703–7.

24 Aronson MD, Bor DH. Blood cultures. *Ann Int Med* 1987;**106**:246–53.

25 Isaacman DJ, Karasic RB, Reynolds EA, Kost SI. Effect of number of blood cultures and volume of blood on detection of bacteremia in children. *J Pediatr* 1996;**128**:190–5.

26 Leventhal JM. Clinical predictors of pneumonia as a guide to ordering chest roentgenograms. *Clin Pediatr* 1982;**21**:730–4.

27 AAP Subcommittee on UTI. Practice parameter: the diagnosis, treatment, and evaluation of the initial urinary tract infection in febrile infants and young children. *Pediatrics* 1999;**103**:843–52.

28 Black S, Shinefield H, Fireman B *et al.* Efficacy, safety and immunogenicity of heptavalent pneumococcal conjugate vaccine in children. *Pediatr Infect Dis J* 2000;**19**:187–95.

29 McCracken GM Jr. Emergence of resistant *Streptococcus pneumoniae*: a problem in pediatrics. *Pediatr Infect Dis J* 1995;**14**:424–8.

30 Tan TQ, Mason EO, Kaplan SL. Systemic infections due to *Streptococcus pneumoniae* relatively resistant to penicillin in a children's hospital: clinical management and outcome. *Pediatrics* 1992;**90**:928–33.

31 McCabe KM, Khan G, Zhang Y *et al.* Amplification of bacterial DNA using highly conserved sequences: automated analysis and potential for molecular triage of sepsis. *Pediatrics* 1995;**95**:165–9.

32 Zhang Y, Isaacman DJ, Wadowsky RM *et al.* Detection of *Streptococcus pneumoniae* in whole blood by PCR. *J Clin Microbiol* 1995;**33**:596–601.

28 Seizures associated with fever

Martin Offringa

Case scenario

A 19-month-old boy is rushed to the emergency department after being found unconscious at home by his mother. As she went to wake him from his afternoon nap she heard a short cry. She found him lying on his back, rigid and unresponsive, apparently not breathing and with blue lips. When she took him in her arms he grunted and shook. She immediately dialed the local emergency number and the boy was transported to hospital by ambulance. You examine him on arrival in the emergency room. His breathing and circulation are adequate, his pulse rate is 110 per minute, blood pressure 100/60 mmHg, and temperature 39·9°C and there is no cyanosis. The boy is lethargic but can be woken. He is uncooperative and appears confused but seems to recognize his mother. There is a mild generalized hypotonia. Apart from a slightly red pharynx there is no obvious focus of infection and no rash or lymphadenopathy. Neck rigidity is difficult to evaluate since he actively resists examination and refuses to sit. The previous history is unremarkable. The boy's mother and her elder brother suffered two or three short episodes of loss of consciousness under the age of 4, but it is unclear if these were associated with fever. At present they are in good health and no relatives are known to have epilepsy or febrile seizures. You wonder how likely it is that this boy has meningitis and whether lumbar puncture would be helpful? If this event is a simple febrile seizure, what is the likelihood of future febrile seizures, epilepsy, or brain damage? You wonder whether treatment with anticonvulsants should be initiated.

Background

A febrile seizure is defined as a seizure occurring in a neurologically healthy child between 6 months and 5 years of age. Simple febrile seizures are brief (< 15 minutes) and generalized, and occur with fever no more than once during a 24-hour period.[1] Children whose seizures are attributable to a central nervous system infection and those who have had a previous afebrile seizure or central nervous system abnormality are not considered to have simple febrile seizures.

Seizures occurring in association with fever are the most common neurologic disorder in pediatrics, and affect 2–4 of all children in Great Britain and the United States.[2] Despite the frequent nature of these seizures, debate continues regarding their management.

In the acute situation, the pediatrician must judge whether there is an underlying illness that requires immediate, specific treatment. The most urgent diagnostic decision is whether a lumbar puncture is necessary to exclude meningitis. Lumbar puncture is not totally devoid of risk, and undergoing the procedure is a traumatic experience for any toddler. Therefore, in each individual case the physician must weigh the potential harm of failing to diagnose meningitis against the adverse effects of lumbar puncture.

After the acute episode has resolved, the pediatrician must address the possibility of recurrent febrile seizures, and whether the child is at increased risk of frequent or complicated seizures, for which prophylactic medication might be considered. However, such treatment is controversial as the benefits are uncertain, and treatment may have adverse effects on the child's behavior and cognitive development.

Framing answerable clinical questions

The formulation of structured "answerable" questions will help you to design a search strategy.

Questions

1. In young children with a seizure associated with fever (*population*), what is the probability of bacterial meningitis (*outcome*)? **[Baseline Risk/Prognosis]**
2. In young children with a seizure associated with fever (*population*), can an unremarkable physical examination and history (*exposure*) reliably exclude bacterial meningitis (*outcome*)? **[Diagnosis]**

3. In children with a first febrile seizure (*population*), can prophylactic treatment with antiepileptic drugs (*intervention*) as compared with no therapy (*comparison*) decrease the likelihood of future febrile seizures (*outcome*)? **[Therapy]**

4. In children (*population*), with a first febrile seizure (*exposure*), what is the likelihood of future febrile or afebrile seizures (*outcome*)? **[Prognosis]**

Searching for evidence

A variety of search methods are available. As most textbooks are likely to be out of date on the management of seizures with fever you perform a search of the electronic literature. The aim of the search is to identify the "best" evidence by the simplest and most efficient means.

Using "Convulsions-febrile*" as the MeSH heading, you find no systematic reviews in the Cochrane Database of Systematic Reviews (CDSR) but two systematic reviews are listed in the Database of Abstracts of Reviews of Effects (DARE). You find 18 articles in the Central Cochrane Controlled Trials Register (CENTRAL/CCTR). A search of MedLine using *Convulsions-febrile* as a major MeSH heading and *meta-analysis* as a text word nets no additional studies. For the remainder of the questions for which high quality systematic reviews are not available, you decide to make a "clinical query" on the National Library of Medicine's PubMed site (http://www.ncbi.nlm.nih.gov/PubMed/). The searches are shown with the individual questions.

Critical review of the evidence

Question

1. In young children with a seizure associated with fever (*population*), what is the probability of bacterial meningitis (*outcome*)? **[Baseline Risk/Prognosis]**

Search criteria

● MedLine (PubMed) Clinical Queries: "fever seizures meningitis/etiology/sensitivity"

You are looking for cross-sectional studies or follow up studies of children with seizures and fever that identify children who developed meningitis. You make a "clinical query" in PubMed. Your search nets 31 articles, of which 26 are informal reviews and letters, and two concern children

from Nigeria, Africa, in whom – as you can read from the abstract – up to 20% have cerebral malaria.[3,4]

You screen the abstracts of the three remaining articles. One describes a retrospective study based on a case note review of patients with simple, first-time seizures associated with fever who had visited five community hospital and two tertiary pediatric hospital emergency departments between July 1995 and December 1997.[5] Of 455 children identified, 135 (30%) had cerebrospinal fluid cultures performed. None of these cultures grew a bacterial pathogen (prevalence 0%; 95% CI 0·0–2·2%). Although this prevalence is reassuringly low, it is not clear if a diagnosis of meningitis was excluded in the 70% who did not undergo lumbar puncture. In another retrospective, consecutive case series of patients who presented to an urban tertiary care pediatric emergency department for evaluation of febrile seizures during a 12-month period, the prevalence of bacterial meningitis in the absence of initial laboratory evidence of meningitis was estimated.[6] Children who had known seizure disorders, chronic neurologic disease, or documented immunodeficiencies were excluded. Cerebrospinal fluid analysis was performed during the study period in 66 of 243 (27·2%) patient encounters among 218 patients. Of these, none of the cultures grew a bacterial pathogen (meningitis prevalence 0%, 95% CI 0·0–4·5%). Obviously, the least ill children were selected in this study, and, again, how meningitis was excluded in the 72% who did not undergo lumbar puncture is unclear.

You now focus on the remaining article entitled "Which children with febrile seizures need lumbar puncture? A decision analysis approach"[7], but first you click on the "related articles" hyperlink next to this reference, all from the early 1980s. This new search yields 255 titles, most of which are again opinion-based and non-systematic reviews about febrile seizures and letters to the editor. Based on their title, abstract and apparent study design (survey), you select two articles for appraisal.[8,9]

In 1986, Wears *et al.* summarized seven studies performed in urban hospital emergency rooms in the United States.[8] All studies were retrospective surveys of charts documenting the disease outcome after a seizure with fever. Among a total of 2100 cases of seizures associated with fever, an overall meningitis prevalence of 1·2% was found, ranging from 0–4% within the seven studies. However, you do not know whether all children underwent lumbar puncture in these emergency rooms, or whether meningitis was excluded on clinical grounds at follow up.

In the second study published in 1992, 7% of 309 children who visited the emergency room of two Dutch hospitals with a first seizure associated with fever had either bacterial or viral meningitis.[9] As this study was done in the hospital setting in a country where general practitioners manage up to 50% of all seizures with fever,[10,11] it is likely that those included in the study had abnormal clinical findings prompting referral to hospital. The risk of meningitis in these children is therefore likely to be higher than in children who do not have access to a family physician or general practitioner and who therefore present direct to the hospital.

From these two studies,[8,9] it can be concluded that the prevalence of meningitis among children with seizures and fever in North American pediatric emergency wards is between 0% and 2%, and can be as high as 7% in children evaluated by a GP and considered to require referral to hospital. These figures indicate that a large number of "unnecessary" lumbar punctures would be done if you were to perform a lumbar puncture in all children with a seizure associated with fever. You now wonder whether it is safe to rely on the absence of clinical signs of meningitis, and you formulate the second question.

Question

2. In young children with a seizure associated with fever (*population*) can an unremarkable physical examination and history (*exposure*) reliably exclude bacterial meningitis (*outcome*)? **[Diagnosis]**

The question here is whether a seizure can be the sole manifestation of meningitis in an otherwise well-appearing child. This seems unlikely, because one would expect that meningitis cases that are complicated by seizures only entail children who are already in an advanced stage of a potentially debilitating disease. Is there any evidence?

Search criteria

● MedLine (PubMed): "fever AND seizures AND meningitis AND (clinical signs OR diagnosis)"

You are looking for studies that investigate the relationships of various signs and symptoms at presentation in children with a seizure associated with fever and follows them up to determine whether they develop meningitis or not. This search nets 146 hits and identifies many commentaries on the perceived need to perform lumbar puncture as a routine in these children. Only the study from the emergency rooms of two Dutch hospitals provides sensitivity, specificity and likelihood ratios (LR) for the various clinical indicators of meningitis.[9]

This study had tried to identify criteria based on age, specific clinical indicators, and the results of initial blood tests that increased the risk of meningitis. Among 309 consecutive children aged 3 months to 6 years seen with a first seizure associated with fever in the emergency room of two major children's hospitals in the western part of the Netherlands,

23 (7%) cases of meningitis were diagnosed. These were compared with a reference group of 69 children with seizures associated with fever, but without meningitis, selected at random from the remaining 286 children.

Several clinical signs and symptoms were examined for their ability to discriminate between children with and without meningitis. Clinical "risk factors" as postulated in the early study by Joffe *et al.* were confirmed.[7] These factors were: a physician visit within 48 hours before the seizure; the occurrence of seizure(s) at the emergency room; focal, prolonged, or multiple seizures; suspicious findings on physical examination (i.e., petechiae and signs of circulatory failure, or so-called "minor signs"); and abnormal neurological findings on physical examination (i.e., signs of meningeal irritation and various degrees of coma, so called "major signs"). In the absence of meningeal irritation, petechiae, and complex features of the seizure, there were no meningitis cases in the study. The child's age, gender, degree of fever, and results of routinely performed blood tests did not have any diagnostic value.

The accuracy of the clinical indicators for detecting meningitis is shown in Table 28.1. The presence of petechiae, nuchal rigidity, and/or coma identified 16 out of the 23 children with meningitis (70%). In the absence of meningitis, these "major" signs of the disease were not found; the likelihood ratio when any of these signs is present (LR +) is therefore infinite (95% CI 6·0 to infinity) and the risk of meningitis approaches 100% (95% CI 31–100%). Other combinations of indicators (complex features, history features, "minor" signs) had a lower LR+ and therefore yielded a lower posterior probability of meningitis. On the other hand, all indicators had low likelihood ratios when they were absent (LR−), resulting in a very low risk of meningitis given the absence of all these indicators. When looking at nuchal rigidity alone, the sensitivity is 48%, specificity 100%, the LR+ infinite, and the LR− 0·52. With the pretest probability of 7%, the post-test probability of meningitis after a negative test (no nuchal rigidity) is 3%, and the post-test probability of meningitis after a positive test (nuchal rigidity) approaches 100%. All of the meningitis cases (n = 23) had either nuchal rigidity or complex seizures.

The likelihood ratios of the negative and positive test can separate children into different groups: for example, a group in which the risk of meningitis is very high and who should have a lumbar puncture regardless of other history or physical findings, and a group in which the risk of meningitis is very low.

The study described above[9] was a retrospective review of the medical records of children presenting with first episode of seizure and fever. A possible bias is that "children without signs" who were sent home but who developed meningitis and went to a different hospital may have been missed. A further potential problem is that the study population

Table 28.1 Likelihood ratios with 95% confidence interval (95% CI) for the presence (LR+) and absence (LR−) of major and minor clinical signs[9]

Clinical indicators present*	Meningitis Total n = 23 (n %)	No meningitis** Total n = 69 (n %)	LR + (95% CI)
Any major	16 (70)	0 (0)	∞ (6·0 − ∞)
Any minor (no major) or complex or history feature	23 (100)	45 (65)	1·5 (1·3–1·8)
No signs	0 (0)	15 (35)	0 (0–1)

*"Major" signs of meningitis: petechiae, definite nuchal rigidity, coma. "Minor" signs of meningitis: dubious nuchal rigidity, persisting drowsiness, convulsions or paresis or paralysis on examination in the emergency room. Complex seizure features: partial, multiple, or prolonged seizure, i.e., longer than 15 minutes. History features: febrile illness for at least 3 days, vomiting or drowsiness at home, a physician's visit in the previous 48 hours.
**Referent cases were randomly sampled from the list of all 286 children with febrile seizures but without meningitis; three referents were sampled for each case of meningitis.

consisted of children 3 months to 6 years with a first seizure with fever. The mean age was 18 months. It is well known that nuchal rigidity may not be present in children aged 1 year or younger with meningitis, but the study showed that, even in this young age group, children with meningitis had other major or minor signs, even if nuchal rigidity was absent.

This is an example of a highly sensitive "test", which, in the case of a negative test result, rules out the disease. Highly sensitive tests go, in general, with low specificities, which, in this case, would imply that still a lot of children without meningitis will undergo lumbar puncture in case any of the indicators tests positive. Given the likelihood ratio of 1·5 (1·3–1·8) for *"any minor (no major) or complex or history feature positive"* the post-test probability for all children undergoing lumbar puncture would be around 12%; but no meningitis cases would be missed. One has to consider, however, that, as the number of children studied is low, the power to exclude possible cases of meningitis in children without any major and minor signs is low. Yet, this is all the information we can find currently.

In summary, the probability of meningitis in infants and children with a first febrile seizure is close to zero. Meningitis may occur in the absence of nuchal rigidity but will be indicated by other major or minor signs such as prolonged febrile illness, vomiting, drowsiness prior to clinical evaluation, and focal or repeated seizures.

Question

3. In children with a first febrile seizure (*population*), can prophylactic treatment with an antiepileptic drug or an antipyretic (*intervention*), compared to no therapy (*comparison*), decrease the likelihood of future febrile seizures (*outcome*)? **[Therapy]**

Search criteria

- PubMed: "seizures AND fever AND recurrence"
- *Cochrane Library*: "seizures AND fever"

You are looking for studies in which patients with febrile seizures were randomized to different treatment regimens and followed over time to see how many develop subsequent febrile seizures. More than 114 articles come up including 26 randomized controlled trials. You also find the reference to a protocol for an upcoming Cochrane systematic review that should be published in the *Cochrane Library* in 2004 but is not yet available.[12] However, in their abstract, they refer to two meta-analyses on the effect of continuous medication,[13,14] one randomized controlled trial on intermittent diazepam during episodes of fever,[15] and one randomized controlled trial on the effect of intermittent antipyretics.[16]

The first meta-analysis assessed the efficacy of phenobarbitone and valproate for the prophylactic treatment of febrile convulsions by summarizing the results from all eight British clinical trials that had been done before 1988.[13] Data were pooled and analyzed on an intention to treat basis. The overall odds ratio [OR] of recurrent febrile seizures for phenobarbitone was 0·8 (95% CI 0·5–1·1) and for valproate 1·42 (95% CI 0·9–2·0). As neither result was statistically significant the author concluded that neither treatment is to be recommended.

A second meta-analysis summarized four published non-British randomized, placebo-controlled trials that had been done up to 1996 that used phenobarbital as a preventive treatment of febrile seizures.[14] The risk of recurrences was lower in children receiving continuous phenobarbital therapy than placebo (OR 0·54, 95% CI 0·33–0·90). On average, eight children would have to be treated with phenobarbital for 2 years continuously to prevent one febrile seizure (number needed to treat to [NNT] benefit 8, 95% CI 5–27).[17] Yet, because phenobarbital has adverse effects such as irritability, hyperactivity, and somnolence, and even may lower the cognitive development of the toddlers,[18] the authors of this second review concluded that this prophylaxis of febrile seizures cannot be recommended. They wrote:

> The ultimate goal in prevention of febrile seizures is to reduce the risk of epilepsy and to allow normal neurologic and intellectual development for these children. Long-term outcome of children with febrile seizures is good irrespective of whether their febrile seizures were successfully prevented or not. Thus, there appears to be no medical indication to prevent febrile seizures, the merits of prevention being primarily the reduction of parental anxiety.[14]

To avoid the side effects of continuous antiepileptic drugs, rapid-acting anticonvulsants given only during fever periods have been used in an attempt to reduce the risk of recurrent febrile seizures. Phenobarbital at times of fever has not been found to be effective, probably because of the delay in achieving appropriate serum and tissue levels. Thus far, only prophylactic diazepam, given orally or rectally, has been studied in placebo controlled trials.

Rosman *et al.* conducted a randomized, double-blind, placebo-controlled trial among 406 children with a mean age of 24 months who had at least one febrile seizure.[15] Diazepam (0·33 mg kg^{-1} of body weight) or placebo was administered orally every 8 hours during any febrile illness. During a mean follow up of 2 years children in the diazepam group had 675 febrile episodes and 41 febrile seizures, of which seven occurred while the study medication was being given. In the placebo group there were 526 febrile episodes and 72 febrile seizures, of which 38 occurred while the children were receiving the placebo (relative risk of subsequent febrile seizures per person-year 0·56, 95% CI 0·38–0·81). A survival analysis of the length of time to the first recurrent febrile seizure did not show a significant difference between the treatment groups. An analysis restricted to children who had seizures while actually receiving the study medication (a so-called "on treatment analysis" of seven in the diazepam group and 29 in the placebo group) showed an 82% reduction in the risk of febrile seizures with diazepam (RR 0·18, 95% CI 0·09–0·37). However, of the 153 children who took at least one dose of diazepam, 39% had ataxia, lethargy, or irritability, or at least one other moderate side effect.

The authors listed three reasons for using diazepam: reducing anxiety, reducing healthcare expenditures, and preventing severe seizures, and, although the results of their study were mixed, they recommended prophylactic intermittent oral diazepam during febrile illness for all children who had had at least one febrile seizure.[15]

In a series of reactions to this study the point was made that the study had addressed none of these adverse outcomes.[19] The authors of these letters suggested that insistence on the detection of fever is likely to create phobia about fever, and it may increase parental anxiety.[20] "Seizure phobia" may be replaced by "fever phobia". Another point made was that the use of diazepam may impair the clinical assessment during fever or after a subsequent seizure. Between 25% and 30% of the children in the study by Rosman were irritable, lethargic, or had ataxia after taking diazepam, which may interfere with parents and clinicians being able to distinguish benign childhood febrile illness from more serious disease. The number needed to treat to cause these symptoms (the NNT to harm)[17] is 3·5–4. The authors of these letters advocated that the best treatment for children with a first febrile seizure is education and reassurance for the parents.[21–23] Most children need no medication. The child who is at high risk or who lives far from medical care could have diazepam available for rectal administration in the event of a prolonged seizure.[24]

To assess the efficacy of intermittent antipyretic treatment in the prevention of seizure recurrence, a randomized placebo-controlled trial was conducted in the Netherlands.[16] Children aged 1–4 years who had at least one risk factor for febrile seizure recurrence (see below) were enrolled. They were randomly assigned to either ibuprofen syrup, 5 mg kg^{-1} of body weight per dose, or placebo, to be administered every 6 hours during fever, defined as temperature > 38·4°C. Parents were instructed to take the child's rectal temperature immediately when the child seemed ill or feverish and to promptly administer the study medication in case of fever. The primary outcome was the first recurrence of a febrile seizure. Of 230 children, 111 were randomly assigned to ibuprofen syrup and 119 to placebo. Median follow up time was 12 months. Of all children, 67 had a first febrile seizure recurrence, 31 in the ibuprofen group (32% after 2 years) and 36 in the placebo group (39% after 2 years; RR of recurrence 0·9, 95% CI 0·6–1·5). The authors concluded that there was no evidence to show that ibuprofen is effective for the prevention of recurrent febrile seizures.[16]

In summary, there are no effective treatments to reduce the risk of subsequent febrile seizures after an initial febrile seizure and all have serious drawbacks. The best thing to do is to reassure parents, telling them about the good prognosis of febrile seizures.

Question

4. In children with a first febrile seizure (*population*), what is the likelihood of future febrile or afebrile seizures (*outcome*)? **[Prognosis]**

Search criteria

- PubMed Clinical Queries: "seizures AND fever AND epilepsy (prognosis, specificity)"

You are looking for a large cohort of patients who have been followed over time to see how many develop febrile and non-febrile seizures. The search yields 59 articles, but most of them are commentaries and letters. You select two papers based on the information from the title, the abstract, the outcome studied, and the study design.[25,26]

The first study assessed the relationship between risk factors and seizure recurrence after a first febrile seizure using individual patient data from five follow up studies that used similar definitions for febrile seizure.[25] The risk of frequent recurrent seizures and occurrence of complex seizures in previously healthy, untreated children was estimated. Of a total of 2496 children with 1410 episodes of recurrent seizures, 32% had one, 15% had two, and 7% had three or more recurrent seizures after a first febrile seizure; 7% had a complex recurrence. The hazard of recurrent seizures was highest between the ages of 12 and 24 months. After a first and a second recurrence, the risk of further febrile seizures was 2 and 2·5 times higher, respectively. A history of febrile or unprovoked seizures in a first-degree family member and a relatively low temperature at the first seizure were also associated with a doubled risk of subsequent recurrences. Young age at onset (< 12 months), a family history of unprovoked seizures, and a partial initial febrile seizure were all associated with a slightly increased risk of subsequent complex seizures.

Complex features of the first seizure, i.e., partial, multiple, or seizure longer than 15 minutes, have long been thought to predict recurrence. The follow up studies included in this review showed that only multiple initial seizures are associated with a 1·6 fold increase in risk for a first recurrence.[23] Prolonged or focal initial seizures were not associated with an increased risk, as long as they had not led to permanent neurological abnormalities.

This collaborative study found complex recurrences in 7% of all children with a first febrile seizure – mainly multiple seizures. Prolonged recurrences or recurrences with combinations of complex features occurred in 2%. Risk factors for such complex recurrences were an initial focal seizure, age < 12 months at the first febrile seizure and a family history of unprovoked seizures.

The risk of epilepsy after febrile seizures has been studied in population-based cohorts and ranges from 2% to 5%.[1,2] Traditionally accepted predictors of epilepsy following febrile seizures are neurodevelopmental abnormalities, complex febrile seizures, and a family history of epilepsy.[1] In a cohort of 428 children followed prospectively for at least 2 years from their first febrile seizure these factors were assessed.[26] In this hospital-based cohort, unprovoked seizures occurred in 26 (6%), a quite higher incidence than that reported in population based studies.[1,2] Neurodevelopmental abnormalities, complex febrile seizures, and a family history of epilepsy were associated with an increased risk of unprovoked seizures. Recurrent febrile seizures and brief duration of fever before

the initial febrile seizure were also risk factors. A family history of febrile seizures, temperature and age at the initial febrile seizure, sex, and race were not associated with unprovoked seizures.

This high quality evaluation of predictors gives insight into the risk of epilepsy and may be used to counsel patients. However, there are no studies that have examined the possibility of preventing epilepsy with pharmacologic interventions after a first or a second febrile seizure. Therefore, given the low risk of epilepsy, expert opinion currently recommends only treating epilepsy when it occurs.[21]

Resolution of the scenario

Given the history and the physical examination, you consider this child to be at a low risk of meningitis, and decide to observe him without doing a lumbar puncture. After resolution of the acute episode, you reassure the parents and counsel them regarding the risk of future seizures. For this child, the probability of frequently recurring febrile seizures, or of epilepsy, is less than 5%. You decide that the evidence does not support using a daily anticonvulsant like phenobarbital or sodium valproate to prevent recurrence of febrile seizures, nor does it support the use of intermittent diazepam; the harms outweigh the benefits. There is no evidence that antipyretic agents during fever reduce seizure recurrence. You counsel these parents that the risk of recurrence declines rapidly after 6 months from the previous seizure, instruct them to position the child for optimal airway patency in case of a new seizure, which is especially important if the child vomits. You discuss whether they want to have a prescription for rectal diazepam, and, if they do, you instruct them on how to administer it if a seizure goes on for more that 15 minutes.[27] This approach has been suggested to reduce parental fear.[28]

Future research needs

Modern management of children with seizures associated with fever is based on careful medical practice and relevant and valid evidence. The focus is on both the child and the parents. Still, the efficiency of the emergency room decision-making process, i.e., the directness of the route from initial patient contact to formulation of the most likely diagnosis and optimal management plan can be improved. Prospective studies relating the clinical indicators of meningitis shortly after a seizure with fever could confirm the relationships that have been found in retrospective studies, and may further guide clinicians in setting indications for lumbar punctures and hospital admission.

Seizures are a most unpleasant experience for both the child and the parents. Parental fear of fever and recurrent febrile seizures is a major problem with several negative consequences for daily family life.[29–33] Adequate provision of information may reduce parental fear.[22,33] Development and evaluation of an optimal counseling strategy is necessary, and clinical trials comparing different approaches may be considered.

Summary table

Question	Type of evidence	Result	Comment
What is the probability of bacterial meningitis after a seizure with fever?	Cohort or cross-sectional studies of children presenting with a seizure and fever with lumbar puncture or follow up in all to diagnose or exclude meningitis	0–7% depending on population	Pretest probability may be higher in systems where GPs refer only severe cases to hospital
Can an unremarkable physical examination and history reliably exclude bacterial meningitis?	Cohort or cross-sectional study of children presenting with a seizure and fever with diagnosis or exclusion of meningitis in all and a description of physical examination and history items in all	Absence of abnormal signs or symptoms rule out meningitis	The published evidence describes no children with meningitis who present only with a seizure
Can prophylactic treatment with continuous antiepileptic drugs, intermittent oral diazepam, or an antipyretic decrease the likelihood of future febrile seizures?	Two systematic reviews of randomized trials, two randomized trials	Continuous antiepileptic drugs, intermittent diazepam, or antipyretics were not found to reduce the recurrence rate	Two meta-analyses with the same results; lack of effectiveness and side effects limit the use of intermittent oral or rectal diazepam
What is the likelihood of future febrile or afebrile seizures?	Synthesis of five cohort studies with risk factor analyses, and a cohort study	A younger age at the initial seizure, the presence of a first-degree relative with febrile or unprovoked seizures increases recurrence risk	Complex features of the seizure do not predict recurrence of febrile seizures, but are associated with an increased risk of epilepsy

References

1 Nelson KB, Ellenberg JH (eds). *Febrile Seizures*. New York: Raven Press, 1981.
2 Verity CM, Butler NR, Golding J. Febrile convulsions in a national cohort followed up from birth. I Prevalence and recurrence in the first five years of life. *BMJ* 1985;**290**:1307–10.
3 Akpede GO, Sykes RM. Convulsions with fever of acute onset in school-age children in Benin City, Nigeria. *J Trop Pediatr* 1993;**39(5)**:309–11
4 Akpede GO, Sykes RM, Abiodun PO Indications for lumbar puncture in children presenting with convulsions and fever of acute onset: experience in the Children's Emergency Room of the University of Benin Teaching Hospital, Nigeria. *Ann Trop Paediatr* 1992;**12**:385–9.
5 Trainor JL, Hampers LC, Krug SE, Listernick R. Children with first-time simple febrile seizures are at low risk of serious bacterial illness. *Acad Emerg Med* 2001;**8**:781–7.
6 Teach SJ, Geil PA. Incidence of bacteremia, urinary tract infections, and unsuspected bacterial meningitis in children with febrile seizures. *Pediatr Emerg Care* 1999;**15**:9–12.
7 Joffe A, McCormick M, DeAngelis C. Which children with febrile seizures need lumbar puncture? A decision analysis approach. *Am J Dis Child* 1983;**137**:1153–6.
8 Wears RL, Luten RC, Lyons RG. Which laboratory tests should be performed on children with apparent febrile convulsions?

An analysis and review of the literature. *Pediatr Emerg Care* 1986;**2**:1916.
9 Offringa M, Beishuizen A, Derksen-Lubsen G, *et al.* Seizures and fever: Can we rule out meningitis on clinical ground alone? *Clin Pediatr* 1992;**9**:514–22.
10 Offringa M, Hazebroek-Kampschreur AAJM, Derksen-Lubsen G. Prevalence of febrile seizures in Dutch schoolchildren. *Paediatr Perinat Epidemiol* 1991;**5A**:181–8.
11 Verburgh ME, Bruijnzeels MA, van der Wouden JC, *et al.* Incidence of febrile seizures in the Netherlands. *Neuroepidemiology* 1992;**11**:169–72.
12 Offringa M, Newton R. Prophylactic drug management for febrile convulsions in children (Protocol for a Cochrane Review). In: Cochrane Collaboration *Cochrane Library*, Issue 2. Oxford: Update Software, 2003.
13 Newton RW. Randomised controlled trials of phenobarbitone and valproate in febrile convulsions. *Arch Dis Child* 1988;**63**:1189–91.
14 Rantala H, Tarkka R, Uhari M. A meta-analytic review of the preventive treatment of recurrences of febrile seizures. *J Pediatr* 1997;**131**:922–5.
15 Rosman NP, Colton T, Labazzo J, *et al.* A controlled trial of diazepam administered during febrile illnesses to prevent recurrence of febrile seizures. *N Engl J Med* 1993;**329**:79–85.
16 van Stuijvenberg M, Derksen-Lubsen G, Steyerberg EW, *et al.* Randomized, controlled trial of ibuprofen syrup administered

during febrile illnesses to prevent febrile seizure recurrences. *Pediatrics* 1998;**102**:pE51.

17 Altman DG. Confidence intervals for the number needed to treat. *BMJ* 1998;**317**:1309–12.

18 Farwell JR, Lee YJ, Hirtz DG, Sulzbacher SI, Ellenberg JH, Nelson KB. Phenobarbital for febrile seizures–effects on intelligence and on seizure recurrence. *N Engl J Med* 1990;**332**:364–9.

19 Fischbein CA, Berg IJ, Leiner S *et al.* Diazepam to prevent febrile seizures. *N Engl J Med* 1993;**329**:2033.

20 May A, Bauchner H. Fever phobia: the pediatrician's contribution. *Pediatrics* 1992;**90(6)**:851–4.

21 Freeman JM. The best medicine for febrile seizures. *N Engl J Med* 1992;**327**:1161–3.

22 Bethune P, Gordon K, Dooley J, Camfield C, Camfield P. Which child will have a febrile seizure? *Am J Dis Child* 1993;**147(1)**:35–9.

23 Camfield CS, Camfield PR. Febrile seizures: a Rx for parent fears and anxieties. *Contemp Pediatr* 1993;**10**:26–44.

24 Knudsen FU. Rectal administration of diazepam in solution in the acute treatment of convulsions in infants and children. *Arch Dis Child* 1979;**54**:855–7.

25 Offringa M, Bossuyt PMM, Lubsen J *et al.* Risk factors for seizure recurrence in children with febrile seizures: A pooled analysis of individual patient data from five studies. *J Pediatr* 1994:**124**:574–84.

26 Berg AT, Shinnar S Unprovoked seizures in children with febrile seizures: short-term outcome. *Neurology* 1996;**47**: 562–8

27 Dreifuss FE, Rosman NP, Cloyd JC *et al.* A comparison of rectal diazepam gel and placebo for acute repetitive seizures. *N Engl J Med* 1998;**338(26)**:1869–75.

28 Rossi LN, Rossi G, Bossi A, *et al.* Behavior and confidence of parents instructed in home management of febrile seizures by rectal diazepam. *Helv Paediatr Acta* 1989;**43**:273–81.

29 van Stuijvenberg M, de Vos S, Tjiang GCH, Steyerberg EW, Derksen-Lubsen G, Moll HA. Parents' fear regarding fever and febrile seizures. *Acta Paediatr* 1999;**88**:618–22.

30 Miller R. The effect on parents of febrile convulsions. *Paediatr Nurs.* 1996 Nov;**8(9)**:28–31.

31 Shuper A, Gabbay U, Mimouni M. Parental anxiety in febrile convulsions. *Isr J Med Sci* 1996;**32**:1282–5.

32 Huang MC, Liu CC, Huang CC. Effects of an educational program on parents with febrile convulsive children. *Pediatr Neurol* 1998;**18(2)**:150–5.

33 Huang MC, Liu CC, Chi YC, Huang CC, Cain K. Parental concerns for the child with febrile convulsion: long-term effects of educational interventions. *Acta Neurol Scand* 2001;**103**:288–93.

29 Meningitis

Peter McIntyre

Case scenario *On your admitting day for the pediatric service at an urban general hospital, the senior resident in the emergency department telephones for advice concerning a 7-month-old boy with presumptive pneumococcal meningitis. He has been previously well apart from two episodes of otitis media treated with oral amoxycillin, the first at 3 months of age and the most recent completed 7 days ago. He is late for his immunizations, having had a second dose of diphtheria, tetanus, and pertussis (DTP), and Haemophilus influenzae type b (Hib) vaccine 1 week ago. He has now been febrile for just over 24 hours, worsening over the last 8 hours with lack of interest in feeds and, over the last 3 hours, vomiting, which prompted presentation to hospital. His vital signs are a temperature of 39·6°C, respiratory rate of 50 per minute and a pulse of 140 per minute. A full evaluation for sepsis was performed including lumbar puncture after establishing i.v. access and giving a fluid bolus of 10 ml kg^{-1} (half normal saline and 5% dextrose). The cerebrospinal fluid (CSF) microscopy is unequivocally abnormal – 450 leukocytes ($\times 10^9$ per liter) of which 90% were polymorphonuclear cells (PMNs) and Gram stain showing Gram-positive cocci resembling pneumococci. The serum sodium is low at 129 mmol per liter. The resident, who has never seen a case of bacterial meningitis, wants your advice about use of vancomycin and dexamethasone as well as fluid therapy.*

Background

Meningitis is defined by inflammation of the meninges, and is almost always due to an infective cause in children. Clinical signs such as neck rigidity or a tense fontanelle are notoriously unreliable in infants; meningeal inflammation is reliably diagnosed only by lumbar puncture and examination of the CSF. After the neonatal period, normal CSF contains fewer than 10×10^9 leukocytes per liter. In acutely unwell infants over the age of 1 month with abnormal CSF (meningitis), viruses, particularly enteroviruses, and a limited range of bacteria are the most common causes. The CSF becomes turbid in appearance if there are more than 500×10^9 leukocytes per liter or very high numbers of bacteria (purulent meningitis). Purulent meningitis is almost always bacterial.

The optimum evidence for equivalent or superior efficacy of therapy in meningitis comes from well-designed randomized controlled trials, either singly or combined in a meta-analysis (see Chapter 8 on systematic reviews). The outcome measures of greatest importance are mortality and long-term sequelae. The relative rarity of death and severe long-term sequelae from bacterial meningitis in developed countries make it impractical for comparative studies of antibiotic therapy for meningitis to use these outcomes; proxy measures such as bacteriologic response are more commonly reported. In addition, studies comparing third-generation cephalosporins with previous standard therapy were performed at a time when almost all causative organisms of bacterial meningitis were sensitive *in vitro* to all the agents used. The outcomes reported were therefore limited to the rapidity of sterilization of the CSF and pharmacokinetic issues such as dose and dosing frequency.

Although bacterial meningitis has become much less common in countries where routine immunization against *Haemophilus influenzae* type b (Hib) has been introduced, the management of bacterial meningitis continues to generate controversy. The emergence of penicillin-resistant *Streptococcus pneumoniae* (PRSP) and the low probability of Hib meningitis has had a major impact on the baseline probability of bacterial meningitis and empiric antibiotic choice, which in turn impact on the risks and benefits of dexamethasone therapy. As there is substantial regional variation, in the prevalence of pneumococcal antibiotic resistance, even within countries, local data are essential. Furthermore, Hib meningitis still occurs, especially in inadequately immunized children. To add to the difficulty, in some countries, immediate parenteral antibiotic therapy for presumptive meningococcal infection is recommended, which will frequently render cultures sterile. The best answer to these dilemmas will be prevention of pneumococcal and meningococcal meningitis by immunization, as has been achieved for Hib meningitis. Until then and probably occasionally afterwards, clinicians will continue to be faced with scenarios such as the one above.

Framing answerable clinical questions

A number of questions relating to diagnosis and management arise from this scenario. Some are relevant to the immediate management of children in the emergency department and others will help in your personal practice and in framing hospital policy. Questions include:

- What is the most appropriate choice of empiric antibiotic therapy for presumed pneumococcal meningitis?
- What are the indications for dexamethasone as adjunctive therapy for meningitis and the most appropriate timing, dose, and duration if dexamethasone is used?
- What is the most appropriate initial fluid therapy in presumptive bacterial meningitis?

These clinical questions can be reframed into structured questions, which will clarify your thinking and help with your search. Each question should have the following elements:

- the patient/population
- the intervention (event, study factor or exposure), and
- the outcome of interest.

In addition, each question can be mapped to the type of information sought – pertaining to causation, diagnosis, therapy, risk, or prognosis. You frame the following questions:

Questions

1. Among children with meningitis due to *Streptococcus pneumoniae* with reduced sensitivity to third-generation cephalosporins (*population*), how does the addition of vancomycin (*intervention*) affect the probability of short-term adverse events such as delayed resolution of fever, seizures or death, and long-term sequelae, such as hearing loss and neurologic impairment (*outcomes of interest*)? **[Therapy]**

2. In pneumococcal meningitis in children (*population*), how does the addition of dexamethasone (*intervention*) to antibiotic therapy affect the probability of short-term adverse events, such as delayed sterilization of the CSF, seizures, clinically evident gastrointestinal bleeding or death, and long-term sequelae, such as hearing loss and neurologic impairment (*outcomes of interest*)? Among

children with pneumococcal meningitis treated with vancomycin (*subpopulation*), how does the addition of dexamethasone (*intervention*) affect these probabilities? Are these probabilities changed by the timing or duration of dexamethasone therapy? **[Therapy]**

3. In children with bacterial meningitis (*population*), how does the reduction of i.v. fluid administered to two-thirds of maintenance volumes (*intervention*) affect the probability of short-term adverse events, such as delayed resolution of fever, seizures or death, and long-term sequelae such as hearing loss and neurologic impairment (*outcomes of interest*)? In children with bacterial meningitis and hyponatremia at presentation (*subpopulation*) are these probabilities altered? **[Therapy]**

Searching for evidence

You realize that the probability that *S pneumoniae* has reduced sensitivity to third-generation cephalosporins is only answerable with local data. You contact your hospital microbiology department and learn that the proportion of pneumococci showing reduced sensitivity to penicillin has increased to approximately 20%, and that some 5–10% of these resistant strains also have reduced sensitivity to third-generation cephalosporins. Thus the need for additional empiric therapy must be considered.

You decide to look first for systematic reviews or guidelines (see Chapter 8) addressing any of your three questions. Using the *Cochrane Library* database of systematic reviews and the term "meningitis" you find only one on the use of corticosteroids in meningitis is directly relevant to your questions.[1] 'Another 24 protocols for Cochrane reviews are also listed under this topic, of which only "third-generation cephalosporins versus conventional antibiotics for treating acute bacterial meningitis" appears relevant.[2] Thus, you are still interested in pursuing guidelines and other sources of predigested evidence in relation to antibiotic therapy of meningitis. You decide to search using "clinical queries", a feature of PubMed that allows searching using research methodology filters, which also allows you to rapidly search for both high quality primary studies and systematic reviews (http://www.ncbi.nlm.nih.gov/entrez/query/static/clinical.html) (see Chapter 3).

This resource allows selection from a number of categories, including systematic reviews. You may also choose to search primary studies of therapy, diagnosis, etiology, or prognosis. You can then choose to either conduct a wide search (sensitivity) or a focused search (specificity). For dexamethasone, as the topic is specific, you select this search option with the terms meningitis and dexamethasone and click on therapy. This yields 30 references, including one randomized controlled trial (RCT) not mentioned in the Cochrane review – a small trial in adults from India.[3] You are still searching for guidance on empiric antibiotic therapy in pneumococcal meningitis and fluid therapy in bacterial meningitis. For the category therapy and the search terms "pneumococcal meningitis", a sensitive search yields 872 entries, so you decide to do a text word search for "pneumococcal meningitis and empiric therapy", which yields a more managable 23 references. On perusal, three papers appear highly relevant to your question concerning the outcome of therapy for resistant pneumococcal meningitis.[4–6] However, concerned that some relevant reviews of antibiotic therapy may have been missed, you broaden the search terms to "bacterial meningitis, antibiotic AND children", but select only systematic reviews, which yields 31 hits. You find that there are two review papers of interest, one examining antibiotic trials in childhood meningitis in general[7] and the other a guideline from the American Academy of Pediatrics (AAP).[8] Next, you use the search terms "fluid therapy and meningitis". When choosing a specific search produces no hits, you select the "sensitivity" option and this time have 31 hits. Among these are two treatment reviews, downloadable without charge from the *Archives of Disease of Childhood*, one general[11] and one specifically addressing fluid therapy.[12] Most of the articles identified for further review fall under the general category of syntheses of information, but there are a few primary RCTs. The validity of the data syntheses will depend on the quality and comprehensiveness of the literature searches and the process of combining the evidence, for which the Cochrane collaboration has specific quality criteria (see Chapter 8). The methodology section of the practice guideline from the AAP states that 160 articles were selected as being of sufficient relevance and validity for further review, supplemented by material from publications and presentations and the personal files of committee members with final recommendations from the literature or, if this was deemed inconclusive, by a process of group consensus. The AAP recommendations were in turn reviewed by other expert groups before publication. The other review paper is a narrative review,[9] which does not specify a search strategy or quality control mechanisms other than peer review.

Critical review of the evidence

Question

1. Among children with meningitis due to *Streptococcus pneumoniae* with reduced sensitivity to third-generation cephalosporins (*population*), how does the addition of vancomycin (*intervention*) affect the probability of short-term adverse events, such as delayed resolution of fever, seizures or death, and long-term sequelae, such as hearing loss and neurologic impairment (*outcome*)'?
[Therapy]

The American Academy of Pediatrics Guideline outlines the background issues in some detail. The emergence of chloramphenicol-resistant *H influenzae* type b led to selection of a third-generation cephalosporin as the standard empiric therapy for community-acquired bacterial meningitis in children, although the other two important pathogens (*S pneumoniae* and *Neisseria meningitidis*) remained susceptible to penicillin. Subsequently, the fact that third-generation cephalosporins achieved higher CSF levels than penicillin, and were also effective against penicillin-resistant pneumococci, continued to justify their use.

From the review, you feel more familiar with the rationale for vancomycin use. Vancomycin was only indicated for treatment of bacterial meningitis in very specialized settings before the advent of significant pneumococcal resistance to third-generation cephalosporins. This means that trials including vancomycin were not conducted prior to this becoming an issue. The practice guideline discusses the use of vancomycin based on other data. These include *in vitro* studies of bacterial killing of pneumococcal strains with varying levels of resistance to cephalosporins, data from case reports, and pharmacokinetic data on achievable levels of vancomycin in CSF in relation to the concentrations used for laboratory testing. You appreciate that these data are inferior to those from randomized trials, because it is impossible to control for the multiplicity of factors that may be operating in the clinical setting.

On the other hand, randomized controlled trials comparing alternative antibiotic therapy in bacterial meningitis are limited to agents to which the causative organism(s) are sensitive *in vitro*. Thus, clinical as opposed to laboratory data are limited to published observations on the response to therapy of case series, where laboratory data later indicate that their pneumococcal isolate had reduced susceptibility *in vitro*. Recommendations for antibiotic therapy are (implicitly) based on a series of probabilities of:

- pneumococcal meningitis being present, based on Gram stain and other immediately available CSF parameters;
- resistance to cephalosporins at a level where achievement of adequate levels of cephalosporin in the CSF for bacterial killing is unlikely;
- the clinical outcome being inferior when patients with a resistant isolate do not commence vancomycin immediately.

The three papers identified on empiric therapy are case series, one from Australia in a setting of emerging antibiotic resistance[6] and two from the USA in the context of higher levels of pneumococcal resistance.[4,5] The Australian study, which was restricted to proven pneumococcal meningitis, gives some relevant information on the first (diagnostic) probability. With respect to immediately available parameters, all but two (97%) of 57 children with lumbar puncture (LP) prior to antibiotics had a Gram stain consistent with pneumococci. The second probability depends on local levels of antibiotic resistance and the number of cases in a series where the isolate was not sensitive to the initial antibiotic therapy, defined as discordant therapy. The three available case series included relatively small numbers of meningitis owing to pneumococci with reduced sensitivity to penicillin or cephalosporins, and even fewer who received discordant therapy. Thus the power of these accumulated data to address the question of interest is limited, so you are sceptical about the failure of each study to show a statistically significantly worse outcome for cases of discordant therapy. The Australian study recommends that empiric vancomycin be restricted to cases where the Gram stain is suggestive of pneumococcal meningitis, or LP is deferred but bacterial meningitis is suspected. You decide that for your case, where there is clear evidence of pneumococcal etiology, empiric vancomycin is justified. This leads you in turn to the question of whether the success of vancomycin therapy might be influenced by concomitant dexamethasone.

Question

2. In pneumococcal meningitis in children (*population*), how does the addition of dexamethasone (*intervention*) affect the probability of short-term adverse events, such as delayed sterilization of the CSF, seizures, clinically evident gastrointestinal bleeding or death, and long-term sequelae, such as hearing loss and neurologic impairment (*outcomes of interest*)? Among children with pneumococcal meningitis treated with vancomycin (*subpopulation*), how does the addition of dexamethasone (*intervention*) affect these probabilities, when there is or is not resistance to cephalosporins? Are these probabilities changed by the timing or duration of dexamethasone therapy? **[Therapy]**

This Cochrane systematic review of corticosteroids in bacterial meningitis is new, first published in Issue 3, 2003.[1] The review has broad search criteria and identified 28 trials, of which 18 were judged eligible and of sufficient methodological quality. The review includes 18 studies meeting eligibility criteria from 28 identified, of which all but four are confined to children. Overall, in adults and in pneumococcal meningitis, there was significantly lower mortality with corticosteroids. In children, mortality was comparable with (6·2%) and without (6·6%) corticosteroid therapy. With respect to hearing loss, outcome was also significantly improved in the corticosteroid group, both for *H influenzae* and other pathogens, such that 20 children would require treatment to prevent one case of hearing loss. There were too few patients with specified neurologic sequelae and a known causative organism to estimate pathogen-specific effects, but long-term neurologic sequelae

were also reduced overall. Given the need to give dexamethasone before or with antibiotic therapy to derive benefit, it is likely that some children with non-bacterial meningitis will receive it. It is therefore important that adverse effects were equally divided between treatment and placebo groups. The relative risk of gastrointestinal bleeding, an adverse event which has been highlighted as a concern, was not significantly increased. The reviewers concluded that, even after taking into account methodological flaws in the original studies, corticosteroids should be recommended for use in childhood meningitis in settings where prompt diagnosis and treatment can be assured. However, the Cochrane review did not include three recent randomized controlled trials that you found in your search.[3,11,12] The first of these was in adults, but is of interest because it includes a substantial number of pneumococcal cases.[11] Both overall and for pneumococcal meningitis, death and severe disability were significantly lower if dexamethasone was given. This is compelling because the study has been meticulously conducted. However, in the second RCT, conducted in children in Malawi, the findings were very different.[12] Overall, no difference in mortality or sequelae with corticosteroids was found (relative risk [RR] 1·0 and 0·99 respectively), but in a subgroup analysis, children who survived pneumococcal meningitis were more likely to have neurological sequelae (RR 2·0; 95% CI 1·2–3·5). However, the clinical circumstances of children in Malawi differed in many respects from your patient. Prior antibiotics, malaria, and HIV infection were all prevalent and there was a high case fatality rate. In multivariate analysis, death was significantly associated with young age, malnutrition, coma, HIV positivity and causative organism but not with corticosteroid use. This suggests that these factors, rather than corticosteroid use, were the primary determinants of poor outcome. Failure to find any significant benefit from corticosteroid therapy in this study is similar to the findings from another resource-poor country, Pakistan,[13] and consistent with the recommendations of the Cochrane review that steroids only be considered for well-resourced countries. The third RCT, from India, included only 40 adult patients, but in keeping with the Dutch results, neurologic sequelae and hearing loss were significantly less common in the dexamethasone group.[3]

The second part of the question is should dexamethasone be used when vancomycin is given? Unfortunately there is little guidance on this point from either the Cochrane review or the RCTs. From the guideline,[8] you realize that the question of dexamethasone use with vancomycin relates both to concern about the adequacy of CSF penetration of vancomycin, for meningitis from either sensitive or resistant *S pneumoniae*, as well as specific concerns about treatment of resistant pneumococci. In this situation, marginally effective concentrations of vancomycin might be compromised by any reduction in passage of vancomycin across the blood–brain barrier. The guideline refers to data from the rabbit model of pneumococcal meningitis that raise concern about reduced CSF penetration of both cephalosporins and vancomycin in the presence of dexamethasone.[10] This contrasts with the only human data, from children with meningitis, which suggest that CSF levels of both vancomycin and cephalosporins are substantially higher than in the rabbit (20% of serum levels v 3%).[18] These higher levels correlated with greater bactericidal activity of CSF from children receiving dexamethasone who were given vancomycin and ceftriaxone compared with those receiving ceftriaxone alone when incubated with resistant pneumococcal strains in the laboratory. Given the rarity of pneumococcal meningitis and, specifically, use of dexamethasone in the context of resistant pneumococcal meningitis, you realize that answers to these questions are unlikely to be addressed by clinical trials. Reassured by the adequate CSF penetration seen with dexamethasone in a clinical study and the lack of other adverse effects, you decide that the most appropriate regimen is vancomycin with a third-generation cephalosporin plus dexamethasone given just before the first antibiotic dose.

Question

3. In children with bacterial meningitis (*population*), how does the reduction of i.v. fluid administered to two-thirds of maintenance volumes (*intervention*) affect the probability of short-term adverse events, such as delayed resolution of fever, seizures or death, and long-term sequelae such as hearing loss and neurologic impairment (*outcomes of interest*)? In children with bacterial meningitis and hyponatremia at presentation (*subpopulation*) are these probabilities altered? **[Therapy]**

The most appropriate fluid management in bacterial meningitis is also controversial. Recommended i.v. fluid therapy has swung between, on the one hand, recognition that the syndrome of inappropriate secretion of antidiuretic hormone (ADH) could occur, with advice for almost universal fluid restriction,[16] and on the other, recognition that dehydration and circulatory compromise is common in bacterial meningitis and may pose an even greater hazard.[17] The three trials identified in your search are in different settings. The first study was conducted in Rochester, New York, USA[18] and the other two in third world settings in India[19] and Papua New Guinea.[20] The Rochester study randomized 19 children with meningitis (13 bacterial, six aseptic) to receive maintenance fluids (10) or two-thirds maintenance fluids (9). The outcomes evaluated were plasma arginine vasopressin (AVP) concentration and serum osmolality at study entry and at 24 hours. At 24 hours, the

AVP was significantly reduced in children with bacterial meningitis who had received maintenance fluids (-8.7 pg ml^{-1}; $P = 0.01$) but had not changed in the restricted fluids group ($+ 0.5$ pg ml^{-1}). The serum osmolality was also higher in those with bacterial meningitis in the maintenance fluid group (286 mOsmol kg^{-1}) than the comparison group (282 mOsmol kg^{-1}; $P = 0.07$). These changes are the opposite to those expected if the syndrome of inappropriate ADH secretion had been present. The authors argue that maintenance fluids rather than restricted fluids should be the routine practice, with careful follow up evaluation of fluid and electrolyte balance. Although this setting is similar to your own, you note that only 19 of the 74 eligible subjects were included in this study and are concerned about the lack of clinical endpoints. You are also uncertain about the prevalence of the syndrome of inappropriate ADH (SIADH) secretion in bacterial meningitis – how important a problem is SIADH and how likely is it that "close follow up" would necessitate a change in fluid therapy in a typical population of patients?

In the Indian study, 50 consecutively hospitalized children with acute meningitis were stratified into two groups; those with and without hyponatremia, and randomly assigned to receive either normal maintenance or 65–70% of maintenance fluids during the first 48 hours.[5] Total body water, extracellular water (ECW), serum and urinary sodium and plasma and urinary osmolality were measured at admission and after 48 hours. The proportion of children with intact survival was higher (7/11, 64%) in both the hyponatremic and normonatremic group on normal maintenance fluids, compared with those on restricted fluids (6/13, 46% for hyponatremic group, and 5/15, 33% for normonatremic). However, this overall difference was not significant with the sample size in this study. As statistical power is not discussed, you do not know how large a difference the study was able to detect with 95% confidence. When mortality among the fluid-restricted children irrespective of serum sodium (7/28, 25%) was compared with the maintenance group (2/22, 9.1%), this trend was more pronounced ($P = 0.15$). The authors then examined children in either the maintenance or restricted fluid group who had a reduction in ECW of > 10%. When those with large reductions in ECW at 48 hours were compared with others, intact survival was significantly reduced in the group with > 10% reduction in ECW (odds ratio [OR] = 0.52; 95% CI 0.31–0.99).

The largest study is the most recent one, from Papua New Guinea.[20] This trial compared 172 children randomized to restricted fluids (60% maintenance) given as breast milk or by nasogastric tube with 174 children randomized to receive 100% maintenance fluids given as half normal saline intravenously. Overall, an adverse outcome (death or severe neurologic sequelae) was most strongly associated with signs of dehydration at entry (RR 5·7; 95% CI 2·9–11·3). However, children with dehydration were significantly less likely to have an adverse outcome if allocated to intravenous fluids (RR 0·5; 95% CI 0·3–0·). Facial edema at 48 hours after admission was also significantly associated with an adverse outcome (RR 2·5; 95% CI 1·4–4·8) and was much more common in the intravenous group (26%) than the oral group (5%). Overall, an adverse outcome was less likely in the intravenous group and almost reached statistical significance (RR 0·75; 95% CI 0·5–1·04). Despite the largest studies being conducted in different settings from your own, the findings are consistent across all three and suggest that routine fluid restriction is not appropriate. Finally, there is an observational study from Switzerland, a setting similar to your own, which offers some insight into the frequency of hyponatremia in bacterial meningitis.[20] Of 187 children with bacterial meningitis over a 12-year period, 30 (16%) were hyponatremic (plasma sodium < 130 mmol per liter). The authors state that the hyponatremic patients were significantly more likely to be dehydrated than those with normal serum sodium. You decide that normal maintenance fluids are appropriate for your patient.

Resolution of the scenario

Your patient appears to have pneumococcal meningitis. You decide to give a dose of dexamethasone, followed by empirical vancomycin and a third-generation cephalosporin. In light of the evidence about fluid therapy, you choose to provide your patient with normal maintenance fluids.

Future research needs

As bacterial meningitis is becoming progressively rarer, studies of adequate sample size, even if multicenter, are difficult to mount, especially given the need for prolonged follow up and the problems in obtaining informed consent in a timely fashion. The most important question is whether the current, convincing evidence of benefit from dexamethasone in bacterial meningitis in settings with good access to services and low levels of antibiotic resistance is applicable where either of these do not pertain. With respect to access to medical care, it seems likely from the experience in Malawi and Pakistan that most children in resource-poor countries will not benefit from adjunctive dexamethasone and that the emphasis should be on delivering the effective and timely antibiotic therapy. With respect to antimicrobial resistance in pneumococcal meningitis, vancomycin is likely to be an important component of effective therapy where high level resistance is present, and should be combined with a third-generation cephalosporin until antimicrobial sensitivity is known. If dexamethasone is to provide additional benefit, it must be administered before or with the first dose of parenteral antibiotics. To achieve this, even in well-resourced settings, will require well-developed and implemented protocols for emergency management of putative bacterial meningitis. Fluid and electrolyte management remains important in bacterial meningitis but maintenance of adequate circulating volume is of primary importance and will necessitate appropriate replacement and, in most cases, full volume maintenance fluids.

Summary table

Question	Type of evidence	Result	Comment
Addition of vancomycin to third-generation cephalosporins	Laboratory data showing resistance, expert opinion	Vancomycin recommended for cephalosporin-resistant pneumococci, empirically if resistance is high in community	Based on laboratory studies, not human studies
Addition of dexamethasone to antibiotics	Cochrane review	Start dexamethasone before antibiotics	Several small studies conducted before antibiotic resistance was prevalent. Differences between resource-rich and resource-poor countries
Reduction of i.v. fluids to two-thirds maintenance	Two small RCTs, one larger RCT	Higher survival and higher serum osmolality with normal maintenance fluids	Small sample sizes, lack of statistical power. Differences between resource-rich and resource-poor countries

References

1 Beek D van de, Gans J de, McIntyre P, Prasad K. Corticosteroids for acute bacterial meningitis. *Cochrane Library*. Issue 3. Oxford: Update Software, 2003.

2 Prasad K, Coulthard M. Third generation cephalosporins versus conventional antibiotics for treating acute bacterial meningitis (Protocol for a Cochrane Review) *Cochrane Library* Issue 2 Oxford: Update Software; 2003.

3 Gijwani D, Kumhar MR, Singh VB *et al.* Dexamethasone therapy for bacterial meningitis in adults: a double blind placebo control study. *Neurology* (India) 2002;**50**:63–7.

4 Kellner JD, Scheifele DW, Halperin SA *et al.* Outcome of penicillin-nonsusceptible Streptococcus pneumoniae meningitis: a nested case-control study. *Pediatr Infect Dis J* 2002;**21**:903–9.

5 Buckingham SC, McCullers JA, Lujan-Zilbermann J, Knapp KM, Orman KL, English K. Pneumococcal meningitis in children: relationship of antibiotic resistance to clinical characteristics and outcomes. *Pediatr Infect Dis J* 2001;**20**: 837–43.

6 McMaster P, McIntyre P, Gilmour R, Kakakios A, Mellis C. The emergence of resistant pneumococcal meningitis – implications for empiric therapy. *Arch Dis Child* 2002;**87**: 207–10.

7 Krysan DJ, Kemper AR. Claims of equivalence in randomised controlled trials of the treatment of bacterial meningitis in children *Pediatr Infect Dis J* 2002;**21**:753–7.

8 American Academy of Pediatrics Committee on Infectious Diseases. Therapy for children with invasive pneumococcal infections. *Pediatrics.* 1997;**99**:289–99.

9 El Bashir H, Laundry M, Booy R. Diagnosis and treatment of bacterial meningitis. *Arch Dis Child* 2003;**88**:615–20.

10 Duke T. Fluid management of bacterial meningitis in developing countries. *Arch Dis Child* 1998;**79**:181–5.

11 de Gans J, van de Beek D. Dexamethasone in adults with bacterial meningitis. *N Engl J Med* 2002;**347**:1549–56.

12. Molyneux EM, Walsh AL, Forsyth H *et al.* Dexamethasone treatment in childhood bacterial meningitis in Malawi: randomised controlled trial. *Lancet* 2002;**360**:211–18.

13 Qazi SA, Khan MA, Mughal N *et al.* Dexamethasone and bacterial meningitis in Pakistan. *Arch Dis Child* 1996;**75**: 482–8.

14 Paris MM, Hickey SM, Uscher MI, Shelton S, Olsen KD, McCracken GH Jr. Effect of dexamethasone on therapy of experimental penicillin and cephalosporin-resistant pneumococcal meningitis. *Antimicrob Agents Chemother* 1994;**38**:1320–4.

15 Klugman KP, Dagan R, The Meropenem Meningitis Study Group. Randomised comparison of meropenem with cefotaxime for treatment of bacterial meningitis in children. *Antimtcrob Agents Chemother* 1995;**39**:1140–6.

16 Feigin RD, McCracken GH Jr, Klein JO. Diagnosis and management of meningitis. *Pediatr Infect Dis J* 1992;**11**: 785–814.

17 Bianchetti MG, Thyssen HR, Laux-End R, Schaad UB. Evidence for fluid volume depletion in hyponatraemic patients with bacterial meningitis. *Acta Paed* 1996;**85**: 1163–6.

18 Powell KR, Sugarman LI, Eskenazi AE *et al.* Normalization of plasma arginine vasopressin concentrations when children with meningitis are given maintenance plus replacement fluid therapy. *J Pediatr* 1990;**117**:515–22.

19 Singhi SC, Singhi PD, Srinivas B *et al.* Fluid restriction does not improve the outcome of acute meningitis. *Pediatr Infect Dis J* 1995;**14**:495–503.

20 Duke T, Mokela D, Frank D *et al.* Management of meningitis in children with oral fluid restriction or intravenous fluid at maintenance volumes: a randomised trial. *Annls Trop Paediatr* 2002;**22**:145–57.

30 Asthma

Anne Morris, Craig Mellis

Case scenario

A 3-year-old boy presents to the emergency department (ED) with a 24-hour history of cough, wheeze, and increasing shortness of breath, which began shortly after the onset of a low grade fever and rhinorrha. He is agitated and talking in short phrases only, with a respiratory rate of 40 per minute, heart rate of 130, and oxygen saturation in room air of 89%. Examination of the chest reveals moderate intercostal and subcostal retractions. On auscultation, you note reduced breath sounds throughout the lung fields with widespread expiratory wheeze. Other than a clear nasal discharge, the remainder of the physical examination is normal. You diagnose acute asthma and commence nebulized salbutamol (albuterol), and wonder whether the addition of ipratropium bromide would have a beneficial effect. Your staff physician asks whether you would consider using either intravenous salbutamol, theophylline, or magnesium sulfate ($MgSO_4$) if the boy fails to improve. His mother asks what can be done to prevent her son having further attacks but expresses concern re "steroid therapy causing growth stunting". The patient responds well to acute management, and is seen in your office approximately 2 weeks after discharge from hospital. He is now well, with a normal examination. Further history reveals that he has had four or five previous episodes of acute wheeze in the past 18 months. Each episode has followed an upper respiratory tract infection and the episodes seem to be getting progressively worse, both in duration and severity. Also in the past 2 months he has developed persistent night cough and often wakes with wheeze and shortness of breath through the night and in the early hours of the morning. He has been noted to wheeze as well when playing with his older sister. The boy's mother is now approximately 12 weeks pregnant and, although there have been no problems with the pregnancy, she wonders if there is anything she can do to keep the next baby from developing asthma.

Background

Asthma is the most common chronic condition and the most frequent cause of hospital admission in childhood. Determining a precise definition of asthma has been difficult particularly relating to disease in infancy. However, the definition suggested in the Third International Pediatric Consensus Statement on the Management of Asthma for Infancy is: "Recurrent wheezing and/or persistent coughing in a setting where asthma is likely and other rare conditions have been excluded."[1] For older children, the National Heart, Lung and Blood Institute definition, which describes asthma in terms of airway inflammation with prominence of eosinophils and mast cells, bronchial hyperresponsiveness, and reversible airflow limitation resulting in recurrent cough and wheeze, was accepted.[1]

There is objective evidence of increasing rates of asthma in children.[2] Because of the high worldwide burden of childhood asthma,[3] we have available to us a very large body of high-level evidence concerning many aspects of asthma treatment and prevention. Despite this good evidence, there remains considerable mismatching of asthma severity and asthma treatment. Consequently we have evidence of underdiagnosis and undertreatment of some children and overdiagnosis and overtreatment of others.

Framing answerable clinical questions

In order to address the issues of most relevance to your patient and to help in searching the literature for the evidence about these, you should structure your questions as suggested in Chapter 2.

Questions

1. In children with acute asthma (*population*), does oxygen saturation measured by pulse oximetry (*test*) predict the need for hospital admission (*outcome*)? **[Baseline Risk/Prognosis/Diagnostic Test]**

2. In children with acute asthma (*population*), does the addition of a nebulized anticholinergic agent (ipratropium bromide) (*intervention*) to nebulized beta-agonist decrease the risk of admission to hospital compared to treatment with beta-agonist therapy alone (*outcome*)? **[Therapy]**

3. In children with acute severe asthma (*population*), does i.v. salbutamol (*intervention*) in addition to nebulized salbutamol improve rate of recovery (*outcome*)? **[Therapy]**

4. In children with acute severe asthma (*population*), does i.v. magnesium sulfate ($MgSO_4$) (*intervention*) in addition to nebulized salbutamol improve the rate of recovery (*outcome*)? **[Therapy]**

5. In children with acute severe asthma requiring admission to hospital (*population*), does the addition of i.v. theophylline/aminophylline (*intervention*) to beta-agonist therapy improve the rate of clinical improvement (*outcome*)? **[Therapy]**

6. In children with persistent asthma (*population*), does treatment with inhaled corticosteroid (*intervention*) lead to growth impairment (*outcome*)? **[Harm/Therapy]**

7. In a child aged 3 years with asthma (*population*), is metered dose inhaler (MDI) with spacer (*intervention*) an effective means of delivery of inhaled medication (*outcome*)? **[Therapy]**

8. In children with persistent asthma (*population*), does the use of an oral leukotriene antagonist (*intervention*) lead to improved symptom control? (*outcome*) **[Therapy]**

9. In a child at risk of developing asthma (*population*), are primary and secondary prevention strategies (*intervention*) effective in reducing symptoms (*outcome*)? **[Therapy]**

Searching for evidence

You start by searching for evidence syntheses with the *Cochrane Library* and with MedLine (Ovid), looking specifically for meta-analyses. Both sources are rich in systematic reviews of numerous aspects of childhood asthma. When a systematic review is identified, you also search MedLine to identify randomized controlled trials (RCTs) published after the search date of the systematic review.

Searching for evidence syntheses: primary search strategy

- *Cochrane Library*: asthma AND (child OR children)
- MedLine (Ovid): asthma AND (systematic review OR meta-analysis OR meta-analysis) AND (child OR children)

Your search strategy for the *Cochrane Library* identifies systematic reviews addressing questions 2 to 9. Your MedLine search identifies a further two reviews relevant to questions 5 and 6.

For the questions where systematic review or meta-analyses are not available, search terms are outlined with the answer to each question in the following text.

Critical review of the evidence

Question

1. In children with acute asthma (*population*), does oxygen saturation measured by pulse oximetry (*test*) predict the need for hospital admission (*outcome*)? **[Baseline Risk/Prognosis/Diagnostic Test]**

Search strategy

- MedLine (Ovid); asthma AND (oximetry OR oxygen saturation OR SaO_2) AND (child OR children)

To evaluate a risk factor, you are looking for observational studies in which the clinicians who determine or measure the outcome (hospitalization) are not aware of, and will not be affected by, the patient's risk factor status (oxygen saturation). You find several studies that have examined the sensitivity/specificity of oxygen saturation measurement for poor outcome in children with acute asthma (Table 30.1), both at initial assessment and following commencement of therapy, and meet your criteria of independence of the observation from the outcome. In a study of 52 children aged 2–14 years, an initial oxygen saturation of 91% or less was predictive of unfavorable outcome, defined as admission to hospital or re-presentation following discharge from the ED. Of the 11 children with an initial saturation of 91% or less, 10 had an unfavorable outcome, while only one child of the 13 sent home with initial saturation greater then 91% had an unplanned return.[4] The same investigators found initial oxygen saturation (before bronchodilator) of children admitted to hospital was significantly lower than those discharged (SaO_2 admitted 93·0% $\pm$ 2·7 v discharged patients 95·0% $\pm$ 2·2; $P < 0.05$).[5] Five studies have defined oxygen saturation in terms of sensitivity and specificity or likelihood ratio for prediction of poor outcome and all but one clearly stated that clinicians were blinded to oxygen saturation when deciding on the need for admission (see Summary table).[6–10]

Of interest is the finding by Geelhoed *et al.* in 1994[9] that the initial oxygen saturation was predictive of poor outcome independently of other factors, such as duration of symptoms, previous admissions, and use of prophylactic medications. You want to avoid inappropriate discharge from hospital after initial assessment and management, but the low sensitivity of oxygen saturation for prediction of poor outcome means that it cannot be used alone in deciding the need for admission to hospital. Clearly, many children requiring admission would be inappropriately discharged if the decision were made on this measure alone. However, the high specificity means that having a low oxygen saturation is a strong predictor of the need for admission.

Table 30.1 Summary of trials examining oxygen saturation measurement in prediction of outcome

Author	SaO$_2$ pretreatment (%)	SaO$_2$ post treatment (%)	Sensitivity	Specificity	Likelihood ratio [positive test]
Mayefsky and El-Shinaway,1992[6]	< 93		35	92	4·4
Wright *et al.,* 1997[7]	< 91		24	86	1·7
		< 91	34	98	17
Bishop and Nolan, 1991[8]		< 91	42	78	1·9
Geelhoed *et al.,* 1994[9]	< 91				35 (95% CI 11–150)
Keahey *et al.,* 2002[10]	< 91		32	93	4·6

Question

2. In children with acute asthma (*population*), does the addition of a nebulized anticholinergic agent (ipratropium bromide) (*intervention*) to nebulized beta-agonist decrease the risk of admission to hospital compared to treatment with beta-agonist therapy alone (*outcome*)? **[Therapy]**

Additional search strategy

- MedLine (Ovid); asthma AND (ipratropium bromide OR anticholinergic) AND child OR children

You find a systematic review and meta-analysis of RCTs of children and adolescents treated with nebulized anticholinergics added to beta-agonists by Plotnick *et al.* in the *Cochrane Library*.[11] This review included 13 trials involving single or multiple anticholinergic dose protocols. The primary outcome measure for the systematic review was admission to hospital and secondary outcomes included change in respiratory function (determined by forced expiratory volume in 1 second [FEV$_1$], clinical score, oxygen saturation), number of additional bronchodilator treatments, and adverse effects. The addition of a single dose of anticholinergic to nebulized beta-agonist did not reduce hospital admission (odds ratio [OR] 0·93; 95% CI 0·65–1·32). However, in those children with more severe asthma (FEV$_1$, 55% predicted) who received *multiple* doses of anticholinergic, there was a reduction in hospital admission (OR 0·75; 95% CI 0·62–0·82). In terms of respiratory function, the improvement in percentage of predicted FEV$_1$ supported the use of anticholinergics (weighted mean difference 9·68; 95% CI 5·70–13·68). No significant increase in adverse effects was demonstrated.

This systematic review concludes that in children with severe acute asthma (FEV$_1$ 55% of predicted), the addition of multiple doses of inhaled anticholinergic to beta-agonist therapy improves lung function, reduces the risk of hospital admission by 25%, and reduces the need for additional bronchodilator therapy by 19%: 12 children with severe asthma would need to be treated with multiple doses of anticholinergic to avoid one hospital admission. Thus, multiple doses of anticholinergics in addition to inhaled beta-agonist are recommended in the initial management of children with severe acute asthma. There is, however, insufficient evidence for the use of additional anticholinergics in mild to moderate asthma.

Question

3. In children with acute severe asthma (*population*), does i.v. salbutamol (*intervention*) in addition to nebulized salbutamol improve rate of recovery (*outcome*)? **[Therapy]**

Additional search strategy

- MedLine (Ovid): asthma AND (beta-agonist OR salbutamol) AND intravenous AND child OR children

Your search identifies a systematic review in the *Cochrane Library* on the use of intravenous (i.v.) beta-agonists in the management of acute asthma in the emergency department.[12] This review includes 15 trials of which only three involved children. Overall, no benefit in terms of respiratory function or clinical score was found for using i.v. beta-agonists. (increase in PEFR at 60 minutes = 24·7 liters min^{-1} 95% CI 2·9–52·3). The authors state, however, that no conclusion can be drawn for use in children owing to insufficient numbers for subgroup analysis. It should also be noted that in 12 of the 15 trials (including two pediatric trials), participants in the experimental arm received only i.v. beta-agonist and no inhaled therapy. These protocols do not represent the recommended initial management of acute severe asthma in children, which includes nebulized beta-agonist such as salbutamol. The usual dose is 2·5–5 mg either every 20 minutes or continuously, depending on severity of symptoms and response to treatment. Intravenous salbutamol has been used in children failing to respond to nebulized therapy, usually in the intensive care setting.

The single pediatric trial identified in the systematic review comparing the effect of intravenous salbutamol to placebo, in addition to inhaled salbutamol, was published by Browne *et al.*[13] This double-blind RCT involved 29 children aged between 1 and 12 years with acute severe asthma (as defined by the National Asthma Campaign, Australia: the presence of one or more features of the following: altered consciousness, PEFR or $FEV_1 < 40\%$ of predicted value or oxygen saturation of $< 90\%$ at presentation[14]). Participants were randomized to receive either 15 micrograms kg^{-1} i.v. salbutamol or i.v. saline if they had failed to respond by 30 minutes following a first dose of nebulized salbutamol. All patients received i.v. hydrocortisone 5 mg kg^{-1}. Patients receiving i.v. salbutamol had a speedier recovery time, as determined by the following: time to cessation of nebulized salbutamol every 30 minutes (4 hours *v* 11·1 hours; $P = 0·03$); time to discharge from the emergency department (i.e., time to commencement of hourly nebulizations) was 9·7 hours less for the treatment group ($P = 0·02$); a lower clinical asthma severity score at 2 hours (severe or moderate overall severity score, 14/15 in control group *v* 5/14 in treatment group; $P = 0·002$). Control patients were also more likely to require oxygen at 2 hours (OR 5·7; 95% CI 1·06–30). There were no significant side effects reported.

Since the most recent update to the *Cochrane Library* review, Browne *et al.* have published a double-blind RCT comparing three treatment regimens: (a) bolus i.v. salbutamol; (b) nebulized ipratropium bromide, and (c) bolus i.v. salbutamol plus nebulized ipratropium bromide, in addition to standard treatment with inhaled salbutamol.[15] Again, children receiving i.v. salbutamol had a significantly more rapid improvement measured by time to requiring nebulized salbutamol less frequently than every 2 hours compared with those receiving inhalational therapy alone (mean difference 16·6 minutes; 95% CI 2·3–25·5) ($P = 0·008$). The addition of inhaled ipratropium bromide to i.v. salbutamol conferred no additional benefit. Significantly fewer children in the i.v. salbutamol groups required supplemental oxygen at 12 hours post-randomization ($P = 0·0003$). After adjusting for age, there remained a statistically significant reduction in time to discharge from hospital for those receiving i.v. salbutamol (mean difference 28 hours; 95% CI 9·4–46·7) In both studies the authors concluded that a single i.v. infusion of 15 micrograms kg^{-1} of salbutamol over 10 minutes resulted in a clinically relevant response and should be considered in the early management of acute severe asthma for those not responding to nebulized beta-agonists. Further studies in other settings are clearly required to fully determine clinical benefit or adverse effects.

Question

4. In children with acute severe asthma (*population*), does i.v. magnesium sulfate ($MgSO_4$) (*intervention*) in addition to nebulized salbutamol improve the rate of recovery (*outcome*)? **[Therapy]**

Additional search strategy

● MedLine (Ovid): asthma AND (magnesium sulfate OR magnesium sulphate OR $MgSO_4$) AND child OR children

Your first search in the *Cochrane Library* identifies a systematic review of the use of i.v. magnesium sulfate in acute asthma.[16] Of the seven RCTs included, only two were in the pediatric age group, giving a total of 78 patients. Both pediatric trials had similar inclusion criteria, i.e., patients who had failed to respond to initial therapy with nebulized bronchodilator, but differed in the age range of patients (1–12 years and 6–18 years), the dose of magnesium sulfate (100 mg kg^{-1} or 25 mg kg^{-1}) and the additional drug therapy used. (For example, all patients in one trial received i.v. aminophylline in addition to magnesium sulfate.[17])

Overall, when both adult and pediatric patients were considered together, there was no significant difference in rate of admission to hospital between the treatment and control groups (OR 0·31; 95% CI 0·09–1·02). Subgroup analysis of the pediatric trials showed a reduction in hospital admission with use of magnesium sulfate (OR 0·54; 95% CI 0·33–0·87). Those patients (both adult and pediatric) classified as having severe asthma, primarily defined by low PEFR measurements after initial bronchodilator therapy, had a substantial reduction in admission rates (OR 0·10; 95% CI 0·04–0·27). While the two pediatric RCTs were both of high quality, the pooled analysis demonstrated significant heterogeneity so that interpretation of the result must be treated with caution.

Three subsequent studies of the use of intravenous magnesium sulfate in the management of children with acute severe asthma are identified by your MedLine search. The first randomized controlled trial involved 20 children with moderate to severe asthma, clearly defined as PEFR < 60% predicted after three doses of nebulized salbutamol at 20 minute intervals.[18] The treatment group received magnesium sulfate at 40 mg kg^{-1} and the control group the same volume of i.v. normal saline. Thus the severity of asthma and dose of magnesium sulfate used are similar to the studies included in the meta-analysis in the *Cochrane Library*. There was a statistically significant reduction in both clinical score and percentage improvement in PEFR in the treatment group compared with placebo. The conclusion from this study was that children with severe asthma may benefit from magnesium sulfate in addition to beta-2 agonists, consistent with that of the systematic review in the *Cochrane Library*.

The second double-blind RCT involved 30 children with a mean age of 10·9 (+ 0·9) years with moderate to severe asthma (defined as PEFR < 70% of predicted value after three nebulized bronchodilator treatments).[19] The treatment dose of magnesium sulfate was 40 mg kg^{-1}. Patients in the treatment group had a significant improvement in PEFR and FEV at 110 minutes post infusion and were significantly more likely to be discharged home from the emergency department.

The third RCT of 54 children used a higher dose of magnesium sulfate (75 mg kg^{-1}) in the treatment group after a single dose of inhaled bronchodilator.[20] In contrast to the two previously discussed studies, children in this trial were classified as having moderate to severe asthma *prior* to receiving *any* bronchodilator treatment. At 120 minutes after entry to the trial no significant difference in Pulmonary Index score was found between treatment and placebo groups and there was no difference in admission rates between groups. The authors concluded that the addition of i.v. magnesium sulfate was not beneficial in the treatment of acute asthma in children.

The conclusions drawn from the systematic review and subsequent RCTs are that the evidence currently does not support the routine use of i.v. magnesium sulfate in all patients with acute asthma. However, magnesium sulfate may be beneficial in those children with severe exacerbations not responding to nebulized bronchodilators.

Question

5. In children with acute severe asthma requiring admission to hospital (*population*), does the addition of i.v. theophylline/aminophylline (*intervention*) to beta-agonist therapy improve the rate of clinical improvement (*outcome*)? **[Therapy]**

Additional search strategy

- MedLine (Ovid): asthma AND (aminophylline OR theophylline) AND child OR children

Theophylline has been used extensively for the treatment of both acute and chronic asthma of childhood, and is included in published guidelines for the management of acute asthma.[1] You find three meta-analyses addressing this question. A meta-analysis published in 1988 on the use of theophylline in severe asthma concluded that there was insufficient evidence to either "support or reject" its use.[21] However, the applicability of this meta-analysis to children

was limited as a single trial in children only was included. More recently (in 1996) a meta-analysis by Goodman *et al.* included six published trials with a total of 164 subjects aged from 18 months to 18 years.[22] The mean age of subjects in five of the six trials was between 7 and 12 years. Their search strategy was for the period 1966 to February 1995 on MedLine only, and was limited to English language publications. All subjects had acute asthma requiring hospitalization assessed either clinically or after failed ED treatment with subcutaneous adrenaline or nebulized salbutamol/albuterol. In the four most recently included randomized trials of i.v. theophylline (or aminophylline), severely ill subjects were excluded (those who failed to respond to three nebulized doses of salbutamol, patients requiring intensive care management, or those in whom respiratory failure was imminent). The outcome measures were varied, but included measures of lung function (FEV$_1$, FVC, PEFR), change in clinical score, number of doses of bronchodilator, and duration of hospital admission. This, together with the differences in treatment regimens, used made pooling of results for analysis difficult.

The meta-analysis found a significant increase in number of doses of bronchodilator required for the theophylline group (pooled effect size −0·18 SD units; 95% CI −0·3 to −0·1) and also longer hospital stay (pooled effect size −0·18; 95% CI −0·3 to −0·05). This equated to 0·31 days in hospital longer in the theophylline-treated group. There was greater improvement in measures of lung function (FEV or PEFR) in the theophylline group but this failed to reach significance (pooled effect size + 1·6 SD units; 95% CI −2·6 to + 5·9). The overall conclusion was that there is no significant benefit from the use of theophylline in children hospitalized with asthma. The authors also suggested that the slightly longer admission time and greater number of doses of nebulized bronchodilator required in the group receiving theophylline may actually represent weak detrimental effects of this therapy. You wonder about the generalizability of this review to your population because very few young children were included and children with severe or life-threatening asthma were excluded.

The third meta-analysis is published in the *Cochrane Library*.[23] This review includes four of the trials in the Goodman review and three additional trials published since 1996. In this review the authors found that at 6−8 hours there was a significant improvement in the theophylline-treated group in percentage predicted FEV$_1$ (weighted mean difference [WMD] 8·4%; 95% CI 0·82−15·92%) and a significant reduction in respiratory symptom score (WMD −0·71; 95% CI −0·82 to −0·60). However, intravenous aminophylline did not reduce the length of hospital admission and was associated with an increased risk of vomiting (RR 3·69; 95% CI 2·15−6·33). Even though children requiring intensive care admission were excluded from most of the included trials, the authors state that the included children met criteria for acute severe asthma. Their recommendations are that i.v. aminophylline should be considered in hospitalized children with acute severe asthma when there is suboptimal response to inhaled therapy.

A further two trials are identified by your MedLine search. The first randomized controlled trial included 43 children with moderate asthma, defined as failure to respond to three doses of nebulized beta-2-agonist.[24] With the use of outcome measures of clinical score and discharge rates, there was no significant benefit with the addition of i.v. aminophylline. This is consistent with other studies of children with mild to moderate asthma.

Ream *et al.* conducted the first RCT restricted to children admitted to the intensive care unit with status asthmaticus.[25] All 47 children received standard therapy of inhaled beta-agonist, anticholinergic and intravenous steroids, with the treatment group receiving additional intravenous theophylline on arrival in the Pediatric Intensive Care Unit. Outcome measures were time to recovery (i.e., time taken to achieve a clinical asthma score of ≤ 3, correlating with clinical state safe to be managed outside of an ICU) and duration of admission to ICU. Children not requiring mechanical ventilation who received theophylline had a significantly more rapid recovery in clinical asthma score ($18 \cdot 6 \pm 2 \cdot 7$ hours v $31 \cdot 1 \pm 4 \cdot 5$ hrs; $P < 0 \cdot 05$) but no difference in length of stay in the ICU. Vomiting occurred significantly more frequently in the treatment group, but interestingly, tremor occurred more frequently in the control group. In summary, the role of aminophylline in children with mild to moderate asthma is limited, particularly in view of the risk of adverse effects. However, there is some evidence that it still has a role in the management of children with very severe asthma in whom standard therapy has failed to produce clinical improvement, particularly those likely to go to intensive care units.

Question

6. In children with persistent asthma (*population*), does treatment with inhaled corticosteroid (*intervention*) lead to growth impairment (*outcome*)? **[Harm/Therapy]**

Additional search strategy

● MedLine (Ovid): asthma AND (steroid OR corticosteroid OR glucocorticoid OR budesonide OR beclomethasone OR fluticasone) AND child AND growth

Your search reveals a meta-analysis published in 1994 which included 810 children in 21 studies in whom the effects on linear growth of both oral and inhaled corticosteroids in the treatment of childhood asthma were measured.[26] The conclusion by the authors was that corticosteroids lead to a small tendency for treatment to be associated with lower final height. However, inhaled beclomethasone diproprionate was associated with a normal stature even when children with longer duration of therapy, high dose, and severe asthma were included.

While this meta-analysis had the strengths of a large number or patients and prolonged duration of treatment, some limitations have been described.[27] A systematic review in the *Cochrane Library* addresses the effects of an inhaled steroid (beclomethasone) on linear growth in children with asthma.[27] The review includes three studies involving children with mild to moderate asthma taking beclomethasone 200 micrograms twice daily. The conclusion was that beclomethasone at that dose resulted in a decrease in linear growth of $1 \cdot 54$ cm per year (95% CI $-1 \cdot 15$ to $-1 \cdot 94$).

The same authors have published a similar meta-analysis where the type of inhaled steroid was not confined to beclomethasone.[28] In this review, four trials involving treatment with beclomethasone were included and showed a decrease in linear growth velocity of $1 \cdot 51$ cm per year (95% CI $1 \cdot 15 – 1 \cdot 87$). Only one trial of children receiving fluticasone was identified and this showed a reduction in growth velocity of $0 \cdot 43$ cm per year (95% CI $0 \cdot 01 – 0 \cdot 85$). The maximum duration of follow up in both meta-analyses was 54 weeks, so the authors state that it is not possible to make any conclusion about the effect on growth beyond 1 year.

In your MedLine search you identify a number of additional reviews of the effect of inhaled steroids on growth in children with asthma. In assessing the effect of inhaled corticosteroids on growth, a key factor is the choice of the most appropriate outcome measure. Most studies determine short to medium term growth by way of height velocity (or growth rate) or by comparison with normal centiles or height standard deviation scores. These cohort studies have been summarized in a systematic review by Lipworth.[29] From the patient's perspective, it is the final adult height that is more relevant. A recent review identified by your search specifically summarizes the results of long term outcome studies.[30] Five studies were included in this summary and, although the results were not combined in a meta-analysis, all trials demonstrated that, despite exposure to inhaled corticosteroids, there was attainment of normal predicted adult height.

A further trial using different methodology in terms of height measurement also confirmed the finding of normal adult height.[31] The only prospective trial followed a cohort of 142 children with asthma.[32] The children received budesonide at mean daily dose of 412 micrograms. Final adult height was compared with 18 control patients with asthma who have never received inhaled corticosteroids and 51 healthy siblings of patients in the budesonide group. The mean length of follow up was $9 \cdot 2$ years The main result from this cohort study was that there was no significant difference in the mean differences between measured adult height and target height for children treated with budesonide or either of the control groups. There was, however, a significant reduction in mean growth rate of 1 cm during the *first* year of treatment with budesonide compared with the run-in period ($P < 0.001$). The mean growth rate in the run-in period was 6·1 cm (95% CI 5.7–6·5) and during the first year of treatment was 5.1 cm (95% CI 4·7–5.5). Other important results were that there was no significant association between sex, age at commencement of budesonide treatment, duration of treatment, or cumulative dose and the difference between final and target adult height. The results are limited by the lack of clear definition of how the severity of asthma was determined and how the severity of asthma itself may affect growth rate. While a lack of adequate power because of small numbers was acknowledged, the study does have the advantage of the long duration of follow up of children using inhaled steroids for many years.

Thus while we await the results of trials of the more recently introduced inhaled corticosteroids and long-term prospective follow up studies, some reassurance regarding final adult height can be gained from the data currently available.

Question

7. In a child aged 3 years with asthma *(population)*, is MDI with spacer *(intervention)* an effective means of delivery of inhaled medication *(outcome)*? **[Therapy]**

Additional search strategy

● MedLine (Ovid): asthma AND (spacer OR spacing device OR holding chamber OR metered dose inhaler) AND child OR children

In the *Cochrane Library* you find a systematic review addressing the efficacy of metered dose inhaler plus spacer device in delivery of inhaled bronchodilator medication in comparison with nebulized therapy in children with acute asthma ("Holding chamber versus nebulizers for beta-agonist treatment of acute asthma").[33] Only trials where the mean age of participants was > 2 years were included and patients already hospitalized or with very severe asthma were excluded. In total, 21 trials were included involving 880 children. The outcome measures included rate of admission to hospital, measures of lung function, duration of stay in the ED, and rate of adverse events. The reviewer's conclusion was that in children with acute asthma, no outcome measure was significantly worse with use of metered dose inhaler (MDI) and spacer compared to nebulizer. Indeed, the time spent in the ED was less and there were fewer side effects with the spacer. Thus, the MDI and spacer can successfully be used in children in the acute management of asthma and may have some advantages. This conclusion is supported by two further RCTs identified by your MedLine search.[34,35]

Although the evidence presented relates only to children with acute asthma symptoms receiving bronchodilator therapy, it should be applicable to children receiving inhaled prophylactic therapy.

Question

8. In children with persistent asthma *(population)*, does the use of an oral leukotriene antagonist *(intervention)* lead to improved symptom control? *(outcome)* **[Therapy]**

Additional search strategy.

● MedLine (Ovid): asthma AND ((leukotriene antagonist OR anti-leukotriene OR montelukast) AND (child OR children))

Your search identifies three systematic reviews involving the use of leukotriene antagonists for asthma. The first review in the *Cochrane Library* aims to examine the efficacy of daily oral leukotriene antagonists compared with inhaled corticosteroids in the management of persistent asthma.[36] This review included 14 RCTs with predominantly adult subjects. Specifically, only one trial was restricted to children and had equivocal results while another included some adolescents aged 12 years and over. The authors of the review explicitly state that the results of their review can only be generalized to symptomatic adults with mild to moderate asthma. A systematic review published by the same authors in March 2003 differs only by the exclusion of one adult trial following new information on methodology.[37]

The conclusion is unchanged for adult patients in that leukotriene antagonists were shown to be less effective than inhaled corticosteroids for asthma control. There is insufficient evidence based on these systematic reviews to make recommendations on the use of leukotriene receptor agonists instead of inhaled corticosteroids in children with asthma.

The third identified systematic review compared the addition of a leukotriene antagonist to inhaled corticosteroid at either the same or doubled dose of steroid.[38] Again, only one of 13 trials included children. Overall the review found that the small number of trials with short duration of therapy did not provide sufficient evidence to draw firm conclusions on the role of leukotriene antagonists in addition to inhaled corticosteroids in adults or children.

Question

9. In a child at risk of developing asthma *(population)*, are primary and secondary prevention strategies *(intervention)* effective in reducing symptoms *(outcome)*? **[Therapy]**

Additional search strategies

- MedLine (Ovid): asthma AND (smoking OR parental smoking) AND (child OR children) AND (systematic review OR meta–analysis)
- asthma AND (breastfeeding OR breast-feeding) AND prevention
- asthma AND primary prevention

Your initial search of the *Cochrane Library* identifies two systematic reviews to help answer the questions posed by the mother of your patient regarding prevention of asthma in her new baby. The role of maternal antigen avoidance *during lactation* for mothers with infants with a strong family history of atopic disease has been reviewed by Kramer.[39] Two hundred and nine women were included in RCTs and the outcome measured was the incidence of atopic eczema in the first 12–18 months of life, rather than that of asthma. The authors concluded that antigen avoidance might be protective against development of eczema, but that further better quality trials are needed.

The same author has also reviewed the role of maternal antigen avoidance *during pregnancy.* In this review RCTs including mothers whose unborn baby was felt to be at high risk of developing asthma showed that no significant protection was demonstrated with the dietary manipulation. In fact, of some concern was the possibility of adverse effects on fetal weight gain.[40]

Other factors to consider in the prevention of asthma include indoor allergens, parental or passive smoking, and breastfeeding. A meta-analysis of trials addressing the efficacy of house mite elimination methods for prevention of asthma in sensitized patients is published in the *Cochrane Library.*[41] The trials included here involved children and adults with confirmed sensitization to house dust mite, and the meta-analysis examines the efficacy of both chemical and physical methods of elimination. Overall when both elimination methods were combined, no significant improvement in asthma was found (RR 1·04; 95% CI 0·83–1·31). There was also no significant difference in asthma symptom scores, medication usage or peak flow in the morning. The conclusions of the authors were that "currently available evidence from controlled trials of chemical and physical approaches to reducing exposure to house dust mite antigens in the homes of mite-sensitive asthmatics does not provide a secure basis for advice and policy."

Your search in MedLine for a systematic review of the evidence relating to parental smoking and asthma identifies a series of systematic reviews of observational studies by Cook and Strachan examining the health effects of passive smoking. The effect of parental smoking on childhood respiratory symptoms and diseases including asthma is addressed in several of these reviews.[42,43] The pooled OR for either parent smoking and presence of "asthma" was 1·21 (95% CI 1·1–1·34), while for the presence of "wheeze" the OR was 1·24 (95% CI 1·17–1·31). When maternal smoking was considered alone, the pooled OR for wheezing illnesses up to age 6 years was 1·31 (95% CI 1·22–1·41). Although the pooled ORs are small, this result is of clinical significance because of the large number of children who may be exposed to this potentially avoidable known risk factor.

Your search in MedLine for breastfeeding and prevention identifies a systematic review and meta-analysis of breastfeeding and the risk of asthma.[44] The review includes 12 prospective trials examining the possible association between exclusive breastfeeding and development of asthma. While the majority of included trials individually found a protective effect some also reported an increased rate of asthma associated with breastfeeding. However, the summary OR for the protective effect of exclusive breastfeeding for 3 months was 0·70 (95%CI 0·60–0·81) and breastfeeding had a greater protective effect for children with a family history of atopy. (OR 0·51; 95%CI 0·35–0·79).

You also identify several other review articles including a review by Peat and Li.[44] This review presents results of meta-analyses. These include the systematic reviews on house dust mite elimination and smoking identified by your search, and in addition a meta-analysis of 10 observational studies examining the association between breastfeeding and protection from development of asthma. The included studies differed from those in the systematic review by Gdalevich *et al.*[45] but also found that breastfeeding to at least 3 months of age is protective against development of asthma with an OR of 0·80 (95% CI 0·66–0·97).

Finally, you identify from your search for articles on primary prevention a RCT of a combined dietary and environmental intervention.[46] In this study, 545 infants considered high risk for development of asthma, based on family history, were identified prenatally. The infants and their families were randomized to either the multifaceted intervention group or the control group. The intervention included avoidance of house dust mite, pet allergens, and cigarette smoke, and encouragement of breastfeeding (with supplementation with partially hydrolyzed formula as necessary). At 12 months of age there was a modest but statistically significant reduction in risk of possible or probable asthma in the intervention group. (RR 0·66; 90% CI 0·44–0·98) Further RCTs are required to evaluate the efficacy and feasibility of multiple intervention primary prevention strategies.

Resolution of the scenario

Your patient was admitted to hospital where he responded well to the acute management, which included oxygen, nebulized salbutamol with ipratropium bromide and oral corticosteroid.

His frequent interval symptoms of nocturnal cough, early morning wheeze and exercise-induced wheeze indicated the need for prophylaxis, and he was started on inhaled corticosteroid via a spacer device with face mask. After your discussion of the current evidence his mother decided not to alter her diet during the remainder of the pregnancy. Current research data regarding the best choice [between MgSO4, i.v. salbutamol i.v. theophylline] for children with acute asthma failing to respond to "full" therapy is insufficient to make dogmatic recommendation. The choice of therapy in this situation will depend upon the institution's (including ICU and ED resources, nursing staff, medical staff) experience with these individual agents – all of which are potentially harmful interventions. Close monitoring for adverse effects need to be in place for all these additional interventions.

Future research needs

Despite the substantial amount of evidence relating to many aspects of childhood asthma, there are some outstanding deficiencies. These include:

- the role of the leukotriene receptor antagonists in childhood asthma;.
- the specific risks and benefits of low dose inhaled corticosteroids versus non-steroidal agents (particularly sodium cromoglycate, nedocromil, and the leukotriene receptor antagonists) in children with moderately severe asthma;
- further randomized trials to determine whether allergen avoidance during pregnancy or following delivery of an "at risk" infant is of value in primary prevention of asthma;
- further high-quality studies on the role of allergen avoidance measures in reducing asthma symptoms in children with asthma.

Summary table

Question	Type of evidence	Result	Comment
Does oxygen saturation predict need for hospitalization?	5 cohort studies	Sensitivity 24–42% Specificity 78–98%	Low oxygen saturation is poor predictor; high saturation is good predictor of not needing hospitalization
Nebulized ipratropium bromide added to nebulized beta-agonist	Systematic review of RCTs Quality of included studies Mostly high, Jadad[47] score ≥ 4	Improved lung function; decrease in hospitalization	NNT = 13 for acute severe asthma
Salbutamol i.v. added to nebulized salbutamol	Systematic review of RCTs. (includes only 1 pediatric trial, Jadad score > 3) and 1 small RCT	Improvement in acute severe asthma	Only 2 pediatric trials, needs to be replicated
MgSO$_4$ i.v. added to nebulized salbutamol	Systematic review of RCTs. Quality of included studies: overall strong, most had adequate allocation concealment. 3 additional RCTs	Possible decrease in admissions to hospital in subgroup analysis of pediatric patients	Possible role in severe asthma where no response to maximal therapy with bronchodilators
Theophylline i.v. added to nebulized beta-agonist	3 systematic reviews of RCTs Quality of included studies: overall high, mean Jadad score 4·7, all adequate allocation concealment 2 additional RCTs	Meta-analysis showed some benefit in severe asthma but increased side effects	No role in mild to moderate asthma Possible role in very severe asthma with failed standard therapy
Do inhaled corticosteroids cause growth failure?	2 systematic reviews of RCTs Quality of included studies varied, adequate allocation concealment in 2 Systematic review of cohort studies and one prospective long-term follow up study	Meta-analysis shows slight decrease in growth velocity in short term; long-term studies suggest attainment of adult height in normal range	
Is MDI plus spacer as effective as nebulizer to deliver medicaton?	Systematic review of RCTs Quality of included studies widely varied, most had adequate allocation concealment 2 additional RCTs	Meta-analysis found no difference in measure of lung function, and less time in ED and fewer side effects with MDI plus spacer than with nebulizer	
Is leukotriene antagonist as effective as inhaled corticosteroid?	2 systematic reviews of RCTs, only 2 pediatric trials Quality of included studies high (Jadad score ≥ 4)	Meta-analysis shows in adult patients inhaled corticosteroids more effective than currently recommended doses of leukotriene antagonists	Insufficient evidence for recommendations in children
Primary and secondary prevention to reduce symptoms	Systematic reviews of RCTs Quality of included studies varied widely Passive smoking & breastfeeding studies are observational	Antigen avoidance during pregnancy showed no effect, during lactation showed modest decrease in eczema Review of dust mite elimination showed no effect Review of smoke avoidance showed modest effect Breastfeeding showed modest protective effect	

References

1 Warner JO, Naspitz CK, Cropp GJA. Third International Pediatric Consensus Statement on the management of childhood asthma. *Pediatr Pulmonol* 1998;**25**:1–17.

2 Peat JK, van den Berg RH, Green WF, Mellis CM, Leeder SR, Woolcock AJ. Changing prevalence of asthma in Australian school children. *BMJ* 1994;**308**:1591–6.

3 International Study of Asthma and Allergies in Childhood (ISAAC) Steering Committee. Worldwide variation in prevalence of symptoms of asthma, allergic rhinoconjunctivitis and atopic eczema. *Lancet* 1998;**351**:1225–32.

4 Geelhoed GC, Landau LI, Le Souef PN. Predictive value of oxygen saturation in emergency evaluation of asthmatic children. *BMJ* 1988;**297**:395–6.

5 Geelhoed GC, Landau LI, Le Souef PN. Oximetry and peak expiratory flow in assessment of acute childhood asthma. *J Pediatr* 1990;**117**:907–9.

6 Mayefsky JH, El-Shinaway Y. The usefulness of pulse oximetry in evaluating acutely ill asthmatics. *Ped Emerg Care* 1992;**8**:262–4.

7 Wright RO, Santucci KA, Jay GD, Steele DW. Evaluation of pre- and post-treatment pulse oximetry in acute childhood asthma. *Acad Emerg Med* 1997;**4**:114–17.

8 Bishop J, Nolan T. Pulse oximetry in acute asthma. *Arch Dis Child* 1991;**66**:724–5.

9 Geelhoed GC, Landau LI, Le Souef PN. Evaluation of SaO2 as a predictor of outcome in 280 children presenting with acute asthma. *Ann Emerg Med* 1994;**23**:1236–41.

10 Keahey L, Bulloch B, Becker AB, Pollack CV Jr., Clark S, Carmago CA Jr, Multicenter Asthma Research Collaboration (MARC) Investigators. Initial oxygen saturation as a predictor of admission in children presenting to the emergency department with acute asthma. *Ann Emerg Med* 2002;**40**:300–7.

11 Plotnick LH, Ducharme FM. Combined inhaled anticholinergics and beta-2-agonists for initial treatment of acute asthma in children. *Cochrane Library.* Issue 1. Oxford: Update Software, 2003.

12 Travers A, Jones AP, Kelly K, Barker SJ, Camargo CA Jr., Rowe BH. Intravenous beta2-agonists for acute asthma in the emergency department. *Cochrane Library,* Issue 4. Oxford: Update Software, 2002.

13 Browne GJ, Penna AS, Phung X, Soo M. Randomised trial of intravenous salbutamol in early management of acute severe asthma in children. *Lancet* 1997;**349**:301–5.

14 National Asthma Campaign. *Asthma management handbook.* Australia: NAC, 1998.

15 Browne GJ, Trieu L, Van Asperen P. Randomized, double-blind, placebo controlled trial of intravenous salbutamol and nebulized ipratropium bromide in early management of severe acute asthma in children presenting to an emergency department. *Critical Care Med* 2002;**30**:448–53.

16 Rowe BH, Bretzlaff JA, Bourdon C, Bota GW, Camargo CA Jr. Magnesium sulfate treatment for acute asthmatic exacerbations treated in the emergency department. *Cochrane Library.* Issue 1. Oxford: Update Software, 2003.

17 Devi PR, Kumar L, Singhi SC, Prasad R, Singh M. Intravenous magnesium sulfate in acute severe asthma not responding to conventional therapy. *Indian Pediatrics* 1997;**34**:389–97.

18 Gurkan F, Haspolat K, Bosnak M, Dikici B, Derman O, Ece A. Intravenous magnesium sulphate in the management of moderate to severe acute asthmatic children not responding to conventional therapy. *Eur J Emerg Med* 1999;**6**:201–5.

19 Ciarallo L, Brousseau D, Reinert S. Higher-dose intravenous magnesium therapy for children with moderate to severe acute asthma. *Arch Paediatr Adolesc Med* 2000 **154**:979–83.

20 Scarfone RJ, Loiselle JM, Joffe MD *et al.* A randomized trial of magnesium in the emergency department treatment of children with asthma. *Ann Emerg Med* 2000;**36**:572–8.

21 Littenberg B. Aminophylline treatment in severe acute asthma: a meta-analysis. *JAMA* 1988;**259**:1678–84.

22 Goodman DC, Littenburg B, O'Connor GT, Brooks JG. Theophylline in acute childhood asthma: a meta-analysis of its efficacy. *Pediatr Pulmonol* 1996;**21**:211–18.

23 Mitra A, Bassler D, Ducharme FM. Intravenous aminophylline for severe acute asthma in children over 2 years using inhaled bronchodilators. *Cochrane Library.* Issue 1. Oxford: Update Software, 2003.

24 Vieira SE, Lotufo JP, Eizenberg B, Okay Y. Efficacy of i.v. aminophylline as a supplemental therapy in moderate broncho-obstructive crisis in infants and preschool children. *Pulm Pharmacol Therapeut* 2000;**13**:189–94.

25 Ream RS, Loftis LL, Albers GM, Becker BA, Lynch RE, Mink RB. Efficacy of i.v. theophylline in children with severe status asthmaticus. *Chest* 2001;**119**:1480–88.

26 Allen DB, Mullen M, Mullen B. A meta-analysis of the effect of oral and inhaled corticosteroids on growth. *J Allergy Clin Immunol* 1994;**93**:967–75.

27 Sharek PJ, Bergman DA, Ducharme F. Beclomethasone for asthma in children. *Cochrane Library.* Issue 1. Oxford: Update Software, 2003.

28 Sharek PJ, Bergman DA. The effect of inhaled steroids on the linear growth of children with asthma: a meta-analysis. *Pediatrics* 2000;**106**:e8.

29 Lipworth BJ. Systemic adverse effects of inhaled corticosteroid therapy. A systematic review and meta-analysis. *Arch Intern Med* 1999;**159**:941–55.

30 Price J, Hindmarsh P, Hughes S, Efthimiou J. Evaluating the effects of asthma therapy on childhood growth: what can be learnt from the published literature? *Eur Respir J* 2002; **19**:1179–93.

31 Balfour-Lynn L. Growth and childhood asthma. *Arch Dis Child* 1986;**61**:1049–55.

32 Agertoft L, Pedersen S. Effect of long-term treatment with inhaled budesonide on adult height in children with asthma. *N Eng J Med* 2000;**343**:1064–8.

33 Cates CJ, Rowe BH, Bara A. Holding chambers versus nebulisers for beta agonist treatment of acute asthma. *Cochrane Library.* Issue 1. Oxford: Update Software, 2003.

34 Schuh S, Johnson DW, Stephens D, Callahan S, Winders P, Canny GJ. Comparison of albuterol delivered by a metered dose inhaler with spacer versus a nebulizer in children with mild acute asthma *J Pediatr* 1999;**135**:22–7.

35 Delgado A, Chou KJ, Johnson Silver E, Crain EF. Nebulizers vs MDI with spacers for bronchodilator therapy to treat wheezing in children aged 2 to 24 months in a pediatric emergency department. *Arch Pediatr Adolesc Med* 2003; **157**:76–80.

36 Ducharme FM, Hicks GC. Anti-leukotriene agents compared to inhaled corticosteroids in the management of recurrent and/or chronic asthma adults and children. *Cochrane Library.* Issue 1. Oxford: Update Software, 2003.

37 Ducharme FM. Inhaled glucocorticoids versus leukotriene receptor antagonists as single agent asthma treatment: systematic review of current evidence. *BMJ* 2003;**326**:621.

38 Ducharme F, Hicks G, Kakuma R. Addition of anti-leukotriene agents to inhaled corticosteroids for chronic asthma. *Cochrane Library.* Issue 1. Oxford: Update Software, 2002.

39 Kramer MS. Maternal antigen avoidance during lactation for preventing atopic disease in infants of women at high risk. *Cochrane Library.* Issue 2. Oxford: Update Software, 1999.

40 Kramer MS. Maternal antigen avoidance during pregnancy for preventing atopic disease in infants of women at high risk. *Cochrane Library.* Issue 2. Oxford: Update Software, 1999.

41 Hammarquist C, Burr ML, Gotzsche PC. House dust mite control measures for asthma. *Cochrane Library.* Issue 1. Oxford: Update Software, 2003.

42 Cook DG, Strachan DP. Parental smoking and prevalence of respiratory symptoms and asthma in school aged children. *Thorax* 1997;**52**:1081–94.

43 Strachan DP, Cook DG. Parental smoking and childhood asthma. Longitudinal and case control studies. *Thorax* 1998;**53**:204–12.

44 Peat JK, Li J. Reversing the trend. Reducing the prevalence of asthma. J *Allergy Clin Immunol* 1999;**103**:1–10.

45 Gdalevich M, Mimouni D, Mimouni M. Breast-feeding and the risk of bronchial asthma in childhood: a systematic review with meta-analysis of prospective studies. *J Pediatr* 2001;**139**:261–6.

46 Chan-Yeung M, Manfreda J, Dimich-Ward H, Ferguson A, Watson W, Becker A. A randomized controlled study on the effectiveness of a multi-faceted intervention program in the primary prevention of asthma in high-risk infants. *Arch Pediatr Adolesc Med* 2000;**154**:657–63.

47 Jadad AR, Moore RA, Carroll D *et al.* Assessing the quality of reports of randomized controlled trials: Is blinding necessary. *Controlled Clin Trials* 1995;**134**:1–12.

31 Croup

Julie C Brown, Terry P Klassen, Natasha M Wiebe

Case Scenario

A 2-year-old previously healthy, fully immunized boy with a 2-day history of runny nose, cough, and low-grade fever is brought to the emergency department (ED) in acute respiratory distress. On arrival, his vital signs are: respiratory rate (RR) 40, temperature 38·5, pulse 140, blood pressure 90/60, oxygen saturation 95% in room air, 100% in oxygen. He is sitting upright in his mother's lap with a slightly anxious appearance, stridulous, labored breathing, and his neck slightly extended. He has a croupy cough and is not drooling. You confirm diminished breath sounds, without crackles or wheezes. His extremities are pink and warm with brisk capillary refill. The remainder of his examination is non-contributory. As you evaluate this child, your triage nurse begins to administer cool mist approximately 6 inches from the patient's face. She asks you if you wish to treat with steroids and/or racemic epinephrine, and whether or not she should arrange admission. You leave the room considering these questions, and you wonder if you can assume that this patient has croup rather than epiglottitis or a foreign body, or whether confirmatory studies are warranted. Since the patient is in need of urgent medical care, you make a mental note of your unanswered diagnostic questions, and use your best judgement that the clinical presentation is consistent with croup. You decide to give your patient oral dexamethasone 0·6 mg kg^{-1} and nebulized racemic epinephrine. He improves with treatment, and 2 hours afterwards he remains comfortable, with an RR of 20 per minute, no retractions, good air entry bilaterally, and no other abnormalities on examination. You wonder at what point you can consider discharge without worrying about the possibility of subsequent deterioration, whether or not you should prescribe further treatment on discharge, and whether or not follow up care is indicated.

Background

Croup is an acute respiratory illness caused by inflammation and narrowing of the subglottic region of the larynx. It manifests variously as a barking cough, hoarseness, stridor, and respiratory distress, with or without concomitant symptoms of viral upper respiratory infection. The diagnosis of croup is often based on clinical presentation alone, although the symptoms and signs must be differentiated from those of epiglottitis, foreign body aspiration, and anatomical upper airway obstruction. Parainfluenza viruses account for most cases of viral croup, with types 1, 2, and 3 identified in three-quarters of all isolates.[1] Other etiologic agents include respiratory syncytial virus, influenza viruses A and B, and *Mycoplasma pneumoniae*. Treatment of croup has varied over the years, particularly with the development of new pharmacological therapies and increased evidence regarding their effectiveness. Pharmacological therapies generally aim to improve oxygenation, reduce airway narrowing, and/or reverse the inflammatory process. Croup is a common childhood illness, resulting in 30 primary care visits per 1000 children per year in the United States.[1] Fewer than 2% of cases are admitted to the hospital and only 0·5–1·5% of these require intubation. Mortality rates are < 0·5% even in intubated patients.[2] In the United States, emergency visits and hospitalizations resulting from parainfluenza virus types 1 and 2 alone result in annual costs of $US20 million and $US56 million respectively,[3] and about 25% of these visits are due to croup.

Traditionally, researchers emphasized differences between spasmodic (recurrent) croup and laryngotracheitis (viral croup). Some argued that spasmodic croup might be due to an allergic reaction to viral antigens rather than a direct result of a viral infection.[4] However, viral and spasmodic croup are poorly clinically differentiated, can both be associated with recent viral infections, and can have similar clinical presentations. The pathophysiology of the two entities is the same.[5] For these reasons, most authors currently consider these two entities as part of a continual spectrum of disease.[6]

Few clinical trials have differentiated between viral and spasmodic croup, so differences in treatment responsiveness by croup type are impossible to determine.

Framing answerable clinical questions

You consider the questions that arose during the child's emergency center visit, and frame them carefully to help you find the best quality information to answer them (see Chapter 2).

Question

1. In children with acute stridor (*population*), what is the specificity of clinical features (stridor, spontaneous cough, drooling, low grade fever, high grade fever, non-toxic appearance) (*tests*) for differentiating croup from epiglottitis (*outcome*)? **[Diagnosis]**
2. In children with acute stridor (*population*), does a lateral neck radiograph (*test*) increase diagnostic precision (*outcome*)? **[Diagnosis]**
3. In children with clinical features of croup (*population*), does a white blood cell (WBC) count (*test*) provide increased diagnostic precision (*outcome*)? **[Diagnosis]**
4. In children with croup (*population*), is steroid therapy (*intervention*) effective in reducing acute symptoms (*outcome*)? **[Therapy]**
5. In children with MILD croup (*population*) is corticosteroid therapy (*intervention*) effective in reducing acute symptoms (*outcome*)? **[Therapy]**
6. In children with croup (*population*), is single-dose oral dexamethasone 0·6 mg kg^{-1} as effective as intramuscular 0·6 mg kg^{-1} (*intervention*) in reducing acute symptoms (*outcome*)? **[Therapy]**
7. In children with croup (*population*), is single-dose oral dexamethasone 0·15 mg kg^{-1} as effective as 0·6 mg kg^{-1} (*intervention*) in reducing acute symptoms (*outcome*)? **[Therapy]**
8. In children with croup (*population*), is nebulized steroid therapy (*intervention*) as effective as intramuscular steroid therapy in reducing acute symptoms (*outcome*)? **[Therapy]**
9. In children with croup (*population*), is humidified air/oxygen therapy (*intervention*) effective in reducing acute symptoms (*outcome*)? **[Therapy]**
10. In children with croup (*population*), is nebulized racemic epinephrine therapy (*intervention*) effective in reducing acute symptoms (*outcome*)? **[Therapy]**
11. In children with croup (*population*), is a comparable dose of *l*-epinephrine (*intervention*) as effective in reducing acute symptoms (*outcome*) as racemic epinephrine? **[Therapy]**
12. In children with croup who improve following nebulized racemic epinephrine therapy (*population*), is observation for 2 hours (*intervention*) sufficient to demonstrate no "rebound" worsening of symptoms (*outcome*)? **[Prognosis]**

Searching for evidence

Searching for evidence on clinical examination

- Ovid MedLine 1966–2003:
  1. exp *croup/di
  2. exp *epiglottitis/di
  3. 1 or 2
  4. symptom.tw or symptoms.tw
  5. diagnosis, differential/
  6. 4 or 5
  7. 3 and 6
- Article references

Approaches to searching for the evidence to answer these clinical questions are outlined in Chapter 3. In this case, you begin your search by looking at three sources for reviews of the evidence. Using the keywords "croup", "laryngotracheitis", and "laryngotracheobronchitis", you search *ACP Journal Club* and the *Cochrane Library*. *ACP Journal Club* identifies one study and one systematic review evaluating glucocorticoids and croup.[7,8] The Cochrane Database of Systematic Reviews yields the recently updated, comprehensive systematic review on glucocorticoids and croup, which answers many of your clinical questions.[7] You also search *Clinical Evidence*[9] and find a chapter on croup in the eighth edition. You turn to this review before proceeding further, and find that it answers many additional clinical questions. For the remaining questions, you search the *Cochrane Library* Controlled Trials Register, and MedLine. If you wanted to explore this subject more extensively, you could extend your search by perusing the references from the articles you have retrieved and recent review articles. Finally, for a complete systematic review of the evidence, you could contact important researchers in the field.

The critical review that follows began with the sources listed above and continued with more exhaustive literature searching, appropriate for this systematic review.

Diagnosing croup

The first three questions you ask deal with diagnosing croup. Croup must be differentiated from other causes of stridor, including anatomical abnormalities, foreign bodies, and epiglottitis. Anatomical abnormalities often present early, and may have a chronic, progressive course. Children who have inhaled foreign bodies sometimes have a history of either observed aspiration or a choking episode. Symptoms typically begin acutely during the day, and may not include a croupy cough. Epiglottitis is typically a more serious illness and almost invariably requires antibiotics and assisted ventilation. Classically, the affected child is ill and presents with high

Table 31.1 Clinical tests for differentiating croup from epiglottitis in the patient with acute stridor

Symptom or sign	Sensitivity for croup	Specificity for croup	Likelihood ratio for croup	Likelihood ratio for epiglottitis
Spontaneous cough	0·86	1·0	Infinity	0·14
Drooling	0·10	0·33	0·045	2·7
Agitation	0·25	0·17	0·3	4·4

fever, a neck-extending posture, drooling, and stridor. However, severe croup can mimic epiglottitis, and early epiglottitis may mimic croup. Although it would be clinically useful to differentiate croup from all other causes of stridor, you limit yourself to the most clinically important, answerable questions below.

Question

1. In children with acute stridor (*population*), what is the specificity of clinical features (stridor, spontaneous cough, drooling, low grade fever, high grade fever, non-toxic appearance) (*tests*) for differentiating croup from epiglottitis (*outcome*)? **[Diagnosis]**

ACP Journal Club, the *Cochrane Library*, and *Clinical Evidence* do not help answer your questions on diagnosis. You perform two MedLine searches for the clinical exam: the single best search strategy, using sensitivity or specificity, which yields 15 hits, as well as a broader search strategy (shown), which yields 66 hits. You find one prospective cohort study of children presenting to an emergency department with stridor.[10] Patients were diagnosed with either croup (149 children) or epiglottitis (six children), based on clinical findings and confirmed by direct visualization of the epiglottis. The study evaluated the accuracy of three signs (cough, drooling, and agitation) in differentiating croup from epiglottitis in this setting, and found that a diagnosis of croup was more likely in the child with a spontaneous cough, no drooling and no agitation. Sensitivity, specificity, and likelihood ratios for these signs are shown in Table 31.1. The presence of a spontaneous cough was particularly predictive of croup and the absence of drooling and agitation also increased the probability of croup. These findings need to be interpreted with caution, because the small number of cases of epiglottitis increase the error around the estimates of sensitivity and specificity, and because *Haemophilus influenzae* (Hib) was more common when this study was performed. If the study were repeated in the post-Hib era, the even greater preponderance of croup compared with epiglottitis might mean that severe symptomatology is more likely an unusual presentation of croup rather than a classic presentation of epiglottitis. This would result in decreased usefulness of these symptoms and signs for differentiating croup from epiglottitis. Inquiry into the patient's vaccination status could help identify patients at greater risk for epiglottitis. It appears that no single test or clinical feature can adequately confirm the diagnosis of epiglottitis and, when it is strongly suspected, direct laryngoscopy in a controlled setting is warranted.

Question

2. In children with acute stridor (*population*), does a lateral neck radiograph (*test*) increase diagnostic precision (*outcome*)? **[Diagnosis]**

Searching for evidence on radiographs

- Ovid MedLine 1966–2003.

  1. (croup or laryngotracheitis).tw. or exp croup/
  2. epiglottitis.tw. or exp epiglottitis/
  3. 1 or 2
  4. radiograph.tw or radiographs.tw
  5. lateral neck.tw
  6. exp radiology/or exp radiography/
  7. 4 or 5 or 6
  8. 3 and 7

Your MedLine search returns 75 hits. There are no prospective studies evaluating the use of lateral neck radiographs for a population of children with stridor. You find three relevant retrospective studies. These three studies all consider preselected populations who may poorly represent the spectrum of disease being evaluated in either the outpatient or emergency department setting. The selection of patients is probably biased towards those with a less typical clinical course.

There are three retrospective case series evaluating the use of lateral neck radiographs for the diagnosis of croup,

Table 31.2 White blood cell count (WBC) as a test for croup, in patients admitted for croup or epiglottitis

Test	Sensitivity	Specificity	LR+	LR−
WBC < 12 as a test for croup	0·57	0·88	4·8	0·5
WBC > 12 as a test for epiglottitis	0·88	0·57	2·0	0·2

involving a total of 353 patients.[11–13] In two studies, lateral neck radiographs performed well at ruling out a diagnosis of epiglottitis, but in the third study, involving 44 patients, 23% (40/148) of the radiologists' reviews of patients with croup suggested a diagnosis of epiglottitis or "cannot rule out epiglottitis".[11,12]

These studies suggest a limited usefulness of lateral neck radiographs in diagnosing croup, and have variable conclusions regarding their use in diagnosing epiglottitis. Radiographs are usually contraindicated in the presence of suspected epiglottitis, as the stress of the procedure may worsen the clinical course. For the stable patient in whom epiglottitis is still a consideration, or if you are entertaining the possibility of foreign body or anatomical abnormalities, radiography may be useful.

Question

3. In children with clinical features of croup (*population*), does a WBC count (*test*) provide increased diagnostic precision (*outcome*)? **[Diagnosis]**

Searching for evidence on laboratory investigations

- Ovid MedLine 1966–2003

  1. (croup or laryngotracheitis).tw. or exp croup/
  2. epiglottitis.tw or exp epiglottitis/
  3. 1 or 2
  4. exp leukocyte count/
  5. 3 and 4

Laboratory investigations in croup have not been well studied. The above MedLine search yields no pertinent results. From your searches on the clinical exam, you find one retrospective case series of 169 patients admitted with croup and 25 patients admitted with epiglottitis. This study found that a a WBC > 12 000 mm^{-3} was 10 times more common in patients with epiglottitis than patients with croup.[13] If this group is treated as a single cohort, likelihood ratios can be determined based on WBC > or < 12 000. (Table 31.2). You question the usefulness of this test in your

patient population. There are no studies that consider bacterial tracheitis, which may be more common than epiglottitis now that most children are immunized against *H influenza* type b. Applying the positive likelihood ratio of 2·0 to a population with a very low probability of epiglottitis, the change in pretest to post-test probability of epiglottitis would be unlikely to influence management. In addition, since children are very likely to be distressed by venipuncture, this test would be contraindicated for any patient with significant respiratory distress, and thus would have limited usefulness in the circumstances where it might be the most diagnostically useful.

Managing croup

In order to assess the efficacy of treatment, you must first clearly define the measures by which outcome will be assessed. Thus, before we deal with questions of therapy, some methods of assessing outcomes of croup are outlined.

Croup scores allow an objective measure of croup severity, and are used for assessing effectiveness of therapy in clinical trials. Numerous croup scores have been devised, the most commonly used being the Westley and the modified Westley croup scores (Table 31.3).

The validation of croup scores has been considered in four studies[14–17] (see Chapter 10 for a discussion of validation methods). The Geelhoed score was assessed for interrater reliability.[13] In one study, triage nurse versus researcher assessments for 17 randomly selected patients were retrospectively compared; in the other, "worker" assessments for 15 patients were compared.[14,15] The weighted kappas were 0·85 and 0·87 respectively, indicating very good interobserver reliability. The Syracuse croup score was tested prospectively on 165 croup patients in an intensive therapy unit to assess how well scores below 6 predicted suitability of transfer from this unit to the general wards.[17] The authors found that this score had 80% sensitivity and 100% specificity for testing suitability for transfer. The Westley croup score was evaluated with respect to interrater reliability, construct validity (relationship to other means of assessment) and responsiveness to change. It performed well in all cases.[16] Klassen and Rowe evaluated the Westley croup score on 54 patients with croup, none of whom had cyanosis or changes in level of consciousness. Interrater reliability between three

Table 31.3 Croup scores

Name of score	Validated?	Total points	Stridor	Retractions	↓Air entry	Cyanosis	↓LOC	Cough	Dyspnea	↑HR	↑RR
Westley	Y	17	0–2	0–3	0–2	0, 4 or 5	0 or 5				
Modified Westley	N	17	0–4	0–3		0–4		0–3	0–3		
Taussig	N	13	0–2	0–3	0–3	0–3	0–2				
Kristjansson	N	15	0–3	0–3	0–3	0–3	0, 2 or 3				
Muhlendahl	N	18	0–3	0 or 2		0, 4 or 5	0, 4 or 5	0–1		0–1	0–1
Downes and Raphaely	N	10	0–2	0–2	0–2	0–2		0–2			
Geelhoed	Y	6	0–3	0–3							
Kuusela	N	4	0–2						0–2		
Syracuse	Y	11	0–2	0–1		0–2				0–3	0–3

Abbreviations: ↑, increased; ↓, decreased; LOC, level of consciousness; HR, heart rate; RR, respiratory rate.

research assistants was assessed prospectively. The weighted kappa was 0·90 for the total croup score, 0·47 for air entry, 0·93 for stridor, and 0·87 for retractions. Construct validity was assessed by correlating the change in croup score during the course of treatment with other measures, including a parental global assessment of change (correlation coefficient, $r = 0.51$), the treating physician's global assessment of change (0·51), the research assistant's global assessment of change (0·76), length of time spent in the ED (0·44), change in HR (0·19), and change in respiratory rate (0·32). Responsiveness to change was assessed by testing the sensitivity of the change in croup score to final patient disposition (mean [SD] change in croup score was 1·7 [1·7] in patients discharged and 0·3 [1·0] in patients admitted, $P = 0.006$).

Pulsus paradoxus (PP) has been evaluated as a potential objective marker of croup severity. In a prospective, blinded comparison of PP in children with croup versus healthy control subjects, PP was significantly higher in patients with croup than controls (6·1 ± 1·8 [SD] mmHg; [n = 29] in control subjects compared with a mean of 17·8 ± 11·2 [SD] mmHg [n = 28] in patients with croup [$P < 0.00001$]). The mean decrease in PP after racemic epinephrine was 7·5 ± 11·8 (SD) mmHg; ($P = 0.05$; n = 12) (controls were not treated). There was significant concordance between PP and the Westley croup score, both at baseline and following racemic epinephrine (Spearman's rho 0·68 and 0·73 respectively).[18] PP may prove to be a valuable outcome measure in clinical trials, as an adjunct to croup severity scores. Its value in the clinical management of croup is unclear.

Some studies considered HR, RR, and objective measures of oxygen and carbon dioxide levels. None of these measures has been validated as an accurate or sensitive outcome measure. Since deaths and severe complications are rare, these outcomes have not been helpful in comparing treatment modalities.

Question

4. In children with croup (*population*), is steroid therapy (*intervention*) effective in reducing acute symptoms (*outcome*)? **[Therapy]**

Searching for evidence on steroids

- *Clinical Evidence*
- *Cochrane Library*

The croup chapter in *Clinical Evidence* answers this question for two settings (primary care and hospital). Searching the *Cochrane Library* for "croup" yields four systematic reviews, including a Cochrane systematic review and a meta-analysis[8] by the same authors that examined the effectiveness of glucocorticoids in the treatment of croup. The Cochrane systematic review has been recently revised and updated, so you decide that this review will give you the most up-to-date answer to your question.[7]

This Cochrane review employed comprehensive search strategies, including searching MedLine, Embase, and the Cochrane Controlled Trials Register (established through the hand-searching of journals), and writing letters to experts in the field inquiring about additional trials. Two individuals independently selected trials according to predetermined criteria for inclusion in the review. The quality of the trials was assessed according to established criteria and publication bias was assessed. Data were extracted and checked for accuracy by a second individual and meta-analysis was used when appropriate. This review would be considered very high quality evidence (see Chapter 8).

Of the 31 trials included, 25 compared corticosteroids with placebo, some with more than two study arms: 17 assessed

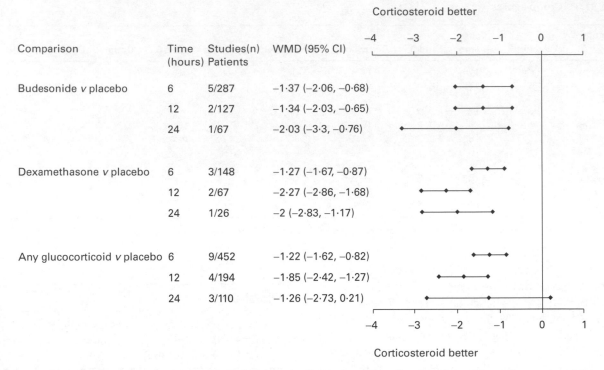

Figure 31.1 Meta-analysis of randomized controlled trials according to type of corticosteroids and time of assessment, for studies using the Westley croup score. The pooled effect sizes of corticosteroids versus placebo are given with the weighted mean difference. (Reprinted with permission.)

dexamethasone, seven assessed budesonide, three assessed prednisone or methylprednisolone, and one assessed fluticasone. The studies tended to be small, with a median of 73 (interquartile range 52–110) participants. Patients ranged in age from 4 months to 12 years. Fifteen trials involved inpatients and 10 trials involved outpatients. Overall, glucocorticoids were associated with a significant improvement in the croup score with an effect size of −0·6 (95% CI −0·8, −0·08) at 6 hours, and of −0·7 (−1·0, −0·3), at 12 hours. By 24 hours this improvement was no longer statistically significant (−0·6 [−1·1, 0]). These results varied according to which croup score was used. For this reason, the 12 studies that used the better validated Westley croup score were evaluated separately. In these studies, the improvement in the Westley croup score at 6 hours was −1·2 (−1·6 to −0·8), at 12 hours was −1·9 (−2·4 to −1·3) and at 24 hours was −1·3 (−2·7 to + 0·2). Detailed results by steroid type and time of assessment are shown in Figure 31.1. There was a 10% (95% CI 1–30%) decrease in the number of epinephrine treatments needed in children treated with glucocorticoids compared with those who did not receive glucocorticoids. Ten (95% CI 5–100) children would need to be treated with glucocorticoids to prevent one epinephrine treatment. In addition, the risk of return visits and/or readmissions were lower in corticosteroid treated patients compared with placebo, with an RR of 0·5 (95% CI 0·4–0·7). There was also

a significant decrease in the length of hospital stay in children receiving glucocorticoids both in the ED (one study), where stay was reduced by a weighted mean difference of −21 (95% CI −35 to −6) hours, and for inpatients (seven studies), where stay was reduced by a weighted mean difference of −10 (95% CI −17 to −3) hours.

The authors of the meta-analysis assessed publication bias by a number of graphical methods including funnel plots and a rank correlation test.[19] This analysis was based on studies that used the Westley croup score, as this score has been better validated, and there was evidence of differences between the Westley score and other croup scores. Contrary to the first edition of this review, the authors of the updated Cochrane review concluded that there was insufficient evidence of publication bias.

You wonder whether or not steroids would still provide benefit for patients with few symptoms at the time of evaluation in the ED.

Question

5. In children with MILD croup (*population*), is corticosteroid therapy (*intervention*) effective in reducing acute symptoms (*outcome*)? **[Therapy]**

The Cochrane systematic review includes one study that evaluated children who present to an ED with mild croup (Westley Croup Score ≤ 2). Eligible children were treated with oral dexamethasone, 0·6 mg kg⁻¹, with a single dose. The study sought to determine if dexamethasone treatment in these children:

1   reduces the rate of return to a healthcare provider for persistent croup symptoms within 7 days of treatment, and
2   reduces croup symptoms in the first 3 days following treatment as measured by the Telephone Out Patient (TOP) Score (a validated tool for assessing croup severity).

All patients were initially discharged home and their primary caretaker was contacted by telephone 1, 2, 3, 7, and 21 days later.

Of 720 children aged 3 months to 9 years with mild croup who were eligible and enrolled in four Canadian pediatric EDs, 26/352 (7·4%) and 53/352 (15·1%) of those treated with dexamethasone and placebo, respectively, returned to a healthcare provider because of persistent symptoms ($P = 0.002$; 95% CI for difference 3·0–12·3%). For every 13 (95% CI 8–33) children treated, one less child will return to a healthcare provider. Children treated with dexamethasone also had significantly lower TOP scores than those treated with placebo ($P = 0.001$).

You conclude that dexamethasone is an effective therapy even for children with mild croup. Treatment reduces croup symptoms and results in fewer return visits to a healthcare provider in the week following treatment.

You conclude that steroids effectively reduce symptoms of acute croup but you have three additional questions regarding their optimal dose and route of administration. Traditionally, dexamethasone was given by intramuscular injection at a dose of 0·6 mg kg⁻¹. This dose is equal to a typical daily dose of dexamethasone for the treatment of meningitis, which is usually given in four divided doses.[20] It has equivalent glucocorticoid activity to approximately 6 mg kg⁻¹ of prednisone,[21] and is arguably a larger dose than is needed for adequate treatment of croup. Recently, many practitioners have considered using lower doses of dexamethasone, and either oral or nebulized routes of administration. To address the efficacy of oral, nebulized and lower dose dexamethasone, you perform the following search.

Searching for evidence route and dosage of steroid administration

● *Clinical Evidence*
● *Cochrane Library* – Systematic Reviews

Question

6.   In children with croup (*population*), is single-dose oral dexamethasone 0·6 mg kg⁻¹ as effective as intramuscular 0·6 mg kg⁻¹ (*intervention*) in reducing acute symptoms (*outcome*)? **[Therapy]**

The croup chapter in *Clinical Evidence* does not address this question and you again turn to the *Cochrane Library*. systematic review.

Two studies have compared oral and intramuscular administration of dexamethasone in the ED setting.[22,23] The first study included all children between 3 months and 12 years of age with moderate croup symptoms and fewer than 48 hours of illness.[22] Moderate croup was defined as a clinical syndrome of hoarseness or barky cough combined with a history of or presence of stridor at rest, and/or retractions. Enrolled children were randomized to receive dexamethasone 0·6 mg kg⁻¹ by either the intramuscular or the oral route. There was allocation concealment at the time of randomization, although nurses and parents were subsequently aware of the medication route used. The physicians remained blinded, and parents were advised not to indicate how the medication was delivered. The primary outcome was the need for further therapy based on telephone follow up at 48–72 hours. Secondary outcomes were caretaker reports of improvement in or resolution of symptoms.

The researchers enrolled 277 children with a median age 2·1 ± 1·8 years. All patients received telephone follow up. Rates of unscheduled return visits in those who received an intramuscular injection (32%) and oral administration (25%) of dexamethasone were not statistically different: RR 0·78 (95% CI 0·54–1·14). Rates of treatment failure (need for additional steroids, racemic epinephrine, and/or hospitalization) were also similar between those who received intramuscular injection (8%) and oral (9%) administration. Caretakers reported resolution of symptoms in 56% and 48% of patients who received intramuscular and oral administration of dexamethasone, respectively. Symptoms were improved in 42% and 47% of patients who received intramuscular and oral administration of dexamethasone, respectively. Oral administration of dexamethasone appears to be as effective for the treatment of croup as intramuscular administration, and is easier and cheaper to administer.

A recent placebo-controlled, randomized trial included all children aged 3–84 months with a history of barky cough or stridor and a Westley croup score of ≥ 2.[23] Enrolled children were randomized to receive dexamethasone 0·6 mg kg⁻¹ by either the intramuscular or the oral route, and a placebo medication by the other route. Providers and families were unaware of the randomization unless the child vomited up the medication, at which time concealment was broken and children who received oral dexamethasone were then given intramuscular dexamethasone. Families were contacted at 24–48 hours and 10 days after the initial visit. The primary outcome was the proportion of patients with symptoms at 24 hours. Secondary outcomes were time to resolution of symptoms and return to the ED.

Ninety-six patients were enrolled, with complete follow up information on 95. At 24 hours, there were no statistical differences between groups in the proportion with stridor, expiratory sounds, barky cough, sleeping patterns or degree of improvement. By report at 10 days, there were no differences in the proportion with continued symptoms, need for additional evaluation and treatment, or duration of symptoms. None of the children discharged from the ED returned for treatment failure.

The authors of both studies concluded that the administration of oral dexamethasone appears to be as effective for the treatment of croup as intramuscular administration, and is easier and cheaper.

Question

7. In children with croup (*population*), is single-dose oral dexamethasone 0·15 mg kg^{-1} as effective as 0·6 mg kg^{-1} (*intervention*) in reducing acute symptoms (*outcome*)? **[Therapy]**

The croup chapter in *Clinical Evidence* identifies one inpatient study comparing dexamethasone doses in the treatment of croup.[15] The *Cochrane Library* systematic review of glucocorticoids for croup also identifies this study, as well as an additional outpatient study.[24] An Ovid MedLine search does not yield additional relevant results.

The two clinical trials[15,24] by Geelhoed suggest that lower doses of dexamethasone are effective in the treatment of croup. In his first randomized trial, Geelhoed[15] evaluated 120 children > 3 months of age admitted for croup, over two separate study periods. He compared dexamethasone 0·6 mg kg^{-1} with dexamethasone 0·3 mg kg^{-1} during the first study period and dexamethasone 0·3 mg kg^{-1} with dexamethasone 0·15 mg kg^{-1} during the second study period. In both study periods there were no differences and no trends towards differences in a six-point croup score at 1, 2, 3, 4 or 8 hours post-treatment, nor were there differences or trends towards differences in duration of hospitalization or need for racemic epinephrine.

Geelhoed also performed a randomized trial of 100 children > 3 months of age who were evaluated in an ED and treated as outpatients for croup with placebo or oral dexamethasone 0·15 mg kg^{-1};[24] 96 children completed follow up. None of the 48 children treated with dexamethasone and eight of the 48 children treated with placebo returned to care with continuing symptoms of croup ($P < 0·01$). Even if the two patients in the treatment group who were lost to follow up had both sought

further treatment, and the two in the placebo group had not, the relative risk of returning to care would be 4·0 times higher for the placebo-treated children compared with the dexamethasone-treated children, although this difference is no longer statistically significant (95% CI 0·89, 17·91). You note that these studies are relatively small and the inpatient studies are underpowered to detect clinically important differences. You conclude that the best evidence, although limited, suggests that lower doses of dexamethasone are as effective as higher doses in reducing acute symptoms of croup for patients with milder disease.

Question

8. In children with croup (*population*), is nebulized steroid therapy (*intervention*) as effective as systemic steroid therapy in reducing acute symptoms (*outcome*)? **[Therapy]**

The croup chapter in *Clinical Evidence* identifies three studies that compared oral or intramuscular dexamethasone with aerosolized budesonide.[14,25,26] The *Cochrane Library* identifies one additional non-English study.[27] The Cochrane Controlled Trials Register and Ovid MedLine searches do not yield any additional relevant studies.

Geelhoed and Macdonald evaluated 80 patients over 3 months of age admitted to the hospital with croup.[14] Patients were randomized to receive oral dexamethasone 0·6 mg kg^{-1} with nebulized saline placebo, nebulized budesonide 2 mg with oral placebo, or double placebo. The Geelhoed croup score was measured at 0, 1, 2, 3, 4, 8, 16, 20, and 24 hours from study entry. Duration of admission and duration of croup score > 1 and use of racemic epinephrine were also measured. Although corticosteroid-treated children had improved outcomes over placebo-treated children for all measured outcomes, there were no statistically significant differences in any outcomes for children between the oral dexamethasone and nebulized budesonide arms of the study.

Johnson et al.[26] randomized 144 children aged 3 months to 9 years and with a Westley croup score of 3–6 to receive intramuscular dexamethasone 0·6 mg kg^{-1}, nebulized budesonide 4 mg, or nebulized placebo. All patients received nebulized racemic epinephrine. Hospitalization rates were measured, as well as change in Westley croup score, and need for additional racemic epinephrine. Rates of hospitalization after treatment were highest in the placebo group (67%), intermediate in the budesonide group (35%), and lowest in the dexamethasone group (17%). Unadjusted rates of hospitalization were not significantly different between the dexamethasone and budesonide groups ($P = 0·18$).

Klassen et al.[25] evaluated 198 children aged 3 months to 5 years presenting to the ED with croup. Patients who had a croup score of ≥ 2 following 15 minutes of mist therapy were randomized to receive oral dexamethasone 0·6 mg kg⁻¹ with nebulized saline placebo, nebulized budesonide 2 mg with oral placebo, or both oral dexamethasone 0·6 mg kg⁻¹ and nebulized budesonide 2 mg. The Westley croup score was measured at baseline and hourly until the patient received racemic epinephrine, had a croup score < 2, had been discharged or had been observed for 4 hours, whichever occurred first. All three therapies were equally effective in reducing the croup score from baseline. The estimated treatment difference between dexamethasone and budesonide was −0·12 (95% CI, −0·53, 0·29). There was no statistical difference in median time to discharge from the ED (127·5 minutes in the dexamethasone group *v* 155 minutes in the budesonide group, *P* = 0·65). Cointervention with racemic epinephrine was evenly distributed amongst the three groups. Physician follow up for croup symptoms after discharge occurred in 27% of patients treated with dexamethasone, 60% of the patients treated with budesonide, and 38% of patients treated with both (*P* = 0·06). Only one patient, from the dexamethasone group, was subsequently hospitalized.

Vad Pedersen *et al.* evaluated 59 children hospitalized for croup, and randomized to receive either two inhalations of budesonide or 0·6 mg kg⁻¹ of intramuscular dexamethasone.[27] Improvements in a modified Westley croup score were similar between groups at 3 hours but favored dexamethasone at 6 and 12 hours (*P* = 0·001 and 0·004 respectively).

You conclude that the evidence suggests that aerosolized budesonide is a reasonable alternative to oral or intramuscular dexamethasone for the management of croup.

Question

9. In children with croup (*population*), is humidified air/oxygen therapy (*intervention*) effective in reducing acute symptoms (*outcome*)? **[Therapy]**

Searching for evidence on humidity

- *Clinical Evidence*
- *Cochrane Library* Controlled Trials Register – "croup," "laryngotracheitis" and "laryngotracheobronchitis"
- MedLine 1966–2003

  1. (croup or laryngotracheitis).tw. or exp CROUP/
  2. clinical trial.pt [best single search strategy]
  3. placebo.tw OR double.tw AND blind.tw [to maximize specificity]
  4. randomized controlled trial.pt [to maximize sensitivity]
  5. meta-analysis.tw
  6. 2 or 3 or 4 or 5
  7. 1 and 6
  8. mist.tw or humidified oxygen.tw or humidity.tw
  9. 1 and 8
  10. 7 or 9

Although humidified air/oxygen therapy receives widespread use, you wonder if evidence supports this treatment. Treatment with moist air probably stems from the late 19th century, when parents used steam from teakettles or hot tubs to treat croup in their children. Hospitals adopted the practice of "croup kettles"[6] long before clinical trials were routine.

The croup chapter in *Clinical Evidence* addresses this question. The authors found no systematic review, and identified one small RCT involving 16 patients, which they believed could not adequately answer the question.[28] Searching the *Cochrane Library* for a systematic review or controlled trial does not reveal any additional results. Searches of both the Cochrane Controlled Trial Register and MedLine identified one additional RCT, which provides the best evidence to address your question.[29]

This recent RCT involved 71 children aged 3–6 years with a Westley croup score of ≥ 2. The authors compared treatment with humidified oxygen via a "mist stick" with no treatment. The study was sufficiently powered to detect a difference in croup score of 1 between the two groups. The two groups were compared using the Westley croup score, pulse rate, respiratory rate, transcutaneous oxygen at 0, 0·5, 1, 1·5, and 2 hours. The groups were comparable at baseline, and both received 0·6 mg kg⁻¹ (maximum 10 mg) of dexamethasone at the onset of mist therapy. Racemic epinephrine and inhaled budesonide were given at the discretion of the treating physician. All patients improved over time. The study failed to demonstrate statistically significant associations between the method of treatment in croup score, oxygen saturation, heart rate, or respiratory rate. Global assessment of change scores by parents, treating physicians, and research assistants were not different between the two groups. There was no difference in lengths of stay in the ED. You conclude that the limited available evidence does not support the addition of humified oxygen to systemic corticosteroids in the treatment of croup.

The next search pertains to your three questions regarding the use of epinephrine.

Question

10. In children with croup (*population*), is nebulized racemic epinephrine therapy (*intervention*) effective in reducing acute symptoms (*outcome*)? **[Therapy]**

Searching for evidence on epinephrine

- *Clinical Evidence*
- Cochrane Database of Systematic Reviews.
- *Cochrane Library* Controlled Trials Register – "croup," "laryngotracheitis" and "laryngotracheobronchitis".

- MedLine 1966–2003.
  1. (croup or laryngotracheitis).tw. or exp croup/
  2. clinical trial.pt [best single search strategy]
  3. placebo.tw OR double.tw AND blind.tw [to maximize specificity]
  4. randomized controlled trial.pt [to maximize sensitivity]
  5. meta-analysis.tw
  6. 2 or 3 or 4 or 5
  7. 1 and 6
  8. exp epinephrine/
  9. 1 and 8
  10. 7 or 9

Clinical Evidence addresses this question, and identifies four randomized trials comparing either racemic epinephrine to placebo[30–32] or no treatment[33] for the management of croup. The *Cochrane Library* does not have any systematic reviews on this subject. By searching the Cochrane Controlled Trials Register you obtain 119 hits and find an additional three studies comparing inhaled racemic epinephrine versus placebo.[34–36] The above MedLine search yields 166 results (many of which were identified during previous searches) and identifies no additional relevant studies. It would be difficult to combine the seven relevant trials given that they all used different croup scores, measured effectiveness at different times, allowed different co-interventions and, in some cases,[33–35] offered repeated epinephrine treatments as needed for continued symptoms. However, all seven studies showed significant improvements in croup score in the treated patients versus the controls, at one or more measured times during the course of the trials. Your conclusions based on extensive searching are not different from what they would have been based on a review of *Clinical Evidence* alone.

Question

11. In children with croup (*population*), is a comparable dose of *l*-epinephrine (*intervention*) *as* effective in reducing acute symptoms (*outcome*) as racemic epinephrine? **[Therapy]**

The use of *l*-epinephrine has been proposed as a less expensive and more readily available treatment for croup. Many practitioners who do not routinely stock racemic epinephrine have *l*-epinephrine available as a resuscitation medication. One randomized controlled trial has compared *l*-epinephrine, 5 mg of a 1:1000 dilution in normal saline with racemic epinephrine 0·5 cc of 2·25% (5 mg) in normal saline.[37] All patients aged 6 months to 6 years presenting with croup were evaluated and those with a Downes and Raphaely croup score of ≥ 6 after 20–25 minutes of mist therapy were included. Patients with a croup score > 8 or oxygen saturation < 95% also received

intramuscular dexamethasone. Sixteen patients were treated with racemic epinephrine and 15 with *l*-epinephrine. Both groups had an initial improvement in croup score following treatment, but repeated measures ANOVA revealed no statistical differences in improvement between the two groups at 5, 15, 30, 60, 90, or 120 minutes following treatment. You conclude that *l*-epinephrine appears to be as efficacious as racemic epinephrine in the outpatient management of severe croup but that, with the small number of patients studied, clinically important differences between the two groups could have been missed.

Question

12. In children with croup who improve following nebulized racemic epinephrine therapy (*population*), is observation for 2 hours (*intervention*) sufficient to demonstrate no "rebound" worsening of symptoms (*outcome*)? **[Prognosis]**

Searching for evidence on prognosis following epinephrine

- Search strategies for epinephrine, as above
- MedLine 1966–1999
  1. exp croup/
  2. exp epinephrine/
  3. exp cohort-studies/ [best one-term strategy]
  4. incidence.tw or mortality or follow up studies/or mo.fs or prognos$.tw or predict$.tw or course.tw [to maximize sensitivity]
  5. prognosis.tw or survival analysis/ [to maximize specificity]
  6. 1 and 2
  7. 3 or 4 or 5
  8. 6 and 7

Your previous searches for epinephrine might answer this prognostic question, as the results of the treatment arm of a randomized trial may provide a cohort followed over time and observed for relapse, although patients who are enrolled in randomized trials are not always representative of the entire population. This search identifies one randomized trial of nebulized racemic epinephrine administration, in which 35% of patients who received racemic epinephrine had a relapse of symptoms within 2 hours of treatment.[36] No child was clinically worse 2 hours after treatment than before treatment. Glucocorticoids were not given during this trial.

A better search strategy for prognosis is outlined above. This search produced 12 hits, including two studies that address outcomes following epinephrine.

One prospective cohort study evaluated 174 children < 13 years of age treated in an ED for moderate or severe croup.[38] Patients met study criteria if they were discharged from the ED after receiving a single dose of racemic epinephrine and dexamethasone 0·6 mg kg^{-1} (maximum 10 mg). Among 82 eligible discharged patients, 11 required follow up within 48 hours of discharge, six for croup and five for either asthma or bronchiolitis. One patient was lost to follow up. Four patients required admission to hospital within 48 hours, two for croup and two for bronchiolitis. The authors used their own croup score, and did not comment on the initial or discharge croup scores for those patients who returned to care.

In an additional prospective cohort study of children aged 3 months to 6 years presenting to the ED with viral croup,[39] all eligible children received mist and intramuscular dexamethasone. Children with continued symptoms after half an hour received racemic epinephrine and were followed. Sixty children received racemic epinephrine, and 20 had continued symptoms and were admitted. All admitted patients who did not receive further racemic epinephrine treatments within 2 hours (16/20) had modified Westley croup scores ≥ 2 at 2 hours. Forty patients who received racemic epinephrine were discharged, 32 with a croup score of 0 or 1, and only one with a croup score of 3 (the remaining seven presumably had a croup score of 2). Thirty-eight patients were followed up. Two patients returned 32–36 hours following racemic epinephrine treatment with worsening symptoms of croup and were admitted. The croup scores of these two patients at discharge were not mentioned. The sensitivity and specificity of the croup score at 2 hours for predicting admission after observation for 4 hours could not be determined from the data provided.

Although these studies are not conclusive, you estimate that roughly 5% of patients discharged from the ED after receiving racemic epinephrine for symptomatic croup will return to care. Relapse within 24 hours is unlikely in patients with minimal symptoms (croup score 0–1) two hours after racemic epinephrine treatment.

Resolution of the scenario

The presence of a barky cough and the history of prior Hib immunization suggests croup rather than epiglottitis in this child. Further evaluation, with radiographs or laboratory tests, is not warranted. Available evidence supports your decision to treat this patient with steroids and epinephrine. You note that lower doses of dexamethasone appear to be as effective for outpatients with croup and that nebulized l-epinephrine is a reasonable alternative to racemic epinephrine. The limited available evidence suggests that, given the absence of respiratory distress and stridor after 2 hours of observation, your patient is unlikely to deteriorate. Although you were unable to directly evaluate the usefulness of further doses of steroids, you note that few patients return to care following single-dose therapy and, after ensuring that the family has good access to medical care if required, you discharge the patient home without medications. You advise the family to return to their usual provider as needed. In follow up, you learn that the patient did well, without further need for treatment.

Future research needs

Many of the above questions were answered based on limited evidence. In particular, studies have not clearly established the roles of humidified oxygen and lower doses of dexamethasone, or the optimal duration of observation following treatment with epinephrine. Further research is also needed to determine the following:

- a decision rule for the diagnosis of croup;
- the efficacy of multidose prednisone versus single-dose dexamethasone for acute croup;
- the efficacy and safety of repeated doses of dexamethasone after 24 or 48 hours, for patients with continued symptoms.

Summary table

Question	Type of evidence	Result	Comment
Clinical features for differentiating croup from epiglottitis	1 prospective cohort study	Spontaneous cough suggests croup; drooling and agitation usually absent	Small number of cases of epiglottitis
Lateral neck radiograph for differentiating croup from epiglottitis	3 retrospective studies: 1 cohort study and 2 case series	Not useful to rule croup in or out; variable conclusions for epiglottitis	Limited data; x ray for epiglottitis not recommended because of risk of airway compromise
Usefulness of WBC	1 retrospective study	LR~5 for WBC <12	Test not likely to be useful
Steroid therapy v placebo	1 meta-analysis of 25 clinical trials	Improvement in croup score, decreased need for epinephrine, decreased hospital stay	Results vary by croup score used
Steroid therapy v placebo, for mild croup	1RCT	Decreased return visits to healthcare provider, lower Telephone Out Patient (TOP) scores	Clinical severity score not directly assessed
Oral v intramuscular dexamethasone	1 RCT	Both routes are effective when evaluated against placebo, and are equally effective when directly compared	Oral dexamethasone is an easier and cheaper alternative to intramuscular dexamethasone
Oral dexamethasone: 0·15 mg kg^{-1} v 0·6 mg kg^{-1}	2 RCTs	No difference in outcome between groups	Larger studies needed
Nebulized v systemic steroids	4 RCTs	Both are effective, largest studies indicate equivalence	Results vary by study
Humidified air	1 RCT	No differences between treatment and control groups	Larger studies needed
Nebulized racemic epinephrine	7 RCTs	All studies showed significant benefit	Differences between studies precludes meta-analysis
L-epinephrine v racemic epinephrine	1 RCT	No difference between groups	Small study, may have missed a true effect
Prognosis for relapse 2 hours after racemic epinephrine	2 cohort studies	Relapse unlikely with low croup score after treatment	5% relapse rate overall. More detailed studies are needed

References

1 Denny FW, Murphy TF, Clyde WA, Jr, Collier AM, Henderson FW. Croup: an 11-year study in a pediatric practice. *Pediatrics* 1983;**71**:871–6.

2 McEniery J, Gillis J, Kilham H, Benjamin B. Review of intubation in severe laryngotracheobronchitis. *Pediatrics* 1991;**87**:847–53.

3 Henrickson KJ, Kuhn SM, Savatski LL. Epidemiology and cost of infection with human parainfluenza virus types 1 and 2 in young children. *Clin Infect Dis* 1994;**18**:770–9.

4 Couriel JM. Management of croup. *Arch Dis Child* 1988; **63**:1305–8.

5 Cherry JD. The treatment of croup: continued controversy due to failure of recognition of historic, ecologic, etiologic and clinical perspectives. *J Pediatr* 1979;**94**:352–4.

6 Skolnik N. Treatment of croup: a critical review. *Am J Dis Child* 1989;**143**:1045–9.

7 Ausejo M, Saenz A, Johnson D, Klassen T, Russell K, Weibe N. Glucocorticoids for croup. Issue 1. *Cochrane Library*. Oxford: Update Software, 1999.

8 Ausejo M, Saenz A, Pham B *et al.* The effectiveness of glucocorticoids in treating croup: meta-analysis. *BMJ* 1999; **319**:595–600.

9 Osmond, M. Croup. *Clin Evid* 2002;**8**:319–29.

10 Mauro RD, Poole SR, Lockhart CH. Differentiation of epiglottitis from laryngotracheitis in the child with stridor. *Am J Dis Child* 1988;**142**:679–82.

11 Walner DL, Ouanounou S, Donnelly LF, Cotton RT. Utility of radiographs in the evaluation of pediatric upper airway obstruction. *Ann Otol Rhinol Laryngol* 1999;**108**: 378–83.

12 Stankiewicz JA, Bowes AK. Croup and epiglottitis: a radiologic study. *Laryngoscope* 1985;**95**:1159–60.

13 Hodge KM, Ganzel TM. Diagnostic and therapeutic efficiency in croup and epiglottitis. *Laryngoscope* 1987;**97**:621–5.

14 Geelhoed G, Macdonald W. Oral and inhaled steroids in croup: a randomized, placebo-controlled trial. *Pediatr Pulmonol* 1995;**20**:355–61.

15 Geelhoed GC, Macdonald WB. Oral dexamethasone in the treatment of croup: 0·15 mg/kg versus 0·3 mg/kg versus 0·6 mg/kg. *Pediatr Pulmonol* 1995;**20**:362–8.

16 Klassen TP, Rowe PC. The Croup Score as an Evaluative Instrument in Clinical Trials. *Arch Pediatr Adolesc Med* 1995;**149**:60–61.

17 Jacobs S, Shortland G, Warner J, Dearden A, Gataure PS, Tarpey J. Validation of a croup score and its use in triaging children with croup. *Anaesthesia* 1994;**49**:903–6.

18 Steele DW, Santucci KA, Wright RO, Natarajan R, McQuillen KK, Jay GD. Pulsus paradoxus: an objective measure of severity in croup. *Am J Resp Crit Care Med* 1998;**157**:331–4.

19 Begg CB, Mazumdar M. Operating characteristics of a rank correlation test for publication bias. *Biometrics* 1994;**50**:1088–101.

20 McIntyre PB, Berkey CS, King SM *et al.* Dexamethasone as adjunctive therapy in bacterial meningitis. A meta-analysis of randomized clinical trials since 1988. *JAMA* 1997;**278**:925–31.

21 Threlkeld DS, ed. *Drug Facts and Comparisons. 51st edn.* 1997, St Louis: Facts and Comparisons.

22 Rittichier KK, Ledwith CA. Outpatient treatment of moderate croup with dexamethasone: intramuscular versus oral dosing. *Pediatrics* 2000;**106**:1344–8.

23 Donaldson D, Poleski D, Knipple E *et al.* Intramuscular versus oral dexamethasone for the treatment of moderate-to-severe croup: a randomized, double-blind trial. *Acad Emerg Med* 2003;**10**:16–21.

24 Geelhoed GC, Turner J, Macdonald WB. Efficacy of a small single dose of oral dexamethasone for outpatient croup: a double-blind placebo controlled clinical trial [see comments]. *BMJ* 1996;**313**:140–2.

25 Klassen TP, Craig WR, Moher D *et al.* Nebulized budesonide and oral dexamethasone for treatment of croup: a randomized controlled trial. *JAMA* 1998;**279**:1629–32.

26 Johnson DW, Jacobson S, Edney PC, Hadfield P, Mundy ME, Schuh S. A comparison of nebulized budesonide, intramuscular dexamethasone, and placebo for moderately severe croup [see comments]. *N Engl J Med* 1998;**339**:498–503.

27 Pedersen LV, Dahl M, Falk-Petersen H, Larsen S. [Inhaled budesonide versus intramuscular dexamethasone in the treatment of pseudo-croup.] *Ugeskrift for Laeger* 1998;**160(15)**:2253–6.

28 Bourchier D, Dawson KP, Fergusson DM. Humidification in viral croup: a controlled trial. *Aust Paediatr J* 1984;**20**:289–91.

29 Neto GM, Kentab O, Klassen TP, Osmond MH. A randomized controlled trial of mist in the acute treatment of moderate croup. *Acad Emerg Med* 2002;**9**:873–9.

30 Gardner HG, Powell KR, Roden VJ, Cherry JD. The evaluation of racemic epinephrine in the treatment of infectious croup. *Pediatrics* 1973;**52**:52–5.

31 Kristjansson S, Berg-Kelly K, Winso E. Inhalation of racemic adrenaline in the treatment of mild and moderately severe croup. Clinical symptom score and oxygen saturation measurements for evaluation of treatment effects. *Acta Paediatr* 1994;**83**:1156–60.

32 Westley C, Cotton E, Brooks J. Nebulized racemic epinephrine by IPPB for the treatment of croup. *Am J Dis Child* 1978;**132**:484–7.

33 Taussig LM, Castro O, Beaudry PH, Fox WW, Bureau M. Treatment of laryngotracheobronchitis (croup). Use of intermittent positive-pressure breathing and racemic epinephrine. *Am J Dis Child* 1975;**129**:790–3.

34 Martinez Fernandez A, Sanchez Gonzalez E, Rica Etxebarria I *et al.* Estudio randomizado doble ciego del tratamiento del crup en la infancia con adrenalina y/o dexametasona. *An Esp Pediatr* 1993;**38**:29–32.

35 Kuusela A, Vesikari T. A randomized, double-blind, placebo-controlled trial of dexamethasone and racemic epinephrine in the treatment of croup. *Acta Paediatr Scand* 1988;**77**:99–104.

36 Fogel JM, Berg IJ, Gerber MA, Sherter CB. Racemic epinephrine in the treatment of croup: nebulization alone versus nebulization with intermittent positive pressure breathing. *J Pediatr* 1982;**101**:1028–31.

37 Waisman Y, Klein B, Boenning D *et al.* Prospective randomized double-blind study comparing L-epinephrine and racemic epinephrine aerosols in the treatment of laryngotracheitis (croup). *Pediatrics* 1992;**89**:302–6.

38 Rizos JD, DiGravio BE, Sehl MJ, Tallon JM. The disposition of children with croup treated with racemic epinephrine and dexamethasone in the emergency department. *J Emerg Med* 1998;**16**:535–9.

39 Kunkel NC, Baker MD. Use of racemic epinephrine, dexamethasone, and mist in the outpatient management of croup. *Pediatr Emerg Care* 1996;**12**:156–9.

32 Bronchiolitis

Maud Meates-Dennis

Case scenario

A 4-month-old infant is seen in your emergency department (ED) with a 2-day history of fever and difficulty in breathing. On examination, he is tachypneic and has widespread wheeze and fine crackles on auscultation. He was born at 32 weeks gestation and had an uncomplicated neonatal course, requiring nasogastric feeding but no oxygen or ventilatory support. He has been well since discharge from the neonatal unit and is on no regular medications. The chest x ray shows evidence of hyperinflation (air-trapping) and some infiltrates in the lower lobes. A diagnosis of viral bronchiolitis is made. This baby's mother is keen to have him discharged after he has been treated in your assessment unit, as it is not convenient for her to stay in hospital with him and he is still breastfeeding. She is concerned, however, that he will now suffer from asthma as he grows up, and has requested more information on this. There is no family history of atopy.

Background

Viral bronchiolitis is a common worldwide disease of infants and young children. The underlying pathophysiology is inflammation of the small airways (bronchioles). This results in distal airway obstruction and air trapping, and may result in respiratory failure and occasionally death. Sixty to ninety percent of bronchiolitis is caused by respiratory syncitial virus (RSV) infection.[1] RSV infects nearly all infants in the first year of life with a peak incidence of hospitalized patients between 2 and 6 months of life.[1] One study showed that 12% of infants developing RSV bronchiolitis required hospital admission.[2] In the United States, it is estimated that there are 100 000 hospitalizations annually with RSV bronchiolitis with a cost of $300 milllion.[3] Mortality runs as high as 0·5% to 1·5% in hospitalized patients.[3]

Epidemics occur in the winter months. Infants with cardiorespiratory disease (congenital heart disease, bronchopulmonary dysplasia and cystic fibrosis) are especially prone to develop severe RSV bronchiolitis.

The clinical features include respiratory distress, wheezing and fine crackles on auscultation, and dehydration. The chest x ray typically shows hyperinflation. Diagnosis can be confirmed by finding evidence of RSV infection from nasopharyngeal aspirates. Therapy is largely supportive, paying attention to hydration and maintaining satisfactory oxygenation. Occasionally, ventilatory support is necessary. Other treatments, such as bronchodilators and steroids, have been used. Ribavirin is an antiviral agent that has been used

in RSV bronchiolitis, but it is expensive and not particularly convenient to administer (aerosolized and given continuously for several hours daily). RSV immune globulin has been used both prophylactically and as treatment in high risk groups. More recently, palivizumab (a monoclonal antibody preparation) has also been used as prophylaxis in high risk groups. Vaccines against RSV are currently being studied.

A significant number of patients subsequently have recurrent episodes of wheeze and may develop asthma later in life.[4] There is evidence that infants who develop RSV bronchiolitis have reduced lung function prior to becoming infected with RSV.[2]

Clinical scoring systems have been developed to assess the severity of bronchiolitis. One example of a clinical scoring system is the Respiratory Distress Assessment Instrument (RDAI) which has undergone validation and reliability measurements and has been shown to have good interobserver reliability (see Table 32.1).[5,6]

Framing answerable clinical questions

A number of questions arise from this scenario, such as whether you should treat with bronchodilators (and if so, which one), steroids, routine antibiotics, or ribavirin? Is there a place for RSV immune globulin or palivizumab in prophylaxis in high risk groups and would this infant have benefited given he was premature? Is there an association with asthma later in life and, if so, can this be prevented? Is there a test

Table 32.1   Respiratory Distress Assessment Instrument (RDAI). Ordinal scale from 0–17

Score	0	1	2	3	4
Wheezing:					
Expiratory	None	End expiratory	½ exp. phase	¾ of exp. phase	All of exp. phase
Inspiratory	None	Part inspiratory	all of insp. phase		
Location	None	≤ 2/4 lung fields	≥ 3/4 lung fields		
Retractions:					
Supraclavicular	None	Mild	Moderate	Marked	
Intercostal	None	Mild	Moderate	Marked	
Subcostal	None	Mild	Moderate	Marked	

(such as the Abbot TestPack), that will diagnose RSV more quickly than your current method (ELISA), which takes more than 12 hours for a result?

As they stand these questions are difficult to answer. Therefore, they each need to be broken down into their three component parts.

Questions

1. In infants with clinical features of bronchiolitis (*population*), does treatment with bronchodilators (*intervention*) compared with no bronchodilators, reduce symptoms or the need for hospital admission (*outcome*)? **[Therapy]**

2. In infants with clinical features of bronchiolitis (*population*), does treatment with glucocorticoids (*intervention*) compared with no glucocorticoids, reduce symptoms or the need for hospital admission (*outcome*)? **[Therapy]**

3. In infants with RSV bronchiolitis (*population*), does treatment with ribavirin (*intervention*) compared with no ribavirin, reduce mortality (*outcome*)? [*As Ribavirin is a very expensive treatment and may be harmful to healthcare workers involved with its administration, the outcome of interest is a reduction in death.*] **[Therapy]**

4. In high risk infants with RSV bronchiolitis, such as those with underlying cardiorespiratory disease or those who are ventilated (*population*), does treatment with ribavirin (*intervention*) compared with no ribavirin, reduce mortality (*outcome*)? **[Therapy]**

5. In infants with RSV bronchiolitis (*population*), does treatment with antibiotics (*intervention*) compared with no antibiotics, reduce bacterial complications or the need for readmission (*outcome*)? **[Therapy]**

6. In infants with clinical features of bronchiolitis (*population*), what is the sensitivity and specificity of the Abbot TestPack for RSV (*exposure*) compared with the ELISA test to correctly diagnose those babies with RSV bronchiolitis (*outcome*)? **[Diagnosis]**

7. In infants with no family history of atopy (*population*), does RSV bronchiolitis (*exposure*) compared with no RSV bronchiolitis, lead to wheeze/asthma later in life (*outcome*)? **[Prognosis]**

8. In infants with RSV bronchiolitis (*population*), does treatment with steroids (*intervention*) compared with no steroids reduce the risk of subsequent wheeze/asthma at ≥ 3 years (*outcome*)? **[Therapy]**

9. In infants with RSV bronchiolitis (*population*), does treatment with RSV immune globulin (*intervention*) compared with no RSV immune globulin reduce symptoms or length of stay (*outcome*)? **[Therapy]**

10. In high risk infants, such as premature infants or those with cardiorespiratory disease (*population*) does prophylactic treatment with RSV immune globulin or palivizumab (*intervention*) reduce serious illness or death due to RSV bronchiolitis (*outcome*)? [*You choose serious illness (i.e., needing intensive care or mechanical ventilation) or death, as these treatments are very expensive.*] **[Therapy]**

Searching for evidence

Your first stop is *Clinical Evidence* (2003, Issue 8). You are pleased to see a chapter on bronchiolitis, which answers many of your questions. Because you have time, you decide to continue your search. The next stop is the *Cochrane Library* where you search the term "bronchiolitis". The 2003/1 library shows you three complete reviews related to questions you have asked; "Bronchodilator therapy in bronchiolitis", "Ribavirin for RSV lower respiratory tract infections", and "Immunoglobulins for preventing respiratory syncitial virus infection". There are also three protocols of interest: "Immunoglobulin for treatment of RSV", "Epinephrine for bronchiolitis" and "Glucocorticoids for acute viral bronchiolitis in hospitalized infants and young children." These topics are currently being reviewed and will appear in the library once complete.

In the Database of Abstracts of Reviews of Effects (DARE) you find three items of interest: "Efficacy of bronchodilator therapy in bronchiolitis: a meta-analysis", "Efficacy of beta-2-agonists in bronchiolitis: a reappraisal and meta-analysis", and "Systemic corticosteroids in infant bronchiolitis: a meta-analysis."

The Cochrane Controlled Trials Register gives nearly 200 references, and you see that many of these will be helpful in answering your intervention questions.

Critical review of the evidence

Question

1. In infants with clinical features of bronchiolitis (*population*), does treatment with bronchodilators (*intervention*) compared with no bronchodilators, reduce symptoms or the need for hospital admission (*outcome*)? **[Therapy]**

The chapter in *Clinical Evidence* lists bronchodilators under unknown effectiveness. It states there may be short-term improvements in clinical scores but no reduction in admission. A study on epinephrine has shown a reduction in admission but this is awaiting confirmation. You decide to look at the literature yourself and examine the systematic reviews.

The Cochrane systematic review[7] is performed in a valid manner (there was a focused clinical question with clear criteria for inclusion; it is unlikely that important relevant studies were missed; validity of included studies was appraised; assessment of the studies was reproducible; results were similar from study to study) (see Chapter 8). Some of the papers included recurrent wheezers, which is not the group of infants that you are interested in. Looking at outpatient management, there are five included studies, four of which include only first time wheezers.

The outcome measures of the studies in which there was sufficient homogeneity to pool results included improved oximetry, reduction in hospital admission (the outcome you are interested in) and improvement in clinical symptoms. When the results of these studies are pooled, only improvement in clinical symptoms is statistically significant. The conclusion of the overview is that there is a modest short-term effect on bronchiolitis from bronchodilators, (including beta-2 agonists, such as salbutamol [albuterol]; anticholinergics, such as ipratropium bromide; and alpha-adrenergic and beta-adrenergic agents, such as epinephrine). The odds ratio (OR) for hospital admission is 0·7. This is < 1 and suggests there may be a benefit, but because the 95% CI (0·36–1·36) includes 1, it does not reach statistical significance. You note that the majority of the included studies where results have been pooled have used salbutamol as the bronchodilator.

You look at the other systematic review by Flores and Horwitz.[8] The authors felt unable to pool results because of the variability of outcome measures used in the studies, in which only beta-2 agonists were included. Their conclusion was that a well-designed multicentre randomized controlled trial examining clinically relevant outcomes is needed.

You believe that perhaps epinephrine, which has both alpha- and beta-adrenergic properties, may have an advantage over salbutamol and other beta-agonists. The alpha-adrenergic effect acts to reduce capillary and postcapillary leakage by constriction of the bronchiolar arterioles, thus reducing airway obstruction. You decide to look for further evidence. The Cochrane Controlled Trials Register (CENTRAL) has two references that might answer your question and you have previously looked at "A randomized trial comparing the efficacy of epinephrine with salbutamol in the treatment of acute bronchiolitis".[9] The study looks at the ED treatment of first time wheezing infants (aged 6 weeks to 1 year) with either nebulized salbutamol (1·5 mg) or nebulized epinephrine (3 mg) with the outcome of interest the rate of admission. The study was randomized (randomization was concealed) and double-blind with complete follow up. The two groups (20 infants in the epinephrine group and 21 infants in the salbutamol group) were similar at the start and were treated equally. The study was therefore valid (see Chapter 6).

The admission rate in the control group (salbutamol) was 81% and the admission rate in the epinephrine group was 33%. The absolute risk reduction in hospitalization with epinephrine compared with salbutamol is 48%. This gives a number needed to treat (NNT) to prevent one hospital admission when treated with epinephrine compared with salbutamol of 2. There were no side effects in the epinephrine group.

A recent audit in your department revealed that 50% of infants were admitted, even if they had received a bronchodilator. This gives your unit a baseline rate of admission of 0·5. The relative risk of admission in the study was 0·4. (0·33/0·81). Extrapolating these results to your unit, you could expect a 20% admission rate with the use of epinephrine, (0·4 × 0·5). Your absolute risk reduction for admissions with epinephrine would therefore be 0·3 (0·5–0·2), giving you an NNT of 4 (1/0·3 rounded up); i.e., four patients would need to be treated with epinephrine to prevent one admission to the hospital.

Luckily you notice that the systematic review on epinephrine[10] (previously found on searching as a Cochrane protocol) has just been published and you decide to look at it more closely. It includes studies that use a variety of outcome measures. The studies are generally not of high methodologic quality. The pooled result (OR) for reduction in admission for epinephrine used in the outpatient setting compared with salbutamol is 0·4 (0·12, 1·33), and compared with placebo is 0·51 (0·18, 1·42). Both results suggest benefit but as the 95%

CIs include 1, they are not statistically significant. The pooled results (weighted mean difference) for epinephrine in inpatients looking at length of stay compared with salbutamol and placebo are −3·96 (−25·55, 17·62) and −5·9 (−16·23, 4·43), respectively. The confidence intervals around these values are so wide it is impossible to know what the effect of epinephrine really is in these patients. The conclusion of the systematic review is that large multicenter trials are required to determine whether epinephrine has a place in the treatment of bronchiolitis. There does appear to be some evidence to support the use of epinephrine in the outpatient setting but insufficient to support its use in inpatients.

Question

2. In infants with clinical features of bronchiolitis (*population*), does treatment with glucocorticoids (*intervention*) compared with no glucocorticoids, reduce symptoms or the need for hospital admission (*outcome*)? [Therapy]

The chapter in *Clinical Evidence* lists corticosteroids as having unknown effectiveness. The authors state that the evidence presented in the systematic review by Garrison *et al.*[11] is difficult to interpret because some of the RCTs included children with recurrent wheezing or who may have had asthma. Some RCTs were not included in the meta-analysis and most of these did not find a benefit of corticosteroids. Benefits found in the systematic review were not thought to be clinically significant.

You find some references in CENTRAL, which look like good studies. In the study by Cade,[12] 161 infants admitted with RSV positive bronchiolitis were enrolled in double-blind RCT and given either nebulized budesonide or placebo twice daily until 2 weeks after discharge. The study was valid (see Chapter 6).

There were no short-term benefits in clinical score or time to discharge with nebulized budesonide, and similar results are seen in studies using oral prednisolone and dexamethasone.[6,13] However, another study by Schuh *et al.*[14] looking at oral dexamethasone given to moderately severe bronchiolitic patients in the outpatient setting did find a reduction in admission (measured 4 hours after administration). The study was a randomized (concealed randomization) double-blind study using an intention-to-treat analysis and was valid (see Chapter 6). There was a 25% reduction in admission rate using dexamethasone 1 mg kg^{-1} compared with placebo, giving an NNT of four. The authors feel that the early administration of dexamethasone in the outpatient setting may be important as most other studies have looked at inpatient treatment. However, the dose used was large and there was a large number of infants with a positive family history of atopy in the group. Further evidence is therefore awaited and you hope the upcoming Cochrane review[15] will provide a more definitive answer.

Question

3. In infants with RSV bronchiolitis (*population*), does treatment with ribavirin (*intervention*) compared with no ribavirin, reduce mortality (*outcome*)? [*As ribavirin is a very expensive treatment and may be harmful to healthcare workers involved with its administration, the outcome of interest is a reduction in death.*] [Therapy]

The chapter in *Clinical Evidence* lists ribavirin as having unknown effectiveness. You refer to the Cochrane review "Ribavirin for respiratory syncytial virus lower respiratory tract infection. A systematic overview".[16] This systematic review is performed in a valid manner (there was a focused clinical question with clear criteria for inclusion; it is unlikely that important relevant studies were missed; validity of included studies was appraised; assessment of the studies was reproducible; results were similar from study to study) (see Chapter 8). No significant reduction in mortality or reduction in length of stay was found. Mortality data were only available for three studies of high risk patients. A more recent RCT by Everard[17] found no difference either.

Question

4. In high risk infants with RSV bronchiolitis, such as those with underlying cardiorespiratory disease or those who are ventilated (*population*), does treatment with ribavirin (*intervention*) compared with no ribavirin, reduce mortality (*outcome*)? [Therapy]

Using the systematic review above, you decide to look more closely at the pooled results from the studies with mortality data.[16] They involve high risk patients who are ventilated. The pooled relative risk is 0·42 with a 95% CI of 0·16–1·34. As the CI includes 1, the result is not statistically significant. The three studies all show a relative risk of < 1 (suggesting benefit) but all have CIs (like the pooled result)that include 1. The conclusion of the systematic review is that a large randomized controlled trial of ribavirin in ventilated and other high risk patients is needed. The fact that there is not statistical significance in this group does not necessarily mean there is no clinical significance. However, the fact that the confidence intervals are so wide means that you just do not know whether ribavirin has any place in the treatment of high risk ventilated patients with RSV bronchiolitis. A recent RCT by Guerguerian *et al.*[18] also fails to show any benefit from ribavirin in ventilated patients. The chapter in

Clinical Evidence notes that a clinically important effect may have been missed. Further studies are required.

Question

5. In infants with RSV bronchiolitis (*population*), does treatment with antibiotics (*intervention*) compared with no antibiotics, reduce bacterial complications or the need for readmission (*outcome*)? **[Therapy]**

In CENTRAL, you find a study by Friis *et al.* [19] that looked at the routine administration of oral antibiotics to infants and children admitted with bronchiolitis. The study was randomized (randomization was concealed), and the two groups (oral antibiotics and no antibiotics) were similar at the start of the study (72 in the antibiotic arm and 64 in the control arm). The results were analyzed on an intention to treat basis and follow up was complete. The study was not blind, but outcome criteria were clearly defined and decided prior to commencement of the study, reducing any bias that may have been introduced because groups were aware of their treatment. You consider that, on balance, the study was valid (see Chapter 6).

The outcome measure of "pulmonary healthy by three days" was seen in 42·2% of the control group and 38·9% of the treatment group. There was clearly no difference between the two groups and the 95% CI around the difference included 0, so was not statistically significant. Looking just at patients who were RSV positive, there were 33·3% "pulmonary healthy" at 3 days in the control group and 32·4% "pulmonary healthy" at 3 days in the intervention group. Again, no difference can be seen. Other outcomes considered included the incidence of bacterial complications and readmission for respiratory illness. For each of these outcomes, there were two patients from each group, meaning no differences were seen. The routine administration of antibiotics to infants with RSV bronchiolitis does not appear to improve the clinical outcome nor do they reduce the incidence of bacterial complications or the need for readmission. As infants who were very ill and required intensive care were excluded from the study, you cannot generalize the evidence from this trial to them. It is likely that infants requiring intensive care would receive intravenous antibiotics. The chapter in *Clinical Evidence* states that the study may have been too small to exclude a clinically important effect.

Question

6. In infants with clinical features of bronchiolitis (*population*), what is the sensitivity and specificity of the Abbot TestPack for RSV (*exposure*) compared with the ELISA test to correctly diagnose those babies with RSV bronchiolitis (*outcome*)? **[Diagnosis]**

Search strategy

For this question about diagnosis, you use the following search strategy on the Ovid interface for MedLine:

1. explode "Respiratory-Syncitial-Viruses"/all subheadings
2. explode "Sensitivity-and-Specificity"/all subheadings
3. 1 and 2
4. Abbott.tw
5. 3 and 4

Results: seven records

Of the seven articles, you choose to look more closely at the study by Krilov *et al.*[20] The gold standard for isolation of RSV was direct fluorescent assay (DFA) and the rapid test was compared with this. The study involved an appropriate spectrum of patients (infants and young children admitted with acute respiratory disease), and compared the rapid test with the DFA in an independent and blind manner, all patients having the DFA as well as the rapid test. Therefore the study was valid (see Chapter 5).

In the laboratory, the rapid test had a sensitivity of 97% (this is very high and will "rule out the disease" if the test is negative; a test with a high sensitivity that is negative rules out the disease: SnNOut), and a specificity of 99% (this is also very high and will "rule in the disease if the test is positive"; a test with a high specificity that is positive rules in the disease: SpPIn). The sensitivity and specificity can be converted to likelihood ratios (see Chapter 5).

The likelihood ratio for a positive test is 97% ÷ 1% = 97. This very high likelihood ratio results in a major increase from pre- to post-test probability of RSV. The likelihood ratio for a negative test is 3% ÷ 99% = 0·03. This result will lead to a vast reduction from pre- to post-test probability of RSV.

This test is useful in a number of ways. Quick diagnosis will enable more accurate information to be given to the parents regarding outcome and you will be able to use isolation facilities more efficiently because you will know within 20–30 minutes which patients are RSV positive and can isolate them accordingly. Similar results for sensitivity and specificity have been found for the Abbott TestPack in other studies (Obel *et al.*[21] and Mackie *et al.*[22] found sensitivities of 98% and 90% with specificities of 95% and 92%, respectively).

Question

7. In infants with no family history of atopy (*population*), does RSV bronchiolitis (*exposure*) compared with no RSV bronchiolitis, lead to wheeze/asthma later in life (*outcome*)? **[Prognosis]**

Search strategy

For a question relating to prognosis, you use the Ovid interface for MedLine and the search strategy:

1. explode "Bronchiolitis"/all subheadings
2. in TI, AB, MESH
3. 1 and 2
4. explode "asthma"/all subheadings
5. 3 and 4

Results: 35 records

Your search reveals a quantitative review by Kneyber *et al.*,[23] which you decide to look at. The review includes data from cohort studies. All studies included infants < 12 months of age hospitalized with virologically confirmed RSV infection compared with controls at follow up. Recurrent wheezing was defined as three or more wheezing episodes. This is a valid study (see Chapter 8).

At 5 years after RSV bronchiolitis, 40% of children had wheezing compared with 11% of controls. This was a significant result. By 10 years, however, the results were not significant with 22% of RSV children still wheezing compared with 10% of controls. You choose to examine some of the original studies. The study by Sigurs *et al.*[24] is a prospective cohort study, the index cases being infants admitted with a diagnosis of RSV bronchiolitis. Each case is matched with two controls from the local health clinic (matched for date of birth, sex, and residence) and then followed up until 3 years of age. The outcome measure of asthma was defined as "doctor-diagnosed bronchial obstruction on at least three occasions", which is objective. Adjustment was made for smoking and family history of atopy. The study was therefore valid (see Chapter 4). In this study, there were 47 cases and 93 controls (one infant had only one control). The relative risk of asthma in patients with bronchiolitis and no family history of atopy compared with patients without bronchiolitis and no family history of atopy was 9·9 with a 95% CI of 1·2–81·27. As the CI does not include 1, this result is statistically significant. Interestingly, some of the control cases had experienced RSV infection, which had not been severe enough for them to attend hospital. It would not be appropriate, therefore, to generalize these data to infants with mild disease who do not require any hospital treatment. The relative risk of asthma in patients with bronchiolitis and a family history of atopy compared with patients without bronchiolitis and no family history of atopy was 38·7 with a 95% CI of 5·14–291·6. Again this result is statistically significant. The 95% CIs are wide and so you cannot be precise about the magnitude of the relative risk. You look at the absolute risk for asthma (as defined above) and find the baseline risk is 1% (in those without bronchiolitis). This is not clinically insignificant so any increase following bronchiolitis is likely to be clinically important.

Another study by Noble *et al.*[25] that followed cases of RSV bronchiolitis for 9–10 years also found an excess of respiratory symptoms in those patients who had RSV bronchiolitis compared with matched controls. The differences were not due to a family history of atopy. In this study, the index cases (RSV bronchiolitis patients) were followed up from their initial admission. At age 5·5 years, controls were recruited for the remainder of the study. There was only 56% follow up in the control group compared with 84% in the bronchiolitis group. These factors may affect the validity, but the results are similar to the Sigurs study.[27]

A study by McConnochie *et al.*[26] followed up 51 infants who had suffered mild bronchiolitis with 102 matched controls, evaluating them at 8 and 13 years. Bronchiolitis was a predictor of wheeze at 8 years, but not such a strong predictor of wheeze at 13 years. There was an increased risk of wheezing if there was a family history of atopy or exposure to passive wheezing.

The individual studies and the review all suggest that the wheezing tendency seen post-bronchiolitis will disappear as the child gets older if there is no family history of atopy. The importance of passive smoking as a risk factor is seen in the studies.

Question

8. In infants with RSV bronchiolitis (*population*), does treatment with steroids (*intervention*) compared with no steroids reduce the risk of subsequent wheeze/asthma at age ≥ 3 years (*outcome*)? **[Therapy]**

The chapter in *Clinical Evidence* has a table[27] that summarizes the evidence for steroids versus placebo in bronchiolitis for both short- and long-term outcomes. Most studies show no benefit. From CENTRAL you find a number of references relating to studies on this subject. Looking at the abstracts, it appears there are conflicting results. You choose to look at steroids given within double-blinded RCTs, which will mean studies least likely to have bias introduced. You also decide to avoid studies where infants with recurrent wheeze are included, (as these infants are likely to respond to steroids) (see Chapter 6).

The study by Bulow *et al.*[13] is a double-blind RCT in 147 patients with RSV infection who were randomized to either oral prednisolone or placebo for 5 days. They were reviewed at 1 year and there were no differences in morbidity or use of medicines. The study by Cade *et al.*[12] looked at 161 infants admitted with RSV positive bronchiolitis who were given nebulized budesonide or placebo twice daily for 2 weeks. There were no differences in respiratory readmission, use of medication, or general practitioner attendances at 12 months. A study by von Woensel *et al.*[28] compared 7 days oral prednisolone with placebo in infants admitted with bronchiolitis. At 5 years follow up, there was no difference in incidence of transient wheezing, persistent wheezing, or late-onset wheezing.

Despite the increased incidence of wheeze post-bronchiolitis and the apparent conflicting evidence about the use of steroids to reduce this, when you look at those studies least likely to introduce bias and those restricted to infants with bronchiolitis (and not recurrent wheeze), there appears to be no benefit in long-term wheeze from steroids given during the acute infection.

Question

9. In infants with RSV bronchiolitis (*population*), does treatment with RSV immune globulin (*intervention*) compared with no RSV immune globulin reduce symptoms or length of stay (*outcome*)? **[Therapy]**

From CENTRAL, you find three studies. The first by Rimensberger *et al.*[29] looks at high risk infants with RSV bronchiolitis who are randomized to receive either aerosolized immune globulin or placebo. The study included 68 infants and follow up was complete. There were no statistically significant differences between the groups in symptom reduction, oxygen requirement, or length of stay. The second study by Rodriguez *et al.*[30] was a randomized double-blind trial involving 102 infants hospitalized for RSV bronchiolitis and considered high risk. They were given either intravenous RSV immune globulin or intravenous albumin. There were no significant differences between the two groups in symptom scores or hospital stay. The RSV Ig group had higher respiratory scores on entry to the study. This may have made it more difficult to show a difference if there was one, and demonstrates that randomization is not perfect at ensuring the two groups are similar at the start of the study (but it is the best method we have).

Another study by Rodriguez *et al.*[31] looked at 98 well infants with RSV bronchiolitis randomized to receive either intravenous RSV immune globulin or intravenous albumin. Again there were no significant differences between the two groups in symptom scores or hospital stay. Subgroup analysis suggested that infants who required intensive care had a modest benefit from RSV immune globulin, having shorter length of stay and need for intensive care. Both of Rodriguez' studies[30,31] demonstrated the safety of RSV immune globulin administration in these infants.

You think a systematic review may be helpful. You remember that the *Cochrane Library* contained a protocol, "Immunoglobulin for treatment of respiratory syncitial virus".[32] As there is no evidence as yet that RSV immune globulin is effective treatment for infants with RSV bronchiolitis, you keenly await the completed systematic review from the *Cochrane Library*.

Question

10. In high risk infants, such as premature infants or those with cardiorespiratory disease (*population*), does prophylactic treatment with RSV immune globulin or palivizumab (*intervention*) reduce serious illness or death due to RSV bronchiolitis (*outcome*)? [*You choose serious illness (i.e., needing intensive care or mechanical ventilation) or death, as these treatments are very expensive.*] **[Therapy]**

The chapter in *Clinical Evidence* categorizes RSV immunoglobulin and palivizumab (monoclonal antibody) for prevention of bronchiolitis as beneficial. It quotes the Cochrane systematic review by Wang and Tang.[33]

The review included four studies with a total of 2598 subjects. The conclusion was that RSV immunoglobulins (including the monoclonal antibody palivizumab) are effective in preventing RSV hospitalizations and admission to intensive care units, but not in preventing mechanical ventilation. There was a non-significant trend towards a higher mortality in infants given RSV immunoglobulin.

Premature infants included in the RCTs were children < 6 months old with gestational age at birth of < 32 or 35 weeks old. Children with bronchopulmonary dysplasia were < 2 years and still requiring treatment. Subgroup analysis, which had been planned, showed that prophylaxis significantly reduced hospital admission in those with prematurity alone (OR 0·27; 95% CI 0·15, 0·49), and in those with bronchopulmonary dysplasia alone (OR 0·54; 95% CI 0·37, 0·80), but not in those with congenital heart abnormalities alone (OR 0·64; 95% CI 0·37, 1·1).

Looking at the results of the randomized-controlled trial of palivizumab,[34] you see that premature infants with chronic lung disease have a hospitalization rate of 12·8% with placebo compared with 7·9% for those receiving palivizumab. This means that there is 4·9% absolute risk reduction, so for every 20 premature infants with chronic lung disease you treat prophylactically with palivizumab, you will prevent one hospital admission. When subgroups of infants are looked at, the number needed to treat comes down to seven for the most high risk groups.

The chapter in *Clinical Evidence* makes the comment that economic analysis suggests that the clinical effect of palivizumab when used in all children who meet the licensed indication is small, and its benefits are likely to be clinically and economically relevant in children at the highest risk. A cost effectiveness analysis by Joffe[35] shows palivizumab to be more cost-effective than RSV immune globulin. It was most cost-effective for infants whose gestational age was < 32 weeks who had required at least 28 days of oxygen in the neonatal unit and had been discharged from September to November (Northern hemisphere). In this group, palivizumab was predicted to cost US$12 000 per hospitalization averted, (or US$33 000 per life year saved), with a number needed to treat to avoid one hospitalization of 7·4. Cost-effectiveness analyses are available for the United Kingdom,[36] Australia,[37] and New Zealand.[38] A systematic review of economic analyses on RSV prophylaxis[39] found that there were estimates ranging from cost savings to considerable incremental costs per hospitalization avoided, and that these divergent results could be explained in part by differences in study methods and assumptions but also by poor methodological quality. Interestingly, studies with some form of pharmaceutical industry funding were more likely to report the possibility of cost-effectiveness or cost savings of prophylaxis in the entire high risk population either in their point estimates or in their sensitivity. As commented by Klassen[40] in his editorial following publication of the systematic review, greater clarity is required if cost-effectiveness analyses are to play a key role in healthcare decision making.

Summary

You have looked at the evidence base behind management of RSV bronchiolitis. You know you can quickly diagnose whether RSV is responsible for symptoms using the Abbott TestPack. You can give the parents information regarding the increased risk of asthma later in childhood and can tell them that, if there is no family history of atopy, their child will likely "grow out" of the asthma by teenage years. You have looked at a number of interventions for the acute illness and for the reduction of post-bronchiolitic wheeze. You now feel confident that as further studies relating to bronchiolitis reach the literature, you will be able to appraise their validity and apply the results as appropriate. You were delighted to find a chapter on bronchiolitis in *Clinical Evidence*, as this has made incorporating the latest evidence into your clinical practice extremely easy. From the Trip Database (http://www.tripdatabase.com) you also found a useful summary from the Agency for Healthcare Research and Quality[41] and an evidence-based guideline.[42]

Resolution of the scenario

A recent audit in your department revealed that 50% of infants were admitted, even if they had received a bronchodilator. This gives your unit a baseline rate of admission of 0·5.

The relative risk of admission in the study using epinephrine was 0·4. (0·33/0·81). Extrapolating these results to your unit, you could expect a 20% admission rate with the use of epinephrine, (0·4 × 0·5). Your absolute risk (of admission) reduction with epinephrine would therefore be 0·30, giving you an NNT of 4 (rounded up). You decide it is worth giving a trial of two doses of nebulized epinephrine (3 ml of 1:1000) 30 minutes apart to the infant while he is in the assessment unit. Further, you decide that there is no evidence to support the use of steroids in this child's management, nor does he need ribavirin or antibiotics. In your unit, you find that 67% of young infants with bronchiolitis are RSV positive. Using the information that you have on likelihood ratios with the rapid test, you know that, if this child has a positive test, you will be 99·5% sure he has RSV (using a pretest probability of 0·67 and the nomogram on page 35, post-test probability = 0·995). If his test is positive, there is no evidence as yet that RSV immune globulin is effective treatment for infants with RSV bronchiolitis. If he has a negative test, his chances of being RSV positive are only 5·7%. You tell the baby's mother that he is more likely to have asthma later in life, (as his disease is at least moderate and has required some hospital intervention), even though there is no family history of atopy. You note that there is no evidence that steroids given prophylactically in patients with RSV bronchiolitis reduce the post-bronchiolitic wheezing episodes or hospital readmission. This child is not in the high risk group that would have benefited most from palivizumab or RSV immune globulin.

Future research needs

- Clear evidence of benefit and cost-effectiveness is needed, particularly for highly expensive treatments, such as ribavirin, RSV immunoglobulin, and palivizumab.
- Benefit for interventions must be seen in outcomes of clinical relevance, such as death or need for intensive care for high cost treatments that are not easy to administer.
- Systematic reviews show bronchodilators have a modest benefit, but clarification is needed as to which type of bronchodilator is most beneficial. Actions other than specific bronchodilation may be important in their effectiveness against bronchiolitis, as suggested with epinephrine.
- Work on RSV vaccination and its benefit.

Summary table: therapy

Study question	Type of evidence	Result	Comment
Bronchodilators	2 systematic reviews[7,8]	Modest clinical benefit; no reduction in admission	Worth giving trial of bronchodilator
Epinephrine	RCTs[9–14] 1 Cochrane review[10]	Benefit seen in symptom reduction and hospital admission (NNT = 2 to reduce one admission)	Full systematic review awaited; appears beneficial
Glucocorticoids – acute treatment or prevention of post-bronchiolitic wheeze	1 systematic review[11] RCTs[6,12,13,14,27,28] 1 Cochrane protocol[11]	Evidence of effect is not strong; some studies include recurrent wheezers	Unlikely to be of benefit ? More study required in outpatient setting looking at reduction in admission
Ribavirin in healthy infants or high risk infants?	1 systematic review[16] RCTs[17,18]	No benefit seen in short or long term	
Routine antibiotics	RCT[19]	No benefit	
RSV immunoglobulin treatment	1 Cochrane protocol[32] RCTs[29,30,31]	No significant benefit seen in RCTs	
RSV immunoglobulin or palivizumab prophylaxis	1 systematic review[33] RCT[34]	Reduction seen in hospitalization but not in ventilation; most effective if used in preterm infants with bronchopulmonary dysplasia, discharged home between September and December	Careful consideration needs to be given to which infants receive prophylaxis

Summary table: diagnostic tests

Test	Sensitivity	Specificity	Likelihood ratios	Comment
Abbott TestPack[20,21,22]	90–98%	92–99%	LR+ 11·25–97 LR– 0·03–0·1	Good test; higher sensitivity and specificity if performed in lab as opposed to near-patient testing

Summary table: prognosis

Study	Index cases	Follow up	Relative risk of asthma
Prospective cohort with two matched controls[24]	RSV positive bronchiolitis	3 years	9·9 if no history of atopy 38·7 if atopic ? No increase if community infection
Prospective cohort Matched controls added at 5·5 years[25]	First wheeze episode	10 years	4·43 (OR)
Prospective cohort with matched controls[26]	Mild bronchiolitis	8 years 13 years	3·24 Nil
Quantative review[23]	RSV bronchiolitis	up to 10 years	Increased at 5 years Nil at 10 years

References

1 Boeck KD. Respiratory syncitial virus bronchiolitis: clinical aspects and epidemiology. *Mondali Arch Chest Dis* 1996; **51**:210–13.

2 Young S, O'Keeffe PT, Arnott J, Landau LI. Lung function, airway responsiveness, and respiratory symptoms before and after bronchiolitis. *Arch Dis Child* 1995;**72**:16–24.

3 Levy BT, Graber MA. Respiratory syncitial virus infection in infants and young children. *J Fam Pract* 1997;**45**:473–81.

4 Jeng MJ, Lemen RJ. Respiratory syncitial virus bronchiolitis. *Am Fam Physic* 1997;**55**:1139–46.

5 Lowell D, Lister G, von Koss H, McCarthy P. Wheezing in Infants: The response to Epinephrine. *Pediatrics* 1987;**79**:939–45.

6 Klassen T, Sutcliffe T, Watters L, Wells G, Allen U, Li M. Dexamethasone in salbutamol-treated patients with acute bronchiolitis: a randomised controlled trial. *J Pediatr* 1997;**130**:191–6.

7 Kellner JD, Ohlsson A, Gadomski AM, Wang EE. Efficacy of bronchodilator therapy in bronchiolitis: a meta-analysis. *Arch Pediatr Adolesc Med* 1996;**150**:1166–72.

8 Flores G, Horwitz R. Efficacy of beta(2)-agonists in bronchiolitis: a reappraisal and meta-analysis. *Pediatrics* 1997;**100**:233–9.

9 Menon K, Sutcliffe T, Klassen T. A randomised trial comparing the efficacy of epinephrine with salbutamol in the treatment of acute bronchiolitis. *J Pediatr* 1995;**126**:1004–7.

10 Hartling L, Wiebe N, Russell K, Patel H, Klassen TP. A meta-analysis of randomised controlled trials evaluating the efficacy of epinephrine for the treatment of acute viral bronchiolitis. *Arch Pediatr Adolesc Med* 2003;**157**:957–64.

11 Garrison MM, Christakis DA, Harvey E, Cummings P, Davis RL. Systemic corticosteroids in infant bronchiolitis: a meta-analysis. *Pediatrics* 2000;**105**:E441–E446.

12 Cade A, Brownlee KG, Conway SP *et al.* Randomised placebo controlled trial of nebulised corticosteroids in acute respiratory syncitial viral bronchiolitis. *Arch Dis Child* 2000;**82**:126–30.

13 Bulow SM, Nir M, Levin E *et al.* Prednisolone treatment of respiratory syncitial virus infection: a randomized controlled trial of 147 infants. *Pediatrics* 1999;**104**:e77.

14 Schuh S, Coates AL, Binnie R *et al.* Efficacy of oral dexamethasone in outpatients with acute bronchiolitis. *J Pediatr* 2002;**140**:27–32.

15 Patel H, Platt R, Lozano JM, Wang EEL. Glucocorticoids for acute viral bronchiolitis in hospitalized infants and young children (Protocol for a Cochrane Review). In: *Cochrane Library*, Issue 1. Oxford: Update Software, 2002.

16 Randolph A, Wang E. Ribavirin for respiratory syncitial virus lower respiratory trract infection. A systematic overview. *Arch Pediatr Adolesc Med* 1996;**150**:942–7.

17 Everard ML, Swarbrick A, Rigby AS, Milner AD. The effect of ribavirin to treat previously healthy infants admitted with acute bronchiolitis on acute and chronic respiratory morbidity. *Resp Med* 2001;**95**:275–80.

18 Guerguerian AM, Gauthier M, Lebel MH, Farrell CA, Lacroix J. Ribavirin in ventilated respiratory syncitial virus bronchiolitis. A randomized, placebo-controlled trial. *Am J Resp Crit Care Med* 1999;**160**:829–34.

19 Friis B, Andersen P, Brenoe E *et al.* Antibiotic treatment of pneumonia and bronchiolitis. A prospective randomised study. *Arch Dis Child* 1984;**59**:1038–45.

20 Krilov L, Lipson S, Barone S, Kaplan M, Ciamician Z, Harkness H. Evaluation of a rapid diagnostic test for respiratory syncitial virus (RSV): potential for bedside diagnosis. *Pediatrics*. 1994;**93**:903–90.

21 Obel N, Andersen HK, Jensen IP, Mordhorst CH. Evaluation of Abbott TestPack RSV and an in-house RSV ELISA for detection of respiratory syncitial virus in respiratory tract aspirates. *APMIS* 1995;**103**:416–8.

22 Mackie PL, Joannidis PA, Beattie J. Evaluation of an acute point-of-care system screening for respiratory syncitial virus infection. *J Hosp Infect* 2001;**48**:66–71.

23 Kneyber MCJ, Steyerberg EW, de Groot R, Moll HA. Long-term effects of respiratory syncitial virus (RSV) bronchiolitis in infants and young children: a quantitative review. *Acta Paediatr* 2000;**89**:654–60.

24 Sigurs N, Bjarnason R, Sigurbergsson F, Kjellman B, Bjorksten B. Asthma and immunoglobulin E antibodies after respiratory syncitial virus bronchiolitis: A prospective cohort study with matched controls. *Pediatrics* 1995;**95**:500–5.

25 Noble V, Murray M, Webb MSC, Alexander J, Swarbrick AS, Milner AD. Respiratory status and allergy nine to 10 years after acute bronchiolitis. *Arch Dis Child* 1997;**76**:315–19.

26 McConnochie K, Roghmann K. Wheezing at 8 and 13 years: changing importance of bronchiolitis and passive smoking. *Pediatr Pulmonol* 1989;**6**:138–46.

27 Lozano JM. Bronchiolitis. *Clin Evid* 2002;**8**:291–303.

28 van Woensel JB, Kimpen JL, Sprikkelman AB, Ouwehand A, van Aalderen WM. Long-term effects of prednisolone in the acute phase of bronchiolitis caused by respiratory syncitial viru. *Pediatr Pulmonol* 2000;Aug:92–6.

29 Rimensberger P, Burek-Kozlowska A, Morell A *et al.* Aerosolized immunoglobulin treatment of respiratory syncitial virus infection in infants. *Pediatr Infect Dis J* 1996;**15**:209–16.

30 Rodriguez W, Gruber W, Weeliver R *et al.* for the Respiratory Syncitial Virus Immune Study Group. RSV immune globulin intravenous therapy for RSV lower respiratory tract infection in infants and young children at high risk for severe RSV. *Pediatrics* 1997;**99**:454–61.

31 Rodriguez W, Gruber W, Groothuis J *et al.* for the Respiratory Syncitial Virus Immune Study Group. RSV immune globulin intravenous therapy for RSV lower respiratory tract infection in previously healthy children. *Pediatrics* 1997;**100**:937–42.

32 Tan D, Wang E, Ohlsson A. Immunoglobulin for treatment of respiratory syncitial virus [Protocol]. In: Douglas R, Bridges-Webb C, Glasziou P, Lazano J, Steinhoff M, Wang E, eds. *Acute Respiratory Infections Module of the Cochrane Database of Systematic Reviews*. Available in the *Cochrane Library*, Issue 2. Oxford:Update Software, 1999.

33 Wang EEL, Tang NK. Immunoglobulin for preventing respiratory syncitial virus infection (Cochrane Review). *Cochrane Library*, Issue 1. Oxford: Update Software, 2002.

34 The Impact-RSV Study Group. Palivizumab, a humanised respiratory syncitial virus monoclonal antibody, reduces hospitalisation from respiratory syncitial virus infection in high risk infants. *Pediatrics.* 1998;**102**:531–7.

35 Joffe S, Ray T, Escobar G, Black S, Lieu T. Cost-effectiveness of respiratory syncitial virus prophylaxis among preterm infants. *Pediatrics* 1999;**104**:419–27.

36 Clark SJ, Beresford MW, Subhedar NV, Shaw NJ. Respiratory syncitial virus infection in high risk infants and the potential impact of prophylaxis in a United Kingdom cohort. *Arch Dis Childh* 2000;**83**:313–16.

37 Numa A. Outcome of respiratory syncitial virus infection and a cost-benefit analysis of prophylaxis. *J Paediatr Child Health* 2000;**36**:422–7.

38 Vogel AM, Lennon DR, Broadbent R *et al.* Palivizumab prophylaxis of respiratory syncitial virus infection in high-risk infants. *J Paediatr Child Health* 2002;**38**:550–4.

39 Kamal-Bahl S, Doshi J, Campbell J. Economic analyses of respiratory syncitial virus immunoprophylaxis in high-risk infants: a systematic review. *Arch Pediatr Adolesc Med* 2002;**156**:1034–41.

40 Klassen TP. Economic evaluations of immunoprophylaxis in infants at high risk for respiratory syncitial virus: shedding light or creating confusion? *Arch Pediatr Adolesc Med* 2002;**156**:1180–1.

41 Evidence Report/Technology Assessment No 69. *Management of Bronchiolitis in Infants and Children.* Agency for Healthcare Research Quality, 2003.

42 Cincinnati Children's Hospital Medical Center. *Evidence based clinical practice guideline for infant with bronchiolitis.* Cincinnati (OH): Cincinnati Children's Hospital Medical Center; National Guideline Clearing House, 2001.

33 Otitis media

Sandi Pirozzo, Chris Del Mar

Case scenario   *Your last patient of the morning is a 3½-year-old girl whose mother brought her straight from preschool because she had a fever and complained that her ear was hurting. She has no significant medical history. The child is not pleased to be in the doctor's office, and has been crying. Her mother explains that she developed a "cold" about 3 days ago with sniffles. Her temperature is raised (37·8°C) and with some difficulty the rest of the physical examination is completed. The only abnormalities are slight redness of the throat, a nose full of thick green mucus, and red tympanic membranes. You wonder what findings other than her red tympanic membranes should lead you to diagnose otitis media, and also consider the recent controversy about whether to treat acute otitis media (AOM) with antibiotics.*

Background

AOM is a disease of infancy and early childhood defined by the presence of inflammation and fluid in the middle ear, accompanied by at least one sign of acute illness.[1] The model of the mechanism for the illness of AOM is based on the observation that AOM commonly follows an upper respiratory illness in children. Excessive secretions of mucus from the nasopharyngeal mucosa, together with edema, may cause temporary obstruction of the eustachian tube. The obstruction causes a build-up of pressure in the middle ear cleft because there is only one exit via the eustachian tube. Air is replaced with fluid (mucus or inflammatory fluid) and the accompanying stasis increases the probability of bacterial infection in the middle ear space.

Support for this model comes from the observation that children with anatomical disorders of the nasopharynx (for example, those with cleft palate or trisomy 21) are more likely to suffer repeated attacks of AOM.[2,3] Studies examining the content of the middle ear cavity during attacks of AOM have found both bacterial and viral pathogens.[4-8] The pathophysiologic model has been used to propose that antibiotics might be useful in the management of the infection. However, there has been dissent to this approach: 12 different case series failed to identify *any* causative infectious agent in the middle ear fluid of 28–62% of cases.[9] In America, the UK, and Australia, standard practice is to use antibiotics promptly on diagnosis.[10] This is not the norm in parts of continental Europe, particularly the Low Countries and Scandinavia.[11] Some have argued that infective or inflammatory fluid in a confined space constitutes an abscess, so tympanocentesis is regarded as the proper method of managing the condition. Perforation of the tympanic membrane (artificial or spontaneous) with accompanying drainage of pus, although frightening for many parents, usually heralds immediate relief of pain and resolution of the episode of illness for the child. Another view altogether suggests that AOM is a "self-limiting" (spontaneously remitting) illness,[12] the normal resolution of which is fast enough to obviate the need for any treatment.[11,13]

Several questions arise from the scenario:

- How many children get otitis media?
- In children suspected of having AOM, what signs and symptoms influence the accuracy of diagnosis?
- In children with AOM, do antibiotics shorten duration of illness?

Phrasing these in the structure suggested in Chapter 2 helps to clarify the issues and guides your search for evidence.

Searching for evidence

Questions

1. In children of preschool age (*population*), what is the incidence (*event*) of otitis media? (*outcome*) **[Baseline Risk]**
2. In children with otitis media (*population*), what is the probability that earache, cold symptoms, fever, vomiting, and diarrhea (*events*) will help in making the diagnosis (*outcome*)? **[Diagnostic Test]**

3. In children with otitis media (*population*), what is the probability that red, cloudy, bulging, retracted, or immobile tympanic membranes (*events*) will help in making the diagnosis (*outcome*)? **[Diagnostic Test]**
4. In children with AOM (*population*), do antibiotics (*intervention*) shorten the course of illness without significant adverse effects (*outcomes*)? **[Therapy]**

You search for summaries of evidence in *Clinical Evidence*, the *Cochrane Library*, and in MedLine. In *Clinical Evidence* (2002, Issue 8), you find one chapter on AOM in the Child Health section. Knowing that this publication addresses only issues of treatment, you are not surprised to find that your fourth question is the only one addressed in the chapter. Similarly, the *Cochrane Library* (2003, Issue 1) reveals three completed reviews; two reviews directly address the question of antibiotic treatment of AOM in children,[14,15] and one assesses the efficacy of decongestants for AOM.[16] The Database of Reviews of Effects (DARE) lists six more reviews, which address the effectiveness of antibiotic therapy.[10,17–21] A search of MedLine using AOM as a major MeSH heading and meta-analysis as a text word nets one additional study,[22] although this is an older version of one of the Cochrane Reviews.[14] For the remainder of the questions for which high-quality systematic reviews are not available, the searches are shown with the individual questions.

Critical review of the evidence

Question

1. In children of preschool age (*population*), what is the incidence (*event*) of otitis media (*outcome*)? **[Baseline Risk]**

Search criteria

- PubMed: acute otitis media AND (incidence OR prevalence OR frequency)
- References of articles obtained from this search and general search

The best study design to answer questions in relation to incidence is a cohort study where a defined population of patients is followed over time to see how many develop the condition of interest, in this case AOM. You could add "cohort study" to your search terms to decrease the number of hits but this would also reduce the sensitivity of the search and you may miss some relevant papers. Your simple search

nets 12 articles relevant to the incidence of AOM, but you quickly exclude four of these – two are duplicate publications, one has not used acceptable criteria to diagnose the cases of AOM, and the cross-sectional design of the fourth does not lend itself to an accurate estimation of incidence. It is clear from your search that AOM is one of the most common reasons for children to make visits to their family doctors.

You are now left with eight studies of the incidence of AOM: five Finnish,[23–27] two American,[28,29] and one British.[30] Half the studies calculate incidence rate as a percentage per year (or per 100 child years)[23,26,28,30] and this ranged from 17% to 32%. The four remaining studies present the cumulative incidence[24,25,27,29], which ranged from 21% to 62% by the end of the first year of life. In most of the studies, the peak incidence occurred during the second six months of life[23–25,27,29]; however, two studies found incidence was greatest after 12 months; either in the 12–24 month period[26] or in the third year of life.[30] Table 33.1 summarizes the incidence rates and cumulative incidences reported in the eight selected epidemiological studies.

You note that study design varied considerably and may have affected the validity of the results. In four of the studies[23,26,28,30] the patients were self-selected, i.e., they were brought to the clinic or doctor's office on the basis of symptoms, and the denominator used in calculating incidence was based on the total number of children in the entire district[23,26] or practice.[28,30] This method of measuring incidence may underestimate the number of cases since infants and children without symptoms would not be diagnosed. Four studies[24,25,27,29] were prospective cohort studies with one of these[25] using a random sample from a larger cohort. The cohort study design is one of the most rigorous designs for determining incidence. However, one of these studies[27] depended, at least to some extent, on parental report of AOM, and thus may have underestimated the cumulative incidence (only 21%). The other three cohort studies,[24,25,29] with cumulative incidences of 45%, 42%, and 62% respectively, employed both a rigorous design and good follow up procedures.

While most of the studies used a combination of symptoms and signs to diagnose AOM, one study[30] based the diagnosis of AOM solely on the degree of redness of the tympanic membrane, which may have overestimated the frequency of disease. Several studies also found a difference in incidence rate between males and females, with males having a significantly higher rate of first occurrence of AOM as well as recurrence.[23,24] The recurrence rate was relatively high with approximately 17–30% of children having two or more episodes of AOM during the first year of life.[24,28]

Despite differences in study design, diagnostic criteria, and study population, the incidence rates were remarkably similar among the studies. The fact that 50% of children had

Table 33.1 Incidence of acute otitis media in population studies

					Overall incidence (%)	
References	Number of children	Follow up period (months)	Age of children	Age at peak incidence (%)	Incidence rate/year	Cumulative incidence
Pukander, 1982[23]	37 570	12	0–5 years	6–11 months (76)	17	
Sipila, 1987[24]	1642	18	First 18 months of life	10 months		45 by 1 year
Alho, 1991[25]	2512	24	First 2 years of life			42 by 1 year
Joki-Erkkila, 1998[26] (1978 data)	2921	12	0–10 years	12–24 months (37)	19	
Joki-Erkkila, 1998[26] (1994 data)	2611	12	0–10 years	12–24 months (63)	32	
Aniansson, 1994[27]	400	12	First year of life	8–12 months (62)		21 by 1 year
Howie, 1983[28]	4602*	12	0–17 years	1st year (21% of all cases)	18	
Teele, 1989[29]	498	84	0–7 years	6–12 months (56)		62 by 1 year
Ross, 1988[30]	334	12	0–3 years	3rd year (30·8)	22	

*Office visits.

experienced at least one episode of AOM before 3 years of age and 75% before the age of 10 years[23] reflects how common this disorder is.

Question

2. In children with otitis media (*population*), what is the probability that earache, cold symptoms, fever, vomiting, and diarrhea (*events*) will help in making the diagnosis (*outcome*)? **[Diagnostic Test]**

Search criteria

- PubMed:

  1. acute otitis media AND (signs OR symptoms)
  2. acute otitis media AND (earache OR pain OR fever OR cough OR irritab* OR catarrh OR vomiting OR diarrhea OR rhinitis OR sign* OR symptom*)

You wonder about the certainty of diagnosing AOM, and consider whether specific symptoms should influence your diagnosis. From experience, you know that common signs and symptoms associated with AOM, such as pulling on the ear and erythema of the tympanic membrane, may be found in children without AOM,[31] while symptoms such as earache and fever, the "classic" findings of AOM, are sometimes absent. You decide to search for studies that examine the frequency and likelihood ratios of various associated symptoms. There are two options to retrieve only diagnostic studies: use the diagnostic emphasis on PubMed Clinical Queries or include diagnostic terms such as "sensitivity or specificity" as search terms.

Your search yields eight studies reporting the frequency of symptoms in children with AOM.[28,30,32–37] All but two[30,33] of the studies performed pneumatic otoscopy on all children and used multiple signs associated with the tympanic membrane (redness, bulging, and immobility) as the gold standard for diagnosis of AOM. One of these[33] performed a mini-tympanometric examination on all children and, if this was abnormal or if the child had an earache, then pneumatic otoscopy was also performed. Study designs varied from prospective cohort studies,[33,34,36] which followed children over a period of time, to studies which enrolled consecutive cases of AOM in a practice setting.[28,30,32,35,37] All studies involved an appropriate spectrum of patients (infants and young children with suspected AOM); however, in three studies,[28,30,35] it was not clear who collected the information about symptoms and whether the person performing the otoscopy was blinded to these. For this reason, you base your evaluation on the five studies that appear to have the most valid methods.[32–34,36,37]

In a prospective Finnish cohort study by Heikkinen and Ruuskanen,[34] 302 children younger than 4 years attending day care centers were followed up and examined during episodes of upper respiratory tract infection. Earache was

Table 33.2 Prevalence of associated symptoms in children with otitis media

References	Percentage of children with acute otitis media (based on signs) with the symptom							
	Earache	Ear pulling	Irritability	Cough	Catarrh/rhinitis	Fever	Vomiting	Diarrhea
Hayden[32]	83	NS	NS	NS	NS	21	NS	NS
Kontiokari[33]	59	NS	39	NS	50	42	NS	NS
Heikkinen[34]	60	NS	NS	83	96	69	NS	NS
Uhari[36]	21	NS	NS	71	67	84	26	18
Niemela[37]	54	42	55	47	24	40	11	8
Summary	21–83	42	39–55	47–83	24–96	21–84	11–26	18

NS, not stated.

reported in 88 (29%) of the 302 children, 73 (83%) of whom had AOM. The likelihood ratios for a positive result (having an earache) and a negative result (not having an earache) are 7·3 and 0·4, respectively. This means that having an earache is seven times more likely to be seen in a child with otitis media as compared with a child without otitis media. Not having an earache is just over one-third as likely to be seen in a child with, as opposed to a child without, otitis media. You note that 40% of the children with AOM in this study had no apparent earache. In other words, earache is more useful as a "rule-in" symptom than a "rule-out" one. Hayden and Schwartz[32] found the age of the child to be a significant factor in determining the predictive value of earache. The younger the child, the less likely that earache will accompany AOM. Whether this is due to a difference in the pathology of AOM or the inability of infants to localize or express pain is not clear. Table 33.2 summarizes the findings from these studies, clearly showing that earache is an inconsistent finding, with a reported frequency between 21% and 83%.

The same studies considered cough and rhinitis, finding them to be relatively common symptoms among children with otitis media. This is not surprising, considering that AOM is associated with an upper respiratory tract infection (URTI) in 76% of cases.[38] Unfortunately, cough and rhinitis are non-specific symptoms. Based on the data from the Heikkinen and Ruuskanen study,[34] the likelihood ratios for a positive test (having a cough or rhinitis) are both 1, indicating that cough and rhinitis are equally likely to be found in a child with, as compared with a child without, otitis media. The likelihood ratios for a negative test (not having a cough or rhinitis) are 1 and 0·5, respectively.

Fever can be considered either as a sign or a symptom. Like earache, fever is also an inconsistent finding in AOM, occurring in 21–84% of cases.[32,36] One of the five selected studies, a case–control study conducted by Uhari *et al.*,[36] compared 197 patients with AOM to hospital age-matched controls and found that fever was a common finding among both groups of children, and there was no significant difference between the two groups. In the prospective cohort study by Heikkinen and Ruuskanen,[34] fever actually

decreased the likelihood of having AOM, with positive and negative likelihood ratios of 0·9 and 1·3, respectively.

Only two of the five studies addressed the frequency of vomiting and diarrhea in children with otitis media.[36,37] Neither study found vomiting and diarrhea to be more common in children with AOM as compared with children with other acute illnesses.

You realize from your review of these papers that the frequency of associated symptoms in children with AOM varies greatly and AOM cannot be reliably differentiated from URTI on the basis of symptoms alone. Only earache has a high specificity with a corresponding likelihood ratio (positive) showing that it is over seven times more likely to be found in children with, as compared to children without, AOM.

Question

3. In children with otitis media (*population*), what is the probability that red, cloudy, bulging, retracted or immobile tympanic membranes (*events*) will help in making the diagnosis (*outcome*)? **[Diagnostic Test]**

Search criteria

- PubMed: acute otitis media AND (clinical sign* OR diagnosis OR otoscop* OR pneumatic otoscop* OR pneumotoscop* OR tympanoscop* OR tympanic membrane). (NOTE: The asterisk (*) is a "wildcard" to search for terms containing the word fragment preceding the asterisk.)

Your search for evidence about the predictive value of clinical signs yields a number of studies, only one of which actually provides sensitivity, specificity, and predictive values for the various tympanic membrane changes seen in AOM.[39] This large Finnish study conducted by Karma *et al.* sought to determine the value of different pneumotoscopic findings in diagnosing middle ear effusion of acute and non-acute otitis media. During almost 12 000 ear-related visits, 2911

Table 33.3 Sensitivity, specificity, positive predictive values, and likelihood ratios of otoscopic findings among children with acute symptoms for middle ear effusion[33]

Tympanic membrane findings	Children examined by otolaryngologist				Children examined by pediatrician			
	Sn (%)	Sp (%)	LR+	LR−	Sn (%)	Sp (%)	LR+	LR−
Red	18	84	1·1	0·98	27	84	1.7	0·87
Distinctly red*	14	91	1·6	0·95	24	92	3.0	0·83
Cloudy	81	95	16·2	0·2	67	90	6.7	0·37
Bulging	61	97	20·3	0·40	41	97	13.7	0·61
Retracted	7	91	0·8	1·02	19	88	1.6	0·92
Impaired mobility	98	79	4·7	0·03	94	72	3.4	0·08

*Hemorrhagic, strongly or moderately red. Sn, sensitivity; Sp, specificity.
Data adapted from Karma *et al.,* 1989[39]

unselected children were examined, half by an otolaryngologist and half by a pediatrician, in two different geographic areas. When middle ear effusion (MEE) was suspected, myringotomy was performed to confirm its presence. While this may be justifiable on ethical grounds, restricting the use of confirmatory myringotomy to those children who were suspected of having middle ear effusion on otoscopy is a particular shortcoming of the study, and may lead to "verification bias". Verification bias is a distortion of the properties of a diagnostic test that occurs when its result influences whether patients undergo confirmation by the "gold" or "reference" standard. The effect would be to improve both sensitivity and specificity. In this case, it is unlikely that many children with MEE were missed by verifying only the positive results, because of the high proportion (20%) of myringotomies that yielded negative results. Table 33.3 summarizes the findings from this study. Since predictive values are dependent on both the accuracy of the test and the pretest probability, they have been replaced by likelihood ratios, which mainly reflect the accuracy of the test.

As is evident in Table 33.3, observed redness of the tympanic membrane has poor sensitivity in AOM, seen in approximately 14–27% of cases.[39] When redness was present, it predicted only about half of the cases with acute symptoms. In children examined by the otolaryngologist, a red tympanic membrane was just as likely to be found in children with AOM as in children without AOM. While redness of the tympanic membrane cannot be regarded as a reliable indicator of AOM, you remember noting from one of the previous studies that you reviewed that a red tympanic membrane is more likely to be associated with severe pain than a yellow or grey one.[32]

A cloudy or opacified tympanic membrane is a strong predictor of AOM with relatively high sensitivity and specificity.[39] The high likelihood ratios for the presence of this sign (16·2 and 6·7) confirm that it is much more likely to be found in children with AOM. However, you know from experience that the tympanic membrane may be rendered

opaque from previous episodes of AOM and glue ear. You also remember reading in one of the articles that you retrieved during your initial search for this question that very young infants (< 4 months of age) may have decreased translucence in the absence of disease.[40] This finding was ascertained in a study by Cavanaugh who examined 81 healthy infants at 3 days and followed them up at well-baby clinics.[40]

Bulging of the membrane shows the highest likelihood ratios for a positive result (20·3 and 13·7) indicating that it is far more likely to be present in children with AOM compared with those without AOM. Unfortunately, the absence of bulging (LR for a negative test: 0·40 and 0·61) does not preclude the diagnosis of AOM.

When present, impaired mobility indicates an increased likelihood of AOM (LR for a positive test: 4·7 and 3·4). Perhaps it is most useful in ruling out AOM when it is absent (LR for a negative test: 0·03 and 0·08). Although not shown in Table 33.3, when cases were classified as having only slight impairment in tympanic membrane mobility, the sign lost its diagnostic value in predicting AOM.

You wish that there were more than one study; however, this one appears to be valid. Based on the findings in this study,[39] it would appear that redness and retraction of the tympanic membrane (with likelihood ratios close to 1) are relatively poor signs on which to base a diagnosis. The presence of cloudiness and bulging (with high LRs for a positive test) helps to rule in the diagnosis of AOM, while the absence of impaired mobility (with low LR for a negative test) helps to rule out AOM. Clearly, reliance on any one sign or symptom is likely to result in many false positives and false negatives.

Question

4. In children with AOM (*population*), do antibiotics (*intervention*) shorten the course of illness without significant adverse effects (*outcomes*)? **[Therapy]**

The ideal evidence for the effectiveness of a treatment (see Chapter 6) comes from well-conducted randomized controlled trials, especially trials using outcomes that are relevant to the patient and his or her family. The outcomes that you are concerned with include *symptoms and complications* attributable to otitis media (pain and deafness, a shorter duration of illness, later episodes of illness, and side effects from antibiotics), rather than *signs*. Meta-analysis of such trials that show a homogeneous effect would represent the best possible evidence.

In your search for evidence summaries, you find three meta-analyses. The chapter in *Clinical Evidence* concludes that evidence on the effectiveness of antibiotics is conflicting, and cites the same three systematic reviews that you found in your search of the *Cochrane Library* (one by Rosenfeld et al.,[10] one by Damoiseaux[17] and one by Glasziou et al.[14]). The Damoiseaux study only looked at children under 2 years. The Glasziou meta-analysis includes studies that more closely fulfil the strict criteria mentioned above and is slightly more stringent in its admission of trials into the analysis. The main difference between the Rosenfeld[10] and Glasziou[14] meta-analyses is that the latter only included data relevant to patient-centered outcomes.

Table 33.4 from the Glasziou meta-analysis shows the size and direction of the effect of antibiotics on AOM in children. You notice that antibiotics have no effect on pain within the first 24 hours; however, there is a 27% reduction in the odds of experiencing pain at 2–7 days if children are given antibiotics at the initial visit. Similarly, there is no effect of early use of antibiotics for the deafness of AOM at 1 month after the episode. Although there is a trend to reduced hearing loss at three months, this may be due to chance alone, as the 95% CI crosses the odds ratio (OR) of 1·0.

The outcomes of pain and hearing loss are difficult to measure in children. Pain and associated symptoms have been measured in a variety of ways. In the meta-analysis these were grouped into those that were early (within 24 hours) and later (2–7 days). This wide spread of days for the later measure was chosen to accommodate the different studies. Deafness is difficult to assess subjectively in children who rarely complain of being deaf even when their hearing is severely compromised; audiometry is used as a proxy measure to estimate the presence of deafness. Although there was no benefit at 1 month from antibiotics for the resolution of deafness, there is a trend evident from Table 33.4 for an improvement at 3 months. However, the effect is too modest, and the number of patients too few, for you to be sure that this is not a chance effect (the 95% confidence intervals cross unity).

Randomized controlled trials and meta-analyses of randomized controlled trials answer questions about reasonably common events so some rare adverse outcomes may not be picked up from the data. The most common major

complication of AOM is mastoiditis. The Glasziou meta-analysis[14] refers to two studies that addressed mastoiditis. One case series from 1954[49] reported an incidence of 17%. If this rate still occurs in modern times, it should be evident among the cases in this meta-analysis, but only one case was reported (in the antibiotic group). In another study of 860 children aged 2–12 years with AOM (not controlled and thus not included in the Glasziou meta-analysis), only two children whose illness was managed without the use of early antibiotics developed mastoiditis (and were successfully treated with oral amoxycillin).[13] Perhaps mastoiditis has become a less common, and less severe, complication with time. The same study[13] reported an incidence of 2% for a severe form of otitis media, defined as causing an illness beyond 3–4 days or discharge from the ear for more than 14 days, which was lower than the rate reported in the meta-analysis.

Other more serious complications of AOM (such as meningitis) occur at a rate so low that even large trials cannot detect them. The number of children who must be treated to prevent such rarities would be astronomical. This concern also applies to the serious complications of orally administered antibiotics. These have been recorded in the literature as causing devastating illness and even death, although also so rarely as to preclude easy estimates of the risk.[50]

Antibiotics can also cause a series of minor and not so minor side effects. The meta-analysis showed a near doubling of the chance of the child experiencing vomiting, diarrhea, or rashes: about one child is affected by side effects for every 18 treated. It would obviously be useful to be able to identify children who are more likely to have a prolonged or complicated course of AOM and thus might benefit relatively more from early prescription of antibiotics. A recent secondary analysis of a randomized controlled trial cohort sought to identify children at greater risk of a poorer outcome and to assess benefit from antibiotics in these children.[51] Factors that might act as markers for having a significantly greater OR of being ill (distressed) at 3 days after diagnosis of acute otitis media were:

- high temperature (adjusted OR 4·5; 95% CI 2·3–9·0);
- vomiting (OR 2·6; 95% CI 1·3–5·0), and
- cough (OR 2·0; 95% CI 1·1–3·8).

Other factors including age, appearance of the eardrum, preceding illness, and satisfaction with the consultation, were not associated with episodes of distress at day 3. Children with high temperature or vomiting were less likely to experience distress at day 3 if antibiotics had been given immediately (number needed to treat [NNT] of about five for distress and three for disturbed nights). However, in children without higher temperatures or vomiting, immediate antibiotics made little difference.

Table 33.4   Summary of the evidence relating to antibiotic treatment for acute otitis media[14]

Study*	Expt n/N	Ctrl n/N	Peto OR (95% CI fixed)	Weight (%)	Peto OR (95% CI fixed)
Pain at 24 hours					
Burke[41]	53/112	56/117		34·4	0·98 [0·58, 1·64]
Thalin[42]	58/159	58/158		44·2	0·99 [0·63, 1·56]
van Buchem a[43]	13/47	11/40		10·5	1·01 [0·39, 2·57]
van Buchem b[43]	17/48	10/36		10·9	1·41 [0·56, 3·55]
Subtotal [95% CI]	141/366	135/351		100·0	1·03 [0·76, 1·39]

Test for heterogeneity chi-square 0·52 (df = 3), $P = 0.91$; test for overall effect $z = 0.17$, $P = 0.9$

Study*	Expt n/N	Ctrl n/N	Peto OR (95% CI fixed)	Weight (%)	Peto OR (95% CI fixed)
Pain at 2–7 days					
Appelman[44]	11/67	10/54		6·7	0·86 [0·34, 2·22]
Burke[41]	20/111	29/114		14·8	0·65 [0·34, 1·22]
Damoiseaux[45]	69/117	89/123		20·9	0·55 [0·32, 0·94]
Halsted[46]	17/62	7/27		5·8	1·08 [0·39, 2·97]
Kaleida[47]	19/488	38/492		20·7	0·50 [0·29, 0·85]
Mygind[48]	15/72	29/77		12·0	0·45 [0·22, 0·90]
Thalin[42]	15/158	25/158		13·5	0·57 [0·29, 1·10]
van Buchem a[43]	4/38	3/46		2·5	1·68 [0·36, 7·87]
van Buchem b[43]	5/48	4/38		3·1	0·99 [0·25, 3·94]
Subtotal [95% CI]	175/1161	234/1129		100·0	0·62 [0·47, 0·82]

Test for heterogeneity chi-square 5·38 (df = 8), $P = 0.72$; test for overall effect $z = -4.02$, $P = 0.00006$

Study*	Expt n/N	Ctrl n/N	Peto OR (95% CI fixed)	Weight (%)	Peto OR (95% CI fixed)
Deafness at 1 month					
Appelman[44]	21/51	25/46		22·2	0·59 [0·27, 1·31]
Burke[41]	41/111	41/116		47·9	1·07 [0·62, 1·84]
Mygind[48]	23/72	25/77		29·8	0·98 [0·49, 1·94]
Subtotal [95% CI]	85/234	91/239		100·0	0·91 [0·63, 1·33]

Test for heterogeneity chi-square 1·51 (df = 2), $P = 0.47$; test for overall effect $z = -0.47$, $P = 0.6$

Study*	Expt n/N	Ctrl n/N	Peto OR (95% CI fixed)	Weight (%)	Peto OR (95% CI fixed)
Deafness at 3 months					
Burke[41]	20/110	31/111		58·9	0·58 [0·31, 1·08]
Mygind[48]	18/72	18/77		41·1	1·09 [0·52, 2·31]
Subtotal [95% CI]	38/182	49/188		100·0	0·75 [0·47, 1·21]

Test for heterogeneity chi-square 1·63 (df = 1), $P = 0.2$; test for overall effect $z = -1.17$, $P = 0.2$

Study*	Expt n/N	Ctrl n/N	Peto OR (95% CI fixed)	Weight (%)	Peto OR (95% CI fixed)
Vomiting, diarrhea, or rash					
Burke[41]	53/114	36/118		90·3	1·96 [1·16, 3·32]
Mygind[48]	3/72	1/77		6·4	2·98 [0·41, 21·58]
Thalin[42]	1/159	1/158		3·3	0·99 [0·06, 15·96]
Total [95% CI]	57/345	38/353		100·0	1·97 [1·19, 3·25]

Test for heterogeneity chi-square 0·40 (df = 2), $P = 0.82$; test for overall effect $z = 2.65$, $P = 0.008$

The next task is to weigh these issues against other considerations such as cost. The cost of antibiotic use can be expressed in terms of the harms or potential harms of treatment, as well as in monetary terms. Some harms are borne by society in general, such as the development of antibiotic resistance. Antibiotics used now (even for minor self-limiting conditions) may be unavailable for use in the future (even for serious life-threatening conditions).

It appears that there is not necessarily a "correct" way to decide on antibiotic use for this condition and that patient choice should be considered. How can you present this information to your patient's mother? The data in Table 33.4 can be described as suggesting that antibiotics provide a *relative* benefit by reducing the risk of pain by 27% (95% CI 13–39%) after day 1. However, the *absolute* benefit of antibiotics will depend on the prevalence of the outcome (for example, pain), as well as the relative benefit conferred by the antibiotics. Pain was present in only 21% of children in control groups after day 1. Therefore the use of antibiotics will reduce the chance of children experiencing pain from 21% to 15% (an absolute risk reduction of only 6%). Thus, the number of children a physician must treat to prevent one child from having pain after day 1 is about 17 (100/6). Since your patient does not have the markers for a more distressing illness (high temperature, vomiting, or cough[51]), a marked response to antibiotics is unlikely. This benefit should be balanced against a similar chance of side effects directly attributable to the antibiotics (number needed to harm [NNH] of 18).

Some families will judge this information as indicating that treatment with antibiotics is worthwhile; others that it is not. This will depend on the values that patients have for different experiences such as pain during the night for their child, the effectiveness of alternatives for pain management such as analgesics, and the complications of antibiotic use. Not all patients (or their parents) want to accept the responsibility of having to decide what to do, and sort through this complicated information, which leaves the physician to make the best informed decision on behalf of the patient.

Resolution of the scenario

Based on an annual incidence rate of 0·3 (30%)[30] and an estimated duration of AOM of 2 days, this 3·5-year-old child has a 0·2% pre-examination probability of having AOM. Since the likelihood ratio for fever is 1, its presence does not have any effect on her post-test probability. Her complaint of ear pain, with a likelihood ratio of 7·3,[34] increases the post-test probability to 1·5%. Her only physical finding is redness of the tympanic membrane, which has a likelihood ratio of 1 and therefore, would not alter the post-test probability. If she had bulging of the tympanic membrane (with a likelihood ratio of 20·3[34]), the post-test probability would be increased to about 4%. (Note: since her ear pain and bulging of the tympanic membrane are unlikely to be independent findings, you cannot use the two likelihood ratios in sequence; see Chapter 5.) You and the child's mother discuss the possible benefits and harms of treating her presumed otitis media with antibiotics, and decide to provide only analgesics for now, but you advise the mother to keep in touch in case her child's condition worsens.

Future research needs

Since antibiotics provide less than expected symptom relief, perhaps a search for effective treatments other than antibiotics could be pursued. These might include analgesics, and preventive measures such as vaccination.

Summary table

Question	Type of Evidence	Result	Comment
Incidence of otitis media in preschool age children	4 prospective cohort studies 4 other observational studies	17–30% have 2 or more episodes by age 1yr 50% by age 3 yrs 75% by age 10 yrs	Variable diagnostic criteria, but consistent results
Usefulness of symptoms for diagnosis	8 studies overall, TM findings as gold standard for diagnosis, 5 studies of high quality	Ear pain – LR+ = 7.3; LR– = 0.4 Cough – LR+ = 1; LR– = 1 Rhinitis – LR+ = 1; LR– = 0.5 Fever – LR+ = 1; LR– = 1 Vomiting & diarrhea – no difference	Symptoms can be suggestive but are not diagnostic; earache is the most useful
Usefulness of TM findings for diagnosis	1 large prospective study; myringotomy performed to confirm presence of fluid	Cloudy, bulging TMs likely to represent otitis media; mobile TMs unlikely to be infected Red – LR+ = 1; LR– = 1 Cloudy – LR+ = 7–16; LR– = 0.2–0.4 Bulging – LR+ = 14–20; LR– = 0.4–0.6 Retracted – LR+ = 1; LR– = 1 Immobile – LR+ = 3–5; LR– 0.03–0.08	Single study, question of verification bias
Usefulness of antibiotic therapy	3 Meta-analyses	NNT for pain at 2–7 days = 17. No evidence of effect on deafness	Treatment benefits are modest. Adverse outcomes of treatment or non-treatment are rare

References

1   Klein JO. Otitis media. *Clin Infect Dis* 1994;**19**:823–33.
2   Sando I, Takahashi H. Otitis media in association with various congenital diseases. Preliminary study. *Ann Otol Rhinol Laryngol* (Suppl.) 1990;**148**:13–6.
3   Davies B. Auditory disorders in Down's syndrome. *Scand Audiol* (Suppl.) 1988;**30**:65–8.
4   Douglas RM, Miles H, Hansman D, Moore B, English DT. Microbiology of acute otitis media with particular reference to the feasibility of pneumococcal immunization. *Med J Aust* 1980;**1**:263–6.
5   Heikkinen T, Thint M, Chonmaitree T. Prevalence of various respiratory viruses in the middle ear during acute otitis media. *N Engl J Med* 1999;**340**:260–4.
6   Karma P, Virtanen T, Pukander J *et al.* Branhamella catarrhalis in acute otitis media. *Acta Otolaryngol (Stockh)* 1985;**99**:285–90.
7   Luotonen J, Herva E, Karma P, Timonen M, Leinonen M, Makela PH. The bacteriology of acute otitis media in children with special reference to *Streptococcus pneumoniae* as studied by bacteriological and antigen detection methods. *Scand J Infect Dis* 1981;**13**:177–83.
8   Trujillo H, Callejas R, Mejia GI, Castrillon L. Bacteriology of middle ear fluid specimens obtained by tympanocentesis from 111 Colombian children with acute otitis media. *Pediatr Infect Dis J* 1989;**8**:361–3.
9   Ruuskanen O, Arola M, Heikkinen T, Ziegler T. Viruses in acute otitis media: increasing evidence for clinical significance. *Pediatr Infect Dis J* 1991;**10**:425–7.
10 Rosenfeld R, Vertrees J, Carr J *et al.* Clinical efficacy of antimicrobial drugs for acute otitis media: metaanalysis of 5400 children from thirty-three randomized trials. *J Pediatr* 1994;**124**:355–67.
11 Froom J, Culpepper L, Grob P *et al.* Diagnosis and antibiotic treatment of acute otitis media: report from International Primary Care Network. *BMJ* 1990;**300**:582–6.
12 Del Mar C. Spontaneously remitting disease. Principles of management. *Med J Aust* 1992;**157**:101–7.
13 van Buchem FL, Peeters MF, van't Hof MA. Acute otitis media: a new treatment strategy. *BMJ* 1985;**290**:1033–7.
14 Glasziou PP, Del Mar CB, Sanders SL, Hayem M. Treatments for acute otitis media in children: antibiotic versus placebo (Cochrane Review). In: *Cochrane Library*, Issue 1. Oxford: Update Software, 2003.
15 Kozyrskyj AL, Hildes-Ripstein GE, Longstaffe SEA *et al.* Short course antibiotics for acute otitis media (Cochrane Review). In: *Cochrane Library*, Issue 1. Oxford: Update Software, 2003.
16 Flynn CA, Griffin G, Tudiver F. Decongestants and antihistamines for acute otitis media in children (Cochrane Review). In: *Cochrane Library*, Issue 1. Oxford: Update Software, 2003.
17 Damoiseaux RA, van Balen FA, Hoes AW, de Melker RA. Antibiotic treatment of acute otitis media in children under two years of age: evidence based? *Br J Gen Pract* 1998;**48**:1861–4.
18 Takata GS, Chan LS, Shekelle P, Morton SC, Mason W, Marcy SM. Evidence assessment of management of acute otitis media: I. The role of antibiotics in treatment of uncomplicated acute otitis media. *Pediatrics* 2001;**108**:239–47.
19 Kozyrskyj AL, Hildes-Ripstein GE, Longstaffe SE *et al.* Treatment of acute otitis media with a shortened course of antibiotics: a meta-analysis. *JAMA* 1998;**279**:1736–42.
20 Bonati M, Marchetti F, Pistotti V *et al.* (Italian Working Group in Paediatric General Practice). Meta-analysis of antimicrobial prophylaxis for recurrent acute otitis media. *Clin Trials Metaanal* 1992;**28**:39–50.
21 Williams RL, Chalmers TC, Stange KC, Chalmers FT, Bowlin SJ. Use of antibiotics in preventing recurrent acute otitis media and in treating otitis media with effusion. A meta-analytic attempt to resolve the brouhaha. *JAMA* 1993;**270**:1344–51.
22 Del Mar C, Glasziou P, Hayem M. Are antibiotics indicated as initial treatment for children with acute otitis media? A meta-analysis. *BMJ* 1997;**314**:1526–9.
23 Pukander J, Karma P, Sipila M. Occurrence and recurrence of acute otitis media among children. *Acta Otolaryngol (Stockh)* 1982;**94**:479–86.
24 Sipila M, Pukander J, Karma P. Incidence of acute otitis media up to the age of 11/2 years in urban infants. *Acta Otolaryngol (Stockh)* 1987;**104**:138–45.
25 Alho OP, Koivu M, Sorri M, Rantakallio P. The occurrence of acute otitis media in infants. A life-table analysis. *Int J Pediatr Otorhinolaryngol* 1991;**21**:7–14.
26 Joki-Erkkila VP, Laippala, Pukander J. Increase in paediatric acute otitis media diagnosed by primary care in two Finnish municipalities – 1994–5 versus 1978–9. *Epidemiol Infect* 1998;**121**:529–34.
27 Aniansson G, Alm B, Andersson B *et al.* A prospective cohort study on breast-feeding and otitis media in Swedish infants. *Pediatr Infect Dis J* 1994;**13**:183–8.
28 Howie V, Schwartz R. Acute otitis media: one year in general pediatric practice. *Am J Dis Child* 1983;**137**:155–8.
29 Teele DW, Klein JO, Rosner B and the Greater Boston Otitis Media Study Group. Epidemiology of otitis media during the first seven years of life in children in greater Boston: a prospective, cohort study. *J Infect Dis* 1989;**160**:83–94.
30 Ross AK, Croft PR, Collins M. Incidence of acute otitis media in infants in a general practice. *J R Coll Gen Pract* 1988;**38**:70–2.
31 Weiss JC, Yates GR, Quinn LD. Acute otitis media: making an accurate diagnosis. *Am Fam Physician* 1996;**53**:1200–6.
32 Hayden GF, Schwartz RH. Characteristics of earache among children with acute otitis media. *Am J Dis Child* 1985;**139**:721–3.
33 Kontiokari T, Koivunen P, Niemela M, Pokka T, Uhari M. Symptoms of acute otitis media. *Pediatr Infect Dis J* 1998;**17**:676–9.
34 Heikkinen T, Ruuskanen O. Signs and symptoms predicting acute otitis media. *Arch Pediatr Adolesc Med* 1995;**149**:26–9.
35 Schwartz RH, Stool SE, Rodriguez WJ, Grundfast KM. Acute otitis media. *Clin Pediatr* 1981;**20**:549–54.
36 Uhari M, Neimala M, Hietala J. Prediction of acute otitis media with symptoms and signs. *Acta Paediatr* 1995;**84**:90–2.

37 Niemela M, Uhari M, Jounio-Ervasti K, Luotonen J, Alho O, Vierimaa E. Lack of specific symptomatology in children with acute otitis media. *Pediatr Infect Dis J* 1994;**13**:765–8.

38 Pukander J. Clinical features of acute otitis media among children. *Acta Otolaryngol (Stockh)* 1983;**95**:117–22.

39 Karma PH, Penttila MA, Sipila MM, Katajs MJ. Otoscopic diagnosis of middle ear effusion in acute and non-acute otitis media. I. The value of otoscopic findings. *Int J Pediatr Otorhinolaryngol* 1989;**17**:37–49.

40 Cavanaugh RM. Pneumatic otoscopy in healthy full-term infants. *Pediatrics* 1987;**79**:520–3.

41 Burke P, Bain J, Robinson D *et al.* Acute red ear in children: controlled trial of non-antibiotic treatment in general practice. *BMJ* 1991;**303**:558–62.

42 Thalin A, Densert O, Larsson A, Lyden E, and Ripa T. Is penicillin necessary in the treatment of acute otitis media? Proceedings of the International Conference on Acute and Secretory Otitis Media, Jerusalem. pp 441–446. In: *Proceedings of the International Conference on Acute and Secretory Otitis Media, Jerusalem*. Amsterdam: Kugler Publications, 1985.

43 van Buchem FL, Dunk JHM, van't Hof MA. Therapy of acute otitis media: myringotomy, antibiotics or neither? A double-blind study in children. *Lancet* 1981;**2**:883–7.

44 Appelman CL, Claessen JQ, Touw Otten FW, Hordijk GJ, de Melker RA. Co-amoxiclav in recurrent acute otitis media: placebo controlled study. *BMJ* 1991;**303**:1450–2.

45 Damoiseaux RAMJ, van Balen FAM, Hoes AW, Verheij TJM, de Melker RA. Primary care based randomised, double-blind trial of amoxicillin versus placebo for acute otitis media in children aged under 2 years. *BMJ* 2000;**320**:350–4.

46 Halsted C, Lepow ML, Balassanian N, Emmerich J, Wolinsky E. Otitis media: clinical observation, microbiology and evaluation of therapy. *Am J Dis Child* 1968;**115**:542–51.

47 Kaleida PH, Casselhrant ML, Rockette HE *et al.* Amoxicillin or myringotomy or both for acute otitis media: results of a randomized clinical trial. *Pediatrics* 1991;**87**:466–74.

48 Mygind N, Meistrup-Larsen K-I, Thomsen J, Thomsen VF, Josefsson K, Sorensen H. Penicillin in acute otitis media: a double-blind placebo-controlled trial. *Clin Otolaryngol* 1981;**6**:5–13.

49 Rudberg R. Sulfonamide and penicillin in acute otitis media. *Acta Otolaryngologica* 1954;**44**(Suppl.):45–65.

50 Lin RY. A perspective on penicillin allergy. *Arch Intern Med* 1992;**152**:930–7.

51 Little P, Gould C, Moore M, Warner G *et al.* Predictors of poor outcome and benefits from antibiotics in children with acute otitis media: pragmatic randomised trial. *BMJ* 2002;**325**:22–7.

34 Gastroesophageal reflux in the infant

Lynnette J Mazur, Holly D Smith

Case scenario

The parents of a 4-month-old infant present to your office because their daughter "spits up". She was exclusively breastfed for 3 months at which time the mother returned to work and began bottle feeding with a whey-based formula. The infant takes 6 oz of formula five to six times a day. She drinks eagerly and seems satisfied but "spits up" a small amount after each feed and when she is put down for a nap. She was born at term by normal spontaneous vaginal delivery. Her height, weight, and head circumference are all at the 75th percentile for age and the rest of the examination, including development, is normal. A urine culture is negative for a UTI. The parents have read about gastroesophageal reflux on the internet and have tried a time-limited trial of a hypoallergenic formula without success.[1] You think the baby has uncomplicated GER. Because she is eating and growing well, and has no respiratory or other symptoms, you do not think that treatment is needed. The parents ask whether thickening the feeds and postural change will work, and whether there are any medications that you would recommend.

Background

Gastroesophageal reflux (GER) is the return of gastric contents into the esophagus. Several factors are involved in the pathophysiology of GER including motility of the esophagus, function of the lower esophageal sphincter (LES), gastric motility and emptying, and gastric acid secretion. GER usually presents in infancy, when it is a normal physiological event, and resolves by 1 year of age. GER may be complicated by failure to thrive, aspiration pneumonia, or esophagitis (manifested by pain, feeding difficulties, or anemia). Complicated GER is referred to as gastroesophageal reflux disease (GERD). The diagnosis of GERD may be based on clinical, radiological, or histological criteria, abnormalities found during esophageal pH monitoring (EpHM) or on response to treatment.[2-5]

GER is common. In one cross-sectional survey, GER (regurgitation of at least once per day) occurred in 50% of infants > 3 months of age, 67% of infants between 4 and 6 months of age, and 5% of infants between 10 and 12 months of age.[6] Most parents perceived regurgitation as a problem only when it occurred four or more times a day and few reported treating the problem: 77 (8·1%) changed the formula, 21 (2·2%) thickened the feeds, 10 (1·1%) stopped breastfeeding, and 2 (0·2%) used medication. Without treatment, 95% were symptom-free by 1 year of age. The same authors performed a case–control study to determine how many infants outgrow GER within 1 year.[7] At follow up, the parents of neither cases nor control subjects described regurgitation as a problem. However, infants with GER were more likely to have frequent feed refusal (odds ratio [OR] = 4·2; 95% CI 1·4–12·0).

Although pediatricians consider that medications are unnecessary for the majority of infants with uncomplicated GER, thickening of the feeds and posturing are often recommended.[1,8] Feed thickeners decrease gastric contractions thereby decreasing GER. By slowing gastric emptying, thickened feeds may maintain a neutral pH in the stomach for a longer period of time after a meal, thus the late postprandial refluxate may be less hazardous to the esophageal mucosa. Two main carbohydrates are used for thickening formula – rice starch and carob bean gum. Rice cereal increases the density of feeds and may cause constipation. Carob bean gum is a soluble fiber with no nutritional value. It passes undigested into the colon where it may be fermented by bacteria and cause abdominal pain, colic, and diarrhea. Less commonly used thickening agents include pectin and cellulose, potato starch, and corn-derived products.

In contrast, most would acknowledge that the infant or child with GERD may require a medical or surgical intervention (fundoplication) to minimize morbidity – failure to thrive or recurrent aspiration. Esophagitis is treated medically using a range of products including alkalis to neutralize gastric acid and agents that inhibit gastric acid secretion, increase gastric emptying, or inhibit the gastric proton pump.

Framing answerable clinical questions

From your reading about evidence-based medicine you know that questions must be clearly formulated to ensure clear answers (Chapter 2). You think in terms of a relationship between the patient, some "exposure" (to a treatment), and one or more specific outcomes of interest and modify your original question as follows:

Questions
1. In infants with uncomplicated GER *(population)*, does feed thickening *(intervention)* compared with placebo or no treatment *(comparison)* alter the frequency of regurgitation or vomiting *(outcome)*? **[Therapy]** **2.** In infants with uncomplicated GER *(population)*, does formula type *(intervention)* affect the frequency of regurgitation or vomiting *(outcome)*? **[Therapy]** **3.** In infants with uncomplicated GER *(population)*, do different postures *(intervention)* alter the frequency of regurgitation or vomiting *(outcome)*? **[Therapy]**

General search for evidence

For questions of therapy you first search for systematic reviews or randomized controlled trials (RCTs) in the *Cochrane Library* using the term "gastroesophageal reflux". In the Cochrane Database of Systematic Reviews in 2003 you find 14 completed systematic reviews of studies of GER in adults but no reviews or protocols specifically for children. In the Database of Abstracts of Reviews of Effects (DARE) you find 12 items and in the Cochrane Controlled Trials Register you find 774 references.

You also search MedLine using PubMed and the following terms: gastroesophageal reflux, children, positioning, and thickening. After excluding letters, editorials, case reports, expert opinions, and narrative review articles you identify articles you think will help you to answer your questions. You first read and evaluate the systematic reviews and a guideline published by the North American Society of Pediatric Gastroenterology and Nutrition on the evaluation and treatment of gastroesophageal reflux in infants and children.[1] You also read the most recent, relevant RCTs.

Question
1. In infants with uncomplicated GER *(population)*, does feed thickening *(intervention)* compared with placebo or no treatment *(comparison)* alter the frequency of regurgitation or vomiting *(outcome)*? **[Therapy]**

The clinical practice guideline was an evidence-based systematic review developed by five gastroenterologists, two clinical epidemiologists, and a general pediatrician. Using the methods of the Canadian Preventive Services Task Force,[9] the quality of evidence of each of the questions as well as the recommendations made by the GER Committee was determined. Consensus was achieved through the Nominal Group Technique.[10] The studies used a combination of EpHM parameters and/or symptom scores to diagnose GER in the study participants. Although the EpHM measures a variety of parameters, the percentage of total time that the esophageal pH is < 4 (the reflux index) is considered the most valid measure of reflux because it reflects the cumulative exposure of the esophagus to acid.

After evaluating the studies on milk thickening agents, the committee found that the thickening agents did not improve reflux EpHM index scores but that they did decrease the number of episodes of visible reflux. Therefore, they suggested that parents and clinicians could consider thickeners for the treatment of uncomplicated GER in infants (happy spitters). Because this is such a common issue in your practice, you decide to review the primary studies.

You find eight trials evaluating the effect of feed thickening on GER,[11–18] one RCT,[11] six randomized cross-over trials, and one before-after study (see the Summary Table at the end of this chapter).[12–17] In the double-blind RCT, Vandenplas[11] used symptoms (reflux diary) and laboratory (EpHM) outcome criteria to study the effect of thickening feeds in 20 term infants (1 week to 4 months of age) with a history of GER for > 5 days and a pH < 4 on EpHM for 10–30% of the time. The number of regurgitations decreased significantly in both the treatment group (formula thickened with carob bean gum, prone positioning, parental reassurance) and the placebo group (the same formula without thickening, prone positioning, parental reassurance). The difference between the groups was not statistically significant, suggesting that factors other than feed thickening were responsible for improvement in symptoms.

In a blinded randomized cross-over trial, Fabiani[12] evaluated the effect of feed thickening with a water-soluble fiber (galactomannans) on gastric emptying time in 47 infants with frequent (≥ 5 episodes/week) regurgitation or vomiting. The mean gastric emptying time was similar with the unthickened and thickened formula (136 minutes *v* 133 minutes). However, vomiting occurred in 18 (38%) infants who received the standard formula and in 6 (13%) who received the fiber-enriched formula ($P < 0.05$).

In a blinded randomized cross-over trial, Orenstein[13] found a decrease in GER in the postprandial period in 20 infants receiving feeds thickened with rice cereal as measured by vomiting episodes per 90 minutes ($P = 0.015$) or volume per 90 minutes ($P = 0.023$). Gastric emptying (18 *v* 22%; $P = 0.04$), time spent crying (11·7 minutes *v* 17·6 minutes;

$P = 0.042$) and total time spent awake (45 minutes *v* 53 minutes; $P = 0.026$) were also significantly decreased in infants receiving thickened feeds. However, when GER was defined by scintigraphy, thickened and unthickened meals were followed by similar amounts of GER. An unexpected finding was that infants fed thickened formula tended to cough more frequently (2·8 times *v* 1·3 times in the postprandial period; $P = 0.075$). A later blinded randomized cross-over study[14] confirmed a relationship between thickened feeds and coughing in 33 infants. However, other clinical outcomes were not considered. Confirmation and definitive explanation of the results await further study, aimed at determining whether the increased coughing represents microaspiration, adherence of the particles of rice cereal to the larynx, or some other effect. Orenstein postulated that non-regurgitant reflux may also lead to esophagitis and/or pulmonary problems.

In a randomized cross-over trial of 19 infants, Sutphen found that infants receiving a higher osmolality feed (D10W compared with D5W), had more GER (measured by postprandial EpHM). Because the osmolalities (mosm kg^{-1} H2O) of D5W (297), D10W (594), breast milk (75), and formula (110–125) are different, the results may not be comparable or applicable to your patients.[15] Also, it is unclear if the observers were blinded to allocation of treatments.

In a non-randomized cross-over trial Wenzl[16] examined the influence of thickening a formula with carob bean gum on acid and non-acid GER: 14 infants who were alternately fed thickened and non-thickened formula during six feeding intervals. Although the formulae were similar, it is unclear if the observers were blinded to treatment groups. GER was documented by simultaneous EpHM and intraesophageal impedance (IMP), which detects bolus movements inside a luminal organ. Clinically significant decreases in regurgitation frequency (15 *v* 68 episodes) and amount (severity score 0·6 *v* 1·8) were noted after feedings with thickened formula. The difference in GER documented by IMP was also pronounced (536 *v* 647 episodes). Mean GER duration and the frequency of acid (pH < 4) GER were not altered.

Bailey reported variable EpHM results in a non-blinded, non-randomized cross-over study in 52 infants who were given apple juice.[17] There was no significant difference between infants receiving thickened and unthickened feedings in the percentage of GER time, frequency, or duration of reflux in the 2 hours after feeds in any position except for the 30-degree prone position. In this position, thickened feeds significantly increased the percent of reflux time, $P < 0.006$. Improvement or worsening of reflux was arbitrarily defined as > 30% change in the time when distal esophageal pH was < 4. Using this definition, GER improved in one-third of patients, was unchanged in one-third, and increased in one-third after thickened feeds. Possible explanations for this "negative" study are that the study lacked power to detect a difference between groups and the use of EpHM, rather than clinical symptoms, was used to determine improvement. It is also possible that apple juice and formula may yield different results and that rice cereal may induce constipation, increase abdominal pressure, and result in GER.

In a before-after study by Vandenplas, the effect of feed thickening varied according to the outcome measure used.[18] Significant clinical improvement was noticed in 25 (80%) of the infants studied and "regurgitation and emesis lessened or disappeared totally" with thickened feeds. However, symptoms were not well defined or quantified and it is not clear whether the observers were blinded to the intervention. When EpHM was used to define GER, treatment decreased the number of reflux episodes (34·5 *v* 15·1; $P < 0.002$) but increased the duration of the longest reflux episode (23·2–56·6; $P < 0.001$). Other indices of reflux and the number of reflux episodes > 5 minutes per 24 hours were similar between groups. Because of the increased duration of the longest reflux episode, Vandenplas concluded that thickening agents might lead to esophagitis or respiratory dysfunction. However, the weak study design and lack of a control group makes you question the validity of these results.[18]

In summary, despite the differences in GER definitions, diagnostic tools, and outcome measures, the overall quality of the evidence is good. Although the RCT by Vandenplas had the strongest design, the magnitude of the power to detect a difference was not addressed. More importantly, however, the study predated the finding of the association between sudden infant death and the prone position. In aggregate, the studies suggest that visible reflux is decreased but that reflux as measured by EpHM is unchanged by thickened feedings.

Question

2. In infants with uncomplicated GER *(population)*, does formula type *(intervention)* affect the frequency of regurgitation or vomiting *(outcome)*? **[Therapy]**

The clinical practice guideline states that there is evidence to support a 1–2 week trial of a hypoallergenic formula in formula-fed infants with GER.[1]

You identify six relevant studies (see Summary Table at end of this chapter). Two were RCTs[19,20] and four were case–control studies.[21–24] One of the case–control studies compared formula with water and/or glucose solution.[24] You question whether the results are applicable to your patient, especially when studies on human milk and formula are available.

The RCT by Sutphen showed no difference in 2-hour postprandial emptying times among 28 infants receiving formulae containing medium chain triglycerides (experimental) and long chain triglycerides.[19] Although MCT formulae are available (Portagen and Pregestimil), they are rarely used in a general pediatric practice. This limits the generalizability of the results to your patient.

In a large RCT, Weisbrod studied regurgitation in over 700 neonates who received either a ready-to-use or powdered formulae. Infants who were given the ready-to-use formulae had significantly more regurgitation than those fed with powdered formulas.[20] It is unclear whether the observers were blinded to the intervention and the size of the effect is not given.

Billeaud's case–control study included 201 infants between birth and 12 months of age with "digestive symptoms". Subjects were divided into case and control groups based on the results of scintigraphy; 111 with positive results (cases) and 90 with negative results (controls). The effects of milk composition and the influence of gastroesophageal reflux on gastric emptying were studied. Gastric emptying time was fastest with human milk, followed by whey-predominant, whey-adapted, casein-predominant, follow up formula, and cow's milk. Contrary to expectations, gastric emptying was slightly more rapid in children with GER, $P < 0.05$.[21]

The aim of the case–control study by Van Den Driessche was to compare the rate of gastric emptying in infants fed formula milk and in those fed breast milk using a new, non-invasive technique (^{13}C-octanoic acid breath test). Results indicated faster gastric emptying with breast milk (47 minutes v 65 minutes, $P < 0.05$).[22]

The case–control study by Hillemeier evaluated gastric emptying and reflux time in patients with varying degrees of illness, but formula types were not compared.[23]

Although results of the case–control studies agree, they provide lower level evidence when compared with RCTs. They are studies done "after the fact" and the results may be subject to bias if the cases and controls are not chosen correctly. However, the RCTs were limited by the use of an experimental formula in one and a time-limited study in neonates in the other. Therefore, you conclude that human milk has the fastest gastric emptying and that whey-predominant formulae are a close second. However, the question of a cause and effect relationship between delayed gastric emptying and GER remains unanswered. Even if gastric emptying time and GER are related, it is difficult to state which came first, reflux or delayed gastric emptying. In a letter to the editor by Dimler, it was suggested that reflux is the cause of delayed emptying, rather than vice versa.[25] On the basis of the work by Wilbur and Kelly, "Gastric emptying of liquid occurs when the intraluminal pressure in the stomach exceeds that in the duodenum…Greater pressures in the stomach have been correlated with faster gastric emptying."[26] Therefore, it would seem possible that the presence of gastroesophageal reflux would supply a "pop-off" valve to keep the pressure in the fundus from achieving adequate levels to empty into the duodenum.

Question

3. In infants with uncomplicated GER (*population*), do different postures (*intervention*) alter the frequency of regurgitation or vomiting (*outcome*)? **[Therapy]**

The clinical practice guideline states: "Prone positioning has been recommended for the treatment and prevention of GER in infants. However, this advice conflicts with the recent recognition that prone positioning is associated with a higher rate of sudden infant death syndrome (SIDS). The Nordic epidemiological SIDS study demonstrated that the odds ratio of SIDS mortality was 13·9 for the prone position and 3·5 for the side position when compared with the supine position."

You identify 11 relevant studies (see the Summary Table at the end of this chapter).[27–38] Two were RCTs,[27,28] four were randomized cross-over trials,[29–32] three were case–control studies,[33–35] and two were case series,[33,37] which you would only consider in the absence of better quality evidence. All showed that prone positioning was better for gastric emptying in the 2-hour postprandial period.

The RCT by Yu[27] studied the effect of body position on gastric emptying in 48 neonates. Results showed that the stomach emptied more rapidly in the prone and right lateral positions than in the supine and left lateral positions.

In the RCT by Tobin[28], 24 infants were randomly assigned to one of the 24 permutations of four positions (supine, prone, right, left). During the first 24 hours the infant was held horizontally, and then the permutation was repeated at 30 degrees head elevation, giving a total of eight study segments for each infant. Gastroesophageal reflux expressed as reflux index (mean %) was significantly less in the prone and left lateral positions (6·72 and 7·69 respectively) than in the supine and right lateral positions (15·33 and 12·02, $P < 0.001$). Head elevation did not affect any variables significantly.[28]

In a randomized, cross-over study, Orenstein[29] compared two types of prone positioning in 100 infants less than 6 months of age to determine whether the effort involved in maintaining the head-elevated position was justified by a significant reduction in GER. She found that in 90 subjects with abnormal reflux, no measurement of reflux was significantly better in the head-elevated position than in the prone position. For all 100 subjects, only two of the 10 EpHM measurements were significantly improved by elevation of the head: the frequency of postprandial episodes ($P < 0.05$) and the frequency of postprandial episodes lasting longer than five minutes ($P < 0.005$). Although statistically significant, the mean number of episodes per 120 minutes in flat prone and head-elevated was 7·5 and 5·9 respectively and the mean number of postprandial episodes lasting longer than 5 minutes was 1·4 and 1·2 respectively. One must question if these are clinically significant. No relative risk reduction is given.[29]

In a smaller randomized cross-over study by Orenstein[30] comparing the upright and prone positions in nine infants with GER, EpHM demonstrated significantly longer exposure to GER in the seated compared with the prone position, $P = 0.023$. Orenstein suggests a number of explanations for the detrimental effect of the infant seat.[30] The same authors' comparison study of the infant seat and prone-elevated positioning showed a reduction of reflux time (shorter individual episodes and fewer episodes) in the prone position.[31]

Orenstein also evaluated the effect of pacifier use (non-nutritive sucking) on GER in 48 infants. She found that pacifier use significantly affected only the frequency of reflux episodes, increasing it in prone infants ($P = 0.04$) and decreasing it in seated infants ($P = 0.003$).[32]

In a case–control study that followed the pacifier study non-pacifier periods for the same 48 were analyzed for the effects on behavior state of prone versus seated positioning: 24 infants were positioned continuously prone and 24 remained seated during a 120-minute postprandial period. The prone position was associated with more sleep time, 83.5 v 43 minutes, $P = 0.01$. The increase in sleep time in the prone position could be largely accounted for by a tendency toward a decrease in crying time.[33]

Meyers studied the effect of position and sleep or awake state on the frequency, percent time, and mean duration of reflux episodes as determined by EpHM in 128 infants (79 with GER, 49 controls).[34] In this case–control study, cases had less reflux during sleep than when awake but, while awake, children in the 30-degree prone position was significantly less reflux than children in the either supine ($P < 0.001$) or upright positions ($P < 0.01$). The control group had no change in reflux with any position or wake/sleep state. Although not statistically compared, the mean age was 11.6 months in cases and 28.8 months in controls. The generalizability of the results to your patient is also limited by the large number of study participants with associated health problems; 11 had neurological disorders, seven had respiratory disease, and four had esophageal dysmotility.[34]

In a case–control study, Vandenplas found that the infants < 10 days of age had less GER in the 30 degree prone position than the head-elevated position,[35] but similar EpHM values. The head-elevated and prone positions were not compared in the same infants. The supine right and left lateral positions appeared to have similar EpHM values but statistical analyses were not performed. The question of power to detect a difference is left unanswered.[35]

All studies used the 2-hour postprandial period because reflux is frequent during this time in normal infants and symptoms are often most severe during the early postprandial period. One could question if the results from a limited period of time are representative of the effects for chronic positioning. One disadvantage of the cross-over study design is that the ability to study late effects of treatment is lost.

Studies of fluid-gas retentions in the stomach in young infants in different positions show that when supine, fluid accumulates in the fundus which is in the most dependent position of the stomach; and the air bubble rises to the highest part, the pyloric antrum. The fluid-filled fundus acts as a barrier to prevent eructation and hence the supine position may predispose to regurgitation and inhalation.[37]

You conclude that position can have a profound effect on gastric emptying time and reflux measurements and that prone position has the best emptying time. However, most of the studies were done before the association of the prone sleep position with the sudden infant death syndrome became known. In 1992 the American Academy of Pediatrics Task Force on Infant Positioning and SIDS stated: "…for the well infant who was born at term and has no medical complications, the Academy recommends that these infants be placed down for sleep on either their side or back." They do however make a qualifying statement for children with GER "For…infants with symptoms of gastroesophageal reflux…prone may well be the position of choice. It should be stressed that, although the relative risk of the prone position may be several times that of the lateral or supine position, the actual risk of SIDS when placing an infant in a prone position is still extremely low".[37] Although the prone position is the single best position for gastric emptying, the lateral position may be the next best.[37]

Summary

GER is a normal physiological event in young infants and uncomplicated GER will usually resolve without treatment over time. However, frequent vomiting is distressing to parents, who frequently ask for therapy. Prone posturing, which has been shown in RCTs to decrease GER is associated with an increase risk of SIDS and should not be recommended in infants with uncomplicated GER. As this chapter indicates, there is a paucity of good quality RCTs evaluating the role of feed thickening and changes to feed composition (including osmolality, protein, triglyseride content) in infants with GER. Education of mothers, carers, and health workers is needed about the benign nature of GER in most infants, the potential benefits of breastfeeding and the symptoms and signs that might indicate complicated GER disease and the need for investigation and therapy.

Resolution of the scenario

You reassure the infant's mother that GER is a developmentally normal event that is usually uncomplicated and significantly improves with time and without treatment. You suggest she continue with the infant's current formula feeds without thickening and advise her against placing the baby in the prone position because of the increased risk of SIDS.

Future research needs

- RCTs are needed to assess a wider range of formula composition in the treatment of uncomplicated as well as complicated GER in infants.

- RCTs are needed to assess the value of thickened feeds, now that the prone position's association with SIDS is known.
- Studies are needed to determine the most effective ways to encourage mothers to breast feed.

Summary table

Question	Type of Evidence	Result	Comment
Feed thickening (carob or rice cereal)	One RCT	No added benefit beyond positioning and parental reassurance	Power not addressed Prone positioning associated with SIDS
	Four randomized cross-over trials	Benefit in 3	Results differed depending on whether symptoms or EpHM measured
	Two non-randomized cross-over trials	Benefit in 1	
	One Before-After	Benefit	
Formula type (variations in osmolality, triglyceride type, long chain triglycerides, milk protein) Infants receiving, powdered milk	Two RCTs Four case–control studies Gastric emptying used as a proxy for symptoms and/or EpHM	No difference Have less GER	Study of neonates limits between medium generalizability
Positioning Supine versus non-supine posture	Two RCTs Four randomized cross-over trials Three case–control studies	GER decreased in prone compared to right and left lateral supine, and seated positions	

References

1 North American Society for Pediatric Gastroenterology and Nutrition. Guidelines for evaluation and treatment of gastroesophageal reflux in infants and children. *J Pediatr Gastroenterol Nutr* 2001;**32**:S1–S31.

2 Cucchiara S, Staiano A, Gobio CL, Boccieri A, Paone FM. Value of the 24 hour intraoesophageal pH monitoring in children. *Gut* 1990;**31**:129–33.

3 Koch A, Gass R. Continuous 20–24 hour Esophageal pH-monitoring in infancy. *J Pediatr Surg* 1981;**16**:109 13.

4 Tolia V, Calhoun JA, Kuhns LR, Kauffman RE. Lack of correlation between extended pH monitoring and scintigraphy in the evaluation of infants with gastroesophageal reflux. *J Lab Clin Med* 1990;**115**:559–63.

5 Gustafsson PM, Tibbling L. 24-hour oesophageal two-level pH monitoring in healthy children and adolescents. *Scan J Gastroenterol* 1988;**23**:91–4.

6 Nelson SP, Chen EH, Syniar GM *et al.* Prevalence of symptoms of gastroesophageal reflux during infancy: a pediatric practice-based survey. *Arch Pediatr Adolesc Med* 1997;**151**:569–72.

7 Nelson SP, Chen EH, Syniar GM *et al.* One-year follow up of symptoms of gastroesophageal reflux during infancy. Pediatrics 1998;**102**:6/e67.

8 Vandenplas Y, Belli D, Banhamou P *et al.* A critical appraisal of current management practices for infant regurgitation–recommendations of a working party. *Eur J Pediatr* 1997; **156**:343–57.

9 Examination Canadian Task Force of Preventive Health. The periodic health examination. *Can Med Assoc J* 1979;**121**:119.

10 McMurray AR. Three decision-making aids: brainstorming, nominal group, Delphi technique. *J Nurs Staff Dev* 1994;**10**: 62–5.

11 Vandenplas Y, Hachimi-Idrissi S, Casteels A, Mahler T, Loeb H. A clinical trial with an "anti-regurgitation" formula. *Eur J Pediatr* 1994;**153**:419–23.

12 Fabiani E, Bolli V, Pieroni G *et al.* Effect of a water-soluble fiber (galactomannans)-enriched formula on gastric emptying time of regurgitating infants evaluated using an ultrasound technique. *J Pediatr Gastroenterol Nutr* 2000;**31**:248–50.

13 Orenstein SR, Magill HL, Brooks P. Thickening of infant feedings for therapy of gastroesophageal reflux. *J Pediatr* 1987;**110**:181–6.

14 Orenstein SR, Shalaby TM, Putman PE. Thickened feedings as a cause of increased coughing when used as therapy for gastroesophageal reflux in infants. *J Pediatr* 1992;**121**:913–15.

15 Sutphen JL, Dillard VL. Dietary caloric density and osmolality influence gastroesophageal reflux in infants. *Gastroenterology* 1989;**97**:601–4.

16 Wenzl TG, Schneider S, Scheele F, Silny J, Heimann G, Skopnik H. Effects of thickened feeding on gastroesophageal reflux in infants: A placebo-controlled cross-over study using intraluminal impedance. *Pediatrics* 2003;**111**:e355–9.

17 Bailey DJ, Andres JM, Danek GS, Pineiro-Carrero VM. Lack of efficacy of thickened feeding as treatment for gastroesophageal reflux. *J Pediatr* 1987;**110**:187–9.

18 Vandenplas Y, Sacre L. Milk-thickening agents as a treatment for gastroesophageal reflux. *Clin Pediatr* 1987;**26**:66–8.

19 Sutphen JL, Dillard VL. Medium chain triglyceride in the therapy of gastroesophageal reflux. *J Pediatr Gastroenterol Nutr* 1992;**14**:38–40.

20 Weisbrod M, Mimouni FB. Feeding tolerance of ready-to-use versus powdered formulas in neonates. *Isr Med Assoc J* 2000 Oct;**2**:787–9.

21 Billeaud C, Guillet J, Sandler B. Gastric emptying in infants with or without gastro-oesophageal reflux according to type of milk. *Eur J Clin Nutr* 1990;**44**:577–83.

22 Van Den Driessche M, Peeters K, Marien P, Ghoos Y, Devlieger H, Veereman-Wauters G. Gastric emptying in formula-fed and breast-fed infants measured with the C-octanoic acid breath test. *J Pediatr Gastroenterol Nutr* 1999;**29**:46–51.

23 Hillemeier AC, Lange R, McCallum R, Seashore J, Gryboski J. Delayed gastric emptying in infants with gastroesophageal reflux. *J Pediatr* 1981;**98**:190–3.

24 Euler AR, Byrne WJ. Gastric emptying times of water in infants and children: Comparison of those with and without gastroesophageal reflux. *J Pediatr Gastro Nutr* 1983;**2**:595–8.

25 Dimler M. Delayed gastric emptying and gastroesophageal reflux. *J Pediatr* 1981;**105**:504.

26 Wilbur BG, Kelly KA. Effect of proximal gastric, complete gastric, and truncal vagotomy on canine gastric electric activity, motility, and emptying. *Ann Surg* 1973;**178**:295.

27 Yu VYH. Effect of body position on gastric emptying in the neonate. *Arch Dis Child* 1975;**50**:500–4.

28 Tobin JM, McCLoud P, Cameron DJS. Posture and gastro-oesophageal reflux: a case for left lateral positioning. *Arch Dis Chil* 1997;**76**:254–8.

29 Orenstein SR. Prone positioning in infant gastroesophageal reflux: Is elevation of the head worth the trouble? *J Pediatr* 1990;**117**:184–7.

30 Orenstein SR, Whitington PF, Orenstein D. The infant seat as treatment for gastroesophageal reflux. *New Engl J Med* 1983;**309**:760–3.

31 Orenstein SR, Whitington PF. Positioning for prevention of infant gastroesophageal reflux. *J Pediatr* 1983;**103**:534–7.

32 Orenstein SR. Effect of nonnutritive sucking on infant gastroesophageal reflux. *Pediatr Res* 1988;**24**:38–40.

33 Orenstein SR. Effects of behavior state of prone versus seated positioning for infants with gastroesophageal reflux. *Pediatrics* 1990;**85**:765–8.

34 Meyers WF, Herbst JJ. Effectiveness of positioning therapy for gastroesophageal reflux. *Pediatrics* 1982;**69**:768–72.

35 Vandenplas Y, Sacre-Smits. Seventeen-hour continuous esophageal pH monitoring in the newborn: Evaluation of the influence of position on asymptomatic and symptomatic babies. *J Pediatr Gastroenterol Nutr* 1985;**4**:356–61.

36 Hood JH. Effect of posture on the amount and distribution of gas in the intestinal tract of infants and young children. *Lancet* 1964;**2**:1007.

37 American Academy of Pediatrics Task Force of Infant Positioning and SIDS. *Pediatrics* 1992;**89**:690–6.

35 Gastroesophageal reflux in the adolescent

Holly D Smith, Lynnette J Mazur

Case scenario

A 16-year-old Hispanic boy presents to your clinic complaining of "heartburn" for the last 3–4 months. The pain occurs several times a week; is worse after meals, is burning in nature and radiates up his mid-chest. At times there is a sour taste in his mouth. He has tried some over-the-counter antacids without relief. You ask about his diet and he says he likes fried foods, chocolate, and drinks several carbonated drinks every day. On weekends, he smokes a few cigarettes and drinks a few beers with his friends. His height is at the 50th percentile, he weighs 85 kg (> 95th percentile), and he has a body mass index of 28 kg m^{-2}. The physical examination is normal. He asks what you can do to help.

Background

Gastroesophageal reflux (GER) is the return of gastric contents into the esophagus. Several factors are involved in the pathophysiology of GER, including the motility of the esophagus, function of the lower esophageal sphincter, gastric motility and emptying, and gastric acid secretion. GER is physiological in infancy and usually resolves by 1 year of age. Complicated GER is referred to as gastroesophageal reflux disease (GERD). This may occur in older children, who may present with heartburn, epigastric pain, regurgitation, or dysphagia. The diagnosis of GERD may be based on clinical, radiological, or histological criteria, abnormalities found during esophageal pH monitoring (EpHM) or on response to treatment.

One survey of over 1700 parents and children determined the prevalence of symptoms consistent with GER in 3 to 17 year old children.[1] The prevalence of symptoms varied with age and depended on how the question was asked and whether the parent or the child answered the question (Table 35.1). In children aged between 10 and 17 years,

heartburn was associated with cigarette use (odds ratio [OR] 6·5; 95% CI 2–21). According to parents of children aged 3–9 years, 0·5% of children used antacid treatment in the past week. In children aged 10–17 years, antacid use in the past week was 1·9% according to parents and 2·3% according to the children. According to parents, none of the children used over-the-counter histamine receptor antagonists. However, when children aged 10–17 answered this question themselves, 1·3% said they used these medications. Thus, although symptoms suggestive of GER are reported in 5–8% of children in late childhood, only a fraction of these children receive treatment.

Treatment of GER often includes recommendations for lifestyle change, including changes to diet (avoidance of alcohol, caffeine, chocolate, fatty foods), weight loss, and avoidance of tobacco. Alcohol decreases lower esophageal sphincter pressure and adults with GER complain of heartburn after drinking alcohol. As a result, physicians often recommend that people with heartburn refrain from alcohol. Caffeine may induce heartburn through its effect on decreasing lower esophageal sphincter pressure (LESP) and

Table 35.1 Prevalence of GER symptoms reported by parents and children

	Parents of children aged 3–9 years	Parents of children age 10–17 years	Children aged 10–17 years
Heartburn	1·8%	3·5%	5·2%
Epigastric pain	7·2%	3·0%	5·0%
Regurgitation	2·3%	1·4%	8·3%

some studies suggest that cigarette smoking has a similar effect on LESP.[2,3]

A range of medical treatments is used to treat symptoms, including alkalis to neutralize gastric acid and agents that inhibit gastric acid secretion, increase gastric emptying, or inhibit the gastric proton pump.

Framing answerable clinical questions

You know that clinical questions must be clearly formulated to facilitate the search for answers (Chapter 2). You think in terms of a relationship between the patient, some "exposure" or intervention (a treatment), and one or more specific outcomes of interest. You modify your original questions as follows:

Questions

1. In adolescents with GER (*population*), do lifestyle and dietary factors increase the risk of GER symptoms (*outcome*)? **[Causation/harm]**
2. In adolescents with GER (*population*), does treatment with a cholinergic agent (*intervention*) compared with placebo or other medications (*comparison*), reduce the frequency of GER symptoms without added risk (*outcome*)*?* **[Therapy]**
3. In adolescents with GER (*population*), does treatment with prokinetic agents (*intervention*) compared with placebo or other medications (*comparison*), reduce the frequency of GER symptoms without added risk (*outcome*)*?* **[Therapy]**
4. In adolescents with GER (*population*), does treatment with proton pump inhibitors (*intervention*), compared with placebo or other medications (comparison), reduce the frequency of GER symptoms without added risk (*outcome*)*?* **[Therapy]**
5. In adolescents with GER (*population*), does treatment with antacids and surface agents (*interventions*), compared with placebo or other medications (*comparison*), reduce the frequency of GER symptoms without added risk (*outcome*)? **[Therapy]**
6. In adolescents with GER (*population*), does obesity increase the risk of GER symptoms (*outcome*)? **[Causation/harm]**
7. In adolescents with GER (*population*), does treatment with H₂ blockers and other acid suppressants (*intervention*), compared with placebo or other medications (*comparison*), reduce the frequency of GER symptoms without added risk (*outcome*)*?* **[Therapy]**

Searching for evidence

When a harmful association between a risk factor and a symptom or disease is observed, it is important to establish that this was causal and not a chance finding or a finding due to confounding or bias in the study. You know that the best study type to establish causation is a randomized controlled trial (RCT) (see Chapter 7). If no RCTs are available, you will look for cohort studies or case–control studies.

For questions of therapy you will search for good quality systematic reviews of RCTs (see Chapter 6). You are most interested in studies that report clinical outcomes, rather than proxy outcomes such as changes to esophageal pH or LESP. Ideally, such studies would compare the therapy under question with placebo and would include adolescent or young adult patients with GER and/or heartburn.

The *Cochrane Library*'s Database of Systematic Reviews lists no completed reviews for "gastroesophageal reflux" in adolescents but lists four reviews that may be relevant for an adolescent. The Database of Abstracts of Reviews of Effects (DARE) lists six items that might be useful. In the Cochrane Central Register of Controlled Trials (CENTRAL), you find 774 references, almost all of which address pharmacological therapy. You also search MedLine using PubMed and the following terms: gastroesophageal reflux, adolescent AND therapy. After excluding letters, editorials, case reports, expert opinions, and narrative review articles you identify a number of articles, you think will help you to answer your questions. For the purpose of this chapter, you decide to read only the best available evidence and to evaluate its quality and applicability to your patient population. You first read and evaluate the systematic reviews and a guideline published by the North American Society of Pediatric Gastroenterology and Nutrition on the evaluation and treatment of gastroesophageal reflux in infants and children.[4] You also read the most recent, relevant RCTs.

Question

1. In adolescents with GER (*population*), do lifestyle and dietary factors increase the risk of GER symptoms (*outcome*)? **[Causation/harm]**

Alcohol

You identify no RCTs but find five relevant cohort studies. Pehl[5] recruited young, healthy volunteers and performed 24 hour-EpHM for 3 days. Fifteen subjects drank white wine (400 ml) on the first day and water (400 ml) on day 2; 11 subjects drank ethanol on day 3 and had 24-hour EpHM. The primary study showed that white wine significantly increased reflux compared with ethanol ($P < 0.001$) and water ($P < 0.001$). In a subset of subjects, the author compared people who drank white wine, beer, 7-Up (pH < 3.2), and water. The lower esophageal pH was checked immediately after drinking and three hours later. The secondary study showed that white wine increased reflux compared with beer ($P < 0.01$), water ($P < 0.001$), and 7-Up ($P < 0.05$). There was no difference in results between 7-Up and water.

Vitale[6] recruited 17 young healthy, volunteers to undergo 20-hour EpHM. After a low fat evening meal, they drank either 120 ml of whisky or 120 ml of water and lay supine 2 hours later. On EpHM, 7 of 17 had prolonged asymptomatic acid reflux (average duration 47.1 minutes) 3.5 hours after drinking whisky but not after drinking water. There was no difference in the number of symptomatic reflux events between groups. One explanation for the lack of symptoms may have been that the subjects were too inebriated to notice.

Using EpHM, Kaufman[7] compared results of 3-hour EpHM in 12 young healthy volunteers who had drank orange juice and vodka with breakfast and volunteers who drank orange juice and water with breakfast. Significantly higher reflux scores were found in those who drank vodka in each of the 3-hour periods ($P = 0.0105$, $P = 0.0034$, and $P = 0.0156$, respectively) and for the entire period ($P = 0.0005$). Comparison with other studies is difficult because the methods in this study varied from those used in more recent studies, in that the pH probes were positioned lower in the esophagus (3 cm above LES) and the threshold for reflux (pH < 5) was higher.

Two other studies addressed alcohol use as a risk factor for GER. In a population-based study Locke[8] showed that intake of more than seven alcoholic drinks per week increased GER symptoms. In contrast, the large National Health and Nutrition Examination Survey (NHANES I)[9] cohort study failed to detect an association between alcohol use and GER. However, this study is not directly comparable because the outcome of interest was risk of hospitalization for GER, rather than symptoms of GER.

You conclude that there is some evidence that alcohol increases acid reflux and GER symptoms. You will recommend to your patient that avoidance of alcohol might reduce his heartburn.

Caffeine

You identify no RCTs but six relevant studies. Four showed a positive association between caffeine and symptoms of GER.[10–13] A double blinded, cross-over study by Brazer[10] included 20 subjects with a minimum 1-year history of heartburn associated with coffee drinking. Over a 1-hour period, participants drank three different coffees (American, European treated, and European untreated). Afterwards, a high fat meal was consumed. EpHM revealed a significant difference between the American coffee and untreated European coffee in terms of symptoms ($P < 0.05$) and acid contact time ($P = 0.005$). There was no difference in the heartburn or regurgitation severity indices between groups.

Differences between coffees were not defined and both the fatty meal and the large fluid volume in a short period of time may be confounding factors.

In the cross-over study by Pehl,[11] 17 patients with GER were randomly given regular coffee on one day and decaffeinated coffee on the next. After each, they had a 3-hour EpHM. The fraction of time with the pH < 4 was significantly greater in participants who drank caffeinated compared with those who drank decaffeinated coffee ($P < 0.001$). Effects on symptoms were not studied.

In a cross-over study by Wendl,[12] 16 young healthy volunteers drank various beverages to assess the effect of caffeine on GER. In the initial study, subjects were randomly allocated to drink regular coffee, decaffeinated coffee, or water on three separate days. After drinking, they had a 3-hour EpHM. Two additional studies with a subset of subjects were also performed. In the first subset, six subjects drank tea, decaffeinated tea, or coffee with caffeine in the same concentration as tea on three consecutive days and EpHM was performed. In the second subset of subjects, eight drank either regular water or water with caffeine. GER, as measured by EpHM, was significantly greater in people who drank caffeinated coffee than decaffeinated coffee or water ($P < 0.05$). There was no difference in EpHM results in those who drank tea, decaffeinated tea, or water. However, caffeinated tea caused significantly more GER than decaffeinated tea ($P < 0.05$). There was no difference between regular water and water with caffeine. The authors concluded that caffeine alone is not responsible for GER but that other components in coffee may contribute to the effect. Effects of caffeine on GER symptoms were not studied.

In a case–control study by Elta,[13] 58 patients with duodenal ulcers, 55 patients with non-ulcer dyspepsia, and 55 asymptomatic controls completed a questionnaire about their intakes of coffee, tea, and caffeinated soda. Caffeine intake was similar for each group. Coffee-induced peptic symptoms were more common in the group with non-ulcer dyspepsia than in the controls ($P = 0.036$).

Studies that show no association between caffeine and GER include one cross-over trial and one cohort study.[9,14] In the cross-over study by Van Nieuwenhoven,[14] young male athletes were given water, a sports drink, or a sports drink with caffeine during 90 minutes of exercise over three separate days. EpHM performed before, during, and after exercise failed to detect a difference between the drinks. Results of a cohort study by Ruhl[9] showed that use of coffee or tea does not increase the risk of hospitalization for GER.

The quality of the evidence to address this question is limited and conflicting and few studies examined clinical outcomes. There is some evidence that caffeine decreases LESP and increases acid reflux and that it may cause "peptic symptoms". You explain this to your patient and suggest he limit his intake of caffeine.

Chocolate

Two studies examining the relationship between chocolate and GER were identified. In a case–control study, Murphy[15] assessed the relationship between chocolate ingestion and esophageal acid exposure using EpHM. Compared with a dextrose control solution of similar volume, osmolality, and calories, the ingestion of chocolate resulted in a significant increase in acid exposure in the first postprandial hour in patients with esophagitis. Clinical outcomes were not reported.

In the case series by Wright,[16] LESP was monitored for a 15-minute basal period and for 60 minutes after ingestion of chocolate syrup alone or of chocolate syrup with either a commercial antacid, oral bethanecol, or subcutaneous bethanecol. After the ingestion of chocolate, the mean basal LESP decreased significantly ($P < 0.01$). An identical response occurred when chocolate was given with antacid. An increased in LESP was observed when chocolate was given with oral or subcutaneous bethanecol ($P < 0.05$). Clinical outcomes were not reported. You advise your patient that there is insufficient evidence that chocolate causes symptomatic GER.

Fatty foods

Fatty foods are commonly considered detrimental in patients with GER. You find eight studies addressing the association between fatty foods and GER.[9,17–23] Six are RCTs or randomized cross-over trials,[17–22] one is a cohort study,[9] and one is a case-control study.[23]

In a randomized cross-over study, Becker[20] evaluated 20 young volunteers who neither smoked nor drank alcohol: 10 patients were healthy and 10 had symptomatic GERD. On consecutive days the subjects were given either a high fat (61%) or low fat (16%) meal. Both meals were from McDonald's, were eaten by mouth, and were of equal volume. Postprandial EpHM was performed in upright and recumbent positions. There was significantly more GER in healthy volunteers in the upright position after a high fat meal. No other differences between groups were noted. Because the meals were not isocaloric, the effect of total caloric count may have confounded the effect of fat on GER.

In a randomized cross-over trial by Colombo,[21] 13 young healthy volunteers were fed a high fat meal (58%), a low fat meal (23%), and a low fat (25%) low calorie meal over 3 separate days. While the subjects ate a ham and cheese sandwich and drank 250 ml of Coca Cola, 300 ml of a high fat, low fat, or low fat low calorie solutions was given through a nasogastric tube. EpHM showed significantly more GER 6 hours after the high calorie than the low caloric meal ($P < 0.05$) but no difference between high and low fat meals. This study adjusted for the effect of meal volume on GER. It also determined that it was the increase in fat calories rather

than fat alone that had a deleterious effect on GER. Clinical symptoms were not studied.

In an RCT by Just,[22] 19 young healthy volunteers were fed a high fat (3·5 oz of potato chips prepared with 100% vegetable oil) and a low fat meal (3·5 oz of potato chips prepared with Olestra) on separate days. Smoking, drinking alcohol or caffeinated beverages, or medication use was not permitted during the study. EpHM results showed that the high fat meal led to significantly more GER ($P < 0.05$). However, because Olestra has no calories, the meals were not isocaloric. Since others have suggested that total calories may be more deleterious to GER than fat, the variation in calories between the meals may have confounded the effect of the fat.

The randomized cross-over trial by Mangano[17] included 11 young healthy volunteers and eight patients with GERD. On separate days, a nasogastric tube was inserted and saline or lipid then hydrochloric acid were infused. After 10 minutes the infusion order was switched. All the patients and five volunteers experienced heartburn after the acid infusion. Symptoms were not affected by the lipid. This negative study is limited by its small sample size – it is possible that the study power was not sufficient to detect a difference in symptoms between groups. Also, it is questionable whether infusion of hydrochloric acid through a nasogastric tube is representative of gastric acid reflux.

Pehl[18] studied 12 young, healthy, non-smoking volunteers who were fed isocaloric and isoosmotic high fat (50%) and low fat (10%) meals 2 days apart. Meals were given by mouth and included 310 ml of liquid. During 1 hour supine and 2 hours upright, no difference in EpHM parameters were noted between groups. Although the authors stated that the study was blinded, the meals may not have tasted the same. The power of this negative study is not addressed.

In an RCT/cross-over trial on 13 young, healthy volunteers and 14 patients with GERD,[19] subjects were randomly allocated to a high fat (52%) or balanced fat (24%) meal. Esophageal pH and LESP were measured over 3 hours. The high fat meal did not increase the rate of reflux episodes or exposure to esophageal acid in either group regardless of body posture (recumbent or sitting). Although the meals were iso-osmotic, the difference in calories may have influenced the results.

In the case–control study by Iwakiri,[23] the effect of meal volume and fat content was studied in asymptomatic healthy volunteers. In each subject, EpHM was performed over a 3-hour postprandial period in the same position (supine or upright). In subjects who remained upright and received the large volume (800 ml) meal, the acid exposure time was significantly greater than in those who received the small-meal volume (500 ml). For patients who remained supine, there was no difference between acid exposure time in groups receiving the large and small volume meals. In the upright position, the air in the stomach collects in the fundus, and the pressure at the fundus is further increased after a large meal. The authors speculate that an increase in intragastric pressure causes a transient decrease in LESP. There was no difference between acid exposure times in the low fat (125 kcal) and high fat (350 kcal) meal groups when subjects remained upright. However, when subjects were supine, acid exposure time in the high fat meal group was significantly greater than that in the low fat meal group. The authors suggest that the delay in gastric emptying in the supine position contributes to a significant increase in acid exposure time.

In the cohort study by Ruhl, multiple risk factors associated with hospitalization for GER were studied.[9] A high fat diet did not influence the risk of hospitalization for GER. Unlike the other studies, details of the diet were self-reported and uncontrolled.

In these studies, differences between results may be explained by the type of subjects studied (healthy volunteers vesus symptomatic subjects with a history of GER) or the type of meal used (solid versus liquid, high fat etc). Gastric emptying of a liquid meal is faster than that of a solid meal. Results of the studies are too variable to confidently state that fatty foods adversely influence GER symptoms.

Based on the inconclusive evidence from small studies that did not report clinical outcomes, you resolve not to recommend a low fat diet for your patient.

Tobacco

Some studies suggest that cigarette smoking lowers LESP.[2,3] However, you know that the specificity of low LESP for diagnosing GER is poor and you need more evidence because your patient challenges the idea that cigarette smoking is related to his heartburn. You identify seven relevant articles.[8,24–29]

In a cross-over study by Kadakia,[24] 14 smokers with heartburn and esophagitis abstained from smoking 48 hours before and during 24 hour EpHM. After resuming their smoking habit for 48 hours or more, they had a second 24-hour EpHM and smoked 20 regular, filtered, Marlboro cigarettes. Cigarette smoking significantly increased the percentage of time that lower esophageal pH was < 4 during a 24-hour period from 7·35% to 11·1%. While smoking, subjects reported a 114% increase in episodes of daytime heartburn that immediately followed a reflux event.

In a cross-over study by Rahal,[25] 20 volunteers (12 smokers and 8 non-smokers) had 24 EpHMs while wearing a placebo patch for 24 hours and a nicotine patch for a subsequent 24 hours. Participants experienced a significant increase in the total acid score ($P = 0.005$), duration of acid exposure ($P = 0.010$), and duration of acid exposure when supine ($P = 0.004$) when wearing the transdermal nicotine versus the placebo patch. In a smaller cross-over study by Waring,[26] eight patients with esophagitis had EpHMs in hospital for two 24-hour periods. On the first day they smoked at least 20 cigarettes and they abstained from smoking on the second day. During the non-smoking period there were fewer reflux episodes, but the total reflux time was not significantly different between periods.

In Smit's case–control study[27] the effect of cigarette smoking in smokers on gastropharyngeal reflux (GPR) and GER was assessed. Double-probe pH monitoring in 15 smokers showed pathological GER in one, pathological GER and GPR in two, and pathological GPR in five while they smoked. Seven, almost half, had no evidence of either GER or GPR. In a case–control study by Locke[8] that addressed multiple risk factors for GER, symptomatic GER was associated with a past, but not present, history of cigarette smoking. In two other case–control studies there was no significant association between cigarette smoking and GER. Kahrilas[28] showed that cigarette smoking increased transient LES relaxation but that this was not associated with GER. Pehl[29] found that being a smoker or actually smoking a cigarette had no influence on GER. You note that all the negative studies have a small sample size and may have limited the power to detect an effect.[26,28] Also, the lack of a nicotine washout period may have affected the ability to detect a difference between smoking and non-smoking periods.[26]

You conclude that smoking tobacco may worsen your patient's reflux symptoms and recommend to your patient that he consider quitting.

Gum chewing

Two case–control studies suggest that gum chewing may have beneficial effects for people with GER.[30,31] Both studies used EpHM to evaluate GER. Avidan showed that chewing gum for at least an hour after a meal reduced the esophageal acid contact time in both groups.[30] Subjects in the second study were asked to chew two sticks of gum during EpHM. Chewing gum consistently increased both esophageal and pharyngeal pH.[31] Although there is no evidence that gum chewing improves GER symptoms, it is unlikely to do harm.

Question
2. In adolescents with GER (*population*), does treatment with a cholinergic agent (*intervention*) compared with placebo or other medications (*comparison*), reduce the frequency of GER symptoms without added risk (*outcome*)? **[Therapy]**

Bethanecol

Bethanecol is a cholinergic agent that has been used in GERD. It is postulated that by increasing esophageal sphincter pressure, bethanecol decreases the duration of reflux episodes, increases esophageal clearance, and decreases the duration of reflux episodes.

Six studies relevant to the question were identified,[32–37] including one randomized controlled trial,[32] one cross-over trial,[33] two case–control studies,[34,35] and two before and after studies.[36,37] In half of the studies, only a single dose of bethanecol was used to determine its immediate effect on LESP and postprandial pH scores.[34–36] Orenstein and Sondheimer documented an increase in LESP after a single dose of bethanecol.[34,35] Sondheimer showed bethanecol decreases the time that esophageal pH is < 4 and the duration of the longest GER episode.[36] However, these studies had methodological limitations. The numbers of children studied were small, the groups were heterogeneous, study power was not addressed in the negative study,[34] and clinical outcomes were not stated.[34–36] Since long-term treatment was not the primary objective of these studies, their applicability to the boy in clinical scenario is limited.

Of the long-term studies, the RCT/cross-over study by Euler[32] showed an improvement in GER symptoms (decreased number of vomiting episodes per day and weight gain) in eight of 15 children while taking bethanecol. EpHM showed a significant difference in the number of episodes of reflux per hour after the oral administration of bethanecol (5·8 *v* 1·8; $P < 0.01$). The duration of episodes was also shorter after bethanecol (4·3 *v* 1·3; $P < 0.01$). Symptoms returned in most (11 of 13) of these patients during the placebo arm of the study. Co-therapies in both therapy and control groups included sleeping with the head of the bed elevated 6 in, fasting after 6 pm, eating six small-volume meals, and avoiding foods that caused chest pain.

In the cross-over study by Levi,[33] bethanecol was compared with an antacid (Maalox) rather than a placebo in 20 infants aged 2–32 months. Improved clinical scores and EpHM measures occurred in both therapy and control groups. Bethanecol was no more effective than the antacid for controlling gastroesophageal reflux (9/10 and 8/10 patients respectively). Clinical improvement preceded the reduction in reflux documented on EpHM in both groups. In this small, unblinded study neither compliance nor power were addressed.

Strickland[37] used a before-after (quasi-case–control) research design to study patients with GER before and during treatment with bethanecol. Total reflux scores measured by EpHM were significantly improved by bethanecol therapy ($P < 0.02$). This improvement resulted primarily from a decrease in the frequency and duration of reflux episodes occurring more than 2 hours after feeding (fasted states). This

was the only study that analyzed the effects of bethanecol in relationship to time of feeding. Four non-compliant patients were used as controls and only one had improvement in the total reflux score. A possible explanation for the non-therapeutic effect of bethanecol in the postprandial period is that the increased salivation and swallowing caused by the drug is also accompanied by lower esophageal sphincter relaxation. Although all the articles addressed efficacy of bethanecol for treating GER, esophagoscopy and biopsy were not performed to confirm or exclude esophagitis. Thus, it is unclear whether the results can be readily generalized to patients with esophagitis. None of the studies addressed the safety of bethanecol, its effect on gastrointestinal strictures, or its cholinergic effect on small airways.

In conclusion, one RCT showed improvement in GER symptoms and EpHM values with bethanecol. However, the risk of side effects such as irritability, tremors, diarrhea and bronchospasm probably outweigh any potential benefit.

Question

3. In adolescents with GER (*population*), does treatment with prokinetic agents (*intervention*) compared with placebo or other medications (*comparison*), reduce the frequency of GER symptoms without added risk (*outcome*)? **[Therapy]**

Cisapride

Cisapride is a prokinetic agent used in GER because it enhances the release of acetylcholine at the myenteric plexus, thus increasing LESP, increasing the amplitude of peristalsis, accelerating gastric emptying, and improving antroduodenal coordination. You identify a Cochrane review on cisapride treatment for gastroesophageal reflux in children.[38] The review included nine RCTs (eight comparing cisapride with placebo) with 236 participants under the age of 5 years and with a diagnosis of GER. The primary outcomes were a change in symptoms, adverse effects of cisapride, complications, and weight gain. Secondary outcomes included change in esophagitis (histological) or physiological measures of reflux. There was considerable heterogeneity between trials and evidence of publication bias (favoring studies in which cisapride had a positive effect). Meta-analysis provided no clear evidence that cisapride improved GER symptoms (OR 0·34, 95%CI 0·10,1·19). Cisapride did reduce the reflux index, or percentage time that the pH was < 4 on EpHM (WMD −6·49; 95%CI −10·13, −2,85). However, the significance of this finding is not clear because there is poor correlation between clinical symptoms and the reflux index. In view of reported adverse effects of cisapride, including sudden death from arrhythmias, the authors concluded that the risks of cisapride treatment outweigh the benefits. You note that the children included in the review were all under five and look at the other studies you identify

You identified 11 primary studies, some of which are included in the review. One reports the cardiac side effects of cisapride[39] and 10 evaluate cisapride as a therapy for GER.[40–49] Eight of the 10 studies were RCTs [40–47] and seven were placebo controlled.[40–42,44–47]

The effect of cisapride treatment depends on the definition used for GER. When outcome is based on clinical symptoms, Cohen and Scott noted no beneficial effect of treatment with cisapride in young children.[40,45] The results of this study may be explained by the large number (40%) of patients who received prior therapy with other medications – the authors state that these patients may have already experienced optimal improvement before treatment with cisapride. Also, the 2-week treatment time was shorter than any of the other studies.[40] In the studies that evaluated EpHM results, all showed a beneficial effect of cisapride.[40–46,48–49]

Patients with endoscopically diagnosed esophagitis were included in several studies.[41–42,45] Two studies had a sufficient number of patients with esophagitis for subgroup analysis.[41,45] Cucchiara found that the histological score for esophagitis was significantly better in the group treated with cisapride but was not changed in the group treated with placebo.[41] Half (four) of the patients on cisapride had totally healed, two had improved, and two had no change.[41] In Scott's study,[45] seven of 11 (64%) of children treated with cisapride had abnormal biopsy findings at the end of treatment, compared with five of nine (56%) of the placebo patients but this difference was not significant. However, the criteria for grading were not given and outcomes were assessed as normal or abnormal, not by scoring or improvement.[45]

Although none of these studies reported on safety issues, adult and pediatric case reports have suggested an association of malignant ventricular arrhythmias with administration of cisapride in conjunction with drugs that inhibit cytochrome P450 metabolism. Hill[39] performed a prospective, double blind, case–control study to evaluate its effect on ventricular repolarization in children being treated with cisapride. Electrocardiograms from 35 children who were currently being treated with cisapride and 1000 normal children who were not taking any medications were compared. There was no statistically significant difference for either QTc or JTc in the cisapride patients versus the control group. However, 11 (31%) of the patients receiving cisapride had prolongation of the QTc ($\geq$ 450 ms) and two had torsades de pointes ventricular tachycardia; both of which are risk factors for malignant ventricular arrhythmias and sudden death. The number of control patients with a prolonged QTc is not given and statistical comparison was not reported.

In June 1998, Janssen Pharmaceutica changed the labeling for cisapride to warn of the association between use of the drug and adverse cardiac events. In response, the North American Society for Pediatric Gastroenterology and Nutrition critically appraised all available published and unpublished reports on cisapride, metoclopramide, bethanecol, and domperidone and developed a position statement.[49] The committee concluded that:

> cisapride does have a place in pediatric therapeutics when used in conditions in which a prokinetic drug is indicated but that cisapride can cause serious dose-related adverse effects (increased QTc interval). It recommended that the list of contraindications outlined in the current package insert be expanded to include pre-existing cardiac conditions (congenital or acquired) that might predispose the patient to ventricular arrhythmias; intraventricular conduction disturbances; and instances of reduced hepatic function.

It also stated that with avoidance of contraindicated drugs, patient counseling, and appropriate patient selection and monitoring, the risk for adverse effects can be reduced. Since July 2000, the use of cisapride has been restricted to pediatric gastroenterologists in the USA and to children participating in clinical trials or safety studies in Europe.

In conclusion, there is poor evidence that cisapride is useful for the treatment of GER symptoms, and its use may be associated with harm. Although histological improvement in esophagitis and improvement in reflux index is reported in some studies, the clinical significance of this is not clear.

Domperidone

Domperidone is a synthetic dopamine-blocking agent that increases antroduodenal motility and gastric emptying. It decreases postprandial reflux time and therefore may decrease regurgitation and vomiting. You find five studies relevant to this question.[50–54] Three were RCTs (comparing domperidone versus placebo), one was a case–control study, and one a before-after study. Four of the five studies showed a "positive" response of GER to domperidone by both clinical and by EpHM criteria. In an RCT, Bines[50] showed EpHM measures improved significantly in the treatment compared with the placebo group. However, there was no difference between groups in symptom reduction. This study included seven children with esophagitis. All the patients in the RCT by Carroccio[51] had esophagitis based on endoscopic and histologic examination and there were significant improvements in symptoms and EpHM measures in the group receiving domperidone. Domperidone plus magnesium hydroxide and aluminum hydroxide was significantly more effective ($P < 0.05$) than domperidone plus alginate-antacid, domperidone alone, or placebo in treating GER/esophagitis. In the RCT by DeLoore,[52] domperidone was compared with metoclopramide and placebo in 47 infants with chronic vomiting. Domperidone was superior to both metoclopramide and placebo in controlling symptoms. A rating of "excellent" was given to 10 of 15 patients in the domperidone group compared with 6 of 17 in the metoclopramide and 0 of 15 in the placebo group. No attempt was made to confirm the clinical diagnosis of gastroesophageal reflux or esophagitis and patients in the domperidone group were considerably older than patients in the other groups. The before-after study by Grill[54] showed significant improvement in both clinical and EpHM measures with domperidone.

In a case–control study related to harm, Deprettere[53] found that patients on domperidone therapy for GER had a 50% increase in prolactin levels over the course of 1 month compared with age-matched controls. No adverse clinical signs were noted, so the clinical significance of this finding is unknown. Domperidone does not readily cross the blood–brain barrier and central nervous system so side effects are uncommon.

In one RCT, domperidone was effective for the treatment of symptoms associated with esophagitis. However, there is uncertainty about harm and this medication is not available in the USA.

Metoclopramide

Metoclopramide is an antidopiminergic agent with mixed cholinomimetic and serotoninergic effects. It increases LESP, promotes rapid clearing of esophageal contents, and accelerates gastric emptying. Unlike cholinergic agents, it produces these changes in gastric activity without stimulating secretion of acid or gastrin.

You identify five relevant articles.[55–59] Because studies with intravenous metoclopramide cannot be used to predict clinical response to oral metoclopramide and because the results can not be generalized to your patient, the studies by Hyman[55,57] you exclude. Although the study by Pons[56] was an RCT, it compared dose responses of metoclopramide over a 2-day period and has little application to your patient. In the cross-over study by Tolia,[58] the effect of metoclopramide on gastroesophageal reflux was evaluated in 30 infants < 1 year of age. After a 1-week period of treatment, patients receiving metoclopramide significantly benefited with regard to measures of reflux on EpHM compared with patients receiving placebo ($P < 0.001$). There were no significant differences in daily symptom count or scintigraphically measured gastric emptying between the placebo and metoclopramide periods. Machida[59] randomized eight patients in a 6-month double blind, placebo-controlled trial of metoclopramide after initial studies indicated metoclopramide increased lower esophageal sphincter pressure. The three patients receiving metoclopramide but none of those receiving placebo, were withdrawn by their parents because of exacerbation of GER symptoms and marked irritability ($P < 0.01$).

There is little evidence of benefit from long-term use of metoclopramide in children with either uncomplicated or complicated GER. Adverse effects are common and include parkinsonian reactions and tardive dyskinesia (rigidity and oculogyric crisis) which may be irreversible. Its use cannot be recommended in children.

Question

4. In adolescents with GER (*population*), does treatment with proton pump inhibitors (*intervention*), compared with placebo or other medications (*comparison*), reduce the frequency of GER symptoms without added risk (*outcome*)? **[Therapy]**

Proton-pump inhibitors

Proton-pump inhibitors (PPIs) are substituted benzimidazoles that include lansoprazole, omeprazole, and pantoprazole. They inhibit acid secretion by inhibition of gastric hydrogen-potassium adenosinetriphosphatase ("the acid pump"), the enzyme responsible for the final step in the secretion of hydrochloric acid by the gastric parietal cell. PPIs bind irreversibility to the enzyme and inhibit acid secretion until more enzyme is synthesized. This accounts for their long duration of action (more than 24 hours).

You identify seven relevant studies, all of which showed a "positive" effect of therapy on esophagitis.[60–66] Patients in four of the studies had GER with esophagitis and had failed medical treatment with an H2 blocker and a prokinetic.[60–62,64]

In the RCT by Cucchiara,[60] standard doses of omeprazole were compared with high dose ranitidine. All patients had GER esophagitis and had failed treatment with prokinetics. Both therapies decreased clinical score, improved esophageal histology, and reduced esophageal acid exposure. No serious adverse events requiring discontinuation of treatment were noted, but 58% of patients relapsed after discontinuing treatment.

All 13 patients in the case–control study by Kato[61] had documented reflux esophagitis and had failed medical treatment with cimetidine or famotidine. They were aged between 3 and 18 years. Serial endoscopies were performed after treatment commenced. The cumulative healing rates on PPI at 2, 4, 6, and 8 weeks of treatment were 46%, 85%, 92%, and 92% respectively. After 8 weeks, patients were considered refractory to treatment. Limitations of the study included non-treatment of *Helicobacter pylori* in the six patients with documented illness. The criteria used to define healing are unclear as biopsy results were not reported.

Alliet[62] performed a before-after study on 12 neurologically normal infants (age 2.9 ± 0.9 months) who did not respond to cimetidine (in addition to positioning, cisapride, and Gaviscon). Significant improvement was noted in symptoms, EpHM, and biopsy results in patients on omeprazole. Although the study design was weak, patients were followed for 1 year, when 83% of patients remained asymptomatic.

De Giacomo[63] studied 10 children with severe esophagitis before and after 3 months of therapy with omeprazole. Significant improvement in symptoms and EpHM was noted in all. The evaluation of histological changes following treatment gave conflicting results – there was no significant difference between pre- and post-treatment scores. The author comments that both American and European gastroenterologists question the value of esophageal histology in monitoring the treatment of children with esophagitis. Although the length of follow up is not given, six children became symptomatic after discontinuing the medication. Three eventually underwent surgery: two for Barrett's esophagus and one for recurrent pneumonia.

Gunasekaran[64] performed a before-after study using omeprazdex in 15 patients with severe esophagitis and had failed prior treatment with histamine blockers and prokinetic agents. Symptoms and signs abated and evidence of esophagitis diminished in all patients by 6 months of follow up. However, the fact that all patients had major associated co-morbidities limits the generalizability of the results to your patient.

Karjoo[65] evaluated the cause of chronic abdominal pain in a series of 153 patients who had undergone endoscopy. Those patients with esophagitis as the cause of their pain were treated with high dose ranitidine followed by omeprazole for those that did not respond: 84% of the patients had esophagitis and 70% responded to an 8-week course of high dose ranitidine. Of the 30% who failed to respond, 87% responded to an 8-week course of omeprazole. One factor that was predictive of response to ranitidine therapy was the degree of esophagitis on endoscopy. Ninety percent of patients with grade 1 (mild) esophagitis responded to ranitidine therapy.

Studies with lansoprazole show similar results. Faure[66] examined the efficacy of lansoprazole in 23 children (3 months to 13 years) with endoscopically confirmed reflux esophagitis. The initial dose of 0.73 mg kg^{-1} was doubled in non-responders after 1 week. Response was defined as a gastric pH > 3 for 65% of the 24-hour EpHM study and esophageal healing upon repeat endoscopy at 28 days. Overall, 15 (64%) children were responders. Of these, 80% had healed on endoscopy by day 28.

You conclude that there is strong and consistent evidence that PPIs are safe and effective for the treatment of reflux esophagitis.

Question

5. In adolescents with GER (*population*), does treatment with antacids and surface agents (*interventions*), compared with placebo or other medications (*comparison*), reduce the frequency of GER symptoms without added risk (*outcome*)? **[Therapy]**

Gaviscon

You identify three placebo-controlled RCTs of Gaviscon.[67–69] Forbes[67] randomized 30 patients to receive metoclopramide, Gaviscon, or placebo. Gaviscon is a preparation containing alginic acid, magnesium trisilicate, aluminum hydroxide, and sodium bicarbonate. Alginic acid reacts with sodium bicarbonate in the presence of saliva in the mouth to form a highly viscous solution of sodium alginate (pH 5–6) which floats on the surface of the gastric contents as a high surface or "raft" thus decreasing reflux of gastric contents. Compared with placebo, neither metoclopramide nor the alginic acid-antacid compound decreased the frequency or duration of gastroesophageal reflux as measured by EpHM. In this small study, no power calculation was given and the length of therapy is not stated (it may have been too short to have had an effect).

Miller[68] compared the efficacy and safety of an aluminum-free formulation of alginate with placebo in infants. For the primary outcome (number of vomiting/regurgitation episodes), alginate was superior to placebo ($P = 0.009$). Patients receiving alginate were assessed as responding clinically to treatment by both investigators ($P = 0.008$) and parent/guardians ($P = 0.002$). The relevance of this study to adolescents is unclear.

In a quasi-RCT,[69] patients were alternately assigned to receive Gaviscon or placebo. Compared with initial values, indicators of reflux on EpHM were significantly reduced by −35% to −61% ($P < 0.05$) 8 days after the onset of Gaviscon treatment.

Gaviscon contains $NaHCO_3$, so there is potential risk for hypernatremia; however, none of the studies presented any data on serum sodium levels. There are also reports of concretions of milk formula, alginic acid, and antacid, known as "Gavisconomas" in infants.[70,71] Their clinical significance is not clear. You conclude that there is insufficient evidence of benefit from Gaviscon for GER treatment in children and potential for harm.

Sucralfate gel

Sucralfate gel acts by adhering to peptic lesions, and protects the esophageal mucosal surface. In the only RCT in children,[72] Arguelles-Martin studied 66 children from 4 months to 12 years of age with peptic esophagitis. Patients received either sucralfate in tablet or liquid form or cimetidine. No other treatments were permitted. After 4 weeks of treatment, 59% in the sucralfate liquid group; 44% in the sucralfate tablet group; and 42% in the cimetidine group showed complete endoscopic remission of reflux esophagitis. Sucralfate is an aluminum complex, and there are currently insufficient data to determine the safety of sucralfate in the treatment of GERD in children.

Question

6. In adolescents with GER (*population*), does obesity increase the risk of GER symptoms (*outcome*)? **[Causation/harm]**

Obesity

It is often assumed that obesity is associated with GERD and that weight loss will help reflux symptoms. You find no RCTs evaluating the effects of weight loss on reflux symptoms but find several cohort and case–control studies applicable to your patient.[9,73–78]

The most important of these is the NHANES I (National Health and Nutrition Examination Survey) cohort study,[9] which included 12 349 people recruited between 1971 and 1975 and followed for 18·5 years. Risk factors for hospitalization with GERD were assessed. In a second analysis (NHEFS), the effect of dietary fat on hospitalization with GERD was evaluated in 9851 people recruited between 1982 and 1983 and followed for 9 years (542 patients with hiatal hernia were excluded). A high BMI increased the risk of hospitalization for GERD. In the NHANES study the age adjusted hazard ratio was $HR = 1·26$ per 5 kg m^{-2} $(CI = 1·22–1·3)$. In the NHEFS study the $HR = 1·19$, $CI = 1·05–1·34$. Each 5 kg m^{-2} increase in BMI increased the risk for GERD-related hospitalization by 22%.

In a large historical cohort study[74] (135 participants with symptomatic GERD and 685 without), there was no association between overweight or obesity and GERD. This study was subject to recall bias (it was questionnaire based and asked about symptoms occurring > 5 years prior to the study) and historical data, for example, weight is likely to be unreliable (participants were asked to provide weight at age 20 years and weight 20 years before the interview).

In a cohort study,[75] a retrospective analysis was conducted on the relationship between BMI and GERD in 70 patients (55 overweight with BMI 28) with GERD symptoms and abnormal 24-hour EpHM. There was a strong correlation between a reflux severity score (EpHM) and BMI $(P < 0·001)$ and between pH < 4 and increasing BMI $(P = 0·03)$. There was no difference in manometric studies (LESP) between normal and overweight patients.

In a study of 30 morbidly obese patients[76] (mostly women, average BMI 51·5) who were being evaluated for surgery, 16 had symptomatic GERD. All 30 had manometry performed and 28 had 24-hour EpHM. There was a significant association between increased weight and BMI and abnormal EpHM $(P < 0·02)$. Increased weight was significantly associated with longer reflux duration $(P < 0·2)$. Neither increased weight nor BMI were significantly associated with more than 72 episodes of pH < 4 over 3 hours. Weight and BMI were significantly

higher in patients with abnormal reflux scores (by EpHM) than in patients with normal reflux scores $(P < 0·03)$. Ultimately, 16 patients underwent surgery for obesity (type not specified) and 15/16 had immediate complete resolution of their reflux symptoms. Thus surgery itself, rather than weight loss improved GERD symptoms.

Kjellin[73] evaluated 20 obese patients (average BMI 31·4) with GERD. They underwent a baseline, mid-study, and end-study questionnaire, 24-hour EpHM, manometry, and endoscopy. With diet and exercise half of the patients lost about 10 kg weight over the first 6-month period and the other half lost the same amount of weight during the second 6-month period. After the intervention there was no difference between groups in reflux symptoms or objective measures of reflux; however, this was a small study and no power calculations had been performed.

A BMI of > 30 has been independently associated with reflux symptoms.[77] However, when 50 massively obese patients (average BMI 42·5, 24-hour EpHM) were compared with 29 age- and sex-matched controls, there was no statistical difference between cases and controls in the number of patients with GERD by EpHM.

In a case–control study,[78] LES pressure was measured in 55 obese people and 20 non-obese controls. Compared with controls, LES pressure was decreased only in obese people > 35 years old $(P = 0·001)$. However, 72% of obese people were symptomatic, nine had reflux on barium study, and four had esophagitis on histology (these assessments were not done in controls).

The strongest evidence of a causal relationship between obesity and GERD comes from the large US cohort study and, taken in association with the other evidence, suggests that weight loss in the obese would decrease GERD symptoms.

Question

7. In adolescents with GER (*population*), does treatment with H_2 blockers and other acid suppressants (*intervention*), compared with placebo or other medications (*comparison*), reduce the frequency of GER symptoms without added risk (*outcome*)? **[Therapy]**

H_2 blockers

Because of their low cost and easy accessibility, histamine-2 receptor antagonists (H_2RAs), including cimetidine, ranitidine, famotidine, and nizatidine, have long been the first-line treatment for acid suppression and are often used to self-medicate heartburn in adults. They inhibit gastric acid secretion, raising the pH of gastric contents so that the refluxate is less irritating and causes fewer symptoms. Tolerance to these compounds may develop over time and increasing dose is required to achieve continued symptom relief and/or acid suppression.

You find 12 RCTs that evaluate H$_2$ blockers in adults and children. In most studies the comparison was a proton pump inhibitor such as omeprazole. Orenstein[79] studied 29 children with ≥ 3 months of reflux symptoms: 19 were given 75 mg of ranitidine and 10 were given placebo in a double-blinded fashion, and EpHM was performed for 6 hours. The maximum serum concentration of ranitidine occurred 2·5 hours after it was given. Gastric pH increased significantly 60 minutes after the dose, was at maximum at 2–4 hours, and stayed high for 5–6 hours. Given its duration of action, ranitidine may need to be given more frequently than every 12 hours. In this study, no clinical outcomes were reported. Further, the pretrial duration of symptoms was longer in the placebo group (46 months) than the treatment group (14 months). This may bias the results by exaggerating the effect of treatment.

In adults,[80] 307 patients with reflux symptoms were randomized to receive pantoprazole or ranitidine in a double-blinded trial (154 received 20 mg of pantoprazole four times a day and 153 received 150 mg of ranitidine twice a day for 12 months). Symptom frequency and severity were assessed at 4 and 8 weeks and at 3, 6, 9, and 12 months. By intention-to-treat analysis, pantoprazole caused more "complete" control of symptoms (71% *v* 56% at 6 months; $P = 0.007$). However, there was no difference in "sufficient" control of symptoms, relapse rate at 12 months, or adverse events between the two groups. The attrition rate was high (184 patients, more than half, dropped out of the study) and drop-out occurred more commonly in the ranitidine group (70 *v* 53) because of lack of effect.

Kawano[81] compared omeprazole and famotidine in 56 patients with reflux esophagitis randomly assigned (but not blindly) to 20 mg of omeprazole four times a day (n = 29) or 20 mg of famotidine twice a day (n = 27) for 8 weeks. Symptom improvement was greater with omeprazole than famotidine at both 2 weeks (67% *v* 29%; $P = 0.005$) and 4 weeks (95% *v* 55% $P = 0.009$). Omeprazole promoted greater healing of esophagitis than famotidine at 4 weeks (72% *v* 32%; $P = 0.025$) and 8 weeks (95% *v* 53%; $P = 0.003$).

Kovacs[82] studied 221 mostly white men with at least grade 2 reflux esophagitis (Hetzel–Dent scale) in a randomized, blinded study in which they were given 20 mg of pantoprazole four times a day, 40 mg of pantoprazole four times a day, or 150 mg nizatidine twice a day for 4 weeks. If esophagitis was not healed at endoscopy, treatment was continued for 4 more weeks; 214 patients completed the study. Significantly more in the pantoprazole group became asymptomatic ($P < 0.05$) and fewer used antacids ($P < 0.001$). Healing of esophagitis occurred more frequently with pantoprazole than nizatidine ($P < 0.001$). Of note, 84% of *H. pylori*-positive patients healed and only 65% of

H pylori-negative patients healed. There was no difference in healing or symptoms in groups receiving 20 mg or 40 mg of pantoprazole and there was no difference in side effects between pantoprazole and nizatidine. The authors comment that one of their reasons for doing this study was because pharmaceutical plans restrict the use of proton pump inhibitors to patients who have failed a histamine blocker. While the study showed that a proton pump inhibitor is clearly superior for patients with grade 2 or worse esophagitis, of the 20 % of the population with GERD, 50% have esophagitis and only a percentage of them have grade 2 or worse esophagitis.

Earnest[83] looked at 155 mostly white men with greater than 3 months of heartburn. They randomly and blindly gave 78 of them calcium carbonate as needed plus placebo, and gave 77 of them 150 mg of effervescent ranitidine twice a day and calcium carbonate as needed for 12 weeks. Each patient was evaluated by symptom diary and endoscopy at baseline, 6 weeks, and 12 weeks. After one day of treatment with ranitine, heartburn scores significantly decreased ($P < 0.015$). Treatment significantly decreased weekly antacid use ($P < 0.001$). Also, of the 47% of patients who had esophagitis at baseline, 55% had healing with ranitidine versus 29% with antacids ($P = 0.022$). These results confirm many earlier studies done in the 1980s on H$_2$ blockers.

A final adult study by Galmiche[84] evaluated 1336 patients with heartburn for at least 3 months. In this randomized, double blinded study, 504 were given 75 mg of ranitidine three times a day or as necessary, 515 were given 200 mg of cimetidine three times a day or as necessary, and 270 were given placebo. The primary endpoint was the relief of 75% of symptoms. They found significantly less discomfort after 15 days in the ranitidine group versus placebo ($P = 0.004$) and no significant difference was found between ranitidine and cimetidine. This was a particularly short trial without any objective evidence of benefit. Also, the doses were more frequent and lower than standard treatment doses for GERD.

In a randomized, double blind study by Simeone[85] on 26 infants and children with reflux esophagitis, they were given either nizatidine (10 mg kg^{-1} bid) or placebo for 8 weeks. Pre- and post-study pH probes and endoscopies were done. There was a significant reduction in symptoms in the treatment group ($P < 0.01$). pH probe performed post-trial (48 hours prior to the end of the study while still on medication) showed significant improvement with nizatidine ($P < 0.01$). If the pH probe is performed while patients are still on medication, it cannot be concluded that the reflux esophagitis is cured or simply controlled. Also, 75% of patients in the treatment group and only 16·7% in the placebo group were cured by endoscopy.

A randomized controlled trial done by Cucchiara[60] compared ranitidine and omeprazole. They studied 25 infants and children with GER and esophagitis who had previously been treated with 8 weeks of cisapride and regular dose ranitidine. Thirteen patients were given 20 mg kg^{-1} per day of ranitidine and 12 were given 40 mg/day of omeprazole for 8 weeks. They found no significant difference between the number of patients with symptomatic improvement or healing of esophagitis by endoscopy between the two treatment groups. While this was a negative study, power was not addressed. This result contrasts with many adult studies where proton pump inhibitors are significantly more effective than H2 blockers.

Lambert[86] conducted a randomized, double blind study on 23 children with GER by pH probe and esophagitis by endoscopy. They gave 5 mg/kg, 7·5 mg/kg, 10 mg kg^{-1} of cimetidine at 8-hour intervals while the gastric pH was measured. Eight of the 23 were also given 15 mg kg^{-1} per dose because of poor response to the lower doses. Four additional patients were given 10 mg kg^{-1} and 15 mg kg^{-1} because they had a poor previous response to the lower doses. When the dose reached 10 mg kg^{-1}, 75 % responded with a pH > 4 for over 2 hours. While no symptomatic outcomes were addressed, this study suggested that we may be using too low of a dose for GER in children.

Cucchiara[89] did a double blind, randomized trial on 32 infants and children with GER by pH probe and esophagitis by endoscopy and assigned 17 to treatment with cimetidine 30–40 mg kg^{-1} per day three times a day and 15 to placebo for 12 weeks. Based on symptoms and endoscopy, 70% of the patients on cimetidine healed versus 20% on placebo ($P < 0·01$).

Another randomized controlled trial by Arguelles-Martin[88] performed in 75 children with GER by *x* ray and esophagitis by endoscopy evaluated the efficacy of sucralfate tabs versus sucralfate suspension versus cimetidine at 20 mg kg^{-1} per day given for 8 weeks. Endoscopy was repeated at 4 weeks and showed that patients were all improved without any difference between the groups (44%, 50%, and 42% respectively). Most of the patients were also asymptomatic after 8 weeks of treatment (68%, 92%, and 79% respectively). There was no placebo control group as the investigators felt that it was unethical to not treat symptomatic patients. This led to a negative study (i.e., no difference found between the groups) yet no power was addressed.

In a third but earlier study by Cucchiara,[87] they did a randomized controlled trial on 29 infants and young children with GER and esophagitis. Fifteen were placed on an antacid and 14 on cimetidine at 20 mg kg^{-1} per day for 12 weeks. There was no placebo group. Approximately half of both groups were cured after 12 weeks as assessed by symptoms, pH probe, and endoscopy. All but three were cured after an additional month of therapy. The authors' basis for no placebo was the fact that all the patients had esophagitis and most of them were failing to thrive, anorexic, anemic, or had respiratory problems. Again this led to a negative study but power was not addressed. The results of this study vary considerably from adult studies in which proton pump inhibitors are required for consistent healing of esophagitis.

Summarizing the studies that you have read on the use of H$_2$ blockers in children and adults, you recommend that your patient try an over the counter H$_2$ blocker at the therapeutic dose (for example, ranitidine 150 mg twice a day).

Resolution of the scenario

Initial treatment for the adolescent consists of education regarding the appropriate lifestyle changes and H$_2$ blocker or PPI therapy. Initial treatment with a PPI results in a more rapid rate of symptoms relief and healing compared with treatment with a H$_2$ RA.[90] You recommend one of the PPIs that his HMO is willing to supply. It is not known whether lifestyle changes have an additive benefit in patients receiving pharmacologic therapy. You also tell them that the long-term adverse effects of PPIs are unknown and that surgical options might be considered if he requires long-term therapy. You arrange to follow him up to assess his symptoms and will perform an endoscopy after 8 weeks of treatment if he does not improve.

Future research needs

- Assess the long-term safety of proton pump inhibitors in children.
- Determine the cost-benefits of long-term therapy with PPIs versus surgery.

Summary table

Question	Type of evidence	Result	Comment
Alcohol	5 cohort studies	Increased GER symptoms and/or EpHM indices in three studies	Difficult to blind
Caffeine	4 cross-over trials	Increased GER by EpHM in three studies	Negative study had limited power; Sports drink, not coffee used
	1 cohort study	No increased risk of hospitalization	Symptoms not studied
	1 case–control study	Increased symptoms in one study	
Chocolate	1 case–control study	Increased GER by EpHM	
	1 case-series	Decreased LESP	
Fatty Foods	6 RCTs cross-over	No change in GER by EpHM or symptoms in four studies	When the studies controlled for calories, there was not an effect
	1 cohort study	No increased risk of hospitalization	Symptoms not studied
	1 case–control study	No effect on GER by EpHM unless patient supine	
Tobacco	3 cross-over studies	Increased GER by EpHM and symptoms	Study methods not comparable
	4 case–control studies	Increased GER by EpHM and symptoms in two studies	Negative studies had limited power
Gum Chewing	2 case–control studies	Decreased GER by EpHM	
Bethanecol	1 RCT	Decreased GER by EpHM and symptoms	Unequal and small feeding volumes
	1 cross-over study	GER by EpHM and symptoms were not different between bethanecol and Maalox	Negative study and power not addressed
	2 case–control studies 2 before-after studies	GER by EpHM improved in one study	Non-compliant patients used as controls in one study
Cisapride	8 RCTs	Decreased GER by EpHM but no change in symptoms	Heterogeneity between trials
Domperidone	3 RCTs	Decreased GER by EpHM and symptoms	Drug not available in US
	1 case–control study	Increased prolactin level but no adverse clinical effects	Study addressed harm only
	1 before-after study	Decreased GER by EpHM and symptoms	
Metoclopramide	1 RCT	Increased GER symptoms	Small study
	1 cross-over study	Decreased GER by EpHM but no changes in symptoms	
Proton Pump Inhibitor	1 RCT	Decreased GER by EpHM and symptoms	Majority relapsed when treatment discontinued
	1 case–control study	Decreased esophagitis by endoscopy	*H pylori* patients not treated
	3 before-after studies	Decreased GER by EpHM and symptoms	
	2 case-series	Decreased endoscopic esophagitis	
Gaviscon	3 RCTs	Decreased GER by EpHM and symptoms in two studies	Power not addressed in negative, small study
Sucralfate Gel	1 RCT	Decreased endoscopic esophagitis	No data on sucralfate aluminum complex in children
Obesity	3 cohort studies	Increased hospitalizations for GERD and GER increased by EpHM in one study	Recall bias in negative study
	4 case–control studies	Half of studies showed increased GER	
H_2 blockers	12 RCTs	3/5 studies showed PPI superior to H_2 blocker 5/7 studies showed H_2 blocker superior to antacid or placebo	

References

1 Nelson SP, Chen EH, Syniar GM, Cristoffel, KK. Prevalence of symptoms of gastroesophageal reflux during childhood: a pediatric practice-based survey. Pediatric Practice Research Group. *Arch Pediatr Adolesc Med* 2000;**154**:150–4.

2 Dennish GW, Castell DO. Inhibitory effect of smoking on the lower esophageal sphincter. *New Engl J Med* 1971;**284**: 1136–7.

3 Stanciu C, Bennett. Smoking and gastro-oesophageal reflux. *BMJ* 1972;**3**:793–5.

4 North American Society for Pediatric Gastroenterology and Nutrition. Guidelines for evaluation and treatment of gastroesophageal reflux in infants and children. *J Pediatr Gastroenterol Nutr* 2001;**32**:S1–S31.

5 Pehl C, Wendl G, Pfeiffer A, Schmidt T, Kaess H. Low proof alcoholic beverages and gastroesophageal reflux. *Dig Dis Sci* 1993;**38**:93–6.

6 Vitale GC, Cheadle WG, Patel B, Sadek SA, Michel ME, Cuschieri A. The effect of alcohol on nocturnal gastroesophageal reflux. *JAMA* 1987;**258**:2077–9.

7 Kaufman SE, Kaye MD. Induction of gastro-oesophageal reflux by alcohol. *Gut* 1978;**19**:336–8.

8 Locke GR 3rd, Talley NJ, Fett SL, Zinsmeister AR, Melton LJ 3rd. Risk factors associated with gastroesophageal reflux. *Am J Med* 1999;**106**:642–9.

9 Ruhl CE, Everhart JE. Overweight, but not dietary fat intake, increases risk of gastroesophageal reflux disease hospitalization: the NHANES I epidemiologic followup study first National Health and Nutrition Survey. *Ann Epidem* 1999;**9**:424–35.

10 Brazer SR, Onken JE, Dalton CB, Smith JW, Schiffman SS. Effect of different coffees on esophageal acid contact time and symptoms in coffee-sensitive subjects. *Physiol Behav* 1995;**57**:563–7.

11 Pehl C, Pfeiffer A, Wendl B, Kaess H. The effect of decaffeination of coffee on gastro-oesophageal reflux in patients with reflux disease. *Aliment Pharmacol Ther* 1997; **11**:483–6.

12 Wendl B, Pfeiffer A, Schmidt T, Kaess H. Effect of decaffeination of coffee or tea on gastro-oesophageal reflux. *Aliment Pharmacol Ther* 1994;**8**:283–7.

13 Elta GH, Behler EM, Colturi TJ. Comparison of coffee intake and coffee-induced symptoms in patients with duodenal ulcer, nonulcer dyspepesia, and normal controls. *Am J Gastroenterol* 1990;**85**:1339–42.

14 Van Nieuwenhoven MA, Brummer RJM, Brouns F. Gastrointestinal function during exercise: comparison of water, sports drink, and sports drink with caffeine. *J Appl Physiol* 2000;**89**:1079–85.

15 Murphy DW, Castell DO. Chocolate and heartburn: Evidence of increased esophageal acid exposure after chocolate ingestion. *Am J Gastroenterol* 1988;**83**(6):633–6.

16 Wright LE, Castell DO. The adverse effect of chocolate on lower esophageal sphincter pressure. *Am J Dig Dis* 1975;**20**: 703–7.

17 Mangano M, Colombo P, Bianchi PA, Penagini R. Fat and esophageal sensitivity to acid. *Dig Dis Sci* 2002;**47**:657–60.

18 Pehl C, Waizenhoefer A, Wendl B, Schmidt T, Schepp W, Pfeiffer A. Effect of low and high fat meals and lower esophageal sphincter motility and gastroesophageal reflux in healthy subjects. *Am J Gastroenterol* 1999;**94**:1192–6.

19 Penagini R, Mangano M, Bianchi PA. Effect of increasing the fat content but not the energy load of a meal on gastro-oesophageal sphincter motor function. *Gut* 1998;**42**:330–3.

20 Becker DJ, Sinclair J, Castell DO, Wu WC. A comparison of high and low fat meals on postprandial esophageal acid exposure. *Am J Gastroenterol* 1989;**84**:782–6.

21 Colombo P, Mangano M, Bianchi PA, Penagini R. Effect of calories and fat on postprandial gastro-oesophageal reflux. *Scand J Gastroenterol* 2002;**37**:3–5.

22 Just R, Katz L, Verhille M, Schlagheck T, Castell D. A comparison of the effect of Olestra and triglyceride on postprandial esophageal acid exposure. *Am J Gastroenterol* 1993;**88**:1734–7.

23 Iwakiri K, Kobayashi M, Kotoyori M, Yamada H, Sugiura T, Nakagawa Y. Relationship between postprandial esophageal acid exposure and meal volume and fat content. *Dig Dis Sci* 1996;**41**:926–30.

24 Kadakia SC, Kikendall JW, Maydonovitch C *et al.* Effect of cigarette smoking on gastroesophageal reflux measured by 24-h ambulatory esophageal pH monitoring. *Am J Gastroenterol* 1995;**90**:1785–90.

25 Rahal PS, Wright RA. Transdermal nicotine and gastroesophageal reflux. *Am J Gastroenterol* 1995;**90**: 919–21.

26 Waring JP, Eastwood TF, Austin JM *et al.* The immediate effects of cessation of cigarette smoking on gastroesophageal reflux. *Am J Gastroenterol* 1989;**84**:1076–8.

27 Smit CF, Cooper MP, van Leeuwen JA, Schoots IG, Stanojeie ID. Effect of cigarette smoking on gastropharyngeal and gastroesophageal reflux. *Ann Otol Rhino Larygol* 2001;**110**: 190–3.

28 Kahrilas, PJ, Gupta RR. Mechanisms of acid reflux associated with cigarette smoking. *Gut* 1990;**31**:4–10.

29 Pehl C, Pfeiffer A, Wendl B, Nagy I, Kaess H. Effect of smoking on the results of esophageal pH measurement in clinical routine. *J Clin Gastroenterol* 1997;**25**:503–6.

30 Avidan B, Sonnenberg A, Schnell TG, Sontag SJ. Walking and chewing reduce postprandial acid reflux. *Aliment Pharmacol Ther* 2001;**15**:151–5.

31 Smoak BR, Koufman JA. Effects of gum chewing on pharyngeal and esophageal pH. *Ann Otol Rhinol Laryngol* 2001;**110**:1117–19.

32 Euler AR. Use of bethanecol for the treatment of gastroesophageal reflux and peptic esophagitis. *Arch Dis Child* 1980;**96**:321–4.

33 Levi P, Marmo F, Saluzzo C *et al.* Bethanecol versus antacids in the treatment of gastroesophageal reflux. *Acta Helv Pediatr* 1985;**40**:349–59.

34 Orenstein SR, Lofton SW, Orenstein DM. Bethanecol for pediatric gastroesophageal reflux: A prospective. Blind, controlled study. *J Pediatr Gastroenterol Nutr* 1986;**5**: 549–55.

35 Sondheimer JM, Mintz HL, Michaels M. Bethanecol treatment of gastroesophageal reflux in infants: Effect on

continuous esophageal pH records. *J Pediatr* 1984;**104**: 128–31.

36 Sondheimer JM, Arnold GL. Early effects of bethanecol on the esophageal motor function of infants with gastroesophageal reflux. *J Pediatr Gastroenterol Nutr* 1986; **5**:47–51.

37 Strickland AD, Chang JHT. Results of treatment of gastroesophageal reflux with bethanecol. *J Pediatr* 1983; **103**:311–15.

38 Augood C, MacLennan S, Gilbert R, Logan S. Cisapride treatment for gastroesophageal reflux in children (Cochrane Reviews). In: *Cochrane Library*, Issue 4. Chichester, UK: John Wiley & Sons, Ltd, 2003.

39 Hill SL, Evangelista JK, Pizzi AM, Mobassaleh M, Fulton DR, Berul CI. Proarrhythmia associated with cisapride in children. *Pediatrics* 1998;**101**:1053–6.

40 Cohen RC, O'Loughlin EV, Davidson GP, Moore DJ, Lawrence DM. Cisapride in the control of symptoms in infants with gastroesophageal reflux: A randomized, double-blind, placebo-controlled trial. *J Pediatr* 1999;**134**:287–92.

41 Cucchiara S, Staiano A, Capozzi C, DiLorenzo C, Boccieri A, Auricchio S. Cisapride for gastro-oesophageal reflux and peptic esophagitis. *Arch Dis Child* 1987;**62**:454–7.

42 Cucchiara S, Staiano A, Boccieri A *et al.* Effects of cisapride on parameters of oesophageal motility and on prolonged intraoesophageal pH test in infants with gastro-oesophageal reflux. *Gut* 1990;**31**:21–5.

43 Greally P, Hampton FJ, MacFadyen UM, Simpson H. Gaviscon and Carobel compared with cisapride in gastro-oesophageal reflux. *Arch Dis Child* 1992;**67**:618–21.

44 Langer JC, Winthrop AL, Issenman RM. The single-subject randomized trial. *Clin Pediatr* 1993;**32**:654–7.

45 Scott RB, Ferreira C, Smith L *et al.* Cisapride in pediatric gastroesophageal reflux. *J Pediatr Gastroenterol Nutr* 1997; **25**:499–506.

46 Vandenplas Y, de Roy C, Sacre L. Cisapride decreased prolonged episodes of reflux in infants. *J Pediatr Gastroenterol Nutr* 1991;**12**:44–7.

47 Van Eygen M, Van Ravensteyn H. Effect of Cisapride on excessive regurgitation. *Clin Therapeut* 1989;**11**:669–77.

48 Brueton MJ, Clarke GS, Sandhu BK. The effects of cisapride on gastroesophageal reflux in children with and without neurological disorders. *Develop Med Child Neurol* 1990; **32**:629–32.

49 Shulman RJ, Boyle JT, Colletti RB *et al.* A Medical Position Statement of the North American Society for Pediatric Gastroenterology and Nutrition: The use of cisapride in children. *J Pediatr Gastroenterol Nutr* 1999;**28**:529–33.

50 Bines JE, Quinlan JE, Treves S, Kleinman RE, Winter HS. Efficacy of Domperidone in infants and children with gastroesophageal reflux. *J Pediatr Gastroenterol Nutr* 1992; **14**:400–5.

51 Carroccio A, Iacono G, Montalto G, Cavataio F, Soresi M, Notarbartolo A. Domperidone plus magnesium hydroxide and aluminum hydroxide: A valid therapy in children with gastroesophageal reflux. Scan J Gastroenterol 1994;**29**: 300–4.

52 DeLoore I, van Ravensteyn H, Ameryckx L. Domperidone drops in the symptomatic treatment of chronic paediatric vomiting and regurgitation. A comparison with metoclopramide. *Postgrad Med J.* 1979;**55**(Suppl.1):40–2.

53 Deprettere AR, van Acker KJ, Du Caju MVL. Increased serum prolactin but normal TSH during prolonged domperidone treatment in children. *Eur J Pediatr* 1987;**146**: 189–91.

54 Grill BB, Hillemeier AC, Semeraro LA, McCallum RW, Gryboski JD. Effects of domperidone therapy on symptoms and upper gastrointestinal motility in infants with gastroesophageal reflux. *J Pediatr* 1985;**106**:311–16.

55 Hyman PE, Abrams C, Dubois A. Gastric emptying in infants: Response to Metoclopramide depends on underlying condition. *J Pediatr Gastroenterol Nutr* 1988;**7**:181–4.

56 Pons G, Duhamel JF, Guillot M *et al.* Dose-response study of metoclopramide in gastroesophageal reflux in infancy. *Fundam Clin Pharmacol* 1993;**7**:161–6.

57 Hyman PE, Abrams C, Dubois A. Effect of Metoclopramide and Bethanecol on gastric emptying in infants. *Pediatr Res* 1985;**19**:1029–32.

58 Tolia V, Calhoun J, Kuhns L, Kauffman RE. Randomized, prospective double-blind trial of metoclopramide and placebo for gastroesophageal reflux in infants. *J Pediatr* 1989;**115**:141–5.

59 Machida HM, Forbes DA, Gall DG, Scott RB. Metoclopramide in gastroesophageal reflux of infancy. *J Pediatr* 1988;**112**:483–7.

60 Cucchiara S, Minella R, Iervolino C *et al.* Omeprazole and high dose ranitidine in the treatment of refractory reflux esophagitis. *Arch Dis Child* 1993;**69**:655–9.

61 Kato S, Ebina K, Fujii K, Chiba H, Nakagawa H. Effect of omeprazole in the treatment of refractory acid-related diseases in childhood: Endoscopic healing and twenty-four-hour intragastric acidity. *J Pediatr* 1996;**128**:415–21.

62 Alliet P, Raes M, Bruneel E, Gillis P. Omeprazole in infants with cimetidine-resistant peptic esophagitis. *J Pediatr* 1988;**132**:352–4.

63 De Giacomo C, Bawa P, Franceschi M, Luinetti O, Fiocca R. Omeprazole for severe reflux esophagitis in children. *J Pediatr Gastroenterol Nutr* 1997;**24**:528–32.

64 Gunasekaran T, Hassall EG. Efficacy and safety of omeprazole for severe gastroesophageal reflux in children. *J Pediatr* 1993;**123**:148–54.

65 Karjoo M, Kane R. Omeprazole treatment of children with peptic esophagitis refractory to ranitidine therapy. *Arch Pediatr Adolesc Med* 1995;**149**:267–71.

66 Faure C, Michaud L, Shaghaghi E, Popon M *et al.* Lansoprazole in children: pharmacokinetics and efficacy in reflux oesophagitis. *Aliment Pharmacol Ther* 2001;**15**: 1397–402.

67 Forbes D, Hodgson M, Hill R. The effects of Gaviscon and Metoclopramide in gastroesophageal reflux in children. *J Pediatr Gastroenterol Nutr* 1986;**5**:556–9.

68 Miller S. Comparison of the efficacy and safety of a new aluminium-free paediatric alginate preparation and placebo in infants with recurrent gastro-oesophageal reflux. *Curr Med Res Opin* 1999;**15**:160–8.

69 Buts JP, Barudi C, Otte JB. Double-blind controlled study on the efficacy of sodium alginate (Gaviscon) in reducing

gastroesophageal reflux assessed by 24h continuous pH monitoring in infants and children. *Eur J Pediatr* 1987;**146**: 156–8.

70 Hewitt GJ, Benham ES. A complication of Gaviscon in a neonate, the Gavisconomas. *Aust Paediatr J* 1976;**12**: 47–8.

71 Keipert JA. The mode of action and complications of infant Gaviscon. *Aust Paediatr J* 1979;**15**:263–5.

72 Arguelles-Martin F, Gonzalez-Fernandez F, Gentles MG, Navarro-Merino M. Sucralfate in the treatment of reflux esophagitis in children. *Scand J Gastroenterol* 1989; **156**(Suppl.):43–47.

73 Kjellin A, Ramel S, Rossner S, Thor K. Gastroesophageal reflux in obese patients is not reduced by weight reduction. *Scand J Gastroenterol* 1996;**31**:1047–51.

74 Lagergren J, Bergstrom R, Nyren O. No relation between body mass and gastro-oesophageal reflux symptoms in a Swedish population based study. *Gut* 2000;**47**:26–9.

75 Wajed SA, Streets CG, Bremner CG, DeMeester TR. Elevated body mass disrupts the barrier to gastroesophageal reflux. *Arch Surg* 2001;**136**:1014–9.

76 Fisher BL, Pennathur A, Mutnick JL *et al.* Obesity correlates with gastroesophageal reflux. *Dig Dis Sci* 1999;**44**: 2290–4.

77 Locke GR III, Talley NJ, Fett SL, Zinsmeister AR, Melton LJ III. Risk factors associated with gastroesophageal reflux. *Am J Med* 1999;**106**:642–9.

78 Hagen J, Deitel M, Khanna RK, Ilves R. Gastroesophageal reflux in the massively obese. *Int Surg* 1987;**72**:1–3.

79 Orenston SR, Blumer JL, Faessel HM *et al.* Ranidine, 75mg, over-the-counter dose: pharmacokinetic and pharmacodynamic effects in children with symptoms of gastro-oesophageal reflux. *Aliment Pharmacol Ther* 2002;**16**:899–907.

80 Talley NJ, Moore MG Sprogis A, Katelaris P. Randomised controlled trial of pantoprazole versus ranitidine for the treatment of uninvestigated heartburn in primary care. *Med J Aust* 2002;**177**:415–19.

81 Kawano S, Murata H, Tsuji S *et al.* Randomized comparative study of omeprazole and famotidine in reflux esophagitis. *J Gastro Hepatol* 2002;**17**:955–9.

82 Kovacs TOG, Wilcox CM, Devault K, Miska D, Bochenek and The Pantoprazole US GERD Study Group. Comparison of the efficacy of pantoprazole *v* nizatidine in the treatment of erosive oesophagitis:a randomized, active-controlled, double-blind study. *Aliment Pharmacol Ther* 2002;**16**: 2043–52.

83 Earnest D, Robinson M, Rodriguez-Stanley S *et al.* Managing heartburn at the 'base' of GERD 'iceberg':effervescent ranitidine 150mg bid provides faster and better heartburn relief than antacids. *Aliment Pharmacol Ther* 2000;**14**: 911–18.

84 Galmiche JP, Shi G, Simon B, Casset-Semanaz, Slama A. On-demand treatment of gastro-oesophageal reflux symptoms: a comparison of ranitidine 75mg with cimetidine 200mg or placebo. *Aliment Pharmacol Ther* 1998;**12**:909–17.

85 Simeone D, Caria MC, Miele E, Staiano A. Treatment of childhood esophagitis: A double-blind placebo-controlled trial of nizatidine. *J Pediatr Gastroenterol Nutr* 1997;**25**: 51–5.

86 Lambert J, Mobassaleh M, Grand RJ. Efficacy of cimetidine for gastric acid suppression in pediatric patients. *J Pediatr* 1992;**12**:474–8.

87 Cucchiara S, Gobio-Casali L, Balli F *et al.* Cimetidine treatment of reflux esophagitis in children: Italian multicentric study. *J Paediatr Gastroenterol Nutr* 1989;**8**: 150–6.

88 Arguelles-Martin F, Gonzalez-Fernandez F, Gentles MG, Navarro-Merino M. Sucralfate versus cimetidine in the treatment of reflux esophagitis in children. *Am J Med* 1989; **86**:73–6.

89 Cucchiara S, Staiano A, Romaniello G, Capobianco S, Auricchio S. Antacids and cimetidine treatment for gastro-oesophageal relux and peptic oesophagitis. *Arch Dis Child* 1984;**59**:842–7.

90 Chiba N, De Gara CJ, Wilkinson JM *et al.* Speed of healing and symptom relief in Grade II to IV gastroesophageal reflux disease: a meta-analysis. *Gastroenterology.*

36 Constipation

Gregory S Liptak

Case scenarios

The parents of two children, a 4-month-old girl and a 3-year-old boy, tell you that both have problems with their bowels. The younger child has hard "rabbit pellet" stools, turns red in the face when she defecates and has recently been irritable, with diminished appetite. She is fed with iron-fortified formula, recently started eating rice cereal and has otherwise been well. She is normal on examination. Her brother has fecal soiling and behavior problems. His family had significant difficulty toilet training him and he now refuses to sit on the toilet. He stands in a corner, rocks back and forth on his toes and fidgets – behaviors that his parents interpret as straining to have a bowel movement. When he does move his bowels the stools are "the size of a tennis ball" and hard. He is described as a picky eater. He eats bananas and oranges but no other fruit, corn and carrots but no green vegetables. He drinks about one liter of cows' milk each day. His family is concerned that he has "psychological problems" that may be related to the birth of his sister. They say he has always had a "difficult" temperament. Abdominal examination reveals a fecal mass in the left iliac fossa but no other abnormality. His parents say he has also been constipated since infancy.

You wonder whether the children's diets have contributed to their constipation or whether they could have a serious underlying condition requiring further investigation. Their parents ask what can be done to relieve the symptoms and whether constipation can be prevented.

Background

Constipation is defined as infrequent stools with difficulty in defecation. Constipated stools are usually hard, may be larger than typical, and painful to pass. Constipation is common, accounting for 3% of all visits to a pediatric practice,[1] and its prevalence may be higher in certain countries.[2] The frequency of stools in healthy children has been studied.[3,4] Infants had a mean of 4 stools per day during the first week of life, which declined to a mean of 1·7 stools per day at 2 years of age and 1·2 stools per day at 4 years of age. However, there is a wide range of normality – some normal breastfed babies did not stool for several days or longer[5] – and healthy 3-year-olds have 3–14 bowel movements per week. There are no well-designed studies examining which aspects of history or physical examination are most useful in the evaluation of a child with constipation, and laboratory tests are of no proven value in the initial evaluation.[6] Van der plas and colleagues[7] compared recall of stooling patterns with diaries in 46 children (5–14 years) who were assigned to three groups: constipated, encopretic, and other. Using diaries as the gold

standard, they found that 83% of children were correctly classified if recall only were used.

Numerous drugs and organic conditions can cause constipation. These include anticholinergic and opiate medications; neuropathic conditions including spinal cord anomalies such as meningomyelocele and tethered spinal cord; intestinal nerve disorders such as Hirschsprung disease; metabolic conditions such as hypothyroidism and hypercalcemia; genetic disorders such as cystic fibrosis; anatomic malformations such as anteriorly displaced anus; toxins such as lead; and developmental disorders such as Down's syndrome and cerebral palsy. Collectively, organic causes account for less than 10% of constipation in children, even in a gastroenterologist's practice.[8]

Most children with constipation require treatment for many months. Many of these children have already been treated for several months by the family before seeking medical attention. There are no randomized controlled trials (RCTs) comparing long-term treatment to placebo but "before–after" studies suggest that, when children stop treatment too early, their symptoms recur. Children who have constipation of more than

6 months' duration and children who also have encopresis have a worse prognosis. In one long-term prospective study, 418 children with constipation (with or without encopresis) who were referred to a gastroenterologist at 5 years of age or older were studied. The cumulative percentage of children in whom treatment was successful was 60% at 1 year, and 80% at 8 years follow up. Treatment was more often successful in children who developed constipation after the age of 4 years compared with children who developed symptoms before their first birthday (relative risk [RR] 1·55; 95% CI 1·11–2·15). Treatment is less likely to be successful in children with encopresis than in children with constipation alone (RR 0·87; CI 0·80–0·94). Even in the children with encopresis who were treated successfully, 50% experienced at least one period of relapse.[9] Boys with constipation are more likely to relapse than girls (RR 1·73; CI 1·15–2·62), as are children who had symptoms for more than 4 months prior to referral. In a study of preschool children with chronic constipation referred to a gastroenterologist, one-third still had constipation 3–12 years after the initial treatment. Children aged 2 years or less at the time of referral had a better prognosis than older children.[10]

While thinking about prognosis, you recall reading that urinary symptoms may be associated with constipation. In one study you reviewed[11] 7% of 5350 children aged 5–19 years with primary nocturnal enuresis were constipated. In a second paper[12] 56 children with severe constipation and urinary tract symptoms were evaluated. Despite resolution or improvement in constipation, urinary symptoms did not resolve, suggesting that a neuropathy affecting both the colonic and lower urinary tract systems might exist.

Framing answerable clinical questions

You make a list of the clinical questions you believe to be most important for the management of these children (see Chapter 2).

Questions

1. In infants and children (*patient/population*), what is the effect of diet (*exposure*), including iron therapy, cows' milk, fruit and fiber on the risk of constipation (*outcome*)? **[Etiology]**
2. In infants and children (*population*), does dietary advice (*intervention*) prevent constipation (*outcome*)? **[Prevention]**
3. In children (*population*) with a history of constipation since birth (*exposure*), what is the risk of a serious underlying condition such as Hirschsprung disease, neurogenic bowel, cystic fibrosis, or depression (*outcome*)? **[Diagnosis]**
4. In infants and children with prolonged constipation (*population*), are enemas, laxatives, and manual evacuation (*intervention*) effective for disimpaction of stool (*outcome*)? **[Therapy]**
5. In children with constipation (*population*), what is the effect of maintenance therapy with increased dietary fiber, osmotic laxatives, stimulant laxatives, or placebo (*intervention*) on the risk of pain, hard stool, soiling, and frequency of stools (*outcome*)? **[Therapy]**
6. In children with constipation (*population*) treated with osmotic laxatives, stimulant laxatives, or enemas (*intervention*), what is the risk of adverse drug effects (*outcome*)? **[Therapy]**
7. In children with constipation (*population*) given behavior therapy (*intervention*) compared with standard care (*comparison*), is there a reduction in the risk of pain, hard stool, and soiling (*outcome*)? **[Therapy]**

Searching for evidence

You begin your search by looking for systematic reviews or clinical guidelines on constipation. In the *Cochrane Library*'s Database of Systematic Reviews you find several citations on constipation in children. In one review the authors state that no randomized controlled trials that compare the administering of stimulant laxatives to children with either placebo or alternative treatment were found.[13] The other review you find[14] relates to the use of biofeedback in the management of constipation and encopresis in children. In the conclusion, the authors state, "There is no evidence that biofeedback training adds any benefit to conventional treatment in the management of encopresis and constipation in children." The Database of Abstracts of Reviews of Effects (DARE) has a review of constipation in pregnant women and an article in Dutch on the use of biofeedback. You then search OVID, which allows access to Evidence-Based Medicine Reviews (*Best Evidence*). Using the keyword "constipation," you find 20 references, two of which relate to children. In one article[15] the use of biofeedback was evaluated. The authors concluded that, "Additional biofeedback training compared with conventional therapy did not result in higher success rates in chronically constipated children." Authors of a double-blind trial of cisapride in pediatric constipation[16] conclude that, "Cisapride was effective in the treatment of children with constipation." You then search MedLine for guidelines and reviews on constipation in children and find "A medical position statement of the North American Society of Pediatric Gastroenterology, Hepatology and Nutrition (NASPGHAN)."[6] Next you consult *Clinical Evidence*, a new handbook published by *BMJ* containing summaries of the best available evidence on treatment. You find a chapter on childhood constipation,[17] where the authors state that, "Medical treatment plus toilet training or biofeedback (compared with medical treatment alone)" is likely to be effective (which contradicts the finding from the Cochrane review). The authors also note that cisapride represents a trade-off between benefits and harms and that biofeedback training, increased dietary fiber, osmotic laxatives, and stimulant laxatives are of unknown effectiveness.

Searching for evidence syntheses

- *Cochrane Library*

  Cochrane database of systematic reviews (CDSR)
  Database of Abstracts of Reviews of Effects (DARE)

- OVID: Evidence-Based Medicine Reviews
- MedLine: "constipation AND guideline"
- *Clinical Evidence*: Chapter on constipation in children

The review article published in 1999 by the NASPGHAN[6] was limited to children who were neurologically normal with no underlying conditions like Hirschsprung disease. Neonates < 72 hours old and premature infants were also excluded from this review. For this review MedLine was searched for articles published between 1966 and 1997 using a search strategy designed to find randomized controlled trials as well as articles on diagnosis and therapy. Given the systematic literature search, you believe that all relevant articles will be included. Articles were reviewed using criteria developed by Sackett.[18,19] The methods used for finding and evaluating the evidence included in *Clinical Evidence* are outlined in its preface and described in Chapter 3. You decide to have a closer look at the references of high quality studies that are relevant to your clinical questions.

You now wish to address each of your questions in turn and search PubMed for articles published since January 1997 when the NASPGHAN reviewers searched. You limit your search to "All Children 0–18 years" and English language and find 257 articles. You eliminate 19 case studies, 54 narrative reviews, six editorials, five letters to the editor, 62 articles with a focus on specific conditions (for example, Hirschsprung disease), one article in which constipation was not the primary focus, and three in which the patients were too old. That leaves 107 articles for you to review if the answers to your questions cannot be found in the systematic reviews or guidelines (see Box).

PubMed search

- Constipation (since 1997, limited by age and English Language) = 257 articles
- Not review, not letter, not editorial = 173
- Not meningomyelocele, not cerebral palsy, not Hirschsprung, not imperforate anus = 107

Question

1. In infants and children (*patient/population*), what is the effect of diet (*exposure*), including iron therapy, cows' milk, fruit and fiber on the risk of constipation (*outcome*)? **[Etiology]**

You find an RCT[20] in which 93 term infants were assigned to receive two similar formulas, one with and one without iron fortification. The study was conducted because many practising pediatricians believed that non-fortified formula would prevent the development of constipation. Infants were given the formula for 42 days while their mothers kept detailed daily records of all gastrointestinal symptoms. No differences were found between groups in the number of stools per day (1.93 v 1.91), the description of the stools, the number of days without stools (4.95 in the non-fortified group v 3.33 in the iron group [power = 54%]), or other gastrointestinal symptoms such as cramps. This study has been widely used to reassure parents regarding the use of iron-fortified formulae.

In a paper from Italy[21] the results of a double-blind, crossover study (comparing use of cows' milk with soy milk in 65 children, aged 11–72 months who had been referred to gastroenterologists) were reported. During the first study period, 21/32 children given soy formula had an improvement in their constipation compared with 0/33 in the group on cows' milk formula. In the crossover period, 23/33 given soy formula improved compared with 0/32 on cows' milk formula. When 44 of the children who had improved with soy were given cows' milk formula a month later, all developed constipation within 5–10 days. As long as the children stayed on a soy-based formula, constipation did not recur. However, 15 children were switched to cows' milk 8–12 months after the study ended and all became constipated. The authors concluded that chronic constipation can be a manifestation of intolerance to cows' milk. In another study[22] cows' milk protein intolerance was suggested as a cause of constipation in children: 25 children (3 months to 11 years) with chronic constipation were given a cows' milk protein free diet for 4 weeks. Constipation disappeared in seven (28%) children and reappeared within 48–72 hours of an open challenge with cows' milk protein. Six of the seven children had a personal or family history of atopy and five of the seven had elevated total IgE levels. Because the study was conducted in children referred to a gastroenterologist, the findings may not be generalizable to children in general. Also, although the intake of cows' milk was restricted, no mention was made of other dairy products like cheese and yogurt. You find no RCTs that demonstrate a proven effect of increasing intakes of fluids, non-absorbable carbohydrates or dietary fiber on stool frequency or consistency in children. However, you find two case–control studies[23,24] in which children who were constipated were found to have a lower intake of dietary fiber than controls who were not constipated. In a random sample of children living in Greece,[23] 299 constipated individuals and 1600 controls were identified. Discriminant analysis demonstrated that only fiber intake independently correlated with constipation and that low fiber intake correctly predicted 70% of constipated children. In the second study,[24] 52 constipated Brazilian children aged 2–12 years were compared with 52 controls. The odds ratio (OR) for being constipated was 4·1 (CI 1·6–10·3) in children whose ingestion of fiber was below the recommended level compared with children with an appropriate intake.

You are familiar with two non-randomized clinical trials in children showing that carbohydrates such as sorbitol (which is found in fruit juices such as prune, pear, and apple) is incompletely absorbed and can increase stool frequency and water content; however, neither mentions the effect on constipation as an outcome.[25,26]

Question

2. In infants and children (*population*), does dietary advice (*intervention*) prevent constipation (*outcome*)? **[Prevention]**

You are unable to find any prospective studies comparing methods of preventing constipation in infants and children. Historically, primary care physicians have used education to maximize parental understanding of the normal variations of bowel function and specific interventions to treat mild constipation and prevent chronic constipation.[27] High-fiber diets have been recommended. However, a non-randomized comparative study of two groups of children (with and without chronic constipation), whose families had been encouraged to eat a high-fiber diet, revealed that neither group received the recommended amount of fiber.[28] However, the group with constipation consumed less than one-quarter of the recommended intake. Without intense and ongoing dietary therapy, it is unlikely that families will change their eating habits. The lack of appropriate studies makes it unclear whether increasing dietary fiber is effective for preventing constipation.[29]

Question

3. In children (*population*) with a history of constipation since birth (*exposure*), what is the risk of a serious underlying condition such as Hirschsprung disease, neurogenic bowel, cystic fibrosis, or depression (*outcome*)? **[Diagnosis]**

A perusal of the documents you have found reminds you that many organic conditions, including intestinal nerve disorders like Hirschsprung disease, metabolic conditions like hypothyroidism, medications like opiates, environmental exposures like lead poisoning, occult neural tube defects that affect the sacral nerves, and anatomic abnormalities like anterior displaced anus can be associated with constipation.[6,30] You find that fever, abdominal distention, vomiting, weight loss, or poor weight gain are not typically described in children who have functional constipation and may warn of a more serious condition. Bloody diarrhea in an infant with a history of constipation could be an indication of enterocolitis complicating Hirschsprung disease, which, if not identified early, may have serious, even fatal, consequences.[31] Constipated children, especially those less than 1 year of age, who present with constipation and a history of delayed passage of meconium, vomiting, bloody diarrhea, failure to thrive, abdominal distension, anal stenosis, or an empty rectum on examination, have a higher probability than those without these features of a serious underlying condition such as Hirschsprung disease or cystic fibrosis.[32,33]

The probability of these conditions is extremely low. The sensitivity and specificity (and likelihood ratios) either for individual signs and symptoms, for combinations of signs and symptoms, or for diagnostic tests to detect organic causes of constipation have not been determined. If Hirschsprung disease occurs in 1 in 7000[34] children but the tests (signs and symptoms) are not 100% specific, then even in a child with constipation since birth, the probability of Hirschsprung disease is extremely low. For example, if constipation since birth (the test) is 95% specific for Hirschsprung disease, the post-test probability of having Hirschsprung disease will be 0·27%. Children with constipation who fail to respond to therapy typically undergo further tests to exclude hypothyroidism and celiac disease. Diagnostic tests including abdominal radiography,[35] anorectal manometry,[36] and studies of transit time[37] may also be performed by specialists, but neither the sensitivity and specificity of these tests for detecting uncommon causes of constipation, nor the prevalence of these conditions is known.

Questions of therapy

To answer your questions on therapy you decide to read the most recent articles related to therapy in children most like your two patients. You are particularly interested in RCTs and systematic reviews which provide the best evidence about a therapy. You are also interested in reports of adverse effects as this will influence your decision to use a medication, even if it is an effective treatment for constipation.

Question

4. In infants and children with prolonged constipation (*population*), are enemas, laxatives, and manual evacuation (*intervention*) effective for disimpaction of stool (*outcome*)? **[Therapy]**

Treatment of constipation is typically divided into three stages: disimpaction, maintenance therapy, and monitoring. Impaction is determined by a hard mass in the lower abdomen on physical examination, a dilated rectum filled with a large amount of stool on rectal examination, or excessive stool in the colon on abdominal radiography. Disimpaction is usually performed so that subsequent treatments can be effective.[38] In your search of the literature you find no blinded RCT that compares the effectiveness of medications for use in disimpaction in children. However, uncontrolled clinical trials have described disimpaction by the oral route, the rectal route, or a combination of the two.[40–42] Mineral oil, polyethylene glycol (PEG) electrolyte solution (Golytely), lactulose, magnesium citrate, senna, and bisacodyl have all been reported as effective oral agents. In one study, Tolia[39] performed a randomized, open-label, prospective study comparing mineral oil with a PEG electrolyte solution. Children receiving the PEG electrolyte solution had more frequent bowel movements and showed more effective clearance of abdominal and rectal lumps ($P < 0.01$) 2 days later. However, these children had more vomiting and were less compliant ($P < 0.01$) compared with children taking mineral oil.

Enemas using phosphate soda, saline, and mineral oil are commonly used and appear to be effective, although they have not been studied using controls.[43,44] In one uncontrolled study, glycerin suppositories were useful in infants for facilitating the excretion of meconium.[45] Manual disimpaction, with or without sedation has been used by many practitioners. No controlled trials have been performed to evaluate its safety or efficacy. One prospective, observational study in 17 adults found that manual disimpaction under general anesthesia was associated with endosonographic evidence of disruption of one or both anal sphincters. The relevance to children of this limited study performed in adults is not clear; however, anal sphincter disruption in young children would be an undesirable harm.[46] In a recent trial of PEG powder[47] (PEG 3350, Miralax), 40 children with constipation for more than 3 months and impaction were randomly assigned to receive one of four doses for 3 days. Observers who were blinded to the dose evaluated the children. Of the children who received the higher doses (1 and 1·5 g kg^{-1} per day), 95% were successfully disimpacted compared with 55% of children who received the lower doses (0·25 and 0·5 g kg^{-1} per day) ($P < 0.005$). Diarrhea and bloating were more common ($P < 0.02$) in the group receiving the higher doses than in those receiving the lower doses. No studies were found to support the use of PEG 3350 in *infants* for disimpaction.

Question

5. In children with constipation (*population*), what is the effect of maintenance therapy with increased dietary

fiber, osmotic laxatives, stimulant laxatives, or placebo (*intervention*) on the risk of pain, hard stool, soiling, and frequency of stools (*outcome*)? **[Therapy]**

Maintenance therapy for constipation begins after a child is disimpacted. Typically, therapy consists of dietary advice, behavior modification, and medications. Medications are often required to help constipated children achieve regular bowel movements. Typically, outcomes are measured in months, not weeks, because relapse after short-term therapy is frequent.

You find no RCTs in children evaluating the effect of dietary fiber intake compared with placebo or standard diet on the duration of constipation. As discussed under question 1, children who are constipated have a lower intake of dietary fiber. However, recommending an increase of fiber as a treatment for constipation may not be effective. First, simply recommending a change may not lead to a change in eating patterns and second, increasing fiber may not be sufficient to treat (as opposed to prevent) constipation.

You find no placebo-controlled RCTs of osmotic laxatives in children. Several open-label studies of PEG evaluated maintenance treatment for constipation and suggest that PEG is safe, effective, and well accepted.[48–52] No study suggests that PEG is superior to other less expensive or more traditional agents. One RCT in 169 children showed that adding laxatives to a baseline of behavior management improved constipation and encopresis. Children were followed for 12 months and outcomes included the frequency of fecal accidents and the nature of the stools.[53] The management consisted of disimpaction with a "microenema" (Microlax) plus both oral and rectal bisacodyl, followed by long-term treatment with a combination preparation (Agarol), which contains mineral oil plus phenolphthalein. However, phenolphthaleins are not usually used in children because of the association between their use and adenomatous colorectal polyps in adults.[54] Published studies of commonly used laxatives such as mineral oil[55,56] and magnesium hydroxide[4] have not included a comparison group. The effects of other laxatives have been studied in two small RCTs, which compared lactitol and lactulose, both disaccharides derived from lactose.[57,58] In these studies the preparations were equally effective for normalizing stool consistency[57] and increasing stool frequency[58] at 2 and 4 weeks respectively.

Stimulant laxatives like senna and bisacodyl are frequently used for long-term treatment of constipation.[59,60] You find no placebo-controlled RCTs in children. In one RCT, constipated children aged 3–12 years were assigned to receive senna or mineral oil. After 6 months, 55% of children treated with mineral oil had successfully discontinued regular medication compared with 22% of those treated with senna.[61]

Studies of children who have been referred to pediatric gastroenterologists[27] indicate that relapses of constipation are common and that maintenance medications should be continued for months. For instance, Sondheimer[61] found at least one recurrence of symptoms occurred in 66% of children randomly assigned to be treated with mineral oil and 89% of children treated with senna for 6 months. A stimulant laxative like bisacodyl or senna is often used in clinical practice for short-term treatment to "rescue" a child whose constipation has worsened while on maintenance therapy (relapse).[62] However, no formal evidence of the value of this treatment has been published. Routine monitoring of children during and after maintenance therapy is useful to determine the ongoing effect of treatment and to identify those who relapse or require longer treatment.

Question
6. In children with constipation (*population*) treated with osmotic laxatives, stimulant laxatives, or enemas (*intervention*), what is the risk of adverse drug effects (*outcome*)? **[Therapy]**

A double-blind RCT by Nurko *et al.*[16] identified in *Evidence-Based Medicine Reviews* shows that cisapride is effective in the treatment of children with constipation. It increases the frequency of bowel movements and decreases episodes of soiling and gastrointestinal transit time.[63] However, because of the cardiac arrhythmias associated with its use, cisapride is no longer available in the USA, except under a special Limited Access Program. On the other hand, an epidemiological study of arrhythmias from cisapride[64] found that the risk from the use of cisapride was equivocal (RR for ventricular arrhythmias 1·60; CI 0·67–3·82).

Your search of the literature also reveals isolated case reports of toxicity from various agents used to treat constipation, which makes it impossible to quantify the risk of toxicity. For example, magnesium given as an enema [65] or as an oral agent to an infant[66] may lead to magnesium toxicity. Soapsuds enema may cause acute colitis,[67] tap water enema may lead to hyponatremia.[68] Chronic use of phosphated enemas can lead to hypocalcemia.[69] Oral mineral oil may lead to aspiration with subsequent lipoid pneumonia in infants and children, especially those who are disabled.[70,71] Concern has been expressed that chronic use of oral mineral oil may lead to diminished absorption of fat-soluble vitamins. One prospective cohort study of children who received mineral oil for 4 months found that serum levels of beta-carotene were reduced but that the treatment had no effect on serum levels of retinol and alpha-tocopherol.[56] In a 6-month follow up of children on mineral oil and laxatives, McClung and colleagues found that biochemical and anthropometric indicators of nutritional status were not adversely affected by

the therapy.[72] Long-term use of stimulant laxatives in adults has been associated with anatomic changes in the colon characterized by loss of folds. This finding suggests neuronal injury or damage to colonic longitudinal musculature.[59] Senna, in particular, has been associated with melanotic deposits in the colon, consistent with cell death.[60] Although these studies of toxicity are not population-based, you conclude that it is wise to avoid long-term use of these agents in children.

The treatment of constipation in infancy is similar to that for older children, with some important exceptions. The addition of fruits and vegetables are recommended for an infant weaning to solid foods.[73,74] Previously, concern was expressed that too much fruit juice could lead either to failure-to-thrive or to obesity.[75,76] However, recent studies have questioned these findings.[77,78] Based primarily on clinical experience and studies of the physiology of carbohydrate absorption in infants,[79] increased intake of juices containing sorbitol (such as prune, pear, and apple) is recommended to treat functional constipation. Based on anecdotal experience, barley malt extract, corn syrup, lactulose, or sorbitol are traditionally used as stool softeners. Mineral oil is not recommended in infants because gastroesophageal reflux and incoordination of swallowing are more common in this age group, increasing the risk of aspiration of mineral oil, which can induce a severe lipoid pneumonia.[69,70] Glycerin suppositories can be useful,[45,80] but laxatives, including PEG, and enemas should be avoided because of lack of evidence regarding their safety in infancy.

Question
7. In children with constipation (*population*) given behavior therapy (*intervention*) compared with standard care (*comparison*), is there a reduction in the risk of pain, hard stool, and soiling (*outcome*)? **[Therapy]**

One RCT identified in the *Cochrane Library*'s controlled trials register evaluated the use of biofeedback.[14] Forty-nine children, mean age 93 months, with chronic idiopathic constipation were randomized to receive biofeedback or conventional therapy (laxatives alone). In the short term (3 months) children in the biofeedback group improved more than the children in the conventional therapy group. However, no long-term differences were found. Traditionally, published studies of behavior modification and toilet training in children have not included a comparison group.[81–83] Historically, physicians have advised families to provide unhurried time for regular toileting for children who are developmentally ready for toilet training.[84] The rationale for this is that provision of information to families regarding the pathophysiology of constipation and soiling may help remove some of the anxiety associated with this condition, especially if fecal soiling is present. Unusual behavior in constipated children has been attributed to attempts to withhold stool by contracting the anal sphincter and gluteal muscles because passage of stool is painful.[85] In most instances, fecal soiling is not wilful behavior and is not helped by scolding or embarrassing the child. Asking families to keep a diary of stools and providing children with rewards for stools passed in the toilet are also frequently used methods of behavioral modification. Neither has been studied scientifically and their efficacy is not established.

Resolution of the scenarios

You tell the parents you believe both their children have constipation but because neither has any signs that suggest a serious underlying condition, you treat them without further investigation. You tell the parents that you do not believe that the iron-fortified formula is contributing to their infant's constipation. You add a lactulose supplement to her formula and ask her parents to keep a log of her bowel movements and contact you in 3 days. They report then that the girl's stools are softer and that she appears more comfortable, so you recommend that they continue this treatment for 4 more weeks and call you after that period.

You suggest an oral electrolyte solution containing polyethylene glycol to disimpact the 3-year-old boy; however, he refuses to take it. You therefore prescribe an enema containing phosphate soda plus high dose oral lactulose. This results in a large bowel movement so you start him on maintenance therapy consisting of a smaller dose of daily lactulose. You ask his parents to keep a diary of his bowel movements and behavior. The boy refuses to take the lactulose, so you switch him to high dose PEG, which he accepts. You explain to his parents that the boy's unusual behavior may represent his attempt to withhold stool by contracting the anal sphincter and gluteal muscles and that he does this because passage of stool is painful. Although no controlled trials have evaluated the effects of diet on constipation in children, you recommend a balanced diet containing whole grains, fruits, and vegetables, since this will not cause harm. You think it is also possible that cows' milk

intolerance is contributing to the boy's constipation. You ask his family to contact your nurse every month and arrange a follow up visit in 3 months. You plan to try a cows' milk-free diet for 2 weeks if the boy does not respond to conventional treatment and becomes constipated again.

Future research needs

Although constipation is an extremely common pediatric concern, good quality evidence to guide treatment is lacking. Few RCTs or systematic reviews have been performed in children; most care is based on case series or expert opinion. There is an urgent need for good research to address this deficit and a number of research questions are listed below:

- What aspects of the history and physical examination are most helpful in diagnosing organic causes of constipation? What is their sensitivity and specificity and likelihood ratio?
- What is the prevalence of organic conditions in children presenting with constipation to a primary care physician's office?
- Is dietary fiber beneficial for prevention and/or treatment of constipation in children? If so, what type and how much is required? Are dietary factors, including fruit juices, useful for treating and/or preventing constipation? Does withdrawal of cows' milk reduce symptoms in constipated children?
- What is the best treatment for initial disimpaction of constipated children? What are the long term risks and benefits of manual disimpaction in children?
- What is the best long-term (maintenance) treatment for constipation in children?
- What role does behavior modification have in the treatment of constipation?
- What is the natural history of constipation in children? Do these children become constipated adults? Do they have a higher risk of colon cancer?

Summary table

Question	Type of evidence	Result	Comments and adverse effects
Does dietary content influence the risk of constipation?	RCT of iron-fortified formula[20] Case–control studies of dietary fiber[23,24] Cross-over trial of cows' milk and soy[21] Cows' milk avoidance[22] Uncontrolled studies of carbohydrates in food, e.g., sorbitol[25,26]	Iron-fortified formula made no difference Low dietary fiber correlated with constipation Cows' milk may cause constipation in susceptible children Sorbitol increases stool frequency	Cows' milk study was done in a referral sample and may not apply to all children
Does dietary advice prevent constipation?	No studies		
Risk of underlying problem in children with constipation "since birth"	Case series[6,13,31–33]	<10% underlying disease in referral population, likely much lower in unselected population	Fever, bloody stools, growth failure, failure to pass meconium may point to specific etiology
Treatment of disimpaction with enemas, laxatives, and manual means	One RCT of PEG electrolyte solution *v* mineral oil[39] Uncontrolled trials describe many effective oral and rectal agents[38,40–44]	Golytely (PEG electrolyte solution) more effective than mineral oil but more vomiting, less compliance	Safety of manual disimpaction questioned in adult studies
Increased dietary fiber compared to no added fiber	No RCT Case–control studies suggest constipated children have lower fiber intake[23,24]	Possible improvement in constipation Possible long-term benefit to prevent GI neoplasias	Abdominal pain and cramps
Osmotic laxatives compared to other agents	RCT[53]	Beneficial effect of laxative in children receiving behavior therapy	Infants susceptible to magnesium poisoning
Lubricants, e.g., mineral oil, magnesium hydroxide	Uncontrolled trials showing efficacy[55,56]	Possible benefit	Aspiration risk with mineral oil in infancy
Stimulant laxatives, e.g., senna, bisacodyl	Uncontrolled trials showing efficacy	Possible benefit	Long-term use associated with structural changes in the colon

References

1 Loening-Baucke V. Chronic constipation in children. *Gastroenterology* 1993;**105**:1557–64.

2 de Araujo Sant'Anna AM, Calcado AC. Constipation in schoolaged children at public schools in Rio de Janeiro, Brazil. *J Pediatr Gastroenterol Nutr* 1999;**29**:190–3.

3 Nyhan WE. Stool frequency of normal infants in the first weeks of life. *Pediatrics* 1952;**10**:414–25.

4 Weaver LT, Steiner H. The bowel habits of young children. *Arch Dis Child* 1983;**59**:649–52.

5 Hyams JS, Treem WR, Etienne NL *et al.* Effect of infant formula on stool characteristics of young infants. *Pediatrics* 1995;**95**:50–4.

6 Baker SS, Liptak GS, Colletti RB *et al.* Constipation in infants and children: evaluation and treatment. A medical position statement of the North American Society for Pediatric Gastroenterology and Nutrition. *J Pediatr Gastroenterol Nutr* 1999;**29**:612–26.

7 Van der plas RN, Benninga MA, Redekop WK, Taminiau JA, Buller HA. How accurate is the recall of bowel habits in children with defaecation disorders? *Eur J Pediatr* 1997;**156**:178–81.

8 Loening-Baucke VJ. Assessment, diagnosis, and treatment of constipation in childhood. *Wound Ostomy Continence Nurs* 1994;**21**:49–58.

9 van Ginkel R, Reitsma JB, Buller HA, van Wijk MP, Taminiau JA, Benninga MA. Childhood constipation: longitudinal follow up beyond puberty. *Gastroenterology* 2003;**125**:357–63.

10 Loening-Baucke V. Constipation in early childhood: patient characteristics, treatment, and longterm follow up. *Gut* 1993;**34**:1400–4.

11 Cayan S, Doruk E, Bozlu M, Duce MN, Ulusoy E, Akbay E. The assessment of constipation in monosymptomatic primary nocturnal enuresis. *Int Urol Nephrol* 2001;**33**:513–16.

12 Lucanto C, Bauer SB, Hyman PE, Flores AF, DiLorenzo C. Function of hollow viscera in children with constipation and voiding difficulties. *Dig Dis Sci* 2000;**45**:1274–1280.

13 Price KJ, Elliott TM. Stimulant laxatives for constipation and soiling in children. Cochrane Inflammatory Bowel Disease Group. In: Cochrane Collaboration. *Cochrane Library.* Issue 3. Oxford: Update Software, 2003.

14 Brazzelli M, Griffiths P. Behavioural and cognitive interventions with or without other treatments for defaecation disorders in children. Cochrane Incontinence Group. In: Cochrane Collaboration. *Cochrane Library.* Issue 3. Oxford: Update Software, 2003.

15 van der Plas RN, Benninga MA, Buller HA *et al.* Taminiau JA. Biofeedback training in treatment of childhood constipation: a randomised controlled study. *Lancet* 1996;**348**:776–80.

16 Nurko S, Garcia-Aranda JA, Worona LB, Zlochisty O. Cisapride for the treatment of constipation in children: A double-blind study. *J Pediatr* 2000;**136**:35–40.

17 Rubin G. Constipation. *Clin Evid* 2002;**7**:292–6.

18 Sackett DL, Haynes B, Tugwell P. *Clinical Epidemiology: A Basic Science for Clinical Medicine, 2nd ed.* Boston: Little, Brown, 1991.

19 Evidence-Based Medicine Informatics Project. *Evidence Based Medicine; Users Guides to the Medical Literature.* http://www.cche.net/principles/content_all.asp/, 1999.

20 Anonymous. Ironfortified formulas and gastrointestinal symptoms in infants: a controlled study, With the cooperation of The Syracuse Consortium for Pediatric Clinical Studies. *Pediatrics* 1980;**66**:168–70.

21 Iacono G, Cavataio F, Montalto G *et al.* Intolerance of cow's milk and chronic constipation in children. *N Engl J Med* 1998;**339**:1100–4.

22 Silva D, Soraia T, Dirceu S *et al.* Cows' milk protein intolerance and chronic constipation in children. *Pediatr Allergy Immunol* 2001;**12**:339–42.

23 Roma E, Adamidis D, Nikolara R, Constantopoulos A, Messaritakis J. Diet and chronic constipation in children: the role of fiber. *J Pediatr Gastroenterol Nutr* 1999;**28**: 169–74.

24 Morais MB, Vitolo MR, Aguirre A, Fagundes-Neto U. Measurement of low dietary fiber intake as a risk factor for chronic constipation in children. *J Pediatr Gastroenterol Nutr* 1999;**29**:132–5.

25 Kneepkens CMF. What happens to fructose in the gut? *Scand J Gastroenterol* 1989;**24**(Suppl. 171):1–8.

26 Gryboski JD. Diarrhea from dietetic candy. *N Engl J Med* 1966;**266**:818.

27 Rappaport LA, Levine MD. The prevention of constipation and encopresis: a developmental model and approach. *Pediatr Clin North Amer* 1986;**33**:859–69.

28 McClung HJ, Boyne L, Heitlinger L. Constipation and dietary fiber intake in children. *Pediatrics* 1995;**96**:999–1000.

29 Mooren GC, van der Plas RN, Bossuyt PM, Taminiau JA, Buller HA. [The relationship between intake of dietary fiber and chronic constipation in children] [Article in Dutch]. *Ned Tijdschr Geneeskd* 1996;**140**:2036–9.

30 Nowicki MJ, Bishop PR. Organic causes of constipation in infants and children. *Pediatr Ann* 1999;**28**:293–300.

31 Reding R, de Ville de Goyet J, Gosseye S *et al.* Hirschsprung's disease: a 20 year experience. *J Pediatr Surg* 1997;**32**: 1221–5.

32 Elhalaby EA, Coran AG, Blane CE, Hirschl RB, Teitelbaum DH. Enterocolitis associated with Hirschsprung's disease: a clinical radiological characterization based on 168 patients. *J Pediatr Surg* 1995;**30**:76–83.

33 Rubinstein S, Moss R, Lewiston N. Constipation and meconium ileus equivalent in patients with cystic fibrosis. *Pediatrics* 1986;**78**:473–9.

34 Russell MB, Russell CA, Niebuhr E. An epidemiologic study of Hirschprung's disease and additional anomalies. *Acta Paediatrica* 1994;**83**:68–71.

35 Benninga MA, Buller HA, Staalman CR *et al.* Defaecation disorders in children, colonic transit time versus the Barrscore. *Eur J Pediatr* 1995;**154**:277–84.

36 Emir H, Akman M, Sarimurat N, Kilic N, Erdogan E, Soylet Y. Anorectal manometry during the neonatal period: its specificity in the diagnosis of Hirschsprung's disease. *Eur J Pediatr Surg* 1999;**9**:101–3.

37 Benninga MA, Buller HA, Tytgat GN, Akkermans LM, Bossuyt PM, Taminiau JA. Colonic transit time in constipated children: does pediatric slowtransit constipation exist? *J Pediatr Gastroenterol Nutr* 1996;**23**:241–51.

38 Tolia V. Use of a balanced lavage solution in the treatment of fecal impaction. *J Pediatr Gastroenterol Nutr* 1988;**7**:299–301.

39 Tolia V, Lin CH, Elitsur Y. A prospective randomized study with mineral oil and oral lavage solution for treatment of faecal impaction in children. *Aliment Pharmacol Therapeut* 1993;**7**:523–9.

40 Gleghorn EE, Heyman MB, Rudolph CD. No-enema therapy for idiopathic constipation and encopresis. *Clin Pediatr* 1991;**30**:667–72.

41 Ingebo KB, Heyman MB. Polyethylene glycol-electrolyte solution for intestinal clearance in children with refractory encopresis. A safe and effective therapeutic program. *Am J Dis Child* 1988;**142**:340–2.

42 Halabi IM. Cisapride in management of chronic pediatric constipation. *J Pediatr Gastroenter Nutr* 1999;**28**:199–202.

43 Nurko SS, Garcia-Aranda JA, Guerrero VY, Woroma LB. Treatment of intractable constipation in children: experience with cisapride. *J Pediatr Gastroenterol Nutr* 1996;**22**:38–44.

44 Cox DJ, Sutphen J, Borowitz S, Dickens MN, Singles J, Whitehead WE. Simple electromyographic biofeedback treatment for chronic pediatric constipation/encopresis: preliminary report. *Biofeedback Self Regulation* 1994;**19**:41–50.

45 Weisman LE, Merenstein GB, Digirol M, Collins J, Frank C, Hudgins C. The effect of early meconium evacuation on early-onset hyperbilirubinemia. *Am J Dis Child* 1983;**137**: 666–8.

46 Gattuso JM, Kamm MA, Halligan SM, Bartram CI. The anal sphincter in idiopathic megarectum: effects of manual

disimpaction under general anesthetic. *Dis Colon Rectum* 1996;**39**:43–59.

47 Youssef NN, Peters JM, Henderson W, Shultz-Peters S, Lockhart DK, Di Lorenzo C. Dose response of PEG 3350 for the treatment of childhood fecal impaction. *J Pediatr* 2002; **141**:410–14.

48 Ferguson A, Culbert P, Gillett H, Barras N. New polyethylene glycol electrolyte solution for the treatment of constipation and faecal impaction. *J Gastroenterol Hepatol* 1999; **31**(Suppl. 3):S249–S252.

49 Gremse DA, Hixon J, Crutchfield A. Comparison of polyethylene glycol 3350 and lactulose for treatment of chronic constipation in children. *Clin Pediatr. (Phila)* 2002; **41**:225–9.

50 Loening-Baucke V. Polyethylene glycol without electrolytes for children with constipation and encopresis. *J Pediatr Gastroenterol Nutr* 2002;**34**:372–7.

51 Pashankar DS, Loening-Baucke V, Bishop WP. Safety of polyethylene glycol 3350 for the treatment of chronic constipation in children. *Arch Pediatr Adolesc Med* 2003;**157**:661–4.

52 Staiano A. Use of polyethylene glycol solution in functional and organic constipation in children. *Ital J Gastroenterol Hepatol* 1999;**31**(Suppl. 3):S260–S263.

53 Nolan T, Debelle G, Oberklaid F, Coffey C. Randomized trial of laxatives in treatment of childhood encopresis. *Lancet* 1991;**338**:523–7.

54 Longnecker MP, Sandler DP, Haile RW, Sandler RS. Phenolphthaleincontaining laxative use in relation to adenomatous colorectal polyps in three studies. *Environ Health Perspect* 1997;**105**:1210–12.

55 McClung HJ, Boyne LJ, Linsheid T *et al.* Is combination therapy for encopresis nutritionally safe. *Pediatrics* 1993;**91**:591–4.

56 Clark JH, Russell GJ, Fitzgerald JF, Nagamori KE. Serum beta-carotene, retinol, and alpha-tocopherol levels during mineral oil therapy for constipation. *Am J Dis Child* 1987;**141**: 1210–12.

57 Martino AM, Pesce F, Rosati U. [The effects of lactitol in the treatment of intestinal stasis in childhood] [Article in Italian]. *Minerva Pediatr* 1992;**44**:319–23.

58 Pitzalis G, Deganello F, Mariani P *et al.* [Lactitol in chronic idiopathic constipation in children] [Article in Italian]. *Pediatr Med Chir* 1995;**17**:223–6.

59 Joo JS, Ehrenpreis ED, Gonzalez L *et al.* Alterations in colonic anatomy induced by chronic stimulant laxatives: the cathartic colon revisited. *J Clin Gastroenterol* 1998;**26**: 283–6.

60 Benavides SH, Morgante PE, Monserrat AJ, Zarate J, Porta EA. The pigment of melanosis coli: a lectin histochemical study. *Gastrointest Endosc* 1997;**46**:131–8.

61 Sondheimer JJ, Gervaise EP. Lubricant versus laxative in the treatment of chronic functional constipation of children: a comparative study. *Pediatr Gastroenterol Nutr* 1982;**1**: 223–6.

62 Nurko SS. Constipation. In: Walker-Smith J, Hamilton D, Walker AW, eds. *Practical Pediatric Gastroenterology, 2nd edn.* Hamilton, Ontario: BC Decker, 1996.

63 Shulman RJ, Boyle JT, Colletti RB *et al.* The use of cisapride in children. The North American Society for Pediatric Gastroenterology and Nutrition. *J Pediatr Gastroenterol Nutr* 1999;**28**:529–33.

64 Enger C, Cali C, Walker AM. Serious ventricular arrhythmias among users of cisapride and other QT-prolonging agents in the United States. *Pharmacoepidemiol Drug Saf* 2002;**11**:477–86.

65 Sutton D, Nielsen M. Severe magnesium toxicity after magnesium sulphate enema in a chronically constipated child. *BMJ* 1990;**300**:541.

66 Alison LH, Bulugahapitiya D. Laxative induced magnesium poisoning in a 6 week old infant. *BMJ* 1990;**300**:125.

67 Pike BF, Phillipini PJ, Lawson EH Jr. Soap colitis. *N Engl J Med* 1971;**285**:217–18.

68 Chertow GM, Brady HR. Hyponatraemia from tapwater enema. *Lancet* 1994;**344**:748.

69 Reedy JC, Zwiren GT. Enema-induced hypocalcemia and hyperphosphatemia leading to cardiac arrest during induction of anesthesia in an outpatient surgery center. *Anesthesiology* 1983;**59**:578–9.

70 Rabah R, Evans RW, Yunis EJ. Mineral oil embolization and lipid pneumonia in an infant treated for Hirschsprung's disease. *Pediatr Pathol* 1987;**7**:447–55.

71 Fan LL, Graham LM. Radiological cases of the month. Lipoid pneumonia from mineral oil aspiration. *Arch Pediatr Adolesc Med* 1994;**148**:205–6.

72 McClung HJ, Boyne LJ, Linsheid T, Heitlinger LA, Murray RD, Fyda JU. Is combination therapy for encopresis nutritionally safe? *Pediatrics* 1993;**91**:591–4.

73 Basch CE, Zybert P, Shea S. 5ADAY: dietary behavior and the fruit and vegetable intake of Latino children. *Am J Publ Hlth* 1994;**84**:814–18.

74 Lifshitz F. Weaning foods: the role of fruit juice in the diets of infants and children. *J Am Coll Nutr* 1996;**15**(Suppl. 5):1S–3S.

75 Smith MM, Lifshitz F. Excess fruit juice consumption as a contributing factor in nonorganic failure to thrive. *Pediatrics* 1994;**93**:438–43.

76 Dennison BA, Rockwell HL, Baker SL. Excess fruit juice consumption by preschool aged children is associated with short stature and obesity. *Pediatrics* 1997 Jan;**99**(1):15–22.

77 Alexy U, SichertHellert W, Kersting M, Manz F, Schoch G. Fruit juice consumption and the prevalence of obesity and short stature in German preschool children: results of the DONALD Study. Dortmund Nutritional and Anthropometrical Longitudinally Designed. *J Pediatr Gastroenterol Nutr* 1999;**29**:343–9.

78 Skinner JD, Carruth BR, Moran J 3rd, Houck K, Coletta F. Fruit juice intake is not related to children's growth. *Pediatrics* 1999;**103**:58–64.

79 Perman JA. Digestion and absorption of fruit juice carboydrates. *J Am Coll Nutr* 1996;**15**(Suppl. 5):12S–17S.

80 Smith MM, Davis M, Chasalow FI, Lifshitz F. Carbohydrate absorption from fruit juice in young children. *Pediatrics* 1995;**95**:340–4.

81 Zenk KE, Koeppel RM, Liem LA. Comparative efficacy of glycerin enemas and suppository chips in neonates. *Clin Pharm* 1993;**12**:846–8.

82 Van der plas RN, Benninga MA, Taminiau JA, Buller HA. Treatment of defaecation problems in children: the role of education, demystification and toilet training. *Eur J Pediatr* 1997;**156**:689–92.

83 Lowery SP, Srour JW, Whitehead WE, Schuster MM. Habit training as treatment of encopresis secondary to chronic constipation. *J Pediatr Gastroenterol Nutr* 1985;**4**: 397–401.

84 Howe AC, Walker CE. Behavioral management of toilet training, enuresis and encopresis. *Pediatr Clin North Am* 1992;**39**:413–32.

85 Partin JC, Hamill SK, Fischel JE, Partin JS. Painful defecation and fecal soiling in children. *Pediatrics* 1992;**89**:1007–9.

37 Acute gastroenteritis

Kate Armon, Elizabeth J Elliott

Case scenario

You are called to the emergency department to see a 2-year-old boy with an 18-hour history of watery diarrhea (nine dirty diapers containing a greenish, liquid stool without blood) and vomiting (five clear vomits containing neither blood nor bile). He is "off his food" and reluctant to drink. He had a glass of flat lemonade an hour ago, but vomited this back immediately. His mother can't say when he last passed urine and is worried that he is lethargic and looks unwell. She asks whether he is dehydrated. On examination, he is listless but cooperative. His temperature is 38°C, pulse 120 beats per minute, and respiratory rate 35 breaths per minute. Peripheral perfusion is normal and blood pressure 85/65 mmHg. His tongue is dry, his eyes are sunken and his skin turgor is diminished. His weight, at 14·1 kg, is 0·9 kg lower than that recorded by the family doctor when he was seen 8 days earlier with a cut forehead. There is no evidence of localized or systemic infection, and his abdomen is soft and non-tender. A number of children at the same day care center have had gastroenteritis, and you think this is his diagnosis. You wonder whether he could be treated at home, but calculate that he has lost 6% body weight and admit him to hospital for rehydration therapy. You wonder whether you should insert an intravenous line. His mother asks whether you are going to prescribe any medications.

Background

Acute gastroenteritis is defined as the rapid onset of diarrhea (< 10 days duration) with or without nausea, vomiting, fever, or abdominal pain.[1] Diarrhea is a change in the frequency and/or consistency of the stools for an individual child.[2] Acute gastroenteritis is caused by a viral agent in 87% of cases, and rotavirus makes up the majority of these.[3–6] Most of the remaining 13% of cases have a bacterial etiology, the most common pathogens in developed communities being *Campylobacter* spp., *Salmonella* spp, *Shigella* spp., and *Escherichia coli*.

Worldwide, acute gastroenteritis is a major health problem. Acute diarrhea affects 3–5 billion individuals per year, and is either directly or indirectly associated with 5–10 million deaths per year.[7] In 1988 the World Health Organization (WHO) estimated that in Asia (excluding China), Africa, and Latin America, 4 million children < 5 years die annually from diarrhea and that 80% of these deaths occur in the first 2 years of life.[8] Although the vast majority of deaths occur in developing communities, gastroenteritis remains a significant cause of morbidity in the developed world. In the UK it accounts for 204 general practitioner consultations per 1000 children aged < 5 years per year.[9] Gastroenteritis leads to hospital admission in 7/1000 children aged < 5 years per year in the UK, and 13/1000 in the USA.[10] In Australia it is the fifth most common cause of hospital admission, and accounts for 5·9% of all admissions of children < 15 years.[11]

The symptoms and signs of gastroenteritis are non-specific and it is important to exclude systemic infections, surgical, and other causes, particularly in young children. Acute gastroenteritis is usually self-limiting and the associated morbidity and mortality results from water and electrolyte losses. The key to management is rehydration and prevention of dehydration. Fluids may either be given by the oral (mouth or nasogastric tube) or intravenous route. Antibiotics have no role in the management of viral gastroenteritis but are occasionally indicated for treatment of some bacterial infections. The use of antiemetics and antidiarrheal agents is contentious.[1]

Framing answerable clinical questions

A number of management issues arise from this case scenario. You structure your clinical questions to clarify your thinking and help direct your search of the literature (see Chapter 2) and focus on issues directly relevant to the management of your patient.

Questions

1. In children with acute gastroenteritis (*population*), what clinical signs (*tests*) are of value in estimating the presence of mild–moderate dehydration (*outcome*)? **[Diagnosis]**
2. In young children with acute gastroenteritis and mild–moderate dehydration (*population*), is admission to hospital *(intervention)* preferable to outpatient/home management (*comparison*) for management of fluid and electrolyte balance (*outcome*)? **[Therapy]**
3. In young children with acute gastroenteritis and mild–moderate dehydration (*population*), are intravenous fluids *(intervention)* more effective than oral fluids (*comparison*) for rehydration without risk of adverse effects (*outcome*)? **[Therapy]**
4. In young children with acute viral gastroenteritis and mild–moderate dehydration (*population*), is a glucose-electrolyte solution (*intervention*) more effective than a cereal-based solution (*comparison*) for oral rehydration (*outcome*)? **[Therapy]**
5. In children with acute gastroenteritis and mild–moderate dehydration (*population*), is a low osmolality solution (*intervention*) more effective than a high osmolality solution (*comparison*) for rehydration, decreasing stool output or decreasing hospital stay (*outcome*)? **[Therapy]**
6. In children with viral gastroenteritis (*population*), is treatment with *Lactobacillus* plus a hypotonic ORS (*intervention*) more effective than treatment with ORS alone (*comparison*) for decreasing stool output or hospital stay (*outcome*)? **[Therapy]**
7. In young children with acute viral gastroenteritis (*population*), does loperamide (*intervention*) decrease the volume or duration of diarrhea (*outcome*)? **[Therapy]**

Searching for evidence

You first search for "predigested" evidence, such as systematic reviews (which may include meta-analyses) and clinical practice guidelines, for information on the management of "acute gastroenteritis" (see Chapters 3 and 8). This is a time-efficient method of obtaining information following its critical appraisal by others. You look for high-quality systematic reviews and guidelines that have been developed using sound methodology. You initially search under "gastroenteritis", which appears as a medical subject (MeSH) heading in the available electronic databases.

In the *Cochrane Library* you find 16 completed systematic reviews of which four (one on immunoglobulin in rotavirus gastroenteritis, one on reduced osmolarity oral rehydration solutions [ORS], one on rice-based ORS and one on the use of antibiotics in gastroenteritis) may be relevant. The Database of Abstracts of Reviews of Effects (DARE) in the *Cochrane Library* has three abstracts of quality assessed systematic reviews, one of which (on the efficacy of glucose-based ORS)

is directly relevant to one of your questions. While in the *Cochrane Library*, you also go to the Cochrane Central Register of Controlled Trials (CENTRAL), knowing you will need a randomized controlled trial (RCT) for questions on therapy for which no systematic review is available. You find over 223 RCTs under gastroenteritis, nine of which look relevant to your questions.

Next you go to the index of *Clinical Evidence*, a new compendium of evidence on the effects of common clinical interventions, and find a chapter on acute gastroenteritis in the section on Child Health with a search date of June 2003.[12] This looks both useful and relevant to your questions.

You then go to MedLine using the PubMed search screen, enter "gastroenteritis AND guideline" and find 55 articles, which you limit to "children 0–18" and "human", yielding 41. You are particularly interested in guidelines based on systematic reviews. You scan the titles and discard those that address virology, vaccinations, gastroenteritis in adults, and evaluations of practice guidelines. The remaining five look very useful. The first is a "practical guideline for the management of gastroenteritis in children,"[13] the second "an evidence and consensus based guideline for acute diarrhea management,"[14] and the third is entitled "guidelines for managing acute gastroenteritis based on a systematic review of published research".[15] The fourth is an article on refeeding in gastroenteritis by the European Society of Paediatric Gastroenterology and Nutrition[16] and the fifth is a practice parameter by the American Academy of Pediatrics (AAP)[1] on the management of acute gastroenteritis in young children.

You then enter the search terms "gastroenteritis AND systematic review", which yields six articles. You have already found two of these,[14,15] two are not relevant, one relates to the use of probiotics,[17] and one looks like a personal practice review.[18] You decide to look at the systematic reviews before searching further.

Searching for evidence syntheses (secondary evidence)*

Cochrane Library: "gastroenteritis"

- Cochrane database of systematic reviews (CDSR): 16 (4)
- Database of Abstracts of Reviews of Effects (DARE): 3 (1)
- Cochrane Central Register of Controlled Trials (CCRCT): 223 (9)

Clinical Evidence: 1 (1)

MedLine: (PubMed)

- "gastroenteritis AND guideline": 55 (5)
- "gastroenteritis AND systematic review": 6 (3)

*Numbers of articles found and (in brackets) number considered relevant and useful

Critical review of the evidence

As with any publication, it is necessary to critically appraise sources of secondary evidence (systematic reviews and clinical practice guidelines) to assess their validity. Guides for evaluating these are found in Chapter 8 and in the relevant Users' Guides to the Medical Literature.[19–21]

The *Practical guideline for the management of gastroenteritis in children*[13] does not have an abstract. The journal is not available on line to non-subscribers, so you order a copy from your local library and read the next review. "An evidence and consensus based guideline for acute diarrhea management" is published in *the Archives of Disease in Childhood*, and the full text is available free.[14] The guideline addresses a clinical problem rather than a diagnosis, namely the assessment, investigation, need for admission, and treatment in the child attending hospital with diarrhea and vomiting. The recommendations in the guidelines are based on a systematic review of the literature and the evidence found is graded according to described methods. The recommendations were also subjected to a Delphi consensus development process.[14] This process involved a multidisciplinary panel of 39 health professionals (medical and nursing staff on pediatric wards, in A&E departments, and including specialist gastroenterology consultants) who look after children with diarrhea. Consensus statements were generated using a three round postal method. For this process to be valid, the views of contributors must remain anonymous. The final recommendations included in the guideline state both the level of published evidence on which they are based and whether or not the panel achieved 83% agreement on the recommendation. Thus, areas where evidence is poor and there is a need for further research are made explicit in the review. An accompanying commentary appraises this paper along with that of Murphy[15] and the American Academy of Pediatrics guidelines.[1] The author of the commentary points out that none of the three reviews included hand searching or looking for unpublished trials, suggesting that important evidence may be missing.[22] Bearing in mind this possible limitation you read on because the paper both addresses your questions and focuses on the same patient population as yours.

The AAP practice parameter[1] was based on a systematic review of the literature addressing the issues of rehydration method, refeeding following rehydration, and use of antidiarrheal agents. The population studied was children aged 1 month to 5 years with acute diarrhea (< 10 days), who live in developed countries and who had no underlying disorder. Specific outcomes studied included success or failure of rehydration, resolution of diarrhea, and adverse effects of antidiarrheal agents. Search strategies were clearly defined. As the patient population is similar to yours, you believe the results will be applicable to your patients. The authors state whether qualitative or quantitative (meta-analysis) data synthesis was used for each question, but do not provide details on critical appraisal of the primary sources. The reader is referred to the "Technical Report" which is available by post from the AAP. An abstract of the report is published with the practice parameter. The technical report is not available on line at the AAP website (http://www.aap.org). However, the abstract provides sufficient information to indicate that the parameter is methodologically sound. The recommendations do not state the level of evidence on which they are based.

Murphy's systematic review[15] clearly defines the population of interest (infants and children with acute gastroenteritis), the search strategy, and the topics addressed (assessment of the risk of dehydration; assessment of the degree of dehydration; use of oral rehydration therapy [ORT]; strategies for rehydration; management of hypernatremic dehydration; nutritional management during and after the illness; and the role of pharmacological agents including antidiarrheals and antimicrobials). The strength of the evidence in support of each recommendation is graded, based on criteria recommended in the north of England evidence-based guidelines development project.[23] You are satisfied that the method of this review was sound and that the results can be applied to your patients.

Your librarian has located a copy of Sandhu's paper.[13] When you read the first few paragraphs, it is clear that the recommendations have been developed by an "expert" panel, the European Society of Paediatric Gastroenterology, Nutrition (ESPGAN) working group on acute diarrhea. Although references are given, there is no evidence to suggest a systematic literature review was performed, neither is there any attempt to explicitly link the recommendations with evidence, or to grade the level of evidence available. The ESPGAN working group states that their recommendations are concordant with those issued by the American Academy of Pediatrics and the World Health Organization, except that the ORS recommended by the WHO has a different composition from that recommended for Europe. In summary, there has not been an explicit attempt to collect all the evidence, published or otherwise, or to appraise the quality of the evidence found. The guidelines could be termed a "narrative review" and you read it aware of these limitations.

You now address each clinical questions in turn and find that for several questions you require more information. Additional search strategies are stated after each question.

Question
1. In children with acute gastroenteritis (*population*), what clinical signs (*tests*) are of value in estimating the presence of mild–moderate dehydration (*outcome*)? **[Diagnosis]**

Search criteria

● MedLine: "gastroenteritis AND dehydration (368) AND child": 243 (2)

Severity of dehydration is most accurately assessed in terms of weight lost as a percentage of total body weight prior to the dehydrating episode. On the advice of a colleague you access the World Health Organization site (http://www.who.org) for their current classification of dehydration. According to the WHO criteria, mild–moderate and severe dehydration correspond to 3–8% and ≥ 9% loss of body weight, respectively.[24] However, you know from your clinical practice that an accurate weight immediately pre-illness is rarely available. You are therefore interested to know whether the clinical signs that you noted in your patient can accurately define the presence and/or degree of dehydration. In this situation the diagnostic tests that you have available include both clinical signs and laboratory tests.

Armon's paper addresses this issue and quotes from two prospective cohort studies.[25,26] You also search MedLine for articles on gastroenteritis and dehydration in childhood. You recognize that the most useful type of study to answer a question about the usefulness of a diagnostic test is a cross-sectional or cohort study in which the test being evaluated is compared with a reference or "gold" standard in an appropriate spectrum of patients. In the comparison group the reference standard should be performed independent of, blind to, and regardless of the test result. You do not find any additional studies. You read Chapter 5 (Assessing diagnostic tests) and use the *JAMA* Users' guides for assessing diagnostic tests to evaluate the two studies found.[27,28]

Mackenzie *et al.*[25] studied a cohort of 102 Australian children aged 3–36 months presenting to an emergency department with acute gastroenteritis. The authors aimed to determine the reliability of clinical signs of dehydration, venous pH, base deficit, and serum urea, in assessing the degree of dehydration, as quantified by an objective measure, namely weight gain following rehydration. Dehydration was assessed clinically by the pediatric admitting medical officer. Clinical signs of dehydration were noted and bare weight was recorded by nursing staff before and after rehydration. Children with no clinical signs of dehydration and those with circulatory failure (judged to have severe dehydration) were excluded from the analysis. Children who had *any* clinical signs of dehydration were included in the study. Children were categorized as having had no dehydration if they had gained <4% body weight (59/102 [58%]) and mild–moderate dehydration if they had gained ≥ 4% of their body weight (43/102 [42%]) during rehydration.

In Mackenzie's study there was an independent blind comparison with the "gold" standard for diagnosis of dehydration. Nurses recording weight gain following rehydration were unaware of the clinical assessment of dehydration and biochemical parameters were recorded before the extent of dehydration (weight gain) was known. The diagnostic tests were evaluated only in children with clinical signs of dehydration and not in those with severe dehydration. In some cases the "tests" were poorly defined, for example, "no urine for many hours" and "increased thirst" are subjective. For some signs data were missing. However, the reference standard was applied regardless of the test result and the children in this study are very similar to your patient population.

The authors examined whether the proportion of children with each clinical sign at presentation differed significantly between those subsequently shown to be < 4% or ≥ 4% dehydrated. The best clinical indicators of mild–moderate dehydration (i.e., indicating weight loss of ≥ 4%) were decreased peripheral perfusion, deep breathing, and decreased skin turgor. The best laboratory investigations were high urea, low pH, and a large base deficit. However, the data were expressed as proportions of each group with each physical sign and no sensitivities or specificities were given for any of the diagnostic tests. You use the raw data from the paper to determine the sensitivity, specificity, and positive and negative likelihood ratios (LR) for each clinical test for predicting those with ≥ 4% dehydration (Table 37.1). The likelihood ratio for a positive test result is calculated as LR+ = sensitivity/[1 − specificity] and for a negative test result is LR- = [1 − sensitivity]/specificity]. The larger the LR, the better the test for diagnosing or excluding a condition. As shown in Table 37.1 the sensitivity/specificity of these signs and tests was generally low and the LR is > 2 only for decreased peripheral perfusion, serum urea > 6·5 mmol liter^{-1}, and capillary pH < 7·35. If a test (for example, decreased peripheral perfusion) has a positive likelihood ratio of 2·5, that means that decreased peripheral perfusion is ~2·5 times more likely to be seen in a child with gastroenteritis and ≥ 4% dehydration, than in a child with < 4% dehydration.

From the data in the paper you calculate that the pretest probability of children in this study population having ≥ 4% dehydration is 42%. You can then use the LR that you have calculated and the LR nomogram (p. 35)[29] to estimate that, for children in your patient population, the post-test probability for ≥ 4% dehydration would be 68%, 68%, and 65%, respectively, for those having decreased peripheral perfusion, serum urea > 6·5 mmol liter^{-1} and capillary pH < 7·35. These tests individually do not increase the post-test probability much above the pretest probability and are therefore not particularly useful on their own (see action threshold in Chapter 5).

You suspect that use of a combination of the clinical signs and tests described would enable you to better predict the degree of dehydration in your patients, but data on children

Table 37.1   Usefulness of clinical signs and other diagnostic tests for detecting ≥4% dehydration in children with acute gastroenteritis (derived from Mackenzie *et al.*[25])

Clinical signs and symptoms and laboratory tests	Sensitivity (%)	Specificity (%)	LR+	LR−
↓ Skin turgor	65	56	1·4	0·6
↓ Peripheral perfusion	35	86	2·5	0·8
Sunken eyes	81	27	1·1	0·7
Pulse > 130 per min	56	49	1·1	0·9
Restless/lethargic	91	10	1·1	0·9
No urine for many hours	41	48	0·8	1·2
Sunken fontanelle	54	25	0·7	2·6
Systolic BP < 100 mmHg	45	62	1·2	0·8
Absent tears	43	66	1·3	0·9
Deep breathing (acidotic)	50	74	1·9	0·7
Respiratory rate < 30 per min	51	69	1·7	0·7
Dry mouth	85	29	1·2	0·5
Increased thirst	66	49	1·3	0·7
Serum urea > 6·5 mmol liter^{-1}	71	71	2·5	0·4
Capillary pH < 7·35	43	80	2·2	0·7
Base deficit > 7	67	52	1·4	0·6

Abbreviations: LR+, positive likelihood ratio; LR−, negative likelihood ratio.

with a combination of positive signs and tests are not available from this study. You know that in practice you take a history, do an examination, then perform a test if indicated, i.e., you do a sequence of diagnostic tests. The advantage of using the LR is that the post-test probability for the first test in the sequence becomes the pretest probability for the next. Thus, the pretest probability of having ≥ 4% dehydration in this study population (42%), becomes 68% in those children with decreased peripheral perfusion, and becomes 72% if they are also restless/lethargic. However, the use of a sequence of diagnostic tests is valid only when tests are independent of each other, i.e., measuring something different. For example, you could not combine decreased perfusion and decreased skin turgor because both reflect depleted intravascular volume. Similarly capillary pH and base deficit are not independent measures.

The other paper you found was a study of the value of clinical signs for estimating dehydration in a cohort of 135 boys 3–18 months of age in Egypt.[26] Boys with five or more watery stools per day for < 7 days were included. You decide the findings are applicable to your patient population, since children with malnutrition and serious non-gastrointestinal illness were excluded. On entry of patients into the study, a clinical estimate of the degree of dehydration was made by one of the three investigators in the presence of the other two. In the event of a disagreement with respect to the presence or magnitude of the various clinical signs, the majority opinion was accepted. Children assessed as mildly or moderately dehydrated were given ORS to replace their fluid

deficit over four hours. Children with severe dehydration received intravenous boluses of 20 ml kg^{-1} until their pulse, perfusion, and mental state returned to normal. Following rehydration children were weighed and the percentage dehydration was calculated.

You evaluate the study.[27,28] Because children were assessed clinically for dehydration before the true extent of dehydration (actual weight gain after rehydration) was known, there was an independent blind comparison with the "gold" standard for diagnosis. The diagnostic test was not evaluated in the full spectrum of patients with gastroenteritis, because children thought not to be dehydrated on clinical examination and children with malnutrition were excluded. However the "test" was well defined and the patients were similar to your population. The reference standard was applied regardless of the test result, and the test was applied in all cases. You are therefore satisfied the results of the study are valid.

All clinical signs tested (except sunken fontanelle) were found more frequently with increasing dehydration, as indicated by subsequent weight gain. "Prolonged skinfold" (decreased skin turgor) correlated most closely with the extent of dehydration. However, the correlation between individual signs and degree of dehydration was low. Multiple linear regression was used to examine the ability of various subsets of clinical signs to predict weight gain. In the final model "prolonged skinfold", dry oral mucosa, sunken eyes, and altered neurological status were selected as the clinical signs that could best explain variability in weight gain.

Table 37.2   Assessment of severity of dehydration*

No dehydration (< 3% weight loss)	Mild–moderate dehydration (3–8% weight loss)	Severe dehydration (≥ 9% weight loss)
No signs	Dry mucous membranes (be wary in the mouth breather)	Signs from the mild–moderate group plus
	Sunken eyes (and minimal or no tears)	Decreased peripheral perfusion (cool/mottled/pale peripheries; capillary refill time > 2 sec)
	Diminished skin turgor (pinch test > 1 sec)	Circulatory collapse
	Altered neurological status (drowsiness, irritability)	
	Deep (acidotic) breathing	

*Modified from WHO classification of dehydration[24]; signs are listed in each column in order of increasing severity.

However, these explained only 24% of the variability. As in Mackenzie's study, deep breathing, decreased skin turgor, and decreased peripheral perfusion were more often seen in children ≥ 4% dehydrated than in those < 4% dehydrated. Unfortunately the raw data are not given, and therefore you cannot calculate the sensitivity, specificity, or LRs for each clinical sign.

The WHO classification of dehydration, which has been modified in Table 37.2,[24] correlates very well with the evidence that you have found, and you therefore decide to continue to use it in your clinical practice.

Question

2. In young children with acute gastroenteritis and mild–moderate dehydration (*population*), is admission to hospital (*intervention*) preferable to outpatient/home management (*comparison*) for management of fluid and electrolyte balance (*outcome*)? **[Therapy]**

Search criteria

● MedLine: "gastroenteritis AND patient admission AND child": 33 (4)

Several studies that you have found suggest that many non-dehydrated children without biochemical or acid-base disturbance are admitted unnecessarily to hospital in developed communities, and that many of these children receive unnecessary intravenous fluids.[11,30–32] At the time of writing the guideline,[14] Armon found no published trials addressing this question. However, the consultative panel did formally agree on some consensus statements using the Delphi method described above. The published statements are in italics, with your thoughts in brackets.

● *Children presenting to hospital with acute gastroenteritis who are severely dehydrated should be admitted to hospital.* (This seems intuitive because it is likely they will require intravenous fluids.)

● *Children with mild–moderate dehydration should be–observed in a hospital pediatric facility for a period of at least 6 hours to ensure successful rehydration (3–4 hours) and maintenance of hydration (2–3 hours).* (This seems reasonable and you decide to review any child with signs of dehydration four hours after you commence oral rehydration, in order to assess the success or not of that therapy. Whether children are admitted to hospital for this period or observed in an emergency setting depends on individual circumstances.)

● *Children at high risk of dehydration on the basis of young age, high frequency of watery stools, or vomits, should be observed in a hospital pediatric facility for at least 4–6 hours to ensure adequate maintenance of hydration.* (Several publications[11,30–34] identify groups of "high risk" patients in whom admission should be readily considered. These include young infants [< 6 months age] and infants or children with high grade fever, a serious underlying condition [for example, diabetes, renal failure], blood in the stool, in whom the diagnosis is in doubt, in whom a surgical diagnosis [for example, appendicitis, intussusception] is being considered or in whom symptoms are worsening. You believe it is sensible to consider children in all these categories for admission, despite the lack of evidence to support these recommendations.)

● *Children whose parents or carers are thought to be unable to manage the child's condition at home successfully should be admitted to hospital.* (Fitzgerald[33] found that for children with the same severity of acute gastroenteritis, children whose mothers report higher levels of psychological distress, were more likely to be admitted. These mothers were also likely to have poor social resources. The influence of these factors on hospital admission is not easy to define, but they are important. In the USA the supply of beds, type of medical facility available (teaching or district general), and distance from home to the hospital have a profound effect on hospitalization rates in children. For example, children with gastroenteritis have a 15% higher chance of admission if they live in an area with a bed supply of 4/1000 rather than 1·9/1000 population.[34] You resolve to take into account social factors in families, including access to medical services, when assessing a child for admission.)

You find no RCTs comparing hospital admission with home management by parent or GP. However you find one RCT,[35] published after Armon's review comparing an acute pediatric "hospital at home" scheme with conventional hospital care. The hospital at home is operated by nurses, who provide a 24 hour a day service 7 days a week until 23·00 hours and an on-call service overnight. The trial included 399 of 464 eligible children with asthma, gastroenteritis, or fever. Of the 125 children with vomiting (with or without diarrhea) who were eligible for randomization, 70 received "hospital at home" and 55 received inpatient care. To be eligible for inclusion in the trial, children with acute diarrhea had to be over 6 months of age, with < 4 stools in 4 hours, with no bloody diarrhea, no dehydration, and adequate urine output. Children also had to be alert and to have tolerated at least 10 ml kg^{-1} of clear fluid without vomiting for 1 hour post-feed. Outcomes included readmission rate (a proxy for parent confidence in dealing with the illness), length of stay/care, and parent/carer satisfaction. Overall, the median number of care days was higher in children treated in the hospital at home versus the hospital (2 [0–9] versus 1 [0–10]; $P < 0.001$) but this outcome was not reported by disease subgroup. The readmission rate for children with diarrhea was lower in those treated at home (5% versus 13%; $P = 0.06$). In a qualitative study using the same sample the majority of parents and children indicated a clear preference for home care. They said that they believe a child recovers more quickly in their own home and that home care is cheaper and less disruptive to the family. Further research needs to be done on this subject.

Question

3. In young children with acute gastroenteritis and mild–moderate dehydration (*population*), are intravenous fluids (*intervention*) more effective than oral fluids (*comparison*) for rehydration without risk of adverse effects (*outcome*)? **[Therapy]**

You recognize that, for a question about therapy, a good systematic review of RCTs or individual RCTs will provide the best evidence. The authors of the article on Gastroenteritis in the Child Health section of the BMJ publication *Clinical Evidence* specifically addresses this question.[12] *Clinical Evidence* provides one of the best sources of regularly updated evidence for therapies for a wide range of conditions. A comprehensive search of the literature is conducted by BMJ staff for systematic reviews and RCTs that address questions asked by the authors. Abstracts of articles found are then sent to the authors for selection and critical appraisal of trials. The process is repeated approximately every 6 months. A systematic review and meta-analysis by Gavin[36] and four additional RCTs[37–40] (three in children with mild to moderate dehydration in developed communities) were critically appraised.

The systematic review,[36] on the "Efficacy of glucose-based oral rehydration therapy," included six RCTs comparing oral with intravenous rehydration (n = 193). It was reviewed in the *ACP Journal Club*[41] and the methods were considered to be sound. The search strategy was comprehensive (including contacting major organizations focusing on diarrhea), and inclusion criteria were specific (only RCTs in children with gastroenteritis in developed communities). The methods for the meta-analysis were described in detail and were appropriate.[42,43] All six trials were sufficiently homogeneous to be included in the meta-analysis. The way in which trial validity was assessed and data was extracted was not explicitly stated. The selection criteria for trial participants specified that only well-nourished children, similar to your own patient population, were included. The primary outcome, overall failure rate of ORT, was defined as the persistence or recurrence of signs of dehydration and other clinical indications requiring the need for intravenous rehydration and was 3·6% (95% CI 1·4–5·8].

Gavin[36] also looked at other outcomes in the six RCTs. Weight gain (between the time when the child was rehydrated and left hospital) was reported in five studies. In three there was no difference between groups and in two weight gain was greater with the ORS than with intravenous fluids, suggesting that nutrition was better maintained in the ORS group. However, neither the oral intake of food nor the weight gain is quantified. In four trials length of hospital stay was reported. In three trials there was no difference, but in one trial a longer stay (not quantified) was observed in the intravenous therapy group. Duration of diarrhea was reported in only two trials. In one there was no difference between groups and in the other diarrhea duration was shorter in the ORS group, but was not quantified. Stool frequency was reported in two studies and was higher in children receiving ORS for the first 24 hours of therapy only. Uncommon adverse events of treatment are often reported in case reports or series and may not be identified in a systematic review. Only one of the studies with an intravenous arm reported any derangement of electrolytes during therapy. There were no other adverse events recorded. The relative costs of intravenous versus oral fluids and adverse treatments including trauma and pain associated with intravenous fluids were not reported in any trial. The risk of iatrogenic hypernatremia and hyponatremia was very low with both intravenous and oral rehydration, regardless of the sodium content. Gavin concluded that there is no significant difference between groups receiving oral and intravenous fluids in the duration of diarrhea, time spent in hospital, or weight gain at discharge.

You now turn to the four additional RCTs listed in the article in *Clinical Evidence*.[37–40] Sharifi *et al*.[40] studied 470 children aged 1–18 months, who were admitted to hospital in Iran with "severe gastroenteritis" with moderate–severe dehydration according to WHO criteria (Table 37.2). In children receiving oral fluids, the duration of diarrhea (4·8 *v* 5·5 days; $P < 0.01$) was less and % weight gain at discharge (9% *v* 7% $P < 0.001$) was greater than in children who received intravenous fluids. ORT failed in only one patient (0·4%). Hospital stay and stool output were not reported. During rehydration therapy, 2/34 (6%) children with hypernatremia (Na > 155) in the ORS group and 6/24(25%) with hypernatremia in the intravenous group developed seizures and required an anticonvulsant (Chi-square test $P < 0.05$); 19% of children receiving ORS vomited in the first 6 hours of treatment, compared with 30% of the intravenous group ($P < 0.001$), but vomiting did not interfere with ORT. There was no difference in mortality rates. Because 33% of children were below the third percentile for weight and 23% were severely dehydrated (a much higher proportion than in your clinical practice), you are concerned that the results may not be applicable to your patients. Although children in this patient population are more severely affected than children in your population, you are reassured by the fact that ORS has nevertheless been demonstrated to be safe and effective.

In the other three RCTs duration of diarrhea, time spent in hospital, and weight gain were no different in groups receiving oral or intravenous rehydration. In one small study (n = 34)[39] children receiving oral rehydration spent significantly less time in the emergency department (225 versus 358 minutes; $P < 0.01$) but the hospitalization rate was similar to the intravenous treatment group. In one trial,[37] rigors and fever were reported in 9/50 (18%) of children receiving intravenous fluids but in no child receiving oral fluids. The quality of these RCTs was difficult to assess because of poor reporting of randomization methods, allocation concealment. and intention-to-treat analysis. Blinding was not possible because of the nature of the treatments.

Question

4. In young children with acute viral gastroenteritis and mild–moderate dehydration (*population*), is a glucose-electrolyte solution (*intervention*) more effective than a cereal-based solution (*comparison*) for oral rehydration (*outcome*)? **[Therapy]**

Your initial search of the *Cochrane Library* identified a systematic review comparing the efficacy of cereal-based versus glucose-based ORS.[44] On closer reading it is clear that all the trials included in this meta-analysis are hospital based, were carried out in developing countries, and included both adults and children with cholera and non-cholera diarrhea. You also find that the glucose-based formula in all the trials was the WHO solution, which has a higher osmolality and sodium content than those recommended for use in developed countries (Table 37.3). You are concerned that these data are not directly applicable to your patient population but nevertheless scan the results. The mean 24-hour stool output was significantly lower in children and adults with cholera or cholera-like diarrhea treated with rice-based ORS compared with children treated with WHO-ORS. However, in children with non-cholera diarrhea the weighted mean difference (WMD) in stool output (−4·3 ml kg^{-1} body weight [95% CI −9·3 to +0·8] and duration of diarrhea (WMD −2 [−5 to +2]) days) between children treated with rice based or glucose based ORS was small and non-significant.

Eighteen studies of cereal-based ORS did not fulfill the inclusion criteria for the Cochrane review.[44] Only one of these was conducted in a developed community. Wall *et al*.[45] studied 100 children aged < 5 years admitted to hospital in Australia with acute watery diarrhea and mild–moderate dehydration (a population very similar to your own). Children were randomized on an open label basis to receive either a rice-based or a glucose-based ORS (both were hypotonic and contained 60 mmol liter^{-1} sodium). Blinding was not undertaken because the ORS were visually very different, but none of the investigators was involved in patient management. Groups were similar at study entry and a standard protocol was used to administer ORS. Little information was given on the comparability of other management. There were no treatment failures or side effects in either group, follow up was complete, and analysis was based on intention to treat. Children receiving the rice-based solution had reduced mean stool volume ($P < 0.02$), reduced duration of diarrhea ($P = 0.03$), and decreased time to resumption of normal diet ($P = 0.01$) and fluids ($P = 0.001$) compared with children receiving the glucose based ORS. Despite these being clinically significant findings suggesting an earlier return to "normal function", the duration of hospitalization did not vary between groups. Since the study

Table 37.3 Composition of oral rehydration fluids recommended by ESPGAN[1] and WHO,[2] and commercially available in Australia,[3] United Kingdom,[4] and USA[5]

	Osmolality (mOsm liter^{-1})	Glucose (mmol liter^{-1})	Sodium (mmol liter^{-1})	Chloride (mmol liter^{-1})	Potassium (mmol liter^{-1})	Base (mmol liter^{-1})
ESPGAN[1]	200–250	74–111	60	Not < 25	20	Citrate 10
WHO ORS[2]	330	111	90	80	20	Citrate 10
Gastrolyte[3]	240	90	60	60	20	Citrate 10
Dioralyte[4]	240	90	60	60	20	Citrate 10
Pedialyte[5]	250	140	45	45	20	Bicarbonate 30

*Glucose given with fructose (1 mmol liter) and sucrose (94 mmol liter^{-1}).

is valid and applicable to your patients, you decide to investigate the cost and availability of ORS-R in your setting and to watch out for additional RCTs in developed communities.

Question

5. In children with acute gastroenteritis and mild–moderate dehydration (*population*), is a low osmolality solution (*intervention*) more effective than a high osmolality solution (*comparison*) for rehydration, decreasing stool output or decreasing hospital stay (*outcome*)? **[Therapy]**

In 1992 the European Society of Paediatric Gastroenterology and Nutrition (ESPGAN)[46] published recommendations for the composition of ORS for children in Europe, based on experimental evidence from intestinal perfusion studies in animals and humans and confirmed in clinical trials. The recommendations were not based on a systematic review and no details were given on the methods used to find and evaluate the evidence.

However, the hypotonic solution recommended by ESPGAN (see Table 37.3) has subsequently undergone further evaluation in children with gastroenteritis. In the Cochrane Database of Systematic Reviews you find a review by Hahn *et al.*[47] entitled "reduced osmolarity ORS for the treatment of dehydration caused by acute diarrhea in children," published in November 2001. The inclusion criteria were RCTs comparing reduced osmolarity ORS with WHO standard ORS in children aged < 5 years with diarrhea for < 5 days. The primary outcome measure was unscheduled use of intravenous rehydration. Secondary outcome measures included duration of diarrhea, vomiting, and asymptomatic hyponatraemia during follow up. You are satisfied with the rigor of the review. Of the 14 trials that met the inclusion criteria, 11 reported the primary outcome and in three of these trials no child required intravenous rehydration. Meta-analysis of the results of the remaining eight trials showed a

statistically significant reduction in the need for an unscheduled intravenous infusion in children who receiving a reduced osmolarity ORS compared with children who received the WHO standard ORS (combined OR 0·59; 95% CI 0·45–0·79). Stool output (11 trials) was reduced in the group receiving reduced osmolarity ORS. This was measured in different ways so is expressed as a standardized mean difference (SMD −0·23; 95% CI −0·33 to −0·44). Risk of vomiting (reported in six trials) was also reduced in the group who received oral fluids (OR 0·7; 95% CI 0·55–0·92). There was no difference in hyponatraemic events in the three of six trials that reported this outcome.

You decide you will use a reduced osmolarity glucose-based ORS with a composition similar to that recommended by ESPGAN for rehydration in patients with viral diarrhea and mild–moderate dehydration. ORS with similar composition are available commercially in Australia, the UK, and USA (Table 37.3).

Question

6. In children with viral gastroenteritis (*population*), is treatment with *Lactobacillus* plus a hypotonic ORS (*intervention*) more effective than treatment with ORS alone (*comparison*) for decreasing stool output or hospital stay (*outcome*)? **[Therapy]**

You are aware of the proposed role of *Lactobacilli* spp. in the management of gastroenteritis and wonder whether it would be of value in your patient. *Lactobacilli* spp. are naturally occurring bacterial commensals with a protective role in the gastrointestinal tract. *Lactobacilli* spp. depletion during viral diarrhea permits overgrowth of pathogenic, urease-producing bacteria which may exacerbate diarrhea. You search the *Cochrane Library* for systematic reviews, then for clinical trials using the term "probiotics" and then "lactobacillus".

In the *Cochrane Library* you find no completed systematic reviews, but one published protocol on the use of probiotics for treating acute infectious diarrhea in adults and children.[48] In DARE two reviews that meet the Cochrane Collaboration's rigorous criteria for inclusion. are listed, for which abstracts are currently being prepared.[49,50] In your previous MedLine search you found another systematic review on "probiotics in the treatment and prevention of acute infectious diarrhea in infants and children.[17]

Search criteria

Cochrane Library

- CDSR (1 relevant protocol)
- DARE (2 relevant reviews; abstracts in preparation)
- CENTRAL (over 350 trials, several of relevance published in the last 5 years)

MedLine

- 1 additional systematic review

The methodology of Szajewska's review is sound.[17] However, the search was limited to MedLine so some trials may have been missed. Only published trials in infants or children that were randomized, blinded, and placebo controlled were included. All but one of the 10 trials on treatment were performed in a developed country, and all but one included exclusively hospitalized children. There was no evidence of trial heterogeneity. The study population included predominantly well-nourished children with viral diarrhea. The primary outcome was duration of diarrhea. Secondary outcomes included number of stools per day, duration of hospitalization, and weight gain. Eight of the 10 trials, involving 731 children, reported on the risk of diarrhea lasting 3 days or more. Children receiving probiotics, compared with placebo, had a significantly reduced risk of diarrhea lasting > 3 days (relative risk [RR] 0·43; 95%CI 0·28–0·57; $P < 0.0001$). *Lactobacillus* GG (LGG) strain was used in three of the trials, in different doses, and showed the most consistent effect in reducing duration of diarrhea. For this outcome, the number needed to treat (NNT) was four. That means that four patients need to be treated with LGG to avoid one additional case of diarrhea lasting > 3 days. A sub-group analysis of children with confirmed rotavirus gastroenteritis and treated with LGG (four studies) showed that LGG resulted in the greatest reduction in diarrhea compared with placebo (WMD −24·8 hours; 95% CI −31·8 to −17·9; $P < 0.001$). The authors concluded that probiotics have a clinically significant benefit in the treatment of acute gastroenteritis in infants and children, and that the effect on duration of diarrhea is most marked when LGG is used in rotavirus diarrhea. No adverse events were reported in any of the included trials. There was significant heterogeneity

between the studies for other outcome measures which were not, therefore reported. Further trials measuring stool output and hospitalization rates are required.

The methods of the review published in *Pediatrics* in 2002[50] are comprehensive and rigorous. Complementary medicine databases were searched and key investigators in the field were contacted. Included trials were restricted to double blind, placebo-controlled trials of lactobacillus (any species or strain). Main outcome measures were the duration, frequency, and amount of diarrhea. Nine studies were included in the review, eight of which included only inpatients and seven of which were part of the systematic review discussed above. Two studies included in that review were excluded from the second review because of "exclusion or reallocation of patients after randomization". The meta-analysis showed a significant reduction in diarrhea duration of nearly 24 hours (0·7 days [CI 0·3–1·2 days]) in children given lactobacillus compared with children given placebo. A dose-response relationship was evident in all trials that reported this outcome.

The third review was also methodologically sound, with a comprehensive search strategy and inclusion of 18 RCTs in children with acute gastroenteritis.[49] There was considerable overlap between RCTs included in this and the other reviews. The primary endpoint was not stated in any trial, but all evaluated the effect of probiotics on duration of diarrhea. A range of probiotics was given in addition to oral rehydration therapy (*lactobacillus* GG was used in 10 trials). Children who received probiotics had a reduced duration of diarrhea (pooled estimate −0·8 days; 95% CI −1·1 to −0·6). This finding was upheld when analysis was restricted to double-blind RCTs, hospitalized children, and use of lactobacilli.

To educate yourself further on the recommended dose and method of administration of *Lactobacillus* spp., you refer a multicenter European study.[51] In this double-blind, placebo-controlled RCT, the effect of lactobacillus GG administered in a hypotonic ORS was evaluated. The trial included 287 children (aged 1 month to 3 years) admitted with acute gastroenteritis. Children received either ORS plus placebo or ORS plus a preparation of live *lactobacillus* GG (at least 10 CFU per 250 ml) for 4–6 hours, then had free access to ORS (plus placebo or *lactobacillus* GG) and normal feeds until diarrhea stopped. Groups were similar at enrolment. Findings were consistent with the systematic reviews. Children receiving *Lactobacillus* spp. had a shorter hospital stay and mean duration of diarrhea (77 [42] *v* 58 [28] hours; $P < 0.05$). This clinically important effect was more marked in rotavirus-positive cases. Diarrhea lasted longer than 7 days in 11% of the placebo and 3% of the treatment group ($P < 0.01$). No adverse effects were reported.

You conclude that the addition of *Lactobacillus* spp. to a hypotonic ORS is safe and effective (particularly in rotavirus diarrhea) for decreasing diarrhea duration and hastening discharge from hospital. You undertake to inquire about its cost and availability in your clinical setting.

Table 37.4   Placebo-controlled RCTs examining the effect of loperamide in acute infectious diarrhea with mild to moderate dehydration*

Intervention (loperamide dose mg kg⁻¹ per day)	Participants	Diarrhea duration	Stool output	Weight gain	Hospital stay
Loperamide (0·4, 0·8) v placebo[53]	315 children (3 m to 3 years)	Risk of diarrhea 24 h; L < P; RR 0·83, 95% CI 0·73–0·94.	NR	L > P	NS
Loperamide (0·2) v placebo[54]	40 children (1–4 years)	NS	NR	NS	NS
Loperamide (0·2) v placebo[55]	100 children (under 2 years)	Duration L < P; 59 v 81 hours	NS	NS	NR
Loperamide (0·4, 0·8) v placebo[56]	53 children (3 m to 3 years)	NR	NR	L > P	NR
Loperamide (0·8) v placebo[57]	185 children (3–18 m)	NR	NR	NR	NS

*Adapted from *Clinical Evidence*.[12]
NS, not significant; NR, not reported; L, loperamide, P, placebo.

Question

7.   In young children with acute viral gastroenteritis (*population*), does loperamide (*intervention*) decrease the volume or duration of diarrhea (*outcome*)? **[Therapy]**

This question is addressed in the systematic review in *Clinical Evidence*[12] and the protocol for a Cochrane Review on the role of antimotility agents in acute diarrhea in children is published by the same authors in the *Cochrane Library*.[52] Five RCTs comparing loperamide with placebo in children with acute infectious diarrhea[53–57] are summarized in Table 37.4, which is modified from *Clinical Evidence*.[12] In two of the three trials in which diarrhea duration was an outcome, loperamide significantly reduced the duration of diarrhea compared with placebo. In one study the risk of having diarrhea at 24 hours was 36% in children receiving loperamide and 55% in children receiving placebo (RR 0·83; 95% CI 0·73–0·94).[53] In the other trial[55] the mean duration of diarrhea was reduced by over 20 hours (59 hours in the loperamide group and 81 hours in the placebo group; $P < 0.05$). Two trials report increased weight gain after 3 days in children receiving loperamide,[53,56] but two trials report no difference between groups.

You look more closely at the largest trial, a multicenter, double blind, randomized, placebo-controlled trial of loperamide, conducted in 315 children (3 months to 3 years) admitted to hospital with acute diarrhea in the UK.[53] The randomization was concealed. Twelve children with underlying disease, chronic diarrhea, or current use of antimotility drugs were excluded after allocation to treatment. The rest, including four children discharged before diarrhea ceased, were analyzed according to intention-to-treat. Children received either oral rehydration and placebo, rehydration and 0·8 mg kg⁻¹ per day loperamide, or rehydration and 0·4 mg kg⁻¹ per day loperamide (given until cessation of diarrhea). Groups were similar with regard to disease severity at the outset of the trial. Stool pathogens (type not given) were isolated in a higher proportion of the placebo than treatment group (0·8 mg kg⁻¹ loperamide). Also, the proportion of children who had no bowel action following admission was higher in both loperamide groups than in the placebo group, suggesting that they may have had milder diarrhea. The rehydration regimen was not specified and varied "in accordance with the routine currently practiced by each center". The proportion of children with persistent diarrhea beyond 24 hours was lower in both treatment groups than in the placebo group (36% v 55%) and the rate of recovery was significantly higher in the treatment groups by about 24 hours (also clinically significant). Weight gain by day 3 after admission was significantly higher in both treatment groups than the placebo group. No adverse effects were noted.

In four RCTs no adverse effects from loperamide were reported. In one trial[56] a significantly higher rate of mild abdominal distension, excessive sleep, and lethargy was reported with loperamide. You also find a non-randomized, non-blinded trial evaluating the effect of loperamide on stool output and duration of acute infectious diarrhea in 60 male infants (aged 6 weeks to 12 months) with moderate dehydration, admitted to hospital in South Africa.[58] The analysis was not on an intention-to-treat basis and children were not given ORS. You are concerned about both the study methodology and the applicability of the results (the population differed from yours as > 50% had bacterial pathogens). However, you are interested in the adverse effects reported, which raise concerns about the safety of loperamide in infants. Two children receiving loperamide were withdrawn from the trial because they developed ileus or persistent severe vomiting. Four others receiving loperamide developed drowsiness which resolved on withdrawal of the drug.

You try to clarify this issue by looking at the clinical guidelines published by the AAP.[1] Ten reports of adverse effects attributed to use of loperamide in children are cited. These include poisoning, necrotizing enterocolitis, toxicity, neurological symptoms, delirium, respiratory depression, coma, and death. Although some trials demonstrate benefits with regard to weight gain and duration of diarrhea, you conclude that the risks of this medication probably outweigh its benefits in a self-limiting and common illness.

Resolution of the scenario

You assess the patient and make a provisional diagnosis of viral (rotavirus) gastroenteritis. You explain to his parents that this is the most likely diagnosis considering the season (spring) and the presentation (watery diarrhea without blood) and that the condition is self-limiting. You note that the boy is moderately dehydrated on the basis of his current and recent weights (6% loss of body weight) and admit him to oversee rehydration therapy. You start him on oral rehydration therapy using a commercially available hypotonic glucose-electrolyte solution (containing 60 mmol liter⁻¹ sodium and citrate as the base) with added lactobacillus GG. You ask the boy's mother to give 5 ml every few minutes and tell her that the volume of fluid can be increased and the frequency decreased if her son does not vomit. You review his progress 2 hours later and find the boy is refusing to drink. The nurse asks you to insert an intravenous catheter but you explain this procedure is often traumatic and is not without risks. You insert a nasogastric tube for ORS administration, the tube is well tolerated and the child does not vomit. Four hours later the boy is well hydrated and asking for a drink. You ask his mother to give the boy fluids by mouth ad libitum, to ensure that he gets at least his required maintenance volume. You explain that medications such as antibiotics and antidiarrheal agents are not indicated and may cause harm.

Future research needs

- Admission criteria need to be established for children with acute gastroenteritis, in view of the evidence that many children are unnecessarily admitted to hospital.
- RCTs are needed to evaluate outpatient (home-based) versus hospital management of gastroenteritis. In addition to clinical outcomes, economic analyses, and parent/carer and child satisfaction should be included.
- Educational interventions (targeting both health professionals and the wider community) about the management of gastroenteritis should be developed and evaluated. These should include information about the use of oral rehydration therapy (and the relative benefits of hypotonic and cereal-based solutions); the role of probiotics (particularly *lactobacillus* GG); and the role of antidiarrheal medications and antibiotics.
- Additional RCTs evaluating the role and acceptability (for example, palatability) of glucose electrolyte versus cereal-based ORS in acute gastroenteritis are required in children with viral diarrhea and in developed countries.

Summary table

Question	Type of evidence	Result	Comment and adverse effects
Value of clinical signs, tests for assessing dehydration	Cross-sectional studies[25,26]	Best predictors are decreased peripheral perfusion, serum urea > 6.5 mmol liter^{-1}, capillary pH < 7.35, decreased skin turgor, deep breathing	LRs low for all tests
Outpatient versus inpatient management	Evidence-based guideline;[14] RCT[36] including children with gastroenteritis Cross-sectional studies, none addressing the specific question	Many non-dehydrated children admitted. This incurs costs and risk of harms, e.g., unnecessary intravenous fluids, cross-infection	Potential for missing children with worsening dehydration treated at home – need to educate parents, primary carers
Oral versus intravenous rehydration therapy	Systematic review of RCTs[36] Review of 4 RCTs in *Clinical Evidence*[12]	ORT rapid, effective, low failure rate ($\sim 4\%$). Potential reduced risk of electrolyte disturbance, infection at injection site, pain, cost	In vomiting ORT can be given by NG tube. Outpatient management or shorter admission possible with ORT
Cereal-based *v* glucose-electrolyte solution	Systematic review with meta-analysis in developing countries[44]	Diminished stool output, duration of diarrhea with cereal-based ORT in cholera. No benefits in non-cholera diarrhea	Limited evidence in well-nourished children with viral diarrhea in developed communities
	Single RCT in developed community[45]	Reduced stool volume, duration of diarrhea, time to commencing normal diet with rice-based ORS	
Low versus high osmolality oral rehydration solution	Systematic review of RCTs[47]	Lower stool output, higher urine output, decreased duration of diarrhea, lower failure rate with hypotonic ORS	Hypotonic solutions are commercially available in UK, USA, Australia
Lactobacillus plus ORS versus ORS alone	Three systematic reviews of RCTs[17,49,50]	Decreased duration of diarrhea	Effect greater in rotavirus than bacterial gastroenteritis
Loperamide	Review of 5 RCTs in *Clinical Evidence*[12] Protocol for systematic review published in *Cochrane Library*[52]	Decreased diarrhea duration, increased weight gain in some trials. Not consistent findings	Different outcomes examined in RCTs. Adverse effects not reported in systematic review but in CCS and case reports

References

1 Anonymous. Practice parameter: the management of acute gastroenteritis in young children. American Academy of Pediatrics. Provisional Committee on Quality Improvement, Subcommittee on Acute Gastroenteritis. *Pediatrics* 1996; **97**:424–36.

2 Baldassano RN, Liacouras CA. Chronic diarrhea: a practical approach. *Pediatr Clin N Amer* 1991;**38**:667–86.

3 Conway SP, Phillips RR, Panday S. Admission to hospital with gastroenteritis. *Arch Dis Child* 1990;**65**:579–84.

4 Finkelstein JA, Schwartz JS, Torrey S, Fleischer GR. Common clinical features as predictors of bacterial diarrhea in infants. *Am J Emerg Med* 1989;**7**:469–73.

5 DeWitt TG, Humphrey KF, McCarthy P. Clinical predictors of acute bacterial diarrhea in young children. *Pediatrics* 1985;**76**:551–6.

6 Person MJ. Hospitalisations for rotavirus gastroenteritis among children under five years of age in New South Wales. *Med J Aust* 1996;**164**:273–6.

7 OPCS. *Mid-1993 population estimates for England and Wales.* London: HMSO, 1994.

8   WHO. *A manual for the treatment of diarrhea.* Programme for the control of diarrheal diseases. WHO/CDD/SER/80·2 Rev.2, 2nd edn. Geneva: WHO, 1990.

9   OPCS. *Morbidity statistics from general practice. Fourth national study, 1991–1992.* London: HMSO, 1993.

10   Glass RI, Lew JF, Gangarosa RE, LeBaron CW, Ho MS. Estimates of morbidity and mortality rates for diarrheal diseases in American children. *J Pediatr* 1991;**118**(Suppl.): S27–S33.

11   Elliott EJ, Backhouse JA, Leach JW. Pre-admission management of acute gastroenteritis. *J Paediatr Child Hlth* 1996;**32**:18–21.

12   Dalby-Payne J, Elliott E. Child Health. Gastroenteritis in children. In: *Clinical Evidence.* Issue 9. London, BMJ Publishing Group Ltd, 2003.

13   Sandhu B for the European Society of Pediatric Gastroenterology and Nutrition. Practical guideline for the management of gastroenteritis in children. *J Pediatr Gastroenterol Nutr* 2001;**33**:536–9.

14   Armon K, Stephenson T, MacFaul R, Eccleston P, Werneke U. An evidence and consensus based guideline for acute diarrhoea management. *Arch Dis Child* 2001;**85**: 132–42

15   Murphy MS. Guidelines for managing acute gastroenteritis based on a systematic review of published research. *Arch Dis Child* 1998;**79**:279–84.

16   Sandhu B, Isolauri E, Walker-Smith J *et al.* Early feeding in childhood gastroenteritis. A multicentre study on behalf of the European Society of Paediatric Gastroenterology and Nutrition working group on acute diarrhea. *J Pediatr Gastroenterol Nutr* 1997;**24**:522–7.

17   Szajewska H, Mrukowicz JZ. Probiotics in the treatment and prevention of acute infectious diarrhea in infants and children: a systematic review of published randomised, double-blind, placebo-controlled trials. *J Pediatr Gatroenterol Nutr.* 2001;**33**:S17–S25.

18   Lifschitz C. Treatment of acute diarrhea in children. *Curr Opin Pediatr* 1997;**9**:498–501.

19   Oxman AD, Cook DJ, Guyatt GH. Users' guides to the medical literature. VI. How to use an overview. Evidence based Medicine Working Group. *JAMA* 1994;**272**:1367–71.

20   Hayward RS, Wilson MC, Tunis SR, Bass EB, Guyatt G. Users' guides to the medical literature. VIII. How to use clinical practice guidelines. A. Are the recommendations valid? The Evidence based Medicine Working Group. *JAMA* 1995;**274**:570–4.

21   Wilson MC, Hayward RS, Tunis SR, Bass EB, Guyatt G. Users' guides to the medical literature. VIII. How to use clinical practice guidelines. B. What are the recommendations and will they help you in caring for your patients? The Evidence based Medicine Working Group. *JAMA* 1995;**274**:1630–2.

22   Baumer H. Commentary on 'An evidence and consensus based guideline for acute diarrhoea management'. *Arch Dis Child* 2001;**85**:141–2.

23   Eccles M, Clapp Z, Grimshaw J *et al.* North of England evidence based guidelines development project: methods of guideline development. *BMJ* 1996;**312**:760–2.

24   Anonymous. *A manual for the treatment of diarrhea. World Health Organisation, Programme for Control of Diarrheal Diseases.* Geneva: World Health Organisation, 1990.

25   Mackenzie A, Barnes G, Shann F. Clinical signs of dehydration in children. *Lancet* 1989;**ii**:605–7.

26   Duggan C, Refat M, Hashem M, Wolff M, Fayad I, Santosham M. How valid are clinical signs of dehydration in infants? *J Pediatr Gastroenterol Nutr* 1996;**22**:56–61.

27   Jaeschke R, Guyatt GH, Sackett DL. Users' guides to the medical literature. III. How to use an article about a diagnostic test. A. Are the results of the study valid? Evidence-Based Medicine Working Group. *JAMA* 1994;**271**:389–91.

28   Jaeschke R, Guyatt G, Sackett DL. Users' guides to the medical literature. III. How to use an article about a diagnostic test. B. What are the results and will they help me in caring for my patients? Evidence-Based Medicine Working Group. *JAMA* 1994;**271**:703–7.

29   Fagan T. Nomogram for Bayes's Theorem. *New Engl J Med* 1975;**293**:257.

30   Conway SP, Newport MJ. Are all hospital admissions for acute gastroenteritis necessary? *J Infect* 1994;**29**:5–8.

31   O'Loughlin EV, Notaras E, McCullough C, Halliday J, Henry RL. Home-based management of children hospitalized with acute gastroenteritis. *J Paediatr Child Hlth* 1995;**31**: 189–91.

32   Jenkins HR, Ansari BM. Management of gastroenteritis. *Arch Dis Child* 1990;**65**:939–41.

33   Fitzgerald M and HM McGee, Psychological health status of mothers and the admission of children to hospital for gastroenteritis. *Family Practice* 1990;**7**:116–120.

34   Goodman DC, Fisher ES, Gittelsohn A, Chang CH, Fleming C. *et al.* Why are children hospitalized? The role of non-clinical factors in pediatric hospitalizations. *Pediatrics* 1994;**93**: 896–902.

35   Sartain SA, Maxwell MJ, Todd PJ *et al.* Randomised controlled trial comparing an acute paediatric hospital at home scheme with conventional hospital care. *Arch Dis Child* 2002;**87**:371–5.

36   Gavin N, Merrick N, Davidson B. Efficacy of glucose-based oral rehydration therapy. *Pediatrics* 1996;**98**:45–51.

37   Singh M, Mahmoodi A, Arya LS *et al.* Controlled trial of oral versus intravenous rehydration in the management of acute gastroenteritis *Indian J Med Res* 1982;**75**:691–3.

38   Oritz A. Rehidratacion oral:Experiencia en el manejo de pacientes con gastroenteritis aguda en la sala de emergencia hospital pediatrico. *Bol Asoc Med PR* 1990;**82**:227–33.

39   Atherly-John YC, Cunningham SJ, Crain EF. A randomized trial of oral vs intravenous rehydration in a pediatric emergency department. *Arch Pediatr Adolesc Med* 2002; **156**:1240–3.

40   Sharifi J, Ghavami F, Nowrouzi Z *et al.* Oral versus intravenous rehydration therapy in severe gastroenteritis. *Arch Dis Child* 1985;**60**:856–60.

41   Feldman W. Meta-analysis: Failure of oral rehydration therapy is infrequent in young, well-nourished children with gastroenteritis. *Evidence-Based Medicine* 1997;**2**:12.

42   Muir Gray JA. *Evidence based healthcare.* London: Churchill Livingstone, 1997.

43 Cook D, Guyatt G, Laupacis A, Sackett D. Rules of evidence and clinical recommendations on the use of antithrombotic agents. *Chest* 1992;**102**:305S–311S.

44 Fontaine O, Gore S, Pierce NF. Rice-based oral rehydration solution for treating diarrhoea. In: *Cochrane Library*, Issue 1. Chichester, UK: John Wiley and Sons Ltd, 2004.

45 Wall CR, Swanson CE, Cleghorn GJ. Rehydration in infants with gastroenteritis. A controlled trial comparing the efficacy of rice-based and hypotonic oral rehydration solutions in infants and young children with gastroenteritis. *J Gastroenterol Hepatol* 1997;**12**:24–8.

46 Booth I, Cunha Ferreira R, Desjeux JF *et al.* Recommendations for composition of oral rehydration solutions for the children of Europe. Report of an ESPGAN working group. *J Pediat Gastroenterol Nutr* 1992;**14**:113–15.

47 Hahn S, Kim S, Garner P Reduced osmolarity oral rehydration solution for treating dehydration caused by acute diarrhoea in children In: Cochrane Collaboration. *Cochrane Library.* Issue 2. Oxford: Update Software, 2003.

48 Allen SJ, Okoko B, Martinez E, Gregorio G, Dans LF. Probiotics for treating infectious diarrhoea (Protocol for a Cochrane Review). In: Cochrane Collaboration. *Cochrane Library.* Issue 4. Chichester, UK, John Wiley and Sons Ltd, 2003.

49 Van Niel CW, Feudtner C, Garrison MM, Christakis DA. Lactobacillus therapy for acute infectious diarrhea in children: A meta-analysis. *Pediatrics* 2002;**109**:678–84.

50 Huang JS, Bousvaros A, Lee JW, Diaz A, Davidson EJ. Efficacy of probiotic use in acute diarrhea in children. A meta-analysis. *Dig Dis Sci* 2002;**11**:2625–34.

51 Guandalini S, Pensabene L, Zikri M *et al. Lactobacillus* GG administered in oral rehydration solution to children with acute diarrhea: a multicenter European trial. *J Pediatr Gastroenterol Nutr* 2000;**30**:54–60.

52 Dalby-Payne J, Elliott EJ. Anti-motility agents for treatment of acute diarrhoea in children. (Protocol for a Cochrane Review). In: Cochrane Collaboration. *Cochrane Library.* Issue 5. Chichester, UK, John Wiley and Sons Ltd, 2003.

53 Diarrhoeal Diseases Study Group (UK). Loperamide in acute diarrhoea in childhood: results of a double blind, placebo controlled multicentre clinical trial. *BMJ Clin Res Ed* 1984;**289**:1263–7.

54 Owens JR, Broadhead R, Hendrickse RG *et al.* Loperamide in the treatment of acute gastroenteritis in early childhood. Report of a two centre, double-blind, controlled clinical trial. *Ann Trop Paediatr* 1981;**1**:135–41.

55 Kassem AS, Madkour AA, Massoud BZ *et al.* Loperamide in acute childhood diarrhoea: a double blind controlled trial. *J Diarrhoeal Dis Res* 1983;**1**:10–16.

56 Karrar ZA, Abdulla MA, Moody JB *et al.* Loperamide in acute diarrhoea in childhood: results of a double blind, placebo controlled clinical trial. *Ann Trop Paediatr* 1987;**7**:122–7.

57 Bowie MD, Hill ID, Mann MD. Loperamide for treatment of acute diarrhoea in infants and young children. A double-blind placbo-controlled trial. *S Afr Med J* 1995;**85**:885–7.

58 Motala C, Hill I, Mann M, Bowie M. Effect of loperamide on stool output and duration of acute infectious diarrhea in infants. *J Pediatr* 1990;**117**:467–71.

38 Appendicitis

Carolyn A Paris, Eileen J Klein

Case scenario

A 5-year-old girl presents to the emergency department (ED) with a 36-hour history of abdominal pain and fever. She had been seen the previous day with a 12-hour history of pain that was attributed to constipation. Today the pain is peri-umbilical and cramping in nature and its location has not changed since onset. The child had four episodes of vomiting immediately after the onset of abdominal pain, but has not vomited in the last 24 hours. Her mother reports she has poor appetite, decreased urination, and decreased activity. There is no history of diarrhea, rash, dysuria, sore throat, or upper respiratory symptoms. On physical examination, the temperature is 38·7° C, heart rate 120 beats per minute, respiration rate 20 breaths per minute, and blood pressure 102/60 mmHg. The patient is tired but does not appear toxic and her skin is well perfused. Abdominal examination reveals significant diffuse abdominal tenderness to deep palpation. There is no rebound; the psoas and obturator signs are negative. There is guarding and the pain does not decrease when the patient is distracted. The rest of the examination is normal. A plain abdominal radiograph reveals stool in the rectum but no other findings. White blood cell count (WBC) is 16·9 K mm^{-3} with 76% neutrophils, 12% bands, 7% lymphocytes, 4% monocytes, and 1% basophils. You consult the surgical team. They are concerned about her elevated WBC, but do not believe she has a surgical abdomen at this time. They recommend a urinalysis but the patient is unable to provide a sample. You give the patient an enema, believing she is constipated. After a large stool is passed, her examination still reveals diffuse tenderness without peritoneal signs. You are concerned that this child might have acute appendicitis and question the value of the history, examination, and preliminary investigations in confirming this diagnosis. You wonder whether an abdominal ultrasound or computed tomography (CT) would provide you with useful additional information.

Background

Appendicitis is among the most serious etiologies of acute abdominal pain and is the most common indication for emergency abdominal surgery in children. The incidence varies depending on the clinical setting in which patients are evaluated and the age and gender of the patient. The reported prevalence of abdominal pain among pediatric patients seen in the ED or outpatient clinic is 3–5·1% for pain of < 3 days duration, and 8·1% for pain of any duration.[1,2] The frequency of admission for abdominal pain of any etiology is only 1·7%, but 32–50% of those admitted will have appendicitis.[1,3] Thus, appendicitis explains 1% of abdominal pain episodes.[1] National Hospital Discharge Survey data for the years 1979–1984 estimate that the incidence of appendicitis peaks in older children and adolescents, with a rate of 23·3 per 10 000 population per year in persons aged 10–19 years. The male to female ratio is 1·4:1.[4] Unfortunately, few studies involve follow up of all patients evaluated for abdominal pain; thus potential cases of appendicitis may be missed in the acute care setting. Furthermore, most studies fail to clearly define the patient inclusion criteria, leaving denominators unclear. As a result, these are only estimates of the true incidence of appendicitis.

Of pediatric patients undergoing appendectomy, 10–40% have a normal appendix, and usually have a non-surgical explanation for their abdominal pain.[5–12] Negative appendectomy occurs more commonly in post-pubertal girls, probably due to the concern of infertility associated with peritonitis, while perforation rates are higher in boys[5,8]: 15–40% of those with acute appendicitis have progressed to perforation at the time of laparotomy.[5,7,9,11,12] This proportion is higher in younger children, being 63–93% in those < 6 years old.[12,13] Mortality rates have declined dramatically since the recognition of appendicitis in the late 1800s; however, it remains a cause of death in 0·02–0·8% of general populations studied.[7,14] Death resulted from undetected appendicitis in early childhood in 4·5 per million children at risk per year in one defined US community.[15] A 10-year study of mortality after appendectomy in Sweden found a case fatality of 2·44 per 1000 appendectomies for all ages and 0·31 per 1000 appendectomies in children < 9 years of age.[16] Prompt and accurate diagnosis of appendicitis remains the key to reducing morbidity and mortality. The pediatric population provides particular challenges. Although the diagnosis of appendicitis has historically been based on the history and physical examination, recent advances have placed a greater emphasis on technology.

Framing answerable clinical questions

Most of your questions relate to making the diagnosis of appendicitis. As this is a very common problem in your setting, you decide to perform a comprehensive search for evidence to guide your daily practice. You develop a number of structured clinical questions on diagnosis to facilitate your search of the literature.

Questions

In children with acute abdominal pain (*patient/population*):

1. Will historical details such as duration of pain and vomiting (*intervention/tests*) help in making a diagnosis of acute appendicitis (*outcome*)? **[Diagnosis]**
2. Will specific findings on physical examination (for example, location of pain, rebound tenderness, guarding) (*intervention/tests*) help in making a diagnosis of acute appendicitis (*outcome*)? **[Diagnosis]**
3. Will laboratory measures of inflammation (for example, ESR, WBC) (*intervention/tests*) help in making the diagnosis of acute appendicitis (*outcome*)? **[Diagnosis]**
4. Will an abdominal ultrasound scan (*intervention/test*) assist in the diagnosis of acute appendicitis (*outcome*)? **[Diagnosis]**
5. Will computed tomography (CT) scanning (*intervention/test*) assist in the diagnosis of acute appendicitis (*outcome*)? **[Diagnosis]**
6. Does clinical scoring (*intervention/test*) facilitate the accurate diagnosis of appendicitis (*outcome*) in children? **[Diagnosis]**

Searching for evidence

You limit your search to the *diagnosis* of appendicitis in both adult and pediatric patients. In general, studies of diagnostic tests compare the test in question with some kind of reference standard on a defined population of people with suspicious symptoms. Occasionally, a diagnostic test is evaluated for its benefit to patients using randomized trials, but these are rare. Search of the Cochrane database for systematic reviews (both Cochrane reviews and reviews in the DARE) and randomized clinical trials (in the Cochrane Controlled Trials Register) relating to the diagnosis of appendicitis reveals one systematic review of the use of ultrasound. As expected, there are no randomized controlled trials (RCTs) or meta-analyses of RCTs related to the diagnostic tests, although there are several randomized trials relating to treatment strategies, which are not relevant to your specific questions. You find no relevant articles in *Best Evidence*. You therefore search MedLine for each individual question. The strategies for these searches are shown with the questions that follow.

Question

1. In children with acute abdominal pain (*patient/ population*), will historical details such as duration of pain and vomiting (*intervention/tests*) help in making a diagnosis of acute appendicitis (*outcome*)? **[Diagnosis]**

● MedLine (Ovid): "Appendicitis: diagnosis AND (explode: abdomen or explode: pain) AND duration AND time factors AND prospective; limit English AND limit Humans"

You are looking for studies that compare findings obtained in the history with a "gold standard" for the diagnosis of appendicitis. A reasonable reference standard would be histologic confirmation of an acutely inflamed appendix removed at appendectomy or good follow up of patients believed not to have appendicitis, to ensure that the diagnosis of appendicitis has not been missed. You also want studies in which the pathologist was blinded to historical findings, and the clinician to pathologic findings, though it is unclear that the literature will provide this information. You concentrate your efforts on duration of pain and vomiting as the features of the history that you want to evaluate.

Duration of pain as a predictor of appendicitis

To address this question you enter the Medical Subject Heading (MeSH) appendicitis and subheading diagnosis and get 3078 listings (see Box). You then put in the MeSH heading of abdominal pain and realize that abdominal pain has only been a MeSH heading since 1990. You therefore search using the heading of "explode: abdomen" and "explode: pain". When you combine these three with an "OR" statement "AND" with "appendicitis: diagnosis" you get 752 listings. Even though you know it can cause bias, you limit your search to English because you do not have translation services easily available. You further define pain duration by typing in the textword "duration" and the MeSH

Table 38.1 Calculation of likelihood ratios for appendicitis based on duration of abdominal pain[11]

Pain duration	Appendicitis	No appendicitis
< 12 hours	7	100
> 12 hours	17	122
Total patients	24	222

Sensitivity = 7/24 = 29%
Specificity = 122/222 = 55%
Likelihood ratio for pain < 12 hours = 0·29/(1−0·55) = 0·64
Likelihood ratio for pain > 12 hours = (17/24)/(122/222) = 1·3

Pain duration	Appendicitis	No appendicitis
< 24 hours	12	134
> 24 hours	12	88
Total patients	24	222

Sensitivity = 12/24 = 50%
Specificity = 88/222 = 40%
Likelihood ratio for pain < 24 hours = 0·5/(1−0·4) = 0·83
Likelihood ratio for pain > 24 hours = (12/24)/(88/222) = 1·2

heading "time factors". You now have 26 listings of which four are prospective studies. Of these, two deal mainly with the appearance of the appendix in delayed diagnosis rather than the typical duration of pain. Another study addresses the differential diagnosis of males with abdominal pain in an ambulatory clinic setting. Only one study specifically reported duration of pain in differentiating appendicitis from other causes of abdominal pain.[11] Fortuitously, this study is specific to the pediatric population.

This prospective study by O'Shea *et al.* involved 246 children from 13–18 years old presenting to an emergency department with abdominal pain of less than 1-week duration,[11] and no history of recent trauma or of recurrent abdominal pain. All families were contacted within 6 days of their ED visit so that missed appendicitis would be unlikely in those discharged from the ED. You evaluate the data on all patients, whether or not they were operated on, because you want to know if duration of pain will help you in the decision whether to operate or not. You compare those with appendicitis verified by pathology report to those without appendicitis (either by pathology report or phone follow up indicating the child was not operated on). In this study, the likelihood ratio (LR) of appendicitis in a patient with pain of < 12 hours was 0·64, compared with a patient with pain for > 12 hours (Table 38.1). When looking at patients with a longer duration of pain, the likelihood ratio of appendicitis in a patient with pain of < 24 hours is 0·83, compared with pain present for > 24 hours (Table 38.1).

You review the bibliographies from other articles and find another pertinent study. Andersson *et al.*[17] prospectively evaluated 502 patients (aged 10–86 years) admitted to the

hospital with abdominal pain and suspected appendicitis. The patient completed a questionnaire and the surgeon recorded physical exam findings and inflammatory measures (WBC and CRP). Of the patients, 259 underwent laparotomy and 194 (75%) of these had appendicitis on pathology. Duration of follow up in the group who did not have an operation is not clear, thus it is not possible to be certain that they did not later present with appendicitis. This could create a selection bias as patients presenting with less severe symptoms and possible appendicitis may have been discharged and gone elsewhere for follow up, and hence been incorrectly classified as not having appendicitis. These authors broke pain duration into 6-hour increments up to 72 hours. The greatest likelihood ratio, at pain duration of 7–12 hours, was 1·7 (95% CI 1·1–2·6). Based on these studies, you conclude that duration of pain at presentation should not influence your decision to evaluate further or operate. However, these studies did not specifically evaluate pain of very short or very long duration so no statement can be made in that regard.

Vomiting as a predictor of appendicitis

To address the value of vomiting as a predictor of appendicitis you search MedLine (Box) using the term appendicitis and subheading diagnosis and obtain 3078 articles. Combined with the MeSII heading "vomiting or nausea" you come up with 33 articles. Three were prospective.[17–19]

- MedLine: "Appendicitis:diagnosis AND (vomiting OR nausea) AND prospective"

The prospective cohort study by Andersson[17] found the likelihood ratio for appendicitis in a patient with vomiting compared with one with no vomiting to be 1·8 (95% CI 1·4–2·4). Given a pretest likelihood of 10%, the presence of vomiting would modify your estimate of the chance of appendicitis very little (to about 15%, see nomogram on page 35). Thus, vomiting does not appear to be a very good predictor of appendicitis in children or adults.

Korner and colleagues prospectively studied vomiting in 544 patients age 2–89 in Norway between 1990–1992.[18] All patients thought to need surgery for acute appendicitis were enrolled and had nine clinical variables documented, including a "classic history" of abdominal pain followed by anorexia and/or vomiting (LR+ = 1·16, LR– = 0·74) or the presence of nausea or vomiting (LR+ = 1·24, LR– = 0·67). Given the weak magnitude of the likelihood ratios, and the fact that this study included only patients thought to need surgery for appendicitis (not the larger group of patients with abdominal pain), who were evaluated by trainees of various levels, you further conclude that neither a "classic history" nor the presence of nausea or vomiting are strong predictors of the presence of appendicitis.

A prospective study by Reynolds and Jaffe[19] included 377 children (aged 2–16 years) with abdominal pain seen in an emergency department. The physician completed a data form, follow up phone calls were made to all families, and pathology reports were reviewed for all patients who underwent surgery. Unfortunately, this study does not give enough information for you to calculate a likelihood ratio for vomiting alone. In this study, a combination of four predictors (vomiting, right lower quadrant pain, abdominal tenderness, and abdominal guarding) maximizes the diagnosis of appendicitis. In fact, 97% of patients with appendicitis had two of these four predictors. With a sensitivity of 0·96 and a specificity of 0·72 for any two of these four predictors, the positive likelihood ratio is 3·4. Even more interesting is the negative likelihood ratio of 0·08. Therefore, a patient with fewer than two of the above predictors is very unlikely to have appendicitis. (A pretest likelihood of 10% is modified by this information to a post-test likelihood of less than 1%.) Since many signs and symptoms occur in patients with appendicitis, it is not surprising that a combination of findings may be most helpful in making a diagnosis. Given the fact that, overall, the pretest probability of appendicitis in a child with abdominal pain is somewhere between 1% and 10%, the negative likelihood ratio is even more compelling.

Question

2. In children with acute abdominal pain (*patient/ population*), will specific findings on physical examination (for example, location of pain, rebound tenderness, guarding) (*intervention/tests*) help in making a diagnosis of acute appendicitis (*outcome*)? **[Diagnosis]**

Pain quality or location as a predictor of appendicitis

Using the search strategy shown in the Box you find 20 articles, and in four of these the main goal was to evaluate pain quality or location as a predictor of acute appendicitis.

- MedLine: "Appendicitis:diagnosis AND exp:pain AND prospective studies; limit children"

The Andersson study[17] specifically evaluated whether pain migrated to the right lower quadrant in patients subsequently determined to have or not have acute appendicitis. If pain migrated to the right lower quadrant, then the positive likelihood ratio for appendicitis was 1·45 (95% CI 1·07–1·99). If the pain did not migrate to the right lower quadrant, then the likelihood ratio was 0·74 (95% CI 0·55–0·95). Based on these results, you conclude that migration of pain to the right lower quadrant alone is not sufficient evidence to diagnose appendicitis.

Golledge *et al.*[20] prospectively evaluated 100 patients aged 4–81 years with right lower quadrant pain and possible appendicitis. Physicians completed a form describing history and physical examination findings. The gold standard for diagnosis of appendicitis was histological evidence in the appendix removed at laparotomy. Those who did not undergo laparotomy were followed up to 1 month after initial evaluation. No mention was made of any missed cases of appendicitis. Fifty-eight patients were operated on and 44 (76%) of these had confirmed appendicitis. The authors specifically evaluated "cat's eye symptom" (pain on going over a bump in the road), the cough sign, right lower quadrant pain to percussion, rebound tenderness, and guarding. The likelihood ratios for these parameters based on the sensitivities and specificities provided in the article are shown in Table 38.2. There were insufficient data to calculate confidence intervals for the likelihood ratios. However, these data suggest that rebound tenderness is a very useful sign in the diagnosis of acute appendicitis, but that the other signs and symptoms listed are not.

Alshehri *et al.*[21] also studied rebound tenderness in 130 patients with suspected appendicitis. Seven were withdrawn from the study as they refused appendectomy and 53 improved within 12 hours and were assumed to not have acute appendicitis; 70 underwent appendectomy and 66 (94%) of these had appendicitis proven by histology. The positive likelihood ratio for rebound tenderness in the diagnosis of acute appendicitis was 1·2 based on a sensitivity of 95% and a specificity of 20%. Of note, the authors found similar likelihood ratios for guarding (LR+ = 1·2), Rovsing sign (LR+ = 1·5), and rigidity (LR+ = 1·7). (The definition of the Rovsing sign in the *Dorland's Medical Dictionary* is: "Pressure on the left side over the point corresponding to McBurney's point will elicit the typical pain at McBurney's point in appendicitis.") Although the authors feel that rebound tenderness is a useful sign, you

Table 38.2 Likelihood ratios for clinical signs and symptoms in predicting acute appendicitis[20]

Signs and symptoms	Likelihood ratio
Pain on going over a bump in the road (cat's eye)	1·7
Cough sign	1·6
Right lower quadrant pain (found in all patients)	1·1
Percussion tenderness in right lower quadrant	4·1
Rebound tenderness	7·4
Guarding	2·9

conclude that all of these signs would only prove useful when there is already a high suspicion of appendicitis. The absence of rebound or other signs may be more useful in ruling out the diagnosis of acute appendicitis. The lack of rebound tenderness gives a negative likelihood ratio of 0·3. Negative likelihood ratios for other findings were guarding (0·06), Rovsing sign (0·76), and rigidity (0·97). The lack of guarding in this case is the most useful finding. Without guarding appendicitis appears to be very unlikely.

O'Shea *et al.*[11] also evaluated whether patients had localized or generalized tenderness on examination and how that related to the diagnosis of appendicitis. The authors do not explain the exact location of tenderness in the "localized" cases. Because of this you believe this study may not be very useful in your clinical practice. Furthermore, including patients without appendicitis who did and did not undergo laparotomy, you note that the likelihood ratio for "localized pain" in the diagnosis of acute appendicitis is 1·1; you conclude this sign is unhelpful.

The study by Reynolds and Jaffe[19] provides insufficient information to determine likelihood ratios, but the authors note that right lower quadrant pain, abdominal tenderness and abdominal guarding were significantly associated with the diagnosis of acute appendicitis. Not enough information is provided in this study to influence your clinical practice and decision making.

You conclude that rebound tenderness may be a useful predictor of appendicitis in a child with a high probability of acute appendicitis. Furthermore, lack of guarding on physical exam may sway you to observe, rather than operate on, a patient with few other findings suggesting appendicitis.

Question

3. In children with acute abdominal pain (*patient/population*), will laboratory measures of inflammation (for example, ESR, WBC) (*intervention/test*) help in making the diagnosis of appendicitis (*outcome*)? **[Diagnosis]**

White blood cell count as a predictor of appendicitis

In MedLine you find 14 studies but only three of these evaluate leukocyte counts at different cut-off points.

- MedLine: "Appendicitis:diagnosis AND exp:leukocyte count AND prospective"

You first look at the article by Andersson *et al.*[17] which also reviewed the usefulness of vomiting and location of pain in making the diagnosis of appendicitis. In this large prospective study the authors found a likelihood ratio for appendicitis of 0·16 for a total WBC < 8000 K mm^{-3}. The likelihood ratio increased with increasing WBC, to a maximum of 7·0 for a WBC of 15 000 or more. Table 38.3 lists the likelihood ratios and 95% confidence intervals for different levels of total WBC.

According to these data, patients with possible appendicitis and a WBC of < 8000 are at substantially decreased risk for acute appendicitis. A WBC of between 8000 and 15 000 does not significantly change the estimate of risk. A WBC of ≥ 15 000 moderately increases the estimated risk of appendicitis. Thus, only at the extremes of WBC does this test appear to be clinically useful.

Dueholm *et al.*[22] report a blinded prospective study evaluating the usefulness of total leukocyte count, neutrophil count, and C-reactive protein (CRP) in 237 patients between the ages of 15 and 45 years with suspected appendicitis. Although the sensitivity of total WBC decreased greatly as the WBC increased, the specificity increases greatly, so that the likelihood ratios increased with rising WBC (Table 38.4).

Izbicki *et al.*[9,23] conducted a retrospective evaluation of 536 patients followed by a prospective evaluation of 150 patients with the presumed diagnosis of appendicitis. They correlated histologic diagnosis of appendicitis (the gold standard), with history, clinical examination, and laboratory investigations. The evaluation of WBC is based on the retrospective portion of this study. A WBC of > 11 000 had a likelihood ratio of 1·9, whereas a WBC of < 8000 had a likelihood ratio of 0·2. All the studies available have consistent results and suggest the diagnosis of appendicitis is unlikely when the WBC is low unless there is a very high pretest probability.

Ultrasound as a predictor of appendicitis

Question

4. In children with acute abdominal pain (*patient/population*), will an abdominal ultrasound scan (*intervention/test*) assist in the diagnosis of appendicitis (*outcome*)? **[Diagnosis]**

Table 38.3 Likelihood ratios for different values of total white blood count in the prediction of acute appendicitis[17]

WBC count	Likelihood ratio	95% CI
< 8000	0·16	0·10–0·26*
8000–< 10 000	0·83	0·53–1·28
10 000–< 12 000	1·12	0·75–1·65
12 000–< 15 000	2·44	1·63–3·65*
≥ 15 000	7·13	4·11–12·15*

*Likelihood ratios are not reported for WBC below 7000.

Table 38·4 Likelihood ratios for different values of total white blood count in the prediction of acute appendicitis[22]

WBC count	Likelihood ratio	95% CI
> 7000	1·2	1·2–1·4
> 9000	1·7	1·2–2·2
> 11 000	2·9	1·7–5·4
> 13 000	3·0	1·0–26·5

Note that WBC is reported by different cut-offs rather than as a range.

- *Cochrane Library:* one meta-analysis
- MedLine: "appendicitis AND diagnosis AND ultrasonography AND prospective studies, limit to English language"

Using the search strategy in the above box, you identify one meta-analysis in *Cochrane Library* and 11 articles from MedLine. Seven of these 11 articles are truly prospective, unique data, and evaluate the accuracy of ultrasound related to the likelihood of appendicitis. Review of references cited identifies an additional five articles that clearly state prospective methodology, which you consider worth reviewing. Two focus on children.

You start by reading the article referenced in the *Cochrane Library*.[24] This is a meta-analysis of 17 studies assessing the role of ultrasound in 3358 adults and children suspected of having appendicitis. The combined prevalence of disease in these studies is 37% (1247 subjects with appendicitis). The review's objective is clear and applicable, the participants, outcomes and search sources are explicit, and the statistical methods are stated. The validity of, and inclusion criteria for, studies assessed was not always stated. The pooled sensitivity of abdominal ultrasound examination for diagnosing acute appendicitis was 84·7% (95% CI 81·0, 87·8) and the specificity 92·1% (95% CI 88·0, 95·2). You calculate the

LR+ = 10·7 and LR− = 0·17. To determine the usefulness of ultrasound in real-world decision making, these LRs can be applied to three hypothetical groups of patients with different pretest probabilities of appendicitis. The authors also used probability calculations for three hypothetical groups of patients: those with definite signs of appendicitis (group 1); those with intermediate signs requiring serial evaluations (group 2); and those with a low probability of appendicitis and usually allowed to go home (group 3). Positive and negative predicative value calculations for the three groups, based on pretest probabilities of 80%, 40%, 2% respectively, are given in Table 38·5. The authors conclude that only those patients with equivocal clinical findings should proceed to ultrasound.

You then read the two articles from your MedLine search that focus on children but were not included in the systematic review. Vignault *et al.*[25] prospectively evaluated 70 children between the ages of 4 and 18 with suspected acute appendicitis. Although you cannot tell exactly how the study population was selected, you note that all children had "abdominal pain believed to be secondary to appendicitis", were evaluated by a surgeon, and received an abdominal ultrasound examination. Furthermore, you note that patients who did not undergo surgery were followed for a minimum of 1 month, thus a potential source of false-negative test results has adequately been accounted for. Thirty-three (47%) of the 70 children evaluated had appendicitis, so you presume this group represents patients with equivocal findings from the history, physical exam, and lab data for a diagnosis of appendicitis (otherwise they would have gone directly to the operating room, or been discharged home). This sounds like a population with a similar probability of appendicitis to your patient. From the article you calculate likelihood ratios of 8·5 for a positive test and 0·07 for a negative test.

In the second pediatric study, Ceres *et al.*[26] report on 368 prospectively collected ultrasound results from patients aged 2–14 years and with a "clinical diagnosis of acute appendicitis". Although a larger study, the findings are less supportive of the role of ultrasound in diagnosing appendicitis (LR+ = 1·8; LR− = 0·11). In the process of calculating likelihood ratios from the study results, you noted that a large number of the patients in this study (349/368 [95%]) had pathologically confirmed appendicitis. You look again at the study population and realize that *all* of the children evaluated were taken to the operating room. By including only those patients with clinical evidence supporting operative intervention regardless of ultrasound findings, the authors have selected a population with a very high pretest probability of having appendicitis. In doing so they have undermined the test's diagnostic accuracy and this is reflected in likelihood ratios much closer to 1 than in the Vignault study.[25]

Table 38.5 Hypothetical ultrasound test performance for populations with different prior probabilities of appendicitis[24]

Group	Pretest probability (%)	PPV (%)	NPV (%)
Group 1: Usually treated with urgent surgery	80	97·6	59·50
Group 2: Usually observed to clarify diagnosis	40	87·30	89·90
Group 3: Usually sent home after initial evaluation	2	19·80	99·70

Three other articles relevant to pediatrics were identified in your search of the literature. Two of these reported findings consistent with Vignault.[25] Ramachandran *et al.*[27] evaluated 452 subjects with clinically suspected appendicitis, aged 1–20 years. Hahn *et al.*[28] report on findings from 3859 patients aged 1–17 years. The pretest probabilities among the study cohorts were 25% and 13% respectively, and you assume this incidence is similar to your patient population. The first study reports LR+ = 30, LR– = 0·1; the second study reports LR+ = 30, LR– = 0·12.

The third article by Pena *et al.*[29] also reports findings on 139 patients suspected of having appendicitis, with a pretest probability of 36%. However the accuracy of ultrasound in this study was lower than in the previous studies: LR+ = 6·3, LR– = 0·6. In this study, patients with a negative or inconclusive ultrasound study also received a limited CT scan with rectal contrast. Of the 139 eligible patients, 108 went on to have a CT scan. You wonder if the availability of a second confirmatory study may have altered their findings on ultrasound, perhaps leading to misclassification bias. Furthermore, although only 13 subjects are reported as having equivocal findings following ultrasound and CT scan, 25 patients were admitted for observation. You decide your concern about misclassification bias is valid. The range of likelihood ratios for the three studies most similar to your population[22,24,25] is LR+ = 8·5 to 30, LR– = 0·1 to 0·07.

Horton *et al.*[30] conducted a prospective, randomized comparison of ultrasound versus CT scan diagnosis of appendicitis. This study enrolled only adult patients (age 18–65) thought after evaluation to have an atypical clinical presentation, or inconclusive presentation for appendicitis. After exclusions, 49 patients were randomly assigned to CT scan and 40 to ultrasound. This study found a LR+ of 1·08 and a LR– of 0·78 for ultrasound. These findings are notably worse than previously reported studies of ultrasound. This is due to a large number of patients with equivocal ultrasound findings (28%), who required reclassification for summary statistics calculation, as described above. Although small in size, this study of adults represents the only randomized study of ultrasound; the findings raise concern as to the usefulness of ultrasound.

In reviewing these studies you recognize several sources of bias. First, technical differences exist between studies. Studies differed by type of ultrasound machine used, the skill level of the radiologist performing the examination (some including senior radiology residents and surgeons), and the criteria used for defining appendicitis by ultrasound (largely from changes over time). Second, few studies clearly state how patients with inconclusive ultrasound results, or findings consistent with an alternative diagnosis, are handled. Third, variability may be due to different follow up times for patients with a purely clinical diagnosis (ranging from duration of hospitalization to several months). Fourth, the population studied, or pretest probability of appendicitis, varied between studies. In some studies only patients who went to the operating room were included, in other studies all patients considered for surgery were included. You are unable to fully control for the first three problems, except for those studies that clearly state that patients with equivocal ultrasound results were excluded. For these studies, you recalculate test performance including these patients as false-negative or false-positive results, recognizing this to be the most conservative method of handling this potential bias in summary measures. Regarding the fourth source of bias, variation in pretest probability (baseline risk), you decide to exclude studies limited to hospitalized patients, presuming that their pretest probability is likely to be higher than your patients. Thus, for adult patients with equivocal clinical findings, you believe the likelihood of appendicitis following ultrasound ranges from 1·08 to 50 for positive results and from 0·78 to 0·001 for negative results. Table 38.6 gives likelihood ratios for ultrasound performed in patients with suspected appendicitis.

On the basis of the available evidence, you conclude that patients with strong clinical evidence of appendicitis should be referred to a surgeon without an ultrasound, given the large number of false-negative results using this as a diagnostic test. Patients with a low probability of appendicitis on clinical grounds should not undergo an ultrasound, given the large number of false-positive results obtained. Those patients with an equivocal clinical diagnosis and a positive ultrasound result should be evaluated by a surgeon. For those patients with an equivocal clinical diagnosis and negative ultrasound results, you will consider a more conservative management plan if ongoing evaluation of the patient and the family situation allow for this.

Table 38.6 Likelihood ratios for ultrasound performed in patients with suspected appendicitis

Study	Year	Subjects (n)	Ages (years)	Pretest probability (%)	LR+	LR−
Karstrup[31]	1986	46	16–80	63	14	0·18
Puylaert*[32]	1987	111	8–86	47	10·7	0·27
Adams*[33]	1988	43	17–72	50	4·1	0·33
Schwerk[34]	1989	532	3–88	24	44·3	0·12
Amland[35]	1989	110	13–33	25	7·8	0·16
Vignault[25]	1990	70	4–18	47	8·5	0·07
Ceres[26]	1990	368	2–14	95	1·8	0·11
Schwerk[36]	1990	857	2–88	23	49·8	0·001
Ramachandran*[27]	1996	452	1–20	25	30	0·1
Chen[37]	1998	191	15–79	75	3·1	0·01
Hahn[28]	1998	3859	1–17	13	30	0·12
Franke**[38]	1999	870	6–?	27	11	0·47
Pena[29]	1999	139	3–20	36	6·3	0·6
Horton[30]	2000	500	18–65	75	1·08	0·78

*Results recalculated such that excluded patients, or those with equivocal findings, are treated as false-positive or false-negative results to give the most conservative estimate.
**Multicenter study.

Computed tomography as a predictor of appendicitis

Question

5. In children with acute abdominal pain (*patient/population*), will computed tomography (*intervention/test*) assist in the diagnosis of appendicitis (*outcome*)? **[Diagnosis]**

● MedLine: "Appendicitis: diagnosis AND computed tomography AND prospective, limit to English language"

The majority of studies evaluating the accuracy of computed tomography (CT) in diagnosing acute appendicitis have been conducted in adult patients. In reviewing these studies you find sources of bias similar to those identified for ultrasound, most notably the different types of contrast used (Table 38.7). Although the pretest probability among studies varies, only one study[39] was limited to patients undergoing surgery. Elimination of this study does not alter the range of likelihood ratios found: LR+ = 5·5–infinity; LR − = 0·1– < 0·001.

The prospective, randomized comparison of ultrasound versus CT scan diagnosis of appendicitis mentioned above enrolled only patients (age 18–65) considered after evaluation to have an atypical clinical presentation, or inconclusive presentation for appendicitis.[30] After exclusions, 49 patients were randomly assigned to CT scan and 40 to ultrasound. This study found an LR+ of 12·1 and an LR− of 0·3 for CT scan. This study restricts evaluation to those patients with equivocal clinical exams, the subset of patients most difficult to evaluate and most likely to benefit from radiographic evaluation. This study, while small and focusing on adults only, supports evaluation with CT scan rather than ultrasound.

The article by Pena and colleagues[29] focuses on pediatric patients and has results consistent with the other studies: 29 of the 108 patients undergoing CT scanning had appendicitis (pretest probability = 27%). CT identified appendicitis in 28 of these patients (true positives); 74 patients without appendicitis had negative CT results (true negatives). The authors, conservatively, treat patients with equivocal CT results as false-positive (if they did not have appendicitis) and false-negative (if they did have appendicitis), for a total of one false-negative result and five false-positive results. Thus, you derive a positive likelihood ratio of 16·2, and a negative likelihood negative of 0·03. You recall your concern about misclassification of ultrasound results, but as no further studies were obtained after the CT, you believe the CT results are less likely to be influenced by misclassification bias. The study's objective was to determine the diagnostic value of a protocol involving ultrasound followed by CT in the diagnosis of appendicitis; a follow up study by the same authors found that implementation of this protocol decreased the perforation rate and the negative appendectomy rates in children with suspected appendicitis.[40] Although you cannot directly compare the accuracy of CT to ultrasound, there appears to be potential benefit in obtaining some radiologic study in equivocal cases of severe acute abdominal pain. The study authors conclude that a CT following ultrasound is highly accurate in diagnosing appendicitis in children;

Table 38.7 Likelihood ratios for computed tomography performed in patients with suspected appendicitis

Study	Year	Subjects (n)	Ages (years)	Pretest probability (%)	LR+	LR−	Notes re contrast
Balthazar*[41]	1991	100	9–87	64	5·5	0·07	Oral + i.v.
Lane[42]	1996	109	≥ 18	38	30	0·1	None
Rao[43]	1997	100	6–75	53	49	0·02	Rectal
Rao*[44]	1997	100	6–84	56	Infinity	< 0·001	Rectal + oral
Funaki[45]	1998	100	6–64	30	16·1	0·03	Rectal and oral
D'Lppolito[39]	1998	52	6–71	77	Infinity	< 0·001	None
Pena[29]	1999	139	4–21	27	16·2	0·03	Rectal
Rao[46]	1999	100	11–63	32	Infinity	< 0·001	Rectal + i.v.
Horton[30]	2000	49	18–65	76	12·12	0·03	None
Cakirer[47]	2002	130	16–67	72	11·9	0·05	None

*Results recalculated such that excluded patients, or those with equivocal findings, are treated as false-positive or false-negative results.

however, you are concerned that additional tests involve diagnosis delays, radiation exposure, discomfort from rectal contrast, and possibly an adverse event related to sedation. Therefore you conclude that, when choosing a test in truly equivocal cases, you will need to consider the referral radiologist's experience with performing the two tests, as well as family preferences related to discomfort and risk from radiation and contrast exposure.

Clinical scoring as a predictor of appendicitis

Question

5. In children with acute abdominal pain (*patient/ population*), does clinical scoring (*intervention/test*) facilitate the accurate diagnosis of appendicitis (*outcome*)? **[Diagnosis]**

You recall the improved likelihood ratios for appendicitis obtained by combining signs and symptoms in the study by Reynolds, and decide to evaluate studies of clinical scoring systems. Using the search strategy shown in the Box you find 13 articles; three of these evaluate a scoring system as a predictor of acute appendicitis in children, with only two prospectively applied.

- MedLine: "Appendicitis: diagnosis AND computer-assisted AND prospective, limit to English language"

Various clinical and computer-assisted scoring systems for diagnosing appendicitis have been developed over the past 30 years. These were generally developed from adult databases, with poor performance when applied to children. Tests of performance vary, although accuracy tends to improve with increased complexity. Reviewing the articles

generated in your search, you find a single clinical scoring system developed from the assessment of children alone; since the differential diagnosis of abdominal pain and the presentation of appendicitis is distinct in the pediatric age range, you consider this article the most relevant.

A 5-year prospective study of 1170 children with acute abdominal pain aged 4–15 years was used to develop an 8-variable diagnostic score.[48] A uniform prospective data form included 14 variables (including symptoms, signs, laboratory findings, and demographic data) was completed at two hospitals in England and used to develop an 8-variable, 10-point Pediatric Appendicitis Score (PAS) (Table 38.8). The authors report a sensitivity of 1 and specificity of 0·92. You decide not to bother calculating the likelihood ratios from these numbers, given that the validation of the diagnostic tool was performed on the same set used to derive the rule; hence the sensitivity is 1 by definition.

You recognize the PAS as very similar to the Alvarado score, originally reported in 1986 under the mnemonic MANTELS (Migration, Anorexia-acetone, Nausea-vomiting, Tenderness in the right lower quadrant, Rebound pain, Elevation of temperature, Leukocytosis, Shift to the left). Macklin *et al.*[49] prospectively evaluated a modified version of this scoring system (omitting the left shift of neutrophil maturation) in 118 children aged 4–14 years. They report a sensitivity of 76·3% and a specificity of 78·8 (representing an LR+ = 3·6 and LR− = 0·31), and concluded that clinical assessment was more accurate than the modified Alvarado score. The final pediatric study you found developed and evaluated computer-aided diagnosis of appendicitis in 677 children under the age of 15 years on a prospectively derived data set.[3] Although the authors do not describe the computer program's complicated system, they similarly conclude, "its sensitivity was equivalent to that of inexperienced clinicians".

It appears that no single tool has been found or developed which has the 100% sensitivity required of a screening tool

Table 38.8 Pediatric appendicitis score

Diagnostic indicants	PAS (10)
Cough/percussion/hopping tenderness	2
Anorexia	1
Pyrexia	1
Nausea/emesis	1
Tenderness in the right lower quadrant	2
Leukocytosis (WBC $\geq$ 10 000 (10^9 per liter)	1
Polymorphonuclear neutrophilia	1
Migration of pain	1

for a disease with as serious an outcome as an appendicitis. However, you recognize that efforts have been made to optimally combine the multiple features of appendicitis that work together to contribute to a clinical diagnosis. Combining clinical features with the highest likelihood ratios makes sense; however, for now you decide to rely on your own interpretation of the results. You have a renewed appreciation of the importance of very careful and complete data collection when making the diagnosis of appendicitis.

Resolution of the scenario

Given the history of vomiting, abdominal pain and high WBC, you believe acute appendicitis is possible in this 5-year-old girl. There is no evidence of an alternative diagnosis: she does not have diarrhea or dysuria although you would have liked a urine sample from the patient. The absence of localized tenderness

makes the diagnosis of acute appendicitis less likely, although there is no specific mention of the presence or absence of rebound tenderness. You are concerned by her persistent pain following the enema and arrange an abdominal ultrasound. This reveals a dilated tubular structure in the right lower quadrant consistent with acute appendicitis. You do not request a CT scan. You again consult the surgeon, who takes the child to the operating room where a non-perforated, thickened, inflamed appendix is removed. The patient recovers without complication.

Future research needs

- Epidemiologic studies to establish the true incidence of acute appendicitis. Population-based studies are required to more clearly define those at highest risk, especially amongst populations of young children with abdominal pain.
- Evaluation of the predictive value of traditional signs and symptoms of acute appendicitis in children.
- Evaluation of the predictive value of additional signs (for example, whether or not the patient can jump) and symptoms (for example, unable to eat favorite food) used by pediatricians and pediatric surgeons.
- Prospective evaluating of the role of radiological studies (including ultrasound and CT) in children with suspected appendicitis.
- Evaluation of the interrater reliability of signs and symptoms of appendicitis and implications for designing a clinically useful scoring system.

Appendicitis

Summary table

Diagnostic question	Type of evidence	Clinical usefulness	Comment
Duration of pain	2 prospective cohort studies	LR 0·6–1·7	Not clinically useful
Vomiting	3 prospective cohort studies	LR 1·8–3·4 for vomiting LR 0·08–0·7 for no vomiting	Combination of factors including history of no vomiting helpful in excluding diagnosis
Localized pain	2 prospective cohort studies	LR 1·1–1·5 for RLQ pain LR 0·7 for no RLQ pain	Helpful only if other signs/symptoms are also present
Rebound tenderness	2 prospective cohort studies	LR 1·2–7·4 for rebound LR 0·3 for no rebound	Helpful if there is a high pretest probability
WBC	2 prospective cohort studies	LR 7·1–7·5 for WBC > 15 000 LR 0·2 for WBC < 8000	High WBC should increase suspicion for acute appendicitis
Ultrasound	8 prospective cohort studies and 1 meta analysis	LR+ 1·08–50 LR– 0·6–0·001	Most helpful for ruling appendicitis out
Computed tomography	8 prospective cohort studies	LR+ 5·5–infinity LR– 0·07–< 0·001	Possibly helpful ruling appendicitis in or out; further research required
Scoring system	2 prospective cohort studies	LR+ 3·6 LR– 0·31	Possibly helpful ruling appendicitis out; await more research before applying

References

1. Scholer SJ, Pituch K, Orr DP, Dittus RS. Clinical outcomes of children with acute abdominal pain. *Pediatrics* 1996;**98**: 680–5.
2. Reynolds SL, Jaffe DM. Children with abdominal pain: evaluation in the pediatric emergency department. *Pediatr Emerg Care* 1990;**6**:8–12.
3. Dickson JA, Jones A, Telfer S, de Dombal FT. Acute abdominal pain in children. *Scand J Gastroenterol Suppl* 1988,**144**: 43–6.
4. Addiss DG, Shaffer N, Fowler BS, Tauxe RV. The epidemiology of appendicitis and appendectomy in the United States. *Am J Epidemiol* 1990;**132**:910–25.
5. Gilmore OJ, Browett JP, Griffin PH *et al.* Appendicitis and mimicking conditions. A prospective study. *Lancet* 1975; **2**:421–4.
6. Bell MJ, Bower RJ, Ternberg JL. Appendectomy in childhood. Analysis of 105 negative explorations. *Am J Surg* 1982;**144**: 335–7.
7. Berry J, Jr, Malt RA. Appendicitis near its centenary. *Ann Surg* 1984;**200**:567–75.
8. Irvin TT. Abdominal pain: a surgical audit of 1190 emergency admissions. *Br J Surg* 1989;**76**:1121–5.
9. Izbicki JR, Knoefel WT, Wilker DK *et al.* Accurate diagnosis of acute appendicitis: a retrospective and prospective analysis of 686 patients. *Eur J Surg* 1992;**158**:227–31.
10. Nauta RJ, Magnant C. Observation versus operation for abdominal pain in the right lower quadrant. Roles of the clinical examination and the leukocyte count. *Am J Surg* 1986;**151**:746–8.
11. O'Shea JS, Bishop ME, Alario AJ, Cooper JM. Diagnosing appendicitis in children with acute abdominal pain. *Pediatr Emerg Care* 1988;**4**:172–6.
12. Savrin RA, Clatworthy HW, Jr. Appendiceal rupture: a continuing diagnostic problem. *Pediatrics* 1979;**63**: 36–43.
13. Graham JM, Pokorny WJ, Harberg FJ. Acute appendicitis in preschool age children. *Am J Surg* 1980;**139**:247–50.
14. Howie JG. Death from appendicitis and appendicectomy. An epidemiological survey. *Lancet* 1966;**2**:1334–7.
15. Neuspiel DR, Kuller LH. Fatalities from undetected appendicitis in early childhood. *Clin Pediatr (Phila)* 1987;**26**: 573–5.
16. Blomqvist PG, Andersson RE, Granath F, Lambe MP, Ekbom AR. Mortality after appendectomy in Sweden, 1987–1996. *Ann Surg* 2001;**233**:455–60.
17. Andersson RE, Hugander AP, Ghazi SH *et al.* Diagnostic value of disease history, clinical presentation, and inflammatory parameters of appendicitis. *World J Surg* 1999;**23**:133–40.
18. Korner H, Sondenaa K, Soreide JA, Nysted A, Vatten L. The history is important in patients with suspected acute appendicitis. *Dig Surg* 2000;**17**:364–9.

19 Reynolds SL, Jaffe DM. Diagnosing abdominal pain in a pediatric emergency department. *Pediatr Emerg Care* 1992;**8**:126–8.

20 Golledge J, Toms AP, Franklin IJ, Scriven MW, Galland RB. Assessment of peritonism in appendicitis. *Ann Roy Coll Surg Engl* 1996;**78**:11–14.

21 Alshehri MY, Ibrahim A, Abuaisha N *et al.* Value of rebound tenderness in acute appendicitis. *East Afr Med J* 1995;**72**:504–6.

22 Dueholm S, Bagi P, Bud M. Laboratory aid in the diagnosis of acute appendicitis. A blinded, prospective trial concerning diagnostic value of leukocyte count, neutrophil differential count, and C-reactive protein. *Dis Colon Rectum* 1989;**32**:855–9.

23 Izbicki JR, Wilker DK, Mandelkow HK *et al.* [Retro- and prospective studies on the value of clinical and laboratory chemical data in acute appendicitis]. *Chirurg* 1990;**61**:887–94.

24 Orr RK, Porter D, Hartman D. Ultrasonography to evaluate adults for appendicitis: decision making based on meta-analysis and probabilistic reasoning. *Acad Emerg Med* 1995;**2**:644–50.

25 Vignault F, Filiatrault D, Brandt ML, Garel L, Grignon A, Ouimet A. Acute appendicitis in children: evaluation with US. *Radiology* 1990;**176**:501–4.

26 Ceres L, Alonso I, Lopez P, Parra G, Echeverry J. Ultrasound study of acute appendicitis in children with emphasis upon the diagnosis of retrocecal appendicitis. *Pediatr Radiol* 1990;**20**:258–61.

27 Ramachandran P, Sivit CJ, Newman KD, Schwartz MZ. Ultrasonography as an adjunct in the diagnosis of acute appendicitis: a 4-year experience. *J Pediatr Surg* 1996;**31**:164–9.

28 Hahn HB, Hoepner FU, Kalle T *et al.* Sonography of acute appendicitis in children: 7 years experience. *Pediatr Radiol* 1998;**28**:147–51.

29 Pena BMG, Mandl KD, Kraus SJ *et al.* Ultrasonography and limited computed tomography in the diagnosis and management of appendicitis in children. *JAMA* 1999;**282**:1041–6.

30 Horton MD, Counter SF, Florence MG, Hart MJ. A prospective trial of computed tomography and ultrasonography for diagnosing appendicitis in the atypical patient. *Am J Surg* 2000;**179**:379–81.

31 Karstrup S, Torp-Pedersen S, Roikjaer O. Ultrasonic visualisation of the inflamed appendix. *Br J Radiol* 1986;**59**:985–6.

32 Puylaert JB, Rutgers PH, Lalisang RI *et al.* A prospective study of ultrasonography in the diagnosis of appendicitis. *N Engl J Med* 1987;**317**:666–9.

33 Adams DH, Fine C, Brooks DC. High-resolution real-time ultrasonography. A new tool in the diagnosis of acute appendicitis. *Am J Surg* 1988;**155**:93–7.

34 Schwerk WB, Wichtrup B, Rothmund M, Ruschoff J. Ultrasonography in the diagnosis of acute appendicitis: a prospective study. *Gastroenterology* 1989;**97**:630–9.

35 Amland PF, Skaane P, Ronningen H, Nordshus T, Solheim K. Ultrasonography and parameters of inflammation in acute appendicitis. A comparison with clinical findings. *Acta Chirurg Scand* 1989;**155**:185–9.

36 Schwerk WB, Wichtrup B, Ruschoff J, Rothmund M. Acute and perforated appendicitis: current experience with ultrasound- aided diagnosis. *World J Surg* 1990;**14**:271–6.

37 Chen SC, Chen KM, Wang SM, Chang KJ. Abdominal sonography screening of clinically diagnosed or suspected appendicitis before surgery. *World J Surg* 1998;**22**:449–52.

38 Franke C, Bohner H, Yang Q, Ohmann C, Roher HD. Ultrasonography for diagnosis of acute appendicitis: results of a prospective multicenter trial. Acute Abdominal Pain Study Group. *World J Surg* 1999;**23**:141–6.

39 D'Lppolito G, de Mello GG, Szejnfeld J. The value of unenhanced CT in the diagnosis of acute appendicitis. *Rev Paul Med* 1998;**116**:1838–45.

40 Pena BM, Taylor GA, Fishman SJ, Mandl KD. Effect of an imaging protocol on clinical outcomes among pediatric patients with appendicitis. *Pediatrics* 2002;**110**:1088–93.

41 Balthazar EJ, Megibow AJ, Siegel SE, Birnbaum BA. Appendicitis: prospective evaluation with high-resolution CT. *Radiology* 1991;**180**:21–4.

42 Lane MJ, Katz DS, Ross BA, Clautice-Engle TL, Mindelzun RE, Jeffrey RB, Jr. Unenhanced helical CT for suspected acute appendicitis. *Am J Roentgenol* 1997;**168**:405–9.

43 Rao PM, Rhea JT, Novelline RA, Mostafavi AA, Lawrason JN, McCabe CJ. Helical CT combined with contrast material administered only through the colon for imaging of suspected appendicitis [see comments]. *Am J Roentgenol* 1997;**169**:1275–80.

44 Rao PM, Rhea JT, Novelline RA *et al.* Helical CT technique for the diagnosis of appendicitis: prospective evaluation of a focused appendix CT examination. *Radiology* 1997;**202**:139–44.

45 Funaki B, Grosskreutz SR, Funaki CN. Using unenhanced helical CT with enteric contrast material for suspected appendicitis in patients treated at a community hospital. *Am J Roentgenol* 1998;**171**:997–1001.

46 Rao PM, Feltmate CM, Rhea JT, Schulick AH, Novelline RA. Helical computed tomography in differentiating appendicitis and acute gynecologic conditions. *Obstet Gynecol* 1999;**93**:417–21.

47 Cakirer S, Basak M, Bolakoglu B, Mankaoglu M. Diagnosis of acute appendicitis with unenhanced helical CT: a study of 130 patients. *Emerg Radiol* 2002;**9**:155–161.

48 Samuel M. Pediatric appendicitis score. *J Pediatr Surg* 2002;**37**:877–81.

49 Macklin CP, Radcliffe GS, Merei JM, Stringer MD. A prospective evaluation of the modified Alvarado score for acute appendicitis in children. *Ann Roy Coll Surg Engl* 1997;**79**:203–5.

39 Wound repair and tissue adhesives

Martin H Osmond

Case scenario

An 18-month-old male is brought into your emergency department with a laceration on his forehead. He was playing at home when he fell and hit his head on the corner of a coffee table. He did not lose consciousness. He has had no vomiting and his mother states that he is acting and playing normally now. His immunizations are up to date. On examination his only physical finding is that of a 2-cm horizontal laceration on his forehead. It is a full-thickness skin laceration through to the subcutaneous fat. It is not actively bleeding. The mother is extremely concerned about both the potential discomfort in closing this laceration and the eventual cosmetic outcome. She has heard of a new "skin glue" and wants to know if that would be better than stitches for her child. You have tried tissue adhesives for laceration closure in the past but are unsure of how to answer her questions.

Background

Traumatic wounds are one of the most common reasons for children to seek care in emergency departments.[1] Traditionally these lacerations have been closed with sutures. Although effective, the technique of suturing usually involves the injection of a local anesthetic, which is painful and may further distress an already frightened child. Wound repair by suturing is also relatively time consuming, both at the time of repair and in the need for a follow up visit for suture removal.

Over the last 15 years physicians have worked on many fronts to try to minimize the discomfort of pediatric laceration closure. Much work has been done to make the delivery of analgesia less painful with the development of buffered lidocaine, and topical analgesics such as TAC (tetracaine-adrenalin-cocaine) and LAT (lidocaine-adrenalin-tetracaine). Others have refined protocols of conscious sedation to be used for laceration closure. This chapter will deal with the significant work that has been done recently in the development of cyanoacrylate tissue adhesives for laceration repair.

Cyanoacrylate adhesives were first synthesized in 1949 but not used clinically until the late 1950s. The early derivatives, methyl-2- and ethyl-2-cyanoacrylate, polymerized rapidly on contact to make a tremendously strong bond. These adhesives became extremely popular as commercial "super glues" such as Krazy Glue. Unfortunately, these products could not be used clinically as they were found to degrade rapidly into cyanoacetate and formaldehyde which caused histotoxicity in the form of acute and chronic inflammation in the wound. It was not until cyanoacrylate tissue adhesives with longer alkyl chains were synthesized that histotoxicity was reduced and clinical use of tissue adhesives for wound closure started.

Butylcyanoacrylates were the first tissue adhesives to be widely studied and used clinically. They have now been in use for over 25 years and have a strong safety record.[2] They have shown no toxicity when applied topically for skin closure, but have had variable toxicity when implanted in vascular wounds.[3] Like all tissue adhesives, they are supplied as a liquid monomer in a sterile plastic vial. In the presence of basic substances, such as skin moisture or tissue fluid, they polymerize rapidly to form a strong bond with the skin. This process is an exothermic reaction with heat being momentarily generated as the adhesive hardens. This heat is felt as a slight burning sensation by the child. The amount of heat released is directly related to the amount of tissue fluid (or blood) present and the amount of adhesive applied. This becomes important for the clinical situation where, to minimize pain, only a small amount of the tissue adhesive should be applied to a relatively dry wound.

Early studies describing the use of *N*-butyl-2-cyanoacrylate for pediatric laceration closure came from Europe[4] and Israel.[5] They revealed, in non-controlled studies of over 1500 children, that the product Histoacryl Blue could be used safely to perform a quick and relatively painless wound closure with very good cosmetic results. Other case series in adults described the same findings.[6–10]

A new generation of tissue adhesive, called octylcyanoacrylate, has recently been developed. It is a longer-chain cyanoacrylate with a three-dimensional breaking strength that is four times that of *N*-butyl-2-cyanoacrylate. It is supplied in a single-use vial with a porous applicator tip from which the tissue adhesive is painted in several coats over the opposed skin edges. It has the advantage of producing a less brittle and stronger, more flexible bond than butylcyanoacrylate.

The technique of wound closure with tissue adhesives is easy to learn and simple to perform.[11] After the wound has been thoroughly cleaned and debrided (if necessary), hemostasis must be obtained with pressure or epinephrine-containing topical anesthetics. As mentioned earlier, the polymerization reaction releases some heat which is felt momentarily by the patient. The drier the wound edges, the less heat that is released. The wound edges are then opposed with fingers or forceps and the tissue adhesive is either dropped onto the opposed skin edges to form a thin film of glue (in the case of most tissue adhesives) or painted over the opposed skin edges in three coatings (in the case of the octylcyanoacrylate, Dermabond – see Figure 39.1). Apposition of the wound edges should be maintained for 30–60 seconds. Full strength will occur by 2 minutes. The wound should be covered with a protective dressing and kept dry for 48 hours. After 48 hours, patients may shower but should avoid soaking or scrubbing the area. Routine medical follow up is not necessary as there are no sutures to remove, but patients and parents should be instructed to return immediately should there be signs of dehiscence or infection. The tissue adhesive will gradually fall off in 1–2 weeks.

During tissue adhesive application care must be taken to avoid complications. Cyanoacrylates are recommended as topical agents that bond to the top layer of the epithelium. It is important to make sure that the glue does not enter the wound where it may impair wound healing and cause a mild foreign body giant cell response (see Figure 39.1). The operator must also be sure to avoid sticking his/her fingers to the patient. If this occurs, you can unstick the fingers by rolling them off the surface of the patient's skin. As some adhesives are not very viscous, the wound should be positioned in such a way that if the adhesive does run, it does not run into unwanted areas such as the eye. In general, with careful technique, tissue adhesives are very easy and safe products to use.

You think of several questions that are suggested by the scenario:

- How effective are tissue adhesives in closing facial lacerations in children?
- Is tissue adhesive closure more or less painful than suture closure?
- Which tissue adhesive is most effective and easiest to apply?

You reframe the questions in a structured way to assist you with your search for evidence (see Chapters 2 and 3).

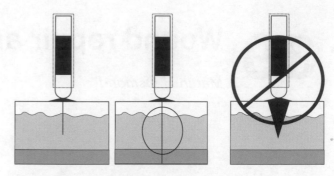

Figure 39.1 Left and center: proper topical use of octylcyano-acrylate tissue adhesive. Right: improperly used, the adhesive acts as a foreign body and a barrier to wound healing. Reproduced with permission.[15]

Framing answerable clinical questions

In this case we are concerned with the *population* of children with facial lacerations. The *intervention* of interest is the repair of the laceration by tissue adhesive or suture closure. The *outcomes* that we would like to assess are long-term cosmetic outcome and pain of the procedure. Focusing the question helps guide the literature search and allows the physician to effectively screen the titles and abstracts of the articles that are located. Thus the questions can be phrased as follows.

Questions

In pediatric facial lacerations (*population*), which method of laceration closure, tissue adhesive or sutures, (*intervention and comparison*) is superior with respect to (*outcomes*):

1 long-term cosmetic outcome?
2 pain during the procedure?
3 time required to complete the procedure?
4 complications?

Searching for evidence

Having posed your focused questions, you need to be able to find the best available evidence in the most efficient manner. There are three ways in which you may proceed:

- look up references in a textbook;
- ask a colleague; and
- search a database, such as MedLine.

In general, recent textbooks may provide a starting point in order to summarize the evidence surrounding a particular question. They may also provide references of specific studies of interest. Unfortunately, a review of your most recent pediatric emergency procedure text published in 1997[12] reveals only three sentences on the use of tissue adhesives for laceration closure and provides only one reference (Quinn *et al.*, 1993).[13] This illustrates one of the drawbacks of textbooks in that they are only as up to date as their most recent reference. In general with the rapid development of new knowledge from research, most standard textbooks are unable to be of dependable help. In addition you cannot be sure that the experts who have written the chapter have taken all the available evidence into account when arriving at their conclusions.

Asking a colleague can be a very time-efficient way of finding the answer to a clinical question. However, the appropriate colleague may not be easily available to give advice. In addition, once the advice is given, you must be sure that the opinion is based on a fair evaluation of the existing evidence.

The third route is searching the relevant medical literature through access to a medical database. It is helpful to first search for a comprehensive literature review or a meta-analysis of the area in question. This should provide a synthesis of the evidence to date and can save the time of having to search original trials. You start by searching *Clinical Evidence* (Issue 8, December 2002). Unfortunately, the area of laceration closure by tissue adhesives has not yet been addressed. Next you search the *Cochrane Library* looking specifically for systematic reviews.

Searching for evidence synthesis

- *Clinical Evidence.*
- *Cochrane Library*: Tissue Adhesive.

Your search of the *Cochrane Library* (Issue 1, 2003) reveals one completed systematic review by Farion *et al.* entitled, "Tissue adhesives for traumatic lacerations in children and adults".[14] Although you have identified a current systematic review, you should also search MedLine for any randomized controlled trials (RCTs) published after the search date in the systematic review. The search strategy for finding trials on tissue adhesive closure of skin lacerations is shown in the Box.

MedLine search strategy (on Ovid) for identifying studies relating to tissue adhesive use in laceration closure

- 1 Exp "wounds AND injuries"
- 2 Exp *tissue adhesives
- 3 1 AND 2
- 4 limit 3 to human

This simple search strategy uncovers all articles dealing with human subjects with a major focus on tissue adhesives and any type of wound or injury. It is a relatively broad search but as the tissue adhesive literature is small the number of citations retrieved can easily be scanned to see if they are trials that address the question and are published after the most recent meta-analysis.

You find four RCTs and one systematic review that were published after the Cochrane review. One RCT compares a new "hair apposition" tissue adhesive technique to sutures in scalp lacerations.[15] This you pass over, as it does not concern facial lacerations. Another trial, by Singer *et al.*,[16] contains data on emergency department patients previously reported in two RCTs that were included in the Cochrane systematic review.[17,18] In this publication the emergency department data are combined with data from patients having incisions closed as part of an elective procedure. You decide not to use this RCT as its data are already reported in the systematic review. The other two RCTs are original studies on the use of tissue adhesives for general laceration closure and you choose to examine these more closely.[19,20]

The systematic review you uncover is by Farion *et al.*[21] This is the Cochrane review that you found earlier, now published in the journal *Academic Emergency Medicine*. You decide to use the Cochrane review as it should be regularly updated as new information becomes available and you have access to the *Cochrane Library* on-line.

Critical review of the evidence

Before returning to your questions you decide to start with an appraisal of the systematic review from the *Cochrane Library*.[14] This Cochrane review used a very complete search strategy including MedLine, Embase, the Cochrane Controlled Trials Register and the Cochrane Wounds Group Specialized Trials Register. In addition, in an effort to find further trials, they did citation searches of all selected articles, contacted the primary author of selected studies and contacted the manufacturers of tissue adhesive products. Two reviewers independently examined articles for inclusion in the systematic review and the quality of the selected trials was assessed by a validated scoring system. Data were extracted by one reviewer and checked for accuracy by a second reviewer and meta-analysis was used when appropriate. After reviewing the methodology, you are confident that this is a high quality systematic review (see Chapter 8).

You then look for a description of the RCTs included in the systematic review. Eight studies compared a tissue adhesive (TA) versus standard wound closure (SWC), four with butyl-cyanoacrylate (Histoacryl),[13,22–24] and four with octylcyano-acrylate (Dermabond).[17,18,25,26] The standard wound closure method was sutures in five studies,[13,22–25] adhesive strips in one study,[26] and a mixture of closure methods in the remaining two studies,[17,18] though the majority of patients received sutures. Five of the eight studies were limited to pediatric patients,[13,18,23,24,26] one was limited to adults,[25] and the remaining two studies included all ages.[17,22] Two of the pediatric studies[13,26] and one of the studies without age restriction[22] were limited to facial lacerations. Three studies[13,22,24] excluded deep suture lacerations. The remaining studies did not stratify their results by extent of laceration. The final included study[27] compared butyl-cyanoacrylate and octylcyanoacrylate for the closure of pediatric facial lacerations not requiring deep sutures. It was the only study available that compared two tissue adhesives.

You note that most studies excluded long lacerations (> 5 cm), bite wounds, crush wounds or highly contaminated wounds, stellate wounds, wounds under high tension, or wounds crossing the mucocutaneous junction. The results therefore cannot be extrapolated to patients with these types of lacerations.

You then assess the two new RCTs.[19,20] Two key guides in assessing RCTs are determining whether the assignment of patients to treatment groups was truly random and whether all patients who were enrolled in the trial were accounted for at its conclusion.[28] Secondary guides include assessing whether patients, health workers and study personnel were "blind" to treatment, whether groups were similar at the start of the trial, whether allocation of study participants were adequately concealed up to the point of treatment, and whether, aside from the intervention, the groups were treated equally. See Chapter 6 for a complete discussion of how to critically appraise studies of therapeutic interventions.

The first trial, by Mattick *et al.*[19] compares Dermabond (octyl-2-cyanoacrylate) to adhesive strips (Steristrips) in children (1–14 years) with simple, low-tension lacerations. This is a small study with 60 children entering the trial and 16 of these being lost to follow up. The patients were adequately randomized and the primary outcome measure, cosmetic outcome at 3–12 months, was assessed by a blinded plastic surgeon. Unfortunately, a healing scar can change significantly from 3 to 12 months post-closure and the authors do not report which children were assessed at what time in this 9-month period. It is unclear if this may have affected study results.

The second trial, by Karcioglu *et al.*[20] is a comparison of Histoacryl Blue (*N*-butyl-2-cyanoacrylate) versus suturing in the repair of simple lacerations (≤ 5 cm in length) in adults. The 92 enrolled patients appear to have been well-randomized. As with all wound closure trials the study physicians, nurses and parents were not blinded to the procedure being performed; however, the physicians assessing cosmetic outcome at 10 and 90 days were blinded. Unfortunately, there was a significant loss to follow up with 75% returning at 10 days and only 57% returning at 90 days.

Although the two new RCTs are small and have lost a significant number of patients to follow up, you decide to consider their data in your search to answer your questions. However, you decide to give much more weight to the evidence of the high quality Cochrane systematic review. Armed with the most recent evidence in the literature you are now ready to return to your questions.

Question

1. In pediatric facial lacerations (*population*), which method of laceration closure, tissue adhesive or sutures, (*intervention and comparison*) is superior with respect to long-term cosmetic outcome (*outcome*)?

Long-term cosmetic outcome is accepted to be the most critical factor in assessing wound closure technique. In the Cochrane systematic review,[14] cosmesis was the primary outcome reported by all selected studies. Many studies used a 100 mm Cosmetic Visual Analog Scale (CVAS) that has been shown to be a reliable and valid outcome measure of long-term cosmesis with excellent intra- and interrater agreement.[29] This was performed by a blinded assessor (often a plastic surgeon) who assessed the scar either in person or, more commonly, from a photograph. Other studies used a Wound Evaluation Score (WES) that reported a dichotomous outcome as either optimal or suboptimal wound closure. See Chapter 10 for a discussion of how to assess the usefulness of a clinical measure such as the WES.

Six studies with a total of 469 patients compared tissue adhesives (TAs) with standard wound closure (SWC) using CVAS. Overall, no significant difference in cosmetic outcome was found at any of the time points examined. At 1–3 months the weighted mean difference (WMD) was 0·6 (95% CI = − 5·1–6·3). An exploratory power analysis, using a minimum clinically important difference (MCID) of 12 mm, showed that an independent two-sample t test, given this sample size, would be sufficiently powered (power > 99%) to detect a difference if one truly existed. At 9–12 months the WMD was 4·3 (95% CI = −5·8–14·4; two studies with 109 lacerations). For those studies reporting WES, there was no significant difference between the treatment groups for any of the time periods examined.

There was also no difference in cosmetic outcome in any of the subgroups examined by the Cochrane systematic review. These subgroups included age of patient (pediatric *v* adult), glue type (butylcyanoacrylate *v* octylcyanoacrylate), RCT quality as determined by the Jadad score, and funding sources (private, public, or not stated). There was insufficient detail in the included studies to determine whether laceration size or location might influence cosmetic outcome between TAs and SWC.

You next turn to the recent RCTs not included in the systematic review. The study by Mattick *et al.*[19] showed no difference in the CVAS score between TAs and adhesive strips at a follow up between 3 and 12 months as scored by both parents and a plastic surgeon. The study by Karcioglu *et al.*[20] showed no difference in the CVAS score between TAs and sutures at 10 days and 3 months.

After reading the Cochrane systematic review and the more recent RCTs, you conclude that there is no difference in the short- or long-term cosmetic outcome between lacerations closed with TAs and SWC.

Question

2. In pediatric facial lacerations (*population*), which method of laceration closure, tissue adhesive or sutures, (*intervention and comparison*) is superior with respect to pain during the procedure (*outcome*)?

The Cochrane systematic review addresses this question in its reporting of "secondary outcomes".[14] All pain scores were recorded on visual analog scales (VAS) either by the patient experiencing the procedure, the physician performing the procedure, or the parent or nurse observing the procedure. In all cases the pain score results favored the TA intervention. The pain outcome with the most studies, the parent-reported VAS, had a WMD of -15.7 (95% CI $= -21.9$ to -9.5; four studies with 390 lacerations). The patient-reported VAS WMD was -10.8 (95% CI $= -17.1$ to -4.5). The physician-reported VAS WMD was -12.6 (95% CI $= -20.1$ to -5.1). The nurse-reported VAS WMD was -14.9 (95% CI $= -22.5$ to -7.3).

In reviewing the more recent RCTs, you note that Mattick *et al.*[19] found that parents recording their child's pain on a 100 mm VAS showed no difference in degree of distress suffered by their children when comparing TA to adhesive strips. However, physicians performing the technique (necessarily unblinded) found the technique of applying TA more distressing to the child than adhesive strips (median VA score; 91 *v* 95, *P* = 0.07). The study by Karcioglu *et al.*[20] did not specifically assess the pain of the procedure.

You conclude that the use of TA results in less pain to the patient than the use of sutures. Although the existing evidence is weak, it is possible that adhesive strips result in similar or less pain experienced by the patient.

Question

3. In pediatric facial lacerations (*population*), which method of laceration closure, tissue adhesive or sutures, (*intervention and comparison*) is superior with respect to time required to complete the procedure (*outcome*)?

Time is a precious resource in your emergency department and you are very interested to know whether the application of TAs will save time for both you, and your young patient who will need to be restrained for the procedure. The Cochrane systematic review[14] found five studies representing 487 lacerations in which time was reported. Time to complete the procedure in minutes favored the tissue adhesive interventions. Tissue adhesives, on average, were about 5.7 minutes faster to apply than SWC (WMD -5.7 95% CI $= -8.2$ to -3.1). No study in this review reported on the outcome of ease of the procedure. You note that the recent RCTs by Mattick *et al.*[19] and Karcioglu *et al.*[20] do not report on the time taken to perform the procedure. You are happy to conclude that the use of a TA should shorten the procedure time for both you and your patient.

Question

4. In pediatric facial lacerations (*population*), which method of laceration closure, tissue adhesive or sutures, (*intervention and comparison*) is superior with respect to complications (*outcome*)?

You are encouraged that TAs in comparison to SWC seems to result in less pain, take less time, and result in an equal cosmetic outcome. However, your willingness to adopt this new technique will be affected by the rate of complications. Particularly, you are concerned with the dehiscence rate, as you know that a TA bond is not as strong as sutures in the first few days after the procedure.

The Cochrane systematic review[14] looked specifically for the complications of dehiscence, erythema, infection and discharge. No individual RCT has been able to show a significant difference in any complication comparing TA to SWC. This could be due to insufficient power to detect rare outcomes. However, in pooling the eight trials that compared TA to SWC, Farion *et al.* found that significant fixed-effects differences were found for dehiscence (favoring SWC) and erythema (favoring TA).

The small but significant increased risk of dehiscence was found with TAs using the fixed-effects model. The estimate of this risk difference (RD) is 0.04 (95% CI $= 0.01–0.07$) favoring SWC (see Figure 39.2).[21] This results in a number needed to harm (NNH) of 25 (95% CI $= 14–100$). In other words approximately 25 patients would have to be treated with a TA to result in one excess wound dehiscence. The baseline risk of dehiscence for the SWC arm was 1.8% (95% CI $= 0.3–3.2$). The clinical significance of this finding is unclear. Factors that could determine dehiscence rates include the characteristics of the wound, the physician's skill level, different tissue adhesive properties or patient characteristics. Further research will have to uncover the role

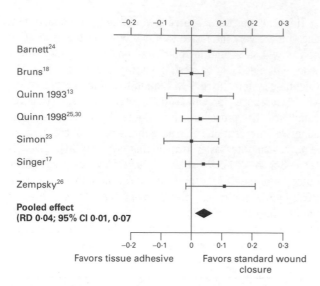

Figure 39.2 Risk difference (RD) for dehiscence, tissue adhesive versus standard wound closure point estimates and 95% CIs (fixed-effects model). (Reprinted from Farion KJ, Osmond MH, Hartling L, *et al*. Tissue adhesives for traumatic lacerations: a systematic review of randomized controlled trials. *Acad Emerg Med* 2003;**10**:110–118. Copyright 2003, with permission from Society for Academic Emergency Medicine.)

that each factor may play. You note with interest that, despite the difference in dehiscence rate, the Cochrane review found that the final cosmetic outcome between the two groups is equal. You decide to discuss this increased dehiscence rate with the parents prior to deciding on which method of laceration closure to use.

Erythema was significantly more likely to occur in wounds closed by SWC. The fixed effects RD for erythema was -0.12 (95% CI $= -0.23$ to -0.01), favoring tissue adhesives. Eight patients would need to be treated with tissue adhesive to prevent one incident of erythema using SWC (NNH $= 8$; 95% CI 4, 100). The baseline SWC risk is 19.5% (95% CI $= 11.6$–27.4). Again, the clinical significance of this erythema is not known.

No difference was found for infection or discharge between the two groups. This may be due to the fact that these are rare complications, and even greater numbers of patients will need to be pooled to detect significant differences in these areas.

Both recent RCTs were small and therefore would contribute little information about rare complications. The study by Mattick *et al*.[19] did not report on any complications, although they did exclude five patients initially from their trial for being unable to close the laceration (four in the TA group and one in the adhesive strip group). The study by Karcioglu *et al*.[20] found no wound infection in either group but did not specifically comment on wound dehiscence, erythema, or discharge.

You conclude that there is a small but statistically significant increase in the dehiscence rate with TAs

(NNH $= 25$). You make a note to explain this to parents prior to choosing which method of laceration closure to use.

Economic analysis

You have heard that tissue adhesives can be expensive. Before adopting this method of laceration closure you are interested to read a study by Osmond *et al*. that is an economic comparison between non-absorbable percutaneous sutures, absorbable percutaneous sutures, and multi-use Histoacryl Blue in a Canadian emergency department (ED) setting, using 1993 costs.[31] At the time this study was done it was assumed that ED overhead costs, cosmetic results, and complications were equal across the three groups. The major comparison was between personnel time, supply costs, and parental costs. Absorbable sutures were found to be 2.4 times more costly than TAs, while non-absorbable sutures were 6.8 times more costly, due to the need for a repeat visit.

Although this is encouraging for tissue adhesives, you realize that an updated cost analysis is needed to include newer TAs, such as Dermabond, and the cost of conscious sedation, which is being used more often for pediatric lacerations repaired with sutures. The higher rate of dehiscence associated with TAs may also affect the conclusions.

Summary

- Tissue adhesives are an acceptable alternative to stitches in closing simple traumatic lacerations.
- The short-term (1–3 month) and long-term (9–12 month) cosmetic outcome is not significantly different between wounds closed with tissue adhesives and those closed with sutures.
- The pain of the tissue adhesive procedure is significantly less than sutures as rated by parents, patients, physicians, and nurses.
- The time for wound closure is approximately 5 minutes faster with tissue adhesives.
- A small but significant increased risk of dehiscence was found with tissue adhesives (NNH $= 25$).
- The infection rate is not significantly different between groups.
- Cyanoacrylate tissue adhesives have most frequently been studied in simple, uncomplicated facial lacerations in children. They may be used in conjunction with deep sutures. They are not intended for closure of wounds under high tensile stress (for example, over joints) or in areas of high friction (for example, fingers). Closure of animal bites, vermilion border lacerations, and stellate, crush wounds is also contraindicated.
- There may be a cost advantage to using certain tissue adhesives.

Since both the butyl- and octylcyanoacrylate tissue adhesives have been studied, you may wonder which is preferable if both are available for use. A RCT by Osmond *et al.*[27] compared the two tissue adhesives in the closure of simple, low-tension, facial lacerations in 94 children < 18 years of age. They found no difference in time to complete the procedure, pain of the procedure, infection, or cosmetic outcome at 3 months. In addition physicians found no difference in the ease of use of the two tissue adhesives. There were two dehiscences (both in the butylcyanoacrylate group) but this did not reach statistical significance. Again, the patient numbers are relatively low to rule out the presence of rare complications and further trials with larger study populations are needed. However, it seems that for selected simple facial lacerations, either tissue adhesive could be used, and that the choice of which to use may be based on other factors such as cost and physician preference.

Resolution of the scenario

After completing this review and combining the results, you are now able to confidently inform parents of children with simple facial lacerations that, compared with sutures, tissue adhesives are faster to apply, cause less pain to the child and have an equivalent cosmetic outcome. There is no significant increase in complications such as infection or discharge, but there is a very small increase in the dehiscence rate for children treated with tissue adhesives. You are reassured that this information is likely to be true as it is based on a high quality Cochrane systematic review.

Future research needs

- The efficacy of tissue adhesives in the closure of extremity lacerations in children needs to be studied.
- New tissue adhesive applicators are needed, designed specifically for use in children.
- Further research is required to evaluate the contribution of wound characteristics, patient characteristics, operator factors, and tissue adhesive type, to wound dehiscence and ultimate cosmetic outcome.
- An economic evaluation of wound closure methods is needed that takes into account the costs of the various tissue adhesives, the time and costs of conscious sedation, and the higher rate of dehiscence associated with tissue adhesives.

Summary table
Tissue adhesives compared with to standard wound closure

Question	Type of evidence	Result	Comment
Short- and long-term cosmetic outcome?	8 RCTs	No difference in short- or long-term cosmetic outcome	Insufficient detail to comment on effect of laceration size or location on cosmetic outcome
Pain during the procedure?	8 RCTs	Significantly less pain with tissue adhesive closure as reported by patients, parents, and healthcare providers	Adhesive strips may result in similar or less pain as tissue adhesives All assessments are non-blinded
Time required to complete the procedure?	5 RCTs	Tissue adhesives were 5·7 minutes faster	Ease of procedure has not been evaluated
Complications?	10 RCTs	Increased risk of dehiscence with tissue adhesives (NNH = 25) Increased risk of wound erythema with standard wound closure (NNH = 8) No difference in infection or discharge	Insufficient detail to determine if wound characteristic, physician skill level, or different tissue adhesives may play a role

Abbreviation: NNH, number needed to harm

References

1 Sibert JR, Maddocks GB, Brown BM. Childhood accidents – an endemic of epidemic proportions. *Arch Dis Child* 1981; **56**:225–7.

2 Kung H. *Evaluation of undesirable side effects of the surgical use of histoacryl glue with special regard to possible carcinogenicity.* Basel, Switzerland: RCC Institute for Contract Research, 1986. Project 064315.

3 Toriumi DM, Raslam WF, Freidman M *et al.* Variable histotoxicity of histoacryl when used in a subcutaneous site: an experimental study. *Laryngoscope* 1991;**101**:339–43.

4 Watson DP. Use of cyanoacrylate tissue adhesive for closing facial lacerations in children [see comments]. *BMJ* 1989;**21**: 1014.

5 Mizrahi S, Bickel A, Ben-Layish E. Use of tissue adhesives in the repair of lacerations in children. *J Pediatr Surg* 1988;**23**: 312–13.

6 Applebaum JS, Zalut T, Applebaum D. The use of tissue adhesion for traumatic laceration repair in the emergency department. *Ann Emerg Med* 1993;**22**:1190–2.

7 Ellis DA, Shaikh A. The ideal tissue adhesive in facial plastic and reconstructive surgery. *J Otolaryngol* 1990;**19**:68–72.

8 Elmasalme FN, Matbouli SA, Zuberi MS. Use of tissue adhesive in the closure of small incisions and lacerations. *J Pediatr Surg* 1995;**30**:837–8.

9 Kamer FM, Joseph JH. Histoacryl. Its use in aesthetic facial plastic surgery. *Arch Otolaryngol Head Neck Surg* 1989;**115**: 193–7.

10 Keng TM, Bucknall TE. A clinical trial of tissue adhesive (Histoacryl) in skin closure of groin wounds. *Med J Malaysia* 1989;**44**:122–8.

11 Quinn JV. *Tissue adhesives in wound care.* Hamilton, Ontario: BC Decker Inc, 1998.

12 Heretig FM, King C (eds). *Textbook of pediatric emergency procedures.* Baltimore: Williams & Wilkins, 1997.

13 Quinn JV, Drzewiecki A, Li MM *et al.* A randomized, controlled trial comparing a tissue adhesive with suturing in the repair of pediatric facial lacerations. *Ann Emerg Med* 1993;**22**:1130–5.

14 Farion K, Osmond MH, Hartling L *et al.* Tissue adhesives for traumatic lacerations in children and adults (Cochrane Review). In: *Cochrane Library,* Issue 1. Oxford: Update Software, 2003.

15 Hock MO, Ooi SB, Saw SM, Lim SH. A randomized controlled trial comparing the hair apposition technique with tissue glue to standard suturing in scalp lacerations (HAT study). *Ann Emerg Med* 2002;**40**:19–26.

16 Singer AJ, Quinn JV, Clark RE. Hollander JE. TraumaSeal Study Group. Closure of lacerations and incisions with octylcyanoacrylate: a multicenter randomized controlled trial. *Surgery* 2002;**131**:270–6.

17 Singer AJ, Hollander JE, Valentine SM, Turque TW, McCuskey CF, Quinn JV. Prospective, randomized, controlled trial of tissue adhesive (2-octylcyanoacrylate) versus standard wound closure techniques for laceration repair. *Acad Emerg Med* 1998;**5**:94–9.

18 Bruns TB, Robinson BS, Smith RJ *et al.* A new tissue adhesive for laceration repair in children. *J Pediatr* 1998;**132**: 1067–70.

19 Mattick A, Clegg G, Beattie T, Ahmad T. A randomised, controlled trial comparing a tissue adhesive (2-octylcyanoacrylate) with adhesive strips (Steristrips) for paediatric laceration repair. *Emerg Med J* 2002;**19**:405–7.

20 Karcioglu O, Goktas N, Coskun F, Karaduman S, Menderes A. Comparison of tissue adhesive and suturing in the repair of lacerations in the emergency department. *Eur J Emerg Med* 2002;**9**:155–8.

21 Farion KJ, Osmond MH, Hartling L *et al.* Tissue adhesives for traumatic lacerations: a systematic review of randomized controlled trials. *Acad Emerg Med* 2003;**10**:110–18.

22 Schultz A, Olesgaard P. [Tissue glue in minor skin lesions. A prospective controlled comparison between tissue glue and the suturing of skin minor lesions]. *Ugeskr Laeger* 1979; **141**:3106–7.

23 Simon HK, McLario DJ, Bruns TB, Zempsky WT, Wood RJ, Sullivan KM. Long-term appearance of lacerations repaired using a tissue adhesive. *Pediatrics* 1997;**99**:193–5.

24 Barnett P, Jarman FC, Goodge J, Aickin R. Randomised trial of histoacryl blue tissue adhesive glue vs suturing in the repair of pediatric lacerations. *J Pediatr Child Health* 1998;**34**: 548–50.

25 Quinn J, Wells G, Sutcliffe T *et al.* Tissue adhesive versus suture wound repair at 1 year: randomized clinical trial correlating early, 3-month, and 1-year cosmetic outcome. *Ann Emerg Med* 1998;**32**:645–9.

26 Zempsky WT, Grem C, Nichols J, Parrotti D. Prospective comparison of cosmetic outcomes of simple facial lacerations closed with Steri-Strips or Dermabond. *Acad Emerg Med* 2001;**8**:438–43.

27 Osmond MH, Quinn JV, Jaramuske M, Klassen TP. Randomized, controlled trial of octylcyanoacrylate vs butyl-2-cyanoacrylate in the management of pediatric facial lacerations. *Acad Emerg Med* 1999;**6**:171–7.

28 Guyatt GH, Sackett DL, Cook DJ, for the Evidence based Medicine Working Group. Users' guides to the medical literature, II: how to use an article about therapy or prevention. A: Are the results of the study valid? *JAMA* 1993;**270**:2598–601.

29 Quinn JV, Drzewiecki AE, Stiell IG, Elmslie TJ. Appearance scales to measure cosmetic outcomes of healed lacerations. *Am J Emerg Med* 1995;**13**:229–31.

30 Quinn J, Wells G, Sutcliffe T *et al.* A randomized trial comparing octylcyanoacrylate tissue adhesive and sutures in the management of lacerations. *JAMA* 1997;**277**:1527–30.

31 Osmond MH, Klassen TP, Quinn JV. Economic evaluation comparing a tissue adhesive with suturing in the repair of pediatric facial lacerations. *J Pediatr* 1995;**126**:892–5.

40 Iron deficiency anemia

Kent Stobart

Case scenario

A 15-month-old Caucasian girl is seen in your office for her routine well child visit. She is currently well and her growth has been normal. This full-term toddler was breastfed until 7 months of age, when she was weaned onto whole cows' milk. Her current diet consists of puréed fruit and vegetables with the occasional jar of meat or poultry junior baby food. She drinks at least three 8 oz (250 ml) bottles of whole milk daily. Her mother has read that increased cows' milk intake may be associated with a learning disability. On physical examination the child is irritable and difficult to examine. The heart rate is 120 beats per minute. Her conjunctivae are pale but anicteric. You tell the mother you think the child probably has anemia from iron deficiency and that you want to do some tests. She asks whether testing is really necessary.

Background

Iron deficiency is the most prevalent single nutritional deficiency worldwide. It is estimated that one-third of the world's population suffers from iron deficiency anemia.[1,2] Those at greatest risk are infants, adolescent girls, young women, and the elderly.[3] Infants are at particular risk of iron deficiency anemia because of high requirements for iron to support their growth, low iron stores, and diets low in highly available forms of iron. Although children in undeveloped countries are disproportionately affected, a substantial number of infants in industrial countries also suffer from iron deficiency anemia.[3,4] In developed countries, there is an increased prevalence of iron deficiency anemia in the socially disadvantaged.[5] Middle class children rarely suffer from iron deficiency, and if they do the problem is generally mild.[6]

Mild anemia may be asymptomatic, but with decreasing hemoglobin there may be signs of increasing fatigue, weakness, and palpitations, eventually progressing to headache, vertigo, anorexia, and cold intolerance. Iron deficiency anemia in childhood differs in many ways from that in adults. The non-hematological, but clinically important presentations are more clearly defined in infants than in adults. Harmful, non-hematological consequences of iron deficiency include poor weight gain, anorexia, malabsorption, and irritability.[7]

A 1986 World Health Organization (WHO) technical report defined nutritional anemia as "a condition in which the hemoglobin content of blood is lower than normal as a result of deficiency of one or more essential nutrients, regardless of the cause of such deficiency".[8] The WHO diagnostic criteria for iron deficiency anemia are a hemoglobin < 110 g liter^{-1}, and a serum ferritin < 12 micrograms liter^{-1}.[9] The WHO recommendation is not age-specific, covering all age groups from infancy to geriatrics. However, hematologic values vary with age, hemoglobin being relatively high at birth and subsequently declining before rising again to reach adult levels in puberty. Also, the serum ferritin is an acute phase reactant. It may be falsely elevated during infections, which are frequent in childhood, thereby obscuring the diagnosis of iron deficiency anemia. Thus, the WHO definition may not be appropriate for infants and anemia in infancy and early childhood should be defined by age-specific normal values.[10]

Body iron is distributed in two major fractions. The functional component consists mainly of hemoglobin and the storage component provides a buffer against sudden iron demands from blood loss. Most storage iron is contained in a highly specialized protein-iron complex called ferritin. Iron is unique among metals in that its body level is almost entirely regulated by the absorptive cells in the proximal small intestine, which regulate iron absorption to match body losses of iron. Iron is vital for all living organisms, as it is essential for many metabolic processes, including oxygen transport, DNA synthesis, and electron transport. Altered iron equilibrium resulting from diminished absorbable dietary iron, excessive loss of body iron stores, or rapid growth may lead to iron deficiency anemia in infancy.[11]

Inadequate iron intake leads to a sequence of well characterized changes in storage iron, transport iron and eventually metabolic functions that depend on iron. The earliest evidence of inadequate iron intake is the absence of iron stores, which is characterized by a decline in serum ferritin. Although there are no functional consequences of depleted iron stores, there is a lack of iron reserves to meet increased needs during peak periods of growth, or as intake buffer. The next stage, iron deficient erythropoiesis, is characterized by sub-optimal delivery of iron to the erythroid marrow. In the final stage, erythropoiesis decreases, leading to changes in red cell structure with smaller than normal (microcytic) red blood cells that contain less hemoglobin and look pale (hypochromic), and ultimately a decrease in circulating red cell mass.[12]

Framing answerable clinical questions

Several questions arise from the clinical scenario:

- How likely is iron deficiency in this child?
- Does having iron deficiency anemia interfere with development?
- How do clinical findings or laboratory tests help in the diagnosis of iron deficiency anemia?

Reframing these questions into a structured format (see Chapter 2) will help you find the best available evidence with which to answer them.

Questions

1. In children 6–24 months of age (*population*), what is the prevalence of iron deficiency anemia (*outcome*)? **[Baseline Risk]**
2. In children 6–24 months of age (*population*), does iron deficiency anemia (*exposure*) adversely affect child development (*outcome*)? **[Harm]**
3. In children 6–24 months of age (*population*), can the clinical history and physical examination (*intervention*) predict iron deficiency anemia (*outcome*)? **[Diagnosis]**
4. In children 6–24 months of age (*population*), does the complete blood count (including red cell indices) (*intervention*) accurately diagnose iron deficiency anemia (*outcome*)? **[Diagnosis]**
5. In children 6–24 months of age (*population*), do the iron studies (serum ferritin, serum iron, transferrin, transferrin saturation, total iron-binding capacity (TIBC), iron saturation, or transferrin receptor) (*intervention*) accurately diagnose iron deficiency anemia (*outcome*)? **[Diagnosis]**
6. In children 6–24 months of age (*population*), do measures of hemoglobin synthesis (erythrocyte protoporphyrin) (*intervention*) accurately diagnose iron deficiency anemia (*outcome*)? **[Diagnosis]**

Searching for evidence

Search for evidence syntheses

- Cochrane Database of Systematic Reviews: iron deficiency anemia AND infant
- EBM Reviews – *ACP Journal Club*: iron deficiency anemia AND infant

You start with a search for "quality-filtered" evidence syntheses, such as systematic reviews and evidence-based practice guidelines. An evidence synthesis provides a summary of high quality evidence, and may decrease your reliance on single experimental studies. Your search for evidence syntheses yields 21 articles on the *treatment* of iron deficiency anemia in infancy and one article on the *diagnosis* of iron deficiency anemia in children. There are 12 articles on the *risks of not treating* infant iron deficiency anemia, one of which is a highly relevant systematic review in the Cochrane Database of Systematic Reviews. Although this initial search addresses your concerns about the harm of having untreated iron deficiency anemia, you perform specific searches for primary studies to help answer the questions on baseline risk and diagnosis.

Critical review of the evidence

Question

1. In children 6–24 months of age (population), what is the prevalence of iron deficiency anemia (outcome)? **[Baseline Risk]**

Search

- PubMed: iron deficiency anemia AND epidemiology AND infant AND review

Your question addresses the baseline risk (or probability or prevalence) of iron deficiency anemia and you want to find articles that report risk in a patient population similar to yours. Your search yields two relevant articles from developed communities. Looker analyzed a nationally representative cross-sectional health survey in the USA, which included venous blood measurements of iron status.[13] The study design meets validity criteria for studies of baseline risk (see Chapter 4). Iron deficiency anemia was defined as low hemoglobin, with an abnormality of at least two of three laboratory tests (erythrocyte protoporphyrin [EP], transferrin saturation or serum ferritin). Almost 25 000 people were surveyed in this third National Health and Nutrition Examination Survey (1988–1994), of which 1339 were toddlers aged 1–2 years. The incidence of iron deficiency anemia in toddlers was 3%. The use of a geographically representative sample of patients suggests that these results should be valid. Hercberg evaluated European epidemiological data to determine the prevalence of iron deficiency anemia in infants.[14] He summarized five cross-sectional surveys of small numbers of toddlers from Denmark, Italy, Spain, and France during the late 1980s through the early 1990s. Although these surveys are probably not as representative as the Looker study, the conclusions offer a similar prevalence of iron deficiency anemia of 2% to 4%.

Question

2. In children 6–24 months of age (*population*), does iron deficiency anemia (*exposure*) adversely affect child development (*outcome*)? **[Harm]**

To effectively evaluate an article about harm resulting from an exposure, you need to know that all other determinants of outcome were similar in children with and without the exposure, that the outcomes were measured in the same way in groups being compared, and that follow up was adequately long for the outcome of interest to develop. In this case, the minimum time period would be infancy as defined by an age from 0 to 23 months. Questions about harm are most often answered with cohort or case–control studies, since patients are seldom randomized to potentially harmful exposures. However, randomized controlled trials (RCTs) that evaluate the benefit of minimizing potentially harmful exposures can also be used to determine whether an exposure is harmful.

Search

- Quality-filtered Literature Search: iron deficiency anemia AND development
- PubMed Systematic Reviews: iron deficiency anemia AND development

You complete a quality-filtered literature search using the Cochrane Database of Systematic Reviews and EBM – ACP Journal Club and find one article in the Cochrane Database of Systematic Reviews.[15] The specific question asked in the systematic review is: "In children < 3 years of age with iron deficiency, does treatment with iron improve psychomotor development and cognitive function?" Martins scoured databases for RCTs comparing treatment with either oral or intramuscular iron to placebo in children < 3 years of age, to determine whether the outcome of psychomotor development or cognitive function was altered by treatment.[15] Seven RCTs met the selection criteria. Five examined short-term

effects of iron treatment (30 days) and two evaluated long-term effects of treatment (2–4 months). In the short term, infant development assessed by the Bayley Scales of Infant Development did not differ between groups with and without iron therapy. At 2–4 months, one study showed no difference in outcome using the Denver Development Screening Test. The other study reported a greater improvement from the baseline score (using the Bayley Psychomotor Development Index and Motor Development Index scales) in the group receiving iron therapy. Martins concluded that there was no convincing evidence that iron treatment for young children with iron deficiency anemia improved psychomotor development or cognitive function in the short term.[15] Conversely, failure to treat is unlikely to have any detrimental effects in the short term. The benefits of longer-term treatment were conflicting, although one study showed a clinically significant benefit.

Diagnosis of iron deficiency and iron deficiency anemia

Your remaining questions address the diagnosis of iron deficiency and iron deficiency anemia. Although anemia is recognized by a decreased hemoglobin and hematocrit, the bone marrow aspirate is the criterion (gold) standard for the determination of iron deficiency.[16] Perls' stain may demonstrate micronormoblastic hyperplasia of the erythroid elements and decreased or absent stainable iron. The bone marrow aspirate has largely been displaced for the diagnosis of iron deficiency anemia by other tests including serum ferritin, erythrocyte protoporphyrin (EP), mean corpuscular volume (MCV), or response to oral iron treatment.[12] Because invasive diagnostic tests (such as bone marrow aspiration) are generally avoided in infants, most studies of diagnostic tests for iron deficiency use alternative "working" gold standards. In geriatric adults, the serum ferritin is the most sensitive test when compared to the gold standard of bone marrow aspiration.[17] However, serum ferritin is an acute phase reactant and is elevated during infections, and the most common reason for anemia in infancy is either infection or inflammation.[18] Therefore, serum ferritin may not be an appropriate "working" gold standard to measure iron deficiency anemia in children.[19] Another potential "working" gold standard is the response to a therapeutic trial of oral iron. Because there is a paucity of easily applied gold standards, most clinical studies of iron deficiency anemia in children use criterion standards that are imperfect. Under these circumstances, study results (sensitivity and specificity, for example) are likely to be not completely accurate and should be viewed as estimates to aid your thinking rather than exact parameters of these tests.

Questions about diagnostic tests are best answered by studying a population in which there is significant uncertainty about whether the disease process or outcome of interest is present.[20] The diagnostic test under consideration should be assessed against the gold standard (or the "working" gold standard), and should be independent and uninfluenced by the gold standard. For your questions, the outcome of interest is iron deficiency anemia, which is generally determined by use of a "working" gold standard for the reasons mentioned above. As the prevalence of iron deficiency anemia decreases, other common causes of anemia become more likely.[13] In order to avoid having the prevalence of disease influence the outcome of interest, you avoid using predictive values to assess diagnostic tests and concentrate where possible on calculating the likelihood ratios (LR) for diagnostic tests. A large positive LR would assist you in ruling *in* the diagnosis of iron deficiency anemia (see Chapter 5).

General search strategy

- PubMed Clinical Queries (diagnosis + specificity): iron deficiency anemia AND infant

For articles about diagnostic tests you complete a general literature search using PubMed. You enter the term "iron deficiency anemia" in the Clinical Queries screen, and select the radio buttons for "diagnosis" and "specificity". This preformatted search strategy for diagnostic tests yields 20 articles. You perform additional searches for each individual question.

Question

3. In children 6–24 months of age (*population*), can the clinical history and physical examination (*intervention*) predict iron deficiency anemia (*outcome*)? **[Diagnosis]**

Search

- PubMed Clinical Queries (diagnosis + specificity): iron deficiency anemia AND (medical history taking OR physical examination)
- References of articles obtained from the search

To answer this question you are looking for well-designed studies evaluating the clinical history or physical examination as a diagnostic test for iron deficiency anemia. A clinical history should provide an opportunity to assess the dietary intake of iron, potential reasons for iron loss, and whether the child is in a rapid growth period. You run your search and find five relevant articles.

Mira studied 121 Australian children in an urban setting using a case–control design.[21] Almost 500 children were screened with serum ferritin. The 76 children found to have low values (< 10 micrograms liter^{-1}) were presumed to be iron deficient and serum low ferritin was used as the "working" gold standard for this study. The iron deficient infants were matched with 68 iron replete children for gender and age within 6 months. Parents of both cases and controls participated in a 3-day weighed dietary intake and completed identical questionnaires. The cases and control groups were similar except for iron deficiency and the criteria for measuring dietary intake were identical. Two risk factors were significant for development of iron deficiency: low intake of dietary heme iron (odds ratio [OR] = 3·0; 95% CI = 1·3–6·8) and introduction of cows' milk before 12 months of age (OR = 2·44; 95% CI = 1·09–5·44). Multivariate analysis showed these risk factors to be independent.

In a retrospective chart review of 305 primarily African-American children aged 15–60 months from an urban academic primary care clinic, Boutry and Needlman studied the dietary history as a potential tool to determine iron deficiency.[22] Patients with acute illness, premature birth, hemoglobinopathies, elevated lead levels, or recent medicinal intake of iron were excluded. Information was obtained from a standard brief nutritional history that was part of a broader review of health and psychosocial issues that was incorporated into all health supervision visits.[23] Iron deficiency anemia was defined by hemoglobin (< 110 g liter^{-1}) and MCV (< 73 femtoliters). Dietary deficiency was defined as fewer than five servings each of meat, grains, vegetables, and fruit per week, > 16 ounces (480 ml) of cows' milk per day, or a daily intake of fatty snacks, sweets, or > 16 ounces (480 ml) of soft drink. Data were abstracted retrospectively from clinical charts in which the nutrition history had been recorded without a standardized questionnaire or data extraction form. The prevalence of microcytic anemia was 8%. Of 24 infants with a positive dietary history, 17 had microcytic anemia. Of 288 non-anemic infants, 59 had a positive dietary history.

Using the formula LR+ = sensitivity/(1–specificity), you calculate the LR for positive dietary history as LR = 3·4). If the pretest probability of iron deficiency anemia in this population is ~ 3%, then using the likelihood ratio nomogram on page 35 with an LR of 3·4 the post-test probability of iron deficiency anemia is ~ 10%. Thus obtaining a positive dietary history will result in a modest change in your estimate of the probability of iron deficiency.

Bogen conducted a prospective cross-sectional study of 282 mainly African-American children aged 9–30 months in inner city Baltimore.[4] The diagnostic test was a 5-minute parent-completed dietary questionnaire designed to be similar to other standardized questionnaires and completed at a scheduled visit for routine anemia screening. Iron deficiency anemia was defined by a hemoglobin < 110 g liter^{-1}, and either a serum ferritin level < 10 micrograms liter^{-1} or an MCV < 70 femtoliters^{-1} and a red cell distribution width (RDW) > 0·145. The LR for iron deficiency anemia in the presence of abnormal dietary history ranged from 1·0 to 1·1, depending on the laboratory test chosen. With an LR of ~ 1 the pretest and post-test probability are the same. Thus the results of this dietary questionnaire did not predict the risk of iron deficiency anemia.

At the beginning of the 20th century, Osler suggested that blue sclerae were diagnostic of iron deficiency anemia.[24] In a prospective Swiss study of 100 hospitalized children aged 2 months to 17 years, two independent observers determined whether the patients had blue sclerae using a 3-point scale.[25] Children with congenital syndromes associated with blue sclerae were excluded. The observers were not aware of the child's admission diagnosis. Iron deficiency was defined by a serum ferritin < 10 micrograms liter^{-1}. From the data in the article, you extract the relevant values for children < 2 years of age and calculate the LR as 1·4 (95% CI 0·9–2·2). Thus, blue sclerae do not predict iron deficiency anemia.

In a prospective case–control study, Hogan and Jones studied the physical finding of koilonychia (spooning of the fingernails and toenails) in 400 primarily Caucasian infants at a well baby clinic for low-income families in West Virginia.[26] A diagnosis of iron deficiency was based on a serum iron level of < 35 micrograms dl^{-1}, measured independently from physical examination. The overall prevalence of koilonychia in the well baby clinic was 5%. Of 22 infants with koilonychia, 10 were iron deficient, and among 15 infants without koilonychia matched for age, three had low serum irons. The calculated LR = 1·5 (95% CI 0·9–2·5) so you conclude that the presence of koilonychia does not predict iron deficiency.

In all of the above studies, the patient populations are similar to yours, and the test and the gold standard were independent of each other, so you believe the results of the studies are likely to be valid and applicable to your patients. The likelihood ratios calculated from these studies suggest that a history of poor iron intake and physical findings of blue sclerae and koilonychia are not likely to affect your estimate of the risk of iron deficiency anemia. None of the studies addressed pallor or tachycardia in relation to iron deficiency anemia.

Question

4. In children 6–24 months of age (*population*), does the complete blood count (including red cell indices) (*intervention*) accurately diagnose iron deficiency anemia (*outcome*)? **[Diagnosis]**

Search

- PubMed Clinical Queries (diagnosis/specificity): iron deficiency anemia AND (blood count OR hematocrit OR erythrocyte indices) AND infant
- Reference articles obtained from search

The World Health Organization established hemoglobin < 110 g liter^{-1} as one of the criteria for iron deficiency.[9] With the advent of electronic cell counting, red cell indices such as the mean corpuscular volume, mean corpuscular hemoglobin concentration (MCHC), and RDW can be measured quickly and accurately. The RDW, a quantitative measure of variation in the size of red blood cells, has been shown to be the first index of the routine blood cell count to become abnormal during the development of iron deficiency.[27]

You want to determine if there is one single erythrocyte index that is helpful in the diagnosis of iron deficiency anemia. You review your search and quickly critique the abstracts for validity issues of diagnostic tests. Six articles have satisfactory blinding and independence of the test from the working gold standard definition for iron deficiency, and the test and gold standard were independently measured in all six studies.

Demir studied eight erythrocyte indices as potential tools to differentiate between thalassemia trait and iron deficiency anemia.[28] Both thalassemia and iron deficiency anemia may have a low MCV and microctyic hypochromic red cells on the peripheral smear. Twenty-six of 63 Turkish children aged 2–16 years participating in the study had a hemoglobin level between 87 g liter^{-1} and 110 g liter^{-1}, and were diagnosed with iron deficiency anemia based on MCV < 72 femtoliter^{-1}, serum ferritin < 10 micrograms liter^{-1}, and serum transferrin saturation < 12. The other 37 children had beta thalassemia trait as defined by RBC hypochromia and microcytosis and elevated levels of hemoglobin HbA$_2$. Of the eight erythrocyte indices, only the RDW met the validity criteria for a diagnostic test. The LR+ was 1·5 (95% CI 1·2, 2·0). Choi and colleagues prospectively studied the RDW as a diagnostic test for iron deficiency anemia at the 12-month well-baby examination.[29] Of 970 consecutive healthy infants born at a US Army hospital, 62 had low hematocrit (< 0·33). Iron deficiency anemia was defined by an increase in the hemoglobin of greater than 10 g liter^{-1} after 1 month of oral iron therapy. From the data presented, for children with iron deficiency anemia as defined by response to oral iron therapy, the calculated LR+ was 4·56 (95% CI 1·5, 13·9). Kim retrospectively studied 1028 South Korean infants aged 6–24 months admitted to a general pediatric hospital in Korea.[30] All infants with a hemoglobin < 100 g liter^{-1}, a serum ferritin < 10 micrograms liter^{-1} or a transferrin saturation < 12% were classified as having iron deficiency anemia. The LR+ for RDW > 0·15 was 1·96, and the LR+ for MCV < 70 femtoliter^{-1} was 1·94. Mahu studied iron status of 384 randomly sampled children aged 6 months to 6 years in the region of Reunion, France in 1984.[31] The study was designed to compare various parameters of iron status, using serum ferritin < 12 micrograms liter^{-1} as the definition of iron deficiency. In this study, for a RDW > 0·18 the LR was 2·5.

Serdar, in a case–control design, studied the roles of red cell indices, serum ferritin, and EP as a diagnostic test.[32] The cases included 98 Turkish children without chronic diseases aged 7 months to 4 years, admitted to the pediatric service of a general hospital. Iron deficiency anemia was defined by reticulocyte response to 14 days of oral iron therapy. Using the reported sensitivity and specificity, for an MCV < 80 femtoliter^{-1} you calculate an LR of 1·3. A newer test, the reticulocyte concentration of hemoglobin (measured in picograms by flow cytometry), is believed to be an early indicator of iron-restricted erythropoiesis. Brugnara collected 210 blood samples left over from complete blood count and lead levels ordered in a general pediatric clinic.[33] The average age of the children was 2·9 years. Iron deficiency anemia was defined by transferrin saturation < 20% and hemoglobin < 110 g liter^{-1}. The LR for iron deficiency anemia with a low reticulocyte concentration of hemoglobin was 3·3.

In summary, the likelihood ratios for RDW are better with a higher cut-off value, but there may be a trade-off in loss of sensitivity (and thus some missed cases) if the higher cut-off is used; none of these values suggest that RDW will greatly alter your estimate of the probability of iron deficiency anemia. The reticulocyte concentration of hemoglobin has the best LR of the tests that you found, but these results have not been duplicated by other investigators.

Question

5. In children 6–24 months of age (*population*), do the ferric parameters (serum ferritin, serum iron, transferrin, transferrin saturation, total iron-binding capacity (TIBC), iron saturation, transferrin receptor saturation) (*intervention*) accurately diagnose iron deficiency anemia (*outcome*)? **[Diagnosis]**

Search

● PubMed Clinical Queries (diagnosis + specificity): iron deficiency anemia AND iron-binding proteins AND infant
● References of article obtained from the search

You find seven pertinent articles evaluating the use of serum ferritin, serum iron, transferrin, and transferrin saturation, and total iron-binding capacity as diagnostic tests for iron deficiency anemia. Serum iron has a normal diurnal variation, which may limit its usefulness as a diagnostic test. While a low serum ferritin is virtually diagnostic of iron deficiency, a normal serum ferritin can be seen in patients who are deficient in iron and have coexisting diseases (hepatitis, anemia of chronic disorders). A possible new tool to be considered is the serum transferrin receptor saturation. This test is used to assess functional iron status and

erythropoietic activity in adults, but there are few studies available on its role in children.

In the previously mentioned study, Serdar used a case–control design of 98 Turkish children to study serum ferritin as a diagnostic test[32] Iron deficiency anemia was defined by response to oral iron therapy after 14 days of treatment. The reported sensitivity and specificity can be used to calculate an LR+ for serum ferritin of 14·2. In another study described above, 146 of 1028 pediatric patients admitted to a general hospital in Korea were found to be anemic (hemoglobin < 100 g liter^{-1}), and 120 of those had iron deficiency anemia, based on the serum ferritin < 10 micro-grams liter^{-1}.[30] In this study, the LR+ for transferrin saturation was 3·9. Because serum ferritin was used as part of the definition of iron deficiency anemia, and was thus not independent of the gold standard, the sensitivity and specificity of serum ferritin could not be evaluated in this study.

In a prospective cohort study to measure the effectiveness of an iron-fortified cereal in the prevention of iron deficiency anemia in urban Santiago, Chile, Olivares looked at 716 blood samples obtained from 515 well nourished healthy infants aged 8–15 months.[34] Iron deficiency was defined by abnormalities in two indicators of iron status (hemoglobin, MCV, serum transferrin receptor saturation (STFR), and erythrocyte protoporphyrin). The LR for serum ferritin was 1·6, and the LR for a serum transferrin receptor saturation > 13·5 mg liter^{-1} was 8·7.

The LR for serum ferritin varied greatly between the two valid studies. Serdar[32] only excluded infants using a clinical history of infection, while Olivares[34] used a C-reactive protein (CRP < 10 mg liter^{-1}) to exclude children with potential infections. It is possible that the higher LR in Sedar's study is partially attributable to the undiagnosed infection or inflammation. The LRs for transferrin receptor saturation would not greatly alter your estimate of iron deficiency anemia. This study has not been replicated.

Question

6. In children 6–24 months of age (*population*), do measures of hemoglobin synthesis (erythrocyte protoprophyrin) (*intervention*) accurately diagnose iron deficiency anemia (*outcome*)? **[Diagnosis]**

Search

● PubMed Clinical Queries (diagnosis + specificity): iron deficiency anemia AND protoporphyrin AND infant
● Reference articles obtained from search

EP accumulates when there is inadequate iron to bind in the penultimate step of hemoglobin production, so it can be a direct indicator of inadequate iron nutrition. However, elevated lead levels also block conversion of protoporphyrin to heme. Other measures of EP include the zinc protoporphyrin (ZPP), when a trace of zinc rather than iron is incorporated in the protoporphyrin during the final stage of heme biosynthesis. A very slight decrease in availability of iron, as in the stage of iron depletion, causes an increased ZPP binding. A further diagnostic test is the zinc protoporphyrin/ hemoglobin ratio, which reflects iron states in the bone marrow during hemoglobin formation.

Siegel evaluated use of the zinc protoporphyrin/hemoglobin ratio as a diagnostic test for iron deficiency anemia over a 1-year period in well children from Mississippi aged 9–36 months.[35] Iron deficiency anemia was defined by the 1-month response (hemoglobin increase > 10 g liter^{-1}) to oral iron therapy (ferrous sulfate 3 mg Fe kg^{-1} per day). Of 458 prospectively enrolled children, 181 had an elevated zinc protoporphyrin/hemoglobin ratio and all had blood lead levels measured. Toddlers with elevated lead levels had the test repeated and if the lead level remained elevated the infant was investigated for lead poisoning and removed from the study. The calculated LR for iron deficiency was 1·4 (95% CI 1·2, 1·7) for an elevated zinc protoporphyrin/hemoglobin ratio. Major study limitations include the fact that children were not screened for mild viral illness, which could have affected results both before and after therapy.

Serdar also evaluated EP, and found an LR for iron deficiency of 2·5 with an elevated EP.[32] Yip and his group compared EP to age-normed hemoglobin and serum ferritin (< 15 micrograms liter^{-1}) among 4160 Minnesota children between 6 months and 12 years over a 30-month period.[36] Children with an elevated blood lead level were excluded from the study, but only children with an elevated EP were tested for a blood lead level. The LR+ for EP < 35 micrograms dL^{-1} was 8·6 (95% CI 7·8, 9·6). Olivares also evaluated free EP, using a cut-off of 2·12 micromol liter^{-1} RBC at age 8 months and 1·77 micromol liter^{-1} RBC at age 12–15 months.[34] For these cut-off values the LR for iron deficiency was 1·9. Hinchliffe studied 213 UK children undergoing investigation for microcytic anemia.[37] Iron deficiency anemia was defined as microcytosis and a low serum ferritin. The calculated LR for iron deficiency with an increased zinc protoporphyrin/ hemoglobin ratio was 1·5 (95% CI 1·2,1·9).

In summary, none of the diagnostic tests measuring erythrocyte protoporphyrin would greatly modify your initial estimate of the risk of iron deficiency anemia in a toddler.

Resolution of the scenario

You explain to your patient's mother that her infant has clinical features consistent with anemia. You tell her that iron deficiency (owing to inadequate iron intake and often associated with introduction of cows' milk before 12 months of age) is the most likely explanation in an otherwise well child, occurring in ~ 3% of well, middle-class infants. You explain that the diagnosis of iron deficiency cannot be confirmed by history and clinical examination alone and that no single blood test will provide the answer. However, you say that a blood count that shows a low hemoglobin with small, pale red blood cells would be supportive of the diagnosis. You explain that it is important to confirm the diagnosis of iron deficiency anemia and to treat with oral iron because long-term iron deficiency anemia may impair development.[15] Together you agree that the girl will have a complete blood count, blood film, and serum ferritin. The hemoglobin is 75 g liter^{-1} and the red blood cells are microcytic and hypochromic. You commence oral ferrous sulphate therapy and arrange to review the child in 1 week to assess the reticulocyte count. You warn the mother that you will need to repeat the hemoglobin in 1 month and that therapy will be continued for at least 3 months. The mother agrees to decrease the infant's intake of cows' milk.

Future research needs

There is no single ideal diagnostic test for defining iron deficiency anemia in infants. A well-designed study in well infants could encompass several diagnostic laboratory tests along with a therapeutic trial of oral iron against the outcome iron deficiency anemia using age-appropriate norms for hemoglobin and serum ferritin, as defined by the modified WHO criteria. This would be helpful in answering the majority of clinical questions around the diagnostic test.

- As the primary function of the red cell is to deliver and release adequate quantities of oxygen to the body's tissues to meet their metabolic demands, hemoglobin concentration alone may be insufficient to judge whether a patient is functionally anemic. Children with cyanotic congenital heart disease, chronic obstructive pulmonary disease, or with mutant hemoglobin that alters the hemoglobin's affinity for oxygen may have hemoglobin values that are considerably higher, and yet may be anemic when their hemoglobin values are within the normal range for unaffected children. Therefore a measure of both oxygen metabolism and accompanying cardiovascular compensation may be required to complement the current laboratory definition of iron deficiency anemia.
- More research needs to be done on the harmful effects of iron deficiency and iron deficiency anemia. The etiology studies are limited by their short follow up, and the small size of studies may have precluded an ability to find a difference because of underpowering of the randomized controlled trials. Concern is now being raised about the incidence of hemochromatosis and the risk of iron overload in these persons. It would therefore be important to know the prevalence of hemochromatosis in the population at risk to determine if iron deficiency anemia is a greater risk than the risk of premature iron overload.

Summary table of likelihood ratios

Diagnostic test	Likelihood ratio (+)	95% CI	Reference
Dietary history	3·4	2·4, 4·8	22
Dietary questionnaire	1·0	NA	4
Blue sclerae	1·4	0·9, 2·2	25
Koilonychia	1·5	0·9, 2·5	26
RDW > 0·14	1·5	1·2, 2·0	28
RDW > 0·14	4·5	1·5, 13·9	29
RDW > 0·15	2·0	NA	30
RDW > 0·18	2·5	NA	31
MCV < 70 fL	1·9	NA	30
MCV < 80 fL	1·3	NA	32
CHr	3·3	NA	33
Serum ferritin	14·2	NA	32
Serum ferritin	1·6	NA	34
Transferrin saturation	3·9	NA	30
Serum transferrin receptor saturation	8·7	NA	34
ZPP/Hgb	1·4	1·2, 1·7	35
ZPP/Hgb	1·5	1·2, 1·9	37
EP	2·5	NA	32
EP < 35 micrograms dl^{-1}	8·6	7·8, 9·6	36

Abbreviations: EP, erythrocyte protoporphyrin; MCV, mean corpuscular volume; RDW, red cell distribution width; ZPP, zinc protoporphyrin

Summary of evidence

Question	Type of evidence	Result	Comment
In young children 6–24 months of age:			
What is the prevalence of iron deficiency anemia?	Population surveys	2–4%	Data derived from European and USA national health surveys
What are the risks of iron deficiency anemia for child development?	Cochrane Database of Systematic Reviews	No convincing evidence that iron treatment improved psychomotor development or cognitive function	Studies may have been underpowered to detect a difference
Can the clinical history and physical examination predict iron deficiency anemia?	• Case–control study • Retrospective cross-sectional study • Prospective cross-sectional study	Dietary history may be of limited value in children who consume whole cows' milk before 12 months of age, and had low intake of iron rich foods Blue sclerae and koilonychia were not helpful physical signs	Risk of bias in dietary history based on retrospective data
Does the complete blood count accurately diagnose iron deficiency anemia?	• Prospective case series	RDW has some value in specific situation. No single red cell index is helpful in the diagnosis of iron deficiency anemia	Lack of test against a determined "pediatric" gold standard for iron deficiency anemia
Do the ferric parameters accurately diagnose iron deficiency anemia?	• Prospective case series • Randomized controlled trial	Serum ferritin had the strongest LR+ 14·2, but this was not consistent in the RCT	Lack of consistency of results across different types of studies
Do measures of hemoglobin synthesis accurately diagnose iron deficiency anemia?	• Prospective case series • Case–control study	Large prospective case series the LR+ for EP was 8·7	Variety of EP measures, not all similar. Variable results across different studies

References

1 Wu AC, Lesperance L, Bernstein H. Screening for iron deficiency. *Pediatr Rev* 2002;**23**:171–8.

2 Pappas D. In Brief: iron deficiency anemia. *Pediatr Rev* 1998;**19**:321–2.

3 Dallman PR, Yip R, Johnson C. Prevalence and causes of anemia in the United States, 1976 to 1980. *Am J Clin Nutr* 1984;**39**:437–45.

4 Bogen DL, Duggan AK, Dover GJ, Wilson MH. Screening for iron deficiency anemia by dietary history in a high-risk population. *Pediatrics* 2000;**105**:1254–9.

5 Emond AM, Hawkins N, Pennock C, Golding J. Haemoglobin and ferritin concentrations in infants at 8 months of age. *Arch Dis Child* 1996;**74**:36–9.

6 Yip R, Walsh KM, Goldfarb MG, Binkin NJ. Declining prevalence of anemia in childhood in a middle-class setting: a pediatric success story? *Pediatr* 1987;**80**:330–4.

7 Booth IW, Aukett MA. Iron deficiency anemia in infancy and early childhood. *Arch Dis Child* 1997;**76**:549–54.

8 Stoltzfus RJ. Iron-deficiency anemia: reexamining the nature and magnitude of the public health problem. Summary: implications for research and programs. *J Nutr* 2001;**131**:697S–700S.

9 WHO (World Health Organization) group of experts. *Nutritional anemia*. WHO Technical Report Series No. 503, Geneva: WHO, 1972.

10 Dallman PR, Siimes MA. Percentile curves for hemoglobin and red cell volume in infancy and childhood. *J Pediatr* 1979;**94**:26–31.

11 Sherriff A, Emond A, Hawkins N, Golding J, the ALSPAC Children in Focus Study Team. Haemoglobin and ferritin concentrations in children aged 12 and 18 months. *Arch Dis Child* 1999;**80**:153–7.

12 Oski FA. Iron deficiency in infancy and childhood. *N Engl J Med* 1993;**329**:190–3.

13 Looker AC, Dallman PR, Carroll MD, Gunter EW, Johnson CL. Prevalence of iron deficiency in the United States. *JAMA* 1997;**277**:973–6.

14 Hercberg S, Preziosi P, Galan P. Iron deficiency in Europe. *Public Health Nutr* 2001;**4**:537–45.

15 Martins S, Logan S, Gilbert R. Iron therapy for improving psychomotor development and cognitive function in children under the age of three with iron deficiency anemia. *Cochrane Database Syst Rev* 2003;CD001444.

16 Patterson C, Guyatt GH, Singer J, Ali M, Turpie I. Iron deficiency anemia in the elderly: the diagnostic process. *CMAJ* 1991;**144**:435–40.

17 Guyatt GH, Patterson C, Ali M *et al.* Diagnosis of iron-deficiency anemia in the elderly. *Amer J Med* 1990;**88**:205–9.

18 Abshire TC. The anemia of inflammation. A common cause of childhood anemia. *Pediatr Clin North Amer* 1996;**43**:623–37.

19 Domellof M, Dewey KG, Lonnerdal B, Cohen RJ, Hernell O. The diagnostic criteria for iron deficiency in infants should be reevaluated. *J Nutr* 2002;**132**:3680–6.

20 Jaeschke R, Guyatt GH, Lijmer Jeroen. Diagnostic Tests. In: Guyatt GH, Rennie D, eds. *Users' Guides to the Medical Literature*. AMA Press, 2002.

21 Mira M, Alperstein G, Karr M *et al.* Haem iron intake in 12–36 month old children depleted in iron: case–control study. *BMJ* 1996;**312**:881–3.

22 Boutry M, Needlman R. Use of diet history in the screening of iron deficiency. *Pediatrics* 1996;**98**:1138–42.

23 Boutry M, Needlman R. Screening for iron deficiency by dietary history in a high-risk population. *Pediatrics* 2001;**108**:823.

24 Agnoletto A. Blue sclerotics in iron deficiency. *Lancet* 1971;**2**:1160.

25 Beghetti M, Mermillod B, Halperin DS. Blue sclerae: a sign of iron deficiency anemia in children? *Pediatr* 1993;**91**:1195–6.

26 Hogan GR, Jones B. The relationship of koilonychia and iron deficiency in infants. *J Pediatr* 1970;**77**:1054–7.

27 McClure S, Custer E, Bessman JD. Improved detection of early iron deficiency in nonanemic subjects. *JAMA* 1985;**253**:1021–3.

28 Demir A, Yarali N, Fisgin T, Duru F, Kara A. Most reliable indices in differentiation between thalassemia trait and iron deficiency anemia. *Pediatr Int* 2002;**44**:612–16.

29 Choi YS, Reid T. Anemia and red cell distribution width at the 12-month well-baby examination. *South Med J* 1998;**91**:372–4.

30 Kim SK, Cheong WS, Jun YH, Choi JW, Son BK. Red blood cell indices and iron status according to feeding practices in infants and young children. *Acta Paediatr* 1996;**85**:139–44.

31 Mahu JL, Leclercq C, Suquet JP. Usefulness of red cell distribution width in association with biological parameters in an epidemiological survey of iron deficiency in children. *Int J Epidemiol* 1990;**19**:646–54.

32 Serdar MA, Sarici SU, Kurt I *et al.* The role of erythrocyte protoporphyrin in the diagnosis of iron deficiency anemia of children. *J Trop Pediatr* 2000;**46**:323–6.

33 Brugnara C, Zurakowski D, DiCanzio J, Boyd T, Platt O. Reticulocyte hemoglobin content to diagnose iron deficiency in children. *JAMA* 1999;**281**:2225–30.

34 Olivares M, Walter T, Cook JD, Hertrampf E, Pizarro F. Usefulness of serum transferrin receptor and serum ferritin in diagnosis of iron deficiency in infancy. *Am J Clin Nutr* 2000;**72**:1191–5.

35 Siegel RM, LaGrone DH. The use of zinc protoporphyrin in screening young children for iron deficiency. *Clin Pediatr* 1994;**33**:473–9.

36 Yip R, Schwartz S, Deinard AS. Screening for iron deficiency with the erythrocyte protoporphyrin test. *Pediatrics* 1983;**72**:214–9.

37 Hinchliffe RF, Lilleyman JS, Steel GJ, Bellamy GJ. Usefulness of red cell zinc protoporphyrin concentration in the investigation of microcytosis in children. *Pediatr Hematol Oncol* 1995;**12**:455–62.

41 Nocturnal enuresis

Jonathan HC Evans, Cathryn MA Glazener

Case scenario

A 10-year-old boy has come to see you with both his parents because of bedwetting. The only specific treatment he has had was desmopressin nasal spray when he was away from home at a camp for 2 nights. He was dry both nights but, as he slept very little, the parents are not sure whether the desmopressin was responsible for his dry nights or not. The remainder of the time he is wet most nights. His parents have a caring and sensible attitude towards the problem but realize that the wetting is now beginning to upset their son, and both he and they are requesting help. You find nothing of note on examination and urine culture and urinalysis are normal.

Background

Bedwetting is a common symptom with numerous causes. Nocturnal enuresis is the most frequent cause of bedwetting, yet this term means different things to different people. In common usage, nocturnal enuresis is the frequent occurrence of wetting during sleep, in a child > 5 years of age, without identifiable organic diseases of the urinary tract or nervous system. While such a definition has helped to distinguish the small percentage of children with obvious abnormalities such as neurogenic bladder or an ectopic ureter (who have incontinence, not enuresis), and is useful for epidemiological studies, it is no longer an adequate definition when applied to individual patients. This is because several functional disturbances of the urinary system have now been identified in children with "enuresis". The definitions and terminology in the Box are recommended by the International Children's Continence Society[1]:

- *Urinary incontinence.* The involuntary loss of urine.
- *Enuresis.* A normal void occurring at a socially unacceptable time or place.
- *Nocturnal enuresis.* Voiding in bed while asleep that is socially unacceptable.
- *Primary nocturnal enuresis.* Monosymptomatic (no other urinary symptoms) bedwetting, in an individual who has never been dry at night for an uninterrupted period of 6 months.

- *Onset nocturnal enuresis.* Monosymptomatic bedwetting, in an individual who has been dry at night for an uninterrupted period of 6 months or more.
- *Urge syndrome and urge incontinence.* The frequent attacks of imperative urge to void that may be accompanied by incontinence (the most common cause of daytime wetting).
- *Dysfunctional voiding.* Functional disturbances of voiding owing to overactivity of the pelvic floor during micturition. Dysfunctional voiding is characterized by variable urinary stream, prolonged voiding, and incomplete bladder emptying, and may be accompanied by daytime incontinence.
- *Diurnal enuresis.* This is daytime enuresis characterized by normal voiding but at a socially unacceptable time or place. Voiding is complete.

Framing answerable clinical questions

One of the therapeutic options that you are considering for this child is an alarm. You judge that his parents are supportive and that the most important outcome for the whole family is for the child to become dry in the long term. Other options available include simple reward systems (for example, star charts), desmopressin, desmopressin combined with alarm, imipramine and other drug. You formulate these questions in a structured format (see Chapter 2) to help with your search.

Questions

1. In school-age children with nocturnal enuresis (*population*), does an enuresis alarm compared with no alarm (*intervention*) lead to fewer wet nights in the long term (*outcome*)? **[Therapy]**. If so, is one type of alarm better than another?
2. In school-age children with nocturnal enuresis (*population*), does using star charts (*intervention*) lead to fewer wet nights in the long term (*outcome*)? **[Therapy]**
3. In school-age children with nocturnal enuresis (*population*), do imipramine or desmopressin (*intervention and comparison*) lead to fewer wet nights in the long term (*outcome*)? **[Therapy]**
4. In school-age children with nocturnal enuresis (*population*), does combination therapy with drug and enuresis alarm compared to alarm alone (*intervention* and comparison) lead to fewer wet nights (*outcome*)? **[Therapy]**
5. In school-age children with nocturnal enuresis (*population*), do drugs other than desmopressin and tricyclic antidepressants (*intervention*) lead to fewer wet nights in the long term (*outcome*)? **[Therapy]**

Searching for evidence

As you want evidence for the effectiveness of different interventions for enuresis, ideally you want to find a systematic review of randomized controlled trials (RCTs). You search the *Cochrane Library* using the search term "enuresis". You find completed recent reviews on the following interventions in children with nocturnal enuresis:

- enuresis alarms[2]
- simple behavioral and physical interventions[3]
- desmopressin[4]
- desmopressin combined with enuresis alarm[4]
- imipramine and related tricyclics[5]
- drugs other than desmopressin and tricyclic antidepressants.[6]

Critical review of the evidence

The Cochrane reviews all included only randomized or quasi-randomized trials since studies that used other trial designs were excluded. (Quasi-randomized trials use subadequate methods of concealment of allocation such as alternate numbers or odd/even dates of birth, which might introduce bias as the next allocation could be known or predicted.) They used comprehensive search strategies to identify all possible RCTs of interest, including those from a previous systematic review.[7] You thus feel confident that you have found high quality evidence for your questions.

Alarms

Question

1. In school-age children with nocturnal enuresis (*population*), does an enuresis alarm compared with no alarm (*intervention*) lead to fewer wet nights in the long term (*outcome*)? **[Therapy]**. If so, is one type of alarm better than another?

Sixteen trials compared an alarm with no treatment. Three of these trials (involving 85 children) provided adequate data about wet nights during treatment; on average there were nearly four fewer wet nights per week using the alarm (weighted mean difference [WMD] −3·65; 95% CI −4·52 to −2·78). About one-third of children failed to become dry using an alarm in 13 trials (98/304, 32% *v* 239/248, 96% in controls; relative risk [RR] 0·36; 95% CI 0·31–0·43). The duration of treatment was <2 months in about a third of the trials, between 2 and 3 months in another third, and over 3 months in the remainder, although children often stopped earlier if they became reliably dry.

Five trials provided data on the number of children who were dry after treatment was completed with a duration of follow up varying from 44 days to 12 months. About half of the children failed to become dry during treatment or relapsed after treatment compared to almost all of the control group (45/81, 55% *v* 80/81, 99%). Thus, the alarm appears to be a successful approach for one in two children. The RR of treatment failure was 0·56 (95% CI 0·46–0·68). There were no data on the number of wet nights at follow up. There was insufficient evidence to draw conclusions about different types of alarm, or about how alarms compare to other behavioral interventions.

The use of enuresis alarms was often associated with a high drop-out rate, because of the complexity and effort of treatment, or the effect on disrupting other family members. Side effects were otherwise minor and mostly limited to false alarms or failing to wake the child.

Star charts

Question

2. In school-age children with nocturnal enuresis (*population*), does using star charts (*intervention*) lead to fewer wet nights in the long term (*outcome*)? **[Therapy]**

You are aware that star charts are widely used as a motivational tool in enuresis management, as well as in many areas of childhood behavioral management. You want to know how effective they are in the treatment of enuresis. Two small trials provided limited information comparing star charts to no treatment. In one study involving 20 children, fewer children failed to become dry or relapsed compared to controls (RR 0·22; 95% CI 0·06–0·78). There was no comparison of wetting at baseline. In another study of 40 children there were fewer wet nights per week during treatment compared to controls (WMD −4·63; 95% CI −6·41 to −2·85) but there was no information after treatment was completed. Star charts with or without lifting or waking were associated with significantly fewer wet nights while on treatment and fewer children failing or relapsing than untreated control groups, but each finding was based on single very small trials of limited quality. However, it is likely that these measures are used at home by parents before they seek professional help, hence it is unknown how many children respond before seeking professional help. In their favor, simple methods have minimal unwanted adverse events other than those relating to failure (either intrinsic or because it was too demanding) or family disruption.

Question

3. In school-age children (*population*), does imipramine or desmopressin (*intervention and comparison*) lead to fewer wet nights in the long term (*outcome*)? **[Therapy]**

Desmopressin

In total, 28 trials compared desmopressin with placebo or no treatment, 15 of which used a crossover design. During treatment, desmopressin reduced bedwetting by at least one night per week compared with placebo (for example, 20 micrograms: 1·34 fewer wet nights per week; 95% CI 1·11–1·57), and about a fifth of the children became dry (for example, RR for failure to achieve 14 dry nights with 20 micrograms 0·84; 95% CI 0·79–0·91). However, there was insufficient reliable information about the outcome of treatment after treatment was finished: there was little subsequent difference in the numbers of wet nights in four small trials, and all the children in another trial relapsed. There was no clear dose-related effect of desmopressin, but the evidence was limited. Data comparing oral and nasal administration were too few to be conclusive.

Tricyclic antidepressants

Several different tricyclic antidepressants have been used for enuresis. There were 16 RCTs that compared tricyclics to placebo: treatment with most tricyclic drugs (such as imipramine, amitriptyline, viloxazine, nortriptyline, clomipramine and desipramine) was associated with a reduction of about one wet night per week while on treatment in four trials (e.g. imipramine compared with placebo, WMD −1·19; 95% CI −1·56 to −0·82). About a fifth of the children became dry while on treatment (for example, RR for failure with imipramine 0·77; 95% CI 0·72–0·83), but almost all the children relapsed

after treatment stopped (for example, imipramine *v* placebo, RR 0·98; 95% CI 0·95–1·03). There was not enough information to assess the relative performance of one tricyclic against another, except that imipramine was better than mianserin.

Imipramine compared to desmopressin

The evidence comparing desmopressin with tricyclics was unreliable or conflicting in two small trials, but in one of them all the children failed or relapsed after stopping active treatment with either drug. Based on this one small trial, and since both types of drugs reduce bedwetting by one night per week compared with placebo, you draw the tentative conclusion that desmopressin and imipramine have similar effectiveness during treatment. You decide to look for data on adverse effects in order to decide which is the better drug.

RCTs of treatment give some information about adverse effects but often, for rare outcomes, the trials are simply not big enough to detect adverse events. Ideally, large-scale cohort studies of treated children are used to describe adverse effects. Alternatively you may have to resort to interpreting case reports of adverse events – which is difficult because you want to know the risk of an adverse event, and case reports provide no information on the population treated (*denominator*). There are no large-scale cohort studies for imipramine or desmopressin.

In the controlled trials reviewed, there were no instances of serious (for example, life-threatening) events or death with either treatment. Adverse events were, however, much more frequently reported in tricyclic-treated children (in 25/31 trials, which mentioned the presence or absence of adverse effects) than in those receiving desmopressin (in 13/28 trials, although, in a further three, side effects were equally common on active or placebo treatment). There were also differences in the nature of adverse effects. For desmopressin the most common problem was nasal irritation or nosebleed associated with the use of intranasal desmopressin; this accounted for half of the specified adverse effects. This adverse effect does not occur with oral desmopressin. Desmopressin has one rare but serious adverse effect, namely water intoxication causing impaired consciousness and seizures. There are no studies that report the frequency of this event but one report identified 21 cases of this literature up until 1992.[8]

With imipramine, central nervous system effects such as drowsiness, lethargy, agitation, depression, and sleep disturbance accounted for more than half the adverse effects, gastrointestinal upsets accounting for the remainder. These adverse effects appear, on the face of it, more severe. Furthermore, there are reports of rare adverse effects such as seizures, cardiac arrhythmias, and accidental deaths by overdose in the literature. There is a further danger to other family members (for example, siblings) of accidental overdose. It is difficult to estimate the frequency of these rare events, as there may well be underreporting because imipramine is a very old drug and these side effects are well known.

Combination and other therapies

Question

4. In school-age children with nocturnal enuresis (*population*), does combination therapy with drug and enuresis alarm compared to alarm alone (*intervention and comparison*) lead to fewer wet nights (*outcome*)? **[Therapy]**

Three trials addressed this issue. Although there were fewer wet nights during alarm treatment supplemented by desmopressin compared with alarms alone (WMD −1·35; 95% CI −2·32 to −0·38), the data are inconclusive about whether this is reflected in lower failure (RR 0·88; 95% CI 0·52–1·50) or subsequent relapse rates (RR 0·58; 95% CI 0·31–1·10). There were no trials comparing alarms alone to alarms supplemented by tricyclics.

Question

5. In school-age children with nocturnal enuresis (*population*), do drugs other than desmopressin and tricyclic antidepressants (*intervention*) lead to fewer wet nights in the long term (*outcome*)? **[Therapy]**

In 32 randomized controlled trials, a total of 1225 out of 1613 children received an active drug other than desmopressin or a tricyclic. In all, 28 different drugs or classes of drugs were tested, but the trials were generally small or of poor methodological quality (five were quasi-randomized and the remainder failed to give adequate details about the randomization process). Only three of the drugs, reported in four small trials, were shown to be better than placebo during treatment. Indomethacin, diclofenac and diazepam reduced the numbers of wet nights during treatment in comparison to placebo (indomethacin, WMD 3·06; 95% CI −3·89 to −2·23; diclofenac, WMD −4·21; 95% CI −5·76 to −2·66; diazepam, WMD −4·87; 95% CI −6·25 to −3·49). Furthermore, fewer children failed to achieve 14 dry nights during active treatment (indomethacin, RR 0·36; 95% CI 0·16–0·79; diclofenac, RR 0·52; 95% CI 0·38–0·70; diazepam, RR 0·22; 95% CI 0·11–0·46). None of these trials provided information about relapse rates once treatment had stopped.

In one trial, desmopressin was better than indomethacin (WMD for wet nights during treatment 1·45; 95% CI 0·53–2·37) and in another was better than diclofenac (RR for failure to achieve 14 dry nights 1·94; 95% CI 1·13–3·33),

suggesting that indomethacin and diclofenac would not be appropriate treatments for children with enuresis. In the remaining drug comparisons with placebo, the numbers were too small to draw reliable conclusions, and none of the drugs, except oxybutynin, are used in current practice in the UK for children with enuresis.

In one trial of oxybutinin versus placebo in 30 children, the trialists concluded that it was not effective but did not present data suitable for analysis. However, oxybutynin is commonly used to treat an organic cause of wetting (detrusor overactivity), which would normally result in daytime as well as night-time enuresis. Children with daytime wetting were specifically excluded from this trial although the trialists did not seek organic causes. If the children had been shown to have an organic cause for their enuresis, the trial would have been excluded from this review.

Resolution of the scenario

Your patient has primary nocturnal enuresis. He has no daytime wetting, appears to have no psychological problems, and has supportive parents. All these points are good prognostic factors for the use of desmopressin and the alarm. You may wish for further information to be sure of these initial impressions. A detailed voiding history, supported by a frequency/volume chart, would enable you to determine with confidence that he does not have bladder instability, dysfunctional voiding, or a small functional bladder capacity. A more detailed discussion of the patient and family's concerns and wishes would also be helpful.

- *What are their beliefs about medications and alarms?*
- *What is their main priority? (Is it for their child to be dry as soon as possible for some specific occasion, in which case medication would probably be better, or are they taking a longer view and aiming for cure, in which case the alarm would be more suitable?)*
- *If the alarm is to be used, then are the current home circumstances suitable?*

Assuming that your initial impressions are correct, your choices are:

- ***Enuresis alarm.*** *He and his parents are motivated and he has at least a 50% chance of becoming and remaining dry after treatment is completed. The treatment will, however, require considerable effort and persistence.*
- ***Desmopressin.*** *He is likely to improve on desmopressin but he has only a small chance of remaining improved after treatment.*
- ***Desmopressin plus alarm.*** *He is very likely to do well with an alarm and therefore adding desmopressin is unlikely to improve the long-term outcome.*
- ***Imipramine.*** *He is more likely to improve on imipramine than without treatment but again the chance of remaining improved is small. There is a high chance of CNS or gastrointestinal side effects.*

The choice is thus between desmopressin for short-term benefit and the alarm for long-term benefit. This choice is one for the child and parents to make. The two treatments could be used sequentially with desmopressin to provide short-term dryness for a special occasion followed by alarm treatment at a time of the family's choice, in order to try for a cure.

With increasing understanding of the physiology of nocturnal enuresis, several distinct mechanisms for wetting are being identified including sleep abnormalities, polyuria associated with abnormalities of vasopressin secretion, and occult detrussor instability. It is therefore likely that trials of treatment applied to these subgroups of children will become more important.

Future research needs

High-quality controlled trials of the following interventions:

- alarms versus desmopressin
- desmopressin versus imipramine
- star charts versus no treatment

Summary table

Question	Type of evidence	Positive effects	Negative effects
No treatment	Control groups in 2 systematic reviews	About 10% become dry (within weeks), 1–4% remain dry in short term	Poor self-esteem
Enuresis alarm	1 systematic review; total of 16 RCTs	Beneficial in the short and long term	Hard work; poor motivation and adverse family circumstance reduce effectiveness
Alarm and desmopressin	3 RCTs	Probably better than alarm alone during treatment but inconclusive for outcome after stopping treatment	Involves drug and alarm
Star charts	3 small RCTs	Modest benefit during and after treatment	None
Desmopressin	1 systematic review; total of 28 RCTs	Moderate benefit while taking it;? no long-term benefit after stopping drug	Relapse usual when treatment finishes; adverse effects rare; nasal irritation (1·5%) more common
Imipramine	1 systematic review; total of 16 RCTs	Moderate benefit while taking drug; long-term benefit uncertain	Relapse usual when treatment finishes; important CNS side effects common (10%) and can be lethal in overdose
Desmopressin *v* imipramine	3 small RCTs	No reliable evidence of difference in effectiveness	Adverse effects more serious with imipramine
Other drugs	Single small RCTs for most drugs	Limited evidence of short-term improvement with indomethacin, diclofenac and diazepam	Potentially serious adverse effects and lack of reliable evidence of effectiveness
		Limited evidence of **no** benefit with oxybutinin	

References

1 Norgaard JP, van Gool JD, Hjalmas K, Djurhuus JC, Hellstrom AL. Standardization and definitions in lower urinary tract dysfunction in children. *Br J Urol* 1998;**81**(Suppl. 3):1–16.

2 Glazener CMA, Evans JHC, Peto RE. Alarms for nocturnal enuresis in children (Cochrane Review). *Cochrane Library*, Issue 2. Oxford: Update Software, 2003.

3 Glazener CMA, Evans JHC. Simple behavioural and physical interventions for nocturnal enuresis in children (Cochrane Review). *Cochrane Library*, Issue 2. Oxford: Update Software, 2003.

4 Glazener CMA, Evans JHC. Desmopressin for nocturnal enuresis in children (Cochrane Review). *Cochrane Library*, Issue 3. Oxford: Update Software, 2002.

5 Glazener CMA, Evans JHC, Peto RE. Tricyclics and related drugs for nocturnal enuresis in children (Cochrane Review). *Cochrane Library*, Issue 3. Oxford: Update Software, 2003.

6 Glazener CMA, Evans JHC, Peto RE. Drugs (other than desmopressin or tricyclics) for nocturnal enuresis in children (Cochrane Review). *Cochrane Library*, Issue 4. Oxford: Update Software, 2003.

7 Lister-Sharpe D, O'Meara, Bradley M, Sheldon TA. *A systematic review of the effectiveness of interventions for managing childhood nocturnal enuresis, CRD Report 11.* York: University of York, NHS Centre for Reviews and Disseminations 1997.

8 Robson W, Noorgaard J, Leung A. Hyponatraemia in patients with nocturnal enuresis treated with desmopressin. *Eur J Paediat* 1996;**155**:959–62.

42 Acute urinary tract infection

Virginia A Moyer, Jonathan Craig

Case scenario

An 18-month-old girl presents to your office having had high fever off and on for the last 2 days. She has been a little fussy, with slightly decreased appetite and increased sleepiness, but her parents have noticed no change in her bowel movements or urination. She has had no previous illnesses other than occasional coughs and colds. On examination, you find a febrile (39°C), unhappy, but alert child in no obvious distress. The rest of your examination is unrevealing. Among other considerations, you wonder if she might have a urinary tract infection. Right away, the mother asks whether she could be treated with just one dose of antibiotic as she herself was treated this way for a recent urinary tract infection. She then asks whether her daughter should be tested to see if something is wrong with her kidneys.

Background

Urinary tract infections (UTIs) are important because they cause acute morbidity and may reflect an underlying anatomic abnormality of the urinary tract. Recurrent acute UTI is associated with long-term medical problems, including hypertension and reduced renal function, although empirical evidence that the infections are the cause of these problems is lacking. Even if UTI could be shown to lead to these outcomes, there is little evidence supporting the effectiveness of interventions such as prophylactic antibiotics, although these are widely used. Management of children with UTI can involve repeated patient visits, use of antimicrobials, exposure to radiation, and significant cost. Infants and young children with UTI are of particular concern because the risks of underlying pathology are higher and diagnosis is frequently challenging: the clinical presentation tends to be non-specific, and obtaining valid urine specimens for culture usually requires invasive methods.

UTI is the invasion of the bladder and/or kidneys with bacteria, which often causes an inflammatory response and is frequently symptomatic. The number of cultured organisms that must be present in order to diagnose UTI is controversial. Specimens obtained by a sterile method such as suprapubic bladder tap should not have any growth, while specimens obtained by urethral catheter may contain some organisms, which are collected at or around the meatus during the catheterization procedure. Specimens collected by urinary bag are most likely to be contaminated, but are the easiest to collect and the least traumatic to the patient. Hoberman found that among 2181 specimens collected by urinary catheter, those with $\geq 50\,000$ cfu ml^{-1} were more likely to yield pure growth of a single known pathogen.[1] Other authors have used $\geq 10\,000$ cfu ml^{-1} or $\geq 100\,000$ cfu ml^{-1} of a single organism to define UTI from a voided urine sample or catheter sample.[2,3] The most widely used threshold for UTI is $\geq 100\,000$ cfu ml^{-1} for a voided urine sample, ≥ 10–$50\,000$ cfu ml^{-1} for a catheter sample, and any growth of a urinary pathogen from a bladder tap sample. Like any diagnostic threshold, there will be some children with true UTI who do not reach these criteria (false negatives) and so these definitions should be only a clinical guide. The significance of asymptomatic bacteriuria is unclear but it is likely to be a benign problem. For example, children with asymptomatic bacteriuria did better in controlled trials when randomized to receive placebo rather than antibiotic treatment, and children treated with antibiotics during an asymptomatic infection were more likely to later develop symptomatic UTI with virulent organisms than the placebo treated children.[4]

Framing answerable clinical questions

A number of questions arise from the scenario above. You wonder:

- How likely is it that this girl has a UTI?
- Will urinalysis be helpful in confirming the diagnosis?
- How should this girl be treated if she does have a UTI?
- Could she have an underlying abnormality of the renal tract?
- Might she have infections at a later time?

These clinical questions can be reframed into structured questions, which will clarify your thinking and help with your search. Each question should have the following elements:

- the patient/population
- the intervention, event, or exposure (and comparison, if relevant)
- and the outcome of interest.

In addition, the type of information that is sought – information about causation, diagnosis, therapy, risk, or prognosis – can classify each question. See Chapter 2 for further discussion of framing clinical questions. You formulate the following questions.

Questions

1. In young children (*population*) with fever but a normal physical examination and no apparent focus of infection (*exposure*), what is the probability that urinary tract infection is present (*outcome*)? **[Baseline Risk]**
2. In febrile young children (*population*), will urinalysis (*intervention*) reliably detect urinary tract infection (*outcome*)? **[Diagnosis]**
3. In young children with acute urinary tract infection (*population*), is single dose antibiotic therapy (*intervention*) as effective as standard duration therapy (*comparison*) in clearing urinary tract infection (*outcome*)? **[Therapy]**
4. In young children (*population*) with acute UTI (*exposure*), what is the likelihood that an anatomic abnormality of the urinary tract is present (*outcome*)? **[Baseline Risk]**
5. In young children (*population*) with acute UTI (*exposure*), what is the likelihood of another infection occurring (*outcome*)? **[Prognosis]**

Searching for evidence

Evidence to assist you in managing your patients can be sought either for each individual question or in documents that summarize evidence on the condition, such as systematic reviews or practice guidelines. The most efficient source of evidence will be high quality evidence summaries. The quality of evidence found in summaries or syntheses can be critically appraised, just as individual studies are appraised. The criteria for appraising evidence syntheses are reviewed in Chapter 8.

Searching for evidence syntheses

- *Clinical Evidence*: one chapter on Acute UTI in Children
- *Cochrane Library*: urinary tract infection AND child
- *MedLine*: "urinary tract infection" limited to "all child 0–18" AND "practice guideline", "meta-analysis"

You start with the most concise evidence summary you know, the BMJ publication *Clinical Evidence*.[5] In spite of a very short child health section, you are pleased to find that UTI is one of the topics addressed in Issue 2 of 2003. Although this brief summary will likely be helpful in the acute situation, UTI is common in your practice and you would like to find in-depth answers to more of your questions. You decide to search further.

Next you examine the *Cochrane Library* (Issue 2, 2003) for information on UTI in children. Entering the search terms "urinary tract infection AND child" nets 33 completed reviews and four protocols. Two of the reviews specifically address UTI in children: one on short versus standard duration of antibiotics for acute UTI and one on long-term antibiotics to prevent recurrence of UTI.[6,7] Two other reviews address the use of cranberry juice to prevent and treat UTI in unspecified populations (both find no supporting evidence), and the rest of the reviews address topics tangential to acute UTI in children. The database of abstracts of reviews of effects (DARE) in the *Cochrane Library* cites six reviews on the topic of UTI in children. Two address duration of therapy[8,9] and two address diagnostic testing.[10,11]

Next, you go to MedLine, to be sure you have not missed any high quality evidence syntheses, since this, rather than trying to seek out and synthesize all the evidence yourself, is an efficient way to practise evidence-based medicine. Knowing that the American Academy of Pediatrics (AAP) has been developing guidelines for common conditions, you start by looking for a practice guideline on UTI in children. On the PubMed search screen, you enter the search terms "urinary tract infection" and limit the search to "all child 0–18" and "practice guideline" and get nine citations. You also try limiting by "meta-analysis" as a publication type, which nets 19 citations. In addition to the six reviews you have already found, two other citations from these two searches appear relevant: The American Academy of Pediatrics practice parameter on the diagnosis, treatment, and evaluation of the initial UTI in febrile infants and young children,[12] and the technical report that accompanied that practice parameter.[13] The AAP practice parameter appeared in hard copy in the April 1999 issue of *Pediatrics*, but is also available on line at the *Pediatrics* website. The technical report (all 60 pages of it!) is available only on line. The full text of one of the meta-analyses on screening tests is also published in the electronic pages of *Pediatrics*.[11] You decide to review these evidence summaries carefully to determine whether they answer your questions using valid evidence or whether you will need to look further to answer some or all of your questions.

Critical review of the evidence

You use these syntheses of evidence as your starting point for looking at the evidence to answer each of your questions. You begin by considering the criteria for appraising a practice guideline, which are discussed in Chapter 8 and in more depth in *the JAMA Users' Guides to the Literature VIIA and VIIB*.[14,15] The critical issues in judging practice guidelines are their relevance, their currency, and the quality of the evidence on which their recommendations are based. The AAP guideline appears to address many of your questions and is quite recent. The technical report provides the evidence the Subcommittee used in the development of its recommendations. Both the AAP technical report and the summaries in *Clinical Evidence* fall under the general category of syntheses of information, as do the meta-analyses of screening tests. For these, the validity of the conclusions will only be as good as the comprehensiveness of the search for evidence, the quality of the process of culling and combining the available evidence, and the quality of the primary research data, as discussed in detail in Chapter 8. As noted in Chapter 3, the general methods for finding and evaluating the evidence found in *Clinical Evidence* are described in its preface. No further details of the process are offered in individual chapters, so the reader must take the quality of the process on faith and on the track record of the organizations involved. In the practice parameter, the methods that were used are briefly outlined; however, you must go to the technical report to get greater detail regarding the specifics of the process of identifying, assessing, and combining the evidence so that you can make your own independent judgment of its quality. You consider each question separately, referring to the technical report, the meta-analysis and the *Clinical Evidence* chapter, and seeking other evidence when these sources are inadequate.

Question

1. In young children (*population*) with fever but a normal physical examination and no apparent focus of infection (*exposure*), what is the probability that UTI is present (*outcome*)? **[Baseline Risk]**

This first question is about prevalence: in a febrile young child. Chapter 4 describes in detail how to assess studies of prevalence. In the absence of high quality local data, this question is best answered by cross-sectional or cohort studies of large groups of patients similar to yours in settings similar to yours. The chapter in *Clinical Evidence* makes a statement about prevalence in the background section, referencing a single article on UTI in girls. The AAP practice parameter presents the conclusions from the literature search, but you must go to the technical report to see the studies on which these conclusions were based. Although the criteria for inclusion of articles about prevalence are not explicitly stated, a quality score is assigned and the citations are arrayed in a table by quality and relevance. Given the clear description of a thorough search and an assessment of quality, you are reasonably confident that the results are valid. It is also reassuring that the prevalence data are consistent across studies. The pooled prevalence of UTI in febrile infants and young children was 5%. The AAP practice parameter goes on to provide estimates of prevalence in subgroups of patients based on age, gender, and circumcision status, although these are based on a limited number of studies; this means that the estimates of prevalence in these subgroups will be less dependable and less precise than the overall results. Among febrile children with no obvious focus of infection the prevalence of UTI was 3%, 2%, 7%, and 8% in males < 1 year, in males > 1 year, in females < 1 year, and in females > 1 year respectively. Studies of the effect of circumcision on risk of UTI, although retrospective, were consistent in showing marked risk reduction in circumcised boys. The estimate of prevalence among circumcised infant boys is about 0·2%.

Question

2. In febrile young children (*population*), will urinalysis (*intervention*) reliably detect UTI (*outcome*)? **[Diagnostic Test]**

Obtaining a urine specimen in the young (non-toilet trained) child can be a difficult and time-consuming process. You want to avoid both missing the diagnosis because of a false-negative test and overdiagnosing UTI based on a false-positive test. Questions about the validity and reliability of a diagnostic test are best answered by studies that independently and blindly compare the test to a reference standard of diagnosis for the disease (see Chapter 5). *Clinical Evidence* does not address diagnosis of UTI except to define it as the presence of a pure growth of a urinary pathogen in a concentration of 10^5 per ml of urine. The AAP technical report does specifically address the use of dipstick and microscopic examination of the urine in making the diagnosis of UTI. The reference standard chosen for UTI by the guidelines committee was any bacterial growth on a specimen obtained by suprapubic aspiration, but the text notes that many of the included studies used other reference standards that are known to have poorer test characteristics. Thus the estimates of the usefulness of other tests may be less accurate. A thorough search was done for relevant studies, and quality assessment was performed. You note, however, that the quality of the studies, both according to the quality score (as assessed by the methodologist) and according to the subjective quality judgments made by other committee members, are variable and often less than good. Since the results of an evidence synthesis are only as good as the primary studies on which it is based, you expect that recommendations based on these studies will have to rest in part on expert opinion rather than solid evidence.

The meta-analysis by Gorelick and Shaw[11] is readily available to you on line, and you obtain a copy of the Huicho

Table 42.1 Means[12] and/or summary estimates[11] of sensitivity and specificity for specific screening tests for UTI

Test	Sensitivity (%)	Specificity (%)	Range of positive likelihood ratios
WBC:			
> 5/hpf (centrifuged)	73[12], 79[11]	81[12], 67[11]	2·5–3·9
> 10/cc³ (uncentrifuged)	77[11]	89[11]	7
Gram stain, any organisms	93[11]	95[11]	18·6
Microscopy, bacteria seen	81[12]	83[12]	4·8
Leukocyte esterase (LE)	83[12], 83[11]	78[12], 84[11]	3·8–5·2
Nitrite	53[12], 50[11]	98[12], 98[11]	25–26·5
Nitrite or LE+	93[12], 88[11]	72[12], 93[11]	3–13·3

et al. meta-analysis[10] on your next visit to the library. Gorelick and Shaw's study is based on a search of MedLine as well as a bibliographic search and canvassing of experts for relevant studies. Only published studies in English were included, which the authors note has the potential to lead to overestimate of the usefulness of the tests that they were evaluating. Huicho *et al.* did not limit their search by language, and included a search in a Spanish language database as well as MedLine to 2001. Studies in all three reviews were included based on the essential methodological standards that are discussed in Chapter 5: most importantly, independent comparison to a gold standard performed on all subjects, in a broad spectrum of patients. The technical report includes 31 studies, the Gorelick and Shaw meta-analysis 26 studies, and the Huicho meta-analysis 48 studies (see Table 42.1). You note that the results of the three evidence syntheses are quite similar. The method of urine collection varied in these studies. The summary table from the AAP technical report shows that "any item positive" on the urinalysis has an extremely high sensitivity (median 100%, mean 99·8%), while the best specificity was obtained with positive nitrite (median 99%, mean 98%). The Gorelick and Shaw meta-analysis found the summary estimate of sensitivity for "nitrite OR leukocyte esterase positive" to be 88%, and the sensitivity of positive Gram stain (on an unspun specimen) to be 93%. They found the specificity of positive nitrites to be 98%. When a test with very high sensitivity is negative, it is useful in ruling out disease since there are very few false negative tests. Therefore, a patient with a completely negative urinalysis (or, if only Gram stain were done, with a negative Gram stain) would have a very low probability of UTI. For this reason, some clinicians choose to obtain the initial specimen for urinalysis using the least invasive method, the external urine bag, and go no further if the urinalysis is completely negative. On the other hand, the nitrite test (at 98%) and the Gram stain of unspun urine (at 95%) are both highly specific. Since tests with very high specificity rarely have false positive results, a positive nitrite test or a positive Gram stain would very substantially raise the

probability of UTI. Some clinicians would treat empirically without culture in this situation. Simple pooling of data on sensitivity and specificity can be problematic. Huicho *et al.* used the technique of summary ROC curves to identify the single test with the best ability to distinguish affected from unaffected children. A ROC curve plots the sensitivity of a test on the *X* axis against the 1-specificity (or specificity from 100 to 0) on the *Y* axis since there is always a trade-off between the two as the threshold for a positive test is raised or lowered. The best tests have steep curves with a breaking point near the upper left corner of the plot. In their multivariate analysis (accounting for differences in age of patients, collection method, and whether or not the sample was centrifuged), the test with the best overall curve was neutrophils ≥ 10 per high power field *and* any bacteria seen on microscopic examination of the urine.

Other elements of the urinalysis have a much wider range of measured sensitivities and specificities, regardless of quality score (in the technical report), gold standard, or age group (evaluated by subgroup analysis in the Gorelick and Shaw study). Differences in the performance of these tests in different sites suggest that you consider the range of values that may apply to your site when you apply these estimates. Using estimates of the sensitivity and specificity of each of these tests, you can calculate their likelihood ratios (LR for a positive test = sensitivity/(1-specificity)) and use the likelihood ratio nomogram to estimate the probability of UTI given a positive test (see page 35).

Question

3. In young children with acute UTI (*population*), is single-dose antibiotic therapy (*intervention*) as effective as standard duration therapy (*comparison*) in clearing UTI (*outcome*)? **[Therapy]**

Questions about therapy are best answered with randomized controlled trials in which the investigators are unaware of patient assignment and follow up is complete. For a complete discussion, see Chapter 6. The AAP technical report addresses the evidence regarding short-term therapy. The tables listing studies about both the agents and duration of therapy do not list quality scores for the articles. Furthermore, the text does not specify whether only randomized controlled trials were included in the tables or in the pooled estimates of efficacy. You decide that the quality of the evidence synthesis about therapy in the AAP practice parameter is inadequate for your purposes. *Clinical Evidence* focuses almost exclusively on questions about therapy and makes a point of noting, for each question, what kinds of studies were found in the search. For this topic, *Clinical Evidence* found the same systematic reviews of short versus standard duration of therapy that you found in your search, although one is the paper publication of the Cochrane review on the same topic.[16] Two of the three systematic reviews included only studies comparing different durations of the same antibiotic, one of which excluded studies of single-dose regimens, and one included studies of different antibiotics. Based on these systematic reviews, *Clinical Evidence* concludes that a single-dose course of amoxicillin is likely to be ineffective compared to a longer course, but that no conclusion can be drawn about other antibiotics or antibiotic duration longer than a single dose. You consider that you have not found evidence to convince you that you should change your standard duration of therapy, but recognize that short courses (longer than single dose) may be as effective as longer courses.

Question

4. In young children (*population*) with acute UTI (*exposure*), what is the likelihood that anatomic abnormality of the urinary tract is present (*outcome*)? **[Baseline Risk]**

If an anatomic abnormality is present, and it is likely to lead to further infections or to renal damage, you want to know about it. In the background section on UTI in *Clinical Evidence*, the statement is made that obstructive anomalies are found in 0–4% and vesicoureteral reflux (VUR) in 8–40% of children being investigated for their first UTI, with a reference to a systematic overview of diagnostic imaging by Dick and Feldman.[17] The technical report of the AAP practice parameter addresses only VUR, listing 77 studies evaluating this issue. There is considerable scatter in the estimates, but studies with larger patient populations had similar results, suggesting a stable estimate somewhere around 30–40%, higher at younger ages and decreasing with increasing age at first UTI. The presence of anatomic abnormalities, including reflux, is important only if there is an association with risk for renal damage or other adverse outcomes, and if there is an effective intervention which can be offered (for example, prophylactic antibiotics) to prevent such damage. Although

there is an association between vesicoureteral reflux and renal scarring, it is not clear whether the reflux actually causes the scarring. Long-term cohort studies would help to answer this question, but have not been done. Hence, only circumstantial evidence is available to suggest that imaging of children with UTI will prevent future renal damage or other adverse outcomes, and, of course, imaging may lead to more studies and interventions that may not be needed. The systematic review by Dick and Feldman was intended to address the usefulness of imaging studies, rather than the prevalence of anatomic abnormalities *per se*. They performed a comprehensive search and found 63 descriptive studies, most of poor quality, and concluded that there was no direct evidence showing that children who have routine diagnostic imaging after a first UTI are better off than those who do not. The AAP committee chose to recommend imaging for the population they addressed (the < 2-year-olds) but note that this recommendation is based on only "fair" evidence.

Question

5. In young children (*population*) with acute UTI (*exposure*), what is the likelihood of another infection occurring (*outcome*)? **[Prognosis]**

Studies of prognosis, in order to be valid, must follow a representative group of patients from a similar point in the progression of disease forward in time to the outcome of interest, with a high rate of follow up. (See Chapter 4 for a discussion of prognosis studies.) As expected, *Clinical Evidence* presents information about prognosis in the background section (unreferenced) but does not address the quality of the evidence underlying the statements that are made. The AAP technical report also does not address the risk of recurrence, except in the context of the discussion of imaging. In the absence of a high quality evidence summary that addresses this question, you look for this information by going to the *Clinical Queries* screen of the National Library of Medicine's PubMed website; here you click on the question type (*prognosis*) and enter "urinary tract infection AND recurrent AND (infant OR child)". This screen uses a tested set of methodologic filters, search terms that have been demonstrated to have good sensitivity and specificity for specific study types. Using the "specificity" approach (expected to net fewer total articles but avoiding some that are not relevant), you find 23 articles, one specifically addressing your question. The "sensitivity" approach (152 articles) yields one other relevant study.[18]

The first study you find, by Nuutinen, is a retrospective study of all children under 1 old year in one hospital in Finland over a specified time period.[19] Since this is the only pediatric hospital in the region, this may represent a reasonable inception cohort. About 30% of children experienced a recurrence within 3 years, most within the first

6 months, and recurrence was more likely in the presence of severe vesicoureteral reflux. This study is not strong, and does not address patients the age of your patient. You consider the second study, in which 290 consecutive children < 5 years of age presenting to a children's hospital emergency center with a first UTI were followed up for 1 year.[18] This cohort sounds very similar to your patient, and follow up in this study was 90% at a year. The management of these children included imaging studies and prophylactic antibiotics for the 29% of children with any degree of vesicoureteral reflux. The recurrence rate in this population was only 12%. You cannot be sure that this rate was not decreased because of the prophylactic antibiotics, although compliance was only fair by the 6-month follow up visit, and less than one in three of the chidren in the sample were affected by this. These authors found that young age (< 6 months) and high grade reflux predicted recurrence.

Another source of the data you want may be textbooks and review articles that reference original studies addressing recurrence of UTI in children. You look at the recent general pediatric texts that you find in the hospital's library. One makes an unreferenced statement that urinary tract infections tend to recur,[20] and the other does not address the probability of recurrence at all.[21] In the 4th edition of *Pediatric Nephrology*, the recurrence rate for girls with first-time infection is said to be 30% within 1 year, including both symptomatic and asymptomatic recurrences.[22] The chapter in *Pediatric Kidney Disease* (2nd edition), citing the same reference as well as others by the same authors, makes a similar statement. The references for these statements are quite old (1967–1975)[23–27] and you suspect that they will not add much to the information you already have.

A number of issues addressed by *Clinical Evidence* or the AAP practice parameter are not addressed in this chapter. These include:

- the role of prophylactic antibiotics to prevent recurrence of UTI;
- surgical correction for obstructive anomalies or for vesicoureteric reflux;
- whether to obtain a urine sample in the non-toxic child;
- other methods of obtaining the urine sample;
- parenteral versus oral antibiotics;
- the need for reculturing after treatment;
- the need for prophylactic antibiotics while imaging studies are being done.

Resolution of the scenario

Between them, Clinical Evidence, *the AAP technical report, and the meta-analysis of screening tests address some of your questions. For the rest, you have gone to references from these publications,* MedLine *and to textbooks for the references found there. Applying the evidence that you have found to the clinical scenario:*

An 18-month-old girl with fever without focus has a probability of having a UTI of about 8%. With the use of the likelihood ratios listed in Table 42.1 and the likelihood ratio nomogram found on page 35 it is possible to estimate the likelihood of UTI given the results of her urinalysis. In this case, the dipstick was positive for nitrites, and urine microscopy showed 20–50 WBC/hpf and bacteria. The likelihood of this child having a UTI given these findings is 80% based on the dipstick. No studies reported on the sensitivity and specificity of a value of 20–50 WBC in the urine; however, it would be assumed to be more specific than > 5 WBC, which again increases the likelihood of a UTI. You cannot combine these findings or use them in sequence because they are not independent of each other. Given this substantial likelihood that she has an acute UTI, you decide to culture her urine and treat her presumptively. Her mother has requested that she be given single-dose therapy. However, you do not feel comfortable with this change from your current approach. Your next concern is whether the UTI that this child has may be the result of an underlying anatomic abnormality. The likelihood of vesicoureteral reflux is expected to be around 30% based on this child's age. Since the causal chain between VUR and long-term renal damage has not been clearly established, you plan to discuss the possibilities with the parents and determine whether they would rather their daughter undergo imaging now or instead be on the alert for future infections and consider imaging at that time. This decision depends not only on your knowledge of the evidence but also on the value that they place on avoiding the imaging procedure and on watching closely for future infections. Since the risk of recurrence appears to be between 12% and 30% (and probably closer to 12%), you plan to monitor this child's febrile illnesses regardless of whether you and the parents decide to perform imaging studies.

Future research needs

Although we have done reasonably well in providing valid and applicable answers to questions concerning the acute management of children with UTI, we would not do so well if we were asked questions such as:

- "Is it serious?"
- "What will happen to my child long term?"
- "Will she develop hypertension or kidney failure?"
- "Does any intervention reduce the risk of long-term sequelae?"

Unfortunately these questions are largely unanswered, as was noted by Dick and Feldman.[17] Long-term prospective cohort studies of children with first-time UTI are needed, as are randomized controlled trials designed to determine whether children investigated following UTI do better than those who are not, and whether children given long-term antibiotics to prevent UTI really do have a reduction in risk of UTI.

Summary table

Question	Type of evidence	Result	Comment
Risk of UTI in febrile young child (2–24 months)	Cohort studies, mostly of febrile children in emergency room settings	Females: < 1 year 7%; > 1 year 8% Males: < 1 year 3%; > 1 year 2% + circumcision 0·2%	Estimates fairly stable across studies
Will UA reliably detect UTI?	Comparison with urine culture results	Nitrite or LE+: 88–93% sensitivity Nitrite+: 98% specificity Gram stain+: 93% sensitivity; 95% specificity	Other components of the UA were less useful on an individual basis
Single dose *v* standard duration of therapy	Randomized trials, systematic review of RCTs	No difference clearly shown, direction of effect favors standard therapy	All studies underpowered to show a difference
Probability of VUR in patients with acute UTI	Cross-sectional studies	Estimate centers around 30–40%, higher in younger infants, decreasing with age	Very wide variation in estimate
Likelihood of recurrence of UTI after first acute UTI	2 cohort studies	Boys: 30%; girls: 30% in 1 year; 40% overall	One study is > 40 years old, both from Scandinavian countries

Abbreviations: UA, urinalysis; VUR, vesicoureteral reflux; LE, leukocyte esterase.

References

1 Hoberman A, Wald ER. Pyuria and bacteriuria in urine specimens obtained by catheter from young children with fever. *J Pediatr* 1904;**124**:513–19.

2 Lohr JA, Portilla MG, Geuder TG, Dunn ML, Dudley SM. Making a presumptive diagnosis of urinary tract infection by using a urinalysis performed in an on-site laboratory. *J Pediatr* 1993;**122**:22–5.

3 Weinberg AG, Gan VN. Urine screen for bacteriuria in symptomatic pediatric outpatients. *Pediatr Infect Dis J* 1991; **10**:651–4.

4 Cardiff-Oxford Bacteriuria Study Group. Sequelae of covert bacteriuria in school girls. *Lancet* 1978;**1**:889–93.

5 BMJ Publishing Group and American College of Physicians– American Society of Internal Medicine. *Clinical evidence*. London: BMJ Publishing Group (Issue 9), 2003

6 Michael M, Hodson EM, Craig JC, Martin S, Moyer VA. Short versus standard duration oral antibiotic therapy for acute urinary tract infection in children (Cochrane Review). In: *Cochrane Library*, Issue 2. Oxford: Update Software, 2003.

7 Williams GJ, Lee A, Craig, JC. Long term antibiotics for preventing recurrent urinary tract infection in children. *Cochrane Library*, Issue 2. Oxford, Update Software, 2003.

8 Tran D, Muchant DG, Aronoff SC. Short-course versus conventional length antimicrobial therapy for uncomplicated lower urinary tract infections in children: a meta-analysis of 1279 patients. *J Pediatr* 2001;**139**:93–9.

9 Keren R, Chan E. A meta-analysis of randomized, controlled trials comparing short- and long-course antibiotic therapy for urinary tract infections in children. *Pediatrics* 2002; **109**:E70.

10 Huicho L, Campos-Sanchez M, Alamo C. Metaanalysis of urine screening tests for determining the risk of urinary tract infection in children. *Pediatr Infect Dis J* 2002;**21**:1–11.

11 Gorelick MH, Shaw KN. Screening tests for urinary tract infection in children: a meta-analysis. *Pediatrics* 1999; **104**:54 [http://www.pediatrics.org/cgi/content/full/104/ 5/e54].

12 American Academy of Pediatrics Committee on Quality Improvement. Subcommittee on Urinary Tract Infection. Practice parameter: the diagnosis, treatment, and evaluation of the initial urinary tract infection in febrile infants and young children. *Pediatrics* 1999;**103**:843–52 [http://www. pediatrics.org/cgi/content/full/103/4/843].

13 Downs SM. Technical report: urinary tract infections in febrile infants and young children. *Pediatrics* 1999;**103**. [URL: http:// www.pediatrics.org/cgi/content/full/103/4/e5412].

14 Hayward RSA, Wilson MC, Tunis SR, Bass EB, Guyatt G. Users' guides to the medical literature VIII. How to use clinical practice guidelines. A. Are the recommendations valid? *JAMA* 1995;**274**:570–4.

15 Hayward RSA, Wilson MC, Tunis SR, Bass EB, Guyatt G. Users' guides to the medical literature VIII. How to use clinical practice guidelines. B. What are the recommendations and will they help you in caring for your patients? *JAMA* 1995;**274**:1630–2.

16 Michael M, Hodson EM, Craig JC *et al.* Short compared with standard duration of antibiotic treatment for urinary tract infection: a systematic review of randomised controlled trials. *Arch Dis Child* 2002;**87**:118–23.

17 Dick PT, Feldman W. Routine diagnostic imaging for childhood urinary tract infections: a systematic overview. *J Pediatr* 1996;**128**:15–22.

18 Panaretto K, Craig JC, Knight JF, Howman-Giles R, Sureshkumar P, Roy LP. Risk factors for recurrent urinary tract infection. *J Paediatr Child Health* 1999;**35**:454–9.

19 Nuutinen M, Uhari M. Recurrence and follow up after urinary tract infection under the age of 1 year. *Pediatr Nephrol* 2001;**16**:69–72.

20 Urinary tract infections. In: Behrman R, ed. *Nelson textbook of pediatrics, 15th edn.* Philadelphia: WB Saunders, 1996.

21 Gonzales ET, Roth DR. Urinary tract infection. In: McMillan JA, DeAngelis CD, Feigin RD, Warshaw JB, eds. *Oski's pediatrics principles and practice, 3rd edn.* Baltimore: Lippincott Williams and Wilkins, 1999.

22 Hansson S, Jodal U. Urinary tract infection. In: Barratt MT, Avner ED, Harmon WE, eds. *Pediatric Nephrology, 4th edn.* Baltimore: Lippincott Williams and Wilkins, 1999.

23 Jones KV, Asscher AW. Urinary tract infection and vesic-our-eteral reflux. In: Edelmann CM, ed. *Pediatric Kidney Disease, 2nd edn.* Little, Brown and Company, 1992.

24 Bergstrom T, Lincoln D, Orskov F, Orskov I, Winberg J. Studies of urinary tract infections in infancy and childhood VIII. Reinfection vs. relapse in recurrent urinary tract infections. Evaluation by means of identification of infecting organisms. *J Pediatr* 1967;**71**:13–20.

25 Bergstrom T. Sex differences in childhood urinary tract infection. *Arch Dis Child* 1972;**47**:227–32.

26 Winberg J, Andersen HJ, Bergstrom T, Jacobsson B, Larson H, Lincoln K. Epidemiology of symptomatic urinary tract infection in childhood. *Acta Pediatr Scand* 1974;S252:1–20.

27 Winberg J, Bergstrom T, Jacobsson B. Morbidity, age and sex distribution, recurrences and renal scarring in symptomatic urinary tract infection in childhood. *Kidney Int* 1975; (Suppl. 4):S101–106.

43 Diabetes

Margaret L Lawson

Case scenario   *A 10-year-old boy presents to your office with a 3-week history of polyuria and polydipsia and a 3 kg weight loss. There is no family history of diabetes. Physical examination is unremarkable except that he is moderately overweight. Urinalysis shows 2 + glucose but no ketones. A random blood glucose level is 14·2 mmol liter⁻¹. You think the boy has diabetes mellitus and explain to his parents that he will require treatment for this. You wonder whether you should do an oral glucose tolerance test to confirm the diagnosis and whether there are tests which can differentiate type 1 and type 2 diabetes in youths. You also wonder whether it is really necessary to admit the boy to hospital. You have not seen a child with new onset diabetes for some time and you are unsure of the most appropriate treatment. When you next see this patient, his mother asks whether her son's hypoglycemic episodes could cause permanent brain damage.*

Background

Diabetes mellitus is a metabolic disorder characterized by hyperglycemia; it results from abnormalities in insulin secretion, insulin action, or both. There are two main types of diabetes mellitus:

- Type 1 diabetes (previously known as insulin-dependent or juvenile-onset diabetes) is a disease with onset primarily during childhood. It is caused by destruction of the insulin-producing islet cells of the pancreas, which ultimately leads to complete insulin deficiency. Most cases of type 1 diabetes are autoimmune in origin. Although genetics play a role in the pathogenesis of type 1 diabetes, only 5–10% of children with this type of diabetes have a positive family history of the disease.[1]

- Type 2 diabetes (previously known as non-insulin-dependent or adult-onset diabetes) most commonly develops in adults, and adolescents of Aboriginal, Hispanic, Asian, or African descent, and there is frequently a positive family history.[2] Type 2 diabetes is closely linked to obesity, and its prevalence in children and adolescents in developed countries has increased with the increase in obesity. With the exception of these high risk populations, the majority of children with new-onset diabetes have type 1 diabetes.

The incidence of type 1 diabetes varies 40-fold worldwide from 0·6 per 100 000 per year in China and Venezuela to 36·5 per 100 000 per year in Finland.[3] Furthermore, type 1 diabetes is much more common in Caucasians than in African-Americans, Asians, or Hispanics, and the incidence is higher in northern hemisphere countries than in the southern hemisphere.[3] In North America, type 1 diabetes affects 1 in 300–600 children under age 20.[4]

The child presenting with diabetes may be asymptomatic, have mild non-specific symptoms, or present in coma. At presentation, most children and adolescents with type 1 diabetes are thin and have experienced weight loss, polyuria (including new onset of nocturnal enuresis in children), polydipsia, and fatigue. Although unrecognized or untreated type 1 diabetes will progress to life-threatening diabetic ketoacidosis (DKA), only 25% of children and adolescents with type 1 diabetes present with DKA.[5] Recent evidence indicates that children and adolescents with type 2 diabetes may also present with DKA making it difficult to distinguish these two types of diabetes.[6]

The goal of diabetes management is to achieve the most physiologic glucose levels possible, at the same time minimizing the occurrence of both hypoglycemia and hyperglycemia. Although most children and teens with diabetes are healthy, they are at high risk for developing long-term diabetes-related complications during their young adult years. Historically, 30–40% of adults with childhood-onset diabetes developed kidney failure, 20–30% developed visual impairment from diabetic retinopathy, 20–30% developed neuropathy, and 50% developed coronary artery disease.[7] More recent studies suggest that the risk of these complications is decreasing, probably related to better control of blood glucose levels and blood pressure, and reduced prevalence of smoking.[8] The fundamental goal in the management of children and adolescents with diabetes is the prevention of these complications or, failing that, early identification and intervention to prevent long-term damage, while at the same time minimizing the risks from hypoglycemia. However, it should be recognized that the struggle to achieve and maintain optimal blood glucose control can lead to significant stress for children and adolescents and their families.

Framing answerable clinical questions

Clinical questions must be posed in a way that makes them answerable. Ideally, each question should include: the patient or population; the intervention (with or without comparison), event, diagnostic test or exposure; and the outcome of interest (see Chapter 2). Framing questions will make it easier to search for the evidence.

Questions

1. In children with symptomatic hyperglycemia (*patient/population*), is an oral glucose tolerance test (*diagnostic test*) required to diagnose diabetes mellitus (*outcome*)? **[Diagnosis]**
2. In children with newly diagnosed diabetes mellitus (*patient/population*), can autoimmune markers (*diagnostic test*) be used to differentiate type 1 and type 2 diabetes mellitus (*outcome*)? **[Diagnosis]**
3. In children with newly diagnosed type 1 diabetes mellitus, who are not in diabetic ketoacidosis (*patient/population*), is outpatient management as effective as inpatient management (*intervention and comparison*) for diabetes education, preventing rehospitalization and achieving optimal metabolic control (*outcome*)? **[Therapy]**
4. In prepubertal children with newly diagnosed type 1 diabetes (*patient/population*) do three or more, rather than two insulin injections daily (*intervention and comparison*) improve metabolic control (*outcome*), as indicated by hemoglobin A_{1c}? **[Therapy]**
5. What is the risk of long-term cognitive impairment (*outcome*) associated with hypoglycemia (*event*) in children with type 1 diabetes (*patient/population*)? **[Prognosis]**

Searching for evidence

A variety of methods are available to search for the information needed to manage this case (see Chapter 3). Discussion with your local specialist in adult diabetes regarding the need for an oral glucose tolerance test reveals that clinical practice guidelines (said to be evidence-based) on the diagnosis and management of diabetes have been developed in Canada. Looking for these specifically, you go to the National Library of Medicine's PubMed site and perform a search.

Search for evidence synthesis

- PubMed
- "diabetes clinical practice guidelines in Canada"

Thirty-two references are retrieved including the 1998 clinical practice guidelines for the management of diabetes in Canada.[9] The guidelines are published in the *Canadian Medical Association Journal* and the full text can be found on line (http://www.cmaj.ca/cgi/data/159/8/DC1/1). You note that there is a section on diabetes in children and adolescents, so you start with this.

Critical review of the evidence

Question

1. In children with symptomatic hyperglycemia (*patient/population*), is an oral glucose tolerance test (*diagnostic test*) required to diagnose diabetes mellitus (*outcome*)? **[Diagnosis]**

Examination of the Canadian guidelines for diabetes management reveals a methods section describing the membership of the expert committee, which was appropriately broad and experienced. The principles used for developing the clinical practice guidelines, assigning levels of evidence, and making and grading recommendations were based on the *JAMA* guidelines.[10,11] However, no information is provided about search strategies so you cannot be certain that the review of the available literature was complete. The guidelines include a section on the diagnosis of diabetes, including diagnostic criteria and the evidence upon which these are based. The article tells you that these criteria are consistent with those of the American Diabetes Association and the World Health Organization. You decide to apply the diagnostic criteria to your patient.

The guidelines state that diabetes should be diagnosed when:

- there are symptoms of diabetes (fatigue, polyuria, polydipsia, or unexplained weight loss) plus a casual (random) plasma glucose of $\geq 11 \cdot 1$ mmol liter^{-1}, *or*
- there is a fasting plasma glucose $\geq 7 \cdot 0$ mmol liter^{-1}, *or*
- a plasma glucose value of $\geq 11 \cdot 1$ mmol liter^{-1} in the 2-hour sample of the oral glucose tolerance test.

The guidelines further state that: "a confirmatory test must be done on another day in all cases in the absence of unequivocal hyperglycemia accompanied by acute metabolic decompensation." The guidelines don't explain what is meant by unequivocal hyperglycemia and thus this is subject to individual interpretation. You interpret this to mean hyperglycemia in the range that is unlikely to be due to causes other than diabetes (for example, laboratory error, hyperglycemia induced by stress). You are confident that your patient has diabetes and that an oral glucose tolerance test is not required to confirm this. However, this child is overweight and you have heard that type 2 diabetes is on the rise in children and adolescents. You wonder whether this child has type 1 or type 2 diabetes and whether autoimmune markers can be used to differentiate type 1 from type 2 diabetes.

Question

2. In children with newly diagnosed diabetes mellitus (*patient/population*), can autoimmune markers (*diagnostic test*) be used to differentiate type 1 and type 2 diabetes mellitus (*outcome*)? **[Diagnosis]**

Search strategy

- PubMed
- "type 2 diabetes AND autoimmune markers AND diagnosis"

You look for information about this in the guidelines, but this topic is not covered. So you search PubMed limiting the search to English publications and the age group "all child (0 to 18 years)". Eight references are retrieved including one that examined whether clinical and autoimmune characteristics can be used to distinguish between type 1 and type 2 diabetes in childhood.[6] The authors evaluated 48 children with type 2 diabetes diagnosed on the basis of clinical factors (high risk ethnic group, family history of type 2 diabetes, obesity, and/or acanthosis nigricans) and compared them with 39 children with type 1 diabetes who were randomly selected from their clinic population. The children with type 2 diabetes were older, more likely to be overweight and were more likely to be from a high risk ethnic group (predominantly Hispanic). However, presence or absence of autoimmune markers or diabetic ketoacidosis at diagnosis, the degree of hyperglycemia, or amount of endogenous insulin production (fasting C-peptide level) could not be used to differentiate type 1 from type 2 diabetes in these children. Daily insulin requirements were lower (mean of 0·33 units kg⁻¹ per day) at 1-year post-diagnosis in those diagnosed with type 2 diabetes.

This study is evaluating a diagnostic test (autoimmune markers) and comparing it to the clinical criteria they used to classify their patients as type 1 or type 2 diabetes (their gold standard). The problem is that the clinical criteria are not the gold standard for differentiating type 1 from type 2 diabetes. In fact, if clinical criteria were sufficient to diagnose type 2 diabetes in childhood, the biochemical markers would not be needed. Nevertheless, this article does tell you that autoimmune markers are common in children and adolescents with diabetes and that neither their presence nor absence can reliably differentiate type 1 from type 2 diabetes. Instead, the best indicator that a child has type 2 diabetes is the need for lower-than-expected insulin doses with good metabolic control beyond the time at which this might reasonably be attributed to the "honeymoon period".

Your patient is Caucasian, has no family history of type 2 diabetes, and does not have clinical evidence of insulin resistance (acanthosis nigricans). Although he is overweight, he does not have other clinical risk factors for type 2 diabetes. You conclude from the literature that you have reviewed that autoimmune markers and measures of endogenous insulin secretion will not help you in managing this patient. Based on his clinical presentation, you decide that he most likely has type 1 diabetes, autoimmune in etiology, but that, if insulin requirements are lower than expected at 1-year post diagnosis (< 0·5 units kg⁻¹ per day), you will reconsider the diagnosis of type 2 diabetes. You wonder whether hospitalization is required for children with type 1 diabetes who are not in diabetic ketoacidosis at presentation.

Question

3. In children with newly diagnosed type 1 diabetes mellitus but who are not in diabetic ketoacidosis (*patient/population*) is outpatient management as effective as inpatient management (*intervention and comparison*) for diabetes education, preventing rehospitalization and achieving optimal metabolic control (*outcome*)? **[Therapy]**

The section on children and adolescents in the Canadian guidelines[9] recommends that "in children and adolescents with new-onset diabetes, initial outpatient education and management should be considered if appropriate personnel and a 24-hour telephone consultation service are available in the community." The guidelines do not specifically state whether this recommendation refers to children without DKA at presentation. This recommendation is graded C (which means it is based on non-randomized clinical trials or cohort studies plus consensus) with a 1992 cohort study provided as the reference.[12] You wonder whether better evidence is available in the literature now.

Table 43·1   Outpatient therapy in new onset type 1 diabetes mellitus

Therapy question	Type of evidence	Benefits (positive effects)	Harms (negative effects)
Outpatient *v* inpatient management/education	l RCT (abstract only) 1 non-systematic review 4 retrospective cohorts 2 retrospective case series	Beneficial Reduced healthcare costs Similar or better metabolic control Lower or similar rates of future DKA, rehospitalization and severe hypoglycemia	None identified

Search strategy

- *Cochrane Library*: (CDSR and DARE) "diabetes mellitus AND insulin dependent AND child OR Adolescent"
- PubMed
- "diabetes mellitus AND insulin dependent AND newly diagnosed AND hospitalization AND outpatient"

You begin by searching the *Cochrane Library* for "diabetes mellitus AND insulin dependent AND child OR adolescent" and identify 15 completed systematic reviews and 15 protocols for systematic reviews, plus six systematic review abstracts in the Database of Abstracts of Reviews of Effects (DARE). One of these addresses the topic of hospitalization versus outpatient management for children with newly onset diabetes but this is an incomplete protocol.[13] You contact the author and determine that it is still incomplete. Next, you search PubMed, limiting the search to English publications and the age group "all child (0 to 18 years)". Nine references are retrieved.

There are no randomized controlled trials (RCTs) comparing outpatient to inpatient management for children with new onset diabetes. Your search identifies several retrospective studies including the one cited in the Canadian guidelines and one review article published in 1997.[14] You obtain the review article, hoping that it will be a systematic review of the literature, and that it may list references which your search failed to identify. You know this is likely because even a properly done MedLine search can miss up to 50% of relevant references.[15]

The review article is not a systematic review and neither the methods for retrieval of studies nor the criteria for inclusion are reported. You conclude that there may be significant bias in the selection of studies included. The article reports on six retrospective studies (four cohort and two case series), describes the methods and results of each individual study, and the gaps and limitations in the methods of these studies, particularly the potential for selection bias when deciding which children should be admitted to hospital and which can be safely managed on an outpatient basis. Some of the studies included children with DKA who were admitted

to hospital, stabilized within 1–2 days, and then received their diabetes education on an outpatient basis. Each study concluded that outpatient education for new onset diabetes in children was less expensive and associated with similar or slightly better outcomes in terms of metabolic control, rates of rehospitalization, DKA and severe hypoglycemia compared to an inpatient education, program. You review the article's reference list and find only one study not identified through your PubMed search. It is a randomized controlled trial of 60 children which concludes that outpatient education is cheaper and does not alter metabolic control, but the study has only been published in abstract form.[16] You return to PubMed, search for the authors and find that it is still unpublished. You wonder whether this is because of publication bias whereby negative studies are much less likely to be submitted, to be positively reviewed, and to be published than are positive studies.[17]

The review article does not meet criteria for an unbiased comprehensive review of the literature or systematic review (see Chapter 8), because it does not report explicit inclusion and exclusion criteria for the studies reviewed and provides no evidence that a comprehensive literature review was conducted.[18] However, your own search and that of the authors of the Canadian guidelines failed to identify any additional relevant studies. You feel it unlikely that there are additional studies that contradict the review article and, as your patient does not have ketoacidosis, you elect to manage him completely as an outpatient. The evidence for outpatient therapy in new onset type 1 diabetes mellitus is summarized in Table 43.1.

Question

4. In prepubertal children with newly diagnosed type 1 diabetes (*patient/population*) do three or more, rather than two insulin injections daily (*intervention and comparison*) improve metabolic control (*outcome*), as indicated by hemoglobin Ac1? **[Therapy]**

The Canadian guidelines do not address this question except to state that "multiple daily injections (3 or 4 per day) or the use of subcutaneous insulin infusion (CSII) as part of an intensified diabetes management regimen are usually required to achieve target glucose levels in adults or adolescents with diabetes."[9] This is a Grade A, level 1 recommendation (i.e., based on at least one randomized controlled trial with adequate power plus consensus). This statement does not refer specifically to children or adolescents with new onset diabetes.

Search strategy

- *Cochrane Library*: (CDSR, DARE and CCTR) "diabetes mellitus AND insulin dependent AND child OR adolescent"
- PubMed diabetes AND insulin injections AND metabolic control AND random*

As systematic reviews and RCTs provide the best quality evidence to address questions of therapy, you look through the articles found in your earlier search of the *Cochrane Library* and find that none addresses this question nor are there any relevant trials in the Cochrane Clinical Trials Register. You then access PubMed via the internet, limit the search to the age group "all child (0–18 years)" and retrieve 26 articles. You do not identify any RCTs comparing different insulin injection regimens in children with newly onset diabetes. However, you do find three studies (four publications) that are relevant to your question. Methods and findings of these studies are summarized in Table 43.2.

The first study, a randomized controlled trial of insulin pump therapy versus conventional insulin therapy demonstrates the efficacy and feasibility of initiating intensive insulin therapy with insulin pumps in children at onset of diabetes.[19] However, it doesn't address the increased costs associated with pump therapy, which are considerable.[20] More importantly, if pump therapy isn't readily available in your community because of lack of expertise and resources to provide the necessary education, these study results won't really help you in caring for your patient. Furthermore, the study doesn't answer the question that you have posed regarding the most appropriate initial insulin injection regimen in children with newly diagnosed diabetes.

The second study is a cross over trial which compared different insulin injection regimens in adolescents with established diabetes.[21] It demonstrated a small treatment effect in terms of blood glucose levels. However, you cannot exclude the possibility that there was no difference between the treatment groups. Furthermore, the study did not include children or adolescents with newly diagnosed diabetes.

The "DCCT" trial[22] meets most of the criteria set out in Chapter 6 and the *JAMA* Users' Guides,[23,24] but unfortunately does not include children, or individuals with new onset diabetes. The primary criticism of the trial is that the intensive therapy that was practised involved much more than more frequent insulin injections (three to four per day) or use of an insulin pump. It also involved more frequent blood glucose tests by the patient (four per day), more frequent clinic visits (monthly), and regular biweekly telephone contact between the patient and a diabetes nurse educator to assist with insulin adjustment. In contrast, the patients receiving conventional therapy (one to two injections per day) only performed blood glucose or urine monitoring twice daily and attended clinic every 3 months.

The DCCT trial also published a sub-group analysis,[25] which examined the effect of intensive diabetes therapy on residual beta cell function (i.e., the ability to produce insulin in response to a concentrated carbohydrate load). Subjects were termed beta-cell responders if at baseline they had a C-peptide level of 0·2–0·5 pmol liter^{-1} after ingestion of a standardized, mixed meal. The authors concluded from their analysis that intensive therapy helps sustain endogenous insulin secretion and should be initiated as early as possible after diagnosis. Although the treatment effect is large and the estimate of treatment effect is precise, the findings are based on subgroup analyses, with post-hoc stratification.[26] Although patients were not stratified by age, these findings suggest that for adolescents and adults there is a greater benefit from intensive diabetes management (note that this means more than just more frequent injections or delivering insulin by pump) when it is initiated early, before complete loss of beta-cell function. However, this study did not include any subjects with new onset diabetes (all had had diabetes for at least 1–5 years, at study entry) and only 135 of the subjects were adolescents at study entry. Furthermore, it does not distinguish between the effects of an intensive diabetes management program and frequency of insulin injections. Therefore, you question the generalizability of the study's results to your 10-year-old patient.

The majority of prepubertal children in developed countries remain on twice daily insulin injections. There are several reasons for this:

- Insulin pump therapy is much more expensive than insulin injection regimens.[20]
- Teenagers as well as parents of prepubertal children often refuse to initiate intensive insulin therapy when it requires lunchtime injections and/or blood glucose tests.[28]
- There is evidence that factors other than the frequency of injections or method of insulin delivery have an impact on metabolic control. These include frequency of self blood glucose monitoring, frequency of clinic visits, and compliance with diet.[29-31]

Further research is needed to evaluate the acceptability, benefits, and risks of intensive insulin regimens, as well as other means of optimizing control, particularly in children with new onset diabetes.

Table 43·2 Insulin therapy in newly onset type 1 diabetes mellitus

Therapy question: optimal insulin regimen	Population	Type of evidence	Potential bias	Positive effects	Negative effects
Continuous insulin infusion v 1–2 daily s.c.[19]	n=31 Aged 1–16 years New onset diabetes	RCT Unblinded Follow up was complete Intention to treat analysis was used Does not compare injection regimens	Children randomized to pump therapy were slightly older than those randomized to injection therapy (9.5±4.2 v 7.0±3.6 years)	Statistically and clinically significant improvement in HbA$_{1c}$ in pump group from 2–24 months post-diagnosis No increase in adverse events Regimen well accepted with only one child assigned to pump therapy discontinuing at the end of the study[27]	Increased costs and healthcare resources No effect on endogenous insulin secretion
Thrice daily (breakfast, supper, bedtime) in which the evening intermediate-acting insulin was moved from supper to bedtime v twice daily mixed injections of intermediate and fast-acting insulin[21]	n=18 Aged 10.8–15.9 years Diabetes duration of 2–14 years No new onset diabetes	Cross-over study Unblinded randomization of treatment order Study groups were similar at entry Small study, low power	One subject was excluded for failing to comply with the protocol	On the three times daily regimen, subjects had higher morning ($P=0.03$) and nocturnal blood glucose ($P<0.03$) and less hypoglycemia during the night (P value not given) Inadequate power to detect a change in hemoglobin A$_{1c}$	Acceptance of regimen at diagnosis not known Quality of life (QOL) not assessed
The Diabetes Control and Complications Trial[22] Multicenter Intensive therapy (insulin infusion or ≥3 injections per day), with intensive monitoring and follow up v 1–2 daily s.c. injections, routine monitoring and follow up	n=1441 adults and adolescents Diabetes duration of 1–15 years No new onset diabetes	Randomized with good allocation concealment Blinding was used for the primary outcome measures 99% completed study (average 6.5 years follow up) 95% of scheduled examinations completed Intention to treat analysis Treatment groups were similar at the start of the trial	Low	HbA$_{1c}$ was significantly lower amongst those who received intensive therapy compared with patients who received conventional therapy ($P<0.001$) Intensive therapy slowed the development of: retinopathy (OR 0.22; 95% CI 0.14–0.36; NNT 5 [4–7]) nephropathy (OR 0.50 [0.39–0.63]; NNT 7 [6–11]) neuropathy (OR 0.36 [0.24–0.54], NNT 13 [11–18])	Increased cost and use of healthcare resources No effect on QOL Acceptance of regimen at diagnosis not known 3-fold increase in severe hypoglycemia 2-fold increased risk of becoming overweight
Subgroup Analysis of the Diabetes Control and Complications Trial[25] Multicentre intensive therapy (insulin infusion or ≥3 injections per day), with intensive monitoring and follow up v 1–2 daily s.c. injections, routine monitoring and follow up	n=855 adults and adolescents Diabetes duration of 1–5 years No new onset diabetes	Same as DCCT plus post-hoc analysis – intensively treated and conventionally treated cohorts divided into those with or without baseline evidence of residual beta-cell function	Subgroup post-hoc analysis No age stratification	Intensively treated responders had a greater likelihood of maintaining beta-cell function ($P<0.001$) Intensively treated responders had lower hemoglobin A$_{1c}$ ($P<0.001$), a reduced risk for retinopathy progression (RR 50%; 95% CI 12–72%), and a lower risk for hypoglycemia (RR 65%; 95% CI 53–74%)	Increased cost and use of healthcare resources No effect on QOL Acceptance of regimen at diagnosis not known 3-fold increase in severe hypoglycemia 2-fold increased risk of becoming overweight

Question

5. What is the risk of long-term cognitive impairment (*outcome*) associated with hypoglycemia (*event*) in children with type 1 diabetes (*patient/population*)? **[Prognosis]**

The Canadian guidelines[9] state that "extreme caution is required to avoid severe hypoglycemia in children under 5 years of age, because of the permanent cognitive deficit that may occur in this age group". This is a Grade D, level 4 recommendation, meaning it is based on the lowest level of evidence, mainly supported by consensus. The references cited are from 1985 and 1987.[32,33] Looking for more recent evidence, you proceed to a search of the Cochrane Database of Systematic Reviews (CDSR) and DARE but find nothing on hypoglycemia and type 1 diabetes. Next you perform a MedLine search using PubMed and identify six studies, four of which specifically address this question.

Search strategy

- *Cochrane Library*: (CDSR and DARE) "diabetes mellitus" and "hypoglycemia" and "child or adolescent"
- PubMed "diabetes mellitus, insulin-dependent" AND "hypoglycemia AND "longitudinal studies OR "prospective studies AND "mental processes" AND "all child (0 to 18 years)

Of the four studies identified, three are cohort studies and one is an RCT that monitored hypoglycemia and included psychometric assessments as an outcome. You start with the RCT. Hershey *et al.*[34] examined performance on memory tasks in 16 non-diabetic children and 25 children with type 1 diabetes who at the time of diagnosis (at 7–17 years) had been randomly assigned to either intensive diabetes therapy (n = 13) or conventional therapy (n = 12). The intensively treated children (who were receiving three to four insulin injections per day or on an insulin pump) performed less accurately on spatial declarative memory task and more slowly, although not less accurately, on a pattern recognition task than the conventionally treated children with diabetes. Both groups of children with diabetes were significantly impaired on a motor speed task compared with their non-diabetic peers. Rates of severe hypoglycemia were three-fold higher among the intensively treated children but the numbers of children were too small to detect an association with the performance on memory tasks.

Because the small sample size of the RCT prevented interpretation of information in a way that would answer your question, you read the cohort studies you found. Rovet and Ehrlich performed a 7-year longitudinal study of 16 children with newly diagnosed type 1 diabetes.[35] After 7 years of diabetes, the children who had had hypoglycemic seizures were more likely to decline in verbal intelligence and to have deficits on perceptual, motor, memory, and attention tasks than those who had had no seizures. Although the sample size was small, subjects were recruited at the time of diagnosis and received similar diabetes management. The authors examined the effect of age at diagnosis and found greater effects in those with early-onset diabetes (< 5 years). It is not clear whether the psychological tests were performed in a blinded fashion.

In a similar study, Golden *et al.* studied 23 children diagnosed with type 1 diabetes < 5 years of age and followed them for 6–78 months.[36] All but six of the subjects entered the study at diagnosis. Again, it is not clear whether those performing the psychological tests were blinded to the clinical data. The authors found that those children with frequent asymptomatic hypoglycemia had lower scores on the abstract/visual reasoning scale than those with infrequent episodes, suggesting that hypoglycemia, even if mild or asymptomatic, may result in neuropsychological changes in the young child with diabetes.

Northam *et al.* reported on a 6-year follow up in 90 children who were < 12 years of age at diagnosis of type 1 diabetes, and had been previously assessed soon after diagnosis and 2 years later.[37] The neuropsychologic profiles of these children were compared with those of a community control group assessed at similar intervals. There is no mention of whether the tests were performed in a blinded fashion with respect to clinical condition. Six years after disease onset, children with diabetes performed more poorly than the non-diabetic controls on measures of intelligence, attention, processing speed, long-term memory, and executive skills, with the lowest scores amongst those diagnosed before 6 years of age and those with a history of severe hypoglycemia.

On the basis of these four studies, you conclude that there is a relationship between the frequency and severity of hypoglycemia and performance on psychological tests of cognitive function in children with type 1 diabetes. Furthermore, this relationship appears to be strongest in those with diabetes onset before age 6 years. The RCT is small and unable to directly link early initiation of intensive diabetes therapy with adverse cognitive effects in school-aged children. However, you are concerned by the authors' suggestion that there may be permanent cognitive effects from the increased rates of hypoglycemia experienced with intensive diabetes regimens in school-aged children. The clinical significance of reduced scores on psychological tests is not clear from these studies nor their relationship with school performance or functional capabilities. Nevertheless, you conclude that efforts should be made to minimize the frequency and severity of hypoglycemia in your patient, and you plan to take this into account when deciding when and how to intensify diabetes management.

Resolution of the scenario

You decide that your 10-year-old patient with typical symptoms of diabetes and a random plasma glucose of 14·2 mmol liter⁻¹ fulfils the criteria for diagnosis of diabetes and that neither an oral glucose tolerance test nor repeat measurement of plasma glucose is required to confirm this. Although he is moderately overweight, he does not have a family history of type 2 diabetes, is not from an ethnic group at high risk for type 2 diabetes, and has no clinical features of insulin resistance. Therefore, you decide that he most likely has type 1 diabetes and that this is most likely autoimmune in etiology. You recommend outpatient management based on the best available evidence and the resources in your area. You arrange for outpatient diabetes education and organize a visiting nurse to administer insulin in the child's home. You tell your call service that this family may contact you 24 hours a day for the next week or two for advice regarding their child's insulin dose.

You decide to prescribe twice daily insulin injections because there is insufficient evidence that more frequent insulin injections are required to achieve optimal glucose control in the first few years of diabetes, and you are concerned about the potential adverse effects of more frequent injections on quality of life in a 10-year-old child. You are also concerned about the evidence linking intensive diabetes therapy at diagnosis with subsequent impaired performance on memory tasks – was this from the hypoglycemia? You advise the family that the best way of preventing long-term microvascular complications is to maintain good blood glucose control. You will consider more frequent insulin injections or an insulin pump if he is not well controlled on two injections daily.

In answer to the mother's question about the risks of hypoglycemia for her son, you tell her that there is no evidence that mild infrequent hypoglycemia affects brain development in children > 6 years of age. However, you advise her that attempts should be made to minimize the frequency and severity of hypoglycemia. Furthermore, you tell her that it is important to strike a balance between hypo- and hyperglycemia to ensure optimal health for her son, both now and in the future.

Future research needs

Randomized trials are needed to investigate:

- outpatient versus inpatient management in children with newly onset diabetes;
- two versus three insulin injections daily in children with newly onset diabetes (study in progress at Children's Hospital of Eastern Ontario – presented in abstract form, publication in progress);
- insulin infusion versus injections in children with newly onset diabetes;
- the effect of different insulin regimens at diagnosis on quality of life in children;
- other means of optimizing metabolic control (for example, more frequent clinic visits, different types of insulin).
- the relationship between intensity of diabetes treatment, frequency and severity of hypoglycemia and the effect on cognitive function in school-aged and younger children. Cohort studies are needed to investigate:
- the long-term risk of recurrent hypoglycemia on cognitive function in school-aged children.

Summary table

Question	Type of evidence	Result	Comment
1. In children with symptomatic hyperglycemia, is an oral glucose tolerance test (OGTT) required to diagnose diabetes?	Evidenced-based clinical practice guidelines	An OGTT is not required in the symptomatic child with unequivocal hyperglycemia	Unequivocal hyperglycemia is not defined
2. In children with newly diagnosed diabetes, can autoimmune markers be used to differentiate type 1 and type 2 diabetes?	Retrospective cohort study	Autoimmune markers are not useful in differentiating type 1 from type 2 diabetes in childhood	There is currently no gold standard test for diagnosing type 2 diabetes in childhood although clinical risk factors may be helpful (high risk ethnic group, family history of type 2 diabetes, obesity, acanthosis nigricans). The clearest indicator of type 2 diabetes in youths is low insulin requirements 1–2 years post-diagnosis
3. In children with newly diagnosed type 1 diabetes who are not in diabetic ketoacidosis, is outpatient management as effective as inpatient management for diabetes education, preventing rehospitalization, and achieving optimal metabolic control?	1 RCT (abstract only) 1 non-systematic review 4 retrospective cohorts 2 retrospective case series	Outpatient management is less expensive and associated with similar or slightly better outcomes in terms of metabolic control, rates of rehospitalization, DKA and severe hypoglycemia	Although the type of evidence isn't as strong as desired, the available studies have consistent findings. Publication bias may have played a role in the lack of published studies in this area
4. In prepubertal children with newly diagnosed type 1 diabetes, do three or more, rather than two insulin injections daily improve metabolic control as indicated by hemoglobin A_{1c}?	RCT of CSII v s.c. injections in new onset diabetes Cross-over study of 2 v 3 daily injections in adolescents with 2–14 years of diabetes RCT of intensive therapy (3–4 injections or CSII) in adults and adolescents with 1–15 years of diabetes	More intensive therapy improves metabolic control and delays or prevents microvascular complications in those with established diabetes. CSII is effective and well accepted in children with new onset diabetes More intensive therapy increases the risk of severe hypoglycemia and weight gain	There are no published studies of 2 v 3 daily injections in new onset diabetes. Caution must be taken when initiating intensive therapy in young children with diabetes because of the increased risk of hypoglycemia and the potential for long-term effects on cognitive function (see question 5)
5. What is the risk of long-term cognitive impairment associated with hypoglycemia in children with type 1 diabetes?	RCT of intensive therapy in newly diagnosed children, which examined the relationship between hypoglycemia and cognitive function 3 prospective cohort studies	Frequent and severe hypoglycemia is associated with long-term adverse effects on cognitive function assessed by psychological tests, particularly in children <6 years of age at diabetes onset	Steps should be taken to minimize both the frequency and severity of hypoglycemia in young children with diabetes. The relationship between cognitive function and performance, and deficits identified through psychological testing is not clear

References

1 Wagener DK, Sacks JM, LaPorte RE, Macgregor JM. The Pittsburgh study of insulin-dependent diabetes mellitus. Risk for diabetes among relatives of IDDM. *Diabetes* 1982;**31**: 136–44.

2 Rosenbloom AL. Increasing incidence of type 2 diabetes in children and adolescents: treatment considerations. *Paediatr Drugs* 2002;**4**:209–21.

3 Karvonen M, Viik-Kajander M, Moltchanova E, Libman I, LaPorte R, Tuomilehto J. Incidence of childhood type 1 diabetes worldwide. Diabetes Mondiale (DiaMond) Project Group. *Diabetes Care* 2000;**23**:1516–26.

4 Drash AL. The epidemiology of insulin-dependent diabetes mellitus. *Clin Invest Med* 1987;**10**:432–6.

5 Pinkey JH, Bingley PJ, Sawtell PA, Dunger DB, Gale EA. Presentation and progress of childhood diabetes mellitus: a prospective population-based study. The Bart's-Oxford Study Group. *Diabetologia* 1994;**37**:70–74.

6 Hathout EH, Thomas W, El Shahawy M, Nahab F, Mace JW. Diabetic autoimmune markers in children and adolescents with type 2 diabetes. *Pediatrics* 2001;**107**:102.

7 Krolewski AS, Warram JH, Freire MB. Epidemiology of late diabetic complications. A basis for the development and evaluation of preventive programs. *Endocrinol Metab Clin N Am* 1996;**25**:217–42.

8 Hovind P, Tarnow L, Rossing K *et al.* Decreasing incidence of severe diabetic microangiopathy in type 1 diabetes. *Diabetes Care* 2003;**26**:1258.

9 Meltzer S, Leiter L, Daneman D *et al.* 1998 clinical practice guidelines for the management of diabetes in Canada. Canadian Diabetes Association. *CMAJ* 1998;**159**(Suppl. 8):S1–29.

10 Hayward RS, Wilson MC, Tunis SR, Bass EB, Guyatt G. Users' guides to the medical literature. VIII. How to use clinical practice guidelines. A. Are the recommendations valid? The Evidence-Based Medicine Working Group. *JAMA* 1995;**274**: 570–4.

11 Wilson MC, Hayward RS, Tunis SR, Bass EB, Guyatt G. Users' guides to the Medical Literature. VIII. How to use clinical practice guidelines. B. what are the recommendations and will they help you in caring for your patients? The Evidence-Based Medicine Working Group. *JAMA* 1995; **274**:1630–2.

12 Chase HP, Crews KR, Garg S *et al.* Outpatient management vs in-hospital management of children with newly onset diabetes. *Clin Pediatr (Phila)* 1992;**31**:450–6.

13 Clar C, Compton N, Waugh N, Schulga J. Routine hospital admission versus outpatient or home care in children not acutely requiring admission to hospital at diagnosis of type 1 diabetes mellitus (Protocol for a Cochran Review). *Cochrane Library.* Issue 2. Oxford: Update Software, 2002.

14 Charron-Prochownik D, Maihle T, Siminerio L, Songer T. Outpatient versus inpatient care of children newly diagnosed with IDDM. *Diabetes Care* 1997;**20**:657–60.

15 Adams CE, Power A, Frederick K, Lefebvre C. An investigation of the adequacy of MEDLINE searches for randomized controlled trials (RCTs) of the effects of mental health care. *Psychol Med* 1994;**24**:741–8.

16 Simell T, Putto-Laurila A, Nanto-Salonen K *et al.* Randomized prospective trial of ambulatory treatment and one-week hospitalization with newly diagnosed IDDM (Abstract). *Diabetes* 1995;(Suppl. 1):594A.

17 Easterbrook PJ, Berlin JA, Gopalan R, Matthews DR. Publication bias in clinical research. *Lancet* 1991;**337**:867–72.

18 Oxman AD, Cook DJ, Guyatt GH. Users' guides to the medical literature. VI. How to use an overview. Evidence-Based Medicine Working Group. *JAMA* 1994;**272**:1367–71.

19 de Beaufort CE, Houtzagers CM, Bruining GJ *et al.* Continuous subcutaneous insulin infusion (CSII) versus conventional injection therapy in newly diagnosed diabetic children: two-year follow up of a randomized, prospective trial. *Diabet Med* 1989;**6**:766–71.

20 Resource utilization and costs of care in the diabetes control and complications trial. *Diab Care* 1995;**18**:1468–78.

21 Hinde FR, Johnston DI. Two or three insulin injections in adolescence? *Arch Dis Child* 1986;**61**:118–23.

22 The Diabetes Control and Complications Trial Research Group. The effect of intensive treatment of diabetes on the development and progression of long-term complications in insulin-dependent diabetes mellitus. *N Engl J Med* 1993;**329**:977–86.

23 Guyatt GH, Sackett DL, Cook DJ. Users' guides to the medical literature. II. How to use an article about therapy or prevention. A. Are the results of the study valid? Evidence-Based Medicine Working Group. *JAMA* 1993;**270**: 2598–601.

24 Guyatt GH, Sackett DL, Cook DJ. Users' guides to the medical literature. II. How to use an article about therapy or prevention. B. What were the results and will they help me in caring for my patients? Evidence-Based Medicine Working Group. *JAMA* 1994;**271**:59–63.

25 The Diabetes Control and Complications Trial Research Group. Effect of intensive therapy on residual beta-cell function in patients with type 1 diabetes in the diabetes control and complications trial. A randomized, controlled trial. *Ann Intern Med* 1998;**128**:517–23.

26 Yusuf S, Wittes J, Probstfield J, Tyroler HA. Analysis and interpretation of treatment effects in subgroups of patients in randomized clinical trials. *JAMA* 1991;**266**:93–8.

27 Slijper FM, de Beaufort CE, Bruining GJ *et al.* Psychological impact of continuous subcutaneous insulin infusion pump therapy in non-selected newly diagnosed insulin dependent (type 1) diabetic children: evaluation after two years of therapy. *Diabet Metab* 1990;**16**:273–7.

28 Tercyak KP Jr, Johnson SB, Kirkpatrick KA, Silverstein JH. Offering a randomized trial of intensive therapy for IDDM to adolescents. Reasons for refusal, patient characteristics, and recruiter effects. *Diab Care* 1998;**21**:213–15.

29 Littlefield CH, Craven JL, Rodin GM, Daneman D, Murray MA, Rydall AC. Relationship of self-efficacy and binging to adherence to diabetes regimen among adolescents. *Diab Care* 1992;**15**:90–4.

30 Schiffrin A, Belmonte M. Multiple daily self-glucose monitoring: its essential role in long-term glucose control in insulin-dependent diabetic patients treated with pump and multiple subcutaneous injections. *Diab Care* 1982;**5**:479–84.

31 Kaufman FR, Halvorson M, Carpenter S. Association between diabetes control and visits to a multidisciplinary pediatric diabetes clinic. *Pediatrics* 1999;**103**:948–51.

32 Rovet JF, Ehrlich RM, Hoppe M. Intellectual deficits associated with early onset of insulin-dependent diabetes mellitus in children. *Diab Care* 1987;**10**:510–15.

33 Ryan C, Vega A, Drash A. Cognitive deficits in adolescents who developed diabetes early in life. *Pediatrics* 1985;**75**: 921–7.

34 Hershey T, Bhargava N, Sadler M, White NH, Craft S. Conventional versus intensive diabetes therapy in children with type 1 diabetes: effects on memory and motor speed. *Diab Care* 1999;**22**:1318–24.

35 Rovet JF, Ehrlich RM. The effect of hypoglycemic seizures on cognitive function in children with diabetes: a 7-year prospective study. *J Pediatr* 1999;**134**:503–6.

36 Golden MP, Ingersoll GM, Brack CJ, Russell BA, Wright JC, Huberty TJ. Longitudinal relationship of asymptomatic hypoglycemia to cognitive function in IDDM. *Diab Care* 1989;**12**:89–93.

37 Northam EA, Anderson PJ, Jacobs R, Hughes M, Warne GL, Werther GA. Neuropsychological profiles of children with type 1 diabetes 6 years after disease onset. *Diab Care* 2001; **24**:1541–6.

44 Short stature

Shayne P Taback, Heather J Dean

Case scenario

You are a primary care physician seeing a 12-year-old girl for the first time. The mother is concerned about her daughter's height. It seems that the whole family is short, but she believes that her daughter is too short even in comparison to other family members. Your patient has not had a height measurement in the past 3 years but her mother estimates that she has grown only 3 cm in the past 18 months. She also confides that when she was 12 years of age, she was bothered by her short stature and wonders if her daughter needs growth hormone, which the mother read about in a newspaper. The daughter had a normal birth weight, has no significant past medical illness or family history of disease that might be associated with short stature and no alarming symptoms at present. She is a good student and she denies being physically or verbally bullied at school. Her father is 170 cm tall (10th percentile for adult males) and her mother is 160 cm tall (25th percentile for adult females). Neither was a "late bloomer". Your physical examination confirms that your patient is prepubertal (Tanner stage I) with no signs suggesting a genetic syndrome, a central nervous system lesion, or a chronic disease of the cardiorespiratory, gastrointestinal, renal, or endocrine systems. Your patient's height is 133 cm (< 3rd percentile); her weight is 36 kg (20th percentile); her body mass index, therefore is 75th percentile for age. You conclude the clinical encounter by informing the mother and child that you find no sign of any disease, that the clinic nurse will be contacting them to arrange some tests to be more certain, and that you will discuss the use of growth hormone in more detail at your next visit, when you review the results of the investigations with them.

Background

Height is a human characteristic that varies within and between ethnic groups. Short stature is not a disease but rather a statistically defined height threshold that includes some children who are completely healthy, other children who have a known medical condition associated with short stature, and still other children for whom short stature is secondary to an undiagnosed illness. Obviously, an important goal of medical care is to differentiate those who are healthy from those with undiagnosed illness. The parent and child consulting a physician for short stature may be concerned either about the possibility of an underlying disease or about perceived social discrimination, such as bullying in school or decreased future socioeconomic success, because of short stature itself.

The Hall report on child health surveillance in the United Kingdom (*Health For All Children*)[1] considered the rationale for growth monitoring to detect disorders affecting height. Acknowledging limitations to the evidence base, they recommended that the public health program measure height at 18–24 months of age, around 3·5 years of age, and at school entry or 5 years of age, followed by either selective or universal screening in schools around 8 years of age with further research to evaluate the results of continuing growth monitoring into adolescence. Suggested indications for referral to a physician included height less than the 0·4 percentile on the recently revised British growth charts[2] or decreased growth velocity as evidenced by crossing lines on the growth chart over time.[1] More recently, the American Academy of Pediatrics has recommended annual height and weight measurements for all children in order to calculate body mass index percentile for age.[3]

Growth assessment is complex because of special considerations for valid measurements, selection of appropriate population reference standards, and the need to integrate patient-specific information.[1,4,5] Parental heights are used to compute an estimated target height and range by averaging the heights of the biologic parents, adding 6·5 cm if the patient is male, or subtracting 6·5 cm if the patient is female, and drawing a target range around this point on the growth chart to represent ±10 cm. Pubertal staging is performed using Tanner staging of breasts and pubic hair, and by physical examination of testicle size. Height velocity is based on two accurate height measurements taken at least 6 months apart and compared with height velocity curves constructed from longitudinal population data. Infants establish their specific height percentile by having a faster or slower growth rate than others in the first 2 years of life. The standard accepted technique for height measurement is described in many pediatric textbooks; the essential points are to use a stable wall-mounted device that has been accurately installed and is regularly calibrated, and to ensure standard patient positioning by trained personnel. Repetition of the measurement and its recording and plotting reduces error. Weights are relatively easy to measure accurately, although even an electronic scale should be regularly calibrated. When needed, radiographic bone age should be determined in comparison to standards by an individual practised in the methodology.

The manipulation of human stature has become an area of intense biological and psychological research, controversial clinical practice, significant commercial interest, and important ethical debate. An important finding is that, although distinctions based on medical treatment versus prevention versus enhancement are useful, they are imperfect and ultimately the ethical debate moves beyond the goals of medicine to the goals of society at large.[6] However, to the extent that increasing a person's adult height is advantageous for competitive (social or economic) reasons, such treatment has been termed a "self-defeating" enhancement from a societal viewpoint, owing to the fact that, if everyone received the same treatment, then no one gains anything. Since societal resources are limited, the more likely outcome would be a shift from any putative height advantage being conferred to those from families genetically destined to be naturally taller to those from families with greater socio-economic resources.

Framing answerable clinical questions

In response to your patient and her mother, you choose to review the evidence on the baseline risk of underlying diseases in short stature to inform your diagnostic work-up, the psychological effects of short stature, and on the use of growth hormone treatment to increase height. The first question is primarily about baseline risk, the second prognosis, and the third is primarily about treatment effect, although considerations of side effect harm and costs are related.

Questions

1. What is the frequency of underlying disorders (*outcome*) in children (*population*) presenting with short stature or growth failure (*exposure*)? **[Baseline Risk]**

2. Is short stature (*exposure*) during childhood (*population*) associated with psychological disability (*outcome*)? **[Harm]**
3. For children with short stature for various reasons (*population*), does the use of growth hormone (*intervention*) increase adult height or quality of life (*outcome*)? **[Therapy]**

Searching for evidence

- *Cochrane Library:* short stature

To be as efficient as possible, you will search general concise sources first. You log into the *Cochrane Library* and search for "short stature". You find separate Cochrane reviews for growth hormone in children with chronic renal failure awaiting transplant and for Turner syndrome; there are Cochrane review protocols in progress for Prader–Willi syndrome, and Crohn's disease, while the *Cochrane Library* Health Technology Assessment Database contains a review that seems to be comprehensive: "Clinical effectiveness and cost-effectiveness of growth hormone in children: a systematic review and economic evaluation".[7] You note from the online abstract that the five patient populations studied were growth hormone deficiency, Turner syndrome, chronic renal failure, Prader–Willi syndrome, and idiopathic short stature. You request it from the medical library and plan a more specific search strategy for the questions about diagnostic work-up and psychological outcome of short stature. Further searches for the individual questions are included below.

Critical review of the evidence

Question

1. What is the frequency of underlying disorders (*outcome*) in children (*population*) presenting with short stature or growth failure (*exposure*)? **[Baseline Risk]**

PubMed:

- short stature AND mass screening
- growth hormone deficiency AND mass screening
- short stature AND growth hormone deficiency AND prevalence

Finding information on baseline risk can be difficult. Your three searches combining disease terms and epidemiologic terms produce 20–40 records each, several of which are potentially relevant. You note a large British study that had data on the clinical question of disease frequency in short stature, the Wessex Growth Study,[8] and an even larger study from Beijing on the prevalence of growth hormone deficiency.[9]

The Wessex Growth Study[8] attempted to measure all children at 5 years of age (school entry) between 1985 and 1987 in two adjacent health districts in Wessex; those detected by the nurses to have short stature (height less than 3rd percentile according to the Tanner–Whitehouse standards) had measurements of thyroid hormone levels, some blood chemistry, and a bone age radiograph followed by referral to a specialist pediatrician if the results were abnormal. In total, 14 346 children were screened and 180 (1·3%) were found to have short stature. Of these 180 children, 25 had a known diagnosis that was consistent with short stature (such as Down's syndrome), five children belonged to ethnic groups for which the growth standards were deemed inappropriate, three families declined further participation, and eight children were diagnosed with a disease as a result of the screening program. The remaining 140 children with short stature were followed for an additional year. This study exemplifies the validity criteria for a study of disease probability.[11] The study patients are representative of the full spectrum of those who would present to a primary care practitioner. Although not all criteria for each of the final diagnoses were explicitly stated, most of the diagnoses are routinely diagnosed by highly credible and specific tests (for example, karyotype for Turner syndrome, thyrotropin (TSH) level for primary hypothyroidism, lead level for lead poisoning). Growth hormone deficiency was the exception (see below). The diagnostic work-up was fairly comprehensive and consistently applied, with follow up of undiagnosed patients for an additional year. The data from these study patients should apply to the developed world even 15 years later. This large study indicates that 5% (95% CI 0–14%) of the shortest 1·3% of children at school entry have an undiagnosed underlying medical condition.

Growth hormone deficiency was not well studied in the Wessex study, so you decide to look at the study of the prevalence of growth hormone deficiency by X-iu-lan *et al.*[9] This study is another good example of a study of disease probability. The study patients are representative of the full spectrum of those who would present to a primary care practitioner. School doctors measured all 103 753 students in two districts of Beijing that were aged 6–15 years. The diagnostic work-up was comprehensive and consistently applied and the diagnosis of growth hormone deficiency was credible. Specifically, those 202 children confirmed to have short stature (below 3rd percentile for age by northern Chinese standards but in fact the 0·2 percentile for the Beijing population) had a physical examination, bone age measurement, specific tests to rule out hypothyroidism and Turner syndrome, as well as urinalysis, chest radiograph, and liver function tests. In total 13 children (6%) were diagnosed

with conditions other than growth hormone deficiency. The criteria for growth hormone deficiency were highly credible as those patients suspected to have growth hormone deficiency were followed for 6 months to measure height velocity. The children were diagnosed with "total" growth hormone deficiency if they had a subnormal growth velocity, delayed bone age, and peak result on growth hormone stimulation testing < 5 micrograms liter^{-1} on three separate occasions. This strict definition is in accordance with the clinical and biochemical criteria originally used to select children for growth hormone therapy in developed countries[12,13], later shown to have a high frequency of a specific pituitary defect[14]. The children who had a peak growth hormone measurement between 5·0 and 9·9 micrograms liter^{-1} were diagnosed as having partial growth hormone deficiency, a less well established diagnosis.[15] Seven patients (prevalence 1/15 000; 3·5% [95% CI 1·0–6·4%]) of Beijing children < 0·2 percentile were found to have "total" growth hormone deficiency.

Finally, you create a list of potential diagnoses (see Box), using the two journal articles, and a pediatric textbook,[16] consulted to include the rare diseases that are important to diagnose due to severe prognosis or responsiveness to treatment. You note that you have found no single concise summary of evidence on the diagnostic properties of tests for these underlying disorders. The common variants seem to be defined clinically; some of the rarer diagnostic possibilities have very sensitive and specific tests easily available (for example, TSH level for primary hypothyroidism; karyotype for Turner syndrome), while for others (for example, gastrointestinal diseases), the specific tests are invasive. You also notice that, when the height standards label fewer children with short stature, the prevalence of specific disease in the group increases.

Diagnostic possibilities for patients presenting with short stature

A. *Common possibilities (no disease was found in > 95% of short children):*

   1. Familial short stature
   2. Constitutional delay of growth and puberty
   3. Combined constitutional delay of growth and puberty with familial short stature

B. *Rarer possibilities (disease is found in < 5% of short children):*

   1. Subtle genetic syndromes

      a. Turner syndrome
      b. Hypochondroplasia
      c. Pseudohypoparathyroidism
      d. Intrauterine growth retardation including Russell-Silver syndrome

2. Gastrointestinal disease

   a. Celiac disease
   b. Inflammatory bowel disease

3. Endocrine disease

   a. Acquired primary hypothyroidism
   b. Growth hormone deficiency
   c. Steroid-induced growth failure

4. Renal disease

   a. Renal failure
   b. Renal tubular acidosis

Question

2. Is short stature (*exposure*) during childhood (*population*) associated with psychological disability (*outcome*)? **[Harm]**

- PubMed: short stature AND psychol* AND review

If you can find a valid review, you will be able to avoid searching for and appraising individual cohort and case–control studies. A recent review has in fact been done[10] and you order it as well.

The review by Sandberg and Voss[10] does not meet the definition of a systematic review, although it does appraise several large population-based and clinic-based studies. The findings of the review are that, while short stature may confer psychosocial stress on an affected child and family, the psychological adaptation and quality of life in childhood, adolescence, and adulthood is on average normal. As this conclusion does not change your current practice, you proceed to work on the final question on treatment effect that you need answered for your patient, while making a note to search again for a systematic review in the future.

Question

3. For children with short stature for various reasons (*population*), does the use of growth hormone (*intervention*) increase adult height or quality of life (*outcomes*)? **[Therapy]**

You find one systematic review.[7] After confirming from Chapter 1 of the systematic review that it addresses your question, you read the brief methods sections to verify that the potential for bias is minimized. You find that a diligent search strategy was adopted (Appendix 2) and the process for examining the search strategy results for relevant citations was logical and transparent (Chapters 2 and 3). Finally, you wish to ensure that the included primary studies were themselves valid. You note that several observational studies (not randomized trials) have been included in the review because the reviewers stated that these contained much of the data for some of the indications. Since your patient does not have chronic renal failure or Prader–Willi syndrome (and you will follow her height velocity over time to exclude or decide to test further for the rare diagnosis of growth hormone deficiency), you decide for now to read only the chapters on idiopathic short stature, Turner syndrome, and side effects. Given the variability of adult height in the population, the imprecision of height prediction methods, and the potential for observational studies to be subject to confounding, you will restrict your reading for therapeutic effect to the evidence from the randomized controlled trials, while accepting the use of all information contained on side effects.

In Chapter 5 of the review, you read some background information about Turner syndrome and discover that growth hormone supplementation is now widely used to try to increase adult height of girls with Turner syndrome.[7] You read further that the Canadian Growth Hormone Advisory Committee has published an interim analysis of a randomized study to final height results.[17] Details are given in Appendix 13. This study recruited 154 girls aged 7–13 years. Of these, data were available on 69 (40 treated and 29 controls). The trial used randomization to initially create the two groups; however, the loss of 45 of 154 (29%) subjects could have influenced results if the losses were associated with the results of the treatment. The mean growth hormone effect on adult height (controlling by regression analysis for the difference in baseline height between the two groups) was 6·5 cm ± 1·1 cm. No categorical data were abstracted so the number needed to treat (NNT) could not be computed. Completion of the trial and replication of these results by a second trial in progress[18] are important.

In Chapter 8, you read that McCaughey *et al.* have published the only randomized studies of the use of growth hormone to increase adult height in healthy short children.[19] Details are given in Appendix 19. This study recruited 18 girls (mean age 8 years) out of 40 eligible. Of these 18, data were available on the 13 who completed the trial (seven treated subjects and six control subjects). The mean duration of treatment was 6·2 years. The trial used randomization to initially create the two groups; however, the loss of 5 of 18 (28%) of subjects could have influenced results if the losses were associated with the results of the treatment. The difference between the two groups was 7·5 cm. No categorical data were abstracted so the NNT could not be computed. There are three statistical concerns with adopting this evidence, all of which may be removed by replication. First, this is the only study of its kind. Second, the sample size is small, leading to large confidence intervals, especially when dichotomizing results in order to calculate the NNT. Finally, the original study recruited males and females.[20] While it is understandable that the female patients could be analyzed while the males were still growing, because females tend to mature earlier, the results from the male patients will be needed to show whether the effect of growth hormone supplementation is similar in both genders. If the results are not as positive in the males, the outstanding possibilities will be either that there is an interaction meaning that growth hormone supplementation is only effective in females or that this subgroup analysis was a spurious result which should not replace the overall average. Only completion and replication of the study can distinguish between these possibilities.

Resolution of the scenario

Your history and physical examination allow you to be somewhat reassuring about your patient's health as there are no symptoms or signs to suggest an underlying endocrine, genetic, renal, or gastrointestinal disease, or an intracranial space-occupying lesion, and there is no evidence of psychological difficulties associated with this child's short stature. The undocumented report of poor linear growth recently leads you to perform diagnostic tests for the rare causes of short stature that would be important not to miss: you order an 8:00 a.m. sample for cortisol and thyroxine to assess for panhypopituitarism, a TSH level for primary hypothyroidism, a karyotype for Turner syndrome, and screen for celiac disease with antigliadin, endomysial, and transglutaminase antibodies, and for inflammatory bowel disease with a hemoglobin, platelet count, and sedimentation rate. You exclude renal disease with electrolytes including serum calcium and phosphate, urea and creatinine, a capillary or venous blood gas, and urinalysis and pseudohypoparathyroidism with a PTH level. You schedule a repeat appointment in 6 months to remeasure height and calculate height velocity and assess

pubertal development. You also order a bone age x ray which will be significantly delayed if the patient has either constitutional delay or some of the rarer diseases. You consider that, if the child has a normal height percentile for target height range and you can demonstrate a normal growth velocity, a bone age x ray is not necessary unless there is a need to give a height prediction. If the patient does not have a normal height velocity, further evaluation, including growth hormone stimulation testing, will be necessary. With respect to the question of treatment, you decide that it is appropriate to be prudent and not pursue growth hormone for healthy children with idiopathic short stature, but will discuss the option and actual evidence on growth hormone supplementation if your patient is diagnosed with Turner syndrome.

Future research needs

- Systematic review on how sensitive and specific are the items from the medical interview, clinical signs, and laboratory tests in detecting the underlying health problems contained in the differential diagnosis along with primary studies to close the gaps in the diagnostic evidence
- Qualitative and quantitative research to understand the real concerns of specific groups of patients with short stature and on the ethical implications of attempts to enhance height along with a systematic review
- High quality controlled trials that are designed to provide randomized evidence directly on the true clinical outcomes for specific groups of patients

Summary table

Question	Type of evidence	Result	Comment
Diagnostic work-up for short stature	2 cohort studies	> 95% of children with short stature have no pathology; growth hormone deficiency is very rare, 1/15 000, 3·5% in a group of children with significant short stature	Documentation of a normal height velocity is critical in deciding that no pathology is present; limited investigations can rule out chronic disease (see scenario resolution)
Psychological outcomes of short stature	Cohort studies in the general population and in subjects referred for growth evaluation	Short stature during childhood, adolescence, or adulthood is generally not associated with any psychological disability	Teasing and babying may present challenges to the child with short stature
Use of growth hormone in non-growth hormone-deficient patients with short stature	1 RCT in girls with Turner syndrome, an interim analysis in abstract form; 1 very small published RCT in girls with short stature but no underlying illness	Studies report average treatment effects of 6·5 cm (Turner syndrome) and 7·5 cm (girls with idiopathic short stature). Treatment effects stated to be variable between patients	RCT in healthy girls was very small and 5/18 lost to follow up, replication needed as insufficient evidence to change practice policies. No results on psychosocial outcome or quality of life available from these trials

References

1 Hall DMB, editor. Health for all children. *Report of the Third Joint Working Party on Child Health surveillance. 3rd edn.* Oxford: Oxford University Press, 1996.

2 Freeman JV, Cole TJ, Chinn S, Jones PRM, White EM, Preece MA. Cross sectional stature and weight reference curves for the UK, 1990. *Arch Dis Child* 1995;**73**:17–24.

3 Committee on Nutrition. American Academy of Pediatrics. Prevention of pediatric overweight and obesity. *Pediatrics* 2003;**112**:424–30.

4 Goldbloom RB, editor. *Pediatric Clinical Skills. 2nd edn.* New York: Churchill Livingstone, 1997.

5 Tanner J. Auxology. In: Kappy MS, Blizzard RM, Migeon CJ, eds. *The diagnosis and treatment of endocrine disorders in childhood and adolescence. 4th edn.* Springfield USA: Charles C Thomas, 1994.

6 Parens E. Is better always good? The Enhancement Project. *Hastings Center Report 1998*; Supplement (January–February 1998):S1–S17.

7 Bryant J, Cave C, Mihaylova B *et al.* Clinical effectiveness and cost-effectiveness of growth hormone in children: a systematic review and economic evaluation. *Hlth Technol Assess* 2002;**6**(No. 18).

8 Voss LD, Mulligan J, Betts PR, Wilkin TJ. Poor growth in school entrants as an index of organic disease. *BMJ* 1992;**305**:1400–2.

9 X-iu-lan B, Yi-fan S, Yong-chang D, Rong L, Jie-ying D, Su-min G. Prevalence of growth hormone deficiency of children in Beijing. *Chin Med J* 1992;**105**:401–5.

10 Sandberg DE, Voss LD. The psychosocial consequences of short stature: a review of the evidence. *Best Pract Res Clin Endocrinol Metab* 2002;**16**:449–63.

11 Richardson WS, Wilson MC, Guyatt GH, Cook DJ, Nishikawa J, for the Evidence-Based Medicine Working Group. Users guide to the medical literature. XV. How to use an article about disease probability for differential diagnosis. *JAMA* 1999;**281**:1214–19.

12 Guyda HJ, Friesen HG, Bailey JD, Leboeuf G, Beck JC. Medical Research Council of Canada therapeutic trial of growth hormone: first five years of therapy. *CAMJ* 1975;**112**:1301–9.

13 Taback SP, Dean HJ, and members of the Canadian Growth Hormone Advisory Committee. Mortality in Canadian children with growth hormone (GH) deficiency receiving GH therapy 1967–1992. *J Clin Endocrinol Metab* 1996;**81**:1693–6.

14 Hamilton J, Blaser S, Daneman D. MR imaging in idiopathic growth hormone deficiency. American *J Neuroradiol* 1998;**19**:1609–15.

15 Taback SP, Van Vliet G, Guyda HJ. Pharmacologic manipulation of height: qualitative review of study populations and designs. *Clin Invest Med* 1999;**22**:53–9.

16 Reiter EO, Kaplan S. Growth and disorders of growth. In: Rudolph AM, Hoffman JIE, Rudolph CD, eds. *Rudolph's Pediatrics.* Stamford: Appleton and Lange, 1996.

17 Canadian Growth Hormone Advisory Committee. Growth hormone treatment to final height in Turner syndrome: a randomized controlled trial. *Horm Res* 1998;**50**(Suppl. 3): 25(Abs P7).

18 Ross JL, Feuillan P, Kushner H, Roeltgen D, Cutler Jr. GB. Absence of growth hormone effects on cognitive function in girls with Turner syndrome. *J Clin Endocrinol Metab* 1997;**82**:1814–17.

19 McCaughey ES, Mulligan J, Voss LD, Betts PR. Randomised trial of growth hormone in short normal girls. *Lancet* 1998;**351**:940–4.

20 Walker JM, Bond SA, Voss LD, Betts PR, Wootton SA, Jackson AA. Treatment of short normal children with growth hormone – a cautionary tale? *Lancet* 1990;**336**: 1331–4.

45 Attention deficit hyperactivity disorder

James P Guevara, Martin T Stein

Case scenario　*Your first patient of the morning is brought in by his parents for evaluation of school problems. By history, he has always been described as "on the go". When he was 4 years old, a preschool teacher expressed concern that, at times, his activity level limited play with some of the other children. Now, in the middle of the second grade, he is underachieving and not keeping up with either reading or arithmetic lessons. His teacher reports that he moves constantly, and he cannot keep his hands off the other children. Friendships are limited and not sustained. His teacher suggested that he be evaluated by his primary care clinician, so his parents have come to you for this and to discuss treatment options.*

Background

Attention deficit hyperactivity disorder (ADHD) is among the most common disorders that affect children and adolescents.[1] The hallmarks of this disorder are hyperactivity, impulsivity, and inattention that are beyond normal developmental expectations for a child's age, occur across multiple settings, begin prior to the age of 7 years, and are associated with clinically significant impairment.[2] The diagnostic criteria for ADHD from the *Diagnostic and statistical manual of mental disorders, 4th edition* (DSM-IV) are displayed in the Box. According to DSM-IV, children should meet diagnostic criteria in order to receive a diagnosis of ADHD.

Diagnostic criteria for ADHD (DSM-IV)*

A. Either (1) or (2):

(1) Six (or more) of the following symptoms of inattention have persisted for at least 6 months to a degree that is maladaptive and inconsistent with developmental level:

Inattention

(a) Often fails to give close attention to details or makes careless mistakes in schoolwork, work, or other activities

(b) Often has difficulty sustaining attention in tasks or play activities

(c) Often does not seem to listen when spoken to directly

(d) Often does not follow through on instructions and fails to finish schoolwork, chores, or duties in the workplace (not due to oppositional behavior or failure to understand instructions)

(e) Often has difficulty organizing tasks and activities

(f) Often avoids, dislikes, or is reluctant to engage in tasks that require sustained mental effort (such as schoolwork or homework)

(g) Often loses things necessary for tasks or activities (e.g., toys, school assignments, pencils, books, or tools)

(h) Is often easily distracted by extraneous stimuli

(i) Is often forgetful in daily activities

(2) Six (or more) of the following symptoms of hyperactivity-impulsivity have persisted for at least 6 months to a degree that is maladaptive and inconsistent with developmental level:

Hyperactivity

(a) Often fidgets with hands or feet or squirms in seat

(b) Often leaves seat in classroom or in other situations in which remaining seated is expected

(c) Often runs about or climbs excessively in situations it is inappropriate (in adolescents or adults, may be limited to subjective feelings of restlessness)

(d) Often has difficulty playing or engaging in leisure activities quietly

(e) Is often "on the go" or often acts as if "driven by a motor"

(f) Often talks excessively

Impulsivity

    (g) Often blurts out answers before questions have been completed

    (h) Often has difficulty awaiting turn

    (i) Often interrupts or intrudes on others (e.g., butts into conversations or games)

B. Some hyperactive-impulsive or inattentive symptoms that caused impairment were present before age 7 years

C. Some impairment from the symptoms is present in two or more settings (e.g., at school (or work) and at home)

D. There must be clear evidence of clinically significant impairment in social, academic, or occupational functioning.

E. The symptoms do not occur exclusively during the course of pervasive developmental disorder, schizophrenia, or other psychotic disorder, and are not better accounted for by another mental disorder (e.g., mood disorder, anxiety disorder, dissociative disorder, or a personality disorder)

*Reprinted with permission from the *Diagnostic and statistical manual of mental disorders, 4th edn.* Copyright 1994 American Psychiatric Association.[2]

For those children who don't meet DSM-IV criteria for ADHD, the *Diagnostic and statistical manual for primary care, child and adolescent version* (DSM-PC) was developed to guide clinicians.[3] The DSM-PC provides a description of common behavior problems followed by characteristic symptoms. These symptoms describe a spectrum from normal childhood variations to the disorder level found in DSM-IV. The intent of the DSM-PC is to classify common behavior problems and provide a guide for primary care clinicians in their evaluation of behavior problems in children and adolescents. However, limited empirical work has been performed to confirm the validity of the DSM-PC format.

ADHD is frequently diagnosed in children who present to primary care providers with behavioral problems or academic underachievement.[4] Although the diagnosis of ADHD can be made reliably in children using a standardized approach,[5,6] concerns regarding the validity of the diagnosis of ADHD often arise. Evidence supporting the validity of ADHD as a diagnosis comes from multiple sources[7]:

- cohort studies that consistently show similar long-term outcomes for children identified with ADHD;
- twin studies that demonstrate higher concordance rates of ADHD among monozygotic twins than among dizygotic twins or related siblings;
- genetic studies that show higher rates of gene alterations involving dopamine neurotransmission in those with ADHD;

- brain imaging and physiological studies that show a greater proportion of abnormalities among those with ADHD than similar controls.

At present there is no biological marker that reliably identifies those with ADHD. It is unclear whether the symptoms of ADHD represent a unique disorder or merely one end of the continuum of age-appropriate behavior.[7,8]

Framing answerable clinical questions

You wonder how likely it is that a school-age boy with academic difficulties and disruptive behaviors has ADHD, what tests will help you diagnose ADHD, whether stimulant medications or other treatments might work, and what this child's prognosis is, if he really has ADHD. These questions can be framed in a way that ensures they address the target population, the intervention, the event or exposure, and the specific outcome of interest. In addition, each question can be classified according to the type of information that is sought: causation, diagnosis, therapy, risk, or prognosis. You develop five specific questions to address:

Questions

1. In school-aged children (*population*), what is the likelihood of ADHD (*outcome*)? **[Baseline Risk]**
2. In school-age children (*population*) with ADHD (*exposure*), what is the likelihood of additional psychiatric disorders (*outcome*)? **[Baseline Risk]**
3. In school-age children (*population*) suspected of having ADHD (*exposure*), what is the usefulness of behavior rating scales and other tests (*intervention*) in the diagnosis of ADHD (*outcome*)? **[Diagnostic Test]**
4. In school-age children (*population*) with ADHD (*exposure*), what is the effectiveness of stimulant medications, other psychotropic medications, and/or behavioral treatments (*intervention*) on ADHD behaviors (*outcome*)? **[Therapy]**
5. In school-age children (*population*) with ADHD (*exposure*), what is the long-term risk of persistence of ADHD symptoms, delinquency, school failure, or development of substance abuse disorders (*outcome*)? **[Prognosis]**

Searching for evidence

You start your search by looking for evidence in three locations: the Cochrane Database of Systematic Reviews (CDSR),[9] *Clinical Evidence*,[10] and the Centre for Evidence-Based Mental Health (CEBMH).[11] You recognize that these sites contain high quality evidence summaries. You use the online search engines for CDSR and CEBMH by typing in the search terms below without limits. For *Clinical Evidence*, you scan the table of contents and find one chapter devoted to ADHD with available references. Finally, you perform a search of electronic databases using Ovid to identify additional high quality syntheses or clinical trials. You type in the search terms below for each database and limit your search to children and to studies published between 1996 and 2003. You scan the resulting titles and abstracts for systematic reviews, meta-analyses, and clinical guidelines.

Searching for evidence syntheses

- *Cochrane Library:* attention deficit disorder with hyperactivity (14 hits)
- *Clinical Evidence:* attention deficit hyperactivity disorder in children (4 hits)
- *Center for Evidence-based Mental Health:* attention deficit hyperactivity disorder (98 hits)
- MedLine (Ovid), CINAHL, HEALTHstar, EMBASE, PsycINFO: limit to years 1998–2003

   Attention deficit disorder with hyperactivity AND child AND diagnosis (245 hits)

   Attention deficit disorder with hyperactivity AND child AND (drug therapy OR behavior therapy OR cognitive therapy) (98 hits)

   Attention deficit disorder with hyperactivity AND child AND prognosis (47 hits)

Your search of the *Cochrane Library* nets no systematic reviews from the CDSR but 14 abstracts from the Database of Abstracts of Reviews of Effects (DARE) of which seven appear relevant to your questions. Four are systematic reviews of stimulant medications and behavioral interventions, one is a systematic review of clonidine, one is a systematic review of carbamazepine, and the last is a systematic review concerning continuous performance testing in ADHD. The systematic review of carbamazepine, however, includes children with other behavioral disorders, so you decide to exclude it. Of the four reviews of stimulant medications and behavioral interventions, one was commissioned by the Canadian Coordinating Office for Health Technology Assessment (CCOHTA) in Ottawa,[12,13] one was sponsored by the Agency for Healthcare Research and Quality (AHRQ) in the United States,[14,15] one was commissioned by the National Coordinating Centre for Health Technology Assessment in the United Kingdom,[16] and one was published by a group of Canadian investigators.[17] One of the systematic reviews addresses the efficacy of a non-stimulant medication, clonidine, for the treatment of ADHD.[18] The final systematic review examined errors on continuous performance tests

between unmedicated children with and without ADHD and may address your question on the utility of various diagnostic tests.[19]

You search the latest edition of *Clinical Evidence* and find a section devoted to the treatment of ADHD in children. This section contains evidence on the efficacy of stimulant medications, clonidine, and behavioral interventions for the treatment of ADHD from three systematic reviews and one large randomized clinical trial. You previously identified the three reviews from the DARE database.[12,14,18] The randomized trial, known as the Multimodal Treatment Study of Children with ADHD (MTA), was a large multicenter trial in the US that compared the long-term effects of stimulant therapy, behavioral therapy, combination therapy, and usual care on outcomes in children with ADHD.[20]

Next, you search the website for the CEBMH and find that it contains an online journal with evidence-based reviews of the published literature concerning mental health disorders in children and adults. The journal is published quarterly and dates back to 1998. The reviews are organized by volume and study type, such as prevalence, treatment, or prognosis. Using its online search engine, you obtain 98 references, of which five appear relevant. One is a long-term trial of amphetamines versus placebo in children with ADHD.[21] One is a meta-analysis of the effects of stimulant medications on aggression in ADHD.[22] One is a cohort study of the educational prognosis of children with attentional difficulties.[23] The remaining two were previously identified in your search of the *Cochrane Library*.[17,18]

Finally, you search electronic databases to supplement your search to date. After reviewing the long list of titles and abstracts, you find three reviews, a meta-analysis, and two clinical guidelines that appear relevant. The first review is too brief to be of much help in addressing your questions on diagnosis or treatment, so you exclude it. Of the remaining two reviews, one is a qualitative systematic review of psychosocial interventions for children with ADHD,[24] while the other is qualitative review of drug therapy and prognosis in children with ADHD.[25] The meta-analysis is a quantitative synthesis of cohort studies of children with ADHD for the later development of substance abuse.[26] Your search also identifies two clinical practice guidelines from the American Academy of Pediatrics (AAP) concerning the diagnosis and treatment of ADHD in children.[6,27] Since clinical guidelines are often based on evidence reports or technology assessments, you decide to examine these two papers closely. The guideline on ADHD diagnosis refers to a systematic review of the prevalence of ADHD, prevalence of coexisting disorders, and the utility of diagnostic tests for ADHD among school-age children.[28] Meanwhile, the guideline on ADHD treatment refers to one of the systematic reviews of stimulant therapy and behavioral interventions that you previously identified from the DARE database.[14]

Critical review of the evidence

Question

1. In school-age children (*population*), what is the likelihood of ADHD (*outcome*)? **[Baseline Risk]**

You look for population-based studies that address this question, since referral samples may overestimate prevalence. In the systematic review by Green *et al.*,[28] a description of the search strategy indicates that the authors undertook a comprehensive search for evidence using multiple electronic databases, hand-searches of the reference lists of articles and a published clinical guideline on ADHD, and requests for additional citations from American Academy of Pediatrics (AAP) members. The inclusion criteria for the review limited studies to those which included children ages 6–12 from non-referred samples in communities, schools, or clinics. No scoring system was used to grade the quality of the included articles, so you wonder whether studies of poor quality may have influenced their findings.

Ten of the 14 articles included in this review were published between 1982 and 1996, and made determinations of prevalence based on either DSM-III or DSM-IIIR criteria. All 10 articles reported data by gender, age, and setting with a range of overall prevalence between 4% and 12%. With the use of a random effects model to pool data due to significant heterogeneity (in measurement methods, populations, and informants), the pooled prevalence estimates were 6·8% (95% CI 5·0%, 9·0%) with DSM-III criteria and 10·3% (95% CI 7·7%, 13·4%) with DSM-IIIR criteria. A single study published in 1998 using DSM-IV criteria reported a similar prevalence rate of 6·8%. The prevalence of ADHD was 3-fold higher for males (9·2%; 95% CI 5·8%, 13·6%) than for females (3·0%; 95% CI 1·9%, 4·5%) but not significantly higher in community settings (10·3%; 95% CI 8·2, 12·7) than school settings (6·9%; 95% CI 5·5, 8·5). The results did not vary by age. Two additional studies reported the prevalence of ADHD in clinic settings as 2·0% and 4·8%. Parents reported higher prevalence rates than physicians or teachers.

In summary, prevalence estimates of ADHD vary widely from 2% to 12%, as a result of differences in the setting (school, community, or clinic samples), diagnostic criteria (DSM-III, DSM-IIIR, or DSM-IV), gender of subjects, or type of informants (parent, physician, or teacher). Ideally, you would like to examine baseline risk among school-aged boys who present with academic difficulties or disruptive behaviors similar to your patient, since you suspect that baseline risk will be higher, but you are unable to identify such studies.

Question

2. In school-age children (*population*) with ADHD (*exposure*), what is the likelihood of additional psychiatric disorders (*outcome*)? **[Baseline Risk]**

This question concerns the prevalence of co-occurring psychiatric disorders. The systematic review by Green *et al.* includes a section on the prevalence of co-occurring psychiatric disorders among children ages 6–12 years with ADHD and can be used to answer this question.[28] Prevalence data are reported for oppositional-defiant disorder, conduct disorder, depressive disorder, anxiety disorder, and learning disabilities. The results were combined across age and gender categories, so you will be unable to determine age and gender-specific prevalence rates. No overall combined estimate of the prevalence of all coexisting psychiatric disorders is given.

The review cited five studies that met inclusion criteria and reported prevalence rates of various psychiatric disorders with DSM-III or DSM-IIIR criteria. Four of these studies used unscreened populations, while one study used a screened population. In the latter study, the study population completed a screening instrument, and only those who had elevated scores were evaluated further for psychiatric disorders. The authors pooled the rates for each disorder using a random-effects model. Results indicated that coexisting psychiatric disorders were relatively common in children with ADHD, with pooled prevalence estimates of 35% for oppositional-defiant disorder (95% CI 27·2, 43·8%), 25% for conduct disorder (95% CI 12·8, 41·3%), 18% for depressive disorders (95% CI 11·1, 26·6%), and 25% for anxiety disorders (95% CI 17·6, 35·3%). A single study reported on the prevalence of learning disabilities and found a rate of 12%. Over 28% of children had more than one coexisting disorder (95% CI 7·6, 56·3%). One additional study reported prevalence figures using DSM-IV criteria. The results from this study were consistent with the pooled estimates, except for a lower rate of conduct disorder at 10%. Prevalence of coexisting disorders from the two clinic samples varied widely from 8% to 59% depending on the specific disorder. No confidence intervals were given here.

In summary, coexisting psychiatric disorders appear to be frequently diagnosed in children with ADHD, ranging from 8% to 59%. Published prevalence data on these disorders in children with ADHD vary due to differences in study setting, diagnostic criteria, and methodologies. No information on other important coexisting disorders, for example substance abuse disorders, was given.

Question

3. In school-age children (*population*) suspected of having ADHD (*exposure*), what is the usefulness of behavioral

Table 45.1 Summary of sensitivity, specificity, and likelihood ratios for ADHD diagnostic tests

Diagnostic test	Sensitivity (%)	Specificity (%)	LR+
ADHD-specific scales			
Conners ADHD Index	94	94	15·7
Conners DSM-IV Scale	95	95	19·0
Barkley School Situation	85	85	5·7
ACTeRS Subscales	85	85	5·7
DSM SNAP Checklist	97	97	32·3
Broadband checklists			
Global Scales	80	80	4·0
Externalizing Scales	80	80	4·0
Internalizing Scales	70	70	2·3
Adaptive Functioning	72	72	2·6
Continuous performance tests	70	70	2·3

rating scales and other tests (*intervention*) in the diagnosis of ADHD (*outcome*)? **[Diagnostic Test]**

This question concerns the validity and reliability of diagnostic tests in the evaluation of children with ADHD. You seek to address whether these tests can reliably distinguish children with ADHD from those without. Studies that independently and blindly compare each test to a gold standard, in this case the DSM criteria, will be able to answer this question. A good starting point is to peruse the AAP clinical practice guideline on the diagnosis of ADHD.[6] You recall that this guideline was informed by the systematic review by Green *et al.*, which contains a section on diagnostic testing for ADHD.[28] This section examines the accuracy of behavioral screening tests and medical screening tests in the diagnosis of ADHD in children aged 6–12 years from any clinical setting. A second systematic review by Losier *et al.* examined the usefulness of continuous performance tests in differentiating unmedicated children with and without ADHD.[19] This latter review undertook a systematic search of MedLine and PsychLIT databases and hand-searches of the reference lists of included studies to identify relevant trials. Only high quality studies were eligible. However, the authors restricted the analysis to studies published in English, so you wonder whether there were relevant studies published in other languages or non-published studies that were excluded.

Behavioral rating scales were designed as tools to screen for psychiatric disorders. In general, these scales use a checklist format, which can be quickly scored. Behavioral rating scales fall into two general categories: ADHD-specific and broadband checklists. ADHD-specific checklists contain items relevant to specific ADHD-associated behaviors, while broadband screens contain items relevant to a number of common behavioral disorders of which ADHD is one. The systematic review by

Green *et al.* examined 10 ADHD-specific checklists including subscales and seven broadband checklists. Other published checklists were not included in the review, because data on their sensitivity and specificity could not be found. The pooled results from these studies were reported as effect sizes, which represent the number of standard deviations separating the ADHD and non-ADHD populations. Effect sizes were converted into sensitivity and specificity, although the methods for this conversion are unclear.

ADHD-specific checklists adequately discriminate between children with and without ADHD (Table 45.1). The combined effect size for all the ADHD-specific checklists including subscales was 2·9 (i.e., a difference of 2·9 standard deviations on average between children with and without ADHD). This was translated into a sensitivity and specificity of approximately 94% (each), or a likelihood ratio for a positive test of > 15. ADHD-specific checklists were divided into overall scales and subscales that measure hyperactivity or inattention and impulsivity components of the disorder. Of the overall scales, the Conners DSM-IV Symptoms Scales, both teacher and parent versions, performed best, and Barkley's School Situations Questionnaire performed worst. The combined effect size for the hyperactivity subscales was 3·4; the DSM-III SNAP Hyperactivity Subscale performed best, while the ACTeRS-Parent Version Hyperactivity Subscale performed worst. Effect sizes were not combined for the inattention and impulsivity subscales, but effect sizes ranged from 2·0 for the ACTeRS-Parent Version Attention subscale to 5·5 for the DSM-III SNAP Checklist Impulsivity Subscale. Reliability may be limited, however, because effect sizes for each checklist were calculated from single studies.

Next, you look at the broadband checklists. The outcome measure for the analysis was ability to discriminate between populations referred and not referred to mental health for ADHD evaluation, rather than ability to discriminate between populations with and without ADHD. You feel that they do not sufficiently discriminate between these populations, with likelihood ratios of 2–4.

Continuous Performance Tests (CPT) were developed to provide an objective measure of inattention, impulsivity, and vigilance, and take up to 30 minutes to administer. Green *et al.* evaluated 12 studies of this type of test in children with ADHD. Despite heterogeneity in types of tests and measurement methods, the data from the studies were pooled and reported as effect sizes. All 12 studies found statistically significant differences in errors of commission or omission in many of the subscale areas measured between children with and without ADHD. When the data were pooled, the combined effect sizes were small, ranging from 0·49 (95% CI 0·03, 0·96) for vigilance to 0·62 (95% CI 0·10, 1·14) for inattention. Effect sizes < 1·0 were converted into sensitivities and specificities of < 70% or likelihood ratios of < 3 for a positive test. The systematic review by Losier *et al.* also calculated effect sizes for the difference in CPT measures between unmedicated children with and without ADHD. They found similar effect sizes of 0·67 for omission and 0·73 for commission. Unlike the previous review, they did not convert effect sizes into likelihood ratios.

Next, you evaluate the use of imaging studies of the central nervous system (CNS). Green *et al.* evaluated nine imaging studies. In two studies, no differences were found in the CNS between children with and without ADHD by computerized tomography. In the other seven studies, several differences in the CNS architecture were noted. These differences involved the size, shape, symmetry, and volume of various CNS structures. However, these differences were not consistent from study to study, and it is not clear whether these differences are unique to ADHD. You wonder whether they may occur in other neurodevelopmental disorders.

Finally, you examine the evidence for electroencephalographic (EEG) studies in the diagnosis of ADHD. Eight studies were abstracted and reviewed by Green *et al.* No significant EEG abnormalities were discovered in children with ADHD in any of the eight studies. Although seven studies found significant EEG differences between children with and without ADHD, these differences were not consistent from study to study.

In summary, you decide that the evidence supports the inclusion of ADHD-specific checklists in the assessment of children for ADHD. ADHD-specific rating scales can reliably discriminate between children with and without ADHD, while broadband checklists and Continuous Performance Tests do not. Neuroimaging and EEG tests are of little assistance in the evaluation of children for ADHD.

Question

4. In school-age children (*population*) with ADHD (*exposure*), how effective are stimulant medications, other

psychotropic medications and/or behavioral treatments (*intervention*) on ADHD behaviors (*outcome*)? **[Therapy]**

Stimulant medications

Stimulant medications have been the mainstay of treatment for ADHD for the past sixty years.[1,25] They are the most commonly used class of medication for ADHD and account for 80–90% of all psychotropic medications prescribed for children with ADHD.[29] Recent estimates have shown a 2·5 fold increase in the use of stimulants in the USA from 1990 to 1995.[30] Answers to questions regarding the effectiveness of therapy are best derived from RCTs in which patients and study investigators are blinded to treatment assignments. Systematic reviews or meta-analyses in which the results of randomized trials are pooled together also provide solid evidence.

To address the short-term effectiveness of stimulant medications on ADHD, you examine the systematic reviews by Miller *et al.*,[12,13] Gilmore and Milne,[16] Schacter *et al.*,[17] and Connor *et al.*[22] The first three syntheses examined the short-term effect of stimulant medications on ADHD-specific behaviors, while the latter synthesis examined the short-term effect of stimulants on aggression. The authors of all of these reviews undertook comprehensive searches of multiple electronic databases, hand-searches of the reference lists of key articles and book chapters, made requests for data from drug manufacturers, and/or contacted experts in the field to identify potential trials. All restricted inclusion to randomized clinical trials. You are concerned that relevant studies may have been excluded by Miller *et al.*, Schacter *et al.*, and Connor *et al.*, since these reviews only selected published English-language trials. All the reviews incorporated a quality assessment scale to evaluate study quality. You regard all four as high quality syntheses to address your questions on short-term therapy.

To determine the long-term effect of stimulants, you examine the systematic review by Jadad *et al.*[14,15] The authors of this review undertook a comprehensive search to identify relevant trials including a systematic search of electronic databases from 1966, a search of the *Cochrane Library*, hand-searches of the bibliographies of eligible articles, and searches of the personal files of the research team. Trials were included if they were published in peer-reviewed journals in any language, evaluated a treatment for ADHD in children or adults, and were randomized trials. The authors used a quality score based on randomization procedures, blinding, and withdrawals to evaluate for bias. Because of significant heterogeneity among the included trials, the authors did not pool results but rather reported outcomes qualitatively. You regard this as a high quality synthesis to address your question regarding long-term therapy.

Short- and long-term systematic reviews show consistent benefits of stimulants over placebo across studies (Table 45.2).

Table 45.2 Summary of sudies for ADHD interventions versus placebo

Intervention	Comparison*	Studies (n)	Outcomes	Effects (95% CI)
Stimulants				
Miller[12,13]	M, A, P	18	Behavior rating scales	Parents: 0·86 (1·14, 0·58) Teachers: 1·03(1·21, 0·84)
Gilmore and Milne[16]	M	11	QALYs	5·7 QALYs gained by M
Schacter[17]	M	62	Behavior rating scales	Parents: 0·54 (0·40, 0·67) Teachers: 0·78 (0·64, 0·91)
Connor[22]	M, A, P	28	Overt/covert aggression scales	Overt: 0·84 (0·70, 1·02) Covert: 0·69 (0·21, 1·29)
Jadad[14,15]	M, A	12	Behavior rating scales Academic performance Social behavior	M, A >placebo (4/6 studies) M, A >placebo (3/7 studies) M, A >placebo (6/9 studies)
Non-stimulants				
Jadad[14]	I, D	9	Behavior rating scales	D >placebo (6/6 studies) I = placebo (3 studies)
Connor[18]	C	11	Vigilance measures Behavior rating scales	Overall: 0·58 (0·27, 0·39)
Behavioral therapy				
Pelham[24]	B, Cog	68	Behavior rating scales	B >placebo Cog = placebo
Miller[12,13]	B, Cog	2	Behavior rating scales	Teachers: 0·40 (−0·48, 1·28) Parents: 0·49 (−0·29, 1·27)
Combination therapy				
Miller[12,13]	Com	2	Behavior rating scales	Teachers: 3·78 (−0·51, 8·06) Parents: 7·35 (2·40, 12·29)
Jadad[14,15]	Com	20	Behavior rating scales Aggression scales	Com = Meds (6 studies) Com = B (15 studies)

Abbreviations: A amphetamine; B, behavioral training; C, clonidine; Cog, cognitive behavioral training; Com, combination therapy; D, desipramine; I, imipramine; M, methylphenidate; P pemoline; QALYs, quality adjusted life years.

Effect sizes on behavior rating scales and aggression scales were in the moderate to large range. Overall, the results stood up when the analysis was restricted to high quality studies. One trial in particular, the MTA study, contributed over 40% of all the subjects to the Jadad review on long-term efficacy and was considered a high quality trial.[20] This trial found that stimulants given by strict protocol were superior to behavioral therapy or usual care. However, in two subpopulations from the MTA study, those with comorbid anxiety disorders and those on public assistance, stimulant medications were not superior to behavioral therapy.[31]

The review by Gilmore and Milne estimated that long-term treatment with methylphenidate would result in 5·7 quality adjusted life years (QALY) gained when compared with placebo. These authors assumed an increase in QALY associated with treatment of 0·086, a drop-out rate of 6% per year, and a response rate of 70%. Results were relatively insensitive to differing assumptions regarding response rates and drop-out rates. There was little evidence for improvement in academic performance associated with stimulant therapy.

To address the question of relative effectiveness between stimulants, the systematic review by Jadad *et al.* compared stimulant medications directly.[14,15] Of 18 studies included, two studies compared different isomers of either methylphenidate or amphetamine, and reported conflicting results: *d*-methylphenidate was better than l-methylphenidate in improving attention, while *d*-amphetamine and *l*-amphetamine were not significantly different. Three studies compared sustained release versus regular methylphenidate and found no differences. Nine studies compared methylphenidate versus dextroamphetamine. Of these nine studies, eight reported no statistically significant difference between the two, while one reported an advantage of methylphenidate over dextroamphetamine. Two studies compared methylphenidate versus pemoline and showed no statistically significant differences between the two. One study of dextroamphetamine versus pemoline found no significant differences between the two. Finally, one study compared all three medications and found them to be generally equivalent. Case reports of fatal hepatotoxicity associated with pemoline, however, may limit its use.[32]

Non-stimulant medications

The systematic review by Jadad *et al.* examined the evidence for the effectiveness of tricyclic antidepressants (TCAs).[14] The synthesis included nine studies that compared the effectiveness of TCAs to placebo: six of desipramine and three of imipramine. Five of the six studies showed a benefit of desipramine over placebo on parent and teacher ratings of behavior. Only one of the three studies of imipramine reported a beneficial effect over placebo on parent and teacher ratings of behavior. Jadad *et al.* also compared the relative effectiveness of stimulants versus TCAs. Four studies

met criteria for head-to-head comparisons between stimulants and TCAs. One study found benefits in favor of stimulants, while another found benefits in favor of imipramine. It appears that more rigorous studies are needed to help resolve this dilemma. Reports of sudden death in patients receiving TCAs may limit their use.[33]

Bupropion, another antidepressant, has been found to have beneficial effects on ADHD-specific behaviors relative to placebo.[34] No comparisons have been made to stimulants, and there are no systematic reviews that have reviewed its effects. The AAP treatment guideline lists it as a second-line medication for the treatment of ADHD along with TCAs.[27]

The meta-analysis by Connor *et al.* compared clonidine, a central-acting adrenergic agonist, to placebo for the treatment of ADHD.[18] The authors of this study likewise undertook a comprehensive search of electronic databases and non-peer reviewed research reports and book chapters – so-called gray literature – to identify eligible studies. However, their search was limited to English-language papers, so you wonder whether relevant studies published in other languages were excluded. Eligibility criteria included studies with adult patients as long as the mean study age was < 18 years. The authors included 11 trials in their meta-analysis, only eight of which were randomized. You again decide to restrict your focus to only the randomized studies to limit the influence of bias. In these studies, clonidine was superior to placebo on parent, teacher, and clinician behavioral ratings (weighted effect size = 0·58). No comparison was made to stimulants. However, most studies reported greater adverse effects, notably sedation and irritability, in clonidine-treated patients. In addition, one study reported clinically-significant brady-cardia in a single child on clonidine.

A novel non-stimulant, atomoxetine, has recently been introduced. This drug is an inhibitor of the presynaptic norepinephrine transporter and has a similar side effect profile as stimulants. In randomized double-blind clinical trials, atomoxetine was superior to placebo on ratings of behavior in children with ADHD.[35,36] Trials of these sort are considered best to guard against bias. A single open-label study compared atomoxetine to stimulants and found it equivalent on ADHD-specific behaviors, but you are concerned that bias may have influenced the results.[37] You conclude that this drug has not been studied rigorously vis-à-vis stimulants, so you are unsure of its relative effects. A potential advantage of atomoxetine is its long duration of action with a single dose and its non-controlled substance status as compared to stimulants.

Behavioral treatments

Psychosocial treatments are commonly used in the treatment of ADHD, either alone or in combination with medications. Psychosocial treatments used in the treatment of ADHD include cognitive-behavioral therapy, parent and teacher behavior modification therapy, and intensive contingency management therapy. Pelham *et al.* systematically reviewed the evidence for the effectiveness of such treatments.[24] The authors undertook a comprehensive literature search and included articles that met the requirements of the Task Force on the Promotion and Dissemination of Psychological Procedures. However, these requirements are not clearly specified. Few details are given of the search strategy, inclusion/exclusion criteria, or details of the studies identified, so you are left to wonder whether important studies were overlooked or excluded. Fifty-eight articles were selected for inclusion in the review. The data were not pooled, but instead were examined qualitatively. The results of this review indicated that there is little evidence that cognitive-behavioral therapies improve the behavior or academic performance of children with ADHD. On the other hand, behavior modification and contingency management consistently demonstrated a beneficial effect on parent and teacher ratings of behavior across studies. A quality score was not used, so you are unsure whether the findings would hold up among higher quality studies.

Combination therapy pairs medications with psychosocial interventions. Intuitively, you think this intervention may be better adapted to address the wide array of problems in children with ADHD. The systematic review by Miller *et al.* reviewed the short-term efficacy for combined medical and psychological/behavioral treatments on teacher and parent ratings of behavior and identified three studies that met their criteria.[12,13] The results indicated that combination therapy may be more efficacious than placebo or no treatment but was not significantly different from medication alone. Jadad *et al.* also reviewed the published literature on combination treatments for ADHD.[14,15] The results, although qualitative in nature, are similar to the results of the review by Miller. Six studies compared combination treatments with stimulants alone, and showed little difference between combination treatments and stimulants alone on parent and teacher ratings of ADHD-specific behaviors. This suggests that psychosocial treatments add little to the effect of stimulant medications in general.

The MTA study, which was published after most of the reviews above, compared the long-term effects of stimulant therapy, behavioral therapy, combination therapy, and usual community care.[20] The MTA study randomized 579 children ages 7–10 years to one of the treatment arms for a period of 14 months. Follow up was excellent and intention-to-treat analysis was used. However, you are concerned that the strict medication titration regimen may not be feasible in your clinical setting. Combination and medication-only treatments were superior to behavior treatments and community care in reducing ADHD symptoms, but were not different from each other on this and other individual measures. However, combination therapy was superior to medications alone when individual behavioral measures were combined into a single composite score.[38] Combination therapy was also superior to medications alone among children with comorbid anxiety

and among those on public assistance. Finally, combination therapy was superior on measures of parental satisfaction.[20,31]

In summary, stimulant medications are efficacious in improving ADHD-specific behaviors and aggression when compared to placebo. There appears to be little difference among types or formulations of stimulants. Among non-stimulant medications, TCAs, bupropion, clonidine, and atomoxetine may have beneficial effects in children with ADHD, but they have not been studied as extensively as stimulants. Adverse effects associated with clonidine and TCAs may limit their usefulness. Psychosocial interventions, namely behavioral modification and contingency management, demonstrate positive effects on ADHD-specific behaviors. The addition of psychosocial interventions to medications does not show a benefit over medications alone on most outcome measures, but combination therapy may provide modest benefits over medications alone among children on public assistance and those with comorbid anxiety and on composite measures of behavior and on parental satisfaction.

Question

5. In school-age children (*population*) with ADHD (*exposure*), what is the long-term risk of persistence of ADHD symptoms, delinquency, school failure, or substance abuse (*outcome*)? **[Prognosis]**

This question concerns the long-term risk of adverse outcomes for young school-age children with ADHD. Studies of prognosis are best answered by prospective cohort studies that follow children with ADHD and a comparable group of children without ADHD over time until relevant outcomes occur. Systematic reviews and meta-analyses of cohort studies may best answer your question, since they systematically search and pool the results of all relevant studies.

The review by Elia *et al.*, which included nine studies that prospectively followed cohorts of children with ADHD from school age until adolescence or early adulthood, may answer your question.[25] The search strategy and inclusion criteria were not stated in the article, so you are concerned about bias in the selection of studies. In addition, baseline characteristics of the children in each of the studies are not listed, so you are concerned that the studies may have preferentially enrolled children from referral populations. Data from the various studies were not pooled but reported in a qualitative fashion. In addition, no quality measure was used, so you wonder whether the results hold up among higher quality studies.

The results from Elia *et al.* indicated that symptoms of ADHD abate over time, but a significant number still met criteria for ADHD as adults. The proportion of older adolescents who continued to meet criteria for ADHD ranged from 22% to 71%, and the proportion of young adults who continued to meet diagnostic criteria ranged from 4% to 50%. In addition, of those who did not meet explicit criteria for

ADHD, many still exhibited residual symptoms of ADHD as young adults (up to 66%).

Elia *et al.* also found that the prevalence of conduct disorder and substance abuse disorders was significantly greater among adolescents and young adults with ADHD than peers without ADHD. Among studies that followed children from adolescence into young adulthood, the proportion with conduct disorder diminished, while the proportion with substance abuse disorder did not. The proportion with conduct disorder in late adolescence ranged from 27% to 42%, and in early adulthood from 10 to 18%. In the two studies that looked at the prevalence of substance abuse, the data were conflicting, with one study showing a smaller proportion with substance abuse disorder and the other study showing no change.

To determine the risk for development of substance use disorders associated with stimulant therapy, you examine the meta-analysis by Wilens *et al.*[26] This study systematically reviewed the published literature using PubMed and the proceedings of scientific meetings to identify published and unpublished retrospective and prospective cohort studies of children with ADHD that contained information on substance use outcomes in adolescence or adulthood. Inclusion criteria were not explicitly stated, so you wonder whether the included studies contained children similar to yours. In addition, no quality assessments were performed, so you are unsure whether the results hold up in more rigorously conducted studies. The authors pooled results using a random-effects model and evaluated for publication bias. The authors found that stimulant therapy increased the odds of not having a substance use disorder (odds ratio 1·9; 95% CI 1·1–3·6) compared to no stimulant therapy, suggesting a protective effect of stimulants.

To determine the risk of academic failure among children with ADHD, you examine the prospective cohort study by Fergusson *et al.*, which you found on the CEBMH web site.[23] This study followed a birth cohort of 1265 children born in an urban region of New Zealand until age 18 years. Children were not formally diagnosed with ADHD, but were divided at age 8 into five groups of increasing attentional difficulties based on a combined behavioral rating scale. You suspect that children in the highest percentiles of attentional difficulties (96–100%) may be most likely to have ADHD. Children in this highest group of attentional difficulties incurred the highest proportion of school failures (60%) by age 18. This proportion was statistically significantly greater than the group with the lowest percentiles of attentional difficulties, even after adjusting for conduct problems, demographic factors, school factors, and family factors.

In summary, the available evidence regarding prognosis may be limited by bias, but results suggest that symptoms of ADHD diminish over time. However, up to 50% of adolescents and young adults may still meet criteria for ADHD, and a significant number of others may exhibit symptoms compatible with ADHD. While the prevalence of conduct and substance abuse disorders appears greater in children with ADHD, this may

diminish as children grow older. The risk of school failure in children with attentional difficulties is significantly greater than in those without attentional difficulties. Evidence suggests that stimulant therapy decreases the risk of substance abuse, but there is no evidence that treatment alters the risk of persistence of ADHD, delinquency, or school failure.

Resolution of the scenario

The baseline prevalence of ADHD in school-age boys is 9%, and likely to be higher for children with academic or behavioral problems, so you decide to evaluate your patient for this disorder. You decide to incorporate into your evaluation ADHD-specific checklists, specifically the Conners Parent and Teacher Rating Scales, since they have likelihood ratios in excess of 15 and use DSM-IV diagnostic criteria. If his rating scales are elevated and he meets diagnostic criteria for ADHD, you estimate his post-test probability of ADHD to be approximately 65% using the LR nomogram. Owing to insufficient evidence, you decide against the use of Continuous Performance Tests, neuroimaging, or EEGs in the evaluation. Given a diagnosis of ADHD, you estimate that he has a probability of between 18% and 35% of having one or more of the following additional disorders: oppositional-defiant, conduct, anxiety, or depression so you decide to screen for these disorders. Since the evidence for the effectiveness of stimulants is strong and consistent across studies, you recommend these as first-line medications. You inform parents that behavioral treatments, namely behavior modification and contingency management, may be added, but the combination treatment may not be any better than stimulants alone for improving ADHD-specific behaviors but may be superior on overall functioning and parental satisfaction. Following the evaluation, you inform the parents that ADHD is a chronic disorder that may persist into adolescence and young adulthood, and therefore regular monitoring will be necessary.

Future research needs

- The baseline risk of ADHD for school-age children who present with academic difficulties or behavior problems to their clinicians is unknown. Knowing this information would help you to adjust your baseline risk estimates more precisely.
- The relative effects of non-stimulant medications compared to stimulant medications are unclear. Future studies that compare non-stimulant medications directly with stimulants may help to clarify the relative effectiveness of these medications.
- The prognosis for substance abuse may be ameliorated by stimulant therapy, but the effects of treatment on prognosis for persistence of symptoms, academic failure, or delinquency are largely unknown. Decisions to initiate and maintain treatment can be influenced heavily by the potential for improvements in these long-term risks.

Summary table

Question	Type of evidence	Result	Comment
Prevalence (baseline risk) of ADHD in the general population	Systematic review of population-based surveys (10 studies published between 1982 and 1996)	6·8% (CI, 5·0–9·0) using DSM-III 10·3% (CI, 7·7–13·4) using DSM-IIIR Male rate 3 x higher than female No variability by age	Significant heterogeneity among studies owing to measurement methods, setting, and informants
Risk of comorbid psychiatric disorders	Systematic review of population-based surveys (5 studies)	Oppositional-defiance: 35% Conduct disorder: 25% Depressive disorders: 18% Anxiety disorders: 25% Learning disabilities: 12% Multiple disorders: 28%	Only 1 study reporting learning disabilit es. Significant heterogeneity among studies owing to measurement methods, setting, and informants
Usefulness of tests in diagnosis of ADHD	Systematic review of studies using DSM criteria as gold standard	Behavioral rating scales: LR >15 for ADHD-specific scales; LR = 2–4 for broadband checklists; LR < 3 for continuous performance tests; EEG, CNS imaging not useful in diagnosis	Connors DSM-IV Symptom Scales and SNAP subscales performed best
Effectiveness of medications and behavioral treatments	Systematic reviews of RCTs using behavior rating scales as outcome	Methylphenidate, dextroamphetamine, and pemoline all equally effective; tricyclics, bupropion, clonidine, and atomoxetine also appear effective; Behavioral treatments effective; Combination therapy not better than medications alone	Stimulants are best studied, while non-stimulants have limited evidence for effectiveness without rigorous comparisons to stimulants; fatal hepatotoxicity associated with pemoline and sudden death with tricyclics; combination therapy superior to medications alone among children on public assistance and those with anxiety and on measures of satisfaction and overall functioning
Long-term prognosis for children with ADHD	Systematic reviews of cohort studies	ADHD symptoms abate but 21–70% still have symptoms as older adolescents, 4–50% meet diagnostic criteria as adults. Risk of conduct disorder but not substance abuse decreases in adulthood. Up to 60% may experience academic failure by age 18	Few studies, results vary widely, most studies draw from referral populations. Stimulants may decrease later risk of substance abuse

References

1 Goldman L, Genel M, Bezman R, Slanetz P. Diagnosis and treatment of attention-deficit/hyperactivity disorder in children and adolescents. *JAMA* 1998;**279**:1100–7.

2 American Psychiatric Association. *Diagnostic and statistical manual of mental disorders. 4th edn.* Washington, DC: American Psychiatric Association, 1994.

3 American Academy of Pediatrics. *The classification of child and adolescent mental diagnoses in primary care. diagnostic and statistical manual for primary care (DSM-PC).* Elk Grove Village, IL: American Academy of Pediatrics, 1996.

4 Mulhern S, Dworkin P, Bernstein B. Do parental concerns predict a diagnosis of attention-deficit hyperactivity disorder? *J Dev Behav Pediatr* 1994;**15**:348–52.

5 American Academy of Child and Adolescent Psychiatry. Practice parameters for the assessment and treatment of children, adolescents, and adults with attention-deficit/hyperactivity disorder. *J Am Acad Child Adolesc Psychiatr* 1997;**36**(Suppl.):85S–121S.

6 American Academy of Pediatrics, Committee on Quality Improvement, Subcommittee on Attention-Deficit/ Hyperactivity Disorder. Clinical practice guideline: diagnosis and evaluation of the child with attention-deficit/hyperactivity disorder. *Pediatrics* 2000;**105**:1158–70.

7 Anonymous. Diagnosis and treatment of attention deficit hyperactivity disorder (ADHD). NIH Consensus Statement. 1998 Nov 16–18:1–37.

8 Carey W. Problems in diagnosing attention and activity. *Pediatrics* 1999;**103**:664–6.

9 The Cochrane Collaboration. The *Cochrane Library* of Systematic Reviews. http://www.cochranelibrary.com/cochrane/

10 BMJ Publishing Group. *Clinical evidence.* London: *BMJ* Publishing Group, 2002.

11 Centre for Evidence-based Mental Health. Department of Psychiatry, University of Oxford, UK. http:/cebmh.warne.ox.ac.uk/cebmh/

12 Miller A, Lee S, Raina P, Klassen A, Zupancic J, Olsen L. *A review of therapies for attention-deficit/hyperactivity disorder.* Ottawa, Canada: Canadian Coordinating Office for Health Technology Assessment (CCOHTA), 1998.

13 Klassen A, Miller A, Raina P, Lee SK, Olsen L. Attention-deficit hyperactivity disorder in children and youth: a quantitative systematic review of the efficacy of different management strategies. *Can J Psychiatr* 1999;**44**:1007–16.

14 Jadad A, Boyle M, Cunningham C, Kim M, Schachar R. *Treatment of attention-deficit/hyperactivity disorder. Evidence report/technology assessment No. 11*, AHRQ Publ No. 00-E005. Rockville, MD: Agency for Healthcare Research and Quality, 1999.

15 Schachar R, Jadad AR, Gauld M, *et al.* Attention-deficit hyperactivity disorder: critical appraisal of extended treatment studies. *Can J Psychiatr* 2002;**47**:337–48.

16 Gilmore A, Milne R. Methylphenidate in children with hyperactivity: review and cost-utility analysis. *Pharmacoepidemiol Drug Safety* 2001;**10**:85–94.

17 Schachter HM, Pham B, King J, Langford S, Moher D. How efficacious and safe is short-acting methylphenidate for the treatment of attention-deficit disorder in children and adolescents: a meta-analysis. *CMAJ* 2001;**165**:1475–88.

18 Connor DF, Fletcher KE, Swanson JM. A meta-analysis of clonidine for symptoms of attention-deficit hyperactivity disorder. *J Am Acad Child Adolesc Psychiatr* 1999;**38**:1551–9.

19 Losier BJ, McGrath PJ, Klein RM. Error patterns on the continuous performance test in non-medicated and medicated samples of children with and without ADHD: a meta-analytic review. *J Child Psychol Psychiatr* 1996;**37**:971–87.

20 The MTA Cooperative Group. A 14-month randomized clinical trial of treatment strategies for attention-deficit/hyperactivity disorder. *Arch Gen Psychiatr* 1999;**56**:1073–86.

21 Gillberg C, Melander H, Von Knorring A, *et al.* Long-term stimulant treatment of children with attention-deficit hyperactivity disorder symptoms: a randomized, double-blind, placebo-controlled trial. *Arch Gen Psychiatr* 1997;**54**:857–64.

22 Connor DF, Glatt SJ, Lopez ID, Jackson D, Melloni RH. Psychopharmacology and aggression. I: a meta-analysis of stimulant effects on overt/covert aggression-related behaviors in ADHD. *J Am Acad Child Adolesc Psychiatr* 2002;**41**:253–61.

23 Fergusson D, Lynskey M, Horwood L. Attentional difficulties in middle childhood and psychosocial outcomes in young adulthood. *J Child Psychol Psychiatr* 1997;**38**:633–44.

24 Pelham W, Wheeler T, Chronis A. Empirically supported psychosocial treatments for attention deficit hyperactivity disorder. *J Clin Child Psychol* 1998;**27**:190–205.

25 Elia J, Ambrosini P, Rapoport J. Treatment of attention-deficit-hyperactivity disorder. *N Engl J Med* 1999;**340**:780–8.

26 Wilens TE, Faraone SV, Biederman J, Gunawardene S. Does stimulant therapy of attention-deficit/hyperactivity disorder beget later substance abuse? a meta-analytic review of the literature. *Pediatrics* 2003;**111**:179–85.

27 American Academy of Pediatrics, Subcommittee on Attention-Deficit/Hyperactivity Disorder, Committee on Quality Improvement. Clinical practice guideline: treatment of the school-aged child with attention-deficit/hyperactivity disorder. *Pediatrics* 2001;**108**:1033.

28 Green M, Wong M, Atkins D, *et al. Diagnosis of attention-deficit/hyperactivity disorder. Technical Review No. 3.* AHCPR Publication No. 99–0050. Rockville, MD: Agency for Health Care Policy and Research, 1999.

29 Safer D, Krager J. A survey of medication treatment for hyperactive/inattentive students. *JAMA* 1988;**260**:2256–8.

30 Safer D, Zito J, Fine E. Increased methylphenidate usage for attention deficit disorder in the 1990s. *Pediatrics* 1996;**98**:1084–8.

31 The MTA Cooperative Group. Moderators and mediators of treatment response for children with attention-deficit/hyperactivity disorder: the Multimodal Treatment Study of Children with Attention-Deficit/Hyperactivity Disorder. *Arch Gen Psychiatr* 1999;**56**:1088–96.

32 Sheveli M, Schreiber R. Pemoline-associated hepatic failure: a critical analysis of the literature. *Pediatr Neurol* 1997;**16**: 14–16.

33 Biederman J, Thisted RA, Greenhill LL, Ryan ND. Estimation of the association between desipramine and the risk for sudden death in 5- to 14-year-old children. *J Clin Psychiatr* 1995;**56**:87–93.

34 Connors CK, Casat CD, Gauitieri CT, *et al.* Bupropion hydrochloride in attention deficit disorder with hyperactivity. *J Am Acad Child Adolesc Psychiatr* 1996;**35**:1314–21.

35 Michelson D, Faries D, Wernicke J, *et al.* Atomoxetine in the treatment of children and adolescents with attention-deficit/hyperactivity disorder: a randomized placebo-controlled, dose-response study. *Pediatrics* 2001;**108**:e83.

36 Biederman J, Heiligenstein JH, Faries DE, *et al.* Efficacy of atomoxetine versus placebo in school-age girls with attention-deficit/hyperactivity disorder. *Pediatrics* 2002;**110**:e75.

37 Kratochvil CJ, Heiligenstein JH, Dittmann R, *et al.* Atomoxetine and methylphenidate treatment in children with ADHD: a prospective, randomized, open-label trial. *J Am Acad Child Adolesc Psychiatr* 2002;**41**:776–84.

38 Conners CK, Epstein JN, March JS, *et al.* Multimodal treatment of ADHD in the MTA: an alternative outcome analysis. *J Am Acad Child Adolesc Psychiatr* 2001;**40**: 159–67.

46 Cerebral palsy

Adam Scheinberg, Maureen E O'Donnell, Robert Armstrong, Katrina Williams

Case scenario

A 12-month-old boy who was born prematurely is brought to see you by his parents. They are concerned with his slow development, in particular that he is not yet sitting. On examination, motor delay is confirmed. Increased tone in both arms and legs is noted, greater in his legs with brisk tendon reflexes bilaterally. His hips are not dislocatable. A provisional diagnosis of cerebral palsy (CP) of spastic diplegia type is made. He has just started in a therapy program but the parents want to know whether starting the program sooner would have made a difference in his physical development. Twelve months later his parents bring him for further review. They would now like to know if it is likely that he will walk. He is sitting independently. When he is 4 years old you see him again. His parents are keen to improve his ability to walk. So far he has been treated with ankle foot orthoses and has been consistent about wearing them. They report that they have been faithfully completing their home stretching and strengthening program. On physical examination he can walk approximately 20 meters with a hand held aid, before he appears fatigued.

Background

Cerebral palsy has been defined as a symptom complex rather than a specific disease.[1] The more common definition is that of "a disorder of movement and posture that is non-progressive in nature".[2] However, the many definitions of CP in use today attest to the variability of presentation.

The symptom complex was first described in a lecture to the London Obstetrics Society in 1862 by the English surgeon William Little.[3] At that time, and into the recent past, it was believed that CP was caused by a difficult delivery. Freud, however, had suggested that CP may be caused by an abnormality in the fetus prior to delivery.[4] This suggestion has been strengthened by more recent epidemiological studies,[5–7] particularly in those children born at term who later develop CP.

The motor signs associated with CP are normally seen within the first 2–3 years of life. However, making a diagnosis early in life can be problematic because of the possibility that the abnormal motor signs are either a feature of a less severe disorder, such as transient dystonia in the first year of life, or another metabolic, genetic, or neurological disorder that is not yet apparent. In addition, although the cerebral insult resulting in CP is non-progressive, the motor signs may evolve and change over time. This makes both diagnosis and reports of prevalence and incidence problematic. Furthermore, agreement between clinicians on the classification and severity of CP has been noted to be poor.[8]

The clinical classification systems for CP are numerous,[8–10] with the majority classifying according to the extremities involved, and the form of tone abnormality. The groupings include diplegia, tetraplegia (quadriplegia), hemiplegia, dyskinetic, and ataxic CP, as well as spastic, hypotonic, dystonic, athetoid, or a combination of these. Associated disabilities may include impaired cognition and visuoperceptual disturbance, vision and hearing impairment, oromotor problems, and seizure disorder. The complications of the motor disorder, such as muscle contracture, bony abnormalities (scoliosis, hip dislocation), and loss of bone density with easy fractures also affect the function of the affected child and his or her family.

The prevalence of CP has remained relatively constant over time,[1] despite the increase in occurrence of spastic diplegia within the broader diagnostic group. The relatively large numbers of children with a diagnosis of CP coupled with the heterogeneity of presentation and problems have encouraged the development of widely varying therapeutic interventions. Some interventions are targeted at the motor impairment while others have been developed to address the secondary disabilities associated with the disorder.

To date, motor interventions have mainly focused on remediation of spasticity. Interventions have included oral and intrathecal medication administration, physiotherapy and occupational therapy, neurological and orthopaedic surgery, and methods to achieve motor end plate paralysis (botulinum toxin A and phenol).

This chapter aims to answer some of the questions commonly asked by care-givers of children with CP, using an evidence-based approach.

Framing answerable clinical questions

The issues that arise from the scenario can be reframed into structured questions that will clarify your thinking and help with your search. You frame the following questions:

Questions

1. In children with CP (*population*), does early intervention (*intervention*) improve function (*outcome*)? **[Therapy]**

2. How likely is it that children with CP (population), who are able to sit at 2 years (*exposure*), will be able to walk with or without assistive devices (*outcome*)? **[Prognosis]**

3. In young children with spastic diplegia, who have bilateral lower limb spasticity but can ambulate 10 m with or without aids (*population*), are oral antispasticity medications such as oral baclofen, diazepam, and dantrolene (*intervention*), effective in improving gait (*outcome*)? **[Therapy]**

4. In young children with spastic diplegia, who have bilateral lower limb spasticity but can ambulate 10 m with or without aids (*population*), is intrathecal baclofen treatment (*intervention*) effective in improving gait (*outcome*)? **[Therapy]**

5. In young children with spastic diplegia, who have bilateral lower limb spasticity but can ambulate 10 m with or without aids (*population*), is botulinum toxin injection (*intervention*) effective in improving gait (*outcome*)? **[Therapy]**

6. In young children with spastic diplegia, who have bilateral lower limb spasticity but can ambulate 10 m with or without aids (*population*), does selective dorsal rhizotomy (*intervention*) improve gait (*outcome*)? **[Therapy]**

Searching for evidence

Searching for evidence syntheses

- *Cochrane Library*, *Best Evidence* and *ACP Journal Club*
- "spastic diplegia"
- "cerebral palsy"
- "baclofen", "diazepam", "dantrolene", "botulinum toxin", "rhizotomy"
- Further sources of evidence

MedLine, Embase, Cinahl, American Academy of Cerebral Palsy and Developmental Medicine, article reference lists, discussion with key informants in the field

- Further search strategies

  "spasticity" (limited to children)
  clinical trial (in combination with one of the terms related to CP)
  cohort studies (in combination with one of the terms related to CP)

You begin your search by looking at sources of evidence where a critical appraisal will already have been completed. First you search *Best Evidence*, then EBM reviews at the *ACP Journal Club* and finally the Cochrane Database of Systematic Reviews. You begin using only the key word "spastic diplegia" but find limited numbers of studies. You then decide to broaden your search to "cerebral palsy". *Best Evidence* still only yields two results, both papers on pregnancy and childbirth. The ACP Journal Club yields four abstracts; however, these again are on the subject of pregnancy and risk factors for CP. In the *Cochrane Library* 73 abstracts are displayed; however, when you review them, 69 refer to CP as an outcome of pregnancy, early delivery, or neonatal incidents. You do find two abstracts for reviews, which may be of interest in answering your questions. They are both in children with CP and include the use of botulinum toxin in the lower limbs and selective dorsal rhizotomy. During your Cochrane search you also note that several studies were selected in the Database of Abstracts of Reviews of Effects (DARE) section, of which at least six are relevant. You decide to come back to these when looking at the specific questions.

You recall hearing that the American Academy for Cerebral Palsy and Developmental Medicine (AACPDM) has established a "Treatment Outcomes Committee" whose responsibility it is to lead the critical review of the evidence supporting many of the common therapies and treatment used for children with CP. You decide to visit their website at http://www.aacpdm.org and you click on the "Committees" button and then the "Treatment Outcome Committee" page. At this site you find a number of valuable resources that will assist in critical review, as well as the four reports that have been posted to the site to date. One of these is relevant and you note that this was also listed in your DARE search.

You now decide to look for the relevant literature for each question by searching on MedLine (1966–present), and will include Embase (1988–present) and/or Cinahl (1983–present) if you find insufficient studies. You design a search strategy for each of your questions. The search strategies used for each question are shown below.

Critical review of the evidence

Question

1. In children with CP (population), does early intervention (*intervention*) improve function (*outcome*)? **[Therapy]**

MedLine (Ovid 1966 to present)	Number found
● Exp Cerebral Palsy/	7714
● Exp Early Intervention	3230
● Clinical Trial.pt.	351 564
● 1 AND 2 AND 3	7
● 1 AND 2	34

Your first strategy only yields seven papers, while the second (without restricting the publication type) yields a total of 34 papers. You review the abstracts of those papers and find that six are relevant articles. One of these is a systematic review; you decide to start with this paper by Turnbull,[11] but first you return to the Cochrane Database. Entering the search strategy above into the Cochrane Database yields five papers in the Controlled Trials sections, of which one paper published after Turnbull's review article is of interest. You also note two other studies that are listed from your MedLine search, also published after Turnbull's.

Early intervention for children with suspected cognitive and physical impairment has been recommended for several years and is a significant cost to the child, the family and the community. Parry[12] describes three broad groups of children for whom early intervention is offered. They are infants at environmental risk (owing to socioeconomic circumstances), infants with established developmental disability and infants at increased biological risk. You are interested in the evidence supporting intervention for the last two of these groups for your patient, although you are also aware that early intervention is a term used for a collection of different physical, educational and behavioral treatments. The hypothesis driving physical early intervention has been that early sensory input affects motor programming in children with underlying CP,[13] although the benefits of this intervention were questioned in the literature as early as 1984.[14] Despite the large cost in terms of time, money and emotional input, Turnbull[11] notes qualitative and quantitative analyses of valid scientific studies are lacking in the area of early intervention therapy for children at risk or with known CP. The research question is complicated, as it needs to differentiate between "motoric advances attributable to intervention and those that occur as a natural result of maturation".

You are aware that review articles may contain bias and therefore check to see whether it meets the aims of a meta-analysis (see Chapter 8 on systematic reviews, as well as Henry and Wilson[15]). In Turnbull's paper,[11] both quantitative (meta-analysis) and qualitative analyses of the known studies in the area were sought. Turnbull performed a systematic review of early intervention studies and no meta-analyses of early education intervention specifically for children with CP were found. However, reviews of 44 studies were reported. Six of those identified met minimum design standards and only one reported a positive effect of intervention.

The search strategy used for the meta-analysis is documented (MedLine and Psychlit and articles from previous reviews). To be included, subjects had to be children at risk or known to have motor disorders who were started on a clinically accepted therapy prior to 3 years of age. In addition, studies had to have outcome assessments performed using an objective test relevant to the stated aims of the therapy. A total of 17 studies met the author's criteria. The quantitative meta-analysis estimated a negligible effect size (weighted mean *d* index 0·16) and the author noted, with simple inspection, that the least scientifically rigorous studies had contributed the greatest effect sizes. There are also problems interpreting the clinical meaning of the summary statistic used.

As the second stage of his review, now more commonly the first phase, Turnbull scored each of the intervention studies included in the meta-analysis for methodological rigor. Two studies were excluded because they used neither a control nor a contrast group. Of the remaining fifteen studies only six scored > 8 using the Sackett scoring guidelines.[16] Of these, only one reported early intervention to be effective and that study was unblinded to treatment allocation. None of the studies that scored > 8 and looked specifically at early intervention for "at risk" infants reported a positive effect.

You read the more recent papers by Weindling,[17] McCormick,[18] and the abstract from Yi's paper[19] (as you are unable to obtain the journal). Both Weindling[17] and Yi[19] reported no difference in outcome in randomized controlled trials of early physiotherapy for high risk infants, and premature infants, respectively. McCormick's randomized trial (RCTs) assessed early education (home visits, center-based education, and parent support groups) in very low birth weight infants. The study did find some improvements in cognitive development scores and behavior, but no differences in functional status or general health rating. This information, coupled with the information from Turnbull's review, suggests that there is little evidence to support the efficacy or effectiveness of early intervention (physical therapy in particular) for children with, or suspected of having CP.

Questions

2. How likely is it that children with CP (*population*), who are able to sit at 2 years (*exposure*), will be able to walk with or without assistive devices (*outcome*)? **[Prognosis]**

MedLine (Ovid 1966 to present)	Number found
● Exp Cerebral palsy	7714
● (Walking OR gait).mp	6118
● Prognosis.tw OR exp survival analysis/	38 621
● 1 AND 2 AND 3	4

Table 46.1 Walking outcome for sitting at age 2 from Molnar's study

	Eventual walkers	Non walkers	
Sitting by 2	141	0	141
Not sitting by 2	46	46	92
Total	187	46	233

To answer the second question you are keen to find a prospective cohort study, which monitors the outcome of walking in relation to age of sitting. Your MedLine search yields 14 papers of which five are relevant. The first paper listed is a review article on the subject.[20] You decide to try different strategies to ensure that you are not missing other papers on the topic. You scan the reference list of the review and find two other relevant papers. From the combined searches you have seven papers that you are able to access from your library.

Clinicians seeing children with CP on a regular basis are frequently asked, "Will my child walk?" This important clinical question of whether it is possible to predict eventual ambulatory status in a child with CP has only been researched by a handful of studies.[21-27] On closer review of the articles you find that three were conducted retrospectively[22-24] and in one there is no reference to sitting as an exposure.[26]

Sala and Grant review the literature over the past 50 years regarding the prognosis for ambulation in children with CP.[20] They discuss three prognostic categories: primitive reflexes, gross motor skills, and type of CP. The reviewers did not report their search strategy or assessment procedure for the studies reported and no meta-analysis was performed. However, a MedLine search as detailed above did not uncover further relevant studies. The reviewers found that persistence of primitive reflexes (ATNR, STNR, Moro, tonic labyrinthine, and positive supporting) and absence of postural reactions were associated with poor prognosis for ambulation. The critical age for examining children for these signs was 2 years. Independent sitting at 2 years was found to be associated with a good prognosis for ambulation; however, not sitting by 2 years did not exclude ambulation. Children with hemiplegic CP were found to be most likely to achieve ambulation, with children with spastic diplegia being the next most likely group to walk.

You decide to look at the two remaining original studies. Molnar followed 233 children with CP from the age of 12 months until they were between 3 and 11 years.[21] The children included in this study were selected from a larger potential group of unknown number on the basis that they had been adequately followed up and had been prospectively observed. No information about children not included in the study is presented. This selection of children for the study is of concern because it is possible that the children followed up were systematically different to the population from which they were drawn. For instance, the ability to walk (*outcome*) might affect clinic attendance, with carers of children who walk being less likely to attend follow up because they do not perceive a need for ongoing support. If follow up decreased for walkers, then the pretest probability calculated from this data would be an underestimate of the true probability for the population. There might also be factors related to clinic attendance that have a systematic effect the relationship between age of sitting and eventual walking. This is particularly likely in a condition such as CP where the etiology is heterogeneous. This would alter likelihood ratios for both positive and negative tests.

You extract the raw data from Molnar's study so you can make sense of it for clinical work (Table 46.1). From it you calculate a positive and negative likelihood ratio (LR) using sitting by 2 as the "test" and eventual walking as the gold standard outcome, as shown (see Box). You remain concerned that these values may not be applicable to all children with this range of problems.

Pretest probability and likelihood ratios calculated from Molnar's study

- Pretest probability $187/233 = 0.80$
- Likelihood ratio for + test $(141/187) \div (0/46) =$ infinity
- Likelihood ratio for − test $(46/187) \div (46/46) = 0.25$

Because of your concerns about the representativeness of Molnar's sample of children, you also read Watt's study. They have complete follow up of 74 children[25] who were selected from a neonatal follow up cohort because a diagnosis of CP was made before the age of 2 years. You are concerned that neonatal intensive care unit survivors with CP may not be representative of all children with CP. With this reservation about generalizability in mind you decide to extract the data from the study (Table 46.2) and calculate LRs again (see Box) to compare them to the figures you generated from the Molnar paper.

Pretest probability and likelihood ratios calculated from Watt's study

- Pretest probability $47/74 = 0.64$
- Likelihood ratio for + test $(46/47) \div (1/27) = 26$
- Likelihood ratio − test $(1/47) \div (26/27) = 0.02$

Table 46.2 Walking outcome for sitting at age 2 from Watt's study

	Eventual walkers	Non-walkers	
Sitting by 2	46	1	47
Not sitting by 2	1	26	27
Total	47	27	74

You note that a slightly lower proportion of neonatal intensive care unit graduates walk eventually (0·64) than in the Molnar study (0·80). The positive likelihood ratios for both studies are very high, suggesting that children who are able to sit at age 2 are very likely to walk. The negative likelihood ratios are rather different in the two studies. In Watt's study, very few of those not sitting by 2 years walked later, while in Molnar's population half of those not sitting at 2 years became ambulant. These differences are greater than can be accounted for by chance and suggest that the predictiveness of failure to sit by 2 years will vary depending on the clinical situation. This problem of lack of applicability of tests is common in situations where the underlying condition is heterogeneous.

Question

3. In young children with spastic diplegia who have bilateral lower limb spasticity but can ambulate 10 m with or without aids (*population*), are oral antispasticity medications such as oral baclofen, diazepam, and dantrolene (*invervention*), effective in improving gait (*outcome*)? **[Therapy]**

MedLine (Ovid 1966 to present)	Number found
● Exp cerebral palsy	7714
● Exp baclofen/ OR exp dantrolene/ OR exp diazepam/	24 158
● Clinical trial.pt.	351 564
● 1 AND 2 AND 3	28

Using the search term "clinical trial.pt." is often the best single search strategy for study type when looking for articles on intervention, particularly in CP, as using only the search term "randomized trials" tends to give a low yield. In total, you are successful in finding one reference to oral baclofen, five references to dantrolene, and five references to diazepam. However, you note that the most recent of these studies is from 1980. You also are aware that a protocol has been listed on Cochrane for antispastic medication for spasticity in CP.[28] The protocol lists the reviewers' email addresses so you contact them, but continue your search while awaiting their reply.

Having completed the searches, you realize that some key articles are missing. You rerun the above searches using "child" and "muscle spasticity" instead of "cerebral palsy". You also try searching by each agent and the term "spasticity", which yields additional adult studies, including RCTs. This search reminds you that the phenomenon of "cerebral palsy" can be described by authors in many ways, and that multiple search strategies must be used, a situation that differs from a more well-defined or delineated disease where only one term clearly describes the condition.

Pharmacologic management of spasticity has been promoted as having a number of potential advantages over other treatments, such as surgical management. The ability to titrate dose with relative ease and effectiveness and to reverse the effect are possible important advantages. Pharmacologic intervention may reduce or even eliminate the amount of time spent in the hospital, away from daily activities.

A variety of pharmacologic agents are available to the clinician managing children with spasticity. Many drugs have been reported as having potential antispasticity effects, including diazepam, dantrolene, baclofen (oral and intrathecal), botulinum toxin A, tizanidine, and clonidine. Appropriate and effective use of these drugs is based not only on an awareness of the patient's condition, but also on the clinician's understanding of the drugs. Understanding of the principal mechanisms of action, potential side effects, short- and long-term adverse outcomes and the efficacy and effectiveness of such agents is essential.

In reviewing this literature, you must consider the quality of the evidence, including its applicability to your particular patient of interest. Consideration of the studies' patient populations is important in the review of spasticity management literature, as many efficacy studies have been completed in adults with spinal spasticity and may not be applicable to children. The outcome measures used must be reliable and valid, and reflect outcomes of interest to the child, family, and clinicians, the latter being a particular problem with early studies. Your consideration of the outcome measure in relation to the National Center for Medical Rehabilitation Research (NCMRR) Model of Dimensions of the Disabling Process's five dimensions (Table 46.3) will assist in assessment of the value and relevance of the evidence to the individual patient.

Diazepam

Diazepam (valium) was reported for use in CP in the early 1960s.[29] You remember that diazepam, a benzodiazepine, acts by enhancing presynaptic inhibition of primary afferent input in the spinal cord by facilitating or potentiating the effects of gamma-aminobutyric acid (GABA). The overall effect is a reduction in the release of excitatory neurotransmitters.

Table 46.3 National Center for Medical Rehabilitation Research Model of Dimensions of the Disabling Process

Dimension	Definition
Pathophysiology	The cellular and molecular processes of injury or disease pertinent to a particular condition
Impairment	Involves dysfunction of the organ system level resulting from a disease process or injury. Examples of impairment level outcomes include tone, spasms, or strength
Functional limitation	Defines limitation to the set of skills required to perform specific activities, either of the whole body or body segments. Examples include motor performance, self-care, activities of daily living
Disability	Defines difficulties in carrying out the role or function expected for an individual such as attending school, returning to work, partaking in age-appropriate recreation, improved quality of life
Societal limitations	Represents the barriers placed by society which limit full participation by people with disabilities. These barriers may be physical or attitudinal

You discover that the first randomized clinical trial of diazepam[29] for children with CP was a double-blind, randomized, placebo cross-over study of 25 children aged 1–14 years, with moderate to severe CP. The treatment group received diazepam in a dose of 0·4–0·5 mg lb^{-1} per day (which approximates 1 mg kg^{-1} per day) in addition to their established therapeutic regimen. Improvement was noted in 36%, primarily with respect to disruptive behavior rather than a change in tone. Side effects of lethargy and imbalance were found which caused difficulties with the children's meaningful participation in programs.

In contrast, you find that studies of diazepam's effectiveness in treating spasticity in adults with spinal cord lesions suggest a decrease in spasms and spasticity.[30–32] It is postulated that diazepam's antispastic effects occur centrally and directly at the spinal cord level, perhaps explaining this discrepancy in effectiveness in the two populations.[31–32]

In summary, for the group of children with spasticity of cerebral origin, you realize that the best quality evidence suggests that the effects of diazepam are essentially limited by unwanted side effects. You are also disappointed that no randomized clinical trials have gone beyond assessing diazepam's effect in the impairment dimension to the domains of functional limitations, disability or societal limitations.

Dantrolene

Dantrolene has been available and considered for use in spasticity management since the early 1970s and acts at the level of the muscle by decreasing calcium influx from the sarcoplasmic reticulum after membrane depolarization. This reduced calcium flux decreases the excitation-contraction coupling and essentially weakens the muscle,[33] particularly skeletal muscle.

You find three randomized clinical trials of dantrolene in children with CP. In 1973, Chyatte *et al.*[34] reported the use of dantrolene for 17 children and adults (age 7–38 years) with athetoid, not spastic, CP. Patients received between 5 and 25 mg four times daily, increased during the study to a maximum of 100 mg four times daily. A number of outcomes measures were assessed, including spasticity (through tendon reflexes, range of motion, and resistance to passive stretch), motor performance (active range of motion, time required for walking and stair climbing, muscle strength), and subjective assessment of functional performance, as indicated by activities of daily living (ADL). In analyzing their results, the authors found their objective tests lacked reliability. The subjective results, however, suggested that patients felt more motor control and better relaxation on dantrolene. Reported side effects included drowsiness and fatigue, with occasional mention of nausea. The authors concluded that, although results were subjectively measured, dantrolene had shown some benefit. It should be noted, however, that because of the concerns regarding the primary outcome measure, this evidence is weaker than one would expect from an RCT.

Haslam *et al.*[35] reported on the efficacy of dantrolene in a double-blind cross-over study of 23 children aged 1·5–17 years with spasticity thought to be related to perinatal events. Subjects received dantrolene (1 mg kg^{-1} per dose to a maximum of 12 mg kg^{-1} per day) or placebo. Spasticity was evaluated by reviewing ankle clonus, passive range of motion, spontaneous range of motion, reflexes, muscle tone, and scissoring. Dantrolene was associated with improvement in all outcomes except clonus. However, the improvement was statistically significant only for reflexes and scissoring. Tests of self-help skills were also reported as improved with dantrolene, but unfortunately the outcome measure used was not described well enough to allow an assessment of its reliability and validity. No serious side effects were documented, although strength was not assessed.

Denhoff *et al.*[29] gave dantrolene or placebo to 28 children with CP during a double-blind cross-over trial. Dantrolene was given in a dose between 4 mg kg^{-1} per day and 12 mg kg^{-1} per day. Neurological, motor, cognitive, and behavioral assessments were completed. Approximately half the patients showed some improvement while on dantrolene. Anecdotal subjective opinions of observers in the study were that none of the children had definite clinical improvement. However, this study was significantly weakened by concerns regarding the interrater reliability of the outcome measures and questions regarding adequate power.

In the adult rehabilitation literature, a number of studies have examined dantrolene-related outcomes such as strength and function, in addition to spasticity. Katrak[36] studied the effects of dantrolene (to a maximum dose of 200 mg per day) on adults who had spasticity of cerebral origin, secondary to a cerebrovascular accident. The analysis demonstrated reduced strength in the unaffected limb but unaltered strength in the paretic limb. There were no alterations in clinical tone, functional outcome, biochemical, or hematologic outcomes. This study is one of few that used controls, blinding, and objective measurable outcomes.

The side effects of dantrolene are potentially important. Weakness is the most common side effect, having secondary negative impact on function. Drowsiness, dizziness, general malaise, and fatigue can also occur. Nausea and gastro-intestinal upset have been noted. Liver dysfunction, as evidenced by blood chemistry, appears in 0·7–1·0% of patients, and deaths from dantrolene-associated hepatic injury have been reported in adults.[33]

In summary, the trials to date have not provided strong evidence of an effect of dantrolene on spasticity of cerebral origin, perhaps because of inadequate outcome measures and low study power. The adult studies, which suggest a beneficial effect on supraspinal spasticity, show that this effect often occurs in the presence of muscle weakening. In addition, the studies do not provide adequate evidence that dantrolene has a positive impact on the NCMRR domains beyond impairment, such as the domains of functional limitation, disability, or societal limitations. It is suggested, therefore, that perhaps dantrolene be used only for the treatment of spasticity for patients whose daily care is made difficult because of increased tone, and when the patient will accept the loss in voluntary power that may occur.[31]

Oral baclofen

Baclofen (beta-[4-chlorophenyl]-GABA) is a synthetic GABA agonist that acts selectively on GABA-B and has its effect at the spinal level. Different mechanisms have been suggested including an inhibitory effect on presynaptic transmitter release through the restriction of calcium influx into the presynaptic terminal[37] and an action at postsynaptic terminals, causing decrease in neuronal activity by increasing potassium conductance.[38] GABA-B receptors are concentrated in layers II and III of the dorsal gray matter of the spinal cord and at various other sites in the central nervous system, especially the thalamus.[39] Current thinking suggests that baclofen's effect may be potentiated by its ability to reduce the release of excitatory transmitters like substance P that can produce flexor spasm when activated, from nociceptive afferent nerve endings.[31]

You find few studies that examine the efficacy of baclofen in children with CP. A number of pediatric studies[40–43] suggest that baclofen is more effective than placebo in reducing spasticity. However, few controlled trials evaluate baclofen's effects on functional limitations. McKinley *et al.*[44] reported a double-blind cross-over trial of baclofen (up to 60 mg per day) compared to placebo for 20 children aged between 7 and 16 years with CP, attending a day school for children with physical disabilities. There is very little description of the reliability and validity of their outcome measures. No significant differences between baclofen and placebo were observed in muscle tone, clonus, extra-pyramidal symptoms, cerebellar symptoms, manual dexterity, speed of tongue movements, articulation speed, or respiratory function. Similarly, no change in the quality of gait was observed. Side effects of drowsiness, dizziness, and nausea were noted.

Although it is not an RCT, the only other pediatric study that looked at functional outcomes was a case–control study of 15 children (age 4–15 years) with hemiplegic CP and age- and sex-matched controls.[45] In this study, baclofen caused a significant decrease in hip and knee flexion at the toe-off phase in both legs. However, clinical and/or goniometric improvement in gait occurred in only 5/15 (33%) hemiplegic children. Side effects were evident, including sedation and deterioration of behavior and concentration. You recognize that the nature of this study design makes it lower level evidence.

The best evidence you can find to support the use of baclofen comes from clinical trials in adult patients with spinal cord injury, rather than children with spasticity of cerebral origin. For the most part, these studies have focused on the effect of baclofen on impairment-related outcomes. A number of double-blind placebo-controlled trials of baclofen in adult subjects with spasticity of spinal origin have been reported.[29,46–49] All examine outcomes related to spasticity, using the Ashworth Scale (Table 46.4). Patients were started on 5 mg twice or three times daily and increased to a maximum of 80 mg per day. With doses of 30–75 mg per day orally, a significant improvement in tone-related measures was noted.

You find other contradictory information, which suggests that approximately 25% of adults with spinal cord injury are unresponsive to oral baclofen[50] and that weakness and other side effects are commonly noted.[32]

In summary, you realize that there is some evidence in the literature from adult and pediatric randomized clinical trials for oral baclofen decreasing tone and spasticity. However, the evidence for a functionally significant effect appears to be

Table 46.4 Ashworth scale for grading spasticity

Score	Definition
0	no increase in muscle tone
1	slight increase in tone giving a "catch" when the limb is moved
2	more marked increase in tone but the limb is easily moved
3	considerable increase in tone, passive movement difficult
4	Limb rigid in flexion or extension

greatest for spasticity of spinal origin. You cannot find any evidence that suggests that reduced muscle tone results in improved motor function. No studies in children with CP have demonstrated a statistically significant, clinically important improvement in functional limitations, disability or societal limitation domains.

Question

4. In young children with spastic diplegia, who have bilateral lower limb spasticity but can ambulate 10 m with or without aids (*population*), is intrathecal baclofen treatment (*intervention*) effective in improving gait (*outcome*)? **[Therapy]**

MedLine (Ovid 1966 to present)	Number found
● Exp cerebral palsy	7714
● Exp infusion pumps, Implantable/ OR exp injections, Spinal/OR exp baclofen/OR intrathecal baclofen.mp	12 386
● Clinical Trial.pt.	351 564
● 1 AND 2 AND 3	14
● 1 AND 2	69

Intrathecal baclofen has received much attention in recent years as one of the newer treatments for spasticity. You discover that, although many papers have been published examining its use in spasticity, most are reports of case series with relatively few cohort studies or randomized clinical trials. Your attention is drawn, however, to an abstract of an evidence report by the AACPDM, which is available on their website. Having checked the Cochrane Collaboration previously, you remember that there is also a meta-analysis of intrathecal baclofen listed in the DARE section but your library does not hold the journal. Because of the ease of reviewing the AACPDM report on line, you start there.

Intrathecal administration of the drug was considered in an attempt to achieve a more direct effect and minimize the side effects seen with oral administration, as discussed above. With respect to pathophysiologic effects, Kroin et al.[51] observed that intrathecal baclofen (ITB) caused a significant reduction of polysynaptic reflexes in rabbits. In clinical trials, both reduced spasticity and improved clonus have been noted with ITB. Decreases in response to joint movement, H-reflexes, ankle clonus, and defensive reactions are notably suppressed in patients with spinal cord injury on EMG after ITB.[52,53] More recently, Dressandt[54] examined F-waves and demonstrated quantifiable alternations in the F-wave mean and maximum amplitude as well as mean duration following ITB.

The potential advantage of ITB over oral baclofen is a much smaller effective dose. For example, a 75 micrograms bolus dose intrathecally produces CSF levels 10 times those found in serum after a 100 times larger oral dose.[55] It should be noted, however, that individual pharmacokinetics vary significantly, with the elimination half-life ranging from 0·9 to 5·0 hours.[56] You realize that the trade-off of lower required dose and fewer side effects when baclofen is given intrathecally is that the administration involves surgical implantation of a pump delivery system, which has associated risk. The pump sits in a subcutaneous pocket within the abdomen and a catheter, which delivers baclofen, is threaded back and inserted into the subarachnoid space at the T12–L1 level.

During your search, you noted two recent papers[57,58] that reported on longer-term safety of intrathecal baclofen. Both studies found high rates of complications, including infection requiring removal, and device-related problems such as catheter breakage. Despite this, one of the studies reported that care-giver satisfaction with the treatment was high.[57]

You evaluate the AACPDM review by Butler.[59] Their literature search was done on MedLine from 1956 to 2000 searching for intrathecal baclofen and CP; reference lists in studies and review articles were checked, and researchers in the field consulted. The AACPDM classifies evidence into dimensions of disablement and then the level of evidence it represents. Butler found 17 relevant publications, with three subsequently excluded as they only included a few subjects with CP. Butler noted some of the difficulty with doing a systematic review, in finding that 10 of the selected studies consisted of investigations in three pools of subjects, with five of the studies reporting on a total of 137 participants who were not 137 separate individuals. Unfortunately, the probable overlap of the participants could not be determined. The AACPDM evidence reports include tables of evidence for all the relevant studies specifically reporting on interventions, participants, research methods, outcomes, and adverse effects. You note that there is level 1 evidence for only two short-term studies, by Albright[60] and Gilmartin.[61]

Albright's study[60] was of 19 children and four adults with spasticity due to CP, who participated in a randomized multiple cross-over study of bolus doses (not continuous infusion) of intrathecal baclofen. In Albright's study, lower extremity muscle tone as measured with the Ashworth scale was significantly reduced, but a significant change in upper extremity muscle tone could not be demonstrated. Gilmartin's study consisted of two phases, an initial screening and then an open label prospective trial. Results were similar to Albright's for the initial screening phase; however, you note that the second phase of the study was rated as level 5 evidence. There are also two n-of-1 randomized trials[62,63] (also known as single subject trials – randomized controlled trials in an individual patient), which provide some evidence of the treatment's longer-term efficacy. Both studies reported significant changes in ankle clonus and spasms. Almeida's study[62] also showed improvement in range of motion, although this did not persist over time. You note that, while most of the studies reported statistically significant improvements, these were mostly assessing changes in muscle tone. Six studies also evaluated functional limitations, and only one assessed disability/participation with level 5 evidence for the results.

From the AACPDM report, which reports evidence about uniformity of results within treated groups, you can see that there is level 1 evidence only for changes in muscle tone (impairment dimension) and level 5 evidence for functional, disability/participation, and societal dimensions. The AACPDM report importantly includes a table of adverse effects and medical complications. Butler notes that mechanical complications related to catheter and pump were generally reported to be minor and correctable, but that central nervous system effects were documented in at least four studies. Serious side effects occurred including meningitis in two children, and hospitalization was required for three others from somnolence and hypotonia. Butler concluded that intrathecal baclofen suppressed signs of spasticity in the lower extremities but that the level of evidence was generally weak with over three-quarters of the studies producing level 4 or 5 evidence.

In summary, you have found evidence of a reasonable quality to suggest a positive effect of intrathecal baclofen on spasticity, spasm, and exaggerated reflex responses. However, further study is required to delineate the effect of ITB on gross and fine motor function, activities of daily living, and quality of life ("disability" and "societal limitations" dimensions), as well as long-term side effects and complications. As such, you cannot make a strong recommendation to try intrathecal baclofen at this time.

MedLine (Ovid 1966 to present)	Number found
● Exp cerebral palsy	7714
● Exp Botulinum toxins	4916
● (Randomized controlled trial OR meta analysis).pt.	178 997
● 1 AND 2 AND 3	17

You are pleased that your search has uncovered several randomized trials. However, you are aware from speaking with colleagues that relevant systematic reviews have also been published, so you redo your search using "exp evidence-based medicine/ or exp meta-analysis/ or exp randomized controlled trials/ or systematic review.mp or exp review literature/". This yields additional relevant papers, including a systematic review by Boyd in 2001.[64] There is also a complete review listed on the Cochrane database by Hall[65]; however, you note that this was completed in 1999 and has not been updated since. In the introduction to Boyd's review,[64] the authors make the important point that, in studies of CP, subjects are often heterogeneous, so that positive and negative results within the cohort may cancel out if only main results, and not subgroup results, are reported. Many studies of childhood CP, particularly studies of interventions, have limited sample size, making subgroup analysis difficult. Boyd used a comprehensive search strategy using all major databases as well as abstracts from meetings and hand-searches of reference lists. All prospective studies including RCTs were included if they assessed the lower limbs of children with CP who had received botulinum toxin. A total of 116 papers were selected with 10 of them being RCTs. Meta-analysis was used to calculate the magnitude of the treatment effect, showing a pooled risk difference of 0·25 (CI 0·13, 0·37) for BTX-A against placebo, and 0·23 (CI −0·06, 0·527) for BTX-A against casting. This translates to 25% and 23% of the BTX-A treated groups compared to placebo and casting, respectively, improving by 2 or more points on an outcome measure, the Physician Rating Scale. You note that Boyd presents a table of grades of evidence for studies of lower limb botulinum toxin, and find level 1 evidence for BTX-A in "true equinus" (walking on the toes due to calf muscle spasticity) in children with diplegia and hemiplegia. Lower levels of evidence are present for other clinical presentations such as adductor spasticity causing scissoring and hamstring spasticity causing "apparent equinus".

Question

5. In young children with spastic diplegia, who have bilateral lower limb spasticity but can ambulate 10 m with or without aids (*population*), is botulinum toxin injection (*intervention*) effective in improving gait (*outcome*)? **[Therapy]**

Question

6. In young children with spastic diplegia, who have bilateral lower limb spasticity but can ambulate 10 m with or without aids (*population*), does selective dorsal rhizotomy (*intervention*) improve gait (*outcome*)? **[Therapy]**

MedLine Ovid 1966 to present	Number found
● Exp cerebral palsy/	7714
● Exp rhizotomy/ OR dorsal rhizotomy.mp	6203
● Clinical Trial.pt	3 515 644
● Metaanalysis.pt OR (review.pt AND medline.tw)	14 330
● 1 AND 2 AND 3	10
● 1 AND 2 AND 4	1

Selective dorsal rhizotomy is a surgical intervention for spasticity that involves the selective transection of dorsal nerve root tissue. The procedure has been popular in North America since the 1980s, but less so in Europe and Australia.

You begin your search using search terms "cerebral palsy", "rhizotomy", and "clinical trial", which yields a manageable 10 studies. However, you realize a review that you have previous knowledge of is missing. You search again substituting your publication type search strategy with the search term for systematic reviews. This yields a recent meta-analysis by McLauglin[66] and you confirm that no RCTs have been published following that paper. You also check the *Cochrane Library* and find a protocol for a review, which is expected shortly.[67] McLaughlin's meta-analysis was of three randomized trials comparing selective dorsal rhizotomy plus physiotherapy to physiotherapy alone, with the aim being to show whether selective dorsal rhizotomy significantly improves function in children with spastic CP 1 year after the operation. Although all three studies showed a significant reduction in spasticity, there was a difference in the functional outcomes with two studies showing an improvement with rhizotomy and the other showing no difference between the groups. The participants were all children with spastic diplegia without athetosis. For two of the studies the age range was 3–7, and for the other 3–18 years. Strengths of the meta-analysis were the ability to gather unpublished data for all the studies, which allowed pooling, and re-analysis of data, and that similar outcome measures were used for all the studies. McLaughlin reported that the pooled results of the three studies showed a small but statistically significant advantage to selective rhizotomy plus therapy. However, you note that the change on the Gross Motor Function Measure for the pooled studies was only 4%.

You contact a colleague who is familiar with this outcome measure, and are informed that 4% change is only marginally above the expected change with non-invasive treatment. You realize that although a statistically significant difference was noted in the studies, this may not equate to a clinically significant difference, which is more important to the child you are seeing.

Resolution of the scenario

At your first consultation, you were able to tell the family that early intervention was unlikely to have made a significant difference in their child's progress to date. If you were confronted with this question in the future for another child, with the child not yet showing signs of CP, other considerations might include the availability of this sort of intervention in their area and whether or not they can afford it. You would also need to know if early intervention can cause harm or if, alternatively, it has some other positive effect on family function and coping, which is not related to physical or functional outcomes of CP. You would need to discuss these issues with the parents, to assist them in making a decision, which uses the best available evidence along with their judgment about the relative values of the potential harms and benefits.

When you see the family at the 2-year follow up, you are pleased that your patient is sitting. You feel that you are able to confidently tell the parents that he is going to walk. You are pleased that you were able to find studies that presented clinical information that related to real life assessments and outcomes. It was an extra benefit that the clinical signs used did not require special training to elicit and were unlikely to change between observers or over time. However, you are concerned that you cannot tell the parents how functionally effective his walking will be. You are also worried that you cannot answer questions about other, perhaps more important, outcomes such as self-care and independent living. You are also aware that the evidence has not allowed you to estimate accurately the probability of eventual walking for children who are not sitting at age 2.

At later consultation, more specific questions about managing spasticity arise. You are surprised that some of the information you find is not as clinically helpful as you had expected. For the pharmacological agents diazepam, dantrolene, and oral baclofen, the studies are limited in number. There are significant concerns about both outcome measures used and the power of these studies. You are disappointed by the lack of pediatric studies that have adequately explored domains beyond the impairment level. You tell the child's parents that there currently is no information that would lead you to believe that these agents would improve the efficiency of his walking and therefore they are unlikely to reduce his fatigue.

You also explain to the parents that good quality synthesized evidence to answer a couple of the questions about therapies (botulinum toxin, intrathecal baclofen, and selective dorsal rhizotomy) is now available. You explain that all of these therapies are invasive, but that botulinum toxin has been shown to benefit children with CP and equinus gait, and that side effects have been low in multiple studies. Both intrathecal baclofen and dorsal rhizotomy have been shown to reduce spasticity, but little is known about functional improvement for intrathecal baclofen, only a small improvement in function has been seen for dorsal rhizotomy, and quality of life outcomes are mostly unknown for both. His parents decide that they will consider the use of botulinum toxin into his calves to assist with his walking, but would rather wait and have more information about the effectiveness of the other therapies before they discuss them further.

Summary table

Question	Type of evidence	Result	Comment
Effectiveness of early intervention	RCTs	No methodologically rigorous studies have shown effectiveness of early intervention	No evidence to support effectiveness Need studies that consider important non-physical outcomes
Does sitting at 2 years predict walking?	Cohort	Sitting by 2 years increases probability of eventual walking by more than 20-fold	Sitting by 2 can be used to predict eventual walking. Information is still needed about other important outcomes, type of ambulation, and ability to live independently
Do oral agents improve outcome?	RCTs		Studies that explore functional outcomes and quality of life
• Diazepam		• Effects are limited by unwanted side effects	outcomes are needed Await Cochrane review
• Dantrolene		• No strong evidence for functional improvement in spasticity of cerebral origin	
• Baclofen		• Some evidence of decrease of spasticity	
Does intrathecal baclofen improve gait?	Evidence report	Positive effect on spasticity and spasm	Further study is needed to delineate the effect on gross and fine motor function and quality of life outcomes
Is botulinum toxin injection effective in improving gait?	Systematic review/ meta-analysis	Positive effect on spasticity and improved function for children with equinus gait	Further studies required to determine long-term benefits or harms, and benefit to children with other gait abnormalities
Is selective dorsal rhizotomy effective in improving gait?	Meta-analysis	Statistically significant but only marginally clinically significant effect on gross motor function	More information about long-term functional effects, side effects and quality of life

References

1 Kuban KC, Leviton A. Cerebral Palsy (Review). *N Engl J Med* 1994;**330**:188–95.
2 Bax M. Terminology and Classification of Cerebral Palsy. *Develop Med Child Neurol* 1964;**6**:295–97.
3 Little MJ. On the influence of parturition, labour, premature birth and asphyxia neonatorum on the mental and physical condition of the child, especially in relation to the deformities. *Trans Obstet Soc Lond* 1882;**3**:293–344.
4 Collier JS. The pathogenesis of cerebral diplegia. *Proc R Soc Med* 1924;**17**:1–11.
5 Nelson KB, Ellenberg JH. Antecedents of cerebral palsy: multivariate analysis of risk. *N Engl J Med* 1986;**315**:81–6.
6 Blair E, Stanley FJ. Intrapartum asphyxia: a rare cause of cerebral palsy. *Paediatrics* 1988;**82**:240–9.
7 Naeye RL, Peters EC, Bartholomew M, Landis JR. Origins of cerebral palsy. *Am J Dis Child* 1989;**143**:1154–61.
8 Blair E, Stanley F. Interobserver agreement in the classification of cerebral palsy. *Develop Med Child Neurol.* 1985;**27**:615–22.

9 Mutch L, Alberman E, Hagberg B, Kodama K, Perat MV. Cerebral palsy epidemiology: where are we now and where are we going? *Develop Med Child Neurol* 1992;**34**:547–51.
10 Hagberg B, Hagberg G. The origins of cerebral palsy. In: David TJ, ed. *Recent advances in paediatrics XI.* Edinburgh: Churchill Livingstone, 1993:67–83.
11 Turnbull JD. Early Intervention for children with or at risk of cerebral palsy. *AJDC* 1993;**147**:54–9.
12 Parry TS. The effectiveness of early intervention: A critical review. *J Paed Child Health* 1992;**28**:343–346.
13 Low NL. A hypothesis why "early intervention" in cerebral palsy might be useful. *Brain Develop* 1980;**2**:133–5.
14 Parette HP, Hourcade JJ. A review of therapeutic intervention on gross and fine motor progress in young children with cerebral palsy. *Am J Occ Ther* 1984;**38**:462–8.
15 Henry DA, Wilson A. Principles behind practice: 9. Meta-analysis. *Med J Austr* 1992;**156**:31–7.
16 Sackett DL. How to read clinical journals, V: to distinguish useful from useless or even harmful therapy. *CMAJ* 1981; **124**:1156–62.

17 Weindling AM, Hallam P, Gregg J *et al.* A randomized controlled trial of early physiotherapy for high risk infants. *Acta Paediatr* 1996;**85**:1107–11.

18 McCormick MC, McCarton C, Tonascia J, Brooks-Gunn J. Early educational intervention for very low birth weight infants: results from the Infant Health and Development Program. *J Pediatr* 1993;**123**:527–33.

19 Yigit S, Kerem M, Livanelioglu A *et al.* Early physiotherapy intervention in premature infants. *Turk J Pediatr* 2002;**44**:224–9.

20 Sala DA, Grant AD Prognosis for ambulation in cerebral palsy. Review Article. *Develop Med Child Neurol* 1995;**37**:1020–6.

21 Molnar GE, Gordon SU. Cerebral palsy: Predictive value of selected clinical signs for early prognostication of motor function. *Arch Phys Med Rehabil* 1976;**57**:153–8.

22 Barnhart RC, Liemohn WP. Ambulatory status of children with cerebral palsy: a retrospective study. *Percept Motor Skills* 1995;**81**:571–4.

23 Trahan J, Marcoux S. Factors associated with the inability of children with cerebral palsy to walk at six years: A retrospective study. *Develop Med Child Neurol* 1994;**36**:787–95.

24 Campos da Paz A, Burnett SM, Braga LW. Walking prognosis in cerebral palsy: a 22-year retrospective analysis. *Develop Med Child Neurol* 1994;**36**:130–4.

25 Watt JM, Robertson CMT, Grace MGA. Early prognosis for ambulation of neonatal intensive care survivors with cerebral palsy. *Develop Med Child Neurol* 1989;**31**:766–73.

26 Bleck EE. Locomotor prognosis in cerebral palsy. *Develop Med Child Neurol* 1975;**17**:18–25.

27 Badell-Ribera A. Cerebral Palsy: postural-locomotor prognosis in spastic diplegia. *Arch Phys Med Rehab* 1985;**66**:614–19.

28 Howard DC. Antispastic Medication for Spasticity in Cerebral Palsy (Protocol for a Cochrane Review). In: *Cochrane Library*. Issue 1. Oxford: Update Software, 2003.

29 Denhoff E, Feldman S, Smith. Treatment of spastic cerebral-palsied children with sodium dantrolene. *Develop Med Child Neurol* 1975;**17**:736.

30 Verries M, Ashby P, Macleod S. Diazepam effect in reflex activity in patients with complete spinal lesions and in those with other causes of spasticity. *Arch Phys Med Rehab* 1977;**58**:148–53.

31 Young RR, Delwaide PJ. Drug Therapy: Spasticity. *N Engl J Med* 1981;**304**:96–9.

32 Rice GPA. Pharmacotherapy of spasticity: Some theoretical and practical considerations. *Can J Neurol Sci* 1987;**4**:510–12.

33 Pinder RM, Brogden RN, Speight TM *et al.* Dantrolene sodium: A review of its pharmacologic properties and therapeutic efficacy in spasticity. *Drugs* 1987;**13**:3–23.

34 Chyatte SM, Basmajian JV. Dantrolene sodium: Long-term effects in severe spasticity. *Arch Phys Med Rehab* 1973;**54**:311.

35 Haslam RHA, Walcher JR, Lietman PS *et al.* Dantrolene sodium in children with cerebral palsy. *Arch Phys Med Rehabil* 1973;**55**:384–388.

36 Katrak PH, Cole AMD, Poulos CJ *et al.* Objective assessment of spasticity, strength and function with early detection of dantrolene sodium after cerebrovascular accident: A randomized double-blind study. *Arch Phys Med Rehab* 1992;**73**:4–9.

37 Davidoff RA. Antispasticity drugs: mechanisms of action. *Ann Neurol* 1985;**17**:107–16.

38 Zeiglgansberger W, Howe JR, Sutor N. The neuropharmacology of baclofen. In: Muller H, Zierski J, Penn RD, eds. *Local Spinal Therapy of Spasticity*. Berlin: Springer, 1988.

39 Price GW, Wilkin GP, Turnbull MJ *et al.* Are baclofen sensitive GABA-B receptors present in different terminals of the spinal cord? *Nature* 1984;**307**:71–4.

40 Schwartzman JS, Tilberz GP, Kolger E *et al.* Effects of Lioresal in cerebral palsy. *Fohla Medica* 1976;**72**:297–302.

41 Calia RG, Santomauro E, Traldi S. The use of baclofen in children with cerebral palsy. *Fohla Medica* 1976;**3**:199–202.

42 Milla PJ, Jackson ADM. A controlled trial of baclofen in children with cerebral palsy. *J Int Med Res* 1977;**5**:398–404.

43 Ebutt AF, Jukes AM. United Kingdom therapeutic trail of Lioresal in the treatment of spasticity of cerebral origin. In: *Baclofen: Spasticity and Cerebral Pathology*. Cambridge: Cambridge Medical Publications, 1992.

44 McKinley I, Hyde E, Gordon N. Baclofen: a team approach to drug evaluation of spasticity in childhood. *Scott Med J* 1980;**25**:S26–S28.

45 Minford AM, Brown JK, Minns RA *et al.* The effect of baclofen on the gait of hemiplegic children assessed by means of polarized light goniometry. *Scott Med J* 1980;**25**:S29–S35.

46 Hudgson P, Weigthman D. Baclofen in the treatment of spasticity. *BMJ* 1971;**4**:15–17.

47 Duncan GW, Shahani BT, Young RR. An evaluation of baclofen treatment for certain symptoms in patients with spinal cord lesions: A double-blind cross-over study. *Neurology* 1976;**26**:441–6.

48 Whyte J, Robinson KM. Pharmacological management. In: Glenn MB, Whyte J, eds. *The Practical Management of Spasticity in Children and Adults*. Philadelphia: Lea and Febiger, 1990.

49 Hattab JR. Review of European clinical trials with baclofen. In: Feldman RG, Young RR, Koella WP, eds. *Spasticity: Disordered Motor Control*. Chicago: Yearbook Medical Publisher, 1992.

50 Jones RF, Burke D, Marosszeky JE *et al.* A new agent for the control of spasticity. *J Neurol Neurosurg Psychiatr* 1970;**33**:464–8.

51 Kroin JS, Penn RD, Bessinger RL *et al.* Reduced spinal reflexes following intrathecal baclofen in the rabbit. *Exp Brain Res* 1984;**54**:191–4.

52 Latash ML, Penn RD, Corcos DM *et al.* Short term effects of intrathecal baclofen in spasticity. *Exp Neurol* 1989;**103**:165–72.

53 Macdonnell RAL, Talalla A, Swash M *et al.* Intrathecal baclofen and the H. reflex *J Neurol Neurosurg Psychiatr* 1989;**52**:1110–12.

54 Dressandt J, Auer C, Conrad B. Influence of baclofen upon the alpha-motoneuron in spasticity by means of F-wave analysis. *Muscle Nerve* 1995;**18**:103–7.

55 Penn RD. Intrathecal baclofen for severe spasticity. *Ann NY Acad Sci* 1988;**531**:157–66.

56 Sallerin-Cautl B, Lazorthes Y, Monsarrat B *et al*. CSF baclofen levels after intrathecal administration in severe spasticity. *Eur J Clin Pharmacol* 1991;**40**:363–5.

57 Murphy NA, Irwin MC, Hoff C. Intrathecal Baclofen therapy in children with cerebral palsy: efficacy and complications. *Arch Phys Med Rehabil* 2002;**83**:1721–5.

58 Campbell WM, Ferrel A, McLaughlin JF *et al*. Long-term safety and efficacy of continuous intrathecal baclofen. *Develop Med Child Neurol* 2002;**44**:660–5.

59 Butler C, Campbell S. Evidence of the effects of intrathecal baclofen for spastic and dystonic cerebral palsy. Available at http://www.aacpdm.org or *Develop Med Child Neurol* 2000;**42**:634–45.

60 Albright AL, Cervi A, Singletary J. Intrathecal baclofen for spasticity in cerebral palsy. *JAMA* 1991;**265**:1418–22.

61 Gilmartin R, Bruce D, Storrs B *et al*. Intrathecal baclofen for management of spastic cerebral palsy: Multicenter trial. *J Child Neurol* 2000;**15**:71–7.

62 Almeida GL, Campbell SK, Girolami GL, Penn RD, Corocs DM. Multidimensional assessment of motor function in a child with cerebral palsy following intrathecal administration of baclofen. *Phys Ther* 1997;**77**:751–64.

63 Armstrong RW, Steinbok P, Cochrane DD, Kube SD, Fife SE, Farrell K. Intrathecal baclofen for treatment of children with spasticity of cerebral origin. *J Neurosurg* 1997;**87**:409–14.

64 Boyd RN, Hays RM. Current evidence for the use of botulinum toxin type A in the management of children with cerebral palsy: a systematic review. *Eur J Neurol* 2001; **8**(Suppl. 5):1–20.

65 Ade-Hall RA, Moore AP. Botulinum toxin type A in the treatment of lower limb spasticity in cerebral palsy (Cochrane Review). In: The *Cochrane Library*. Issue 1. Oxford: Update Software, 2003.

66 McLaughlin J, Bjornson K, Temkin N *et al*. Selective dorsal rhizotomy: meta-analysis of three randomized controlled trials. *Develop Med Child Neurol* 2002;**44**:17–25.

67 Narayanan U, Howard A. Selective dorsal rhizotomy in the management of children with spastic cerebral palsy (Protocol for a Cochrane Review). In: The *Cochrane Library*. Issue 1. Oxford: Update Software, 2003.

47 Recurrent apnea in the newborn

David J Henderson-Smart

Case scenario

You are called to see a 24-hour-old male infant who has had recurrent episodes of apnea associated with bradycardia and oxygen desaturation. The pregnancy was uncomplicated until 32 weeks' gestation when his mother presented in preterm labor. She was treated with an IV beta-mimetic to suppress labor while corticosteroids were administered, and he was born by vaginal delivery 2 days later when the beta-mimetic was ceased. He did not need resuscitation and had Apgar scores of 6 at 1 minute and 8 at 5 minutes. His birth weight was 1600 g. He was admitted to the neonatal nursery and placed in a humidicrib on a cardiorespiratory monitor. His temperature, heart rate, and breathing rate were normal and he had no signs of respiratory distress while breathing room air. Milk feeds were given every 2 hours via an intragastric tube. The first episode of apnea occurred at 12 hours of age, detected by the cardiorespiratory monitor and confirmed by nursing observation. The apnea was associated with cyanosis and bradycardia to a rate of 80 per minute, which were quickly reversed by cutaneous stimulation. Three more episodes have occurred over the next 12 hours. Between events, he has looked and behaved normally for a preterm infant. You wonder why this particular infant is having apnea, how frequently apnea occurs in preterm infants, how you should monitor and treat the condition, and what is the likely outcome.

Background

Definition of apnea

Clinical apnea is defined as a pause in breathing of more than 20 seconds or a pause of a shorter duration associated with bradycardia or cyanosis.[1] Recurrent apnea is defined as repeated (over three) episodes of apnea after the first hour of age.[2] Apnea at birth, as part of maladaptation to birth for whatever reason, is not included in studies of recurrent apnea unless episodes continue beyond the first hour after birth. Similarly, apnea and cyanosis during initial feeding is not usually considered in the same clinical category as recurrent apnea.

For research purposes, both usual and unusual pauses in breathing require measurement using objective techniques, such as continuous electronic monitoring of breathing, and other variables, which are recorded on a polygraph, tape recorder, or computer. To obtain a normal frequency distribution, all breath intervals should be recorded from infants in a given population. From these data it should be possible to define apnea as an interbreath interval which is longer than the 97th percentile. Although useful for research, this approach has not been helpful to clinicians because there has usually been little attempt to correlate findings with clinical states or long-term outcome.

In order to make more sense of apnea in the clinical setting, bradycardic and hypoxic episodes are also recorded. Continuous measurements of oxygen levels in the infant can be made using transcutaneous Po_2 electrodes or pulse oximetry. Measurements of oxygen levels together with heart rate go some way towards examining the consequences of apnea rather than the phenomenon itself. However, all these are intermediate variables that need to be related to more important outcomes such as neonatal complications and long-term prognosis of infants.

Types of apnea

- Clinical observations have emphasized *central apnea*, where breathing efforts cease, as the most common type. Polygraphic recordings of both breathing efforts and nasal airflow confirm that most short apneas are of the central type[3,4] and that both breathing efforts and nasal airflow cease.
- However, longer apneic events often have an obstructive component, where breathing efforts resume after a

central apnea but there is no airflow for a number of breaths, because of upper airway obstruction. These events are referred to as *mixed apnea*.

- Less commonly, certain infants have continued breathing efforts without airflow throughout an event. This is referred to as *obstructive apnea*. Clinically, these obstructive events are characterized by a continuing fall in oxygen saturation and bradycardia, despite breathing efforts. In infants with some brainstem abnormalities such as the Dandy–Walker malformation, or with anatomical narrowing of the upper airway such as micrognathia, obstructive apnea is the predominant form observed.

Cardiovascular changes during apnea

Bradycardia is the most obvious clinical cardiovascular sign during apnea. This has been defined as an abrupt slowing of the heart rate to below a set level of 80–100 beats per minute, or a decrease of the resting heart rate as a percentage of the baseline (for example, 20–30%). Bradycardia during apnea is thought to represent a chemoreceptor-mediated vagal reflex.[5] Other changes include peripheral vasoconstriction[6] and an increase in pulse pressure.[7] Reflex bradycardia is accentuated in the absence of brainstem inspiratory activity and when there is no phasic inflation of the lungs, as in diving mammals. The main purpose of the cardiovascular changes is to conserve and redistribute oxygen within the body to favor vital organs such as the heart and brain at the expense of others such as the trunk, kidneys, and gut.

Bradycardic episodes, defined as a 30% or greater fall in heart rate were documented during 243 hours of polygraphic recordings in 28 preterm infants.[5] Of the 390 bradycardic episodes; 93% occurred in association with one of the 1520 apneas of > 10 seconds duration, 5% occurred with shorter apneas and the remaining few episodes were associated with shallow breathing, generalized body movements or tube feeding. In sick or intubated preterm infants bradycardia can occur during mechanical ventilation when there is hypoxemia without adequate lung inflation. Bradycardia can also occur with seizures or raised intracranial pressure.

There is a close relationship between oxygen desaturation and bradycardia during apnea.[5,8–10] On average, the fall in heart rate commences 9 seconds into the apneic event and closely follows the fall in oxygen saturation. Bradycardia can occur at the onset of apnea if there is already considerable hypoxic chemoreceptor drive.

Framing answerable clinical questions

You go to the literature to look up the causes and frequency of apnea, the best method for monitoring and treating apnea and its associated bradycardia, and its prognosis. First, you structure the clinical questions as described in Chapter 2.

Questions

1. In newborn infants (*population*), how does clinical monitoring by nurses (*test*) compare with continuously recorded electronic monitoring (*gold standard test*) in the detection of apnea and bradycardia (*outcome*)? **[Diagnosis]**
2. In newborn infants (*population*), what is the frequency of recurrent apnea/bradycardia (*outcome*)? **[Baseline Risk]**
3. In newborn infants (*population*), what are the risk factors (*exposures*) for recurrent apnea/bradycardia (*outcome*)? **[Causation]**
4. In preterm infants (*population*), at what age does apnea first present and how long does the problem continue (*outcome*)? **[Prognosis]**
5. In preterm infants with recurrent apnea (*population*), does treatment with methylxanthines (*intervention*) compared with standard care (*comparison*) reduce apnea and morbidity (*outcome*)? Which methylxanthine is best? **[Therapy]**
6. Are preterm infants with recurrent apnea (*population/ exposure*) at increased risk of sudden infant death syndrome (SIDS) (*outcome*)? **[Prognosis]**
7. In preterm infants (*population*) with apnea (*exposure*), what is the long-term neurodevelopmental outcome (*outcome*)? **[Prognosis]**

Searching for evidence

When you are searching electronic databases such as MedLine, Embase and Cinhal for information about apnea in the newborn, the best search terms are "apnea" OR "apnoea" as text words AND "infant, newborn" as a MeSh heading. Then it depends on the type of question as to which publication type you are seeking. The most sensitive and specific search terms or combination of search terms are shown in Chapter 3. For therapy, the best evidence comes from randomized controlled trials and particularly systematic reviews of randomized controlled trials. The best place to find these is in the *Cochrane Library*. The best place to find information on risk and prognosis is in cohort studies. Many of these studies are difficult to find in MedLine and a check of the reference lists of narrative reviews and other publications can be helpful.

Critical review of the evidence

Question

1. In newborn infants (*population*), how does clinical monitoring by nurses (*test*) compare with continuously

recorded electronic monitoring (*gold standard test*) in the detection of apnea and bradycardia (*outcome*)? **[Diagnosis]**

As outlined in Chapter 3 you search for studies comparing diagnosis by nurses using monitors that detect apnea and bradycardia with diagnosis by continuous electronic monitoring by computer or polygraph (*the gold standard*). Continuous electronic monitoring usually includes more detailed recording of breathing efforts, nasal air flow, heart rate and SaO_2 or $TcPO_2$. Each test must be attempting to detect "clinical apnea" as defined above and should be independent of each other as outlined in the criteria for evaluating a diagnostic test in Chapter 5.

You find a number of reports of case series, of which two are relevant to your question.[4,11] Both show that nursing records of apnea and bradycardia alarms underestimate the incidence. One study[4] showed that, although nurses missed almost half of the events detected by the monitor, they were detectable to prolonged apneas of > 20 seconds and more clinically serious apneas associated with bradycardia. The detection of fewer episodes by nurse monitoring is partly due to nurses ignoring transient "self-reverting" episodes of apnea, bradycardia, and oxygen desaturation, and only recording events that they consider clinically important. Polygraphic studies have, however, been useful to delineate different types of apnea (see Background section above) and to help define what is abnormal in unusual cases, such as term infants.

Questions

2. In newborn infants (*population*), what is the frequency of recurrent apnea/bradycardia (*outcome*)? **[Baseline Risk]**
3. In newborn infants (*population*), what are the risk factors (*exposures*) for recurrent apnea/bradycardia (*outcome*)? **[Causation]**

The best evidence to answer question 2 would come from population-based cohort studies from which incidence/prevalence could be determined. The best evidence to answer question 3 would also come from cohort studies in which independent risk factors are sought using multivariable techniques or well-designed case–control studies. To strengthen the case for causality rather than association, replication in a number of studies, a dose effect, biological plausibility and occurrence of the risk factors before the development of apnea are needed.[12] Unfortunately only hospital-based cohorts using univariate analysis have been reported.

The incidence of apnea, based on clinical records of apnea and bradycardia kept by nursing staff in neonatal nurseries, increases in infants of lower birth weight[13] and gestational age[2] at birth. The latter relationship was obtained from records kept on inborn infants admitted to a tertiary neonatal unit over a 6-year period from 1974–79 when there were 25 154 inborn live births and when methylxanthine treatment was rarely used. Apnea (three or more events) was found to have occurred in over 80% of infants born at < 30 weeks gestation, in 54% of infants born at 30–31 weeks, in 14% of infants born at 32–33 weeks, and in 7% of infants born at 34–35 weeks. These findings have been replicated in another study in which gestational age had a similar dose effect.[14]

Recurrent apnea was recognized as a clinical problem in only 0·08% of term infants. Research studies[15,16] in which breathing movements have been continuously measured for 12–24 hours indicate that 3–12 second pauses in breathing occur frequently in term newborns. The 90th percentile for the longest apnea was 18 seconds at 1 week, 14 seconds at 1 month, and 10–12 seconds at 3–6 months.

Aside from lower gestational age, which is a strong risk factor for apnea, various clinical conditions have been associated with the appearance or accentuation of apnea. Essentially any physiological disturbance or pathological disorder that reduces the infant's vigor can be contributory (see Box). These clinical associations are based on case series of infants with apnea rather than cohort studies, and the causal relationship between the risk factors and apnea have not been rigorously studied.

Risk factors for apnea (adapted from ref 20)

- Immaturity
- Hypoxemia
    - pulmonary
    - anemia
- Central nervous system disturbances
    - asphyxia
    - intracranial hemorrhage
    - seizures
    - drug depression
    - malformations
- Metabolic disturbance
    - hypoglycemia
    - hyponatremia
    - hypocalcemia
    - inborn error
- Systemic illness
    - infection
    - shock (hypovolemia)
    - heart failure
- Thermal disturbance
    - hyperthermia
    - severe hypothermia

- Anatomical narrowing of airways
  choanal atresia
  micrognathia
  macroglossia
  tracheomalacia

- Intervention
  immunization
  anesthesia

In growing preterm infants who have stopped having apnea, apnea may recur if the infant has an intercurrent illness or an intervention such as immunization,[17] general anesthesia,[18] or viral infection.[19]

Question

4. In preterm infants (*population*), at what age does apnea first present and how long does the problem continue (*outcome*)? **[Prognosis]**

There are no population-based studies evaluating the clinical course of recurrent apnea in preterm infants. You find two hospital based cohort studies in which the records of consecutive preterm[2] or very low birth weight[14] infants with recurrent apnea were examined retrospectively. The results are consistent between the studies and show that the first episodes of apnea were detected by 2–4 days of age in 80% of infants, and in all infants who were not ventilated recurrent apnea was evident within 7–10 days. These findings are consistent with the results of a case series in which continuous polygraphic recordings were made[21] and is in contrast to earlier texts suggesting that apnea only appeared after a few days. A delay in onset of apnea may be observed in infants with the respiratory distress syndrome in which apnea/bradycardia usually only appears when the lung disease is abating.

In infants with recurrent apnea and bradycardia, these events continue for days, weeks, or even months. The condition generally persists for longer the lower the gestational age at birth.[2,14] Over 90% infants have no apnea by 37 weeks postmenstrual age (gestational age + postnatal age). There is evidence from studies of brainstem neural maturation that differences in maturation might be an underlying factor in determining the occurrence and duration of recurrent apnea.[22]

These earlier studies contained relatively small numbers of infants born at 24–28 weeks' gestation, who would have had a high mortality rate at that time. Eichenwald and colleagues[23] recently reported a hospital-based cohort of such infants and found that apnea and bradycardia often persisted to term equivalent age and beyond, especially in those born at 24–26 weeks and those with chronic lung disease. This study probably suffers from selection bias since it only included infants who remained in the tertiary center up to term equivalent age and so were more likely to have ongoing clinical problems.

Question

5. In preterm infants with recurrent apnea (*population*), does treatment with methylxanthines (*intervention*) compared with standard care (*comparison*) reduce apnea and morbidity (*outcome*)? Which methylxanthine is best? **[Therapy]**

The best evidence about the effectiveness of therapy would be found in a systematic review of all randomized controlled trials. As outlined in Chapter 5 the results of therapy can be expressed as relative risks (RR), risk difference (RD) and number needed to treat (NNT) calculated from 1/RD (see Glossary). You find a Cochrane systematic review and meta-analysis[24] of five trials which included 192 preterm infants enrolled between 1981 and 1990 (four trials) and in 2000 (one trial). One trial reported on the use of oral theophylline and two used the intravenous equivalent, aminophylline or theophylline. Two trials examined the effects of caffeine. The comparator was a placebo in three trials and no drug therapy in the remaining two. All trials measured apnea/bradycardia consistent with clinical events.[1] These were recorded from clinical monitors in two trials and by chart records of apnea and heart rate in the remaining three. The timing of outcome assessments varied from 48 hours to 10 days after initiation of treatment.

Compared with controls, preterm infants treated with methylxanthine had lower rates of persisting apnea. All trials showed a significant reduction in this adverse outcome and overall the effect size was large (summary RR 0·43 [0·31, 0·60]; RD −40% [−53%, −28%]; NNT 3). No individual trial showed a significant reduction in the use of IPPV. However, when the results were combined in a meta-analysis there was a significant reduction in IPPV in the methylxanthine group (RR 0·34 [0·12, 0·97]; RD −8% [−16%, −1%]; NNT 13). Side effects leading to cessation of treatment were poorly reported. In one trial, two infants in the theophylline group developed tachycardia which led to suspension of treatment. A major concern is the small number of subjects in each study which, while adequate to show the large effect of treatment on apnea, would not be able to detect less common adverse effects.

Outcomes at >10 days after commencing treatment and long-term effects of methylxanthines on growth and development were not assessed in any trial. The long-term safety of caffeine therapy has been suggested in one small cohort study.[25] A more recent retrospective study examined sensorineural development at 14 years of age in a consecutive hospital-based cohort of very low birth weight infants.[26] After adjusting for confounders, theophylline therapy in the newborn period was associated with higher Wechsler Intelligence Scale scores (mean difference) but an increased rate of cerebral palsy (adjusted RR 4·2) in the treated group. Neurodevlopmental outcome is currently being evaluated in an international randomized controlled trial comparing caffeine and placebo.[27]

If treatment with methylxanthines reduces apnea, why not give it prophylactically to spontaneously breathing preterm infants at risk of developing apnea/bradycardia because of their low gestational age? Another Cochrane systematic review of two trials of caffeine given as prophylaxis found no evidence of a beneficial effect.[28]

Which methylxanthine is best? Caffeine and theophylline have been compared in a Cochrane systematic review.[29] Three published trials involving a total of 66 infants were included. There was no difference in the failure rate of treatment (defined as < 50% reduction in apnea/bradycardia) with caffeine or theophylline at 1–3 days (two studies) or 5–7 days (one study) after commencing treatment. The mean rate of apnea was higher in infants receiving standard dose caffeine (compared with infants receiving theophylline) at 1–3 days (three studies) but not at 5–7 days (two studies). Side effects, such as tachycardia or feed intolerance leading to change in dosing, were lower in the groups who received caffeine (summary RR 0·17 [0·04,0·72]; RD −29% [−47%, −10%]; NNT 3). This finding is consistent across the three studies. No trial reported the use of IPPV and no data are available to assess the effects of treatment on later growth and development.

Question

6. Are preterm infants with recurrent apnea (*population/exposure*) at increased risk of sudden infant death syndrome (SIDS) (*outcome*)? **[Prognosis]**

In your search you find a recent publication from the American Academy of Pediatrics, which provides an evidence-based statement on whether apnea is a potential risk factor, the role of predischarge polygraphic recordings and the place of home monitoring.[1] References to the evidence are given and you examine some key ones. In particular, a large case–control study by Hoffman in which 757 SIDS cases are compared with 1514 controls[30] shows that, although preterm birth increases the risk of SIDS, apnea does not. There is no evidence to support the use of predischarge polygraphic recording or home monitoring for the prevention of SIDS. Parents should be encouraged to apply measures known to reduce the risk of SIDS (supine sleeping, safe sleeping environments, and avoidance of exposure to tobacco smoke) whether or not their infant has had apnea.[1]

Question

7. In preterm infants (*population*) with apnea (*exposure*), what is the long-term neurodevelopmental outcome (*outcome*). **[Prognosis]**

There are no population based cohort studies published. Early hospital-based studies report that recurrent apnea places an infant at risk of long-term impairment.[31] These studies used univariate analysis, which failed to differentiate apnea as a cause rather than a symptom of neurological abnormality. Furthermore, in the past, spontaneous apneas were often allowed to continue until the infants were pale, limp, and unresponsive, requiring bag and mask ventilation. More recent reports have suggested that uncomplicated recurrent apnea in preterm infants is not independently associated with a poor neurological outcome.[32–34] In the most extensive study, Tudehope and colleagues[32] reported on the 2-year outcome of 164 of 172 consecutive surviving very low birth weight infants using multivariate analyses to allow for confounding variables that were associated with lowering of the General Development Quotient on the Griffith Scale. They found that the presence of apnea *per se* was not associated with lower developmental scores. However, in this study, apnea was recorded if the monitor alarm registered a pause of > 10 seconds, with bradycardia and cyanosis being also recorded by the nursing staff. Nevertheless, even when the results of infants with moderate or severe apnea were analyzed, there was no effect on overall scores. Analysis of the small group with sensory deficits indicated that there might be an association with apnea, although the authors did not control for confounding variables such as gestational age at birth. Others have stressed the increased risk of developing retinopathy in preterm infants with recurrent apnea and the need to avoid hyperoxia, particularly during bag and mask ventilation resuscitation.[35]

Resolution of the scenario

You examine the infant and find that he is well with normal color, tone, and movements for gestational age, his breathing is regular, and there is no respiratory distress or stridor. Investigations including full blood count, serum electrolytes and calcium, and head ultrasound reveal normal results. Pulse oximeter measurements of his oxygen saturation are in the range of 90–95%. Because of repeated episodes of apnea and bradycardia, you commence therapy with oral caffeine citrate. In the next 24 hours the frequency of apnea decreases. There are only two further episodes and none after that time. The infant's baseline heart rate increases from 130 to 150 beats per minute but there are no episodes of tachycardia and no feed intolerance. One week after the last episode of apnea you cease the caffeine therapy. Apnea does not recur during the next week and to facilitate normalization of parental handling of their infant, including establishment of breast feeding, you cease electronic monitoring. At 4 weeks of age the infant is feeding well and plans for discharge are made. You reassure the parents that the apnea will not influence the infant's development. They ask whether their infant is at increased risk of sudden infant death syndrome (SIDS). You tell them that there is a small increase in the risk of SIDS in preterm infants but that this is not affected by there having been episodes of apnea in the newborn period. You also say that there are general preventive measures that they can take to reduce the risk of SIDS including, placing the infant on his back to sleep.

Future research needs

Evidence is needed on the comparative validity and relevance of apnea detected by nurses using clinical alarm monitors and that detected by continuous computerized or polygraphic recording, both initially in terms of treatment needs, at discharge, and for prognosis. Evidence for the balance between the short-term benefits and long-term outcomes of the use of interventions to treat apnea is also needed. Along this line, caffeine is currently being investigated in a large multicenter randomized controlled trial.[27]

Summary table

Question	Type of evidence	Result	Comment
What is the diagnostic accuracy of clinical monitoring by nurses?	Cross-sectional studies with simultaneous independent evaluation by polygraphic recordings (gold standard)[4,11]	Using apnea/bradycardia alarms, nurses only detect about half of all recorded episodes. They are better at detecting longer more clinically relevant apneas	Infants at high risk should be electronically monitored with apnea and bradycardia alarms
What are the risk factors for apnea in the newborn?	Cohort studies of consecutive admissions of very low birth weight (VLBW) or preterm infants[4,14–16] Case series reporting associations[13,20,23]	Low gestational age at birth is the strongest predictor of apnea. A number of physiological and pathological conditions (particularly those involving the central nervous system) can precipitate or accentuate apnea in a given infant	This information can be used to determine which infants to monitor for apnea and bradycardia
In preterm infants, at what age does apnea present and when do episodes cease?	Cohort studies of consecutive admissions of VLBW or preterm infants[2,14]	In 80% of infants who develop recurrent apnea, the first apnea occurs within 2–4 days of birth. It rarely appears after 7–10 days. Apnea usually ceases by term equivalent age	These results suggest that monitoring should begin soon after birth in infants at risk of apnea
In preterm infants with apnea, is methylxanthine therapy effective?	Cochrane systematic reviews of all randomized controlled trials[24,28,29]	Methylxanthine therapy reduces apnea and use of IPPV 2–10 days after commencement. Caffeine is as effective as theophylline but has fewer side effects. Effectiveness of prophylactic treatment with caffeine has not been demonstrated	Methylxanthine treatment can be used to reduce apnea in the short term. Caffeine is the preferred form of methylxanthine. It is of concern that there is inadequate data on long-term neurodevelopment after methylxanthine treatment
In preterm infants, is apnea predictive of SIDS?	Cohort[15] and case-control[30] studies	Although preterm birth increases the risk of SIDS, apnea does not. There is no evidence to support predischarge polygraphic recording or home monitoring in the prevention of SIDS	Parents should be encouraged to apply the measures known to reduce the risk of SIDS (supine sleeping, safe sleeping environments, and avoidance of exposure to tobacco smoke)
Is recurrent apnea associated with altered neurodevelopmental outcome in childhood?	Hospital-based case–control studies with or without adjustment for confounders[32–35]	Apnea is not independently associated with altered neurodevelopment	Parents can be reassured that apnea does not alter development

References

1 American Academy of Pediatrics. Policy statement. Apnea, Sudden Infant Death Syndrome, and home monitoring. *Pediatrics* 2003;**111**:914–17.

2 Henderson-Smart DJ. The effect of gestational age on the incidence and duration of recurrent apnoea in newborn babies. *Aus Paed J* 1981;**17**:273–6.

3 Butcher-Puech M, Henderson-Smart DJ, Holley D, Lacey JL and Edwards DA. Relation between apnea duration and type and neurological status of preterm infants. *Arch Dis Child* 1985;**60**:634–8.

4 Muttitt SC, Finer NN, Tierney AJ, Rossmann J. Neonatal apnea: diagnosis by nurse versus computer. *Pediatrics* 1988;**82**:713–20.

5 Henderson-Smart DJ, Butcher-Puech MC, Edwards DA. Incidence and mechanism of bradycardia during apnoea in preterm infants. *Arch Dis Child* 1986;**61**:227–32.

6 Storrs CN. Cardiovascular effects of apnoea in preterm infants. *Arch Dis Child* 1977;**52**:534–40.

7 Girling DJ. Changes in heart rate, blood pressure and pulse pressure during apnoeic attacks in newborn babies. *Arch Dis Child* 1972;**47**:405–10.

8 Dransfield DA, Spitzer AR, Fox WW. Episodic airway obstruction in premature infants. *Am J Dis Child* 1983;**137**:441–3.

9 Waggener TB, Stark AR, Cohlan BA, Frantz ID III. Apnea duration is related to ventilatory oscillation characteristics in newborn infants. *J Appl Physiol* 1984;**57**:536–44.

10 Poets CF, Stebbens VA, Samuels MP, Southall DP. The relationship between bradycardia, apnea and hypoxemia in preterm infants. *Pediatr Res* 1993;**34**:144–7.

11 Southall DP, Levitt GA, Richards RM *et al.* Undetected episodes of prolonged apnea and severe bradycardia in preterm infants. *Pediatrics* 1983;**72**:541–51.

12 Lorenz JM, Paneth N. When are observational studies adequate to assess the efficacy of therapeutic interventions. *Clin Perinatol* 2003;**30**:269–83.

13 Miller JC, Berle FC, Smull NW. Severe apnea and irregular respiratory rhythms among premature infants. *Pediatrics* 1959;**23**:676–85.

14 Tudehope DI, Rogers Y. Clinical spectrum of neonatal apnoea in very low birthweight infants. *Austr Paediatr J* 1984;**20**:131–136.

15 Southall DP, Richards JM, Shinebourne EA, Wilson AJ, Alexander JR. Prospective population-based study into heart rate and breathing patterns in newborn infants: prediction of infants at risk of SIDS? In: Tildon JT, Roeder LM, Steinschneider A, eds. *Sudden Infant Death Syndrome*. New York, Acedemic Press, 1983.

16 Stein IM, Fallon M, Mreisalo RL, Kennedy JL. The frequency of apnea and bradycardia in a population of healthy normal infants. *Neuropediatrics* 1983;**14**:73–5.

17 Botham SJ, Isaacs D. Incidence of apnoea and bradycardia in preterm infants following triple antigen immunisation. *J Paediatr Child Hlth* 1994;**30**:533–5.

18 Liu LMP, Cote CJ, Goudsouzian NG *et al.* Life-threatening apnea in infants recovering from anesthesia. *Anesthesiology* 1983;**59**:506–10.

19 Colditz PB, Henry RL, Lakshman MD. Apnoea and bronchiolitis due to respiratory syncytial virus. *Aust Paed J* 1982;**18**:53–4.

20 Henderson-Smart DJ. Recurrent apnoea. In: Yu VYH, ed. *Bailliere's Clinical Paediatrics. Vol 3 No. 1 Pulmonary Problems in the Perinatal Period and their Sequelae*. London: Bailliere Tindall, 1995.

21 Barrington K, Finer N. The natural history of apnea of prematurity. *Pediatr Res* 1991;**29**:372–5.

22 Henderson-Smart DJ, Pettigrew AG, Campbell DJ. Clinical apnea and brainstem neural function in preterm infants. *N Engl J Med* 1983;**308**:353–7.

23 Eichenwald EC, Aina A, Stark AR. Apnea frequently persists beyond term gestation in infants delivered at 24 to 28 weeks. *Pediatrics* 1997;**100**:354–9.

24 Henderson-Smart DJ, Steer P. Methylxanthine for apnea in preterm infants (Cochrane Review). In: The *Cochrane Library*. Issue 4. Oxford: Update Software, 1999.

25 Blanchard PW, Aranda JV. In: Beckerman RC, Brouillette RT, Hunt CE, eds. *Respiratory control disorders in infants and children*. Baltimore: Williams & Wilkins, 1992.

26 Davis PG, Doyle LW, Rickards AL *et al.* Methylxanthines and sensorineural outcome at 14 years in children < 1501 g birthweight. *J Paediatr Child Hlth* 2000;**36**:47–50.

27 Schmidt B. Methylxanthine therapy in premature infants: sound practice, disaster or fruitless byway? *J Pediatr* 1999;**135**:526–8.

28 Henderson-Smart DJ, Steer P. Prophylactic methylxanthine for the prevention of apnea in preterm infants (Cochrane Review). In: The *Cochrane Library*. Issue 1. Oxford: Update Software, 1999.

29 Henderson-Smart DJ, Steer P. Caffeine vs theophylline treatment for apnea in preterm infants (Cochrane Review). In: The *Cochrane Library*. Issue 2. Oxford: Update Software, 1999.

30 Hoffmann HJ, Damus K, Hillman L, Krongrad E. Risk factors for SIDS. Results of the National Institutes of Child Health and Human Development SIDS Cooperative Epidemiology Study. *Ann NY Acad Sci* 1988;**533**:13–20.

31 Jones RAK, Lukeman D. Apnea of immaturity. *Arch Dis Child* 1982;**57**:766–8.

32 Tudehope DI, Rogers YM, Burns YR, Mohay H, O'Callaghan MJ. Apnea in very low birthweight infants: Outcome at 2 years. *Aust Paed J* 1986;**22**:131–4.

33 Levitt GA, Mushin A, Bellman S, Harvey DR. Outcome of preterm infants who suffered neonatal apnoeic attacks. *Early Hum Develop* 1988;**16**:235–43.

34 Koons AH, Mjoica N, Jadeja N *et al.* Neurodevelopmental outcome of infants with apnea of infancy. *Am J Perinatol* 1993;**10**:208–11.

35 Gunn TR, Easdown J, Outerbridge EW, Aranda JV. Risk factors in retrolental fibroplasia. *Pediatrics* 1980;**65**:1096–100.

48 Unconjugated hyperbilirubinemia

Aaron Chiu

Case scenario

A 4-day-old Caucasian baby boy presents to your office with yellow appearance of the face and trunk. He was born at term after an uncomplicated pregnancy, and weighed 3·5 kg. There were no complications during labor or delivery. He was discharged from the hospital at 2 days of age. At that time, his parents were reassured that his mild facial jaundice was a normal finding especially for breastfed newborns. Since discharge, he has been breastfeeding well, has at least four wet diapers a day, and has been passing meconium-type stools at least once per day. Physical examination is normal except for mild yellow appearance to his face and trunk. Laboratory investigation reveals that both mother and infant have blood type O and are Rh positive. The infant's complete blood count shows a white blood count of 12×10^9 liter^{-1}, a hemoglobin of 140 g liter^{-1} and a platelet count of 252×10^9 liter^{-1}. The peripheral smear shows no signs of hemolysis. Total serum bilirubin is 20 mg dl^{-1} (340 micromol liter^{-1}). You decide that the infant should be admitted to hospital for phototherapy. The parents are upset about the need for admission and voice their confusion about the conflicting advice that they have received regarding the risks of jaundice. They ask about the specific risks to their baby and the effectiveness of the proposed treatment.

Background

Kernicterus by strictest definition is a pathologic diagnosis. Elevated levels of unconjugated bilirubin cross the blood–brain barrier to produce pigment deposition and neuronal cell death in characteristic regions of the brain. Acute clinical symptoms include lethargy, increased tone, high pitched cry, opisthotonus, seizures, and even death. Long-term sequelae of kernicterus include dental dysplasia, sensorineural hearing loss, choreo-athetosis, and developmental delay.

The linkage between hyperbilirubinemia and kernicterus in infants with Rh hemolytic disease was forged in the 1950s.[1–3] Prior to the routine use of exchange transfusion, kernicterus affected 15% of liveborn infants with erythroblastosis fetalis.[1,2] It was noted that exchange transfusions decreased the risk of kernicterus when serum bilirubin levels were kept below 20 mg dl^{-1} (342 micromol liter^{-1}).[2,4] Subsequently, the recommendation to keep serum bilirubin below this level was extrapolated to infants with hemolytic disease owing to ABO incompatibility[5] and to infants with non-hemolytic hyperbilirubinemia. Exchange transfusions became the routine to treat bilirubin levels reaching 20–25 mg dl^{-1} (342–428 micromol liter^{-1}) in full-term infants with non-hemolytic jaundice.[6] Vigintiphobia, the clinical fear of a serum bilirubin level of 20 mg dl^{-1}, prevailed.[7]

Much of the published data relating to the risk of neurological sequelae from hyperbilirubinemia originated from the Collaborative Study of Cerebral Palsy, subsequently renamed the Collaborative Perinatal Project (CPP). The CPP was established to follow a cohort of 50 000 pregnant women and their offspring in order to identify causes of cerebral palsy. The study was not designed specifically to test the hypothesis that high bilirubin levels were associated with brain damage.[8]

A preliminary assessment of the CPP data identified a positive correlation between the highest total serum bilirubin levels and both low mental and low motor scores at 8 months of age. The risk did not begin at a level of 20 mg dl^{-1} but was seen to increase and become substantial by 16–19 mg dl^{-1}.[9] Some subsequent analyses of the CPP data identified associations between bilirubin level and lower neurodevelopmental scores,[10–12] while others failed to find any association.[13,14] All had limitations in their design and/or analysis.

The association between hyperbilirubinemia and kernicterus in a healthy term infant with non-hemolytic disease continues to be debated. The aim of this chapter is to examine the evidence available for the management of such infants. The reader is directed elsewhere for a comprehensive review of the pathophysiology of neonatal hyperbilirubinemia.[15–17]

The discovery that sunlight can alter neonatal jaundice is attributed to Sister J Ward who, in 1956, recognized that a premature infant's pattern of dermal jaundice was due to varied exposure to sunlight.[18] Subsequently, blood accidentally exposed to sunlight was found to have a fall in bilirubin level, confirming the idea that light can affect serum bilirubin level.[19] Phototherapy affects the hydrogen bonds of bilirubin in the exposed skin and creates bilirubin photo-isomers which are water soluble and can be excreted in urine and bile.[16] The effect of phototherapy is dependent on the type of light used (blue–green spectrum), the irradiance or light energy used (number of lights and distance from light) and the surface area exposed.[20]

Framing answerable clinical questions

The evidence-based approach begins by using "well-built" clinical questions (see Chapter 2). A "well-built" clinical question has the following components:

- the patient or population
- the intervention or exposure
- the comparison intervention or exposure (if applicable), and
- the outcome of interest

You formulate the following clinical questions relevant to this child:

Questions

1. How accurate is the clinical examination (*test*) in determining whether a jaundiced, healthy, term infant (*population*) has hyperbilirubinemia requiring treatment with phototherapy (*outcome*)? **[Diagnosis]**
2. In a healthy term newborn with a bilirubin level of 20 mg dl^{-1}, whose hyperbilirubinemia is not due to hemolytic disease (*population and exposure*), what is the risk for the development of kernicterus (*outcome*)? Is the infant at any risk? **[Baseline Risk]**
3. In a healthy term newborn with a bilirubin level of 20 mg dl^{-1} and hyperbilirubinemia not due to hemolytic disease (*population and event*), what is the risk for development of adverse sequelae other than kernicterus (*outcome*)? **[Baseline Risk]**
4. In healthy term breastfed newborns with hyperbilirubinemia > 20 mg dl^{-1} (*population*), is phototherapy (*intervention*) effective in reducing the bilirubin level and preventing kernicterus (*outcome*)? **[Therapy]**
5. In a healthy term newborn with hyperbilirubinemia (*population*), is fiberoptic phototherapy (*intervention*) as effective as conventional phototherapy (*comparison*) in reducing the serum bilirubin level (*outcome*)? **[Therapy]**

Searching for evidence

You want to identify the "best" evidence by the simplest and most efficient means. Ongoing collaborative efforts have created a wealth of updated, evaluated evidence (for example, *Cochrane Library*, *Clinical Evidence*). Searches should begin with these resources. Electronic search of MedLine can be used to locate meta-analyses and practice guidelines which may be evidence-based.

Search for synthesized evidence

- Cochrane Database of Systematic Reviews: jaundice-neonatal (MeSH)\
- MedLine (PubMed): neonatal jaundice AND practice guideline

The *Cochrane Library* has two relevant references in the Cochrane Database of Systematic Reviews, one of which will be discussed later.[21] Using PubMed, you find three guidelines from medical societies: Norwegian Medical Society,[22] Netherlands Society of Pediatrics,[23] and American Academy of Pediatrics (AAP),[24,25] but only the last one is in English. You obtain the AAP guideline and the accompanying technical report.[8]

The validity of a guideline can be assessed (see Chapter 8). Generally it is dependent on the thoroughness of the literature search and the quality of the collation. Two independent MedLine searches were performed to identify articles for developing the AAP practice parameter[24] and accompanying technical report.[8] Much of the identified data is of a retrospective nature. Where evidence was lacking, recommendations were based on group consensus. A third literature search with an independent review of the information gathered validated the recommendations of the practice parameter. The methods involved in the literature search, grading of evidence, information synthesis, and decision making were not provided. Furthermore, the guideline is in the process of revision.[25] You decide to use the guideline as a source of references, but to perform your own search and assessment of the literature to address your questions.

Critical review of the evidence

Question

1. How accurate is the clinical examination (*test*) in determining whether a jaundiced, healthy, term infant (*population*) has hyperbilirubinemia requiring treatment with phototherapy (*outcome*)? **[Diagnosis]**

Search strategy

- MedLine (PubMed): ("jaundice, neonatal" [MeSH] AND "bilirubin/blood" [MeSH]) AND ("skin manifestations" [MeSH] OR "skin pigmentation" [MeSH] OR "clinical competence" [MeSH])

The AAP guideline states that "jaundice can be detected by blanching the skin with digital pressure. Dermal icterus is seen first in the face and progresses caudally to the trunk and extremities. As the TSB (total serum bilirubin) level rises, the extent of cephalocaudad progression may be helpful in quantifying the degree of jaundice."[24] The algorithm asks the clinician to define whether the "jaundice is clinically significant by medical judgment" to decide whether a serum bilirubin measurement should be made. To be used as a diagnostic test, this method of examination must accurately identify those infants whose degree of hyperbilirubinemia will need investigation and possibly treatment.

The majority of the 49 retrieved articles deal with transcutaneous bilirubinometry. Three citations specifically deal with the unaided clinical ability to define range of hyperbilirubinemia with the dermal progression of jaundice.[26–28]

The studies by Kramer[26] and by Ebbesen[27] attempted to correlate dermal progression of jaundice with the serum bilirubin level. The overwhelming majority of patients studied were full-term infants without hemolytic disease. In both studies, blanching of the skin with the thumb allowed the evaluation of the underlying skin color. Five dermal zones were arbitrarily created:

1 head and neck
2 trunk to the level of the umbilicus
3 umbilicus to the level of the knees
4 knees to the ankles (arms were also included in the study by Kramer), and
5 feet (Kramer also included hands).

The most caudal limit of dermal jaundice was noted and compared to the gold standard of serum bilirubin level, obtained regardless of the result from the clinical examination.

Both studies found a correlation between degree of hyperbilirubinemia and the most distal zone of dermal icterus. Term infants without hemolytic disease had higher zones of dermal jaundice with higher serum bilirubin levels. Although there was overlap between the ranges of serum bilirubin found in adjacent dermal zones, little overlap was found between zones 1, 3, and 5. For low birth weight infants, the relationship was not consistent.

If treatment with phototherapy is to be initiated once serum bilirubin reaches a level of 15 mg dl^{-1} within the first 24–48 hours of age,[24] then assessment of dermal zone of jaundice will be useful if it changes your estimate of a term infant having a serum bilirubin level ≥ 15 mg dl^{-1} (pretest probability) to a more useful and meaningful post-test estimate (post-test probability).

In the study by Ebbesen, the prevalence of serum bilirubin ≥ 15 mg dl^{-1} was 9% (pretest probability of 9%, pretest odds of 0·1).[27] Sensitivity, specificity, likelihood ratio of a positive test, post-test odds, and post-test probability were calculated from the data provided in the study. If jaundice extends below the knees, the probability of the infant's serum bilirubin ≥ 15 mg dl^{-1} is 22%. If jaundice extends to the feet, the probability of the infant's serum bilirubin ≥ 15 mg dl^{-1} is 53%. This post-test probability suggests that a serum bilirubin level should be done on any infant with this clinical finding. The findings in Kramer's study were similar.[26]

It is important to note that infants with jaundice above the ankle could also have serum bilirubin levels > 15 mg dl^{-1}.[26,27] The study by Moyer *et al.* demonstrated a similar conclusion.[28] In this study of 122 term infants, jaundice seen below the nipple line did not reliably predict which infants would have serum bilirubin ≥ 12 mg dl^{-1}. However, if an infant has no jaundice below the nipple line, this lack of jaundice reliably predicted the infant would have a serum bilirubin < 12 mg dl^{-1}.[28]

Application of this technique is likely limited. Two of the studies were based on clinical assessments by single observers.[26,27] Only Moyer *et al.* used assessments by multiple observers. There was poor interobserver agreement amongst healthcare professionals regarding the presence of jaundice at specific body sites. Experienced nurses and clinicians were in agreement ranging from 0–23% beyond chance.[28]

Question

2. In a healthy term newborn with a bilirubin level of 20 mg dl^{-1} whose hyperbilirubinemia is not due to hemolytic disease (*population and exposure*), what is the risk for the development of kernicterus (*outcome*)? Is the infant at any risk? **[Baseline Risk]**

- MedLine (PubMed): kernicterus AND term infant AND (case report OR case series)

To answer this question you need an estimate of baseline risk or prevalence of kernicterus in healthy term infants. Ideally, a large cohort of healthy term infants with untreated hyperbilirubinemia would be followed from birth to assess development of kernicterus. The number of infants with high bilirubin levels would need to be very large as the disease is so rare. Purposefully not treating significant hyperbilirubinemia would be against current guidelines and unlikely to be performed in a study. However, it is likely any cases of kernicterus in a healthy full-term infant would be reported. Since you want to know whether this occurs at all, you look for case reports of kernicterus developing in any healthy term infant with no hemolytic disease. Despite the fact that an incidence or prevalence cannot be obtained from such cases (we lack the total number of infants at risk), it would be reassuring if no such cases were found.

Fifteen citations are obtained. Of these, 10 reported cases of kernicterus in term infants. Two of the articles refer to a Danish term infant.[29,30] One article[31] is a duplicate reporting of another.[32] Five of the articles report kernicterus in term infants with underlying pathology (G6PD,[33] intestinal obstruction with large cephalohematoma,[34] ABO with hypernatremic dehydration,[35] isoimmune hemolytic anemia,[36] gastroschesis,[37] and congenital nephrotic syndrome[37]). You obtain the two articles in English reporting kernicterus in healthy, term infants.

Penn et al.[32] documented a case of kernicterus in a term infant of unspecified racial background. Although the infant was subsequently diagnosed with *Escherichia coli* sepsis and G6PD deficiency, he had been a healthy breastfed infant prior to presentation with "a 1-day history of jaundice, increasing lethargy, decreased appetite, and fever."[32]

The *MMWR* reported four healthy, term infants who developed kernicterus identified through self-reported survey.[38] Each was a male infant who subsequently developed feeding problems upon discharge. One infant had an ABO incompatibility but it was uncertain whether hemolysis was present. Serum bilirubin level was above 29 mg dl^{-1} for all cases and all were subsequently diagnosed with kernicterus.

Of interest, the *MMWR* refers to a pilot registry which documented 90 cases of kernicterus in 21 states from 1984–2001. Furthermore, it refers to a article by Maisels and Newman[39] who collected 22 cases over a period of 18 years referred by US attorneys for litigation alleging brain damage due to hyperbilirubinemia in healthy full-term infants without hemolytic disease. Six were term, Caucasian, breastfed infants with signs of classic acute bilirubin encephalopathy, chronic bilirubin encephalopathy, normal perinatal and neonatal course, no evidence of hemolytic condition, and no other cause for hyperbilirubinemia.

From these case reports/series, it can be concluded that kernicterus does occur in healthy term infants without hemolytic disease, at a low but unspecified rate. For some, development of jaundice and later signs of bilirubin toxicity revealed the presence of an underlying pathology such as G6PD deficiency, but differentiating between these two groups prior to signs of significant jaundice and neurotoxicity may be difficult.

Question

3. In a healthy term newborn with a bilirubin level of 20 mg dl^{-1} and hyperbilirubinemia not due to hemolytic disease

(*population and event*), what is the risk for development of adverse sequelae other than kernicterus (*outcome*)? **[Baseline Risk]**

● MedLine (PubMed): neonatal jaundice AND neurologic outcome

You find eleven citations, three of which are of particular interest. Hansen et al.[40] evaluated a subgroup of neonatal intensive care unit graduates. The goal was to assess psychosocial outcome and identify any association with neonatal bilirubin exposure. Of the 637 patients invited to participate, only 74 (12%) actually participated. This low rate of patient enrolment casts doubt on the validity of the study outcome. You decide to continue with other articles.

The article by Scheidt[10] provides a preliminary analysis of roughly 27 000 infants enrolled in the Collaborative Perinatal Project, a study from the late 1950s and early 1960s investigating the possible perinatal causes of cerebral palsy. This study was based on an incomplete sample and on a preliminary assessment of neurologic evaluations at 8 months to 1 year of age. Patient follow up was insufficient to provide an accurate assessment of long-term outcome. Sample size of patients with bilirubin level ≥ 20 mg dl^{-1} was small and the lack of differentiation between hemolytic and non-hemolytic causes for jaundice prevents extrapolation to the scenario.

A final analysis of CPP data performed by Newman and Klebanoff[14] was specifically limited to singleton Caucasian or African-American infants with birth weight > 2500 g who survived beyond 1 year of age. They examined the association between serum bilirubin level and three specific outcomes: IQ, neurologic examination (at 7–8 years of age), and hearing.[14] No relationship was found between bilirubin level and IQ, subsequent sensorineural hearing loss or abnormal neurologic examinations at 7–8 years. This study appears valid. A defined, representative sample of patients was assembled at birth, with follow up that was long enough (8 years) to document any sequelae. A total of 41 324 infants were initially enrolled with 20% lost subsequently to follow up. No association was found between neonatal bilirubin level and loss to follow up. It is uncertain whether assessments at 8 years of age were performed by investigators who were blinded to the initial bilirubin levels. However, an assessment protocol was used to limit bias. Subgroup analysis was done to adjust for confounding variables and effect modifiers.

After adjusting for confounding variables and for effect modification by race, there was no relationship between IQ and bilirubin level above or below 20 mg dl^{-1}. A linear association between IQ and bilirubin level was not found. Hearing assessments at 8 years of age were not done on all patients. Only 16 886 patients (50% of patients assessed neurologically at 8 years of age) had a hearing test. Of those tested, 374 (2·2%) had hearing loss. Of the 137 patients with bilirubin ≥ 20 mg dl^{-1}, only three had hearing loss. No association was found between high bilirubin levels and sensorineural hearing loss at 8 years. Because of the small number of patients receiving hearing tests, the validity of this result can be questioned. No relationship between abnormal neurologic examinations at 7 years and bilirubin level was found. The event rate for abnormal neurologic examination was also rare. Of 33 272 patients, 1261 had an abnormal neurologic examination at 8 years of age. Of the 268 infants with bilirubin ≥ 20 mg dl^{-1}, only 12 had an abnormal examination (RR = 1·2 [0·7, 2·1]). Only by including the abnormal neurologic examination group with the "suspicious" neurologic examination group was a significant association found between neurologic outcome and bilirubin level ≥ 20 mg dl^{-1} (RR = 1·5 [1·2, 1·9]). This association remained significant even after adjustments for covariates. Further analysis of the specific aspects of the neurologic examination revealed that increasing bilirubin levels were associated with mostly non-specific items (non-specific gait abnormalities, awkwardness, equivocal Babinski reflexes, abnormal cremasteric reflex, abnormal abdominal reflex, failure at fine stereognosis, unsatisfactory conditions for the examination, vasomotor abnormality, questionable hypotonia, and gaze abnormalities).

General applicability of this conclusion remains problematic. Only 268 infants in the study had serum bilirubin ≥ 20 mg dl^{-1}. Of those, only 66 infants had bilirubin ≥ 25 mg dl^{-1}. Roughly half of the infants in the CPP who had serum bilirubin ≥ 20 mg dl^{-1} received exchange transfusions, thus decreasing the severity of hyperbilirubinemia and potentially affecting the outcome. The use of exchange transfusion in such enrolled patients may underestimate the actual risk of neurologic sequelae for infants with bilirubin ≥ 20 mg dl^{-1}.

Based on your assessment of the identified literature, you conclude that the risk of kernicterus in a healthy term infant with a serum bilirubin level of ≥ 20 mg dl^{-1} is unknown. The CPP study is not capable of assessing the risks for infants with serum bilirubin levels ≥ 20 mg dl^{-1}. The results do suggest that levels of serum bilirubin < 20 mg dl^{-1} have little risk of causing full blown kernicterus in a term Caucasian or African-American infant. Whether the association of increasing serum bilirubin level is associated with subtle neurologic abnormalities remains uncertain but must be considered. Extrapolation to other ethnic groups is not possible.

Question

4. In healthy term breastfed newborns with hyperbilirubinemia (> 20 mg dl^{-1}) (*population*), is phototherapy (*intervention*) effective in reducing the bilirubin level and preventing kernicterus (*outcome*)? **[Therapy]**

● MedLine (PubMed): neonatal jaundice [MeSH] AND phototherapy [MeSH] AND clinical trials [MeSH]

Seven of the 14 articles located by your search were clinical trials investigating the use of phototherapy.[41–46] One study used non-random allocation of patients to treatment arms,[41] and another investigated the use of phototherapy to treat hyperbilirubinemia in infants with G6PD deficiency.[42] One study investigated different types of lamps and configuration to provide most effective phototherapy.[47] The remaining four articles refer to the "NICHD Randomized, Controlled Trial of Phototherapy for Neonatal Hyperbilirubinemia".[43–46] You obtain these four articles.

The NICHD study ran from 1974 to 1976. Its purpose was to assess the effectiveness of phototherapy in preventing brain injury from hyperbilirubinemia as assessed immediately, at 1 year and at 6 years. A total of 1339 infants were enrolled from six US centers. Participants were randomized to 96 hours of phototherapy or no phototherapy and stratified by center and birth weight categories. Exclusion criteria included underlying conditions or anomalies that may be adversely affected by study protocol, and presence of Rh disease that required intrauterine transfusion or presenting with low hemoglobin or high bilirubin at birth. The control and phototherapy groups were treated equally except for the use of phototherapy and an increased fluid intake in the phototherapy group. Protocols were established for the use of exchange transfusions when the bilirubin reached specific levels in either group.

The majority of infants enrolled had birth weights < 2·0 kg (69%). For infants with birth weight categories of 2·0–2·499 kg and ≥ 2·5 kg, there was a decrease in the mean daily serum bilirubin, but there was no change in the number of exchange transfusions required. Subgroup analysis showed a decrease in exchange transfusions only for those infants without hemolysis. There were 134 deaths in study participants during their first year of life, all but two in infants < 2·0 kg birthweight. There were no deaths in infants > 2·5 kg. Of the 85 infants who had an autopsy, only four infants were found to have kernicterus, all of whom weighed < 1500 g.[43]

Study participants were followed to 6 years of age.[48] There were no differences in cerebral palsy, other motor abnormalities, sensorineural hearing loss, development, or intelligence at 1-year and 6-year follow up. No infant in the study developed the full syndrome of posticteric encephalopathy with cerebral palsy, mental retardation, sensorineural hearing loss, and gaze palsy.[48] The sample size was sufficient to identify a moderate effect in dyskinesia, hearing loss, and mental retardation at the 1-year follow up. However, the further loss of patients at both the 1-year (83% returned) and the 6-year follow up (57·9% returned) may have affected the validity of the results.

Phototherapy appears to decrease neonatal hyperbilirubinemia in all infants regardless of birth weight, without immediate or long-term complications. Phototherapy decreases the need for exchange transfusions in all infants except for those with birth weight $\geq 2\cdot0$ kg whose hyperbilirubinemia is secondary to hemolysis. Because so few patients in the study developed kernicterus, it is uncertain whether use of phototherapy can prevent kernicterus.

Question

5. In a healthy term newborn with hyperbilirubinemia *(population)*, is fiberoptic phototherapy *(intervention)* as effective as conventional phototherapy *(comparison)* in reducing the serum bilirubin level *(outcome)*? **[Therapy]**

An important aspect of evidence-based medicine is to identify the "best" evidence by the simplest and most efficient means. The Cochrane Database of Systematic Reviews provides updated, appraised and summarized evidence of therapies.

The review by Mills and Tudehope[21] aimed to review the efficacy of fiberoptic phototherapy in newborn infants with jaundice. Randomized controlled trials that included infants up to 28 days of age with jaundice or elevated serum bilirubin requiring phototherapy were included. The meta-analysis included studies comparing fiberoptic phototherapy to no treatment and studies comparing fiberoptic phototherapy versus conventional phototherapy using halogen or fluorescent lamps. The review was last updated in November 2000.

Thirty-one studies were identified of which seven were excluded due to susceptibility of the study to bias or uncertain eligibility; 24 studies were included in the various analyses. The majority of studies compared fiberoptic versus conventional phototherapy. Conventional phototherapy had a greater percentage change in serum bilirubin level after 24 and 48 hours of therapy (weighted mean difference [WMD] $3\cdot59\%$; 95% CI $1\cdot27$, $5\cdot92$ and WMD $10\cdot79\%$; 95% CI $8\cdot33$, $13\cdot26$). Use of fiberoptic phototherapy was associated with a more likely need for additional phototherapy (RR $1\cdot68$; 95% CI $1\cdot18$, $2\cdot38$). However, there was no difference between the two forms of phototherapy in the need for exchange transfusion, or the need for repeat phototherapy for rebound jaundice. The conclusions were similar after stratifying for the type of conventional phototherapy used (white light or blue light).

The majority of studies excluded infants with hemolysis. No studies specifically investigated the use of fiberoptic phototherapy in infants with hemolysis or provided data on those infants with hemolysis who were included. Furthermore, no study to date has investigated the effects of the different types of phototherapy on parent–child bonding.

Fiberoptic phototherapy appears to be less effective than conventional phototherapy in lowering serum bilirubin levels. The effectiveness of fiberoptic phototherapy in those infants with jaundice due to hemolysis remains uncertain. The beneficial effects of fiberoptic phototherapy on parent–child bonding remains to be proven.

Resolution of the scenario

Your search and appraisal of the literature allows you to reach some conclusions regarding hyperbilirubinemia for the healthy, term infant who is your patient. Clinical assessment of the cephalocaudal progression of jaundice has the potential of being a readily available and inexpensive test to define which infants require further investigation and possible treatment. However, the large interobserver variability seen with this technique and the lack of validation in diverse ethnic populations make you less enthusiastic. There is little evidence regarding the actual risk of kernicterus in a healthy term infant with a serum bilirubin level of ≥ 20 mg dl^{-1}, but it is likely that the risk is very small. Risk of other neurologic sequelae (IQ, CNS abnormalities, hearing) for healthy term infants with serum bilirubin < 20 mg dl^{-1} is also probably small. However, risk of such other neurologic sequelae is unknown for infants with serum bilirubin ≥ 20 mg dl^{-1}. Phototherapy appears to decrease neonatal hyperbilirubinemia and the need for exchange transfusions in all infants except for those with birth weight $\geq 2\cdot0$ kg whose hyperbilirubinemia is secondary to hemolysis. Because so few patients develop kernicterus, it is uncertain whether use of phototherapy can prevent kernicterus. Fiberoptic phototherapy is less effective than conventional phototherapy in reducing serum bilirubin. After making sure that the patient has no underlying abnormalities, you decide to admit your patient to the hospital for phototherapy, and reassure the parents that adverse outcomes are very rare in this situation.

Future research needs

- Better methods of predicting which healthy infants may develop significant jaundice requiring eventual treatment.
- Assessment of non-invasive measures of bilirubin or bilirubin production (photometry, end-tidal CO_2 [ETCO$_2$]) and their ability to predict need for treatment.
- Estimate of the incidence of bilirubin encephalopathy/ kernicterus in the population of newborns with significantly elevated serum bilirubin.
- Assessment of compliance with published guidelines for investigation and treatment of neonatal hyperbilirubinemia.

Acknowledgement

The author would like to thank the editors for the opportunity to write this chapter. The author also acknowledges the invaluable assistance of Dr Molly Seshia and Dr Leslie Simard-Chiu during the development and completion of this chapter.

Summary table

Question	Type of evidence	Result	Comment
Usefulness of clinical assessment to determine need for serum bilirubin test	Cross-sectional studies, mostly single observer	Jaundice to feet: infant likely to have bilirubin > 15 mg dl^{-1} No jaundice below nipple line: infant not likely to have bilirubin > 12 mg dl^{-1}	Very high interobserver variability
Risk of kernicterus in healthy term infant with bilirubin > 20 mg dl^{-1}, not due to hemolytic disease	Case reports	Very rare, but rate cannot be determined	
Risk of adverse neurologic outcome in healthy term infant with bilirubin >20 mg dl^{-1}, not due to hemolytic disease	Cohort study, based on CPP data	No relationship to IQ, hearing loss, abnormal neurologic examination. Possible relationship with "non-specific" neurologic findings	Primary outcome measures are proxies for outcomes of true interest
Effectiveness of phototherapy in preventing kernicterus or other adverse neurologic outcome	Randomized non-blinded trial	Phototherapy decreased biliriubin and need for exchange transfusion, but other outcomes too rare to assess	
Effectiveness of fiberoptic v conventional phototheray	Cochrane Systematic Review: 24 RCTs included	Fiberoptic phototherapy less effective than conventional phototherapy	Infants with hemolysis generally excluded

References

1 Allen SH, Diamond LK, Vaughn VC. Erythroblastosis fetalis: VI. Prevention of kernicterus. *Am J Dis Child* 1950;**80**: 779–91.

2 Hsia DY, Allen FH, Gellis SS *et al.* Erythroblastosis fetalis: VIII. Studies of serum bilirubin in relation to kernicterus. *N Engl J Med* 1952;**247**:668–71.

3 Mollison PL, Cutbush M. A method of measuring the severity of a series of cases of haemolytic disease of the newborn. *Blood* 1951;**6**:777–88.

4 Mollison PL, Walker W. Controlled trials of the treatment of haemolytic disease of the newborn. *Lancet* 1952;**1**: 429–33.

5 Hsia DY, Gellis SS. Studies on erythroblastosis due to ABO incompatibility. *Pediatrics* 1954;**13**:503.

6 Bengtsson B, Verneholt J. A follow up study of hyperbilirubinemia in healthy, full term infants without isoimmunization. *Acta Paediatr Scand* 1974;**63**:70–80.

7 Watchko JF, Oski FA. Bilirubin 20 mg dl-1 = vigintiphobia. *Pediatrics* 1983;**71**:660–3.

8 Smith Z. Technical report. Practice parameter: the management of hyperbilirubinemia in healthy newborns. In: Practice parameters from the American Academy of Pediatrics. American Academy of Pediatrics, 1997.

9 Boggs T, Hardy J, Frazier T. Correlation of neonatal serum total bilirubin concentration and developmental status at age eight months. Preliminary report from the collaborative project. *J Pediatr* 1967;**71**:553–60.

10 Scheidt P, Mellits E, Hardy J, Drage J, Boggs T. Toxicity to bilirubin in neonates. Infant development during first year in relation to maximum neonatal serum bilirubin concentration. *J Pediatr* 1977;**91**:292–7.

11 Naeye R. Amniotic fluid infections, neonatal hyperbilirubinemia, and psychomotor impairment. *Pediatrics* 1978; **2**:497–503.

12 Hardy J, Peeples M. Serum bilirubin levels in newborn infants. Distributions and associations with neurological abnormalities during the first year of life. *Johns Hopkins Med J* 1971;**128**:265–72.

13 Rubin R, Balow B, Fisch R. Neonatal serum bilirubin levels related to cognitive development at ages 4 through 7 years. *J Pediatr* 1979;**94**:601–4.

14 Newman TB, Klebanoff MA. Neonatal hyperbilirubinemia and long-term outcome: another look at the collaborative perinatal project. *Pediatrics* 1993;**92**:651–7.

15 Gartner LM. Neonatal jaundice. *Pediatr Rev* 1994;**15**: 422–32.

16 Gourley GR. Bilirubin metabolism and kernicterus. *Adv Pediatr* 1997;**44**:173–229.

17 Halamek LP, Stevenson DK. Neonatal jaundice and liver disease. In: Fanaroff AA, Martin RJ, eds. Neonatal-perinatal medicine. Disease of the fetus and infant. 6th edn. Philadelphia: Mosby Yearbook, 1997.

18 Dobbs RH, Cremer RJ. Phototherapy. *Arch Dis Child* 1975; **50**:833–6.

19 Cremer RJ, Perryman PW, Richard DH. Photosensitivity of serum bilirubin. *Biochem J* 1957;**66**:60P.

20 Maisal MJ. Phototherapy – 25 years later. In: Fanaroff AA, Klaus MH, eds. The year book of neonatal and perinatal medicine. Philadelphia: Mosby Yearbook, 1996, pp. 29–34.

21 Mills JF, Tudehope D. Fiberoptic phototherapy for neonatal jaundice (Cochrane Review). *Cochrane Library*, Issue 2. Oxford: Update Software, 2003.

22 Bratlid D. [Phototherapy of newborn infants with hyperbilirubinemia. Norwegian Medical Society.] *Tidsskr Nor Laegeforen* 1996;**116**:3207–8.

23 Fetter WP, van de Bor M, Brand PL *et al.* [Hyperbilirubinemia in healthy full-term neonates: guidelines for diagnosis and treatment. Ad-hoc Commission on Hyperbilirubinemia and Phototherapy of the Neonatology Section of the Netherlands Society for Pediatrics] *Ned Tijdschr Geneeskd* 1997;**141**: 140–3.

24 American Academy of Pediatrics Provisional Committee for Quality Improvement and Subcommittee on Hyperbilirubinemia. Practice parameter: management of hyperbilirubinemia in the healthy term newborn. *Pediatrics* 1994; **94**;558–65 [Published erratum in *Pediatrics* 1995;**95**: 459–61].

25 AAP Subcommittee on Neonatal Hyperbilirubinemia. Neonatal Jaundice and Kernicterus. *Pediatrics* 2001;**108**:763–5.

26 Kramer LI. Advancement of dermal icterus in the jaundiced newborn. *Am J Dis Child* 1969;**118**:454–8.

27 Ebbesen F. The relationship between the cephalo-pedal progress of clinical icterus and the serum bilirubin concentration in newborn infants without blood type sensitization. *Acta Obstet Gynecol Scand* 1975;**54**:329–32.

28 Moyer VA, Ahn C, Sneed S. Accuracy of clinical judgement in neonatal jaundice. *Arch Ped Adol Med* 2000;**154**:391–4.

29 Straver B, Hassing MB, van der Knaap MS, Gemke RJ. Kernicterus in a full-term male infant a few days old. *Ned Tijdschr Geneeskd* 2002;**146**:909–13.

30 Semmekrot BA. Kernicterus in a full-term male infant a few days old. *Ned Tijdschr Geneeskd* 2002;**146**:1712–13.

31 Centers for Disease Control and Prevention. Kernicterus in full-term infants – United States, 1994–1998. *JAMA* 2001;**286(3)**:299–300.

32 Penn AA, Enzmann DR, Hahn JS, Stevenson DK. Kernicterus in a full term infant. *Pediatrics* 1994;**93**:1003–6.

33 Akhtar S, Drenovak M, Bantock H, Mackinnon H, Graham J. Glucose 6-phosphate dehydrogenase deficiency with kernicterus: progressive late recovery from profound deafness. *Int J Pediatr Otorhinolaryngol* 1998;**43**:129–40.

34 de Weerd W, Wymenga II, Bergman KA. Bilirubin encephalopathy in an icteric bile-vomiting infant with high intestinal obstruction. *Ned Tijdschr Geneeskd* 1997;**141**: 155–7.

35 Christensen AE. Kernicterus hos et maturt barn. [Kernicterus in a full term infant]. *Ugeskr for Laeger* 1996;**158**:1230–1.

36 Schroeder LL, O'Connor TA. Bilirubin encephalopathy in a term infant after planned home delivery. *Mo Med* 1992; **89**:741–2.

37 Perlman JM, Rogers BB, Burns D. Kernicteric findings at autopsy in two sick near term infants. *Pediatrics* 1997;**99**: 612–15.

38 Centers for Disease Control and Prevention. PMID no. 11428729 MMWR *Morb Mortal Wkly Rep* 2001;**50**: 491–4.

39 Maisels MJ, Newman TB. Kernicterus in otherwise healthy breastfed term newborns. *Pediatrics* 1995;**96**:730–3.

40 Hansen RL, Hughes GG, Ahlfors CE. Neonatal bilirubin exposure and psychoeducational outcome. *J Dev Behav Pediatr* 1991;**12**:287–93.

41 Martin JR. Phototherapy, phenobarbitone and physiological jaundice in the newborn infant. *NZ Med J* 1974;**79**:1022–4.

42 Meloni T, Costa S, Dore A, Cutillo S. Phototherapy for neonatal hyperbilirubinemia in mature newborn infants with erythrocyte G-6-PD deficiency. *J Pediatr* 1974;**85**:560–2.

43 National Institute of Child Health and Human Development. Randomized controlled trials of phototherapy for neonatal hyperbilirubinemia. *Pediatrics* 1985;**75**(Suppl.):385–441.

44 Randomized Controlled Trial of Phototherapy for Neonatal Hyperbilirubinemia. Executive summary. *Pediatrics* 1985;**75** (Suppl.):385–6.

45 Bryla DA. Randomized, controlled trial of phototherapy for neonatal hyperbilirubinemia. *Pediatrics* 1985;**75**(Suppl.): 387–92.

46 Brown AK, Kim MH, Wu PYK, Bryla DA. Efficacy of phototherapy in prevention and management of neonatal hyperbilirubinemia. *Pediatrics* 1985;**75**(Suppl.):393–400.

47 Eggert P, Stick C, Swalve S. On the efficacy of various irradiation regimens in phototherapy of neonatal hyperbilirubinemia. *Eur J Pediatr* 1988;**147**:525–8.

48 Scheidt PC, Bryla DA, Nelson KB *et al.* Phototherapy for neonatal hyperbilirubinemia: six year follow up of the National Institute of Child Health and Human Development clinical trial. *Pediatrics* 1990;**85**:455–63.

49 Neonatal encephalopathy

Nadia Badawi, John M Keogh

Case scenario

You are called to the postnatal ward to see a 6-hour-old male infant who is having seizures. On examination he is irritable and hypertonic. He has not been feeding well. You are told that he was born at 41 weeks gestation by emergency cesarean section for fetal distress, to a primiparous woman aged 39 years. This pregnancy was conceived using in vitro *fertilization and the mother developed late onset pre-eclampsia during the pregnancy. The infant's birth weight was 2·6 kg. His Apgar scores were 2 and 7 at 1 and 5 minutes respectively. The umbilical arterial blood gases showed a pH of 7·2 with a base excess of −8, consistent with mild metabolic acidosis and within the normal range. He was discharged to the postnatal ward following bag and mask resuscitation in the delivery room. The placenta was noted to have several pale areas and was sent for pathological examination. The pediatric resident at the resuscitation has written in the notes that this is a case of "birth asphyxia". The parents ask you what is wrong with their baby, what caused his illness and what will be his outcome.*

Background

Neonatal encephalopathy in the term infant is an important condition with significant mortality as well as short and long-term morbidity. It is defined clinically by an abnormal level of consciousness, seizures, abnormal tone and movement, and an inability to feed or initiate/maintain respiration due to a central neurological cause.[1] This definition requires the presence of either seizures alone or at least two of these features to be present for > 24 hours.[2] Different grading systems have been proposed to classify the severity of neonatal encephalopathy. The best known of these by Sarnat and Sarnat [3] refers to the subgroup with hypoxic ischemic encephalopathy. Badawi *et al.* and others have adapted Sarnat's definition to differentiate between moderate and severe encephalopathy.[2] Criteria for moderate and severe encephalopathy are given in Table 49.1. Mild encephalopathy may be considered to be present when, in the absence of seizures, a baby displays abnormalities of tone, feeding, respiratory drive, or level of consciousness of < 24 hours duration. The diagnosis of mild encephalopathy is notoriously difficult to make because of its very subjective and transient nature.

It is well known that there are many causes for neonatal encephalopathy, including sepsis, inborn errors of metabolism, drugs, and neurological birth defects. There is increasing evidence that most cases of neonatal encephalopathy are not

the result of intrapartum events[4] and that most babies with encephalopathy do not develop cerebral palsy (CP).[5,6] However, despite this there has been a pervasive belief that neonatal encephalopathy is synonymous with intrapartum hypoxia. Until recently the research and publication emphasis has been on the subgroup of newborns with encephalopathy associated with intrapartum hypoxia. This needs to be borne in mind when studies of neonatal encephalopathy are reviewed because they will not necessarily all include infants with the same condition. Furthermore, the assumption that neonatal encephalopathy is caused by hypoxia-ischemia has introduced significant bias into the interpretation of clinical findings.

A proportion of children with neonatal encephalopathy go on to develop cerebral palsy. In the National Collaborative Perinatal Project 70% of term or near term infants who had a 5-minute Apgar score < 3, adverse neonatal signs, and seizures died or had cerebral palsy by age 7 years.[7] However, < 10% of children with cerebral palsy have this cluster of features.[8,9] In both of the international consensus statements that examine the precursors of cerebral palsy, the presence of neonatal encephalopathy is considered an essential criterion for CP due to an intrapartum etiology.[10,11] The causal pathway for CP may have contributions from several events, including events during the intrapartum period, and it is difficult to know if any one event in its own right is sufficient to cause damage in a given infant (Figure 49.1).

Table 49.1   Features of moderate and severe newborn encephalopathy[2]

Criteria for moderate encephalopathy	Criteria for severe encephalopathy
Either seizures alone or two of the following for more than 24 hours: • abnormal level of consciousness • abnormal tone and movement • inability to feed due to a presumed neurological cause • inability to initiate/maintain respiration due to a central neurological cause	Meets the definition of moderate but in addition has at least one of the following features: • being comatose or stuporous • ventilation for > 24 hours • two or more anticonvulsants • death in the neonatal period following encephalopathy

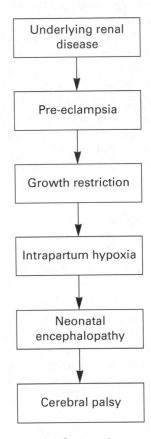

Figure 49.1   An example of a causal sequence for neonatal encephalopathy

In this chapter we discuss the prevalence, risk factors and outcomes of neonatal encephalopathy but have not addressed issues of investigation or treatment.

Framing answerable clinical questions

You decide on clinical grounds that this baby has neonatal encephalopathy. This raises a number of questions:

- How frequent is this problem?
- What causes it?
- Could it be due to "birth asphyxia"?
- Will the infant survive?
- If he survives will he suffer permanent neurological damage?

You frame these clinical questions into a structured form that will help you search for the answers (see Chapter 2).

Questions

1. In term newborn infants (*population/exposure*), what is the incidence/prevalence of moderate or severe neonatal encephalopathy (*outcome*)? **[Baseline Risk]**
2. In term newborn infants (*population*), what are the risk factors (*exposures*) for moderate or severe neonatal encephalopathy (*outcome*)? **[Causation]**
3. In term infants (*population*), does intrapartum hypoxia (*exposure*) cause moderate or severe neonatal encephalopathy (*outcome*)? **[Causation]**
4. In term infants (*population*) with moderate or severe neonatal encephalopathy (*exposure*), what is the short-term and long-term outlook (*outcome*)? **[Prognosis]**

Searching for evidence

For information on prevalence (or baseline risk) as in question 1, you look for cohort studies (preferably population-based birth cohorts) as outlined in Chapter 4. For questions of causation as in question 2, a randomized controlled trial (RCT) provides the most reliable evidence but may not be available. In certain circumstances (Chapter 7) causation can also be inferred from well-designed cohort or case–control analytic studies. Cohort studies provide the best evidence on prognosis as in question 3.

You realize you are unlikely to find summarized evidence to answer your questions in *Clinical Evidence*[12] or the *Cochrane Library,*[13] which have an emphasis on therapy. The

Cochrane Database of Systematic Reviews (CDSR) and the Database of Reviews of Effects (DARE) contain predominantly systematic reviews of randomized controlled trials and the Cochrane Controlled Trials Register (CENTRAL) contains RCTs. However, it is possible these sources may contain randomized trials of exposure to a risk factor such as mode of delivery or treatment for maternal conditions in pregnancy (for example, pre-eclampsia, thyroid disease). Also, narrative reviews and consensus statements may contain data from cohort studies.

Neonatal encephalopathy does not appear as a MeSH term. Therefore it is necessary to search databases using many different terms. You use the terms "neonatal seizures", "hypoxic-ischemic encephalopathy" and "birth asphyxia/ asphyxia neonatorum" as well as "neonatal and newborn encephalopathy"as keywords to search the *Cochrane Library*, *Clinical Evidence*, and MedLine. In MedLine you use combination searches clicking on both MeSH and keyword subheadings and then combining search results using the "AND" operator to join the terms (see Chapter 3 on searching for evidence). You realize it is important to differentiate between neonatal encephalopathy overall and the subgroup of hypoxic ischemic encephalopathy.

In the *Cochrane Library* you find several completed systematic reviews. One (based on pre-eclampsia and neonatal encephalopathy) is indirectly relevant and another by Thacker *et al.*[14] reviews the impact of electronic fetal heart rate monitoring during labor on outcome and considers (amongst other things) the impact on neonatal seizures. DARE contains several abstracts of quality assessed systematic reviews, but none are directly relevant to your questions. In CENTRAL you find one RCT under neonatal seizures and cardiotocographs (CTGs) which has some relevance.

You then go to MedLine using the PubMed search screen, enter "neonatal encephalopathy AND etiology" and find 139 articles. You scan the titles and discard the majority since they either do not relate to your area of interest or consist of small case series and address mainly infants assumed to have "hypoxic ischemic encephalopathy".

You are also aware of several consensus statements published in recent years by multidisciplinary panels of experts and endorsed by various professional organizations. These statements provide useful reviews of the literature and highlight some of the limitations of the current knowledge base. Searching in PubMed under "newborn encephalopathy AND guideline" and "cerebral palsy AND consensus" you find a consensus statement by an international group[10] that touches upon neonatal encephalopathy in the context of cerebral palsy. Searching on the American College of Obstetrics and Gynecology website you find a recent joint statement from the American College of Obstetricians and Gynecologists (ACOG) and the American Academy of Pediatrics (AAP) looking at the etiology of newborn encephalopathy.[11] This includes a comprehensive literature review and assessment of the quality of the evidence. The stated aim of this document is to "consider the current state of scientific knowledge about the mechanisms and timing of possible etiological events which may result in neonatal encephalopathy".

Apart from the systematic reviews mentioned previously the only evidence from randomized controlled trials relevant to term infants relates to intrapartum monitoring[15–16] and "fetal intensive care".[17] All other evidence is from analytical studies with concurrent non-randomized controls (cohort and case–control studies), case series without concurrent controls or opinions of respected authorities (narrative reviews), and consensus reports of expert committees.

Question

1. In term newborn infants (*population/exposure*), what is the incidence/prevalence of moderate or severe neonatal encephalopathy (*outcome*)? **[Baseline Risk]**

You find a number of studies reporting birth prevalence of neonatal encephalopathy. However, comparison between studies is difficult because of the lack of uniform diagnostic criteria used. In some studies inclusive criteria are used while in other studies only subgroups of infants, such as infants with hypoxic-ischemic encephalopathy, are included. Even when a defined subgroup is included, it is not always clear that the population studied really represents the group in question, since assumptions about etiology may lead to misclassification of cases. Therefore the reported birth prevalence of the cluster of conditions covered by the overarching banner of newborn encephalopathy differs widely.

You find one review of three population-based studies of neonatal encephalopathy[18] in term infants. Two of the three studies use broad clinical criteria similar to those outlined previously while the third looks predominantly at hypoxic ischemic encephalopathy. The reported birth prevalence of neonatal encephalopathy was between 1·9 and 3·8/1000 live births.

In the statement from ACOG and AAP,[11] which is based on a systematic review of the literature, the birth prevalence of neonatal encephalopathy is reported as between 1 and 8 per 1000 live births. Prevalence varies according to the definition used and the population in which the study is conducted. The authors conclude that "the best available evidence suggests a rate of pure HIE (i.e., the subgroup of neonatal encephalopathy with intrapartum hypoxia in the absence of any other preconceptional or ante-partum abnormalities) of 1·6/10 000 live births."

Table 49·2   Preconceptional risk factors for neonatal encephalopathy in the Western Australian and Nepalese studies

	Western Australian Study[2,4]	Nepalese Study[19]
Risk factor	**Adjusted OR (95% CI)**	**Adjusted OR (95% CI)**
Family history of seizures	2·55 (1·31–4·94)	Data not available
Infertility treatment (mainly IVF)	4·43 (1·12–17·60)	Data not available
Being unemployed	3·60 (1·10–11·80)	Data not available
Nuliparity	1·81 (0·87–3·73)	2·0 (1·10–3·61)
Maternal age > 35 years	6·01 (1·28–28·15)	4·35 (1·04–18·22)
Maternal short stature*	0·98 (0·57–1·70)	3·16 (1·50–6·66)
No antenatal care**	5·45 (0·47–62·98)	2·05 (1·16–3·66)
Maternal thyroid abnormality	9·7 (1·97–47·91)	2·14 (1·19–3·82)

*Short stature defined as < 160 cm in the Australian population and < 145 cm in the Nepalese population
**No or late antenatal care in the Australian population; no antenatal care in the Nepalese population

Question

2. In term newborn infants (*population*), what are the risk factors (*exposures*) for moderate or severe neonatal encephalopathy (*outcome*)? **[Causation]**

You find two large case–control studies in your search. The first is a population-based case–control study from Australia and the second a large hospital based study from Nepal.[2,4,19] Although both are of interest, you are particularly interested in the one with a patient population that is similar to your own. You take note of the definition of neonatal encephalopathy used in the papers and find that they are both considering the same condition. The definitions are inclusive and make no assumptions about etiology, thus casting a wide net for risk factors. Unlike most earlier studies, both of these included unmatched controls, used a clinical definition without assuming an etiology, and examined risk factors in different epochs of pregnancy. The Australian study is the first population-based study published. In contrast to the Australian study, the authors of the Nepal study included infants with mild encephalopathy and excluded those with neonatal sepsis, congenital malformations or primary hypoglycemia. The authors of the Australian study excluded infants with mild encephalopathy because the clinical features are subtle and likely to be overlooked leading to underascertainment and therefore an incomplete population for study. Furthermore, in developed countries, mild encephalopathy is not associated with adverse outcomes.[20–23]

The most striking feature from the two studies is the wide range of preconceptional and antepartum risk factors identified and the relatively small role of intrapartum hypoxia. Some of the significant independent risk factors identified for neonatal encephalopathy include social class, maternal age, maternal employment status, health insurance status, family history of seizures or neurological disorders, infertility treatment, placental abnormality, maternal thyroid disease, pre-eclampsia, fetal growth restriction, viral illness during pregnancy, postmaturity, pyrexia in labor, and intrapartum emergencies. A negative association was found between neonatal encephalopathy and having an elective cesarean section. In summary, in Western Australia, 69% of infants with neonatal encephalopathy had only antepartum risk factors, 25% had antepartum and intrapartum risk factors, 4% had only intrapartum risk factors, and 2% had no identifiable risk factors.[4] This contrasts with the risk factors in Nepal[19] where 60% of cases had evidence of intrapartum compromise or were born after an intrapartum difficulty likely to result in fetal compromise. The odds ratios (ORs) reported in these papers for a selection of risk factors is shown in Table 49.2 and Table 49.3. It is not clear whether the risk factors identified in these studies act in isolation, or more likely, in unison. The causal pathways to neonatal encephalopathy are difficult to elucidate, but should be the focus of further research. Conditions associated with neonatal encephalopathy that may be amenable to treatment,[24] including metabolic disorders and infection, should also be identified.

You also find several randomized controlled trials looking at the impact of electronic fetal heart rate monitoring during labor on rates of neonatal encephalopathy and neonatal seizures.[14–16] The results of these studies are remarkably uniform and show an approximately 50% reduction in seizures in the monitored group. This has however not been shown to translate into a reduction in cerebral palsy in follow up studies.[25] It is possible that this intervention would also decrease the rate of other forms of neonatal encephalopathy; however, this was not an outcome reported in this study.

Table 49.3 Antepartum and intrapartum risk factors for neonatal encephalopathy in the Western Australian and Nepalese studies

Risk factor	Western Australian Study[2,4] Adjusted OR (95% CI)	Nepalese Study[19] Adjusted OR (95% CI)
Pre-eclampsia	Overall 2·39 (1·31–4·36) Mild 1·62 (0·80–3·27) Severe 6·30 (2·25–17·62)	Overall 1·86 (0·82–4·22)
Bleeding in pregnancy	3·57 (1·30–9·85)	Data not available
Viral illness in pregnancy	2·97 (1·52–5·80)	Data not available
Twins	1·04 (0·11–9·55)	22·11 (3·45–141·47)
Gestational age 42 weeks	13·2 (5·03–34·83)	Data not available
Birth weight < 3rd percentile	38·23 (9·44–154·79)	Data not available
Non-vertex presentation	1·47 (0·35–6·21)	3·35 (1·38–8·11)
Occipito posterior position	4·29 (1·74–10·54)	Data not available
Prolonged rupture of membranes	1·31 (0·69–2·47)	3·84 (1·56–9·47)
Induction of labor	0·97 (0·57–1·68)	5·28 (2·03–13·76)
Intrapartum pyrexia ≥ 37·5° C	3·82 (1·44–10·12)	Data not available
Acute intrapartum event	4·44 (1·30–15·22)	28·16 (2·88–275·6)
Obstructed labor	Data not available	5·73 (2·30–14·23)
Instrumental vaginal delivery	2·34 (1·16–4·7)	Forceps 6·11 (1·005–37·17) Vacuum 7·93 (3·02 to 20·78)
Emergency cesarean	2·17 (1·01–4·64)	3·91 (1·96–7·84)
Elective cesarean*	0·17 (0·05–0·56)	No encephalopathic babies born by elective cesarean section
Probable intrapartum hypoxia**	29%	60%

*Elective cesarean section demonstrated an apparently protective effect
**Using identical criteria

Question

3. In term infants (*population*), does intrapartum hypoxia (*exposure*) cause moderate or severe neonatal encephalopathy (*outcome*)? **[Causation]**

Considerable evidence from animal models demonstrates a causal link between severe hypoxia and encephalopathy.[26,27] While intrapartum hypoxia can clearly cause neonatal encephalopathy, hypoxia is difficult to diagnose. In general, all the criteria used to indicate intrapartum hypoxia, such as an abnormal intrapartum cardiotocograph, an abnormal fetal heart rate, meconium stained amniotic fluid, and low Apgar scores are non-specific. The ACOG taskforce[11] describe a set of essential criteria that must be met in order to support a diagnosis of an intrapartum hypoxic-ischemic event sufficient to cause neonatal encephalopathy, an essential precursor of cerebral palsy due to intrapartum hypoxia (see Box). In their view, "If any one of the four essential criteria is not met, this provides strong evidence that intrapartum hypoxia was not the cause of neurological injury." However they also assert that even "when all four essential criteria outlined are met, it is important to determine whether the hypoxia is attributable to chronic or intermittent hypoxia of long standing duration of days or weeks or whether acute hypoxia has occurred during labor in a previously healthy fetus." They also have criteria which collectively suggest an intrapartum timing but which in themselves, except for a sentinel event, are only weakly associated with acute intrapartum hypoxia, i.e., are non-specific to asphyxial insults. The 1999 international consensus[10] also lists clinical features that make an intrapartum cause less likely. Together these statements provide useful guidelines, in no small part because they require clinicians to positively make a diagnosis rather than an assumption of hypoxia.

These criteria have primarily applied to studies with cerebral palsy rather than neonatal encephalopathy as the outcome. Few studies have addressed the relationship between intrapartum hypoxia and neonatal encephalopathy. In the Australian study,[4] 29% of infants with neonatal encephalopathy had evidence of probable intrapartum hypoxia including 4% who had this as their only identifiable risk factor. In the Nepal study[19] this figure was higher with 60% of case infants demonstrating probable intrapartum hypoxia using similar diagnostic criteria.

Criteria to define an acute intrapartum hypoxic event as sufficient to cause cerebral palsy

1. Essential criteria (must meet all four):

- Evidence of a metabolic acidosis in fetal umbilical cord arterial blood obtained at delivery (pH < 7 and base deficit ≥ 12 mmol liter^{-1})
- Early onset of *severe or moderate neonatal encephalopathy* in infants born at 34 or more weeks of gestation
- Cerebral palsy of the spastic quadriplegic or dyskinetic type
- Exclusion of other identifiable etiologies such as trauma, coagulation disorders, infectious conditions or genetic disorders

2. Criteria that collectively suggest intrapartum hypoxia (within close proximity to labor and delivery, for example, 0–48 hours) but are non-specific to asphyxial insults:

- A sentinel (signal) hypoxic event occurring immediately before or during labor
- A sudden and sustained fetal bradycardia or the absence of fetal heart rate variability in the presence of persistent, late, or variable decelerations, usually after a hypoxic sentinel event when the pattern was previously normal
- Apgar scores of 0–3 beyond 5 minutes
- Onset of multisystem involvement within 72 hours of birth
- Early imaging study showing evidence of acute non-focal cerebral abnormality

Question

4. In term infants (*population*) with moderate or severe neonatal encephalopathy (*exposure*), what is the short-term and long-term outlook (*outcome*)? **[Prognosis]**

The neonatal mortality rate for moderate and severe neonatal encephalopathy is about 10% in Australia[2,5] while in Nepal[19] it is 31%. Death may also occur later on during infancy and childhood; the mortality rate had risen to 13·2% in the Australian study at age 2 years and to 44% in the Nepal study by the age of 1 year. Therefore in both studies most deaths of encephalopathic infants occurred in the neonatal period. In the Nepal study the authors also described a mortality rate of 17% for mild encephalopathy. This highlights the differences in the effects of encephalopathy in developing and developed countries. In developed countries mild encephalopathy has not been associated with death or neurodevelopmental disability.[20–22] Mortality and morbidity in term infants with neonatal encephalopathy are related to the severity of disease. In several case series of the subgroup of hypoxic ischemic encephalopathy the mortality rate has

been reported to be as high as 50% for severe cases and 30% for moderate cases.[22,28] In the Australian study, which is the only population-based case–control study with inclusive diagnostic criteria, 33% of infants with severe newborn encephalopathy died and 16% developed CP compared with 6% and 7% respectively in moderate encephalopathy.[5]

In the Australian study 39% of infants with neonatal encephalopathy had a poor outcome,[18] defined by death, CP, or a significant degree of developmental delay, compared with only 2·7% of controls. Furthermore, 62% of infants with severe encephalopathy had a poor outcome compared with 25% of infants with moderate encephalopathy. In the Nepal study,[28] moderate encephalopathy was associated with a 71% risk of severe impairment or death while severe encephalopathy had a 97% risk of death or severe impairment.

Though most studies have focused on cerebral palsy and death there are many other adverse outcomes of neonatal encephalopathy, including behavioral and learning problems and epilepsy.[5,20–22,29–35] When disabilities such as cognitive impairment and developmental delay have been considered, they have frequently been reported only for infants with hypoxic ischemic encephalopathy.

CP has been the outcome that has received most attention in the medical literature as it is one of the more common, dramatic, and disabling conditions of childhood. In the case–control study from Australia,[5] 10% of children who had neonatal encephalopathy went on to develop CP by 2 years of age compared with 20% of children in the Nepal study,[28] most of whom had spastic quadriplegia.

A recent systematic review of studies published between 1966 and 1997[35] has described the association between Apgar score, umbilical blood pH, or Sarnat grading of encephalopathy, and long-term adverse outcome. The authors identified abstracts of 1312 studies and reviewed 81 articles, 42 of which qualified for inclusion in their meta-analysis. The rate of CP was higher in infants with severe hypoxic ischemic encephalopathy compared with moderate hypoxic ischemic encephalopathy (combined OR 20; 95% CI 6–70). It was also higher for infants with a 20-minute Apgar score between 0–3 compared with infants with a score of ≥ 4 (combined OR 15; 95% CI 5–50).

In the case–control study from Australia, assessment of cases of neonatal encephalopathy who did not have CP at 2 years, showed that 15·5% had developmental delay with a mean developmental score of <85 compared with 2·5% in the control group.[5]

Robertson *et al.* report the outcomes at 8 years of a regional study of infants with hypoxic ischemic encephalopathy[22]: 226 infants were originally enrolled in the neonatal period though results were available on only 174 by 8 years. The mortality rate was 13%. The incidence of impairment, which included CP, blindness, cognitive delay, convulsive disorder, and severe hearing loss, was 16% among those assessed at 8 years (75% of survivors). Intellectual, visual-motor integration, and receptive vocabulary scores, as well as reading, spelling, and arithmetic grade levels were significantly lower in survivors of moderate or severe encephalopathy than in survivors of mild encephalopathy or classroom peers ($P < 0.01$). Non-impaired survivors of moderate encephalopathy were more likely to be delayed by more than one grade level than were children from the mild encephalopathy group or control classroom peers. Severity of encephalopathy was strongly associated with adverse outcome. No children in the mild encephalopathy group who had data available at 8 years had died or had significant disability rates compared with 5% death and 15% disability rates in the moderate and 82% death and 18% disability in the severe encephalopathy groups, respectively.

A number of therapies have been suggested to protect the brain and improve prognosis for infants with hypoxic ischemic encephalopathy in the newborn. These include phenobarbital,[36] head cooling,[37] and magnesium sulfate.[38] Their value is uncertain and further research is required.

Conclusion

In summary, the evidence is limited regarding prevalence, risk factors, and outcomes of neonatal encephalopathy. This in part results from the difficulties in definition and the range of inclusion criteria used. Furthermore the etiology and outcomes seem to differ markedly between developed and developing countries. Clinicians should use data from populations similar to their own to guide their clinical practice and advice to parents. Future investigators should ensure that they use an internationally accepted definition of neonatal encephalopathy. Studies are needed to evaluate causal pathways, identify risk factors amenable to intervention and to assess long-term outcomes of neonatal encephalopathy.

Resolution of the scenario

You tell the parents that the clinical presentation of seizures, irritability, hypertonia, and poor feeding on day one are consistent with a diagnosis of moderate neonatal encephalopathy, and that this occurs in 2–4 of every 1000 live term births. You explain that a number of conditions need to be excluded such as infections and inborn errors of metabolism. You explain that there are several possible factors that might have contributed to the baby's condition, including IVF, older maternal age, pre-eclampsia, and the need for emergency cesarean section. Clinically, you assess the baby as growth restricted even though his birth weight is above 2.5 kg, suggesting some degree of antepartum compromise. This is supported by the placental histology, which shows multiple areas of infarction. The presence of an abnormal intrapartum fetal heart rate trace in labor is likely to be secondary to growth restriction and the abnormal placenta. The arterial cord gases showed a pH of 7.2 with a base excess of −8, consistent with mild metabolic acidosis. In view of the relatively normal cord gases and the MRI findings, you explain that birth asphyxia is unlikely to be a major contributing factor to this baby's encephalopathy. The parents ask you if their baby might die. You tell them that nearly 95% of these babies survive and that if they do 93% will have no evidence of CP at age 2 years. Finally you tell the parents that once the baby has established feeding and the seizures are under control he should be able to go home, usually within a week or two. Moreover the great majority will be on no medication at discharge. You stress the need for long-term neurodevelopmental follow up.

Future research needs

The prevention of neonatal encephalopathy could be addressed by determining the impact of a screening program for the identification and optimal control of thyroid disease prior to pregnancy. A randomized controlled trial of the impact of routine elective cesarean section on neonatal encephalopathy for babies near term who are at high risk of encephalopathy should include those whose mothers have severe pre-eclampsia near term and babies who are growth restricted. Additional information about the prognosis of this condition could come from a comprehensive follow up study (to adulthood) of infants with moderate to severe newborn encephalopathy. A cohort study of the predictive value of magnetic resonance imaging in neonatal encephalopathy would help to direct the appropriate use of this technology. Finally, randomized controlled trials of potential neuroprotective therapies (such as cooling, phenobarbital, magnesium sulfate) for infants with neonatal encephalopathy would assist in managing the cases that cannot yet be prevented.

Summary table

Question	Type of evidence	Results	Comment
In term newborn infants, what is the prevalence of neonatal encephalopathy?	2 case-control studies one of which is population-based[2,19] and 2 reviews[11,17]	For neonatal encephalopathy overall the estimate ranges from 1–8/1000 term live births· Best population prevalence in a developed country suggests 3·8/1000· For hypoxic ischemic encephalopathy without other antepartum risk factors, best estimate is 1·6/10 000	Birth prevalence depends on definition used, in particular the distinction between encephalopathy overall and the hypoxic-ischemic subgroup· Birth prevalence differs markedly between rich and poor countries
In term newborn infants, what are the risk factors for neonatal encephalopathy?	2 well designed case-control studies, one in Australia and one in Nepal[2,19]	The range of risk factors found varies according to the population Intrapartum hypoxia plays a greater role in Nepal	In Australia the role of risk factors in the preconceptional and antepartum periods is of particular note
In term infants, does intrapartum hypoxia cause neonatal encephalopathy?	Animal studies[26,27] 2 case-control studies[2,19]	Intrapartum hypoxia was thought to be present and possibly contributing in 29% of cases in the Australian study and 60% in the Nepal study. Intrapartum hypoxia is an uncommon cause in isolation	Intrapartum hypoxia is difficult to diagnose. Newborn encephalopathy is an intermediate step between intrapartum hypoxia and CP
In term infants with neonatal encephalopathy, what is the short-term and long-term outlook?	2 case–control studies[2,19] and one case–control study of hypoxic ischemic encephalopathy with long-term follow up to age 8[22]	Neonatal mortality in Australia 10% v 31% in Nepal. By age 1 year mortality is 13·2% and 44%, respectively. 10% of case infants in the Australian had CP by age 1 v 20% in Nepal. Developmental delay was present in 12·2% of cases at age 2 in the Australian study	The severity of encephalopathy was strongly linked to the likelihood of an adverse outcome

CP, cerebral palsy.

References

1 Nelson KB, Leviton A. How much of neonatal encephalopathy is due to birth asphyxia? *Am J Dis Child* 1991;**145**:1325–31.

2 Badawi N, Kurinczuk JJ, Keogh JM *et al*. Antepartum risk factors for newborn encephalopathy: the Western Australian case–control study. *BMJ* 1998;**317**:1549–53.

3 Sarnat HB, Sarnat, MS. Neonatal encephalopathy following fetal distress. *Arch Neurol* 1976;**33**:696–705.

4 Badawi N, Kurinczuk JJ, Keogh JM *et al*. Intrapartum risk factors for newborn encephalopathy: the Western Australian case–control study. *BMJ* 1998;**317**:1554–8.

5 Dixon G, Badawi N, Kurinczuk JJ *et al*. Early developmental outcome after newborn encephalopathy. *Pediatrics* 2002; **109**:26–33.

6 Nelson KB, Ellenberg JH. Neonatal signs as predictors of cerebral palsy. *Pediatrics* 1979;**64**:225–32.

7 Ellenberg JH, Nelson KB. Cluster of perinatal events identifying infants at high risk for death or disability. *J Pediatr* 1988;**113**:546–52.

8 Nelson KB, Grether JK. Potentially asphyxiating conditions and spastic cerebral palsy in infants of normal birthweight. *Am J Obstet Gynecol* 1998;**179**:507–13.

9 Yudkin PL, Johnson A, Clover LM, Murphy KW. Assessing the contribution of birth asphyxia to cerebral palsy in term singletons. *Paediatr Perinat Epidemiol* 1995;**9**:156–70.

10 McLennan A. A template for defining a causal relation between acute intrapartum events and cerebral palsy: international consensus statement. *BMJ* 1999;**319**:1054–9.

11 American College of Obstetricians and Gynecologists' Task Force on Neonatal Encephalopathy and Cerebral Palsy and the American College of Obstetricians and Gynecologists and the American Academy of Pediatrics Defining the Pathogenesis and pathophysiology of neonatal encephalopathy and cerebral palsy. *Obstet Gynecol* 2003;**102**:628–36.

12 *Clinical Evidence* 2003 *BMJ* Publishing Group Ltd. http://www.clinicalevidence.com.

13 *Cochrane Library*, Issue 4. Chichester, UK: John Wiley & Sons, 2003.

14 Thacker SB, Stroup D, Chang M. Continuous electronic heart rate monitoring for fetal assessment during labor (Cochrane

Review). In: *Cochrane Library*, Issue 3, 2003. Oxford: Update Software.

15 Wood C, Renou P, Oates J, Farrell E, Beischer N, Anderson I. A controlled trial of fetal heart rate monitoring in a low risk population. *Am J Obstet Gynecol* 1981;**141**:527–34.

16 McDonald D, Grant A, Sheridan-Pereira M, Boylan P, Chalmers I. The Dublin randomized controlled trial of intrapartum fetal heart rate monitoring. *Am J Obstet Gynecol* 1985;**152**:524–39.

17 Renou P, Chang A, Anderson I, Wood C. Controlled trial of fetal intensive care. *Am J Obstet Gynecol* 1976;**126**:470–6.

18 Badawi N, Kurinczuk JJ, Hall D, Field D, Pemberton PJ, Stanley FJ. Newborn encephalopathy in term infants: three approaches to population-based investigation. *Semin Neonatol* 1997;**2**:181–8.

19 Ellis M, Manandhar N, Manandhar DS, de L Costello AM. Risk factors for neonatal encephalopathy in Kathmandu, Nepal, a developing country: unmatched case–control study. *BMJ* 2000;**320**:1229–36.

20 Robertson CM, Finer NN. Term infants with hypoxic-ischemic encephalopathy: outcome at 3.5 years. *Develop Med Child Neurol* 1985;**27**:473–84.

21 Robertson CM, Finer NN, Grace MG. School performance of survivors of neonatal encephalopathy associated with birth asphyxia at term. *J Pediatr* 1989;**114**:753–60.

22 Robertson CM, Finer NN. Long-term follow up of term neonates with perinatal asphyxia. *Clin Perinatol* 1993;**20**:483–500.

23 Adamson SJ, Alessandri LM, Badawi N, Burton PR, Pemberton PJ, Stanley FJ. Predictors of neonatal encephalopathy in full term infants. *BMJ* 1995;**311**:598–602.

24 Felix JF, Badawi N, Kurinczuk JJ, Bower C, Keogh JM, Pemberton PJ. Birth defects in children with newborn encephalopathy. *Develop Med Child Neurol* 2000;**42**:803–8.

25 Grant A, O'Brien N, Joy MT, Hennessy E, MacDonald D. Cerebral palsy among children born during the Dublin randomised trial of intrapartum monitoring. *Lancet* 1989;**2**:1233–6.

26 Myers RE. Brain damage induced by umbilical cord compression at different gestational ages in monkeys. In: Goldsmith EI, Moor-Jankowski J, eds. *Medical primatology conference on experimental medicine and surgery in primates.* New York: Karger, Basel, 1970.

27 Roohey T, Raju TN, Moustogiannis AN. Animal models for the study of perinatal hypoxic-ischaemic encephalopath: a critical analysis. *Early Hum Develop* 1997;**47**:115–46.

28 Ellis M, Manandhar N, Shrestha PS, Shrestha L, Manandhar DS, Costello AM. Outcome at one year of neonatal encephalopathy in Kathmandu, Nepal. *Develop Med Child Neurol* 1999;**41**:689–95.

29 Dennis J. Neonatal convulsions: aetiology, late neonatal status and long term outcome. *Develop Med Child Neurol* 1978;**20**:143–58.

30 Ergander U, Eriksson M, Zetterstrom R. Severe neonatal asphyxia – incidence and prediction of outcome in the Stockholm area. *Acta Pediatr* 1983;**72**:321–5.

31 Finer NN, Robertson CM, Richards RT, Pinnell LE, Peters KL. Hypoxic-ischemic encephalopathy in term neonates: perinatal factors and outcome. *J Pediatr* 1981;**98**:112–17.

32 Hull J, Dodd KL. Falling incidence of hypoxic-ischaemic encephalopathy in term infants. *Br J Obstet Gynaecol* 1992;**99**:386–91.

33 Levene ML, Kornberg J, Williams THC. The incidence and severity of post-asphyxial encephalopathy in term infants. *Early Hum Develop* 1985;**11**:21–6.

34 Thornberg E, Thiringer K, Odeback A, Milsom I. Birth asphyxia: incidence, clinical course and outcome in a Swedish population. *Acta Pediatr* 1995;**84**;927–32.

35 Van de Riet JE, Vandenbussche FP, Le Cessie S, Keirse MJ. Newborn assessment and long-term adverse outcome: a systematic review. [Meta-Analysis] *Am J Obstet Gynecol* 1999;**180**:1024–9.

36 Evans DJ, Levene MI. Anticonvulsants for preventing mortality and morbidity in full term newborns with perinatal asphyxia (Cochrane Review). In: *Cochrane Library*, Issue 4. Chichester, UK: John Wiley & Sons, 2003.

37 Jacobs S, Hunt R, Tarnow-Mordi W, Inder T, Davis P. Cooling for newborns with hypoxic ischaemic encephalopathy (Cochrane Review). In: *Cochrane Library*, Issue 4. Chichester, UK: John Wiley & Sons, Ltd, 2003.

38 Kent A, Kecskes Z. Magnesium sulfate for term infants following perinatal asphyxia (Protocol for a Cochrane Review). In: *Cochrane Library*, Issue 4. Chichester, UK: John Wiley & Sons, Ltd, 2003.

50 Pain in the newborn

Vibhuti Shah, Arne Ohlsson

Case scenario

A 32-year-old primigravida woman with an uncomplicated pregnancy gives birth vaginally to a male infant at 38 weeks gestation. His Apgar scores are 9 at 1 and 5 minutes. He is appropriately grown with a weight of 3810 g, length of 51 cm, and head circumference of 33·5 cm and the clinical examination is normal. During the antenatal classes the parents were informed that their newborn infant would receive an intramuscular injection of vitamin K soon after birth and that a blood sample would be obtained by heel lancing for the newborn-screening test when the baby is one day old. The parents raise the questions, "Will our infant experience pain?" and, if so, "How can we tell that he is in pain?" They ask if we will provide any pain relief. The parents also want their infant to be circumcised and want to know how the pain from the procedure can be reduced or avoided.

Background

The International Association for the Study of Pain defines pain as "an unpleasant sensory and emotional experience associated with actual or potential tissue damage or described in terms of such damage".[1] Identifying and quantifying pain in newborns is difficult because infants cannot verbalize and communicate this subjective phenomenon. Due to these limitations, misconceptions existed amongst healthcare providers until recently that newborns do not feel pain and that there is no need to provide pain relief.

These misconceptions have been put to rest by an extensive body of literature showing that even extremely preterm newborns mount responses to painful stimuli and that these can be relieved with analgesics and other interventions.[2–4] Repeated invasive procedures performed in newborns may also impact on their long-term neuro-development and responses to pain.[5–11] Newborns who undergo circumcision without anesthesia in the first few days of life have an increased response to vaccination pain at 2 months of age.[10] Thus, we have an ethical obligation to relieve/reduce pain, stress and suffering of newborn infants.

The two most common sources of iatrogenic pain in newborns are intramuscular (i.m.) administration of vitamin K soon after birth to prevent hemorrhagic disease of the newborn (a medically indicated intervention) and heel lancing, performed 24 hours after birth, to obtain a blood sample for metabolic screening for a range of conditions including phenylketonuria, hypothyroidism, galactosemia, and cystic fibrosis (a medically indicated test). Heel lancing is

also used to obtain blood for other laboratory investigations in the newborn. The procedure involves cleaning the heel with an antiseptic swab, lancing the heel on the lateral aspect of the foot, squeezing the heel to obtain an adequate amount of blood, and applying pressure once the blood collection is complete.

In addition, circumcision, which is rarely medically indicated in the newborn, is commonly performed on newborns around the world during the postnatal period for social or religious reasons.[12,13] In the USA circumcision rates vary among racial and ethnic groups. Whites (81%) are more likely to be circumcised than Blacks (65%) or Hispanics (54%).[14] The procedure is uncommon in northern Europe, Central and South America, and Asia.[15]

Newborn infants undergoing circumcision mount a physiological response (increases in heart rate and blood pressure, decrease in oxygen saturation), a behavioral response (facial expressions, body movements), and a hormonal response (increase in serum cortisol levels) which are indicative of pain.[15–18]

Although injection, heel lancing, and circumcision are associated with measurable physiological and behavioral responses indicating pain, pain-relieving interventions are not routinely advocated or used. The rationale for not intervening includes the relatively short duration of these procedures, the perceived lack of importance of pain, and concerns about toxicity from currently available agents.

In this chapter we will identify systematic reviews and randomized controlled trials (RCTs) that evaluate the effectiveness of analgesics/anesthetics and non-pharmacological interventions for reducing pain and/or stress in newborns having these common procedures.

Framing answerable clinical questions

In response to the parents' concerns about pain relief for their infant, you structure a number of clinical questions and identify the question type (see Chapter 2) to help you search the literature for the information you need.

Questions

1. In newborn infants (*population*), does the intramuscular administration of vitamin K (*intervention*) cause pain (*outcome*)? **[Causation]**
2. In newborn infants receiving an intramuscular injection (*population*), are topical local anesthetic agents, systemic analgesia, or non-pharmacological interventions (i.e., use of pacifiers, swaddling, holding etc) (*intervention*) compared with no intervention (*comparison*) effective in preventing/reducing pain (*outcome*)? **[Therapy]**
3. In newborn infants (*population*), does heel lancing (*intervention*) performed to obtain blood for the newborn screening test cause pain (*outcome*)? **[Causation]**
4. In newborn infants undergoing heel lancing (*population*), what are the effective interventions (*intervention*) for preventing/reducing pain (*outcome*)? **[Therapy]**
5. In newborn infants undergoing circumcision (*population*), which surgical procedure (*intervention*) is the most effective and the least painful (*outcome*)? **[Therapy]**
6. In newborn infants undergoing circumcision (*population*), which pharmacological and/or non-pharmacological interventions (*intervention*) provide the best pain relief (*outcome*)? **[Therapy]**

Searching for evidence

Although cohort and case–control studies can provide information on risk factors, they are subject to bias and it is therefore more difficult to infer causation from these study types than from RCTs (Chapter 7). However, it is sometimes impractical or unethical to perform an RCT to answer questions of causation (for example, questions 1 and 3). For these questions you look in MedLine (from 1966), EMBASE (from 1980), and CINAHL (from 1982) for cohort or case–control studies or supportive articles that provide a physiological explanation for how an injection or heel lancing might cause pain. For the remaining questions of therapy you want systematic reviews of RCTs or RCTs. You first search the *Cochrane Library* and then the other electronic databases.

For all the searches you use the MeSH heading "infant, newborn OR newborn" and add other headings according to the question. For example, for question 1 "intramuscular drug administration OR injections intramuscular" and for question 3 "heel lancing OR heel prick OR heel stick". To identify clinical trials for example, for questions 2, 4, 5, and 6 you use the publication type "randomized controlled trial OR controlled clinical trial OR clinical trial OR random allocation". You add the following terms/text words: "pain", "pain assessment", "injection pain", "topical anesthesia/creams" and "analgesia" as needed to expand the search. None of the trials you find evaluate pharmacologic or non-pharmacologic interventions for i.m. pain relief in newborns, so you extend the search to adults and children using the following additional MeSH headings: "adult", "children", "infant", "vaccination", "immunization", "pain" and "injection pain". The searches were completed in March 2003.

Critical review of the evidence

Question

1. In newborn infants (*population*), does the intramuscular administration of vitamin K (*intervention*) cause pain (*outcome*)? **[Causation]**

You find an article about the mechanism of pain following i.m. injection. In this situation pain can be attributed both to skin puncture and to infiltration of the medication into the muscle. Studies using intraneural microstimulation have shown that human skeletal muscles are innervated by group III (A-delta fibers, or "fast" fibers) and group IV (C fibers or "slow" fibers) afferent nociceptors, similar to those found in cutaneous tissues.[19] Stimulation of both types of fibers in the muscle is associated with cramping pain. In the skin, stimulation of group III fibers results in sharp pain whereas group IV stimulation results in burning pain. However, it is unclear which fiber type carries the receptive signal for stretching of muscle, the type of stimulus delivered by i.m. injection.[19]

Grunau *et al.*[20] enrolled 36 healthy full-term infants to receive three procedures: (i.m. injection [invasive procedure]; application of triple dye to the umbilical stub; and rubbing the thigh with alcohol [two non invasive procedures]) in a counterbalanced order. Pain assessments were made using the Neonatal Facial Coding System (NFCS) and cry. The mean NFCS score ± standard deviation (SD) was $23\cdot2 \pm 6\cdot4$ in infants receiving an i.m. injection compared with $14\cdot5 \pm 7\cdot6$ in infants whose thigh was rubbed with alcohol. This represents a 60% increase in pain (indicated by facial expression) during i.m. injection compared with a non-invasive procedure. Similarly, the latency of cry was shorter ($1\cdot9$ [$2\cdot4$] v $3\cdot6$ [$2\cdot4$] seconds) and the duration of cry was longer ($20\cdot3$ [$8\cdot3$] v $16\cdot2$ [$5\cdot9$] seconds) in infants who received an i.m. injection compared with infants whose thigh was rubbed with alcohol. These responses indicate that i.m. injection is a painful procedure in newborns.

Question

2. In newborn infants receiving an intramuscular injection (*population*), are topical local anesthetic agents, systemic analgesia, or non-pharmacological interventions (i.e., use of pacifiers, swaddling, holding etc) (*intervention*) compared with no intervention (*comparison*) effective in preventing/reducing pain (*outcome*)? **[Therapy]**

You find that several interventions to reduce pain associated with i.m. vaccination have been evaluated in adults and children. Many of these interventions, such as behavioral and cognitive techniques to divert children's attention cannot be applied to newborns. Interventions relevant to newborns are summarized below.

Topical anesthesia: EMLA versus placebo

You find five RCTs evaluating the use of a topical anesthetic agent lidocaine-prilocaine 5% cream (EMLA) in adults and children. In one RCT 60 adults received one application of ~2·5 g of EMLA cream or placebo 60–90 minutes prior to the administration of influenza vaccine (0·5 ml).[21] Pain from the procedure was assessed using a Visual Analogue Scale (VAS). As compared with placebo, use of EMLA was associated with a statistically and clinically significant decrease in the mean (SD) VAS pain score from needle puncture (4·6 ± 7·8 *v* 15·2 ± 16·5; *P* <0·0002) and injection (9·5 ± 13·7 *v* 18·5 ± 19·6; *P* = 0·0139).

Himelstein *et al.*[22] recruited 40 adult volunteers for an RCT to compare the pain of needle puncture and infiltration of saline into the deltoid muscle after application of EMLA or placebo. Pain was assessed using a VAS. There was a statistically significant reduction in pain from needle puncture (median VAS score, 7·5 *v* 19·5; *P* = 0·0043) and pain from i.m. infiltration (median VAS score, 2·5 *v* 11; *P* < 0·00005) in the group in which EMLA was applied.

Taddio *et al.*[23] in an RCT enrolled 96 infants having their 4- or 6-month diphtheria–tetanus–pertussis (DTP) vaccination; 60 minutes prior to the injection 2·5 g of EMLA or placebo was applied on the infant's thigh. Pain was assessed using the Modified Behavioral Pain Scale (MBPS), latency to cry and duration of cry. The median (range) differences in the prevaccination and post-vaccination MBPS scores were lower for the EMLA compared with the placebo group (5 [1–8] *v* 6 [1–9]; *P* = 0·001]. The latency to first cry was longer (3·3 [1–6·4] *v* 2·4 [0·5–5·5] seconds; *P* = 0·0004), and the total crying time was shorter (10·3 [0–145·1] *v* 25·2 [0–117·4] seconds; *P* = 0·027) for the EMLA-treated group suggesting its effectiveness.

Halperin *et al.*[24] recruited 109 infants at 6 months of age due to receive their third dose of diphtheria–tetanus–acellular pertussis-inactivated poliovirus-*Haemophilus influenzae* type b conjugate (DTaP-IPV-Hib) vaccine and 56 infants from birth to 2 months of age due to receive one of the three primary doses of DtaP-IPV-Hib vaccine in an RCT. The effect of EMLA on the pain associated with vaccination was studied using MBPS. Infants were randomized to receive either an EMLA or a placebo patch. At the 6-month visit, EMLA-treated infants had significantly less pain after vaccination compared with infants who received placebo (total pain score, 6·75 *v* 7·35; *P* = 0·005). Similar effects were seen at 2 and 4 months even though the differences were not statistically significant (attributed to the small sample size). The difference in pain response demonstrated in this study is not likely to be clinically important.

Uhari[25] enrolled 155 infants between the ages of 3 and 28 months to receive either placebo or EMLA at the site of vaccination 60 minutes prior to the procedure. Nurses and parents evaluated the infants' pain, crying, and fear in response to the vaccination using a VAS. The mean pain scores reported by nurses and parents were significantly lower in the EMLA-treated group than the placebo group (2·5 *v* 3·8; *P* < 0·003 and 2·9 *v* 4·8; *P* < 0·001, respectively). Similarly, the mean crying scores reported by nurses and parents were significantly lower in the EMLA-treated group than the placebo group (2·8 *v* 4·0; *P* < 0·003 and 3·6 *v* 5·3; *P* < 0·003, respectively).

In summary, there is good evidence from well designed RCTs that EMLA cream is effective in decreasing pain from i.m. injections in adults and children. All studies show a statistically significant reduction in pain scores. With the exception of one study this reduction was also of clinical significance.

There are theoretical concerns about the risk of methemoglobinemia from prilocaine metabolites in the newborn and this adverse effect has been reported.[26,27] However, several authors have shown that EMLA is safe in both preterm and term newborns. No infant exhibited signs of methemoglobinemia following a single dose application of 0·5–1·0 g.[28–30] There is good physiological evidence that i.m. injections are painful and that parents and nurses also perceive needle injections as painful. Further research is therefore warranted to determine the effectiveness of newer topical anesthetic agents for use in newborns.

Sucrose versus placebo

You identify three RCTs evaluating sucrose for pain relief from i.m. injection in newborns and children. Lewindon *et al.*[31] recruited 110 infants attending clinic for primary (2-, 4-, and 6-month) vaccination. Infants were randomized to receive 2 ml of 75% sucrose solution or sterile water given orally over a period of 15 seconds prior to the injection. Both nurses and parents were blinded to the nature of the solutions that the infant received. *H influenzae* type b vaccine was given in the left leg and within five seconds the DTP vaccine was given in the right leg, In addition to the test solution the nurse used soothing techniques to calm the infant (encouraged parents to cuddle the infant over one shoulder while the nurse employed a distracting, low pitched rattling noise). Infants' distress was assessed using cry. Crying time was defined in three ways: the first cry, defined as the duration of continuous audible crying (seconds) from onset until a crying-free interval of > 5 seconds; the total sum (seconds) of audible cry within 3 minutes from the onset; and the duration (seconds) from the start of crying until the finish of the last cry (maximum of 3 minutes). At the end of the procedure, the nurse and the caregiver assessed their perception of infant distress on an Oucher chart (a VAS from 0 to 100). A score of 0 indicated no distress, whereas a score of 100 was the worst distress possible for the infant. Infants in the sucrose group had a significant reduction in all measures of crying. The mean (SE) duration of first cry was 29 (18) versus 42 (21) seconds, $P < 0.0003$; total crying time was 36 (21) versus 59 (30) seconds, $P < 0.000008$; and duration of crying was 43 (24) versus 69 (34) seconds, $P < 0.00002$, respectively in the sucrose versus the control group. All three measures of crying time demonstrated a 35–40% reduction in infants receiving sucrose solution, which is clinically significant. There was a significant reduction in the nurses' Oucher scores in the sucrose group compared with the controls. Parents' scores were not statistically significantly reduced.

In a longitudinal, randomized controlled trial, Barr *et al.*[32] randomized 66 infants to receive either three 250 microliter doses of 50% sucrose or a water solution by mouth prior to their DTP vaccination at 2 and 4 months of age. The aim of the study was to assess the effectiveness of sucrose in reducing crying time; to detect when sucrose was effective (i.e., at the time of or after the noxious stimulus or both); and to determine whether changes in effectiveness were age-related. Infants who received sucrose (or water) at 2 months received the same intervention at 4 months. Of the original 66 infants, 57 participated at 4 months of age. During the procedure, parents were refrained from comforting their infants but continued to hold them in the same position and talk to them until 1-minute post vaccination. Vaccination was administered after the third dose of sucrose or water and infants were observed for 70 seconds post needle entry. Pain was assessed from videotape recordings as the percentage of time crying during each phase of the procedure (i.e., baseline, injection, and postinjection). No difference was noted in the percentage of time crying during injection in either group. During the postinjection phase, the mean percentage of crying time was significantly reduced in the sucrose group compared with the water group (83% v 69%; $P < 0.05$).

Although the reduction in crying was statistically significant, the clinical effect was small and limited to the postinjection phase. In addition, it appears that even though sucrose has some effect beyond the newborn period, the magnitude of the effect is small.

Allen *et al.*[33] randomized 285 infants between 2 weeks and 18 months of age into one of the following seven different age groupings: 2 weeks old (n = 50), 2 months old (n = 44), 4 months old (n = 50), 6 months old (n = 46), 9 months old (n = 28), 15 months old (n = 30), and 18 months old (n = 37). These groupings were based on the recommended ages at which children receive vaccination. Infants were randomly assigned to receive either no intervention, 2 ml of sterile water or 2 ml of 12% sucrose orally prior to vaccination. Percentage of time spent crying during the procedure was used to assess pain. Oral sucrose administration prior to vaccination did not result in significantly less crying compared with water. Two-week-old infants receiving either sucrose or sterile water had significantly less crying compared with infants of the same age who received no intervention ($P < 0.05$). In older infants, this difference was noted only if infants received one rather than two injections. Thus the age of the child and the number of painful exposures can attenuate calming effects.

The studies by Lewindon *et al.*[31] and Barr *et al.*[32] suggest that sucrose is effective in reducing infant's pain and distress during vaccination. The magnitude of the effect was small in the study by Barr *et al.*[32] In contrast the study by Allen *et al.*[33] suggests that sucrose may not confer any benefits over water when administered orally to reduce pain.

Although sucrose is effective in reducing procedural pain from heel lancing and venepuncture[34] in both preterm and term newborns and for circumcision[35] in term newborns, the use of sucrose for i.m. injection pain has not been proven to be effective.

Behavioral interventions versus no intervention

No reports of randomized controlled trials of behavioral interventions to reduce pain in newborns were identified.

Current best practice for reducing pain associated with i.m. injections

- Apply EMLA (0·5–1 g) 60–90 minutes prior to injection (for single injection)
- Use a pacifier dipped in sucrose

Question

3. In newborn infants (*population*), does heel lancing (*intervention*) performed to obtain blood for the newborn screening test cause pain (*outcome*)? **[Causation]**

As demonstrated in cohort studies newborns undergoing heel lancing cry, exhibit facial expression and body movements, and mount physiological responses suggestive of pain.[36–39]

Question

4. In newborn infants undergoing heel lancing (*population*), what are the effective interventions (*intervention*) for preventing/reducing pain (*outcome*)? **[Therapy]**

You find two systematic reviews relevant to this topic in the *Cochrane Library*. In one the use of sucrose was evaluated for painful procedures in the newborn[34] and in the other the use of venepuncture and heel lancing for blood sampling in newborn term infants were compared.[40] In MedLine you find a systematic review of EMLA use in the newborn[41] and on your bookshelf you find a chapter by Ohlsson *et al.*[42] on neonatal analgesia. Ohlsson *et al.*[42] evaluated the effectiveness of various interventions for managing pain, including warming versus not warming the heel; use of an automated incision device versus a conventional lancet; EMLA cream versus placebo; paracetamol (acetaminophen) versus placebo; sucrose versus placebo; human milk versus no treatment; sweet-tasting solution (Calpol-hydrogenated glucose) versus placebo; and heel lancing versus venepuncture. The review did not include trials that evaluated comfort measures to reduce pain response to heel lancing. Randomized controlled trials published after these reviews were also identified. The available evidence is summarized below.

Warming versus not warming the heel

You find two RCTs, neither of which suggest that warming the heel reduces pain or facilitates blood collection by heel lancing.[43,44]

Automated versus conventional lancets

You find several studies that address this comparison, including some in preterm newborns. Paes *et al.*[45] evaluated an automated incision device (Tenderfoot, International Technidyne Corp, Edison, NJ) for heel lancing. The increase in heart rate from baseline and the time spent crying was not statistically significant in the group in which the automated device was used. The larger volume of blood obtained with this device, the shortened time required for blood collection, and reduced hemolysis makes this a preferred device for heel lancing. Vertanen *et al.*[46] compared a manual lancet (Microlance) with an automatic incision device (Tenderfoot) in preterm infants undergoing repeated heel lancing for blood sampling. The automated device was associated with less

bruising of the heel, ankle, and leg and decreased heel inflammation. The number of punctures required to obtain a sufficient blood sample was also reduced. Kellam *et al.*[47] randomized 40 preterm newborns undergoing heel lancing to either a manual lancet (Monolet lancet) or an automated device (Tenderfoot preemie). Newborns randomized to the automated device required fewer heel punctures and the blood collection time was shorter than with the use of Monolet lancet. Shah *et al.*[48] (study identified from personal files) showed that the use of an automated incision device (BD Quikheel, Becton Dickinson and Company) was associated with less pain as assessed by facial grimacing and cry duration. A reduction in the blood collection time and the number of repeat punctures required to obtain the blood sample was noted.

In summary, the use of automated lancets causes less pain, requires fewer punctures, allows collection of increased volumes of blood, requires less time for blood collection, and reduces hemolysis in the collected blood. Automated lancets are preferred over manual lancets for collecting blood from the heels of preterm and term newborns.

Topical anesthesia versus placebo

EMLA versus placebo. In a systematic review[41] of two RCTs[49,50] EMLA was ineffective for reducing pain associated with heel lancing in both preterm and term neonates.

Amethocaine versus placebo. An RCT demonstrated that amethocaine gel application is ineffective for the prevention of pain from heel lancing.[51]

Lignocaine versus placebo. In a double-blind randomized controlled trial application of 5% lignocaine ointment to the heel 1 hour prior to heel lancing was not effective in reducing the infant's behavioral response.[52]

Paracetamol (acetaminophen) versus placebo

In one RCT oral paracetamol in a dose of 20 mg kg^{-1} was ineffective in decreasing pain from heel lancing in term newborn infants.[53]

Venepuncture versus heel lancing

A systematic review of the literature[40] identified three RCTs[54–56] in which venepuncture was compared with heel lancing to obtain blood sample in newborns. Despite the heterogeneity in pain measures used, statistically significantly lower pain scores were demonstrated for venepuncture compared with heel lancing. A meta-analysis was performed on the need for at least one additional skin puncture to obtain the required amount of blood using venepuncture compared with heel lancing. The relative risk of requiring more than one skin puncture for venepuncture versus heel lancing was 0·30 (95% CI 0·18, 0·49). The risk difference was −39%

(95% CI −50%, −28%). The number needed to treat to avoid one repeat skin puncture was three (95% CI 2, 4). Thus, on average, only three newborn infants need to be sampled by venepuncture compared with heel lancing to avoid one repeat skin puncture. Thus, venepuncture is the preferred method for blood sampling in newborns.

Sucrose versus control (water [sterile, tap, spring, distilled], pacifier or positioning/containing)

In a systematic review,[34] 15 RCTs evaluating the effectiveness of sucrose to reduce pain associated with heel lancing in preterm or term infants were identified. Sucrose was effective for reducing pain associated with heel lancing. Compared with control, sucrose decreased univariate physiological (heart rate) and behavioral (mean percent time crying, total cry duration, duration of first cry, and facial action) pain indicators and a multivariate composite pain score. The dose of sucrose used in these trials varied from 0·012 to 0·12 g (0·05–0·5 of 24% solution). Based on these findings, the routine use of sucrose approximately 2 minutes prior to heel lancing can be recommended.

Glucose versus no intervention

In a blinded RCT, infants were randomly assigned to receive 2 ml of water, glucose 5% or 33% solution, or nothing. Only 2 ml of 33% glucose was associated with reduction in pain with heel lancing.[57]

Breastfeeding versus no intervention

In a prospective RCT, breastfeeding (uniting different components of nursing such as taste, suckling, and skin-to-skin contact) during heel lancing was effective in reducing crying and grimacing, and prevented the marked rise in heart rate seen with heel lancing.[58]

Comforting measures versus no intervention

In RCTs, non-nutritive sucking[59,60] and use of pacifiers and rocking[61] attenuate behavioral responses to pain during heel lancing.

Relative efficacy of oral analgesic interventions

You find six randomized trials that compare the efficacy of different analgesic interventions. Isik et al.[62] showed that 2 ml of 30% sucrose was more effective than 10% and 30% glucose solutions for relieving pain in response to heel lancing. In another study by Guala et al.[63] showed that both glucose and sucrose solutions (33% and 50%) were effective

in reducing the pain response to heel lancing compared with water. Skogsdal et al.[64] evaluated the analgesic effects of two different concentrations of glucose (10% and 30%) and of breast milk in newborns undergoing heel lancing. As compared with controls the duration of crying was significantly reduced in the group given 30% glucose ($P < 0.01$). Newborns given 10% glucose or breast milk also cried less compared with the control group but the differences in duration of crying were not statistically significant.

In a study by Blass[65] the analgesic effect of different formulae and their components (fat, protein, or lactose) was compared with sucrose. Both sucrose and Similac reduced crying during blood collection procedure. Sucrose, fat, protein, and Ross Special Formula reduced crying at 3 minutes after the procedure. Lactose and water were not effective in reducing the pain response.

Ramenghi et al.[66] demonstrated that a sweet-tasting solution (Calpol solution without paracetamol) has analgesic effects equal to the effects of concentrated sucrose solutions (25% or 50%, respectively).

Bucher et al.[67] found that an artificial sweetener (10 parts cyclamate and 1 part saccharin) is an analgesic, that glycine (a sweet amino acid) increases the pain reaction and that breast milk has no effect on the pain reaction to heel lancing.

Skin to skin contact (kangaroo care) versus no intervention

Gray et al.[68] randomly assigned 30 infants to either being held by their mothers in a whole body (kangaroo care) position or to no intervention during a standard heel lancing procedure. Crying was reduced by 82% and grimacing by 65% in the group held in skin-to-skin contact during the procedure compared with the control group. These findings suggest that skin-to-skin contact is an effective and safe intervention, which can be easily implemented.

Combinations of interventions

Bellieni et al.[69] randomized 17 newborns to each receive all five interventions (control, 10% glucose, 10% glucose plus sucking, oral water, and sensorial stimulation) in random order. Sensorial stimulation consisted of tactile, vestibular, gustative, olfactory, auditory, and visual stimuli, and promoted interaction between nurse and infant. Pain was assessed during heel lancing using a validated pain rating scale. Sensorial stimulation and oral glucose plus sucking had the greatest analgesic effect compared with no intervention ($P < 0.001$).

In another study, Bellieni et al.[70] randomized 120 term newborns undergoing heel lancing to one of six groups. The groups were control (no analgesic procedure); 1 ml of 33% oral glucose given 2 minutes before the heel lancing; sucking (water) before, during, and after heel lancing; 1 ml of 33% oral glucose plus sucking; multisensory stimulation including 1 ml of 33% glucose orally; and multisensory stimulation without glucose. Sensory stimulation consisted of massage, voice and eye contact, and smelling perfume during heel lancing. The combination of multisensory stimulation and administration of glucose was found to be the most effective analgesic intervention.

Akman *et al.*[71] compared the analgesic effects of orally administered sweet solutions (dextrose or sucrose 12·5%) with or without pacifiers in newborns subjected to heel lancing. The administration of dextrose or sucrose followed by a pacifier was superior to dextrose or sucrose alone, suggesting that the analgesic effect of sweet solutions can be enhanced with a pacifier.

In a similar RCT, Greenberg[72] demonstrated that the use of a sugar-coated pacifier was more effective in reducing pain behaviors than a water-moistened pacifier, 2 ml of a 12% sucrose solution, or no intervention. Örs *et al.*[73] compared in an RCT the analgesic effect of 2 ml of 25% sucrose and human milk and found that human milk is less effective as an analgesic than sucrose. Gormally *et al.*[74] showed in an RCT that holding the newborn and giving oral sucrose may be a simple and practical method of reducing pain in newborns during heel lancing. Blass and Watt[75] found that the combination of sucrose and non-nutritive sucking was effective in reducing pain associated with heel lancing.

Current best practice for reducing pain associated with heel lancing

- Venepuncture is the preferred method for blood sampling in term newborns
- If heel lancing is used:

  do not warm the heel prior to lancing
  provide sucrose on a pacifier *or*
  encourage the mother to breast or bottle-feed during the procedure
  use an automated lancet
  let the parent hold the infant during the procedure (± skin-to-skin contact)

Searching for evidence: circumcision

In the *Cochrane Library* (Issue 1, 2003) you find one Cochrane review,[76] one abstract in DARE (Database of Reviews of Effects),[41] and 53 RCTs. You also find 90, 76, and 11 potentially relevant RCTs in MedLine, EMBASE, and CINAHL respectively. As expected, there is an overlap among many of the studies that were identified in the different databases. When reviewing all the printouts, you find one additional systematic review[77] and one structured narrative review.[78] In addition, you identify three randomized controlled trials related to pain relief for circumcision that were not included in published reviews.[35,79,80]

Question

5. In newborn infants undergoing circumcision (*population*), which surgical procedure (*intervention*) is the most effective and the least painful (*outcome*)? **[Therapy]**

Three devices are commonly used to perform circumcision in healthy male newborns: the Gomco clamp, the Plastibell device, and the Mogen clamp.[13] Based on one well-designed RCT[81] and one cohort study[82] the Mogen clamp is favored over other devices as it is associated with shorter operation time[35,77] and less pain.[35]

Question

6. In newborn infants undergoing circumcision (*population*), which pharmacological and/or non-pharmacological interventions (*intervention*) provide the best pain relief (*outcome*)? **[Therapy]**

According to a survey in the USA, 45% of physicians performing circumcisions use anesthesia and of these 85% use a dorsal penile nerve block (DPNB).[83] Of respondents who do not use anesthesia, 54% cited "concern over adverse drug effects" and 44% cited that the "procedure does not warrant anesthesia" as the most common explanations.[83] Both the Canadian Paediatric Society and the American Academy of Pediatrics stress that, when circumcision is performed, procedural analgesia should be provided.[12,13] The evidence of effectiveness for different interventions from systematic reviews and RCTs is summarized below.

Paracetamol (acetaminophen)

Based on systematic reviews, paracetamol given orally pre-and postoperatively (15 mg kg^{-1} every 6 hours starting 2 hours prior to circumcision) provides some pain relief postoperatively.[77,78]

Penile nerve block and ring block

Local anesthetic infiltration by injection is considered to be the most effective method of analgesia for circumcision.[77] The best-studied and most commonly used method is DPNB using lidocaine (1%) without epinephrine given as two injections (each of 0·2–0·5 ml) in the subcutaneous tissue at the base of the penis at Buck's fascia. The efficacy/effectiveness of DPNB compared with placebo or no treatment[77] has been reported in 12 published randomized or quasi-randomized trials. Dorsal penile nerve block significantly reduces pain during circumcision. Because the authors of these studies used different outcome measures, meta-analytic techniques could be applied only to subsets of the 12 studies.[77] Pooling of two studies, which measured percentage of time crying during surgery, showed a statistically significant reduction in crying in infants who received DPNB (weighted mean difference, −52·9%; 95% CI, −65·9 −40%).[77] In a meta-analysis of two studies which assessed oxygen saturation during circumcision, there were statistically significantly smaller changes in oxygen saturation in the DPNB group (weighted mean difference, −1·1; 95% CI −1·8 −0·40% oxygen saturation), which is not of any clinical importance. In three studies plasma cortisol levels 30–40 minutes after circumcision were not different between groups (weighted mean difference, −16·7 micrograms liter^{-1}; 95% CI −4·3 micrograms liter^{-1} to 9·7 micrograms liter^{-1}).[77] In a meta-analysis of seven studies, the incidence of injection related adverse events with DPNB (bruising and/or hematoma) were reported to be 6·7% (95% CI 0·5–12·9%).[77]

Buffered lidocaine has not been shown to further reduce pain associated with DPNB compared with regular lidocaine.[77] Ring block is performed by subcutaneous circumferential infiltration of a local anesthetic around the shaft of the penis or distally up to the level of the corona, not at Buck's fascia. Three studies have evaluated the efficacy/effectiveness of ring block compared with no anesthesia. The author of the systematic review could not combine the results of these trials but ring block statistically significantly decreased crying in one study by 36% and decreased changes in heart rate and infant crying in two other studies.[77] Penile nerve block is a safe and efficacious method for neonatal circumcision. Further studies of ring block are required to demonstrate any superiority in efficacy and safety compared with DPNB.[78]

Topical local anesthesia

A single application of EMLA is safe and lessens the pain of circumcision.[41,76–78] EMLA cannot be recommended over proven pain-relieving interventions such as regional nerve block with lidocaine.[41,76,78] Lidocaine is more effective than placebo but less effective than EMLA[79] in reducing stress indicators. *Amethocaine gel* has therapeutic advantages over EMLA, including faster onset and longer duration of action. It is not associated with a clinically significant risk of methemoglobinemia or other systemic effects.[77] It has not been evaluated for circumcision in the newborn.

Sucrose/glucose with or without pacifier

Two systematic reviews and one RCT show that oral sucrose with or without a pacifier provides some analgesia in neonatal circumcision, but that sucrose is not as effective as a dorsal penile nerve block.[77,78] One RCT showed that concentrated glucose (50%) does not provide significant analgesia for neonatal circumcision and is inferior to DPNB.[80]

Non-pharmacological interventions

Swaddling of the upper body of the newborn and padding of the restraint chair reduces behavioral stress in newborns undergoing circumcision.[77,78] Changes to the environment including playing music and intrauterine sounds do not have analgesic effects.[77]

Current best practice for reducing pain associated with circumcision

- Administer 10–15 mg kg^{-1} of acetaminophen within 2 hours before the procedure and every 4–6 hours for 24 hours after the procedure
- Pad the circumcision board (cushioned chair) with blankets
- Offer a sucrose-dipped pacifier to the newborn before the dorsal penile nerve block, during the circumcision procedure, and after
- Administer dorsal penile nerve block using lidocaine (preservative-free and without epinephrine)
- Swaddle the infant's upper body during the circumcision
- Use the Mogen clamp for the procedure

Summary

- Newborn infants experience pain.
- Pain experienced in the newborn period may alter the appreciation of pain or the reaction to painful stimuli later in life.
- Validated pain measures are available to assess pain in the newborn.
- It is not possible to completely avoid stressful/painful events in the routine hospital care of newborn infants.
- A number of comfort measures, pharmacological and non-pharmacological agents are of proven effectiveness and safety. These are readily available and applicable in the clinical setting.
- Proven interventions to minimize pain should be routinely used.

Resolution of the scenario

You tell the parents that their son will experience some pain during the intramuscular injection, the blood taking and the circumcision, but that the pain can be minimized. You will apply EMLA cream at the injection site about 60 minutes before the injection of vitamin K is given. You will also give the infant a pacifier dipped in sucrose and suggest his mother talks to him and rocks him during the procedure. You say you plan to do a venepuncture rather than heel lancing for the metabolic screen because venepuncture has been shown to be less painful in newborn infants and more likely to result in collection of an adequate blood sample and reduce the need for a second puncture. With regard to the circumcision, you discuss why the procedure is not medically indicated. When they insist on having their son circumcised, you tell the parents that you will give their son paracetamol (acetaminophen) within 2 hours before the procedure and every 4–6 hours for 24 hours after the procedure. You will ensure that the circumcision board is cushioned and will offer their son a sucrose-dipped pacifier before giving the preferred anesthesia, a dorsal penile nerve block. The infant's upper body will be swaddled during the circumcision and you will use the Mogen clamp for the procedure.

Future research needs

● Further research is required to find ways to reduce the exposure of newborns to painful stimuli and to refine the pain management for unavoidable, painful, medically indicated procedures.

Summary of interventions to minimize pain from intramuscular injection

Intervention	Type of evidence	Result	Comment and adverse effects
EMLA versus placebo[21–25]	RCTs (n = 5)	EMLA is effective in decreasing pain from intramuscular injection in adults and children	Skin pallor, erythema and methemoglobinemia have been reported. Effectiveness of newer topical anesthetic agents in newborns receiving intramuscular injection should be evaluated
Sucrose versus placebo[31–33]	RCTs (n = 3)	Sucrose is effective in reducing pain response to vaccination in infants	The magnitude of the effectiveness may reduce with increase in age

Summary of interventions to minimize pain during heel lancing

Intervention	Type of evidence	Result	Comment and adverse effects
Warming versus not warming the heel[43–44]	RCTs (n = 2)	Warming the heel does not reduce pain or facilitate blood collection during heel lancing	Unnecessary intervention associated with expenditure of nursing time and hospital resources
Automated versus conventional lancet device[45–48]	RCTs (n = 4)	Automated lancet devices are superior to conventional lancets. They are associated with less pain, reduced need for repeat punctures, shorter procedure time, increased volume of blood collected and reduction in hemolyzed blood samples	
EMLA versus placebo[41] Topical amethocaine versus placebo[51]	Systematic review of RCTs RCT (n = 1)	EMLA is not effective in reducing heel lancing pain Topical amethocaine gel (4%) applied 1 hour prior to heel lancing is not effective in reducing pain response	
Lignocaine versus placebo[52]	RCT (n = 1)	Application of 5% lignocaine gel 1 hour prior to the heel does not reduce pain response from heel lancing	
Paracetamol (acetaminophen) versus placebo[53]	RCT (n = 1)	Oral paracetamol (20 mg kg^{-1}) is not effective for heel lancing pain	
Venepuncture versus heel lance[40]	Systematic review of RCTs	Venepuncture is less painful than heel lancing for blood sampling in newborns	Venepuncture should be the preferred method of blood collection in healthy full term newborns
Sucrose versus control (water, pacifier, or positioning/containing)[34]	Systematic review of RCTs	Sucrose is safe and effective in reducing pain from heel lancing	Routine use of sucrose approximately 2 minutes prior to heel lancing is recommended
Glucose versus no intervention[57]	RCT (n = 1)	2 ml of 33% glucose solution was found to be effective in reducing pain from heel lancing	
Breastfeeding versus no intervent on[58]	RCT (n = 1)	Breast feeding is an effective analgesic during heel lancing as assessed by cry duration, grimacing, and heart rate differences	Breastfeeding should be offered during heel lancing
Comforting measures (use of pacifiers/ non-nutritive sucking or rocking) versus no intervention[59–61]	RCTs (n = 3)	Comforting measures are effective in reducing pain responses	
Oral analgesic interventions (sweet-tasting solutions including glucose, sucrose, lactose, breast milk, formulas, artificial sweeteners versus water or no intervention)[62–67]	RCTs (n = 6)	Except for lactose, sweet tasting solutions reduce pain responses	
Skin-to-skin contact[68]	RCT (n = 1)	Skin to skin contact during heel lancing is effective in reducing pain responses	
Combinations of interventions (sensorial stimulation, sweet tasting solutions with pacifiers versus no intervention or water)[69–75]	RCT (n = 6)	Sensorial stimulation and administration of sucrose with pacifiers are effective in reducing pain responses	

Summary of interventions to minimize pain of circumcision

Intervention	Type of evidence	Result	Comment and adverse effects
Paracetamol (acetaminophen) versus placebo[77,78]	Systematic reviews (n = 2)	Paracetamol is effective in reducing postoperative pain	Benefit was noted only 6 hours after surgery
Dorsal penile nerve block versus no intervention[77]	Systematic review	Dorsal penile nerve block is effective in reducing pain response	Bruising and/or hematoma can occur at the site of injection
Ring block versus no intervention[77]	Systematic review	Ring block is effective in reducing pain response	Further studies of ring block are required to demonstrate any superiority in efficacy and safety compared to dorsal penile nerve block
EMLA versus no intervention[76,78]	Systematic reviews (n =2)	EMLA decreases pain response	EMLA cannot be recommended over local regional nerve block
Lidocaine versus placebo[79]	RCT (n = 1)	Lidocaine is more effective than placebo in decreasing pain response	Lidocaine is less effective than EMLA in reducing stress indicators
Sucrose with or without pacifier compared to water with or without pacifier[77,78]	Systematic reviews (n = 2) and one additional RCT	Oral sucrose with or without pacifier is effective in reducing the pain response	Sucrose is not as effective as dorsal penile nerve block
Glucose versus water[80]	RCT (n = 1)	50% glucose is ineffective in reducing the pain response	
Swaddling versus no intervention[77,78]	Systematic reviews (n = 2)	Swaddling reduces behavioral response	

References

1 Merskey H. Pain specialists and pain terms. *Pain* 1996; **64**:205.
2 Anand KJ, Hickey PR. Pain and its effect in the human neonate and fetus. *N Engl J Med* 1987;**317**:1321–9.
3 Anand KJ, Carr DB. The neuroanatomy, neurophysiology, and neurochemistry of pain, stress and analgesia in newborns and children. *Pediatr Clin N Am* 1989;**36**:795–822.
4 Fitzgerald M, McIntosh M. Pain and analgesia in the newborn. *Arch Dis Child* 1989;**64**:441–3.
5 Porter FL, Grunau RV, Anand KJ. Long-term effects of pain in infants. *J Dev Behav Pediatr* 1999;**20**:253–61.
6 Grunau RV, Whitfield MF, Petrie JH, Fyer EL. Early pain experience, child and family factors as precursors of somatization: a prospective study of extremely premature and full term children. *Pain* 1994;**56**:353–9.
7 Grunau RV, Whitfield MF, Petrie JH, Fyer EL. Children's interpretation of pain producing situations at 8 1/2 years: are they affected by prior nociceptive experiences in the newborn period? *Pediatr Res* 1996;**39**:266.
8 Grunau RV, Whitfield MF, Petrie JH. Pain sensitivity and temperament in extremely low birth-weight premature toddlers and preterm and full-term controls. *Pain* 1994;**58**:341–6.
9 Fitzgerald M, Millard C, McIntosh M. Cutaneous hypersensitivity following peripheral tissue damage in newborn infants and its reversal with topical anesthesia. *Pain* 1989;**39**:31–6.
10 Taddio A, Goldbach M, Ipp M, Stevens B, Koren G. Effect of neonatal circumcision on pain response during vaccination in boys. *Lancet* 1995;**345**:291–2.
11 Taddio A, Katz J, Ilersich AL, Koren G. Effect of neonatal circumcision on pain response during subsequent routine vaccination. *Lancet* 1997;**349**:599–603.
12 Fetus and Newborn Committee, Canadian Paediatric Society (CPS). Neonatal circumcision revisited. *CMAJ* 1996;**154**: 769–80.
13 American Academy of Pediatrics Task Force on Circumcision. Circumcision policy statement. *Pediatrics* 1999;**103**:686–93.
14 Laumann EO, Masi CM, Zuckerman EW. Circumcision in the United States. *JAMA* 1997;**277**:1052–7.
15 Leitch IO. Circumcision: a continuing enigma. *Aust Paed J* 1970;**6**:59–65.
16 Talbert LM, Kraybill EN, Potter HD. Adrenal cortisol response to circumcision in the neonate. *Obstet Gynecol* 1976;**48**: 208–10.
17 Gunnar MR, Fisch RO, Korsvik S, Donhowe JM. The effects of circumcision on serum cortisol and behavior. *Psychoneuroendocrinology* 1981;**6**:269–75.

18 Rawlings DJ, Miller PA, Engel RR. The effect of circumcision on transcutaneous pO2 in term infants. *Am J Dis Child* 1980;**134**:676–8.

19 Simone DA, Marchettini P, Caputi G, Ochoa JL. Identification of muscle afferents subserving sensation of deep pain in humans. *J Neurophysiol* 1994;**72**:883–9.

20 Grunau RV, Johnston CC, Craig KD. Neonatal facial and cry responses to invasive and non-invasive procedures. *Pain* 1990;**42**:295–305.

21 Taddio A, Nulman I, Reid E, Shaw J, Koren G. Effect of lidocaine-prilocaine cream (EMLA®) on pain of intramuscular Fluzone® injection. *Can J Hosp Pharm* 1992;**45**:227–30.

22 Himelstein BP, Cnaan A, Blackall CS, Zhao H, Cavalieri G, Cohen DE. Topical application of lidocaine-prilocaine (EMLA) cream reduces the pain of intramuscular infiltration of saline solution. *J Paediatr* 1996;**129**:718–21.

23 Taddio A, Nulman I, Goldbach M, Ipp M, Koren G. Use of lidocaine-prilocaine cream for vaccination pain in infants. *J Pediatr* 1994;**124**:643–8.

24 Halperin BA, Halperin SA, McGrath P, Smith B, Houston T. Use of lidocaine-prilocaine patch to decrease intramuscular injection pain does not adversely affect the antibody response to diphtheria-tetanus-acellular-pertussis inactivated poliovirus-*Haemophilus influenzae* type b conjugate and hepatitis B vaccines in infants from birth to six months of age. *Paediatr Infect Dis J* 2002;**21**:399–405.

25 Uhari M. A eutectic mixture of lidocaine and prilocaine for alleviating vaccination pain in infants. *Pediatrics* 1993; **92**:719–21.

26 Brisman M, Ljung BM, Otterbom I, Larsson LE, Andreasson SE. Methaemoglobin formation after the use of EMLA cream in term neonates. *Acta Paediatr* 1998;**87**:1191–4.

27 Couper RT. Methaemoglobinemia secondary to topical lignocaine/prilocaine in a circumcised neonate. *J Paediatr Child Health* 2000;**36**:406–7.

28 Law RM, Halpern S, Martins RF, Reich H, Innanen V, Ohlsson A. Measurement of methemoglobin after EMLA analgesia for newborn circumcision. *Biol Neonate* 1996;**70**:213–7.

29 Taddio A, Shennan AT, Stevens B, Leeder JS, Koren G. Safety of lidocaine-prilocaine cream in the treatment of preterm newborns. *J Pediatr* 1995;**127**:1002–5.

30 Essink-Tebbes CM, Wuis EW, Liem KD, van Dongen RT, Hekster YA. Safety of lidocaine-prilocaine cream application four times a day in premature neonates: a pilot study. *Eur J Pediatr* 1999;**158**:421–3.

31 Lewindon PJ, Harkness L, Lewindon N. Randomised controlled trial of sucrose by mouth for the relief of infant crying after immunisation. *Arch Dis Child* 1998;**78**:453–6.

32 Barr RG, Young SN, Wright JH *et al.* "Sucrose analgesia" and diphtheria-tetanus-pertussis immunisations at 2 and 4 months. *J Dev Behav Pediatr* 1995;**16**:220–5.

33 Allen KD, White DD, Walburn JN. Sucrose as an analgesic agent for infants during immunization injections. *Arch Pediatr Adolesc Med* 1996;**150**:270–4.

34 Stevens B, Yamada J, Ohlsson A. Sucrose for analgesia in newborn infants undergoing painful procedures (Cochrane Review). In: *Cochrane Library*, Issue 1. Oxford: Update Software: 2003.

35 Kaufman GE, Cimo S, Miller LW, Blass EM. An evaluation of the effects of sucrose on neonatal pain with 2 commonly used circumcision methods. *Am J Obstet Gynecol* 2002; **186**:564–8.

36 Owens ME, Todt EH. Pain in infancy: neonatal reaction to a heel lance. *Pain* 1984;**20**:77–86.

37 Brown L. Physiologic responses to cutaneous pain in neonates. *Neonatal Netw* 1987;**6**:18–22.

38 Izard CE. *The maximally discriminative facial movement coding system (MAX).* University of Delaware Instructional Resources Centre: Newark DE, 1979.

39 Grunau RV, Craig KD. Pain expression in neonates: facial action and cry. *Pain* 1987;**28**:395–410.

40 Shah V, Ohlsson A. Venepuncture versus heel lance for blood sampling in term neonates (Cochrane Review). In: *Cochrane Library*, Issue 1. Update Software: Oxford, 2003.

41 Taddio A, Ohlsson A, Einarson TR, Stevens B, Koren G. A systematic review of lidocaine-prilocaine cream (EMLA) in the treatment of acute pain in neonates. *Pediatrics* 1998; http://www.*Pediatrics*org/cgi/content/full/101/2/e1

42 Ohlsson A, Taddio A, Jadad AR, Stevens BJ. Evidence-based decision making, systematic reviews and the Cochrane Collaboration: implications for neonatal analgesia. In: Anand KJS, Stevens BJ, McGrath PJ. eds. *Pain in Newborns, 2nd edn. Pain Research and Clinical Management, Vol 10.* Amsterdam: Elsevier Science BV, 2000.

43 Barker DP, Willetts B, Cappendijk VC, Rutter N. Capillary blood sampling: should the heel be warmed? *Arch Dis Child* 1996;**74**:139–40.

44 Janes M, Pinelli J, Landry S, Downey S, Paes B. Comparison of capillary blood sampling using an automated incision device with and without warming of the heel. *J Perinatol* 2002;**22**:154–8.

45 Paes B, Janes M, Vegh P, LeDuca F, Andrew M. A comparative study of heel-stick devices for infant blood collection. *Am J Dis Child* 1993;**147**:346–8.

46 Vertanen H, Fellman V, Brommels M, Viinikka L. An automatic incision device for obtaining blood samples from the heels of preterm infants causes less damage than a conventional manual lancet. *Arch Dis Child* 2001;**84**:53–5.

47 Kellam B, Waller JL, McLaurin C, *et al.* Tenderfoot preemie vs a manual lancet: A clinical evaluation. *Neonatal Netw* 2001;**7**:31–6.

48 Shah V, Taddio A, Kulasekaran K, O'Brien L, Perkins E, Kelly E. Evaluation of a new Lancet device (BD Quikheel lancet) on pain response and success of procedure in term neonates. *Arch Pediatr Adolesc Med* 2003;**157**:1075–8.

49 Larsson BA, Jylli L, Lagercrantz H, Ohlsson GL. Does a local anesthetic cream (EMLA) alleviate pain from heel-lancing in newborns. *Acta Anaesthesiol Scand* 1995;**23**: 1028–31.

50 Stevens B, Johnston C, Taddio A, *et al.* Management of pain from heel lance with lidocaine-prilocaine (EMLA) cream: is it safe and efficacious in preterm infants? *J Dev Behav Pediatr* 1999;**20**:216–21.

51 Jain A, Rutter N, Ratnayaka M. Topical amethocaine gel for pain relief of heel prick blood sampling: a randomised double-blind controlled trial. *Arch Dis Child* 2001;**84**:56–9.

52 Rushforth JA, Griffiths G, Thorpe H, Levene MI. Can topical lignocaine reduce behavioural response to heel prick? *Arch Dis Child* 1995;**72**:49–51.

53 Shah V, Taddio A, Ohlsson A. Randomised controlled trial of paracetamol for heel prick pain in neonates. *Arch Dis Child* 1998;**79**:209–11.

54 Shah VS, Taddio A, Bennett S, Speidel BD. Neonatal pain response to heel stick vs venepuncture for routine blood sampling. *Arch Dis Child* 1997;**77**:143–4.

55 Larsson BA, Tannfeldt G, Lagercrantz H, Olsson GL. Venepuncture is more effective and less painful than heel lancing for blood tests in neonates. *Pediatrics* 1998;**101**:882–6.

56 Eriksson M, Gradin M, Schollin J. Oral glucose and venepuncture reduce blood sampling pain in newborns. *Early Hum Dev* 1999;**55**:211–18.

57 Guala A, Giroletti G. Glucose as an analgesic in neonatology. A blind randomized controlled study. *Pediatr Med Chir* 1998;**20**:201–3.

58 Gary L, Miller LW, Philipp BL, Blass EM. Breast feeding is analgesic in healthy newborns. *Pediatrics* 2002;**109**:590–3.

59 Corbo MG, Mansi G, Stagni A *et al.* Nonnutritive sucking during heelstick procedures decreases behavioral distress in the newborn infant. *Biol Neonate* 2000;**77**:162–7.

60 Field T, Goldson E. Pacifying effects of nonnutritive sucking on term and preterm neonates during heelstick procedures. *Pediatrics* 1984;**74**:1012–15.

61 Campos RG. Rocking and pacifiers: two comforting interventions for heelstick pain. *Res Nurs Health* 1994;**17**:321–31.

62 Isik U, Özek E, Bilgen H, Cebeci D. Comparison of oral glucose and sucrose solutions on pain response in newborns. *J Pain* 2000;**1**:275–8.

63 Guala A, Pastore G, Liverani ME *et al.* Glucose or sucrose as an analgesic for newborns: a randomised controlled blind trial. *Minerva Pediatr* 2001;**53**:271–4.

64 Skogsdal Y, Eriksson M, Schollin J. Analgesia in newborns given oral glucose. *Acta Paediatr* 1997;**86**:217–20.

65 Blass EM. Milk-induced hypoalgesia in human newborns. *Pediatrics* 1997;**99**:825–9.

66 Ramenghi LA, Griffith GC, Wood CM, Levene MI. Effect of non-sucrose sweet tasting solution on neonatal heel prick responses. *Arch Dis Child* 1996;**74**:129–31.

67 Bucher HU, Baumgartner R, Bucher N, Seiler M, Fauchere JC. Artificial sweetener reduces nociceptive reaction in term newborn infants. *Early Hum Dev* 2000;**59**:51–60.

68 Gray L, Watt L, Blass EM. Skin-to-skin contact is analgesic in healthy newborns. *Pediatrics* 2000;**105**. URL:http://www.pediatricsorg/cgi/content/full/105/1/e14

69 Bellieni CV, Buonocore G, Nenci A, Franci N, Cordelli DM, Bagnoli F. Sensorial stimulation: an effective analgesic tool for heel-prick in preterm infants: a prospective randomized trial. *Biol Neonate* 2001;**80**:15–18.

70 Bellieni CV, Bagnoli F, Perrone S, *et al.* Effect of multisensory stimulation on analgesia in term neonates: a randomized controlled trial. *Pediatr Res* 2002;**51**:460–3.

71 Akman I, Özek E, Bilgen H, Ozdgoan T, Cebeci D. Sweet solutions and pacifiers for pain relief in newborn infants. *J Pain* 2002;**3**:199–202.

72 Greenberg CS. A sugar-coated pacifier reduces procedural pain in newborns. *Pediatr Nurs* 2002;**28**:271–7.

73 Örs R, Özek E, Baysoy G *et al.* Comparison of sucrose and human milk on pain response in newborns. *Eur J Pediatr* 1999;**158**:63–6.

74 Gormally S, Barr RG, Werthiem L, Alkawaf R, Calinoiu N, Young SN. Contact and nutrient caregiving effects on newborn infants pain responses. *Develop Med Child Neurol* 2001;**43**:28–38.

75 Blass EM, Watt LB. Suckling- and sucrose-induced analgesia in human newborns. *Pain* 1999;**83**:611–23.

76 Taddio A, Ohlsson K, Ohlsson A. Lidocaine-prilocaine cream for analgesia during circumcision in newborn boys. (Cochrane Review). In: *Cochrane Library*, Issue 1. Oxford: Update Software, 2003.

77 Taddio A. Pain management for neonatal circumcision. *Paediatr Drugs* 2001;**3**:101–11.

78 Geyer J, Ellsbury D, Kleiber C, Litwiller D, Hinton A, Yankowitz J. An evidence-based multidisciplinary protocol for neonatal circumcision pain. *J Obstet Gynecol Neonatal Nurs* 2002;**31**:403–10.

79 Woodman PJ. Topical lidocaine-prilocaine versus lidocaine for neonatal circumcision: A randomized controlled trial. *Obstet Gynecol* 1999;**93**:775–9.

80 Kass FC, Holman JR. Oral glucose solution for analgesia in infant circumcision. *J Fam Practice* 2001;**50**:785–8.

81 Kurtis PS, DeSilva HN, Bernstein BA, Malakh L, Schechter NL. A comparison of the Mogen and Gomco clamps in combination with dorsal penile nerve block in minimizing the pain of neonatal circumcision. *Pediatrics* 1999;**103**. http://www.pediatricsorg/cgi/content/full/103/2/e23

82 Taddio A, Pollock N, Gilbert-MacLeod C, Ohlsson K, Koren G. Combined analgesia and local anesthesia to minimize pain during circumcision. *Arch Pediatr Adolesc Med* 2000;**154**:620–3.

83 Stang HJ, Snellman LW. Circumcision practice patterns in the United States. *Pediatrics* 1998;**101**: http://www.pediatricsorg/cgi/contetnt/full/101/6/e5

51 Neonatal abstinence syndrome

David Osborn, Tracey Burrell

Case scenario

A 29-year-old woman presents for the first antenatal visit, having been referred by her primary practitioner 4 months previously. She thinks she is around 30 weeks' gestation. During the visit she admits to having used heroin for 5 years. She was previously treated with buprenorphine but several months after detoxification started reusing heroin. She currently uses two heroin caps a day. You wonder why the referral letter doesn't mention her drug usage and how this could have been identified earlier.

She appears well but anxious and has numerous scars and red papular areas on her arms. You perform a complete examination. Testing reveals she is HIV, hepatitis B surface antigen, and hepatitis C negative. She asks whether she can go back on buprenorphine; however, after discussing the options with her, you refer her to the drug and alcohol clinic team who start her on methadone.

At 36 weeks' gestation, she presents in labor. She is currently taking methadone 85 mg per day. She delivers a 2·5 kg boy, who appears well, sucks well at the breast and is transferred to the postnatal ward with his mother. At 3 days of age, the nursing staff report that he is irritable, won't settle after feeds and is incessantly sucking. He has posited several times and has watery stools. On examination he is very jittery and has increased tone. His mother is tired and distressed. You diagnose neonatal abstinence syndrome (NAS) and because his NAS score is high you admit him to the newborn nursery. His mother expresses concern when you discuss treating him with an opiate (oral morphine) and asks if this is necessary. The infant settles and feeds well. His mother is shown how to administer morphine safely. The infant is returned to the postnatal ward at 6 days of age and regains his birth weight by 7 days. You wonder, while planning for their discharge, what you can do to support this family at home.

Background

Use of alcohol and drugs during pregnancy is common.[1,2] Drug addiction in pregnant women is associated with detrimental health effects to both the mother and infant. Drug users frequently have poor antenatal and postnatal care and tend to be socially disadvantaged. These are risk factors for adverse pregnancy outcomes including placental abruption, perinatal mortality, and birth of low birthweight infants. Women who use injecting drugs are at increased risk of infection, particularly hepatitis C. Potential pharmacological treatments for opiate dependence include a variety of detoxification and maintenance therapies. Detoxification may be pharmacologically assisted with a partial opiate agonist (buprenorphine), opiate antagonist (naloxone or naltrexone), or a sedative (clonidine). In opiate replacement therapy an opiate agonist (methadone or LAAM) or a partial agonist (buprenorphine) may be used to prevent ongoing illicit drug

use or, after detoxification, an opiate antagonist (naltrexone). However, most trials of these interventions are reported in non-pregnant populations. Methadone maintenance therapy has become standard treatment for pregnant women with an opiate dependence with the goal of reducing risk behaviors in the woman and improving pregnancy and newborn outcomes.

Infants born to mothers with a drug problem, especially to those using opiates, may suffer from neonatal abstinence syndrome (NAS) and require treatment. NAS from opiate withdrawal is characterized by central nervous system hyperirritability, gastrointestinal and autonomic dysfunction, and respiratory distress. Withdrawal occurs in 40–70% of infants born to heroin users and up to 90% of infants born to methadone users. Heroin withdrawal is typically evident within 24 hours of birth, while methadone withdrawal is usually evident between 2 and 7 days after birth. The presence and severity of NAS may be scored using a variety of scoring tools including the Neonatal Abstinence Severity

Score (NASS) and the Lipsitz tool, which are also used to determine need for treatment. Pharmacologic treatments that have been used to ameliorate symptoms and prevent complications in infants with NAS from opiate withdrawal include opiates (paregoric, diluted tincture of opium, morphine, and methadone) and a range of sedatives (phenobarbitone, diazepam, chlorpromazine, and clonidine).[3–5]

Framing answerable clinical questions

A number of clinical questions arise from the scenario above and you structure these and identify the question type to facilitate your search for evidence (see Chapter 2).

Questions

1. In pregnant women (*population*), will a screening questionnaire (*intervention*) compared with an interview (*comparison*) reliably detect drug or alcohol abuse (*outcome*)? **[Diagnosis]**
2. In pregnant women with opiate dependence (*population*), does methadone maintenance (*intervention*) compared with detoxification or continued use of heroin (*comparison*) reduce the risk of placental abruption, low birthweight infants, and decrease perinatal mortality (*outcomes*)? **[Therapy]**
3. In pregnant women using opiates (*population*), does use of buprenorphine (*intervention*) compared with methadone (*comparison*) reduce the severity of NAS (*outcome*)? **[Therapy]**
4. In pregnant women on methadone (*population*), does methadone dose (*exposure*) predict the risk of NAS (*outcome*) in the infant? **[Risk/Prognosis]**
5. In infants with NAS due to opiates (*population*), does the use of a NAS score (*test*) reliably detect infants at risk of complications including poor feeding, excess weight loss, and seizures (*outcomes*)? **[Diagnosis]**
6. In infants with NAS due to opiates (*population*), is an opiate (*intervention*) better than a sedative (*comparison*) for reducing NAS severity and preventing seizures (*outcomes*)? **[Therapy]**
7. In women with a drug or alcohol problem (*population*), does home support (*intervention*) improve pregnancy outcomes and infant development, and reduce the risk of child abuse or neglect (*outcomes*)? **[Therapy]**

Searching for evidence

To answer the questions of therapy you search the most reliable source of secondary evidence – the *Cochrane Library*'s Database of Systematic Reviews (CDSR) and Database of Abstracts of Reviews of Effects (DARE) – for systematic reviews (see Chapter 8). If there is no systematic review (or to find trials published after the review), you search the Cochrane Central Register of Controlled Trials (CENTRAL) and MedLine. You also search MedLine for evidence-based clinical practice guidelines.

General search strategy

*   Searching for evidence syntheses

    Cochrane Library: "substance related disorders" (MeSH) AND "pregnancy" (text word)
    MedLine (Ovid): "substance related disorders" (MeSH) AND "pregnancy" (text) *limit* to "meta-analysis"

*   Searching for evidence-based guidelines

    MedLine (Ovid): "substance related disorders" (MeSH) AND "pregnancy" (text) *limit* to ("guidelines" OR meta-analysis"

You find several systematic reviews[6–10] in the *Cochrane Library* potentially addressing questions 2, 3, and 6. In DARE you find a review[11] that addresses accuracy of alcohol screening in women (question 1). In MedLine you identify some additional meta-analyses[12,13] with the potential to answer question 2. You also find two guidelines from the American Academy of Pediatrics (AAP), one updating the other.[4,5]

To answer questions of risk/prognosis you search MedLine for population-based cohort studies (a MeSH term). For diagnosis or screening questions (see Chapter 5) you look for cross-sectional studies in which the test and the reference or "gold" standard were performed independently in all patients. Assessors conducting one test should be "blind" to the results of the other test.[14] When case–control studies, different reference standards and unblinded assessments are used, a test's accuracy may be overestimated.[15] You use the MeSH term "sensitivity and specificity" because this is the best single search strategy for questions of diagnosis. You start with a specific search strategy to "get rid of the rubbish" using medical subject heading searches (MeSH terms) directed by your structured, focused question. When you do not find any relevant articles using a *specific* search strategy, you use a more *sensitive* search strategy incorporating text word searches, increasing the number of search terms, and looking for specific study types to answer your questions.

Question

1. In pregnant women (*population*), will a screening questionnaire (*intervention*) compared with an interview (*comparison*) reliably detect drug or alcohol abuse (*outcome*)? **[Diagnosis]**

Specific Search strategy

- MedLine (Ovid): "alcohol related disorders" [MeSH] AND "pregnancy" [text] AND "sensitivity and specificity" [MeSH]; "opiate related disorders" [MeSH] AND "pregnancy" [text] AND ("sensitivity and specificity" OR "ROC curve" [MeSH])

In the *Cochrane Library* you find two reviews in DARE, one of which focuses on screening questionnaires for alcohol use in women.[11] In this review the research question is focused, the search strategy and inclusion criteria are documented and a critical appraisal of included studies has been performed. Publication bias is possible because the search strategy was limited to MedLine and the English language, with no mention of an attempt to identify unpublished papers. Two questionnaires ("TWEAK" and "T-ACE"), validated in inner city obstetric populations comprising African-American women, had reasonable sensitivity (T-ACE 83–91%; TWEAK 92%) and specificity (T-ACE 70–75%; TWEAK 67%) for detecting intake of ≥ 2 standard drinks per day in pregnant women. The authors note that these questionnaires may be culturally sensitive and that accuracy may differ depending on race and ethnicity.

You then search MedLine and find five additional reports of four studies validating screening tests for alcohol use in pregnant women.[16–20] In one study[16,17] the T-ACE (with the tolerance being > 2 drinks) correctly identified 65% of current prenatal risk drinkers with a sensitivity of 74% and specificity of 71%. Use of this questionnaire considerably outperformed obstetric staff's antenatal history taking for detecting risk drinking in pregnant women (sensitivity 7%, specificity 89%). In another study[20] the TWEAK questionnaire had 71% sensitivity and 73% specificity for high risk drinking. Self-reported alcohol consumption was used as the reference standard in both studies. You wonder whether self-report may underestimate alcohol consumption. You conclude that the T-ACE (four questions) and TWEAK (five questions) are feasible and have superior accuracy to current antenatal interview of pregnant women (see Table 51.1).

Your search for a screening questionnaire to detect opiate use is more problematic. You expand the search terms to include "pregnancy" as a text word and "ROC curve" (MeSH) and find several studies,[21–24] one of which[24] is potentially relevant to your question. In this study, maternal interview is compared with hair and meconium analysis for opiates. However, only women using drugs were screened, so no true estimate of the accuracy of the maternal interview can be made. You expand the search to include "substance related disorders" (MeSH) and find a large number of articles. In one study[25] the Substance Abuse Subtle Screening Inventory (SASSI), a 78-item questionnaire taking 10–15 minutes to complete, is evaluated. You use the *JAMA* users' guides[26,27] to appraise the article. An independent and probably blinded comparison (urine toxicology) is used and an appropriate spectrum of patients (drug and non-drug using) is included. The SASSI and urine toxicology were performed independently on all 560 women attending an antenatal clinic. The SASSI had 42% sensitivity and 80% specificity for a positive urine toxicological screen in pregnancy (a positive predictive value of only 26%). You are concerned about the potential for causing harm from false positives and that the SASSI will add considerably to the time needed for the antenatal assessment. Given these limitations you decide the SASSI should be subjected to an RCT before you will include it in your clinical practice.[28]

Question

2. In pregnant women with opiate dependence (*population*), does methadone maintenance (*intervention*) compared with detoxification or continued use of heroin (*comparison*) reduce the risk of placental abruption, low birthweight infants, and decrease perinatal mortality (*outcomes*)? **[Therapy]**

Specific search strategy

- *Cochrane Library*: "methadone maintenance" AND "pregnancy" [text]
- MedLine (Ovid): ("methadone" [MeSH] OR "methadone maintenance" [text]) AND "pregnancy" [MeSH OR text] *limit* to "meta-analysis"; "methadone" [MeSH] OR "methadone maintenance" [text]) AND "pregnancy" [MeSH OR text] *limit* to "clinical trial"; "detoxification" [MeSH OR text] AND "pregnancy" [MeSH OR text] *limit* to "clinical trial"

You find two systematic reviews of methadone treatment in the *Cochrane Library*. In the meta-analysis of trials of methadone maintenance,[6] methadone was significantly more effective than non-pharmacological approaches for retaining patients in treatment (relative risk [RR] = 3·1; 95% CI 1·8–5·4) and for suppressing heroin use (RR = 0·3; 95% CI 0·2–0·4). The conclusion of the systematic review of trials of tapered doses of methadone[7] stated that "slow tapering with temporary substitution of long-acting opioids, accompanied by medical supervision and ancillary medications can reduce withdrawal severity. Nevertheless the majority of patients relapsed to heroin use." However, none of the trials in either review included pregnant women, limiting their generalizability.

In a MedLine search limited to "meta-analyses" you find two systematic reviews of observational studies.[12,13] Publication bias is possible because the search was limited to the English language and MedLine. No critical appraisal of

Table 51.1 Brief summary of alcohol and substance abuse screening questionnaires in pregnant women

Alcohol questionnaires

Study	Study type	n	Population	Reference standard	Test	Sn%	Sp%
Budd[19]	Cross-sectional retrospective	56	Inner city high volume prenatal clinic women	CDTect +ve	PAUI ACOG antenatal record	59 19	71 93
Bull[18]	Cross-sectional	208	American-Indian prenatal women	Interview/medical record Any drinking in pregnancy	SAQ	77	93
Chang[16,17]	Cross-sectional	350	Boston prenatal clinic Ethnically/socially diverse	Timeline follow-back ≥ 2 standard drinks/day	T-ACE SMAST	74 11	71 96
Dawson[20]	Cross-sectional	404	Washington antenatal clinic	Self-reported > 1 standard drink/day	Medical record TWEAK	7 71	89 73
Russell[21,22]	Cross-sectional	4743	Inner city antenatal clinic African-American women	Timeline follow-back ≥ 2 standard drinks/day	T-ACE ≥ 1 TWEAK ≥ 1	83–91 92	70–75 67
Sokol[23]	Cross-sectional	971	Inner city antenatal clinic African-American women	Self-reported ≥ 2 standard drinks/day	CAGE ≥ 1 T-ACE ≥ 1	59 76	82 79

Substance abuse questionnaire

Study	Study type	n	Population	Reference standard	Test	Sn%	Sp%
Horrigan[25]	Cohort	560	Literate, English speaking	Self-reported drug use	SASSI	42	80

Tests and reference standards: ACOG record, American College of Obstetricians and Gynecologists Antepartum Record; AUDIT, Alcohol Use Disorder Identification Test; CAGE, Cut down, Annoyed, Guilt, Eye opener; CDTect, Carbohydrate Deficient Transferrin testing; PAUI, Prenatal Alcohol Use Interview; SASSI, Substance Abuse Subtle Screening Inventory; SAQ, Self-administered questionnaire; SMAST, Short Michigan Alcohol Screening Test; T-ACE, Tolerance, Annoyed, Cut down, Eye opener; TWEAK, Tolerance, Worry, Eye opener, Annoy, Kut down.

study quality was performed and no adjustment was made for confounding in the analysis and no sensitivity analysis was performed according to study quality. In women stabilized on methadone, compared with non-drug exposed controls, there was no significant difference in neonatal mortality (RR 1·75; 95% CI 0·60–4·59) or low birth weight, although there was a mean reduction in birth weight of 279 g (95% CI 229–328 g). In women using heroin alone there was no significant difference in neonatal mortality (RR 1·47; 95% CI 0·88–2·33) but there was a significant increase in low birthweight infants (RR 4·61 95% CI 2·78–7·65). Infants of women who failed to stabilize on methadone and continued heroin use had the worst outcomes with substantially increased rates of neonatal mortality (RR 6·37; 95% CI 2·57–14·68) and low birthweight (RR 3·28; 95% CI 2·47–4·39).

The systematic reviews of RCTs of methadone therapy[6,7] do not provide any information concerning pregnant women and the systematic reviews of observational studies[12,13] are open to bias so you search for RCTs in MedLine and Embase. You find one unblinded RCT comparing the severity of NAS in infants whose mothers received either methadone or slow release morphine.[29] Women on slow release morphine consumed fewer benzodiazepines and had fewer visible injection sites, but no significant difference was found for other outcomes including severity of NAS. You find no clinical trials comparing methadone with detoxification or detoxification with any other maintenance therapy.

Question

3. In pregnant women using opiates (*population*), does use of buprenorphine (*intervention*) compared with methadone (*comparison*) reduce the severity of NAS (*outcome*)? **[Therapy]**

Specific search strategy

- *Cochrane Library*: "buprenorphine" and "pregnancy" [text]
- MedLine (Ovid): "buprenorphine" [MeSH] AND "pregnancy" [MeSH OR text] *limit* to "clinical trial". PreMedLine (Ovid): "buprenorphine" [text] AND "pregnancy" [text]

You identify one systematic review in the *Cochrane Library*[8] that includes 13 RCTs of buprenorphine maintenance versus placebo or methadone maintenance for opioid dependence. Trial methodology was generally good and 12 trials were double-blind. Buprenorphine was significantly better than placebo for retaining patients in treatment, but only high and very high dose buprenorphine suppressed heroin use significantly compared with placebo.

Buprenorphine given in flexible doses (unblinded trials) was significantly less effective than methadone in retaining patients in treatment. High dose buprenorphine was not superior to high dose methadone for treatment retention (RR = 0·79; 95% CI 0·62–1·01). High dose buprenorphine was inferior to high dose methadone for suppressing heroin use. The review conclusion states that "buprenorphine is an effective intervention for maintenance treatment of heroin dependence, but it is not more effective than methadone at adequate dosages." No data on other measures of physical and psychological health were included in the review and no trial reported enrolling pregnant women.

You search CENTRAL, MedLine, and PreMedLine (up to July 2003) with a more *sensitive* strategy (including both MeSH and text terms) and *limiting* to "clinical trials". In CENTRAL you find an ongoing prospective, controlled clinical trial of buprenorphine versus methadone use in pregnancy which does not document random allocation to treatment.[30] You find one controlled clinical trial in MedLine[31] and a non-systematic review in PreMedLine.[32] The review[32] does not have a focused objective and does not document a search strategy. Although study type is described, articles are not critically appraised and studies with no control group are incorrectly described as "open-labeled controlled" trials. In a prospective, unblinded cohort study[31] women were allocated treatment according to clinician and/or patient preference to maintenance treatment with buprenorphine (n = 153) or methadone (n = 93). Women receiving buprenorphine were more likely to have a partner, to have opioid replacement therapy before pregnancy and be cared for by a primary care practitioner. However, no adjustment was made for confounding. Buprenorphine-maintained women were less likely to deliver prematurely but there was no difference in the incidence or severity of NAS or any other pregnancy or neonatal outcome.

Question

4. In pregnant women on methadone (*population*), does methadone dose (*exposure*) predict the risk of NAS (*outcome*) in the infant? **[Risk/Prognosis]**

Specific search strategy

- MedLine (Ovid): "methadone" [MeSH OR text] AND "neonatal abstinence syndrome" [MeSH] AND "cohort studies" [MeSH]

In MedLine you find three cohort studies that examine the relationship between methadone dose and occurrence of NAS.[31,33,34] You use the *JAMA Users' guide* for critically appraising an article about prognosis (see also Chapter 4).[35]

None of the three articles was population-based and none documented failure to recruit potentially eligible subjects or losses to follow up of eligible women and infants. A NAS score was used in all studies but blinding to methadone dose was not documented and there was no adjustment for potential confounders (for example, infant prematurity). In all three studies there was a correlation between maternal opiate dose and severity of NAS. In one study[33] infants of mothers taking > 40 mg per day of methadone had a 90% risk of NAS requiring treatment. However, even infants of mothers taking below 20 mg per day of methadone were at risk of having NAS requiring treatment. Although the evidence is potentially biased by the methodological limitations listed above, the relationship between maternal methadone dose and NAS severity was consistent between studies.

Question

5.   In infants with NAS due to opiates (*population*), does the use of a NAS score (*test*) reliably detect infants at risk of complications including poor feeding, excess weight loss, and seizures (*outcomes*)? **[Diagnosis]**

Specific search strategy

●   (*sh = subject heading)
●   MedLine (Ovid): ("substance related disorders" [MeSH] AND "infant newborn" [MeSH]) AND ("sensitivity and specificity" [MeSH OR text] OR "ROC curve" [MeSH] OR "diagnosis" [sh*] OR "diagnostic use" [sh] OR ("predictive" AND "value" [text])

You find no relevant articles in MedLine using PubMed "clinical queries using methodological filters" with "diagnosis" and "specificity" selected. The more recent of the two AAP guidelines[4,5] that you found earlier identifies several NAS scoring systems (including the Lipsitz tool, the Neonatal Withdrawal Inventory, and the Finnegan NAS Score) and recommends use of the Lipsitz tool[36] in view of its sensitivity (77%) and ease of use (11 items). You obtain the original articles referenced in the guidelines and select those reporting data from which sensitivity and specificity or likelihood ratios can be calculated. Two articles meet these criteria[36,37] and you critically appraise them using the *JAMA* guides for how to use a diagnostic test (see also Chapter 5).[26,27]

Lipsitz[36] selected infants of opiate using mothers and used term and low birthweight infants of non-drug users as controls. The reference standard was the ability of the test (Lipsitz tool) to differentiate between infants of opiate dependent mothers from the controls. The test was applied to all infants and assessors were blinded to history of maternal drug use. A Lipsitz score > 4 had 25% sensitivity and 100% specificity for predicting maternal drug use. In the other

study[37] the Neonatal Withdrawal Inventory was compared with the Finnegan NAS Score. The tests were performed simultaneously by two observers, predominantly in infants treated for NAS but it is not clear whether blinding was maintained. The tests had 100% agreement for a Finnegan NAS Score of 8 or more. The Lipsitz tool has high specificity so a positive test (score > 4) should have good "rule-in" value for the diagnosis of NAS. However, you are concerned that the tests have not been validated in an appropriate spectrum of patients or against an appropriate reference standard, especially to determine NAS severity and need for treatment.

Question

6.   In infants with NAS due to opiates (*population*), is an opiate (*intervention*) better than a sedative (*comparison*) for reducing NAS severity and preventing seizures (*outcomes*)? **[Therapy]**

Specific search strategy

●   *Cochrane Library*: "neonatal abstinence syndrome"
●   MedLine (Ovid): "neonatal abstinence syndrome" [MeSH] *limit* to "clinical trial"

You find two systematic reviews in the *Cochrane Library* that were last updated in 2002[9,10] and examine the evidence for using opiates and sedatives for NAS from opiate withdrawal. The review of opiate therapy reports on six studies[38–43] including 511 infants of mothers using opiates and frequently other drugs. Two studies may be sequential reports that include some identical patients (see Table 51.2). There were substantial methodological concerns about studies included in the review. In three studies, quasi-random patient allocation was used and in four studies there were substantial, largely unexplained differences in reported numbers allocated to each group. Meta-analysis of three studies indicated no significant difference in the treatment failure rate in infants receiving an opiate compared with phenobarbitone (RR 0·78; 95% CI 0·46, 1·32). In one study[39] a significant reduction in treatment failure was reported in infants of mothers using only an opiate. As this was a *post hoc* analysis, the authors advise that the result should be interpreted with caution. In one study[41] a reduction in seizures was reported with the use of an opiate compared with phenobarbitone (RR 0·08; 95% CI 0·00, 1·44; risk difference –0·11; 95% CI –0·20, –0·03); however, this was of borderline statistical significance. Meta-analysis of two studies in which an opiate was compared with diazepam found a significant reduction in treatment failure (RR 0·43; 95% CI 0·23, 0·80) in the group given an opiate. No data on neurodevelopmental outcomes were available according to group of assignment.

Table 51.2 Summary of trials of opiate use for infants with NAS born to mothers using opiates

Study	Methods	Participants	Interventions	n	Outcomes RR (95% CI)
Carin[38]	Random, method not reported Blinding not reported No blinding of measurement No losses to follow up	Infants of mothers on methadone Polydrug use 42% Finnegan NASS ≥ 8	1. Paregoric 0·42–2·1 ml kg⁻¹ per day 2. Phenobarbitone 5–16ml kg⁻¹ per day	16 16	Paregoric v phenobarbitone: Days treatment: 22 v 17 days $P < 0.01$ No difference weight gain
Coyle[44]	Quasi-random Blinded treatment Blinded measurement Losses: 3	Infants of mothers using heroin/methadone Finnegan NASS ≥ 8	1. DTO + Phenobarbitone 30 mg kg⁻¹ then maintenance 5 mg kg⁻¹ per day 2. DTO + Placebo	10 10	DTO + phenobarbitone v DTO: Hospitalization: 38 v 79 days $P < 0.001$ % time score >7 : 10 v 15% $P = 0.04$ % time score <5 : 64 v 53% $P = 0.03$
Finnegan[39]	Quasi-random Treatment not blinded Blinded treatment No losses reported	Infants of mothers using opiates ± other drugs Finnegan NASS ≥ 8	1. Paregoric 2. Phenobarbitone 20 mg kg⁻¹ then maintenance 5–10 mg kg⁻¹ per day 3. Diazepam	35 87 20	Paregoric v phenobarbitone: Treatment failure: RR 1·1 (0·5, 2·2) Paregoric v diazepam: Treatment failure: RR 0·4 (0·2, 0·8)
Kaltenbach[40]	Quasi-random Treatment not blinded Blinded treatment No losses reported	Infants of mothers on methadone Polydrug use 95% Finnegan NASS ≥ 8	1. Paregoric 2. Phenobarbitone loading dose then maintenance 3. Phenobarbitone titrated 4. Diazepam	23 20 16 10	Paregoric v phenobarbitone: Treatment failure: RR 0·2 (0·0, 0·6) Paregoric v diazepam: Treatment failure: RR 0·1 (0·0, 0·3)
Kandall[41]	Random, method not reported Blinding not reported Measurement blinding unclear No losses	Infants of mothers with opiate dependence Polydrug use 61% Lipsitz score ≥7	1. Paregoric 0·2 ml every 3 hours, titrated 2. Phenobarbitone 5 mg kg⁻¹ per day IMI	49 62	Paregoric v phenobarbitone: Seizures: RR 0·1 (0·0, 1·4) $P = 0.05$; risk difference –0·1 (–0·20, –0·03)
Khoo[42]	Quasi-random Not blinded Measurement not blinded Losses: 3	Infants of mothers on opiates Finnegan NASS ≥ 8	1. Morphine 0·5 mg kg⁻¹ per day titrated 2. Phenobarbitone 15 mg kg⁻¹ then 6 mg kg⁻¹ per day titrated 3. Supportive therapy alone	46 29 36	Morphine v phenobarbitone: Treatment failure: RR 0·5 (0·2, 1·1) Difference treatment duration: –5 days (–12, 1) Difference hospitalization: –6 days (–13, 2) Difference duration supportive care/day: –35 minutes (–89, 17)
Madden[43]	Random, method not reported Blinding not reported Measurement blinding unclear No losses reported	Infants of narcotic addicted mothers Polydrug use 50% No abstinence score	1. Methadone 0·25–0·5 mg every 6 hours 2. Phenobarbitone 5–8 mg kg⁻¹ per day	18 16	Methadone v phenobarbitone: Treatment failure: RR 0·9 (0·1, 13·0) Difference treatment duration: –3 days (–8, 2)

To update this information, you search MedLine and find an additional study[44] that evaluated the addition of phenobarbitone for infants treated with dilute tincture of opium (DTO) for NAS due to opiate withdrawal. The randomization method was inadequate but participants and assessors were blinded to the treatment (infants were allocated to receive phenobarbitone or placebo according to their Finnegan NAS Score). Three infants were withdrawn after randomization. Infants treated with DTO and phenobarbitone had a reduced duration (and cost) of hospitalization and less time with severe NAS. However, the starting dose of DTO used (0·16 mg kg^{-1} per day morphine) was lower than that reported in several other trials of opiates for NAS included in the systematic review.

Question

7. In women with a drug or alcohol problem (*population*), does support at home (*intervention*) improve pregnancy outcomes and infant development, and reduce the risk of child abuse or neglect (*outcomes*)? **[Therapy]**

Specific search strategy

- *Cochrane Library*: "substance related disorder" [MeSH] AND "pregnancy" AND ("home" [text] "home care services" [MeSH])
- MedLine (Ovid): "substance related disorder" [MeSH] AND ("pregnancy" OR "infant" [MeSH] AND ("home" [text] "home care services" [MeSH]) *limit* to "clinical trial"

You find five reports of four randomized trials.[45–49] Three studies[45–48] enrolled high risk women on the basis of illicit drug use during pregnancy (see Table 51.3). The other study[49] enrolled high risk women with a 15% incidence of illicit drug use in the last month of pregnancy. Interventions in the first three studies included home visits by a community health nurse for two antenatal visits and then up to 18 months postpartum[48]; home visits by a pediatric health nurse for 18 months postpartum;[48] and home visiting by a lay person up to 18 months postpartum.[45,46] Interventions performed by the visitors are briefly summarized in Table 51.3. All studies were randomized although only one reported the method[47] and all had some blinded outcome measures but all had substantial losses to follow up (28–52%). No trial reported perinatal mortality. In one study infant development at 18 months was similar in both groups.[48] There was no significant difference in reported rates of attrition (meta-analysis of three studies, RR 1·04. 95% CI 0·81, 1·35), continued illicit drug or alcohol use, or infants not in the care of their biological mother. One study[45,46] reported a reduction in the use of child protection services in the group that received home

visits (RR 0·38; 95% CI 0·20, 0·74). In individual studies reduced rates of behavioral problems (of borderline statistical significance), parenting stress, and infant abuse potential were reported. In view of potential bias, there is currently insufficient evidence to determine if outreach interventions are effective.

Summary

This case scenario illustrates the complexity of managing pregnancy and newborn care in the context of maternal substance abuse. There is reasonable evidence that a short screening questionnaire is more accurate than clinical history taking and case finding for identifying pregnant women with risk drinking. Questionnaires such as the T-ACE and TWEAK have sensitivities and specificities in excess of 70%.[11,16,17,20] The SASSI is the only questionnaire that has been validated for detecting use of illicit drugs in pregnancy.[25] However, its low positive predictive value (26%) and length (78 questions) limit its clinical usefulness.

Data from observational studies support the use of methadone maintenance in pregnancy.[12,13] In non-pregnant patients, high dose methadone reduces illicit and intravenous drug use. Pregnant women on heroin have smaller babies and women who continue to use heroin while on methadone have increased rates of perinatal mortality and low birthweight babies. Stabilizing women on an adequate dose of methadone to prevent continued illicit drug use seems a reasonable goal of therapy.

In one RCT[29] there was no significant difference in the incidence of NAS in infants of women treated with methadone or SR morphine. There are no RCTs evaluating either opiate detoxification or use of buprenorphine in pregnancy. In one potentially biased cohort study,[31] outcomes were similar for women managed on buprenorphine or methadone and the incidence and severity of NAS in their infants did not differ. Depending on government regulation and patient preference, buprenorphine could be considered an option for treatment of the pregnant opiate-dependent women. However, it would be preferable if such treatment were part of a well-designed RCT.

The cohort studies[31,33,34] documenting methadone dose and risk of withdrawal suggest that the infant in this scenario whose mother is on 85 mg has up to a 90% risk of requiring treatment for NAS. The infant should be monitored for NAS using a validated scoring system. However, the Lipsitz tool is validated against its ability to differentiate between infants of drug-using and non-drug-using mothers (score ≥ 5 had 100% specificity for infants of drug-using mothers).[36] Of concern is that a trial of paregoric versus phenobarbitone that used a Lipsitz score ≥ 7 was the only trial to document seizures.[41] Treatment threshold has not been adequately defined for any

Table 51.3 Summary of studies of home visiting pregnant and/or postpartum women with a substance use problem

Study	Methods	Participants	Intervention visits	Outcomes RR (95% CI)
Black[48]	Random, method not reported Unblinded interventions Blinded measurement Losses 28%	African-American high risk, polydrug using	Pre- and postpartum 2 visits/week for 18 months Community health nurses Support, education, advocacy Carolina Preschool Curriculum Hawaii Early Learning program	Attrition: RR 1·7 (0·7, 4·0) Preterm delivery: RR 0·6 (0·3, 1·5) Low birth weight: RR 0·6 (0·2, 1·6) NAS: RR 0·9 (0·4, 1·7) Improved HOME score ($P = 0.05$) Reduced Child Abuse Potential Index and Parental Stress Index
Butz[47]	Random, computer generated Unblinded interventions Blinded measurement Incomplete data/ losses 52%	Postpartum women, 19-40 years, using opiates and/or cocaine in pregnancy	Postpartum to 18 months Pediatric nurse specialist Support, education, monitoring Parental skills training Carolina Preschool Curriculum Hawaii Early Learning program	Attrition: RR 0·8 (0·6, 1·1) Illicit drug use: RR 1·2 (0·9, 1·7) Not with mother: RR 1·0 (0·6, 1·8) Behavior problem: RR 0·5 (0·2,1·0)
Schuler[45,46]	Random, method not reported Unblinded intervention Blinded measurement Losses: 25% at 6 months, 42% at 18 months	African-American Positive toxicology or self-reported drug use	Postpartum, weekly to 6 months then 2-weekly to 18 months Two African-American lay women Infant health/development program Attended child development center Offered parent group meetings	Attrition: RR 1·3 (0·8, 1·4) Heroin/cocaine use: RR 1·2 (0·8, 1·9) Protective services: RR 0·4 (0·2, 0·7) Maternal competence or child responsiveness: No difference

score although the Finnegan NASS score ≥ 8 (average of three consecutive scores) has been used in several trials as the threshold for treatment.[9,10]

The infant in this scenario has NAS due to opiate withdrawal. In infants whose mothers are on opiates only, the evidence supports the use of an opiate for initial treatment of the infant in addition to appropriate supportive measures.[9] Whether phenobarbitone should be added is unclear in view of the potential for bias, the small size of the only trial and the relatively low starting dose of DTO used.[44]

Finally, improving outcomes of substance abusing women and their infants requires more than just pharmacological therapies. Besides identifying women in need, they need to be engaged in care but are frequently averse to hospitals. One method of engaging this high risk group in care is with outreach programs or home visiting. The trials of home visiting for substance abusing women to date are promising but are yet to replicate the types and timing of interventions (during pregnancy extending up to 2 years) reported in other socially high risk groups that have had a beneficial effect. Because women abusing drugs in pregnancy who have infrequent antenatal care have the worst outcomes,[12] home visiting is an option for those women who fail to engage in hospital based services.

Resolution of the case scenario

You are concerned that drug dependency was not detected until late in pregnancy in this woman. Only the SASSI questionnaire has been validated for detecting illicit drug use in pregnancy. However, because of its low positive predictive value and its length, you do not introduce this as a routine part of your clinical assessment. You continue to ask all women in the antenatal clinic about their use of alcohol, and illicit and prescription drugs, incorporating a short screening questionnaire for alcohol.

When the woman asks to continue on buprenorphine therapy, you explain that there are no good trials evaluating either opiate detoxification or buprenorphine therapy in pregnancy. One potentially biased study suggests that pregnancy and newborn outcomes are similar for women managed on buprenorphine or methadone. However, data from several observational studies support the use of methadone maintenance in pregnancy. In non-pregnant patients, high dose methadone reduces illicit and intravenous drug use. Also, pregnant women on heroin have smaller babies and women who continue to use heroin while on methadone have infants with increased rates of perinatal mortality and low birth weight. You elect to stabilize this woman on methadone with the goal of preventing her continued illicit drug use.

You estimate that this infant has up to 90% chance of developing NAS that requires treatment. You therefore monitor the infant for NAS severity using the Lipsitz tool, being aware of its limitations. When the infant develops symptoms on day 3 you commence him on an opiate (morphine) and, because he responds to treatment, you do not add phenobarbitone. After discharge you arrange for a community nurse to visit mother and infant at home, initially twice a week.

Future research needs

- Development of concise questionnaires is needed that identify risk for and effects of drug abuse in pregnant women, with validation of these questionnaires against appropriate reference tests (for example, a combination of urine, meconium and/or hair toxicology) in observational studies.

- RCTs are needed to compare methadone maintenance with buprenorphine in pregnant women with an opiate dependence.
- Opiate detoxification, including use of clonidine and naltrexone, has been reported in RCTs in non-pregnant populations and in case reports of pregnant women abusing opiates. Pilot studies are required to determine the pharmokinetics and dosage of any new therapies used in pregnant women, followed by the conduct of RCTs to evaluate their efficacy in pregnant women.
- Different NAS severity scores should be evaluated to determine appropriate treatment thresholds. Comparisons between different scoring methods would best be performed as part of a RCT. New objective measures of withdrawal severity are required that eliminate the possibility of inter- and intra-observer variation.
- Methodologically sound RCTs should be conducted to compare opiates versus phenobarbitone for treating NAS due to opiates; to evaluate the effects of adding phenobarbitone to an opiate as initial therapy; and to evaluate the efficacy of clonidine (reported in case series[4]) for infants with NAS.

Summary table

Question	Type of evidence	Results	Comment and adverse effects
Accuracy of screening questionnaires for drug and alcohol abuse in pregnant women	Systematic review of observational studies of screening questionnaires for risk drinking[11]; single observational study of SASSI accuracy[25]	T-ACE and TWEAK have sensitivities and specificities > 70% SASSI has low positive predictive value (26%)	Potential harm with false positive screen
Methadone maintenance *v* continued heroin use *v* methadone and continued illicit drug use in pregnant women	Systematic review of observational studies[6] No RCTs	Pregnant women on heroin have smaller babies, and women who continue to use heroin while on methadone have increased rates of perinatal mortality and low birth weight babies	Stabilizing women on an adequate dose of methadone to prevent continued illicit drug use is a reasonable goal of therapy. High rates of NAS occur in infants of mothers on methadone
Methadone *v* slow release morphine maintenance in pregnant women	Single RCT[29]	No significant difference in incidence or severity of NAS	
Methadone *v* buprenorphine maintenance therapy in pregnant women	No RCT. Single cohort study, potential for bias[31]	No significant difference in incidence or severity of NAS	
Maternal methadone dose and risk of NAS	Several cohort studies[31,33,34]	Increased risk of NAS with high dose methadone	Infants of mothers on low dose methadone still at risk of NAS
Diagnosis of NAS	Two observational studies[36,37]	Lipsitz score > 4 had 25% sensitivity and 100% specificity for predicting maternal drug use Neonatal Withdrawal Inventory has 100% agreement for a Finnegan NAS Score ≥ 8	Treatment threshold not adequately determined for NAS scores
Opiate *v* sedative for NAS from opiate withdrawal	Systematic reviews of RCTs[10]	Meta-analysis of 3 studies indicated no significant difference in treatment failure rate. One study reported a reduction in seizures with use of an opiate compared with phenobarbitone of borderline statistical significance	One study reported a significant reduction in treatment failure in infants of mothers using only an opiate
Home visiting for pregnant substance abusing women	Three RCTs[45-48]	No difference in rates of attrition, continued illicit drug or alcohol use, or infants not in care of their mother. Individual studies reported reductions in use of child protection services, rates of behavioral problems, parenting stress and infant abuse potential	No study provided prolonged, intense antenatal home visiting

References

1   Substance Abuse and Mental Health Services Administration. *Summary of Findings from the 2000 National Household Survey on Drug Abuse*. Office of Applied Studies 2001;NHSDA Series H-13, DHHS Publication No. (SMA) 01-3549. Rockville, MD.

2   Higgins K, Cooper-Stanbury M, Williams P. *Statistics on drug use in Australia 1998*. AIHW cat. no. PHE 16. Canberra: AIHW (Drug Statistics Series) 2000.

3   Bell GL, Lau K. Perinatal and neonatal issues of substance abuse. *Pediatr Clin N Amer* 1995;**42**:261–81.

4   Anonymous. Neonatal drug withdrawal. American Academy of Pediatrics Committee on Drugs. *Pediatrics* 1998;**101**:1079–88.

5   Anonymous. Drug-exposed infants. American Academy of Pediatrics Committee on Substance Abuse. *Pediatrics* 1995;**96**:364–7.

6   Mattick RP, Breen C, Kimber J, Davoli M. Methadone maintenance therapy versus no opioid replacement therapy for opioid dependence (Cochrane Review). In: *Cochrane Library*, Issue 2. Oxford: Update Software, 2003.

7   Amato L, Davoli M, Ferri M, Ali R. Methadone at tapered doses for the management of opioid withdrawal (Cochrane Review). In: *Cochrane Library*, Issue 2. Oxford: Update Software, 2003.

8   Mattick RP, Kimber J, Breen C, Davoli M. Buprenorphine maintenance versus placebo or methadone maintenance for opioid dependence (Cochrane Review). In: *Cochrane Library*, Issue 2. Oxford: Update Software, 2003.

9   Osborn DA, Cole MJ, Jeffery HE. Opiate treatment for opiate withdrawal in newborn infants (Cochrane Review). In: *Cochrane Library*, Issue 2. Oxford: Update Software, 2003.

10 Osborn DA, Jeffery HE, Cole MJ. Sedatives for opiate withdrawal in newborn infants (Cochrane Review). In: *Cochrane Library*, Issue 2. Oxford: Update Software, 2003.

11 Bradley KA, Boyd-Wickizer J, Powell SH, Burman ML. Alcohol screening questionnaires in women: a critical review. *JAMA* 1998;**280**:166–71.

12 Hulse GK, Milne E, English DR, Holman CD. Assessing the relationship between maternal opiate use and neonatal mortality. *Addiction* 1998;**93**:1033–42.

13 Hulse GK, Milne E, English DR, Holman CD. The relationship between maternal use of heroin and methadone and infant birth weight. *Addiction* 1997;**92**:1571–9.

14 Bossuyt PM, Reitsma JB, Bruns DE *et al.* Standards for Reporting of Diagnostic Accuracy steering group. Towards complete and accurate reporting of studies of diagnostic accuracy: the STARD initiative. *BMJ* 2003;**326**:41–4.

15 Lijmer JG, Mol BW, Heisterkamp S *et al.* Empirical evidence of design-related bias in studies of diagnostic tests. *JAMA* 1999;**282**:1061–6.

16 Chang G, Wilkins-Haug L, Berman S, Goetz MA, Behr H, Hiley A. Alcohol use and pregnancy: improving identification. *Obstet Gynecol* 1998;**91**:892–8.

17 Chang G, Goetz MA, Wilkins-Haug L, Berman S. Identifying prenatal alcohol use: screening instruments versus clinical predictors. *Am J Addict* 1999;**8**:87–93.

18 Bull LB, Kvigne VL, Leonardson GR, Lacina L, Welty TK. Validation of a self-administered questionnaire to screen for prenatal alcohol use in Northern Plains Indian women. *Am J Prev Med* 1999;**16**:240–3.

19 Budd KW, Ross-Alaolmolki K, Zeller RA. Two prenatal alcohol use screening instruments compared with a physiologic measure. *JOGNN* 2000;**29**:129–36.

20 Dawson DA, Das A, Faden VB, Bhaskar B, Krulewitch CJ, Wesley B. Screening for high and moderate-risk drinking during pregnancy: a comparison of several TWEAK-based screeners. *Alcohol Clin Exp Res* 2001;**25**:1342–9.

21 Russell M, Martier SS, Sokol RJ, Mudar P, Jacobson S, Jacobson J. Detecting risk drinking during pregnancy: a comparison of four screening questionnaires. *Am J Publ Hlth* 1996;**86**:1435–9.

22 Russell M, Martier SS, Sokol RJ *et al.* Screening for pregnancy risk-drinking. *Alcohol Clin Exp Res* 1994;**18**:1156–61.

23 Sokol RJ, Martier SS, Ager JW. The T-ACE questions: practical prenatal detection of risk-drinking. *Am J Obstet Gynecol* 1989;**160**:863–8.

24 Ostrea EM Jr, Knapp DK, Tannenbaum L *et al.* Estimates of illicit drug use during pregnancy by maternal interview, hair analysis, and meconium analysis. *J Pediatr* 2001;**138**:344–8.

25 Horrigan TJ, Piazza NJ, Weinstein L. The substance abuse subtle screening inventory is more cost effective and has better selectivity than urine toxicology for the detection of substance abuse in pregnancy. *J Perinatol* 1996;**16**:326–30.

26 Jaeschke R, Guyatt G, Sackett DL. Users' guides to the medical literature. III. How to use an article about a diagnostic test. A. Are the results of the study valid? Evidence-Based Medicine Working Group. *JAMA* 1994;**271**:389–91.

27 Jaeschke R, Guyatt GH, Sackett DL. Users' guides to the medical literature. III. How to use an article about a diagnostic test. B. What are the results and will they help me in caring for my patients? The Evidence-Based Medicine Working Group. *JAMA* 1994;**271**:703–7.

28 Barratt A, Irwig L, Glasziou P *et al.* Users' guides to the medical literature: x VII. How to use guidelines and recommendations about screening. Evidence-Based Medicine Working Group. *JAMA* 1999;**281**:2029–34.

29 Fischer G, Jagsch R, Eder H *et al.* Comparison of methadone and slow release morphine maintenance in pregnant addicts. *Addiction* 1999;**94**:231–9.

30 Lacroix I, Berrebi A, Schmitt L *et al. Buprenorphine high dosage in pregnancy: First data of a prospective study. Sixty fourth annual scientific meeting.* Quebec, Canada: CPDD, 2002.

31 Lejeune C, Aubisson S. Simmat-Durand L, Cneude F. Piquet M, Gourarier L. le Groupe d'Etudes Grossesse et addictions. Withdrawal syndromes of newborns of pregnant drug abusers maintained under methadone or high dose buprenorphine:246 cases. [in French] *Ann Med Intern* 2001;**152**(S7):21–7.

32 Johnson RE, Jones HE, Fischer G. Use of buprenorphine in pregnancy: patient management and effects on the neonate. *Drug Alcohol Depend* 2003;**70**(S21):S87–101.

33 Dashe JS, Sheffield JS, Olscher DA, Todd SJ, Jackson GL, Wendel GD. Relationship between maternal methadone dosage and neonatal withdrawal. *Obstet Gynecol* 2002;**100**:1244–9.

34 Doberczak TM, Kandall SR, Wilets I. Neonatal opiate abstinence syndrome in term and preterm infants. *J Pediatr* 1991;**118**:933–7.

35 Laupacis A, Wells G, Richardson WS, Tugwell P. Users' guides to the medical literature. V. How to use an article about prognosis. Evidence-Based Medicine Working Group. *JAMA* 1994;**272**:234–7.

36 Lipsitz PJ. A proposed narcotic withdrawal score for use with newborn infants. A pragmatic evaluation of its efficacy. *Clin Pediatr* 1975;**14**:592–4.

37 Zahorodny W, Rom C, Whitney W *et al*. The neonatal withdrawal inventory: a simplified score of newborn withdrawal. *J Dev Behav Pediatr* 1998;**19**:89–93.

38 Carin I, Glass L, Parekh A, Solomon N, Steigman J, Wong S. Neonatal methadone withdrawal. Effect of two treatment regimens. *Am J Dis Child* 1983;**137**:1166–9.

39 Finnegan LP, Michael H, Leifer B, Desai S. An evaluation of neonatal abstinence treatment modalities. *NIDA Res Monogr* 1984;**49**:282–8.

40 Kaltenbach K, Finnegan LP. Neonatal abstinence syndrome, pharmacotherapy and developmental outcome. *Neurobehav Toxicol Teratol* 1986;**8**:353–5.

41 Kandall SR, Doberczak TM, Mauer KR, Strashun RH, Korts DC. Opiate v CNS depressant therapy in neonatal drug abstinence syndrome. *Am J Dis Child* 1983;**137**:378–82.

42 Khoo KT. *The effectiveness of three treatment regimens used in the management of neonatal abstinence syndrome.* University of Melbourne. PhD Thesis, 1995.

43 Madden JD, Chappel JN, Zuspan F, Gumpel J, Mejia A, Davis R. Observation and treatment of neonatal narcotic withdrawal. *Am J Obstet Gynecol* 1977;**127**:199–201.

44 Coyle MG, Ferguson A, Lagasse L, Oh W, Lester B. Diluted tincture of opium (DTO) and phenobarbital versus DTO alone for neonatal opiate withdrawal in term infants. *J Pediatr* 2002;**140**:561–4.

45 Schuler ME, Nair P, Kettinger L. Drug-exposed infants and developmental outcome: effects of a home intervention and ongoing maternal drug use. *Arch Pediatr Adolesc Med* 2003;**157**:133–8.

46 Schuler ME, Nair P, Black MM, Kettinger L. Mother-infant interaction: effects of a home intervention and ongoing maternal drug use. *J Clin Child Psychol* 2000;**29**:424–31.

47 Butz AM, Lears MK, O'Neil S, Lukk P. Home intervention for in utero drug-exposed infants. *Publ Hlth Nurs* 1998;**15**:307–18.

48 Black MM, Nair P, Kight C, Wachtel R, Roby P, Schuler M. Parenting and early development among children of drug-abusing women: effects of home intervention. *Pediatrics* 1994;**94**:440–8.

49 Marcenko MO, Spence M. Home visitation services for at-risk pregnant and postpartum women: a randomized trial. *Am J Orthopsychiatr* 1994;**64**:468–78.

52 Cognitive outcomes in very preterm infants

Lex W Doyle, Jon E Tyson

Case scenario

You are called to the labor and delivery suite to talk with a 27-year-old mother who is 27 weeks pregnant and in labor. The estimated fetal weight by ultrasound examination is approximately 950 g. Although efforts are being made to stop her labor, it appears likely that she will deliver in the next few days. She and her husband, both school teachers, are very worried about the likely outcome of this delivery. Will the child survive and, if so, is the child likely to have long-term sequelae as a result of a very premature birth? Specifically, they wonder if this child is likely to have normal cognitive development and to be in a regular classroom at school. You reassure the parents that high quality neonatal care is available in the hospital and that the baby has an excellent chance of survival (approximately 90%) – but you are less certain about the long-term outlook for their child. You resolve to find this information and get back to the parents.

Background

Neonatal follow up surveys began to appear in Europe and North America in the early decades of the 20th century. Even early on, investigators wondered what happened to premature infants who survived. How often did survivors develop sensory and motor impairments or disabilities? Were such conditions the consequences of prematurity *per se,* or rather the consequences of specific medical complications that often accompanied a premature birth? These questions were asked perhaps with a greater sense of urgency with the advent of modern neonatal intensive care units (NICUs) in the 1970s. The hallmark of NICUs was the ability to assist ventilation by mechanical means, over and above merely providing additional oxygen to the inspired air. Associated with the introduction of assisted ventilation, mortality rates for low birthweight (LBW) infants (birth weight < 2500 g) and preterm infants (gestational age < 37 weeks) decreased rapidly. Mortality was especially high for very LBW (VLBW) (< 1500 g) and extremely LBW (ELBW) (< 1000 g) infants, and for very preterm infants with gestational ages < 32 weeks or < 28 weeks.

In addition to cognitive outcomes for survivors of NICUs, it is important to note that other adverse neurosensory outcomes occur more frequently than expected. For extremely LBW survivors the rates of cerebral palsy (10%), blindness (2%), and deafness (1–2%) are all much higher compared with rates expected in normal birthweight controls and rates have not changed much over several decades.[1] At this stage the parents of the baby in the scenario are most concerned with cognitive outcomes so we will focus on these in this chapter. Counseling through the baby's neonatal course would however include information on other neurodevelopmental outcomes, as well as other outcomes such as growth, and general and respiratory health.

Framing answerable clinical questions

In response to the concerns of these parents, you frame the following clinical questions.

Questions

1. In infants born at < 30 weeks' gestation (*population/ exposure*), what is the long-term outlook for cognitive development (*outcome*)? **[Prognosis]**
2. In infants born at < 30 weeks' gestation (*population/ exposure*), what is the likelihood that the child will be functioning normally in a regular classroom once she or he is old enough for school (*outcome*)? **[Prognosis]**

Searching for evidence

Answering questions about long-term outcome, or prognosis, requires recruiting an *inception cohort* (a group of subjects identified at a uniform period of time in the natural history of the disorder of interest), and following the cohort as completely as possible, and for as long as necessary to assess the outcomes of interest. For preterm infants, a cohort dating from birth identifies an inception cohort, and is relatively easy to collect. However, the assembled cohort needs to be truly representative of all infants to whom the results might ultimately be extrapolated. Generally, cohorts assembled from geographically-defined regions will be more representative of all preterm infants than cohorts of infants born in high risk tertiary care maternity units or transferred after birth from low risk to high risk neonatal units, in which selection filters may introduce bias. Having assembled a representative cohort, longitudinal follow up is a challenge. Preterm children who are lost to follow up have higher rates of neurosensory impairments, especially in cognition.[2]

Because the survival rate for very preterm infants has increased so dramatically over the past 25 years, the outcome data that you are seeking need to be reasonably contemporary and should come from studies of children born after the introduction of assisted ventilation. The best source of synthesized evidence on therapeutic issues is the Cochrane Database of Systematic Reviews, but you realize that it focuses on synthesizing the results of randomized controlled trials, and it will not provide syntheses of cohort studies examining prognosis of very preterm infants. You thus decide to go directly to MedLine and search for studies of the long-term prognosis for preterm infants. After some preliminary searching, it becomes clear that there have been numerous institution-based follow up studies in which efforts were made to monitor the outcomes of infants (either LBW or premature) discharged from a particular medical center or hospital. Population-based studies tend to be very labor-intensive and expensive to undertake. Unfortunately, there have been only a handful of such studies in which cohorts of LBW or preterm survivors have been followed for long enough to evaluate outcomes at school age.

In pursuit of the information that you need for counseling these parents, you undertake a MedLine search for population-based follow up studies of infants who were LBW and/or premature. Since your questions involve long-term outcome (including school placement), you restrict the MedLine search to studies with follow up assessments at age ≥ 5 years. Finally, you expect that studies comparing normal birth weight or term control groups with preterm cohorts will be most useful.

Your initial MedLine search includes the search terms "low birthweight" or "infant, premature", "follow up" or "outcome," and "population-based." This search fails to identify a couple of studies that had been mentioned by a colleague and a recent review on the topic that you saw in a journal in the library. You search further using pairs of terms such as "low birthweight" and "follow up". You identify a number of studies with marked limitations: follow up durations that are too short to report school-aged outcomes; follow up studies that use qualitative outcome measures; and even some follow up studies from underdeveloped countries (these are likely to be of limited relevance for your population in a developed country). After sifting through the search results (including the reference lists for studies found via the MedLine search), you identify the recent review[3] and a few additional population-based studies that were not included in the review.

Critical review of the evidence

Cognitive outcomes in reports from 1980–2001

Bhutta *et al.*[3] reviewed the literature for reports appearing between 1980 and November 2001, which determined either cognitive or behavioral outcomes at school-age of ex-preterm children. They searched MedLine for English-language articles using many subject headings including *infant-premature* and *infant-low birthweight*, as well as *cognition*. They determined *a priori* that they would include only studies with normal birth weight or term controls, in which the children were at least 5 years of age, and in which the loss to follow up was < 30%. From the 227 studies they reviewed, only 15 studies reporting cognitive data were considered worthy of inclusion and nine of these were from geographically defined regions,[4–12] as distinct from single hospital studies. The quality of the studies was rated on the following criteria: population sampled, study design, sociodemographic data, reporting of other neurosensory impairments, and degree of matching of cases and controls. None of the studies reviewed was given a perfect methodological score.

The years of birth of the children ranged from 1975 to 1988 and they were born in many different countries. In most studies preterm subjects were enrolled on the basis of birth weight, the cut-off for which varied between studies, but was most commonly < 1500 g. The ages of children at outcome assessment ranged from 5 years to 14 years. The types of cognitive tests used varied, but the Wechsler scales were used most commonly. In most studies children with major neurosensory impairments were excluded from cognitive testing.

In all individual studies in the review, the mean IQ for the preterm group was lower than that of the control group and in most studies the difference (see Glossary) between groups was statistically significant. There was little variation between hospital-based and geographically-based studies in the size of the difference between the preterm children and the controls. The overall weighted mean difference between groups was 10·9 (95% CI 9·2, 12·5) IQ points – a difference that is approximately two-thirds of the SD. In most studies the mean IQ for the preterm cohort was within 1 SD of the test mean.

Bhutta *et al.*[3] highlighted some of the limitations of their review, including the fact that they had combined data from many studies over a time when neonatal intensive care was changing rapidly, and that they had combined studies from many different countries and regions. The most recent year of birth of children included in the review, which was reported in 2002, was 1988, or 14 years earlier. There is always a compromise between increasing length of follow up and diminished relevance to contemporary infants in newborn nurseries. On the one hand, the longer the period of follow up the more certain you can be of the outcomes. On the other hand, the longer the follow up, the less relevant are the outcome rates because perinatal care and survival rates have changed dramatically in recent years. However, data from these studies represent the best information available until they are superseded by data from more contemporary cohorts. Bhutta *et al.*[3] did not report on the proportions of children who were in normal classes at school in either the preterm or the term controls because school systems and school class placement vary widely between countries and regions.

Several other regional cohort studies in addition to the studies included in Bhutta's review[3] have been published.

The Victorian birth cohort of 1979–1980

Kitchen and colleagues[13–16] undertook a population-based follow up study in the Australian state of Victoria. The Victorian study focused on ELBW infants with birth weights between 500 and 999 g. Kitchen *et al.*[13] reviewed data from five sources, including public vital statistics records, hospital records, and records from Victoria's neonatal transport service. From 115 973 live births in the State of Victoria during the calendar years 1979 and 1980, 351 ELBW live births were identified. The authors stated that their "ascertainment of all live born extremely LBW infants throughout the state [of Victoria] was satisfactory." Among 351 ELBW live births, the 89 (25·4%) who survived to 2 years of age became the Victorian ELBW follow up cohort, although one child subsequently died between 8 and 14 years of age. The cohorts were assessed and their outcomes have been reported at 2,[13] 5,[14] 8,[15] and 14[16] years of age. It was only at the 14-year assessment, however, that the results were compared with 60 normal birthweight (NBW) peers.[16] The NBW cohort was randomly selected from one of the three level-III perinatal centers in the state and had been followed longitudinally from birth.

Follow up evaluations at each age had certain features in common.

- Neurosensory assessments were performed by a developmental pediatrician.
- Standardized cognitive assessments were performed by trained psychologists using recognized psychometric tests (Bayley Scales of Infant Development at age 2, and Wechsler Scales at each other age).
- Outcome assessors were blinded to results of children's earlier assessments.
- Age was corrected for prematurity at each assessment.
- High follow up rates of ELBW children were achieved at each age, including 90% at 14 years of age.
- The number of individual assessors was remarkably few – a total of four individual psychologists and six individual pediatricians assessed children during the 14-year study.

At all ages the mean cognitive score for ELBW children who were able to be tested was within 1 SD of the standardized test mean.[16] When the cognitive results at all ages were rescored relative to NBW controls, the ELBW group had a mean IQ (95% confidence interval) 15·1 (8·9, 21·3) points below that of the NBW cohort at age 2; 11·7 (5·6, 17·8) points lower at age 5; 13·3 (7·8, 18·8) points lower at age 8, and 13·1 (7·0, 19·2) points lower at age 14. These differences in IQ were of a similar size to those reported in the review by Bhutta *et al.*[3]

A limitation of the Victorian study is that not all ELBW children had a full cognitive assessment, because of severe cognitive, motor, or sensory impairments. Hence the proportions with cognitive scores in the severely impaired ranges would be underestimated in this study. On the other hand, not all NBW controls had cognitive assessments at all ages. Of the 60 NBW controls randomly selected from birth, 80% had testing at age 2 years, 73% at age 5, 87% at age 8, and 68% at age 14. One NBW child was severely disabled at all ages and could not be tested. As cognitive function is lower for preterm children who are difficult to follow up,[2] it might be expected that the NBW children who were not assessed might have lower cognition than children who were assessed. Without testing all children it is difficult to determine the effects of selection bias in this cohort study.

The Liverpool cohort of 1991–92

Foulders-Hughes and Cooke[17] described the outcome of a population-based cohort born in 1991–92 in the eight district hospitals within the Liverpool, UK postal district. This study included all preterm infants < 32 weeks' gestational age. There were 382 survivors, of whom 280 (73%) were attending mainstream schools and were assessed at a mean age of 90 months (not corrected for prematurity). Their IQ results were compared with 210 term controls selected by classroom teachers to be of the same gender and language and closest in birthday to the preterm child. With the use of the Wechsler Intelligence Scale for Children, (third edition), the mean Full Scale IQ was found to be 100.5 (SD 13·7) in controls, significantly higher than the mean IQ of 89·4 (SD 14·2) in the preterm group. The difference in IQ means was approximately two-thirds of an SD as was also noted in the review of Bhutta *et al.*[3]

The major limitations of this study are the relatively low follow up rate of the preterm group, the lack of random selection of the term controls and their low participation rate (in 70 cases a term control could not be found). Both factors may produce misleading results in the term controls, and hence considerably reduce the generalizability of the results.

The Victorian birth cohort of 1991–92

The Victorian Infant Collaborative Study Group[18] assessed another population-based cohort born in 1991–92 in the Australian state of Victoria. This study included both ELBW infants (birth weights between 500 and 999 g) and very preterm infants (23–27 weeks' gestational age). There were 298 survivors at 2-years. Their cognitive function was compared with 262 NBW controls randomly selected from each of the three level-III perinatal centres in the state and matched with the ELBW/very preterm cohort for expected date of delivery, gender, mother's health insurance status, and country of origin (primarily English-speaking or not). Children were assessed at 2, 5, and 8 years of age (corrected for prematurity where appropriate) using methods described for the previous Victorian cohort.

At 8 years of age in the Victorian cohort[18] the follow up rate was 92% for the ELBW/very preterm group and 85% for the NBW group. Differences in follow up rate can potentially bias outcome assessment. For example psychometric tests scores at 2 and 5 years of age were lower for children subsequently not assessed at 8 years of age than those who were assessed. At age 2, the mean difference in the Mental Developmental Index on the Bayley Scales of Infant Development was −4·2 (95% CI −11·7, 3·3). At age 5 the mean difference in full scale IQ was −6·8 (95% CI −13·6, −0·1) using the Wechsler Preschool and Primary Scale of Intelligence-Revised.

The mean Full Scale IQ score on the Wechsler Intelligence Scale for Children (third edition) was 95·5 (SD 16·0) for the 258 ELBW/very preterm children able to be tested. This score was within 1 SD of the standardized mean test but was 9·4 (95% CI 6·7, 12·1) points lower than the mean score in the 220 NBW controls. This represents an improvement in cognitive scores in ELBW from the 1979–80 era, when the mean IQ score was 13·3 (95% CI 7·8, 18·8) points lower than in NBW infants at 8 years of age. Importantly, in 1991–92, 17% of the ELBW/very preterm cohort had mild intellectual impairment and 5% had major impairment. These rates are significantly higher than rates in the NBW controls, of whom 6% had mild and 1% had major intellectual impairment. Including children unable to be tested because of severe cognitive deficits, 10% of the ELBW/very preterm cohort had a major cognitive impairment, compared with 2% of NBW controls.

As with the earlier Victorian study, not all children had full cognitive assessments because of severe cognitive, motor or sensory impairments. Again, follow up rates in the NBW controls were lower than in the ELBW/very preterm group. Adjusting statistically for small imbalances in sociodemographic variables (maternal education, social class, and ethnicity) related to differential follow up rates did not alter the study conclusions. Of interest to the parents in the case scenario above, children from higher social class had an IQ that was on average 5 points higher (95% CI 2, 8) than children from lower social class, and when the mother had completed high school the IQ was another 6 points higher (95% CI 3, 9) than if the mother had not completed high school.

Survivors of lower birth weight (< 750 g) or gestational age (< 26 weeks) had slightly worse cognitive outcomes than those who were heavier at birth (750–999 g) or more mature (26–27 weeks), although only the differences between birthweight groups were statistically significant. Since more very tiny and immature babies survived in the 1991–92 Victorian cohort than in any of the previous studies (either in the review or the 1979–80 Victorian cohort) and because the mean difference in cognitive scores was slightly less than the overall weighted mean difference reported in Bhutta's review,[3] the results from the 1991–92 Victorian cohort might represent a relative improvement over time in the results for ELBW/very preterm children born in the 1990s compared with earlier eras.

Of relevance to the clinical case scenario above, this Victorian cohort also had extensive testing in educational domains at 8 years of age, including the Wide Range Achievement Test. The ELBW/very preterm children performed significantly below the NBW children on tests of reading (mean difference −6·7 [95% CI −9·5, −3·9]); spelling (mean difference −5·6 [95% CI −8·0, −3·3]) and arithmetic (mean difference −8·8 [95% CI −11·3, −6·2]). However, after controlling for IQ, the group differences in reading and spelling were no longer statistically significant (reading: adjusted mean difference −0·8; 95% CI −3·2, 2·4; spelling: adjusted mean difference −0·9; 95% CI −3·0, 1·1). For arithmetic, the ELBW/very preterm cohort performed significantly below the NBW cohort even after controlling for IQ (adjusted mean difference −2·8; 95% CI −4·8, −0·8). In addition to these educational tests, teachers reported that ELBW/very preterm children were not progressing as well as the NBW cohort. Furthermore, significantly more children in the ELBW/very preterm group had repeated a grade level at school (ELBW/very preterm: n = 54, 20·2% versus NBW: n = 16, 7·2%) and required additional educational assistance (ELBW/very preterm: n = 103, 38·7% versus NBW: n = 48, 21·5%). It is important to note, however, that the majority of ELBW/very preterm children had not repeated a grade at school and did not require additional educational assistance.

The strengths of this study are that it represents a complete geographical cohort of ELBW/very preterm children, born in the most recent era and compared with randomly selected NBW controls matched for several important sociodemographic features. The follow up rate was high, and extensive cognitive testing was conducted using robust instruments, by experienced psychologists blinded to the birthweight group and the results of previous assessments. A weakness of the study is that the results may not be readily transferable to others regions or countries, where education systems may differ.

Data on school performance from other cohorts

Several of the regional studies included in the review by Bhutta *et al.*[3] also contained some data on school performance. Lloyd *et al.*[4] studied 45 7-year-old VLBW children born in Wolverhampton, UK, in 1975–1979 and reported that (53%) VLBW children were performing below average compared with 45 (22%) controls. Hall *et al.*[7] studied 8-year-old VLBW children born in Scotland in 1984 and reported that 15% of children of birth weight < 1000 g and 6% of children of birth weight 1000–1499 g were in special schools. Of the remaining children, 36% of the lighter children and 58% of the heavier children were in normal school needing no extra help and 11% and 4% respectively had repeated a grade. In a study of 10-year-old children of < 29 weeks' gestational age born in Sweden in 1985–86, Stjernqvist and Svenningsen[9] reported that 38% of the preterm group were performing below average in school compared with 12% of controls. Saigal *et al.*[11] from Canada reported on the outcome at high school of teenage children of birth weight 501–1000 g born in Ontario from 1977 to 1981. In their study 25% of the preterm group had repeated a grade at school compared with 6% of controls. Of the preterm group, 57% were performing in a normal classroom without special assistance compared with 94% of controls. In summary, very tiny or preterm survivors are more likely to have repeated a grade at school and more are likely to be performing below average at school, or to require special assistance. However, the majority will be in normal school and receiving no special assistance.

Summary

The evidence reported in this chapter estimates the average risk for populations based on cohorts of infants selected by birth weight or prematurity. For the individual infant, additional risk factors related to complications during the pregnancy, birth, or neonatal period could alter outcome. Cognitive function is also influenced by the socioeconomic status and level of education of the parents. Another difficulty in giving a prognosis to an individual infant is that the information available usually derives from studies conducted several years earlier when practice was considerably different.

Resolution of the scenario

With regard to cognitive development, you tell the parents that typically the IQ will be in the low normal range. You reassure them that, although there is an increased risk of a requirement for special educational services, and possibly for repeating school grades, most preterm survivors have neither outcome. Most children who are having difficulties in normal classroom are of normal birth weight and have been born at term, because these latter children greatly outnumber ELBW or very preterm children. You tell them that IQ is also influenced by factors not known to the clinician prior to delivery and that in their case being of higher socioeconomic class and having a mother with a tertiary education will give their baby an IQ advantage. You also tell them that extremely LBW survivors have higher rates of cerebral palsy, blindness, and deafness than normal birthweight infants.

Summary table

Question	Type of evidence	Result	Comment
In infants born at < 30 weeks' gestation, what is the long-term outlook for cognitive development?	Review[3] of 15 studies, 9 of which are population-based. Three additional population-based studies[13–16,17,18]	Typical outcome is within the expected range but mean IQ is approximately two-thirds SD lower than population or control group means	Inclusion criteria mostly based on birth weight. Changing prognosis with advances in neonatal care and wide range of settings limits applicability
In infants born at < 30 weeks' gestation, what is the outlook for school performance?	5 population-based studies [4, 7 0,11,18]	Premature infants are more likely to receive special education services or to have repeated a grade at school, but most are functioning normally in a normal classroom	Wide variability in educational practices limits the usefulness of these data

References

1 Doyle LW and the Victorian Infant Collaborative Study Group. Evaluation of neonatal intensive care for extremely low birthweight infants in Victoria over two decades. 1. Effectiveness. *Pediatrics* (in press).

2 Callanan C, Doyle LW, Rickards AL, Kelly EA, Ford GW, Davis NM. Children followed with difficulty – how do they differ? *J Paediatr Child Hlth* 2001;**37**:152–6.

3 Bhutta A, Cleves M, Casey P, Cradock M, Anand K. Cognitive and behavioral outcomes of school-aged children who were born preterm: A meta-analysis. *JAMA* 2002;**288**:728–37.

4 Lloyd BW, Wheldall K, Perks D. Controlled study of intelligence and school performance of very low birthweight children from a defined geographical area. *Develop Med Child Neurol* 1988;**30**:36–42.

5 Smith AE, Knight-Jones EB. The abilities of very low birthweight children and their classroom controls. *Develop Med Child Neurol* 1990;**32**:590–601.

6 Sommerfelt K, Ellertsen B, Markestad T. Personality and behaviour in eight-year-old, non-handicapped children with birth weight under 1500 g. *Acta Paediatr* 1993;**82**:723–8.

7 Hall A, McLeod A, Counsell C, Thomson L, Mutch L. School attainment, cognitive ability and motor function in a total Scottish very-low birthweight population at eight years: a controlled study. *Develop Med Child Neurol* 1995;**37**:1037–50.

8 Sommerfelt K, Ellertsen B, Markestad T. Parental factors in cognitive outcome of non-handicapped low birthweight infants. *Arch Dis Child Fetal Neonatal Ed* 1995;**73**:F135–42.

9 Stjernqvist K, Svenningsen NW. Ten-year follow up of children born before 29 gestational weeks: health, cognitive development, behaviour and school achievement. *Acta Paediatr* 1999;**88**:557–62.

10 Wolke D, Meyer R. Cognitive status, language attainment, and prereading skills of 6-year- old very preterm children and their peers: the Bavarian Longitudinal Study. *Develop Med Child Neurol* 1999;**41**:94–109.

11 Saigal S, Hoult LA, Streiner DL, Stoskopf BL, Rosenbaum PL. School difficulties at adolescence in a regional cohort of children who were extremely low birth weight. *Pediatrics* 2000;**105**:325–31.

12 Taylor HG, Klein N, Minich NM, Hack M. Middle-school-age outcomes in children with very low birthweight. *Child Devel* 2000;**71**:1495–511.

13 Kitchen W, Ford C, Orgill A *et al.* Outcome in infants with birth weight 500 to 999 g: a regional study of 1979 and 1980 births. *J Pediatr* 1984;**104**:921–7.

14 Kitchen W, Ford G, Orgill A *et al.* Outcome in infants of birth weight 500 to 999 g: a continuing regional study of 5-year-old survivors. *J Pediatr* 1987;**111**:761–6.

15 Victorian Infant Collaborative Study Group. Eight-year outcome in infants with birth weight of 500 to 999 grams: Continuing regional study of 1979 and 1980 births. *J Pediatr* 1991;**118**:761–7.

16 Doyle LW and Casalaz D for the Victorian Infant Collaborative Study Group. Outcome at 14 years and birthweight < 1000 g – a regional study. *Arch Dis Child* 2001;**85**:F159–F164.

17 Foulders-Hughes LA, Cooke RWI. Motor, cognitive and behavioural disorders in children born very preterm. *Develop Med Child Neurol* 2003;**45**:97–103.

18 Anderson PJ, Doyle LW, and the Victorian Infant Collaborative Study Group. Neurobehavioral outcomes of school-age children born extremely low birth weight or very preterm in the 1990s. *JAMA* 2003;**289**:3264–72.

Index

Note: page numbers in *italics* refer to tables and boxes, those in **bold** refer to figures